ESSENTIALS OF PHARMACOLOGY

3RD EDITION Essentials of

Editors

JOHN A. BEVAN
B.SC., M.B., B.S.
CHAIRMAN AND PROFESSOR, DEPARTMENT OF PHARMACOLOGY, UNIVERSITY OF VERMONT, COLLEGE OF MEDICINE; BURLINGTON, VERMONT

JEREMY H. THOMPSON
M.D., F.R.C.P.I.
PROFESSOR, DEPARTMENT OF PHARMACOLOGY, UNIVERSITY OF CALIFORNIA, LOS ANGELES, SCHOOL OF MEDICINE; LOS ANGELES, CALIFORNIA

With 54 contributors

PHARMACOLOGY

Introduction to the Principles of Drug Action

HARPER & ROW, PUBLISHERS
PHILADELPHIA
Cambridge
New York
Hagerstown
San Francisco
London
Mexico City
São Paulo
Sydney
1817

Acquisitions Editor: William Burgower
Sponsoring Editor: Sanford J. Robinson
Manuscript Editor: Leslie E. Hoeltzel
Indexer: Deborah Ziwot
Art Director: Maria S. Karkucinski
Designer: Patrick Turner
Production Coordinator: Susan A. Caldwell
Compositor: Progressive Typographers
Printer/Binder: The Murray Printing Company

The authors and publisher have exerted every effort to ensure that drug selection and dosage set forth in this text are in accord with current recommendations and practice at the time of publication. However, in view of ongoing research, changes in government regulations, and the constant flow of information relating to drug therapy and drug reactions, the reader is urged to check the package insert for each drug for any change in indications and dosage and for added warnings and precautions. This is particularly important when the recommended agent is a new or infrequently employed drug.

Third Edition

3 5 6 4 2

Library of Congress Cataloging in Publication Data
Main entry under title:

Essentials of pharmacology.

Bibliography: p.
Includes index.
1. Pharmacology. I. Bevan, John A., 1930–
II. Thompson, Jeremy H. [DNLM: 1. Pharmacology. WV 4 E78]
RM300.E84 1983 615'.1 82-23996
ISBN 0-06-140462-4

CONTRIBUTORS

MARVIN E. AMENT, M.D.
Professor, Department of Pediatrics, Chief, Division of Pediatric Gastroenterology, Department of Pediatrics, University of California, Los Angeles, School of Medicine, Los Angeles, California
CHAPTER 75

CARL E. ANDERSON, Ph.D.†
Professor Emeritus, Department of Biochemistry and Nutrition, University of North Carolina at Chapel Hill, School of Medicine, Chapel Hill, North Carolina
CHAPTER 73

JAY M. ARENA, B.S., M.D.
Chairman, Department of Pediatrics, Duke University School of Medicine, Durham, North Carolina
CHAPTER 72

JOHN A. BEVAN, B.SC., M.B., B.S.
Chairman and Professor, Department of Pharmacology, University of Vermont, College of Medicine; Burlington, Vermont
CHAPTERS 1, 13, 17, 18, 35

JOSIAH BROWN, M.D.
Professor, Department of Medicine, University of California, Los Angeles, School of Medicine, Los Angeles, California
CHAPTER 46

DON H. CATLIN, M.D.
Chief, Clinical Pharmacology, Departments of Medicine and Pharmacology, University of California, Los Angeles, School of Medicine, Los Angeles, California
CHAPTERS 5, 32

† Deceased.

JACK W. COBURN, M.D.
Professor, Department of Medicine, University of California, Los Angeles, School of Medicine, Los Angeles, California.
CHAPTER 40

SANDRA B. COLVILLE–STEWART, Ph.D.
Associate Librarian, History and Special Collections, Biomedical Library, University of California, Los Angeles, Los Angeles, California
HISTORICAL FOOTNOTES

MATTHEW E. CONOLLY, M.D., M.R.C.P., F.A.C.P.
Professor, Departments of Medicine and Pharmacology, University of California, Los Angeles, School of Medicine, Los Angeles, California
CHAPTER 36

NICHOLAS N. DURANT, B.Sc., Ph.D.
Assistant Professor, Department of Anesthesiology, University of California, Los Angeles, School of Medicine, Los Angeles, California
CHAPTER 19

SIDNEY ELLIS, Ph.D.
Director, Division of Drug Biology, Department of Health and Human Services, Food and Drug Administration, Washington, D.C.
EXAMINATION QUESTIONS AND ANSWERS

DESMOND J. FITZGERALD, M.R.C.P.I.
Research Registrar, Department of Clinical Pharmacology, The Royal College of Surgeons, Dublin, Ireland
CHAPTER 83

HARRISON J. L. FRANK, M.D., Ph.D.
Assistant Professor, Department of Medicine, University of California, Los Angeles, School of Medicine, Los Angeles, California
CHAPTER 46

ROBERT H. GERNER, M.D.
Associate Professor, Department of Psychiatry, University of California at Irvine, Irvine, California; Chief, Psychiatric Research, Long Beach Veterans Administration Medical Center, Long Beach, California
CHAPTER 24

MARK A. GOLDBERG, Ph.D., M.D.
Professor, Departments of Neurology and Pharmacology, University of California, Los Angeles; Chairman, Department of Neurology, Harbor General Hospital, Torrance, California
CHAPTER 29

ISRAEL HANIN, Ph.D.
Professor of Psychiatry and Pharmacology, University of Pittsburgh Medical School, Pittsburgh, Pennsylvania
CHAPTER 21

CHARLES M. HASKELL, M.D.
Director, Wadsworth Cancer Center, Veterans Administration Wadsworth Medical Center, Los Angeles, California
CHAPTER 71

DAN A. HENRY, M.D.
Formerly Assistant Professor, Department of Medicine, University of California, Los Angeles–San Fernando Valley Program, Los Angeles, California
CHAPTER 40

JEROME M. HERSHMAN, M.D.
Professor, Department of Medicine, University of California, Los Angeles, School of Medicine, Los Angeles, California
CHAPTERS 43, 44

LEO E. HOLLISTER, M.D.
Chief of Service, Psychopharmacology, Professor, Departments of Medicine, Psychiatry and Pharmacology, Veterans Administration Medical Center, Palo Alto, California
CHAPTER 26

WYATT R. HUME, B.S., D.D.S., Ph.D.
Senior Lecturer in Dentistry, University of Adelaide, Adelaide, South Australia, Australia
CHAPTER 74

DONALD J. JENDEN, M.B., B.S.
Professor and Chairman, Department of Pharmacology, University of California, Los Angeles, School of Medicine, Los Angeles, California
CHAPTER 9

RICHARD W. JOHNSON, Ph.D.
Formerly, Instructor, Departments of Biochemistry and Pharmacology, University of Arizona College of Medicine, Tucson, Arizona
CHAPTER 25

BENJAMIN M. KAGAN, M.D.
Professor and Chairman, Department of Pediatrics, Cedars–Sinai Medical Center, University of California, Los Angeles, School of Medicine, Los Angeles, California
CHAPTER 7

HAROLD KALANT, M.D., Ph.D.
Professor, Department of Pharmacology, University of Toronto Faculty of Medicine, Toronto, Ontario, Canada
CHAPTER 27

JOHN P. KANE, M.D., Ph.D.
Associate Professor, Department of Medicine, University of California, San Francisco, School of Medicine, San Francisco, California
CHAPTER 37

RONALD L. KATZ, M.D.
Professor and Chairman, Department of Anesthesiology, University of California, Los Angeles, School of Medicine, Los Angeles, California
CHAPTERS 19, 28

BERTRAM G. KATZUNG, M.D., Ph.D.
Professor, Department of Pharmacology, University of California, San Francisco, School of Medicine, San Francisco, California
CHAPTERS 33, 34

BERT N. LA DU, Jr., M.D., Ph.D.
Professor and Chairman, Department of Pharmacology, University of Michigan Medical School, Ann Arbor, Michigan
CHAPTER 6

MORTIMER B. LIPSETT, M.D.
Clinical Professor of Medicine, Uniformed Services University of Health Sciences, Director, National Institute of Child Health and Human Development, Bethesda, Maryland
CHAPTERS 48, 49

PETER LOMAX, M.D., D.Sc.
Professor, Department of Pharmacology, University of California, Los Angeles, School of Medicine, Los Angeles, California
CHAPTERS 20, 41, 42, 66

ALAN G. MALLINGER, M.D.
Assistant Professor of Psychiatry and Pharmacology, University of Pittsburgh School of Medicine, Western Psychiatric Institute and Clinic, Pittsburgh, Pennsylvania
CHAPTERS 22, 23

MARY J. MALLOY, M.D.
Associate Clinical Professor, Department of Pediatrics, University of California, San Francisco, School of Medicine, San Francisco, California
CHAPTER 37

CHARLES H. MARKHAM, M.D.
Professor, Department of Neurology, Reed Neurological Research Center, University of California, Los Angeles, School of Medicine, Los Angeles, California
CHAPTER 30

JOHN C. MCGIFF, M.D.
Professor and Chairman, Department of Pharmacology, New York Medical College, Valhalla, New York
CHAPTER 53

JORDAN D. MILLER, M.D.
Associate Professor, Department of Anesthesiology, University of California, Los Angeles, School of Medicine, Los Angeles, California
CHAPTER 28

DON H. NELSON, M.D.
Professor of Medicine and Physiology, Department of Internal Medicine, The University of Utah College of Medicine, Salt Lake City, Utah
CHAPTER 47

KEVIN O'MALLEY, M.D., Ph.D., F.R.C.P.I., M.R.C.P.
Professor and Chairman, Department of Clinical Pharmacology, The Royal College of Surgeons, Dublin, Ireland
CHAPTER 83

HAROLD E. PAULUS, M.D.
Professor, Department of Medicine, University of California, Los Angeles, School of Medicine, Los Angeles, California
CHAPTERS 10, 31

MICHAEL J. PEACH, Ph.D.
Professor, Department of Pharmacology, University of Virginia School of Medicine, Charlottesville, Virginia
CHAPTER 55

RALPH E. PURDY, Ph.D.
Associate Professor, Department of Pharmacology, University of California, Irvine, College of Medicine, Irvine, California
CHAPTER 39

G. ALAN ROBISON, Ph.D.
Professor and Chairman, Department of Pharmacology, University of Texas Medical School, Houston, Texas
CHAPTER 50

DENIS O. RODGERSON, Ph.D.
Professor, Department of Pathology, University of California, Los Angeles, School of Medicine, Los Angeles, California
CHAPTER 79

FREDERICK R. SINGER, M.D.
Professor, Department of Medicine, University of Southern California Clinical Research Center, Los Angeles, California
CHAPTER 45

I. L. TAYLOR, M.D., Ph.D.
Associate Professor, Department of Medicine, University of California, Los Angeles, School of Medicine, Los Angeles, California; Acting Head, Department of Gastroenterology, Sepulveda Veterans Administration Medical Center, Sepulveda, California
CHAPTER 54

JEREMY H. THOMPSON, M.D., F.R.C.P.I.
Professor, Department of Pharmacology, University of California, Los Angeles, School of Medicine, Los Angeles, California
CHAPTERS 3, 4, 8, 11, 38, 51, 52, 56, 57, 58, 59, 60, 61, 62, 63, 64, 65, 68, 69, 70, 76, 80, 81

MERCEDES TOKORCHECK, Pharm.D.
Formerly Assistant Director, Department of Pharmaceutical Services, University of California, Los Angeles, Hospitals and Clinics, Los Angeles, California
CHAPTER 12

DAVID J. TRIGGLE, Ph.D.
Professor and Chairman, Department of Biochemical Pharmacology, State University of New York, School of Pharmacy, Buffalo, New York
CHAPTER 2

JERROLD A. TURNER, M.D.
Professor, Departments of Medicine, and Microbiology and Immunology, University of California, Los Angeles, School of Medicine, Los Angeles, California; Assistant Medical Director, Harbor UCLA Medical Center, Torrance, California
CHAPTER 67

RAYBURN B. VRABEL, Pharm.D.
Deputy Director, Pharmaceutical Services, University of California, Los Angeles, Hospitals and Clinics, Los Angeles, California
CHAPTERS 77, 78

JOHN H. WALSH, M.D.
Professor, Department of Medicine, University of California, Los Angeles, School of Medicine, Los Angeles, California
CHAPTER **54**

THOMAS C. WESTFALL, Ph.D.
Professor and Chairman, Department of Pharmacology, St. Louis University, School of Medicine, St. Louis, Missouri
CHAPTERS **14, 15, 16**

HENRY I. YAMAMURA, Ph.D.
Professor, Departments of Biochemistry and Pharmacology, Associate Professor, Department of Psychiatry, University of Arizona College of Medicine, Tucson, Arizona
CHAPTER **25**

DIANE ZALBA, Pharm.D.
Assistant Director, Pharmaceutical Services, University of California, Los Angeles, Hospitals and Clinics, Los Angeles, California
CHAPTERS **12, 82**

PREFACE

After being frequently urged to write upon this subject, and as often declining to do it, from apprehension of my own inability, I am at length compelled to take up the pen, however unqualified I may still feel myself for the task.

The use of the Foxglove is getting abroad, and it is better the world should derive some instruction, however imperfect, from my experience, than that the lives of men should be hazarded by its unguarded exhibition, or that a medicine of so much efficacy should be condemned and rejected as dangerous and unmanageable.

(p. vi) It is now about ten years since I first began to use this medicine. Experience and cautious attention gradually taught me how to use it. For the last two years I have not had occasion to alter the modes of management; but I am still far from thinking them perfect.

It would have been an easy task to have given select cases, whose successful treatment would have spoken strongly in favour of the medicine, and perhaps been flattering to my own reputation. But Truth and Science would condemn the procedure. I have therefore mentioned every case in which I have prescribed the Foxglove, proper or improper, successful or otherwise. Such a conduct will lay me open to the censure of those who are disposed to censure, but it will meet the approbation of others, who are the best qualified to be judges.

To the Surgeons and Apothecaries, with whom I am connected in practice, both in this town and at a distance, I beg leave to make this public acknowledgment, for the assistance they so readily afforded me, in perfecting some of the cases, and in communicating the events of others.

The cases related from my own experience, are generally written in the shortest form I could contrive, in order to save time and labour. Some of them are given more in detail, when particular circumstances made such detail necessary; but the cases communicated by other practitioners, are given in their own words.

An Account of the Foxglove, and Some of Its Medical Uses; With Practical Remarks on Dropsy, and Other Diseases
—WILLIAM WITHERING, M.D.

William Withering had a sufficient personal interest and knowledge of botany that he was able to conclude that the medical value of a local folk remedy containing many herbs lay in the foxglove. As a result of his personal observations on the use of this plant in dropsy (congestive heart failure), he learned what it would do and also its limitations. He was commendably slow to generalize and to commit himself in writing conclusions, nor did he try to hide his errors and failures—a most salutary attitude that no doubt was appreciated by his medical colleagues. Unfortunately modern medicine does not encourage such a leisurely practice and wide interests, but we hope that the principles are still followed whenever possible. They are reflected in the general philosophy of this textbook. It is often not the newest and the latest that are most important to master because many of these will be discarded before the student is responsible for his own practice. Rather, since drugs come and go, it is essential that the student-physician learn to ask the right questions and develop the right pattern of thought. A general understanding of pharmacologic principles and problems is the most important thing to be learned.

The dramatic increase in new remedies over the past decade, along with the complexity of the essential knowledge now necessary to use them wisely, has dictated a number of changes since our first two editions. Of greatest importance, the major contributor to the first two editions, Dr. Jeremy Thompson, has become a co-editor. His wide knowledge of medicine, therapeutics, and pharmacology as well as his experience in their intelligent communication is reflected in this new edition. We also welcome back many of our previous contributors and appreciate their suggestions, their support, and their enthusiasm. In addition a number of new and distinguished pharmacologists, physicians, and scientists are on our roster. Some have written completely new topics (*see* below), others have rewritten chapters that have appeared previously, including Prescription Writing; Central Nervous System Neurotransmitter Mechanisms and Psychopharmacology; Antidepressant Drugs; Antimanic Drugs; Neuroleptic Drugs; Sedative—Hypnotics and Antianxiety Agents; Drugs for Rheumatic Diseases; Opioids: Agonists, Antagonists, and Mixed Antagonist—Agonists; Cardiac Glycosides; Antiarrhythmic Drugs; Antihypertensive Drugs; Diuretics; Hormones of the Hypothalamus and Pituitary Gland; Pharmacology of the Thyroid Gland; Pharmacology of the Parathyroid Glands and Calcitonin; Insulin, Hypoglycemic Drugs, and Glucagon; Pharmacology of the Corticosteroids and Adrenocorticotropic Hormone; Pharmacology of Androgens and Estrogens; Oral Contraceptives; Drugs Used to Treat Protozoal Diseases; The Vitamins; Commonly Used Intravenous Solutions and Diagnostic Agents; Prolonged-Action Dosage Forms; Therapeutic Drug Monitoring; and Sources of Information in Pharmacology. At the end of most chapters, a number of examination questions have been introduced. We are indebted to Dr. Sydney Ellis, author of *Pharmacology Review*—a comprehensive review for examination and self-assessment in the Arco medical review series—who has shouldered the responsibilities of this innovation. We hope that these questions will provide our readers the opportunity for self-assessment and lead to their better understanding of the textual material.

Scattered throughout the book are footnotes, small vignettes of historical and scientific interest prepared by Sandra Colville-Stewart, which we anticipate will bring life and flavor to these pages. To keep abreast of new developments, a number of new chapters have been added and others deleted. Specifically new chapters have been included on Principles of Drug-Receptor Interactions; Pharmacokinetics; Drugs That Affect

Uterine Contractility; Cyclic AMP as a Mediator of Drug Action; Prostaglandins; Pharmacology of Gastrointestinal Hormones; Vasoactive Peptides; Oral and Dental Pharmacology; and Parenteral Nutrition. Many of these topics were included in other chapters in previous editions but because of their recent emergence in importance have been designated as separate chapters in this 3rd edition. Because there is a more conservative approach to the approval of new drugs in the United States than in other countries, we have included a reference supplement prepared by Drs. Kevin O'Malley and Desmond Fitzgerald that covers those agents available for use in Europe but not in this country. Because some of these reference drugs may be approved for use in the United States during the lifetime of this edition, this material will be of use to those studying in this country.

Our sincerest thanks go to Nelly Canaan and Michelle Markel-Cohen for their untiring effort to bring together the scattered elements of this text. The patience and administrative skills required to accomplish this task can never be overestimated.

John A. Bevan, B.Sc., M.B., B.S.

PREFACE TO SECOND EDITION

For a perfect sight of the old medicine, let me conduct you to the bedside of Charles II: With a cry he fell. Dr. King, who, fortunately, happened to be present, bled him with a pocket knife. Fourteen physicians were quickly in attendance. They bled him more thoroughly; they scarified and cupped him; they shaved and blistered his head; they gave him an emetic, a clyster, and two pills. During the next eight days they "threw in" fifty-seven separate drugs; and towards the end, a cordial containing forty more. This availing nothing, they tried Goa stone, which was a calculus obtained from a species of Indian goat; and as a final remedy, the distillate of human skull.

Sir Andrew MacPhail
The Source of Modern Medicine, 1933

There is no doubt that the "new medicine" is different. Part of the progress is due to the adoption of a rational drug therapy based upon knowledge of the useful as well as the adverse effects of pharmacologic agents.

Many changes have been made in the second edition of this text. A number of new and distinguished authors have been added to the roster of contributors. The whole text has been revised, brought up to date and expanded, particularly into general pharmacology, the pharmacology of the peripheral and central nervous system and the endocrine glands, and anticancer agents. Completely new chapters have been added, including those on pharmacogenetics, drugs of abuse, poisons, alcohol, pediatric pharmacology and drugs used in the treatment of the hyperlipidemias. I would like to thank all those who made suggestions and gave advice on the reshaping of the contents.

As before, the text is designed primarily for medical and dental students although it would be of considerable value to those in the ancillary sciences of medicine, particularly pharmacy and optometry. Despite its modest increase in length it still remains a relatively short text, a distillate of essential pharmacologic knowledge, a sufficient core of knowledge upon which to base drug therapeutics of the new medicine. An understanding of its contents would be sufficient preparation for the National Boards in Pharmacology.

It is a pleasure to thank those to whom I am greatly indebted for their help in the preparation of this edition. The constructive critical review of various chapters by the following members of the Clinical Staff of the Center for Health Sciences, University of California, Los Angeles, is deeply appreciated: Victor D. Newcomer, M.D., Gary S. Rachelefsky, M.D., Ronald M. Reisner, M.D., Arthur D. Schwabe, M.D., Jerrold A. Turner, M.D., and Lowell S. Young, M.D. Dr. Jeremy H. Thompson has been a continual source of invaluable support, comment, and encouragement. Barbara Friedman has carefully drawn the new figures and helped remedy deficiences in existing ones: Nell Crewe has assisted with typing. The staff of the Medical Department of Harper & Row have redesigned the layout of the text. Partial support for compiling the index was obtained from Roerig Division of Pfizer Pharmaceuticals. Finally, my sincere thanks go to Elizabeth Ainley without whose constant, meticulous help and management of the whole revisionary process this edition would not have been possible.

Los Angeles, California *J.A.B.*

PREFACE TO FIRST EDITION

This textbook is based upon the course in pharmacology for medical and dental students given by the staff of the Department of Pharmacology, The Center for the Health Sciences, University of California at Los Angeles. These students have completed their preclinical studies and are commencing their clinical work. The aim is to present an essential core of pharmacologic knowledge sufficient for those proceeding to clinical clerkships, specific enough to guide others during internship, and yet provide a grounding in basic principles for both that will be valuable during the balance of professional life.

The text has been written within the constraints imposed by a recently adopted shorter curriculum. It has been recognized that although all students should understand the principles of the various basic sciences, and for professional reasons must assimilate and retain an essential compendium of facts, much that has been committed to memory in the past need not have been. Often detailed factual knowledge of a subject has been acquired at the sacrifice of a thorough understanding of its principles. Only the latter will prepare the student to understand and make new claims, developments, and advances. The authors of this book have attempted to effect a compromise between an understanding of the principles of drug action and the pragmatic requirements of practice.

Events of the past few years have drawn the attention of both professional and layman to the price we seem to have to pay for our increasingly bountiful therapeutic cornucopia. New drugs can control and cure disease and make our lives longer and more pleasant. Unfortunately, they cause undesirable adverse reactions, interfere with important laboratory testing procedures, and by their very number, often make the choice of the best drug in any particular instance difficult or impossible. For these reasons the adverse effects of drugs have been given unusual emphasis throughout the book. Until agents with new actions or safer substitutes for those commonly used are found, we must learn to use those we have more circumspectly.

Since this book is designed as a teaching text for students, it is not claimed to be a complete exposition of the discipline, nor to be an *infallible* guide to the clinical indications, uses, limitations, adverse effects, and dosage of drugs. The practicing physician is urged to check the drug package insert and other sources before administration especially if the drug is fairly new or used infrequently.

Los Angeles, California *J.A.B.*

CONTENTS

ONE

General Pharmacology and Pharmacologic Principles

TWO
Systematic Pharmacology

DRUGS ACTING PREDOMINANTLY ON THE PERIPHERAL NERVOUS SYSTEM

DRUGS ACTING PREDOMINANTLY ON THE CENTRAL NERVOUS SYSTEM

ESSENTIALS OF PHARMACOLOGY

ONE

General Pharmacology and Pharmacologic Principles

1

JOHN A. BEVAN

History and General Principles

The idea that there are naturally occurring substances useful in the treatment of disease is very old. Such a belief is reflected in the folklore of many ancient peoples, many of whom discovered a number of effective and useful naturally occurring substances. The Egyptian papyri, the ancient Sanskrit writings, and many other early records, including the Bible, often provide evidence of considerable knowledge and practice. From early times, materials with possible medicinal value were often presumed to have magical associations and properties, an illusion that has persisted to today when so many expect effective medicinals with dramatic properties for every disease. Writings of the Greek physicians, particularly Galen, on the use of drugs were widely read and provided authoritative reference through the centuries. Often in combination with occult overtones, such practice dominated the use of substances of potential medicinal value for more than a millenium.

The rebirth of many of the natural sciences during the Renaissance did not occur in the study of drugs. Rather, this period saw the gradual use of more complex formulations: polypharmacy, mixtures of many often exotic substances considered medicinally worthy. Presumably it was hoped that something in the mixture would be effective. This philosophy was diametrically opposed to our present attempts to find ever more specific agents useful in the treatment of particular diseases. The emergence of pharmacology had to await the development of other sciences that provided the necessary knowledge for the rational use of medicinal formulations. Chemistry, for example, allowed the identification of substances, a systematization of their properties, and the synthesis of both existing and new molecules. Physiology, the study of normal bodily function, and biochemistry allowed the action of chemical substances to be described in useful, functional, mechanistic terms. Botany was often the hobby of physicians, and because most drugs came from plant sources the systematization of plants by those medically conscious was an important contribution. Each basic science, then, combined with the demands of medical practice for the amelioration of symptoms and disease, leading to the emergence of pharmacology as a separate rational science. This dependence on the progress of other sciences probably explains why pharmacology is one of the most recently established disciplines in the medical curriculum.

Professional pharmacology in the United States started in 1893 when the first chair was created at the Johns Hopkins Medical School. J. J. Abel, after completing his medical training in Michigan, Johns Hopkins, and a number of foreign universities that emphasized the sciences of biochemistry and physiology, later returned to the Department of Materia Medica at the University of Michigan in Ann Arbor. At that time the physician had to have detailed knowledge on the source of medical materials, specifically drugs. Two years later, Dr. Abel was appointed to the new chair in Baltimore. Subsequently he founded the American Society for Pharmacology and Experimental Therapeutics in 1908.

In the 1940s, 1950s, and 1960s the rate of introduction of new drugs was phenomenal. Most seemed at the time truly miraculous and a prelude to the golden age of treatment and included analgesics, barbiturates, local anesthetics, sulfonamides, antibiotics such as penicillin, diuretics, and psychotropic drugs. Many drugs, however, were new only in name and did not represent an advancement. Further, new compounds were introduced without adequate testing; in fact, only the most elementary testing procedures existed. The emergence of federal regulatory powers urged on by a series of disasters owing to the use of dangerous formulations—the thalidomide tragedy, for example (*see* Chap. 11)—led to the rather conservative stance seen today. At present, new drugs are released for public use in the United States only after they have been tested exhaustively and found to be better or to have some advantage over existing agents and to be safe in comparison to the consequences of the disease they are used to control and cure (*see* Chap. 10). The recognition of the biologic complexity and diversity of purposes in different types of cells not imagined even a few years ago seems to purport that new, more specific useful agents will continue to become available.

SELECTIVE ACTIVITY

Pharmacology may be defined as the study of the *selective biologic activity* of chemical substances on living matter. A substance has biologic activity when, in small doses, it initiates cellular and subcellular changes; it is selective when the response occurs in some cells and not in others. Pharmacology deals with the nature of these selective changes, the systematization of the responses and the chemicals that cause them, and the mechanism whereby these changes are brought about.

Many chemicals possess selective activity valuable in treating disease. Strictly, these are *drugs,* and their use is part of *therapeutics.* Historically, interest in drugs and their effects has been closely associated with medicine. Today, the need for new compounds with selective activity useful in combating disease is still the strongest and most compelling incentive to further investigative research. Although modern pharmacology is still closely associated with medicine, it draws heavily from the basic physical, chemical, and biologic sciences for theory and technique.

Selectivity of action may be manifest at different levels of biologic organization. Antibiotics, for example, act on one species but not on another; general anesthetics act on one organ-system but not on another; morphine acts on one part of an organ but not on another. Most commonly used drugs, with the major exception of antibiotics, are classified according to the organ-system on which they exert their chief selective action. Provided the selective activity of a compound is therapeutic, the greater the degree of selectivity, the more valuable the drug.

DRUG-RECEPTOR INTERACTION

Because drugs, or selectively active substances, act on some cells and not on others, they must exert their effect at some specific site or system that is unique to, or uniquely associated with, the response. This component of the responsive cell is called a *receptor* and may be loosely defined as the site of attachment of a drug through which it exerts its selective action.

DRUG-RECEPTOR BINDING

The forces that govern the interaction between atoms and molecules underlie the interactions between drugs and their receptors. Four types of bonds have been described, discussed below in order of their increasing strength, decreasing incidence in drug-receptor interaction, and probably decreasing importance in determining selective activity. It is assumed that the receptor is comparatively stable in form and that only the alteration of drug structure will affect pharmacologic selectivity and potency.

VAN DER WAALS' FORCES

Weak binding Van der Waals' forces operate between any atoms brought into proximity. The force of attraction of these bonds is inversely proportional to the seventh power of the distance of separation of the atoms or molecules. When the drug and its receptor can come into contact, these forces become highly significant. The larger and more specific the molecule, the greater the contribution of these forces. They are the main reason why drugs react or bind at one site and not at another.

HYDROGEN BONDS

Many hydrogen atoms on the surface of molecules possess a partial positive charge and can form bonds with negatively charged oxygen and nitrogen atoms. Because these act over greater distances than do Van der Waals' forces, closeness is not as important for their effect. These bonds, together with Van der Waals' forces, represent the basis of most drug-receptor interaction.

IONIC BONDS

Ionic bonds, which form between ions of opposite charge, for example, acetylcholine^{+} and chloride^{-}, act at very high velocity. Their importance can be seen clearly with such neuromuscular blocking agents as *d*-tubocurarine (Ch. 19).

Ionic bonds, hydrogen bonds, and Van der Waals' forces dissociate reversibly at body temperature.

COVALENT BONDS

Formed when the same pair of electrons is shared by adjacent atoms, covalent bonds make organic molecules cohere. Because of their strength and the difficulty of reversal or cleavage, drugs acting in this manner cause a prolonged effect. Chloroquine (*see* Chap. 67), phenoxybenzamine (*see* Chap. 18), and the organophosphorus anticholinesterases (*see* Chap. 15) form such bonds; such compounds tend to be extremely toxic.

Covalent bonds are uncommon in pharmacology.

RECEPTORS, ACCEPTORS, AND BINDING SITES

Not all sites with which drugs bind are necessarily *receptors*. The current concept of a receptor is of a macromolecule with which a drug interacts, leading to a change in cellular function. Chemically similar attachment sites probably do exist with which a drug may combine without resultant biologic change. Thus the concept of a receptor pharmacologically includes both the capacity to bind to or react with a drug and to mediate both positive and negative biologic alteration in function. The connections of the receptor within the cell—its biologic coupling—are an integral part of this important concept. Because the same receptor may be linked with different purposes in the same or different cells, drug selectivity resides not only in the receptor but also with the cellular and intracellular processes to which it is coupled and presumably the mechanisms responsible for such interactions.

The old term *acceptor* has been used to describe sites to which a drug can combine but not cause a biologic change. Evidence suggests that acceptors can be similar to receptors, that is, with the same affinity for the drug or else different in some way, often with a lower affinity. Alternative names for acceptors are silent receptors or sites of drug loss.

Some drugs react with receptors not distributed uniformly over the cell surface but aggregated in discrete areas of the cell membrane. Perhaps the best example is *d*-tubocurarine, which exerts its effects at the synaptic junction between the motor nerves and voluntary muscle by reacting with receptors limited to the end-plate region of the muscle cell. This region represents 0.01% to 1.0% of the surface area of the cell. If the amount of drug effective at the end plate were evenly distributed one molecule thick over this specialized area, it would cover only 1% of its surface. Thus *d*-tubocurarine paralyzes voluntary muscle by its reaction with receptors restricted to 0.0001% to 0.01% of the cell surface. Only a small fraction of the *d*-tubocurarine injected into an animal is actually responsible for its selective biologic action. Much of the drug remains in body fluids, and a considerable proportion reacts with plasma proteins and acceptors in connective and other tissues. Sites of drug binding, therefore, are not necessarily sites of pharmacologic action.

In tissues that comprise similar cells, receptors are not necessarily uniformly distributed throughout their substance. In smaller blood vessels, for example, the receptors with which norepinephrine acts to cause constriction may be congregated toward one surface of the smooth muscle layer, whereas those associated with dilation may be concentrated at the other. Nor are receptor populations the same in histologically or ultrastructurally similar tissue. The vascular muscle of blood vessels contains different proportions of diverse receptor types and, according to present knowledge, different subtypes of the same class of receptor.

STRUCTURE–ACTIVITY RELATIONS

Drugs that exert the same or similar specific biologic activity usually have similar chemical or physicochemical properties. A study of sympathomimetic amines (*see* Chap. 17), voluntary muscle relaxants (*see* Chap. 19), and muscarinic agents (*see* Chap. 14) clearly illustrates this principle. Very small changes of chemical structure can, however, sometimes result in a dramatic loss or reduction of specific activity. For example, *l*-norepinephrine and *d*-norepinephrine are identical except that one is the mirror image of the other. Yet the *l*-form is 50 times more active than is its isomer. Such considerations lead to the rather obvious conclusion that the common denominators for selective activity among a given group of drugs are dictated by the chemical and physical characteristics of the receptor.

Affinity is used to describe the propensity of a drug to bind at a given receptor site; *intrinsic activity* describes its ability to initiate biologic activity as a result of that binding. Presumably because of the complexity of the binding process, a drug may possess affinity, that is, be bound at a receptor site, and yet not initiate specific activity. This is not the same as binding at an acceptor site because other drugs may have affinity for the receptor, be intrinsically active, and still be inactive at an acceptor site. A study of the relation between drug structure and selective activity will help to reveal the nature and characteristics of the receptor site.

Current research is trying to isolate receptors. Progress has been quite remarkable: Receptors have been isolated, then reincorporated into living cell membranes where they seem to make their intracellular connections since, through them, biologic change can be initiated.

The receptors for the anticholinesterases (*see* Chap. 15) and digitalis (*see* Chap. 34) are located on or are enzymes. Many drugs act on the same receptors as those through which physiologically important substances such as the neurotransmitters exert their effects. Many other drugs, however, seem little to resemble known cellular constituents, and the existence of receptors for these drugs must be assumed fortuitous. Recently with the encephalins such arguments were shown to be erroneous (*see* Chap. 32.

Biochemical research has elaborated many of the cyclic and sequential series of chemical reactions that proceed to some final cellular event, whether it be a metabolic change, the shortening of contractile proteins, or mitosis. In a number of instances, the precise site of influence of a drug on such reaction chains is known, as with the sulfonamides (*see* Chap. 57.

DRUG ANTAGONISM

The selective activity of many drugs may be specifically blocked or antagonized by other agents. *d*-Tubocurarine, for example, which antagonizes the effect of acetylcholine at the end plate of the skeletal muscle cell, does not antagonize the effects of acetylcholine at the same dose at other cholinergic sites or those of histamine, serotonin, or epinephrine. Frequently, the antagonism between a drug (agonist) and its selective or specific blocking agent (antagonist) occurs at the same receptor, an interaction known as *pharmacologic antagonism.* Such specific blocking agents have a high affinity for the receptor but little or no intrinsic activity.

Not infrequently antagonists share some of the required structural common denominators as their agonists. Many blocking molecules are more bulky than the molecules of the drugs they antagonize. Perhaps reflecting this similarity of structure, some antagonists at times are also weak agonists. We can only assume that they react with the receptors by virtue of the affinity characteristics they share with their agonists but, because of their more bulky form, that they prevent access of agonist molecules to the receptor. Alternatively, more than one reactive site may be present on a receptor. Ideas of agonist and antagonist action at the same receptors can be incorporated into such a concept. Quantitative studies have shown that when agonist and antagonist molecules, which seem to have no direct influence on each other, compete for the same receptor, they obey physicochemical laws as we know them. True pharmacologic antagonism should be distinguished from physiological antagonism where two drugs may appear to antagonize each other's effects by initiating separate and opposing activities.

DOSE AND POTENCY

Patients vary in their response to drugs even when an attempt is made to select as homogeneous a group as possible. When an unselected group of persons is studied, as is the case in most medical practice, the variation in drug effects is considerably greater. Thus the dose for one person may not be appropriate for another.

The factors that govern the affinity and intrinsic activity of an agonist for the same type of receptor in any one person probably show a variation of properties. Some receptors bind more readily with the selectively active molecule than do others and therefore react with the agonist at a lower concentration. If this is true, then the greater the dose given, the greater the concentration of the drug in the region of the receptors, the greater the number of drug-receptor interactions, and the greater the pharmacologic effect. A dose- or concentration-related effect is an attribute of drug action invariably seen in clinical practice except in those uncommon situations when a dose of a drug producing a maximum effect is administered.

Two chemically similar drugs that initiate the same selective activity probably do so by acting on the same population of receptors. If one is effective at a lower molar concentration than the other, it is said to be more *potent*. If all other factors that influence the concentration of the drug in the region of the receptor (*e.g.*, absorption, distribution, penetration, binding, and metabolism) do not account for this difference in potency, it must be related to the relative affinity of two drugs for the same group of receptors.

The term *potency* is often used to express other ideas. For example, if one drug produces a greater maximum effect than another, irrespective of the dose used, it is often said to be more potent. It might be more correct to say that one drug is more *effective* than another. Alternatively, drugs are sometimes considered to be similarly potent if, when used in recommended doses, they cause similar effects. It might be best to consider the doses therapeutically equivalent in these circumstances.

Drugs of high potency are not necessarily the most valuable therapeutically. The best criterion of the relative value of drugs that produce the same effect is selectivity. Obviously a drug of low potency and high selectivity is fairly easy to measure objectively in the experimental animal but difficult in humans because it depends on measuring the ratio of the dose that produces the desired effect to the dose that causes significant adverse effects. The means used in humans to measure this varies with each class of drug and is one of the important problems for the clinical pharmacologist. Often referred to as the *therapeutic ratio* and varying considerably from one drug to another, it is extremely high for the antibiotic penicillin, usually considered to be a safe drug in patients not hypersensitive to it, and low with digitalis, an indispensable drug in treating heart disease but one that must be used carefully.

ACCESSIBILITY

Selective activity may result from the accessibility to a given drug to some receptors but not others. This is often the result of a diffusion barrier. Certain antibiotics, for example, used to sterilize the gastrointestinal tract appear to be specific in this effect because, when taken by mouth, they are not absorbed. The same drugs administered systemically do not exhibit such specificity. Other drugs that have dramatic effects on the peripheral, but not the central, nervous system are denied access to the latter by the blood–brain barrier. Under certain experimental circumstances when the same drugs are tested in the absence of this barrier, their effect on the central nervous system (CNS) becomes clearly apparent. Many barriers, such as the plasmalemma and lysosomal and mitochondrial membranes, can exist between the extracellular space and the sites of pharmacologic receptors. Such molecular characteristics as lipid solubility, molecular size, ionization constant, molecular shape, and biologic stability influence the ability of a drug to reach its ultimate pharmacologic destination. Access to some cells or parts of cells is sometimes possible by special molecular transport systems.

QUANTITATIVE ASPECTS OF DRUG ACTION

The relation between drug dose and effect is one of the most fundamental in pharmacology. Pharmacologists frequently use simple, isolated preparations of tissues *in vitro* to determine basic drug effects. Such tissues, although isolated from the body, can be maintained in reasonable condition for some time. Under these circumstances, the relation between dose and effect is likely to be more meaningful, although there are still many complicating factors. When response is plotted against dose or log dose, the curve relating response to concentration is typically nearly symmetrical and S shaped. Several features of this curve are important. A *threshold* dose can be recognized. Although difficult to define because ability to measure threshold change varies with circumstances and, possibly, the observer, it is common experience that a certain amount of drug must be given before its effects are apparent. The magnitude of a drug's effect does not increase indefinitely. The *maximum* dose elicits a just-maximum response. Here again, the precision with which this dose can be determined is not very great. In contrast, the drug dose to produce a half-maximum response or effect can usually be determined experimentally with some accuracy. This, the *effective* $dose_{50}$ (ED_{50}), is a measure of drug potency. Finally, the slope of the dose-response curve provides an indication of the rate at which a drug's effect will change with dose.

The shape of a dose-response curve is similar to that obtained when the percentage of a large group of animals showing a particular drug effect is plotted against the drug dose needed to produce that effect (*see* Chap. 9). In this latter case, the change is quantal (all or none), and thus the shape of the curve reflects the variation in sensitivity of the population of animals. It might be argued by analogy that the dose-response curve obtained from experiments on isolated tissues reflects the variation in sensitivity of individual cells that respond in an all-or-none way to the drug and that this population of cells has a Gaussian distribution of sensitivity. Individual variation has, however, many other causes. The many variables that influence the consequence of drug administration and physiological effect suggest that this is a most complex problem and that the variables are almost infinite. Some of the more important factors are discussed in chapter 10.

In the whole animal, the relation between dose and effect often appears simple, although this may well be fortuitous because the final drug-induced change is influenced by a multitude of factors. When epinephrine is injected (*see* Chap. 7), for example, the resultant changes in arterial pressure are the consequence of the effect of the drug on various tissues, including the heart and blood vessels, some of which lead to a rise and others to a fall in arterial pressure. The measured effect is influenced by the drug distribution among various body compartments, its temporary storage in some sites, its metabolism and excretion, and the activity of homeostatic reflexes. Thus any experimentally determined relationship in the whole animal is unlikely to have fundamental significance.

INSTRUCTIONS FOR QUESTIONS AT END OF CHAPTERS

These directions will occur with the set of review questions at the end of chapters.

For the first group of questions in each set, the "stem" of the question is followed by five items lettered A to E. The brief direction "Select the ONE best answer" preceding this group of questions is a condensed version of the following.

DIRECTIONS: Each of these questions or incomplete statements below is followed by five suggested answers or completions (A–E). Select the *one* that is BEST in each case.

For the second group of questions, the "stem" is followed by four items numbered 1 to 4. The brief directions

A = 1,2,3; B = 1,3; C = 2,4; D = 4; E = All

preceding the second group of questions are a condensed version of the following.

DIRECTIONS: For each of the questions or incomplete statements below, *one* or *more* of the answers or completions (1–4) are correct. Select the correct answer (A–E) according to the following.

A, if *only 1, 2, and 3* are correct
B, if *only 1 and 3* are correct
C, if *only 2 and 4* are correct
D, if *only 4* is correct
E, if *all* are correct

There are, after some chapters, a third group of questions. The stem of the question is followed by two items lettered A and B. The brief directions

A = A only; B = B only; C = both A and B; D = neither A nor B

preceding this group of questions are a condensed version of the following.

DIRECTIONS: Each set of lettered drug names or statements below is followed by a numbered word or phrase. For each numbered word or phrase enter

A, if the item is associated with (A) *only*
B, if the item is associated with (B) *only*
C, if the item is associated with *both* (A) and (B)
D, if the item is associated with *neither* (A) nor (B)

2

DAVID J. TRIGGLE

Principles of Drug-Receptor Interactions

Of considerable antiquity is the concept that, central to the therapeutic use of drugs, selectivity of action is involved. Ancient civilizations used many naturally occurring drugs of plant origin, some of which, including atropine, ephedrine, and opium, are used today. Other ancient remedies including ground mummies, antimony, and bats' blood were, one suspects, much less effective. Only in the 20th century, however, has the concept of specific sites of drug action been rationally analyzed and developed. Clearly, with a few notable exceptions, drug actions can now be described in terms of their actions at specific cellular sites or receptors.

Definition of these drug receptors is an extremely important component of the understanding of drug action. In some instances the identity of these receptors is well understood. Enzymes represent one important site of drug action, as, for example, in sulfonamide action at bacterial folate synthesis, neostigmine action at acetylcholinesterase, and digitalis action at the transport enzyme Na^+, K^+-ATPase. In other situations, cell lipids may be important, as in the interaction of general anesthetics, and an additional important site of action is provided by the nucleic acid system with which many anticancer drugs interact. Still other receptors mediate the physiologic roles of endogenous regulatory species, including neurotransmitters, hormones, and neurohormones. Such receptors have proved difficult to analyze but are fundamentally significant to cellular function, since the effective expression of specific cellular potential requires that the cell be responsive to the signals of the extracellular environment.

The term *receptor* thus has a very broad application because it represents the site of action of hormones, neurotransmitters, chemotherapeutic agents, and toxic compounds as well as the site of expression of sensory mechanisms, including taste and smell. An inclusive but compact discussion is difficult, and attention here will be focused primarily on drug-receptor interactions with particular reference to the endogenous regulators—hormones and neurotransmitters.

Drug action at pharmacologic receptors is only one aspect of drug action. Clearly, the several processes that determine availability of a drug at its receptor site, including absorption, metabolism, distribution, and excretion (Fig.

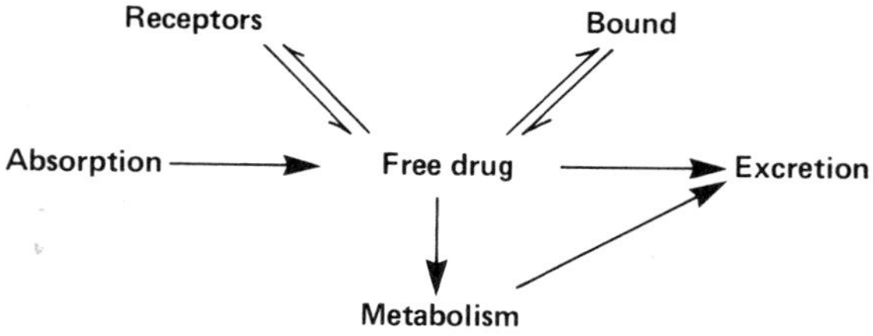

FIG. 2-1. Processes involved in drug distribution and action. After absorption the drug equilibrates with cellular compartments, including those containing specific receptors. The drug may be bound to varying extents in tissues according to its structure and affinity for cell proteins and phospholipids. Additionally, drug may be bound to plasma proteins and thus circulate in bound form. These equilibria are displaced as the drug is metabolized or excreted. The analysis of the interrelations of these several processes is very important in the pharmacokinetic analysis of drug action.

2-1), will obviously contribute to the onset, intensity, and duration of drug action. Further, these same factors and the drug-receptor interaction itself are important in mediating nonconstant expressions of drug action, including the development of resistance, tolerance, and supersensitivity as well as being involved in genetically based and disease-related differences in drug handling and disposition.

RECEPTORS

Our current concepts of receptors, dominant loci of drug action, have their origins in the work of Paul Ehrlich (1845–1912) and J. N. Langley (1852–1926). Ehrlich was much impressed with the high specificity of the antibody–antigen reaction and directed much of his later work toward the design of chemotherapeutic agents that might exhibit a corresponding degree of specificity and thus effectively distinguish between, for example, host and parasitic cells. Ehrlich viewed drug receptors as comprising "protoplasmic side chains," the structures of which differed between cell types. He argued further that drugs were without effect unless bound to such specific cellular entities—"corpora non agent nisi fixata."

Basically the same concept was advanced by Langley during his investigations of the mutually antagonistic actions of atropine and pilocarpine on salivary flow. He wrote,

We may, I think, without much rashness assume that there is some substance or substances in the nerve endings or gland cells with which both atropine and pilocarpine are capable of forming compounds. On this assumption, then, the atropine or pilocarpine compounds are formed according to some law in which their relative mass and chemical affinity are factors.

Subsequently, Langley, from his work on curare and nicotine action on skeletal muscle, defined a specially excitable substance.

. . . I have called it the receptive substance. It receives the stimulus, and by transmitting it, causes contraction.

Both Ehrlich and Langley drew attention, from different perspectives, to a most important feature of drug action—chemical specificity, or the mutual recognition characteristics of drug and receptor. The principles of chemical specificity operate *regardless* of the receptor type. Indeed chemical specificity should be regarded as a fundamental biologic principle, of dominant importance to the expression of biologic function and obviously determinant to processes of molecular evolution. Additionally, Langley drew attention to a feature of the drug-receptor interaction important to pharmacology—the ability of the drug-receptor complex to initiate biologic response. These two aspects of drug-receptor interactions, recognition and activation, and their mutual interrelationship are cornerstones in the contemporary understanding of the pharmacology of drug action. Pharmacologic receptors may be viewed as devices by which a small initial event, the drug-receptor interaction, is greatly amplified to generate a biologic response, very clearly seen

Paul Ehrlich. Born in Silesia in 1854, may very appropriately be called the father of chemotherapy, since he coined the term and defined it as the use of drugs to injure an invading organism without injury to the host. The year 1899 is generally considered to represent the start of Ehrlich's specific interest in chemotherapy, but unquestionably his previous interests in immunity were of fundamental importance. Ehrlich did not receive a great deal of initial encouragement in his pursuit of chemotherapy either from his colleagues or from the government. He received the Nobel prize in 1908 for his work on immunity.

John Newport Langley. Born in Berkshire, England, and graduated from Cambridge in 1874. Originally he intended to enter the Indian Civil Service, but he turned his attention to physiology, becoming Professor of Physiology at Cambridge in 1903. He pioneered in the analysis of the autonomic nervous system, giving to the literature this term. In 1894 he purchased the *Journal of Physiology* and was editor for some 30 years.

in the cascade of events involved in hormone-mediated glycogentolysis (Fig. 2-2).

A classification of receptors based on the biologic response produced is possible but not very helpful because a given response may be initiated by many quite different agents. Thus lipolysis in the fat cell is triggered by many stimuli, including epinephrine, histamine, glucagon, and several other hormones. Such structurally dissimilar species clearly do not act at a common receptor. Conversely, many different responses may result from the interaction of a single agent in different cells. Thus the neurotransmitter acetylcholine can initiate different ion permeability changes (Na^+, K^+, and Cl^-, alone and in various combinations) in excitable tissues ranging from skeletal and cardiac muscle to nerve cells. More usefully, receptors are classified according to the chemical requirements for activation or antagonism of a particular response. Thus acetylcholine interacts with two major classes of receptors at which its actions can be mimicked by muscarine and nicotine and which have been classified as muscarinic and nicotinic acetylcholine receptors, respectively (see Chap. 13). Further, the distinction provided by activator or agonist molecules is paralleled by the actions of antagonist drugs because atropine and curare serve as specific antagonists at the muscarinic and nicotinic receptors, respectively. Such considerations of ligand selectivity have proved fundamental not only to producing primary divisions of receptors, but also in providing subclassifications.

That multiple agents can initiate a common response and a single agonist can initiate distinct responses has important consequences for our general understanding of receptor organization. Such a finding suggests that receptors comprise at least two components that may be functionally, if not structurally, discrete and that subserve the recognition (ligand binding) and amplification (response) components of the drug-receptor interaction (Fig. 2-3).

A further and extremely important aspect of drug-receptor interactions concerns receptor localization. The receptors for neurotransmitters and polypeptide hormones are integral protein components of the plasma membrane. Current views of the plasma membrane depict it as a fluid matrix of proteins and a phospholipid bilayer. The plasma membrane shows considerable dynamic behavior both for mobility and for turnover of membrane components, including receptors. Thus receptors and other membrane components are not permanent entities either in space or time, and changes in receptor population are a component of both physiologic and pathologic cellular states. In contrast, receptors for steroid and thyroid hor-

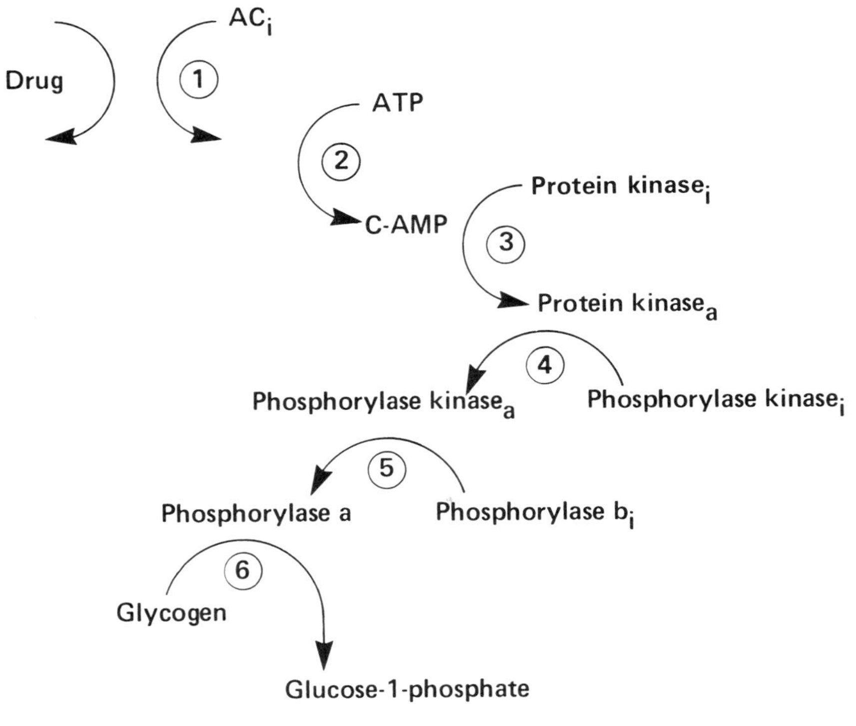

FIG. 2-2. The cascade of events seen in hormone-mediated glycogenolysis. At each step of the sequence (1 through 6), amplification of the original signal occurs. Thus the activation of a very small number of receptors in step 1 results in the generation of a very large response in step 6. This mechanism provides for efficiency and economy in the original signal.

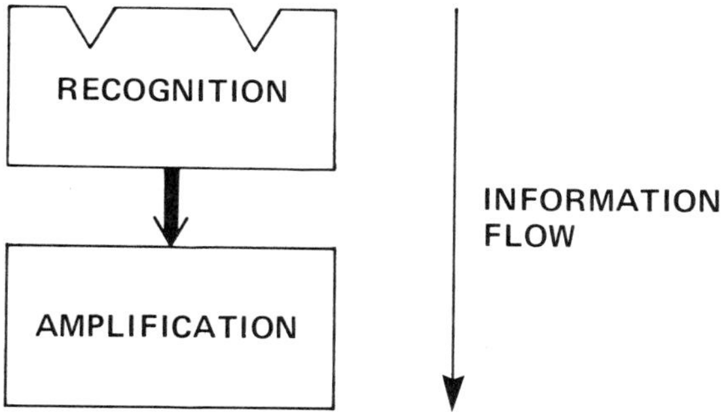

FIG. 2-3. A receptor depicted as two components that separately mediate recognition (drug specificity) and transformation of this signal into biologic activity (amplification). Drug molecules bind specifically to appropriate recognition sites, and the resultant interaction is translated into response.

mones are intracellular entities the function of which is to translocate the hormones to the genetic machinery to initiate changes in genetic expression. These receptors are also subject to regulation.

The above views, although attractive, represent a considerable oversimplification because membrane receptors probably exist to translocate steroid and thyroid hormones to the cell interior. Further, the constant turnover of membrane components indicates that intracellular pools of plasma receptors exist that represent proteins being incorporated into, or being removed from, the cell membrane.

Until recently, characterization of pharmacologic drug receptors has been essentially an indirect process, primarily based on analysis of the biologic response and of the structure–activity relationship underlying drug action. Recent developments using radiolabeled compounds of high specific activity and high affinity have, however, made possible the direct analysis of drug binding to receptors, the localization of receptors, the purification of some receptors and receptor components, and, in some cases, partial reconstitution of receptor activity from isolated components (*see* below, Transduction Processes). These direct approaches to receptor structure and function have increased our understanding considerably.

STRUCTURE–ACTIVITY RELATIONSHIPS

Basic to our understanding of drug-receptor interactions is that there exists a definable mutual molecular complementarity between the drug and its corresponding receptor. The analysis of this complementarity provides the basis of structure–activity relationships. Among the earliest attempts to formulate structure–activity relationships was that of the Edinburgh physicians Crum–Brown and Fraser (1869) who, from their work on the curarelike properties of alkaloids, concluded,

> *There can be no reasonable doubt that a relation exists between the physiologic action of a substance and its chemical composition and constitution.*

The development of structure–activity relationships subsequently has been vitally significant to the development of pharmacology and therapeutics. It has underlain the development of new drugs, has been fundamental to the development of receptor classification and subclassification, and has led to the discovery of new endogenous drug structures.

The original, and daring, postulate by R. P. Ahlquist (1948), based on the differing relative activities of sympathomimetic amines in several catecholamine-sensitive preparations, that two classes of receptor exist, the α- and β-adrenergic receptors, was elegantly confirmed by the later discovery of antagonists, including propranolol, selective for the β-adrenergic receptor. Further developments indicated that β-receptors are subdivided into β_1 and β_2 subcategories and have led to the development of cardioselective (β_1) antagonists and bronchoselective (β_2) agonists. More recently histamine receptors have been divided in H_1 and H_2 categories by an application of structure-activity relationships, leading to the development of H_2 antagonists cimetidine and burimamide, selective for histamine receptors that mediate gastric acid secretion (*see* Chap. 51).

The above examples represent the use of structure–activity relationship to exploit structural clues, often faint and ephemeral and which lead to the development of drugs of novel classes. From the opposite perspective the demonstration of a structure–activity relationship is presumptive evidence for the existence of a specific receptor. Thus the structure–activity relationship for morphinelike structures is consistent with the existence of an opiate receptor and, because morphinelike structures are not brain constituents, pursuit of the receptor concept has led to the discovery of the endogenous receptor specific opiate peptides (*see* Chaps. 17, 18). Other endogenous molecules may exist that interact with receptors defined by the existence of structure-activity relationships. Of particular interest is the search for an endogenous substance that may interact with receptors, defined through structure-activity relationships, for diazepam (Valium) and related benzodiazepines.

Structure–activity relationships can be analyzed at various levels of sophistication. At the simplest level it may be little more than molecular roulette, determining the effects of random molecular variations on the biologic activity of a basic structure. More sophisticated approaches include considerations of the three-dimensional structure of the drug and of the various electronic and steric features of the individual substituents composing the drug structure. Thus the biologic activity of a given series of compounds may be factored into discrete components as

$$\log \text{activity} = a\pi + \gamma\sigma + E_s + c,$$

where π, σ, and E_s represent the hydrophobic (oil:water partition coefficient), electronic (electron withdrawing or releasing), and steric (size) effects of substituents in a given series. A typical, and very simple, example is shown in Figure 2-4, depicting the correlation between atropinelike activity and hydrophobicity in a series of compounds. More subtle expressions of this approach are also possible with the inclusion of molecular variables derived from

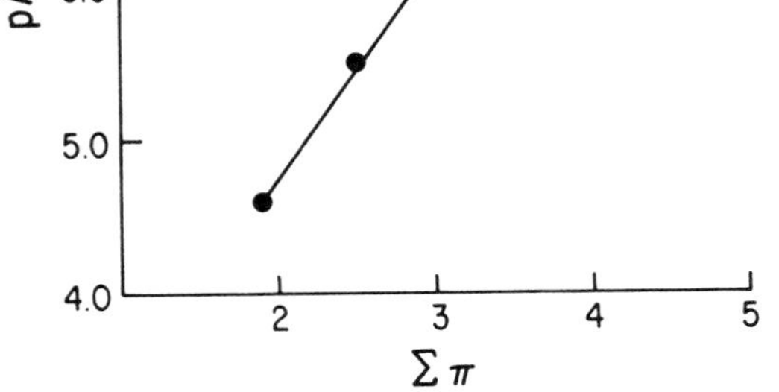

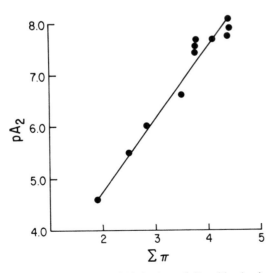

FIG. 2-4. Correlation of biologic activity with physicochemical properties of drug molecules. Biologic activities (pA_2 values) for a series of atropinelike compounds, as antagonists at muscarinic acetylcholine receptors in the gut, are plotted against the hydrophobic properties of the molecule ($\Sigma\pi$). The linear relationship shows that within this series of compounds activity depends on the nonpolar properties of the molecule.

quantum calculations, including electron density and substituent electronegativity.

Steric factors have long been recognized to be fundamentally important to drug-receptor interactions. Indeed, stereoselectivity of drug action is one of the most powerful criteria for the existence of a specific drug-receptor interaction. However, the visualization of three-dimensional molecular structures is difficult. Recent developments in computer graphics have made it possible to display three-dimensional structures from various perspectives and to compare directly structural differences and similarities between different drugs. This is likely to be a major advance in our future interpretation of structure–activity relationships.

KINETICS OF DRUG-RECEPTOR INTERACTIONS

Pharmacology deals essentially with the relationships between drug concentration and biologic effect. Such relationships may be expressed as dose-response curves depicting the (generally) graded relation between drug concentration and effect (Fig. 2-5). The analysis of such relationships is important because it allows quantitative comparisons of drug activities and because of the information gained about fundamental mechanisms of drug-receptor interactions.

Analysis of the basic equation of drug-receptor interaction,

$$A + \text{Rec} \rightleftharpoons A\text{---Rec} \xrightarrow[\text{steps}]{\text{intermediate}} \text{response} \quad 1$$

has, until very recently, been achieved only by indirect procedures. An early and very important approach was that of A. J. Clark (1926), who applied mass action formalism to Equation 1. He made the basic assumption that the magnitude of the biologic response was directly proportional to the concentration of drug-receptor complex, with a maximum response corresponding to complete receptor occupancy. Accordingly,

$$K_A = \frac{[R][A]}{[RA]}, \quad 2$$

where R represents receptor, A the agonist drug, and K_A the dissociation equilibrium constant of the drug-receptor complex. Since

$$[R_{total}] = [R] + [RA]$$
$$= [RA]\left\{1 + \frac{K_A}{[A]}\right\}, \quad 3$$

then if response is directly proportional to receptor occupancy,

$$\text{response} = \frac{[RA]}{[R_{tot}]} = \frac{1}{1 + K_A/[A]} \qquad 4$$

and when 50% of receptors are occupied by drug,

$$K_A = [A]_{50} \qquad 5$$

and the dissociation constant of the drug-receptor interaction is equal to the concentration of drug giving 50% response $[A_{50}]$ (Fig. 2-5). By analogy to the *p*H scale of hydrogen ion concentrations, A_{50} concentrations are sometimes expressed such that

$$pD_2 = -\log [A_{50}]. \qquad 6$$

The analogy between this treatment and that of enzyme-substrate systems is very clear. Equation 4 can be rearranged to show this similarity:

$$\frac{v}{V_{max}} = \frac{[S]}{[S] + K_M} \quad \text{and} \quad \frac{[RA]}{[R_{TOT}]} = \frac{[A]}{[A] + K_A}. \qquad 7$$

On rearrangement,

$$\frac{1}{[RA]} = \frac{1}{[R_{TOT}]}\left\{1 + \frac{K_A}{[A]}\right\} \qquad 8$$

$$= \frac{K_A}{[R_{TOT}][A]} + \frac{1}{[R_{TOT}]} \qquad 9$$

and a plot of $\frac{1}{[RA]}$ (reciprocal of response) against $\frac{1}{[A]}$ should give a straight line, analogous to the Lineweaver–Burke plot in enzyme kinetics (Fig. 2-5). A very obvious difficulty with this simple approach is that it attempts to correlate a primary drug-receptor interaction with a biologic response that may be removed by several intermediate events from its primary interaction.

This treatment can be readily expanded to include antagonist drugs, agents that interact with the receptor but do not initiate a response. Consider an antagonist B competing with agonist A for the receptor with a dissociation constant K_B. It can be shown that

$$\text{response} = \frac{[RA]}{[R_{TOT}]} = \frac{1}{1 + \frac{K_A}{[A]} + \frac{K_A}{[A]} \cdot \frac{[B]}{K_B}}. \qquad 10$$

This, the basic equation for competitive antagonism, indicates that the antagonist B produces an apparent reduction in the affinity of the agonist A for the receptor and that increasing the concentration of A will overcome the antagonism produced by B without reducing the maximum response. The agonist dose-response curve thus undergoes a parallel rightward shift (*see* Fig. 2-6) that can be expressed in a double reciprocal plot entirely analogous to competitive inhibition in enzyme kinetics (Fig. 2-5). Competitive antagonists are very com-

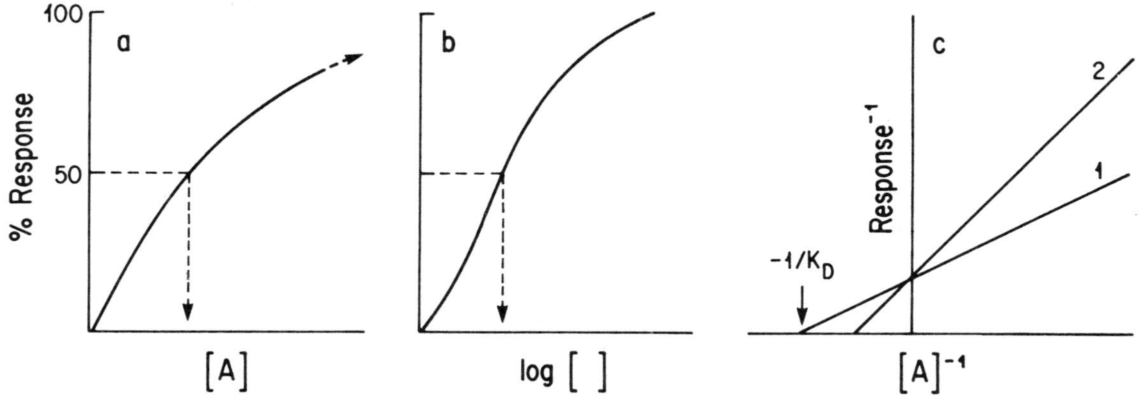

FIG. 2-5. Representation of dose-response relationships. (*a*) A linear representation of the relation between response and drug concentration showing a typical hyperbolic curve. (*b*) A semilogarithmic representation showing the sigmoidal dose-response relationship. (*c*) A double-reciprocal representation of the dose-response curve showing (*1*) response to stimulant alone and (*2*) response to stimulant in the presence of competitive antagonist.

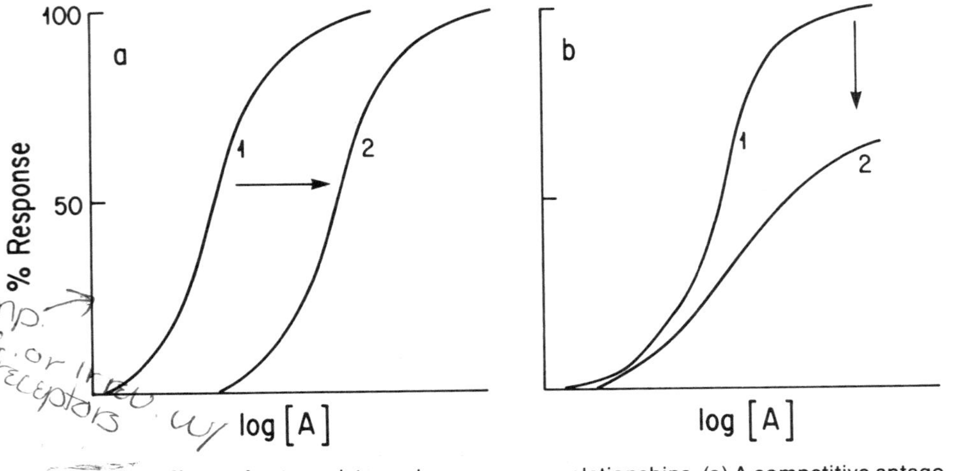

FIG. 2-6. The effects of antagonists on dose-response relationships. (*a*) A competitive antagonist displaces the agonist dose-response curve (*1*) to the right (2) in parallel fashion. No loss of maximum response is seen. An identical displacement can be seen if an irreversible acting antagonist is used in a system that has a receptor reserve. (*b*) A noncompetitive antagonist produces a depression of maximum response without parallel shift to the right. An irreversible antagonist will produce an identical displacement if a receptor reserve does not exist.

mon pharmacologic agents and include atropine and *d*-tubocurarine at muscarinic and nicotinic acetylcholine receptors, respectively, propranolol at the β-adrenergic receptor, and mepyramine at the H_1-histamine receptor.

Not all antagonists belong to this competitive category. An antagonist may function not by competing directly with the agonist at the receptor but by interacting at another site where binding can inhibit response. Such noncompetitive antagonists reduce the maximum response of the agonist (Fig. 2-6).

This simple treatment of drug-receptor kinetics does contain some severe limitations. It offers no mechanistic basis for distinguishing between agonists and antagonists, and both species are presumed to occupy the receptor. Additionally, it is frequently found, when comparing a homologous series of drugs, that a transition occurs between agonist and antagonist with graded molecular change. Some drugs do not produce maximum biologic response (Fig. 2-7). Such compounds are referred to as partial agonists, and their behavior can be described by introducing the term *intrinsic activity*, α, which represents the ability of the drug-receptor complex to initiate response. Clearly for antagonists $\alpha = 0$ and for agonists $\alpha > 0$.

An additional limitation of Clark's treatment is that it is unlikely the basic underlying assumption of complete receptor occupancy needed for maximum response is correct. Evidence for this limitation in Clark's treatment is available from direct and indirect sources. Frequently an irreversibly acting competitive antagonist, an agent that can form a covalent nondissociable bond at the receptor, does not produce the expected reduction in the maximum response of an agonist but behaves rather

FIG. 2-7. Dose-response relationships for a homologous series of compounds showing full agonists (*A*) (*1*, *2*) and the progressive transition to partial agonist behaviour (3, 4, 5). This type of behavior can be observed at virtually all receptor systems.

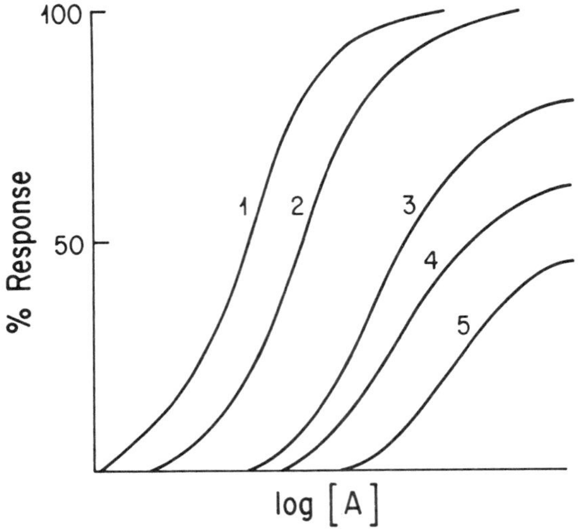

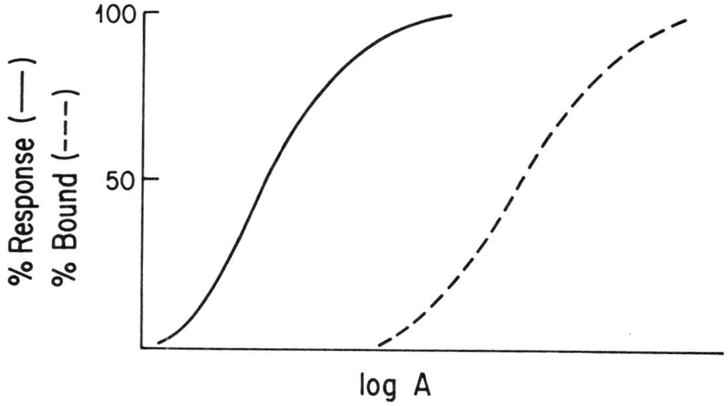

FIG. 2-8. Comparison of dose-response relationship (——) and receptor occupancy relationship (----). In this system the receptor occupancy curve lies to the right of the biologically determined dose-response relationship consistent with occupancy of only a small fraction of receptors necessary for the generation of response.

as a competitive antagonist (Fig. 2-6), suggesting that it is not necessary to occupy all of the receptors to produce maximum response and that "spare receptors" or a "receptor reserve" exists. This conclusion has been supported by more direct evidence where the actual binding of drug to the receptor has been measured and has revealed a discrepancy between the dose-response and the binding curve (Fig. 2-8).

The presence of a receptor reserve has important implications for the analysis of drug-receptor interactions. Agonist dose-response curves cannot be considered as equivalent to saturation curves, and thus K_A values for agonists simply are not equated with the agonist concentration that produces 50% response.

Valid kinetic measurements of competitive antagonist action, obtained from the analysis of dose-response curves, can be shown very simply and demonstrate an important principle in bioassay procedures. If an agonist A and competitive antagonist B interact at the same receptor, and if equal responses are compared in the absence or presence of antagonist, it follows from Equations 7 and 10 that

$$\frac{1}{1 + \frac{K_A}{[A]}} = \frac{1}{1 + \frac{K_A}{[A]_B} + \frac{K_A}{[A]_B} \cdot \frac{[B]}{K_B}}, \qquad 11$$

where [A] and $[A]_B$ are the agonist concentrations producing equal responses in the absence or presence of antagonist. On rearrangement of Equation 11,

$$\frac{[A]_B}{[A]} = 1 + \frac{[B]}{K_B}. \qquad 12$$

Thus by comparing the ratio of agonist concentrations needed to produce an equal response, the dissociation constant for the antagonist K_B

FIG. 2-9. Determination of pA_2 ($-\log_{10} K_B$) value for a competitive antagonist. Shown is the determination for atropine action at muscarinic receptors in intestinal smooth muscle. The dose ratio (*DR*) for an agonist is determined from dose-response curves in the presence and absence of the antagonist. Usually at least three antagonist concentrations are used, allowing graphical evaluation of K_B (↓) and slope of line (= 1.0 for simple competitive antagonism).

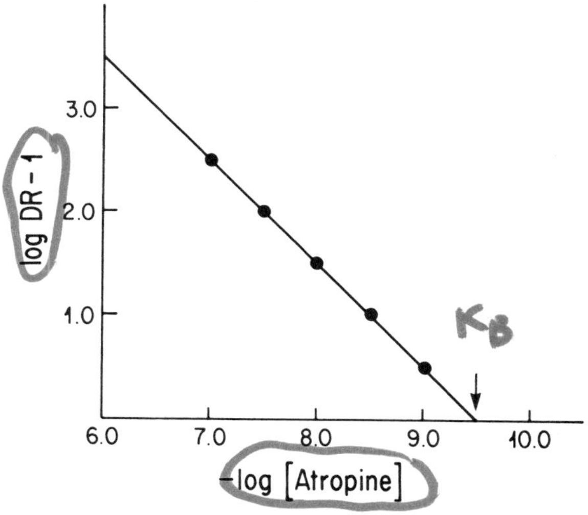

can be measured without any assumption as to the relation between the fraction of receptors occupied by the agonist and the size of the response. For convenience, Equation 12 is usually evaluated graphically:

$$\text{Log}\,\frac{[A]_B}{[A]} = \text{log-dose ratio} = \log\left(1 + \frac{[B]}{K_B}\right) \qquad 13$$

so that a plot of $\log \frac{[A]_B}{[A]}$, usually referred to as dose ratio, against log [B] gives a straight line of unit slope with an intercept of K_B (Fig. 2-9).

By analogy to the notation used for agonists, K_B values obtained by this procedure are often expressed as pA_2 values where

$$pA_2 = -\log_{10} K_B. \qquad 14$$

Whereas pA_2 is a true measure of antagonist affinity, pD_2, because of the uncertain relation between receptor occupancy and response, is usually not a true measure of agonist affinity.

In recent years the essentially indirect approaches to the study of drug-receptor interactions have been aided by approaches in which the binding of agonists and antagonists to drug receptors can be measured directly. These direct approaches are possible because of radiolabeled compounds (usually labeled with tritium or iodine) of high specific activity such that binding to the low concentrations of receptors can be detected. With such techniques drug binding to neurotransmitter, polypeptide, and steroid hormone receptors has been studied. Further, by autoradiographic techniques these compounds have allowed the visualization of receptor localization.

Quite generally, drug binding has both specific and nonspecific components, and in radiodrug studies these can be distinguished because the specific component of binding can be blocked by drugs known from pharmacologic experiments to interact with the receptor system under investigation (Fig. 2-10). Additionally this receptor component of binding has a specificity of drug interaction that parallels the specificity derived from pharmacologic structure–activity data. Thus if binding of ^{3}H-propranolol to β-adrenergic receptors is studied, the specific binding component is sensitive only to drugs, agonists and antagonists, that in-

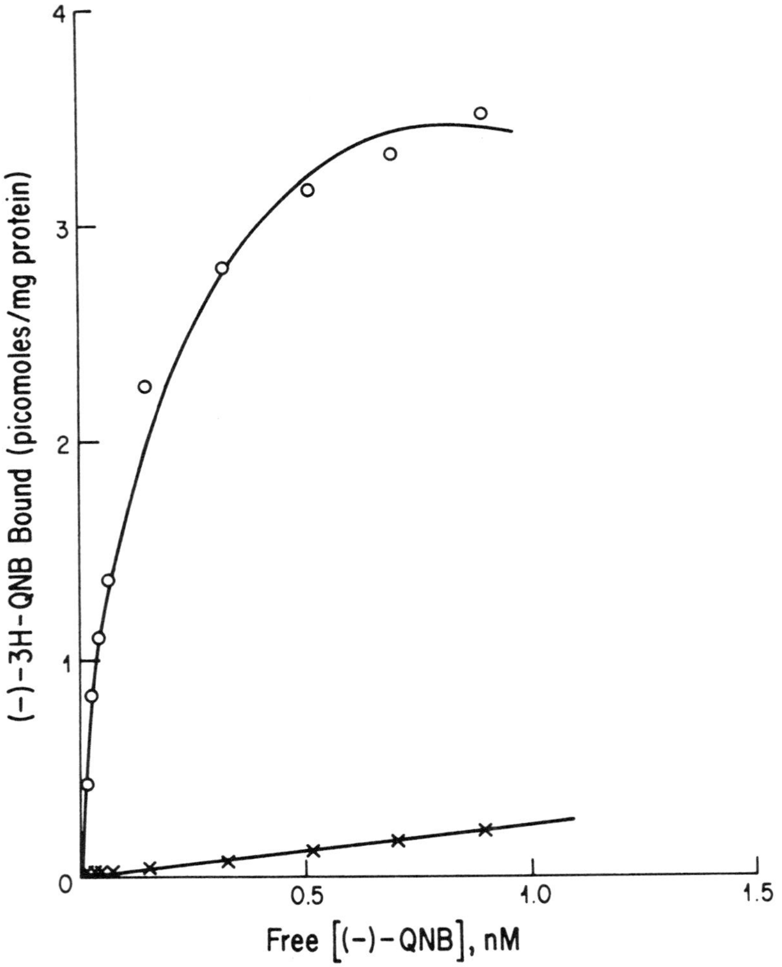

FIG. 2-10. A radioligand receptor-binding experiment. Shown is the binding of a potent atropine-like compound ^{3}H-(−)-quinuclidinyl benzilate (*QNB*) to muscarinic receptors in intestinal smooth muscle. Specific binding to receptors (o-o) is shown relative to nonspecific binding (x-x) to nonreceptor components. Receptor binding is a saturable process, whereas nonspecific binding is typically nonsaturable.

teract with β-receptors and is insensitive to drugs specific for other receptors.

Among the important conclusions derived from direct drug-receptor binding studies is the close agreement found between affinities for antagonists measured both directly and indirectly. A typical example of such a correlation is shown in Figure 2-11 for a series of antagonists active at muscarinic acetylcholine receptors. In marked contrast the affinities of agonists measured by direct binding are usually significantly lower than those determined simply from dose-response curves. Such a discrepancy (Figs. 2-8 and 2-12) is consistent with the existence of a receptor reserve so that occupancy of only a small fraction of receptors is needed to initiate maximum response.

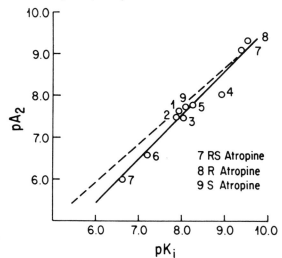

A further, and very important, conclusion drawn from the direct drug-binding studies is that antagonist binding is usually consistent with interaction at a single class of sites of uniform affinity. In contrast, agonist binding often is best described by interaction with two classes of sites of different affinity. Although several different explanations are possible for such behavior, this heterogeneity of agonist binding may be linked to the ability of agonists, but not antagonists, to initiate response.

FIG. 2-11. A typical example of a correlation between affinities of competitive antagonists determined from biologic responses (pA_2) and from radioligand binding (pK_i) experiments. K_i values are determined from inhibition of radioligand binding (in this case ^{3}H-quinuclidinylbenzilate, a potent muscarinic antagonist) and, for direct comparison with pA_2 values, have been presented as $-\log K_i = pK_i$. Shown are data for a series of compounds, including atropine in its racemic (*RS*) and stereoisomeric forms (*R* and *S*), that are muscarinic antagonists. The two sets of data show excellent agreement, pA_2 and pK_i values being almost identical. (The dashed line shows the theoretical 1:1 relationship.) Such agreement is commonly found for antagonist action at many receptor systems.

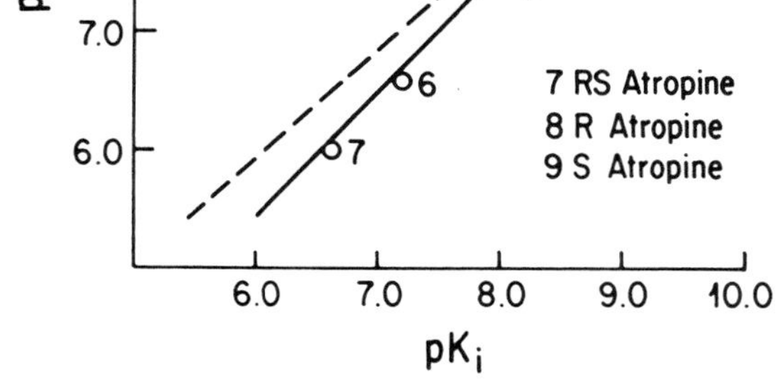

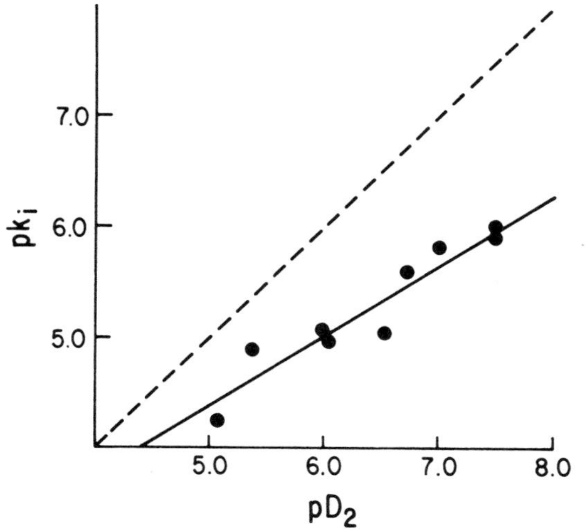

FIG. 2-12. Correlation between affinities of agonists determined from biologic responses (pD_2) and from radioligand binding (pK_i) experiments. Shown are data for a series of muscarinic agonists. In contrast to competitive antagonists (Fig. 2-11), there is a substantial discrepancy between the two sets of data. (The dashed line shows the theoretical 1:1 relationship.) This is consistent with the view that the pD_2 value ($-\log A_{50}$) is not a true measure of the affinity of an agonist for its receptor. Such lack of accord is very commonly found for agonist action in many receptor systems.

TRANSDUCTION PROCESSES

In any study of drug-receptor interactions, the mechanisms by which these interactions initiate the sequence of events leading to biologic response must be classified. This transduction sequence can be a complex series of coupled ionic and biochemical changes by which the initial interation is ultimately amplified to contractile, secretory, and other responses (Fig. 2-13). Elucidating these events is important not only because of the fundamental information gained on drug-receptor interactions, but also because such information is useful for indicating possible new sites of drug intervention and for probing disease-related receptor defects.

The sequence of events subsequent to drug-receptor interaction and the nature of the primary drug-receptor interaction itself are now more clearly known. Many drug (hormone)-re-

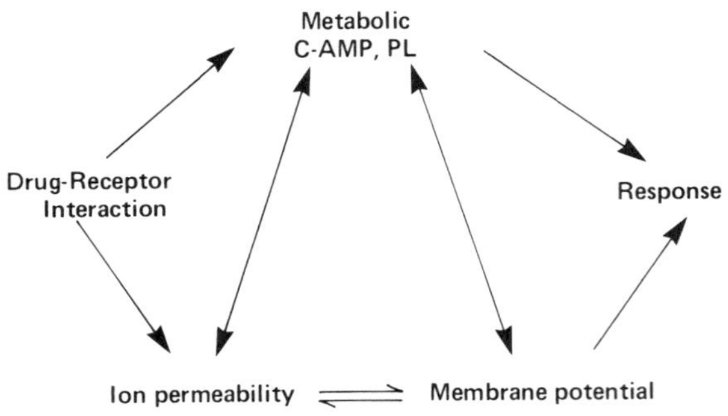

FIG. 2-13. Sequence and interrelationship of events initiated by drug-receptor interaction that serve to generate the biologic response. The initial drug-receptor interaction may generate changes in ionic permeability or changes in some biochemical function (c-AMP formation, phospholipid [*PL*] degradation), which may then interact, either singly or in combination, to generate the final biologic response.

ceptor interactions arise from two general mechanisms: In one, the function of the drug-receptor interaction is to open (or close) an ion channel, thus altering transmembrane ion flow and membrane potential (Fig. 2-14A); in the second mechanism, the drug-receptor complex functions to activate (or inhibit) adenylate cyclase (Fig. 2-14B), thus initiating (or inhibiting) the sequence of c-AMP dependent events (Fig. 2-2). In such systems c-AMP or calcium (for an ionic event) are frequently referred to as second messengers because they execute the instructions of the primary drug-receptor interaction. These processes are not necessarily mutually exclusive, and both may function after a drug-receptor interaction. Both processes indicate, however, that the function of the drug is to facilitate transition between the resting and the activated receptor states.

The hormonally sensitive adenylate cyclase system is activated by a large number of agents, including neurotransmitters, polypeptide hormones, and prostaglandins. Experiments involving cell fusion, mutant cell lines, and receptor reconstitution have shown clearly that hormonally sensitive adenylate cyclase comprises at least three distinct proteins: the R, G, and C proteins that represent recognition (drug binding), guanine nucleotide binding, and catalytic site proteins, respectively. The independence of these three proteins has been shown in cell fusion experiments where two cell lines, one deficient in the R component and the other in the C component, produce a functional drug-sensitive system. Each of the three proteins carries out separate but linked functions (Fig. 2-15) such that binding of drug to R alters the affinity of G for guanine nucleotides (GTP and GDP), and the state of ligation of the G protein determines the catalytic activity of the C protein. The G protein has GTPase activity, and the hormone activation of the G protein

FIG. 2-14. Two representations of primary events in drug-receptor interations depicting the activator drug as promoting conversion of (*A*) an ion channel from an inactive to active state; (*B*) adenylate cyclase from an inactive to active state.

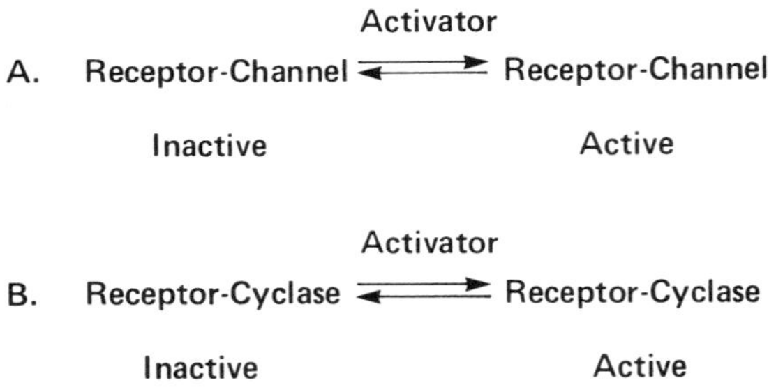

FIG. 2-15. Schematic representation of the events in the activation of hormone-sensitive adenylate cyclase. This receptor system comprises three distinct entities: the recognition (hormone binding) unit ((R)); the guanine nucleotide binding unit ((G)); and the catalytic (adenylate cyclase) unit ((C)). The following sequence of steps is shown: association of hormone A with (R) forms A (R), which then interacts with the G component to form (R) (G). This is depicted as binding guanosine diphosphate (*GDP*). Formation of (R) (G) $_{GDP}$ causes an exchange of GDP with guanosine triphosphate (*GTP*) and a concomitant dissociation to (R) and (G) $_{GTP}$. The latter can activate the inactive adenylate cyclase C_i with hydrolysis of GTP to GDP. Thus the system can be viewed as interlocking cyclic sets of events involving association and dissociation of hormone with receptor, exchange of GDP and GTP, hydrolysis of GTP to GDP, and conversion of adenylate cyclase from the inactive to active state.

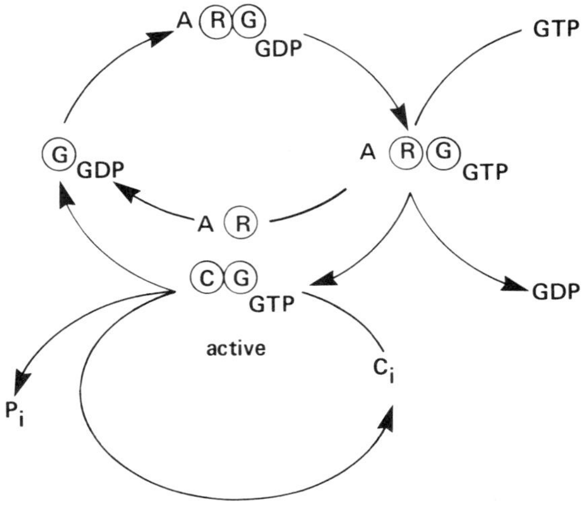

is terminated by this hydrolytic activity. Agents that inhibit GTPase activity, including cholera toxin, thus produce a persistent stimulation of adenylate cyclase. Other agents, including catecholamines (α-adrenergic receptors), opiates and muscarinic cholinergic agonists, are inhibitory toward adenylate cyclase and may prevent association of the G and C protein components.

A second major pathway of drug-receptor activation is exemplified by the receptor-activated ion channel processes, which have been particularly well studied for the nicotinic acetylcholine activated ion channels of skeletal muscle. Ion channel opening allows a flow of Na^+ and K^+ ions, and the resultant depolarization propagates along the muscle fiber to activate the contractile process. The ion conductance changes associated with the activation by agonists of single ion channels can be measured directly. These single conductance events vary in duration but not in magnitude, consistent with the agonist-receptor interaction that facilitates the transition between the closed- and open-channel states.

Despite their obvious differences, both drug-receptor activation processes may be considered as having receptor-effector systems that exist in an equilibrium between two states—resting (shut) and activated (open). The biologic activity of a drug will then depend on its relative affinity for the two receptors states (Fig. 2-16). A drug with high affinity for the activated state will perturb the equilibrium in favor of receptor activation. A drug, perhaps a structural homologue, that has only slightly greater affinity for the activated state than for the resting state will obviously cause a smaller perturbation of equilibrium and will thus be a partial agonist. Finally, a drug that has no selective affinity for either state will cause no change in equilibrium and can function as an antagonist. Such a model explains the fundamental differences between agonists and antagonists but is only a very simple model of drug-receptor interactions. More sophisticated treatments are available. Such models are needed to accommodate cooperative behavior of drug binding in which more than one molecule of drug may bind to the receptor and to accommodate allosteric behavior in which drug binding to a site remote from agonist binding may nonetheless influence the receptor activation process.

FIG. 2-16. Drug action viewed in terms of two-state models of receptor activation. The receptor is assumed to be able to exist in two states: inactive (R_i) and active (R_a). Without a stimulating drug, the equilibrium favors the inactive state. A drug may have differential affinity for these two states: A drug with high relative affinity for R_a will cause the receptor equilibrium to shift in the direction of the active state. Such a drug will be a powerful agonist. A drug with no selective affinity will not shift the equilibrium and hence will be an antagonist. Drugs with intermediate levels of selective affinity will function as partial agonists because they will promote varying degrees of formation of D. R_a, which are less than those promoted by powerful or full agonists.

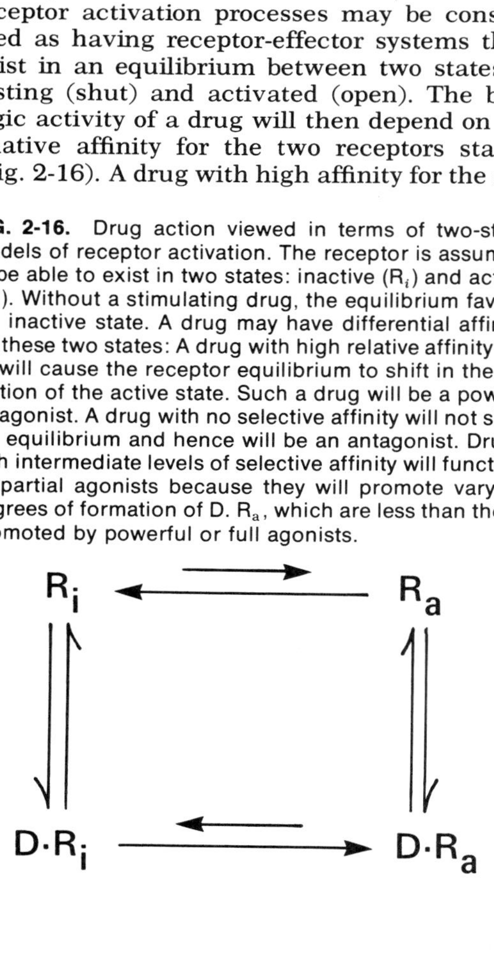

RECEPTOR-RELATED PROCESSES

Initiation or inhibition of biologic response is the primary consequence of the drug-receptor interaction, but the biologic consequences of the drug-receptor interaction are not invariant. States of diminished or increased responsiveness occur during, or after, drug action.

The phenomenon of diminished response, variously described as tachyphylaxis, tolerance, refractoriness, or desensitization, has various origins. At the nonreceptor level, desensitization may occur through increased drug metabolism as, for example, a component of barbiturate tolerance or through substrate depletion as in tachyphylaxis to indirectly acting (norepinephrine release) sympathomimetic amines. However, the direct study of drug-receptor binding has shown that changes in receptors and their drug binding properties play a major role in desensitization phenomena. Self-regulation of receptors, whereby chronic increases or decreases in agonist concentration mediate decreases ("down regulation") or increases ("up regulation"), respectively, in the concentrations of the corresponding receptors, has been established for many hormones, neurotransmitters, and their analogues, including insulin, growth factors, releasing hormones, catecholamines, and angiotensin. Typically, these changes and their recovery have a time-course ranging from hours to days. Such changes in receptor concentration lead to reciprocal changes in agonist sensitivity. Receptor regulation appears to be a general feature of membrane receptor systems and is a consequence of the dynamic character of the plasma membrane.

These homologous regulation processes are paralleled by heterologous regulation whereby cross-regulation of receptors occurs. Thus uterine catecholamine receptors are regulated by steroid hormones and cardiac catecholamine receptors by thyroid hormone.

Clearly such regulation processes represent one component of cellular homeostasis whereby cellular sensitivity adjusts to chronic changes in hormone or neurotransmitter traffic. Desensitization can also occur, however, in an acute form whereby brief exposure to an agonist can reduce the response, frequently with a time-scale of seconds to minutes. Such processes may also serve a regulatory role to terminate a cell signal.

Different mechanisms probably are involved in acute and chronic desensitization. Acute desensitization probably represents events in which the receptor is rendered insensitive to a drug by conversion to an inactive state (Fig. 2-17) or in which the receptor is uncoupled from the amplification unit so that subsequent drug binding is without effect. In contrast, chronic desensitization probably represents changes in the receptor population. The process of actual receptor loss has been described for a number of receptors and involves a dominant role for receptor clustering in membrane-coated pits. From these specific areas, receptor endocytosis occurs with subsequent degradation and delivery to intracellular organelles. Chronic receptor occupancy increases the rate

FIG. 2-17. A cyclic model of desensitization in which rapid formation of the initially active drug receptor complex (*AR*) is followed by a slow transition to the inactivated state (AR_D), from which recovery of the receptor to the activatable state is slow.

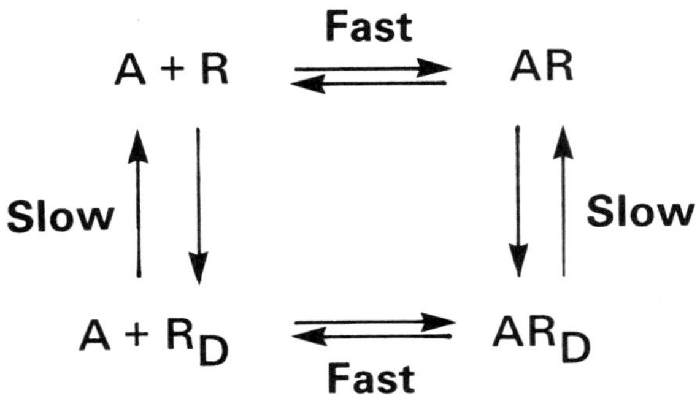

of this process above that of incorporation of newly synthesized receptor into the membrane, and a net receptor loss occurs. Coated pits, in addition to regulating receptor concentration, also facilitate cellular uptake of specific proteins. Low-density lipoprotein (LDL), bound to specific LDL receptors, is taken into the cell and broken down to generate cholesterol, thus regulating cholesterol biosynthesis.

Various mechanisms probably are involved in short-term or acute desensitization. Such mechanisms include uncoupling of the recognition and amplification components of the receptor, conversion of the receptor to an inactive state, and production of a metabolite that may serve to inhibit the function of one or the other receptor components. One such process is the acetylcholine-induced densitization of the nicotinic acetylcholine receptor. For this system desensitization can be represented as a cyclic scheme (Fig. 2-17) in which an equilibrium exists between two receptor states, resting (R) and desensitized (D), the latter state being in slow equilibrium with other receptor states and having a higher affinity for acetylcholine (A) than does the resting state.

Although specific desensitization may be seen as the obvious consequence of receptor-induced changes, nonspecific desensitization also occurs. Such processes are typically seen in multiply sensitive systems and, in contrast to specific desensitization, are presumed to involve alterations in a common pathway distal to the specific (receptor) components (Fig. 2-18).

The importance of desensitization processes is that they are exerted at physiologic, pharmacologic, and pathologic levels. Receptor desensitization may be associated with the generation of rhythms of cellular responses, as in the pineal gland rhythm of adrenergic β-receptor concentrations and in the changes in ovarian luteinizing-hormone receptors as a component of the cellular signals of the estrus cycle. The importance of receptor internalization in the regulation of cholesterol biosynthesis has already been noted, and such internalization processes may facilitate entry of hormones, insulin, and growth factors known to exert long-term effects on cellular responses.

Receptor desensitization is probably also important in some therapeutic situations, as in the loss of isoproterenol sensitivity after repeated use of aerosol bronchodilators to treat asthma or the loss of decongestant activity

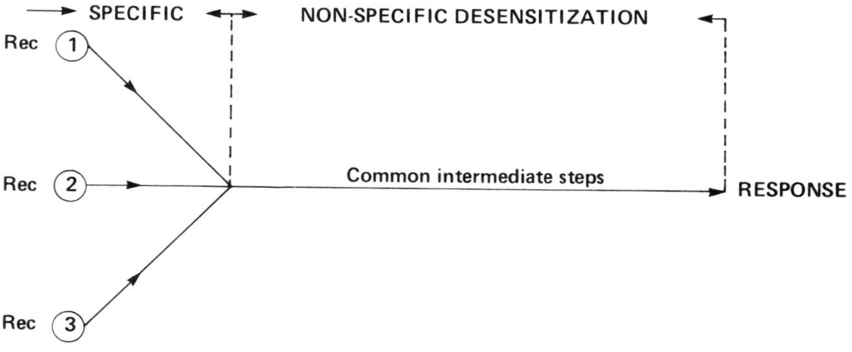

FIG. 2-18. Specific and nonspecific desensitization in a multiple receptor system.

after repeated use of nasal sprays. Chronic receptor occupancy by antagonists may lead to an increased receptor concentration and to the development of supersensitivity on drug withdrawal. The "rebound" phenomena subsequent to rapid withdrawal of propranolol, and probably other antagonist drugs, represent therapeutically important examples of this process.

A further consequence of the dynamic state of receptors is that changes in receptor concentration and organization occur during development and aging. Such changes are likely to have important consequences for drug therapy in both the very young and the aging patient.

Receptor loss or inhibition of receptor function is associated with a number of pathologic states. This has been particularly well described for myasthenia gravis where circulating receptor-directed antibodies (autoantibodies) increase the rate of degradation of nicotinic acetylcholine receptors in skeletal muscle and lead to the impaired neuromuscular transmission characteristic of this disease (*see* Chap. 16). The insulin resistance of obesity is accompanied by elevated basal insulin levels and a reduced insulin receptor concentration; normalization occurs both by suppression of insulin release and by a hypocaloric diet. Autoantibodies have been described in patients suffering from acute insulin-resistant diabetes, accompanied by a decrease in monocyte insulin receptor concentration. Circulating antibodies have been detected against β_2-adrenergic receptors in several patients with allergic rhinitis and asthma, suggesting a basis for the adrenergic hyporesponsiveness seen in such persons. Circulating autoantibodies are found also in Graves' disease, the most common form of hyperthyroidism, directed against the thyroid stimulating hormone (TSH) receptors of thyroid cells. In this case, however, the autoantibodies are stimulatory in nature, leading to overproduction of thyroid hormone (*see* Chap. 44).

In addition to the receptor changes mediated by drug exposure or through antibody action in autoimmune states, genetically linked receptor deficiencies occur associated with a number of disease-states. These deficiencies are not limited to changes in receptor concentration but can include changes in the several steps that link drug-receptor interaction and biologic response. Thus three distinct defects of the LDL receptor have been associated with familial hypercholesteremia: a functional LDL receptor present in greatly reduced concentrations, a nonfunctional receptor unable to bind LDL, and an LDL receptor that, although it can bind LDL, cannot be internalized. All of these receptor-related defects lead to the impairment of cholesterol metabolism characteristic of familial hypercholesteremia.

A number of other clinical disorders are associated with receptor defects: pseudohypoparathyroidism (defect in renal parathyroid hormone receptors); nephrogenic diabetes mellitus (defect in antidiuretic hormone receptors); Laron dwarfism (defective growth hormone receptors); and hypothyroidism (defective TSH and T3 receptors).

FURTHER READING

1. Goldstein A, Aronow L, Kalman SM: Principles of Drug Action, 2nd ed. New York, John Wiley & Sons, 1974
2. Albert A: Selective Toxicity, 6th ed. New York, John Wiley & Sons, 1978
3. Schulster D, Levitzki A (eds): Cellular Receptors for Hormones and Neurotransmitters. New York, John Wiley & Sons, 1980

CHAPTER 2 QUESTIONS

(See **P. 7** **for Full Instructions)**

Select the One Best Answer

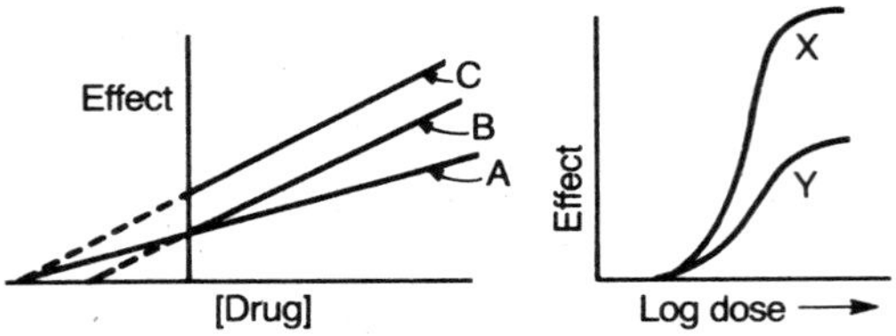

1. On the basis of the Lineweaver–Burk plot above, the following could be true.
   - A. If drug A is an agonist, B could represent the effect of the agonist in the presence of a noncompetitive antagonist.
   - B. Drug C has a greater affinity for the receptor than does drug A.
   - C. If drug A is represented on the log dose-effect graph as curve X, C could correspond to curve Y.
   - D. Drugs A and B could be agonists with similar affinity for the receptor, but different efficacies.
   - E. If drug A is an agonist, C could represent the agonist in the presence of a competitive antagonist.

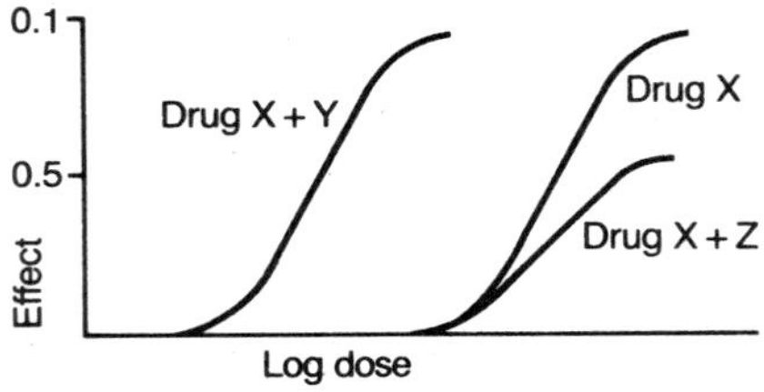

2. With regard to the above graph, all of the following are true EXCEPT
   - A. if drug X is norepinephrine, drug Y could be cocaine.
   - B. if drug X represents an agonist, drug Z could be a noncompetitive antagonist.
   - C. if drug X is acetylcholine, drug Y could be neostigmine.
   - D. if drug X is acetylcholine, drug Z could be atropine.
   - E. if drug X is norepinephrine, drug Z could be phenoxybenzamine.

A = 1,2,3; B = 1,3; C = 2,4; D = 4; E = All

3. Which of the following statements about drug-receptor interactions are correct?
   1. Antagonists are always structural analogues of the drugs that they block.
   2. An agonist is a drug that has both affinity and efficacy.
   3. A noncompetitive antagonist must antagonize all receptors before a significant blocking effect is achieved.
   4. A competitive antagonist will shift the log dose-response curve for an agonist to the right with no depression of the maximum response.

4. The term "competitive reversible inhibition" implies that
   1. the two drugs are interacting at the same receptor site.
   2. increasing the dose of the antagonist will result in a parallel shift to the left of the log dose-response curve of the agonist.
   3. the end-organ response is more a function of the agonist-receptor combination rather than the actual drug concentrations.
   4. both agonist and antagonist must be closely related in chemical structure.

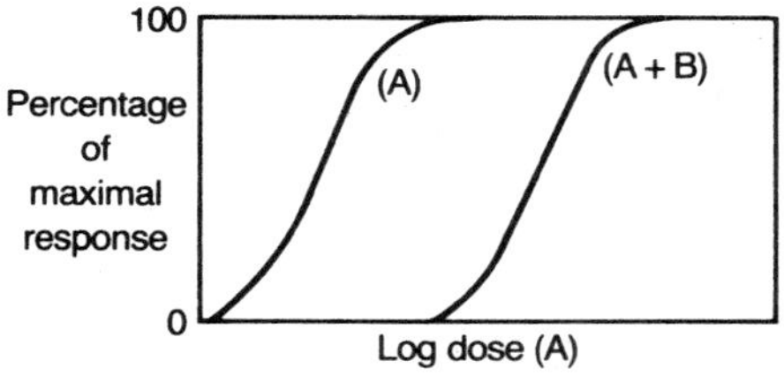

5. The dose-response curves above represent the effect of drug A alone and the effect of drug A in the presence of drug B. Which of the following statements apply?
   1. Drug B is probably a competitive antagonist of drug A.
   2. The intrinsic activity (efficacy) of drug A has been altered by drug B.
   3. If drug A is acetylcholine, drug B could be atropine.
   4. Drugs A and B most likely exert their effects on different receptors.

JEREMY H. THOMPSON

3

Drug Absorption, Distribution, and Excretion

The nonpharmacologic events that occur after a drug is absorbed into the bloodstream, distributed throughout the body, and eliminated either by conversion to another compound or by excretion are described in this chapter. These events are important because they determine the quantity of drug that reaches its site of action and the length of time available to interact with its receptor.

ROUTES OF DRUG ADMINISTRATION

Drugs may be given by various routes (Table 3-1). Clinically the route selected is governed by a drug's physical and chemical properties (*see* later in this chapter); its desired site of action (local or systemic); the general state of the patient (for example, does the patient have vomiting or diarrhea that might preclude using the oral route, or is there a patent, readily accessible vein that allows intravenous (i.v.) injection); the drug volume and dosage interval; the required rapidity of response and the duration of effect; other drugs given concomitantly (*see* Chap. 8); and convenience. The most important and generally safest route for systemic therapy is oral; subcutaneous (s.c.), intramuscular (i.m.), or i.v. injections are also widely used.

A drug can be introduced as a gas, in solution, as a suspension, or as a solid. In the last two states, the rate at which it disintegrates and dissolves or is extracted into biologic fluids is significant in its rate of absorption (its bioavailability). Formulation factors, and the number and order of adding excipients during formulation, influence drug disintegration and dissolution markedly and may lead to altered bioavailability (*see* Chap. 11).

The four most important factors that influence the rate and degree of drug absorption at any given site are blood flow, surface area, length of time a drug is present, and pH at the site of absorption.

TOPICAL

Drugs applied topically are generally given for a local effect since they are rarely absorbed sufficiently to produce systemic effects owing to the thick barrier of the stratum corneum. However, absorption may be excessive from exten-

TABLE 3-1. Routes of Drug Administration

Route	Tissue	Drug Examples for Local (L) or Systemic (S) Effect
Topical (local)	Skin, conjunctivae, otic canal, vagina	Cortisone (L), antibacterials (L), cosmetics (L), nitrite creams (S)
Inhalation	Nose	Decongestants (L), pituitary snuff (S)
	Lungs	Cromolyn sodium (L), anesthetic gases (S)
Enteral (into the digestive tract)	Buccal	Antiseptic lozenges (L)
	Sublingual	Nitrites (S)
	Gastrointestinal tract for intralumenal effect	Poorly absorbed drugs such as nonsystemic antacids (L) Group 4 sulfonamides (L)
	Gastrointestinal tract for a systemic effect	Most drugs given by mouth (S)
	Rectal	Suppositories (glycerine) (L), sedatives, tranquilizers (S)
Parenteral (by injection)	Intradermal	Skin test antigens (L)
	Subcutaneous	Local anesthetics (L), insulin (S)
	Intramuscular	Antibiotics (S)
	Intravenous	Antibiotics (S)
	Intraarterial	Anticancer agents (L)
	Intralymphatic	X-ray contrast media to outline local lymphatics (L)
	Intrathecal	Air (in x-ray studies) antibiotics (L; but usually with systemic therapy
Miscellaneous	Subdural	Some local anesthetics for spinal-type local anesthesia
	Specific cavities (pleura, peritoneum, joints, bladder)	Drugs for a local effect, usually antibiotics, x-ray contrast media, antiinflammatory agents

sive burns or if a drug is applied in dimethyl sulfoxide (DMSO) or some other nonapproved solvent.

INHALATION

Some drugs are formulated for either a local effect in the respiratory passages (*e.g.*, decongestants) or for a systemic effect (*e.g.*, the inhalation anesthetic gases). Drug absorption is rapid from the lungs because of their large surface area and extensive blood flow.

ENTERAL

The mucous membrane of the oral cavity has a thin, richly vascular epithelium conducive to rapid absorption. One advantage of this route of administration is that once absorbed, the drug enters the general circulation directly without first passing through the liver. When absorbed from the stomach or intestines, a drug must pass through the hepatic portal system before entering the general circulation. Because the liver is a major site of drug metabolism, a substantial amount of drug can be metabolized on "first pass" (*see* Chaps. 4 and 8). Examples of drugs subject to extensive loss on first pass are the organic nitrites (*see* Chap. 35) and propranolol (*see* Chap. 18).

Neutral and acidic drugs are readily absorbed from the stomach (*see* below). The gastric mucosa has an extensive blood supply and, as a consequence of its rugae, a large surface area. The low pH prevents significant absorption of basic drugs (*see* below), but they are absorbed more effectively from the oral cavity ($p\text{H} \sim 6.0$) or the intestine ($p\text{H} > 7.8$).

The physiological role of the intestine is to absorb end-products of food digestion. The large surface area, rich vascularity, near-neutral pH, and length of time that end-products stay in the intestine all promote absorption. Enteric coating and various special formulation devices (*i.e.*, "time release" preparations) (*see* Chap. 78) are important in delivering certain drugs to the small intestine or in producing sustained plasma levels (*see* Chap. 78).

Parenteral

A parenterally administered drug is usually injected subcutaneously, intramuscularly, or intravenously. Other routes are less common and involve administration for local effects.

The absorption of drugs from s.c. and i.m. sites is usually quite rapid. These routes are especially important for drugs such as insulin and some penicillins that decompose in the gastrointestinal tract or drugs that are poorly absorbed, such as the aminoglycosides. Modifications of a drug's physical state have been used to retard absorption from these sites in an attempt to prolong the drug's T½. Steroid-containing pellets, for example, have been implanted subcutaneously, and drugs may be formulated in an oily vehicle (for example, hormones) or complexed with other poorly soluble agents such as benzathene (*i.e.*, penicillin G) to form a depôt of the active drug. A more pharmacologic approach for s.c. injections is to include a small volume of epinephrine, a vasoconstrictor (*see* Chap. 18) that reduces local blood flow at the site of administration.

Drugs prepared for intravenous (i.v.) administration must be suitably diluted. Intravenous administration may involve direct injection as a *bolus* (a very rapid injection) or as an *infusion* (an injection over minutes to hours, usually in a large volume parenteral). "*Piggy back*" administration (a fairly rapid injection into the tubing of a large-volume parenteral infusion set followed by a flushing of the system with the infusion solution), is also common.

Intravenous administration has the distinct advantages of speed, precision, and complete "absorption." However, i.v. bolus injections may cause adverse cardiovascular effects such as hypotension and cardiac arrhythmias. Thus i.v. infusions, piggy back injections, or administration from large-volume parenteral solutions are often preferred. Additional problems from the intravascular injection and the high plasma concentration of drug that results include thrombophlebitis, anaphylaxis (which is usually more severe because of the rapid and intense antigen–antibody reaction), and CNS effects, for example, stimulation after procaine (*see* Chap. 22).

PROPERTIES OF ORGANIC MOLECULES THAT GOVERN ABSORPTION, DISTRIBUTION, AND EXCRETION

Most drugs are organic molecules, made up of carbon-containing backbones with different functional groups. The nature of functional groups and the arrangement of the hydrocarbon backbone impart to the organic molecule its *specificity* for a given site of action or receptor and its ability to penetrate tissues and cells. To discuss logically the absorption, distribution, and excretion of drugs, one must recognize the role of the functional groups of drugs in these processes. Because new drugs are continuously being developed, it is important to understand the chemical basis for the pharmacokinetic properties of drugs so that potential distribution and absorption problems may be predicted.

POLARITY

The most important general property of a drug is its *polarity* or ability to dissolve in water. The polarity of a drug will determine its biologic activity (for example, whether it enters the brain), its duration of action, and its route of elimination. The *partition coefficient* (K_p) is used as a measure of polarity and is defined as the equilibrium ratio of concentrations (C) of a drug after it has distributed itself between two immiscible solvents, that is,

$$K_p = \frac{C_{org}}{C_{aq}}.$$

The solvents are usually an aqueous solution (aq) and an oillike organic (org) or lipophilic solvent. Typically the partition coefficient of a substance between water and olive oil, or between water and *l*-octanol, is determined and recorded. Thus the K_p of an organic compound is a measure of its relative affinity for a polar, aqueous medium versus its affinity for a nonpolar, oillike medium.

The affinity of an organic molecule for aqueous media depends on its ability to solvate with water. Functional groups such as $-OH$, $-NH_2$, $-SH$, and $-COOH$ that can form hydrogen bonds impart to a molecule a greater solubility in aqueous media, whereas groups such as alkyl, phenyl, other hydrocarbons, or halogens impart greater solubility in organic solvents. A compound, then, such as inositol would have a smaller oil–water K_p than would cyclohexanol because of its greater number of OH groups.

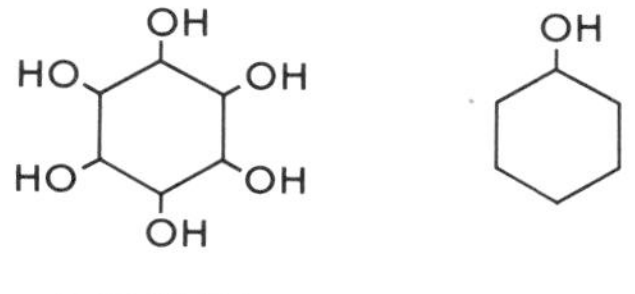

INOSITOL CYCLOHEXANOL

IONIZATION

Carboxyl (COOH), amino ($-NR_2$), and phenolic (ArOH) functional groups also increase solubility in water by ionization. A carboxylic acid ionizes to give a hydrogen ion and conjugate base:

$$CH_3COOH \leftrightarrows CH_3 - COO^- + H^+.$$

An amino group ionizes by accepting a hydrogen ion:

$$CH_3 - NH_2 + H_2O \leftrightarrows CH_3 - NH_3^+ + OH^-$$

and a phenolic group ionizes by losing a hydrogen ion:

$$ArOH \rightleftarrows ArO^- + H^+.$$

Organic acids and bases are weak electrolytes, and at physiologic *p*H the polar (ionized) and the nonpolar (neutral) forms exist in equilibrium, which has important consequences in the distribution and elimination of drugs with ionizing groups. Because of their greater water solubility in the ionized state, drugs such as salicylic acid (a weak acid) and diphenhydramine (an organic base) are used as their sodium or hydrochloride salts, respectively (Fig. 3-1).

PENETRATION OF MEMBRANES

Membranes that separate tissue and cellular compartments are primarily semipermeable owing to their lipid character. Thus membranes can be viewed as a lipid bilayer with a protein coat on each surface and with proteins that extend through the bilayer to provide sites of interaction with intracellular and extracellular polar substances. The mechanisms discussed below are involved in the passage of drug molecules through tissue compartments.

PASSIVE DIFFUSION

In passive diffusion, the most common mechanism of membrane penetration, molecules move from an aqueous extracellular or cytoplasmic medium to the lipid medium of the membrane; from there, depending on partition, they can enter or leave the cell by diffusing through the membrane. The driving force for passive diffusion is the concentration gradient between the compartments. Molecules will move from an area of high concentration to one of low concentration at a rate proportional to the concentration difference between the two areas. The *concentration difference* refers to the diffusable species, which for weak electrolytes such as acids and bases is the neutral (nonpolar) species. Therefore the state of the ionization equilibrium is important in determining the rate of diffusion.

CARRIER-MEDIATED TRANSPORT

Polar compounds such as sugars and amino acids cannot penetrate membranes by passive diffusion but are moved by *carrier systems* present on the membrane surface. A recognition site (carrier) forms a complex with the substrate which, in turn, moves intracellularly across the membrane by one of several different processes: Carriers can move substrates along their concentration gradient (*facilitated diffusion*) or in opposition to an established electrochemical gradient (*active transport*). In both cases, the process is limited by saturation of the carrier at high substrate concentration. Carrier-mediated transport thus displays behavior analogous to enzyme substrate interaction.

Drugs can function as substrates for carriers if they resemble endogenous chemicals. Tyramine, for example, which is chemically similar to norepinephrine and dopamine, has an affinity for the norepinephrine and dopamine carriers (*see* Chap. 13). Tyramine gains access to the nerve cells by complexing with carriers on

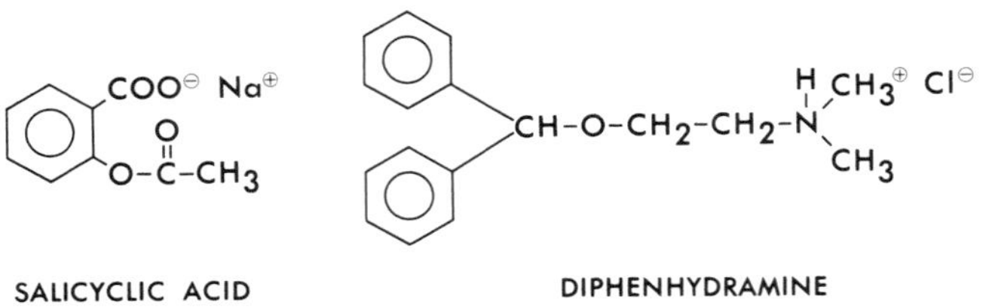

FIG. 3-1. Chemical structures of salicyclic acid and diphenhydramine.

the outside surface and by being transported into the noradrenergic neuron.

MISCELLANEOUS MECHANISMS

Some tissues do not have "tight junctions" but have gaps between adjacent cells, and others have small pores on their surfaces. These gaps and pores allow small molecules such as water or ethanol or small ions to pass freely without having to penetrate the lipid barrier. Large molecules such as proteins and polypeptides move intracellularly by *pinocytosis*, a process in which the solution containing the large molecule is engulfed by the cell.

ABSORPTION OF DRUGS

A drug is usually introduced into an organism at locations remote from its site of action, and, unless the drug is given intravenously, it must enter the circulation if a systemic effect is required. This process, movement into the circulation, is called *absorption*. Two key factors affecting the rate of drug absorption are the *p*H at the site of absorption and the route chosen for its administration.

EFFECT OF *p*H

When the *p*H difference is substantial between the site of absorption and the blood, the rate of absorption of weak electrolytes varies with the nature of the ionized species. The gastric contents, for example, are usually quite acidic (*p*H ~ 1) so that the state of ionization of acids and bases in the stomach will be markedly different from that in the plasma (*p*H 7.4). If a weak electrolyte is introduced into either side of the two compartments, it will diffuse across the separating membranes only in the neutral, nonpolar form and approach an equilibrium where the concentration of neutral species is equal on both sides (Fig. 3-2). The rate at which it will attain equilibrium and the rate at which the drug will move from one compartment to the other will depend on the concentration of the diffusable form. Thus conditions that favor the neutral form of the drug will enhance drug movement. On the other hand, conditions that favor ionization will favor nontransfer of the weak electrolyte, since the proportion existing as the diffusable form will be low. This phenomenon is called *ion trapping* and is illustrated below for a carboxylic acid of pKa 5 and an amine of pKa 9.4 (Equations 1 through 5).

In Figure 3-2, the plasma and the stomach are shown separated by a barrier representative of the mucous membranes between the two compartments. The barrier is permeable only to the neutral form of each electrolyte that diffuses across the membrane along its concentration gradient. The rate of diffusion is

$$\text{rate} = K\Delta X \qquad (1)$$

where ΔX is the difference in concentration of the diffusing species and K is a constant.

In the absorption of a weak acid, the propor-

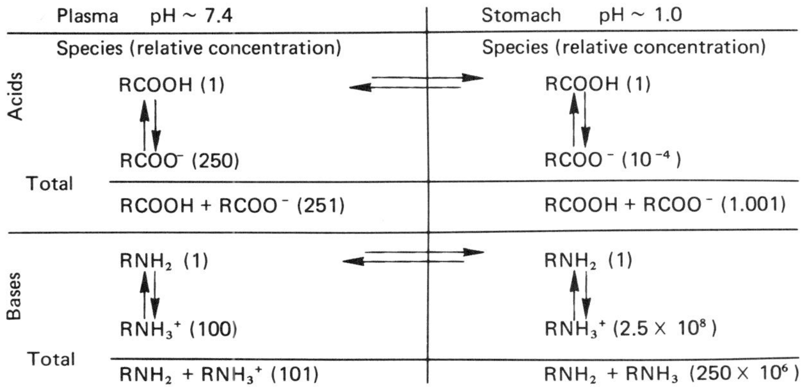

FIG. 3-2. The partition of weak electrolytes between plasma and stomach. The plasma and stomach compartments are separated by a barrier representing a membrane or a series of membranes. Only the neutral, nonpolar form of weak electrolytes can penetrate the barrier so that the equilibria indicated are established, with only the neutral form at equal concentrations across the membrane barrier. The total drug in each compartment is given by the sum of neutral and ionized species.

tion in the diffusable, neutral form (f_{HA}) is given by the expression

$$f_{HA} = \frac{[HA]}{[HA] + [A^-]} \qquad 2$$

where [HA] is *conjugate acid* and $[A^-]$ is *the conjugate base*. [HA] and $[A^-]$ are related by the Henderson–Hasselbach equation so that

$$[A] = [HA] \cdot 10^{pH-pKa}. \qquad 3$$

Then, if intragastric pH = 1 and weak acid's pKa = 5,

$$f_{HA} = \frac{1}{1 + 0.0001} = 0.999. \qquad 4$$

Thus 99.99% of the weak acid in the gastric lumen is in the diffusable form. In the plasma compartment, however, the ratio is quite different:

If plasma pH = 7.4 and the drug's pKa = 5, then

$$f_{HA} = \frac{[HA]}{[HA](1 + 10^{2.4})}$$

$$= \frac{1}{1 + 251.2} = 0.004. \qquad 5$$

Thus only 0.4% of the weak acid in the plasma is in the diffusable state.

These equilibria show that a weak acid introduced into the stomach will move into the plasma rapidly because essentially all of the acid is in the diffusable state. In the plasma, the acid is essentially all in the nondiffusable state. Thus there is a maximal concentration gradient of the diffusable species in the direction of the plasma, and once in the plasma the acid is trapped because of the small proportion that can diffuse back into the stomach.

This relation is reversed in the absorption and distribution of organic bases. For a weak base, the fraction of the neutral species, f_A, is given by

$$f_A = \frac{(A)}{(HA)(A)} = \frac{A}{A(1 + 10^{pKa-pH})}. \qquad 6$$

K. A. Hasselbach. Copenhagen scientist. Developed a formula for the determination of the pH of blood (1912).

Lawrence Joseph Henderson, 1878–1942. Boston biochemist. Worked on the determination of urinary pH (1913) and on blood acid–base equilibria.

For a weak base of pKa = 9.4 in the stomach (pH = 1),

$$f_A = \frac{1}{1 + 10^{8.4}}$$

$$= \frac{1}{1 + 2.5 \times 10^8} = 4 \times 10^{-9}, \qquad 7$$

whereas in the plasma (pH = 7.4),

$$f_A = \frac{1}{1 + 10^2} = \frac{1}{101} = 9.9 \times 10^{-3}. \qquad 8$$

Although the weak base is predominantly ionized in both compartments, the ratio of the neutral species between the stomach and the plasma is

$$\frac{[RNH_2]\text{stomach}}{[RNH_2]\text{plasma}} = \frac{4 \times 10^{-9}}{9.9 \times 10^{-3}} = 4 \times 10^{-7},$$

indicating that a much greater proportion of neutral species exists in the plasma. These calculations show that diffusion will proceed from plasma to stomach, and therefore that amines (or weak bases) are poorly absorbed from the stomach. Any basic drug will be ion trapped in the more acidic compartments, a property sometimes useful in identifying unknown drugs in the stomach contents of a patient who has taken an overdose. Many abused drugs, such as the narcotics, amphetamines, and phencyclidine, are basic compounds and accumulate in the stomach.

DISTRIBUTION

Once absorbed into the bloodstream, a drug is distributed to all organs, including those not relevant to its pharmacologic or therapeutic actions (Fig. 3-3). Thus a drug is reversibly associated with its site of action, with plasma proteins, and with tissues not involved in its primary action.

Three major factors control the entry of a drug into a tissue and its retention there: the blood flow or perfusion rate; the ease of penetration into the tissue; and special cellular mechanisms for drug retention. The wide range of perfusion rates for different organs is shown in Table 3-2. Highly perfused tissues will tend to accumulate more of a drug because they have a greater opportunity to equilibrate with plasma.

The ease of drug penetration into a given tis-

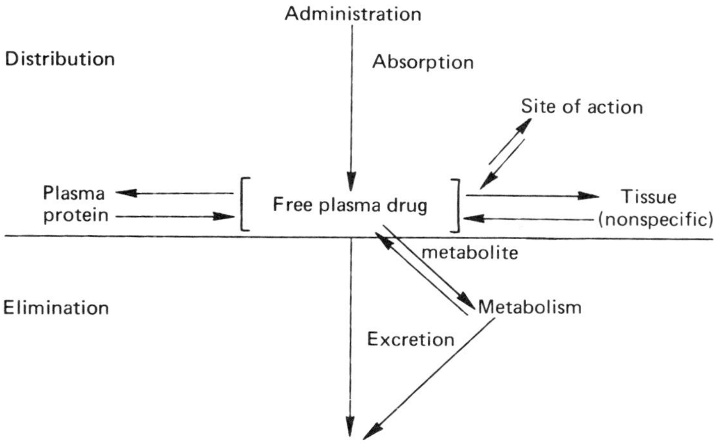

FIG. 3-3. Pathways of drug movement. After absorption, drug in the plasma moves reversibly into the different compartments indicated. The two unidirectional processes are metabolism, where the drug is converted to another compound, and excretion, where the drug is removed from the body.

sue varies with the organ as well as with the drug. Certain tissues are less permeable than others; for example, the brain is separated from the general circulation by the *blood–brain barrier*, and an analogous barrier separates the fetal from the maternal circulation. In general, lipophilic neutral compounds will readily penetrate tissue barriers, whereas polar, charged compounds will not.

Many drugs accumulate within cells—their intracellular concentration becomes higher than their concentration in plasma or extracellular water—because of the *p*H difference between the inside and outside of the cell. Most cells have intracellular *p*H values lower than 7.4, so that basic drugs would be expected to accumulate within the cell. The stomach is an extreme example of an organ with this *p*H difference (*see* above).

Alternatively some drugs (closely related to a physiologically occurring substrate) are localized in specific tissues because they serve as competitive substrates for a specific carrier. The sympathomimetic amines metaraminol and tyramine, for example, are transported into the presynaptic adrenergic nerve ending by the carrier normally involved in the reuptake of *l*-norepinephrine. They are retained in this tissue in opposition to a concentration gradient that would predict much lower tissue levels (*see* Chap. 13).

The distribution of selected drugs is shown in Table 3-3. Chlorpromazine is a highly lipophilic substance, methylatropine is a highly polar hydrophilic, quaternary amine, and meperidine is intermediate in polarity. The highly perfused organs have higher tissue drug levels. Chlorpromazine is extensively concentrated in tissues, whereas antipyrine is not localized at all. The ionic compound methylatropine does not cross the blood–brain barrier although it does accumulate in peripheral tissues in about the same tissue-to-plasma ratio as meperidine. The 0.2 tissue-to-plasma ratio of methylatropine for brain reflects the amount of material in the cerebral vascular bed.

TABLE 3-2. Blood Perfusion Rates in Adult Humans

Organ	Percentage of Cardiac Output	Percentage of Body Weight	Perfusion Rate
			ml · min⁻¹ · 100 g tissue⁻¹
Lungs	100	1.5	400
Kidney	20	0.5	350
Liver	24	2.8	85
Heart	4	0.5	84
Brain	12	2.0	55
Muscle	23	40.0	5
Skin	6	10.0	5
Adipose tissue	10	19.0	3

TABLE 3-3. Localization of Drugs in Various Organs

Organ	Chlorpromazine*	Meperidine†	Antipyrine‡	Methylatropine§
		(concentrations relative to plasma)		
Brain	68.0	5.5	0.95	0.2
Heart	6.7	4.2	0.98	2.1
Lung	52.0	5.6	0.91	3.3
Liver	15.5	3.9	0.98	1.2
Kidney	23.0	4.9	1.04	0.6
Muscle	4.7	1.8	0.98	—
Plasma	1.0	1.0	1.0	1.0

* Salzman NP, Brodie BB: J Pharmacol Exp Ther 118:46, 1956
† Burns JJ et al.: J Pharmacol Exp Ther 114:289, 1955
‡ Brodie BB et al.: J Biol Chem 179:31, 1949
§ Albanus L et al.: Acta Pharmacol Toxicol 27:97, 1969

THE BLOOD–BRAIN BARRIER

The endothelial cells of capillaries in muscle are separated by gap junctions 50Å to 100Å wide that allow molecules that are unable to diffuse through the membranes of the endothelial cell to pass into extracellular space. The morphologic basis of the blood–brain barrier is an essentially continuous layer of endothelial cells with tight gap junctions in cerebral capillaries.

The blood–brain barrier prevents or restricts the entry and exit of polar molecules so that permanently charged molecules such as methylatropine cannot readily enter the brain (Table 3-3), whereas lipid soluble compounds such as meperidine and chlorpromazine are found in brain-to-plasma ratios approximating those of the lungs. Thus most drugs that have effects on the CNS are nonpolar lipophilic compounds, whereas those whose action is primarily peripheral are generally polar or charged. Methylatropine, for example, is used as a peripheral anticholinergic; its nonquaternary analogue, on the other hand, has been used to treat Parkinson's disease (*see* Chap. 30). Lipid soluble drugs do not, however, affect only the CNS. Because of their wide distribution, these types of agents can affect all organ-systems.

The blood–brain barrier also prevents the passive entry of polar physiological substrates such as sugars and amino acids, which must enter the brain by carrier-mediated transport systems. One of these transport systems is used in the treatment of Parkinson's disease with L-dopa (*see* Chap. 30). This disease can also be ameliorated by increasing the brain concentration of dihydroxyphenylethylamine (dopamine). Dopamine does not, however, penetrate the blood–brain barrier so that its administration peripherally will have no effect on brain dopamine levels. The therapeutic approach is to administer L-dihydroxyphenylalanine (L-dopa), an amino acid that can enter the brain by an existing carrier mechanism, where it is decarboxylated to dopamine.

The greater analgesic potency of heroin over that of morphine (*see* Chap. 32) may be explainable in terms of distributional differences. Thus heroin (diacetyl morphine) has a much higher oil/water partition coefficient than does morphine (0.2 vs. 0.016), allowing a more rapid equilibration between plasma and brain and a more rapid entry of heroin into the brain. The relative amounts of brain uptake have been determined to be 68 for heroin and 2.6 for morphine.

ANDEAS JONAS ÅNGSTRÖM, 1814–1874. Swedish physicist and astronomer. One of the founders of spectroscopy, discovered hydrogen in solar atmosphere (1862). Ångström unit named in his honor in 1905.

THE PLACENTAL BARRIER

The maternal circulation is separated from the fetal circulation by several placental layers, resulting in a barrier that restricts the passive diffusion of compounds between the two circulations. The substances that penetrate the placental barrier, like those that enter the CNS, are lipophilic, nonpolar compounds. Thus obstetric anesthetics might also be expected to enter the fetus. Fortunately, however, there is a significant time-delay in the equilibration between the two circulatory systems so that the high initial levels of CNS depressants found in the maternal blood are not immediately achieved in the fetus, and vigorous infants are delivered by mothers under anesthesia. If anesthesia is prolonged 1 hour or more, longer-acting drugs such as meperidine may equilibrate and depress the neonate (*see* Table 81-25). The practical significance of these findings is that the protection afforded the fetus from drugs given to the mother is temporary and depends on the rate of equilibration between the two circulatory systems. The rate of equilibration depends, of course, on the physical properties of the drug, so that highly lipophilic compounds such as thiopental (*see* Chap. 28) can reach pharmacologically effective levels in fetal plasma within 7 minutes of maternal administration.

DRUG BINDING IN PLASMA

Drug distribution is affected by the development of drug/plasma protein complexes. Protein-bound drug behaves like a macromolecule so that its permeability characteristics are markedly different—that is, it remains in the vascular compartment. Thus the complexed drug is not filtered at the glomerulus and does not enter cells. Albumin is the protein most often involved, but globulins and lipoproteins also form complexes. The characteristics of this drug–protein interaction lead to complex dose-effect and drug-drug relationships. Drugs also bind to, or are taken up by, blood cellular elements, but little is known of these processes.

The *reversible binding* of small molecules by proteins may be expressed by the relationship

$$B = \frac{nK[A]}{1 + K[A]},$$

where B equals the number of moles of drug A bound; n is the number of binding sites available; K is the binding constant; and [A] is the concentration of drug A. Binding is thus characterized by a constant (n) that reflects the capacity of the protein to bind A and K, a measure of the affinity of A for that protein. At high [A], the protein will become saturated; increasing [A] further will not increase B. Therefore, with the increase in [A], the proportion of bound drug becomes smaller and smaller. Because the pharmacologic effect of drug A depends on the unbound (free) fraction, protein binding can cause nonlinear dose-effect relationships; for example, at low plasma concentrations where $K[A] \ll 1$, a high proportion of A will be bound and B will increase in proportion to A. Thus only a small fraction of administered A will be available for pharmacologic action. When $K[A] \gg 1$, however, the protein will be saturated and B will be fixed at its maximal value; under those circumstances an increase in [A] will result in a direct increase of free pharmacologically active drug. Therefore the dose of a drug that is significantly protein bound cannot be increased continuously without the danger of a dramatic, possibly toxic response after a relatively small change in dose.

Another way of eliciting this toxic response is to administer two drugs that bind to the same site on proteins. In this situation, the binding sites become saturated at much lower concentrations of either drug, and the resulting increase in free drug will cause its attendant pharmacologic effect to be observed at a much lower dose of each agent. Both warfarin and phenylbutazone, for example, are extensively bound to albumin at the plasma concentrations attained by therapeutic doses. When phenylbutazone is administered to a person taking warfarin, some warfarin is displaced from albumin binding sites and made available for pharmacologic action. As a result, the prothrombin time (a measure of clotting time) of a given dose of warfarin is decreased in the presence of phenylbutazone. Another example of this phenomenon is sulfonamide-induced kernicterus (*see* Chap. 11). Drug effects usually differ immediately after displacement and when new steady-state is achieved (*see* Chap. 8).

Other substances that bind to plasma proteins include hormones such as cortisone and thyroxine. The protein complexes of these substances act as reservoirs in that they maintain a low concentration of free hormone by reversible dissociation of the complex. As the free drug in the plasma is taken up by tissues or eliminated, the protein complex dissociates to liberate more drug.

ADIPOSE TISSUE

Although adipose tissue has a high affinity for lipophilic drugs, it is poorly perfused so that it slowly equilibrates with drugs in the plasma. Once accumulated in fat, however, adipose tissue acts as a reservoir from which the drug is only slowly released back into the circulation. Chlorinated insecticides such as DDT are highly lipophilic, and tissue-to-plasma ratios of 306:1 have been found in autopsy specimens.

VOLUME OF DISTRIBUTION

A quantitative estimate of the tissue localization of a drug may be obtained from its volume of distribution (Vd), the volume in which it would have to be dissolved to give the plasma concentration obtained if no elimination occurred. Vd is a hypothetical number calculated from the total dose given (Q) and the extrapolated initial plasma concentration (C_0):

$$\text{Vd(ml/kg)} = \frac{\text{Q(mg/kg)}}{C_0\text{(mg/liter)}}.$$

The extrapolated initial plasma concentration is obtained experimentally from plots of plasma concentration versus time. When the plasma level of the drug decays with first-order kinetics [log (C) versus time is a straight line] (Fig. 3-4), (C_0) can readily be extrapolated. It is obvious from the above equation that the lower the plasma concentration the larger the Vd.

Table 3-4 lists the volume of distribution of some drugs and other compounds used to measure different body compartments. The theoretical plasma concentration attained immediately after administration of 10 mg/kg of drug is also given. A difference of three orders of magnitude in the Vd occurs. Lipid soluble compounds such as meperidine and chlorpromazine have a large Vd, whereas polar, permanently charged molecules such as decamethonium have a much smaller Vd and, like methylatropine (Table 3-3), do not penetrate tissues easily.

The Vd values of reference compounds are given for comparison; labeled albumin is retained in the plasma, mannitol enters only the extracellular space, and the Vd of labeled water is a measure of total body water. Thus decamethonium is restricted to the extracellular space, whereas chlorpromazine is highly localized in different tissues so that a low plasma concentration results (Table 3-3).

The Vd of a drug varies between persons and with pathologic states, so that a given dose can yield widely varying plasma concentrations in different patients. These differences should result in a wide range of responses to a given dose. In studies of 25 patients given a standard dose of nortriptyline, investigators found a tenfold difference in plasma drug levels. The therapeutic results were also variable but correlated with the plasma levels; low levels were without effect, and high levels were sufficient

TABLE 3-4. Volumes of Distribution of Various Drugs and Reference Compounds

	Volume of Distribution (ml/kg body weight)	Theoretic Plasma Level After 10 mg/kg Dose (μg/ml)
Reference compounds		
^{131}I Albumin (plasma volume)	40	
Mannitol (extracellular volume)	200	
$^{3}H_2O$ (total body water)	600	
Drugs		
Decamethonium	180	55.0
Antipyrine	515	19.5
Clonidine	12,500	0.8
Meperidine	20,000	0.05
Chlorpromazine	100,000	0.01

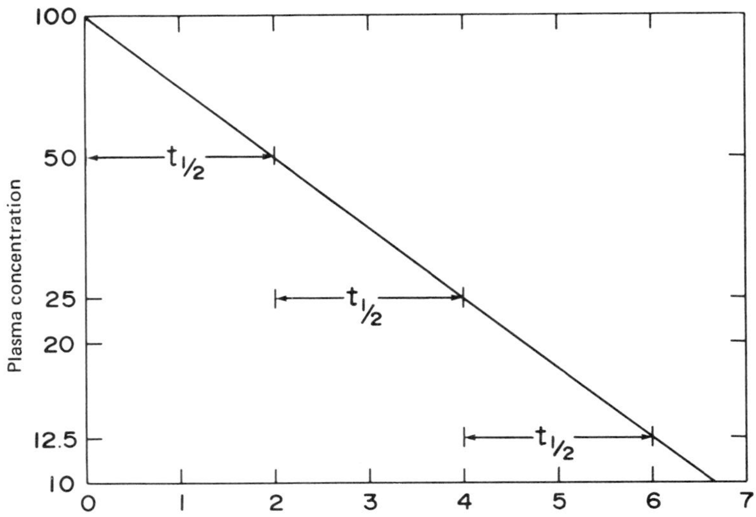

FIG. 3-4. First-order decay. Graphic representation of a first-order decay process. Note that the ordinate is a logarithmic scale. When plotted this way, the time necessary for the plasma concentration to decrease by half is constant.

to cause side-effects. Other causes of individual differences in response to drugs are described in Chapter 8. Pathologic states can also alter the Vd; for example, the Vd of lidocaine is significantly decreased in patients with heart failure as compared to patients with other cardiovascular problems. The result of this lower Vd is a higher plasma concentration that could account for the higher incidence of side-effects from lidocaine in patients with heart failure (*see* Chap. 34). This change in Vd may result from a decreased tissue perfusion rate because of the failing heart.

EXCRETION

RENAL EXCRETION

The most important route of drug excretion is through the kidney. Urine is formed from the plasma by the processes of glomerular filtration; absorption and secretion subsequently occur in the nephron. Filtration is a physical process in which the blood is fractionated according to the molecular size of its components. Most drugs have molecular weights less than 500 and are readily filtered *unless bound to plasma proteins.* The glomerular filtrate is acted on by mechanisms in the proximal and distal tubules that involve removal (reuptake) from the filtrate of physiologically useful materials such as inorganic ions, sugars, amino acids, and water. In the proximal tubule, glucose, amino acids, and sodium ions are removed by carrier-transport systems. Chloride ion is passively reabsorbed to maintain electrical neutrality, and water is absorbed to maintain isotonicity. The proximal tubule also secretes substances from the peritubular capillaries into the ultrafiltrate, including organic anions such as salicylates and penicillins and cations such as the quaternary ammonium anticholinergics. The blood in the peritubular capillaries has ample opportunity to equilibrate with the glomerular filtrate so that nonpolar compounds can move freely back and forth.

As the ultrafiltrate proceeds through Henle's loop, water and sodium ions are removed, concentrating those components not actively transported. The water removed is about 99% of that filtered so that the concentration of a drug in the urine increases substantially as it proceeds through the nephron. This results in a concentration gradient of drug between plasma and urine in favor of the urine. Thus if the drug can readily penetrate the membranes that separate the two fluids, it will diffuse back into plasma; lipophilic compounds are extensively reabsorbed by this mechanism.

Polar compounds that are not substrates for carrier systems are removed from plasma by filtration, whereas substrates for the secretory transport systems are removed from the plasma by filtration and transport. The osmotic diuretic mannitol is filtered and not reabsorbed and reduces the reabsorption of water along the tubules because of its osmotic effect. The penicillins are carboxylic acids and are removed from the plasma by filtration and anion transport. Therefore renal clearance of penicillin G approximates total renal plasma flow. In contrast, a compound such as chlorpromazine that is highly protein bound and lipid soluble is incompletely filtered at the glomerulus because of protein binding and extensively reabsorbed from the filtrate because of its ability to diffuse through membranes that separate plasma and urine.

When the drug is a weak electrolyte, its reabsorption is affected by the *p*H differences between the ultrafiltrate and plasma. The excretion of a basic drug will be favored in acidic urine, in which it will be ion trapped (*see* above), whereas the excretion of an acidic drug will be favored by an alkaline urine. The *p*H of the urine can vary with diet or drug treatment (*see* Chap. 8). High doses of ascorbic acid, for example, decrease urine *p*H, whereas bicarbonate increases it. Ion trapping is used to hasten barbiturate elimination in overdose (*see* Chap. 72).

BILIARY EXCRETION

The liver secretes 0.5 to 1.0 liter of bile daily. Many of the substances present in bile are reabsorbed from the small intestine, but highly polar compounds are not and are excreted through the feces.

Three classes of materials are present in the bile: inorganic ions and sucrose in concentrations equal to those in plasma; and organic compounds, molecular weight about 400, in bile in concentrations 10 to 100 times those in plasma. Most of the drugs excreted through the bile are in this last category; they usually contain large hydrocarbon radicals with a polar

---

FRIEDRICH GUSTAV JACOB HENLE, 1809–1885. German anatomist and pathologist. Often named as the founder of histology. Described Henle's loop in the kidney tubules (1861). Earlier he had discovered epithelial tissue (1837) and arterial wall smooth muscle.

functional group and frequently are conjugates of drugs or their metabolites (*see* Chap. 4).

The compounds of the third group are concentrated in the bile by transport processes; separate carriers for anions, cations, and glycosides appear to exist in the liver. These systems are responsible for the biliary excretion of such drugs as, for example, the barbiturates (*see* Chap. 25), the quarternary antimuscarinics (*see* Chap. 16), and the cardiac glycosides (*see* Chap. 33). Conjugates of other drugs such as the phenothiazines, morphine, and steroids are also excreted in significant amounts in the feces, since these polar compounds are not readily reabsorbed through the intestines after biliary excretion.

ENTEROHEPATIC CIRCULATION

Substances such as bile acids may be conserved after biliary excretion through reabsorption from the intestine into the portal blood, and then back to the liver. This cycle is called the *enterohepatic circulation*. Drugs can also be reabsorbed through the enterohepatic circulation. Indomethacin, for example, is excreted into bile as the glucuronide conjugate (*see* Chap. 4). The intestinal flora, however, hydrolyze the conjugate back to indomethacin, which is reabsorbed. This "recycling" process that prolongs a drug T½ may be inhibited by antibiotic therapy (*see* Chaps. 8 and 61).

MISCELLANEOUS ROUTES OF EXCRETION

Other excretory routes of lesser importance include the breath, saliva, sweat, and milk. The excretion of drugs into these fluids largely depends on passive diffusion and, for weak electrolytes, the *p*H difference between plasma and the secretion. The excretion of drugs in the milk becomes an important consideration in nursing mothers because the breast-fed infant may receive drugs or metabolites of drugs taken by the mother (*see* Chap. 11). Volatile anesthetics and other low molecular-weight compounds that arise by degradation of drugs can be eliminated through the lungs.

FURTHER READING

1. Schmucker DM: Age related changes in drug disposition. Pharmacol Rev 30:445–456, 1978
2. Brodie BB, Gillette JR (eds): Concepts in Biochemical Pharmacology: Part 1. Handbook of Experimental Pharmacology, Volume 28. Berlin, Springer-Verlag, 1971
3. LaDu BN, Mandel HG, Way EL (eds): Fundamentals of Drug Metabolism and Drug Disposition. Baltimore, Williams & Wilkins, 1971

CHAPTER 3 QUESTIONS

(*See* P. 7 for Full Instructions)

Select the One Best Answer

1. A dose of 150 mg of drug X is administered to a 75-kg man. Before sufficient time has elapsed for appreciable metabolism or excretion to occur, his plasma concentration is found to be 10 mg/liter. From the apparent volume of distribution, one would assume that drug X is
   A. likely to have a half-life greater than 16 hours.
   B. highly concentrated in tissues.
   C. distributed with total body water.
   D. distributed with extracellular fluid.
   E. concentrated in the intracellular space.
2. Thiopental anesthesia, produced by a single intravenous dose, terminates rapidly because thiopental is
   A. metabolized.
   B. eliminated by the kidneys.
   C. redistributed from the brain to other tissues.
   D. insoluble in adipose tissue.
   E. eliminated by way of the lungs.
3. Assuming that the unionized forms of the following drugs are equally lipid soluble, which will be more rapidly absorbed from the small intestine (*p*H 6.0)?
   A. Phenobarbital, acid $pK_a = 7.3$
   B. Amphetamine, base $pK_a = 9.9$
   C. Lidocaine, base $pK_a = 7.9$
   D. Caffeine, base $pK_a = 0.8$
   E. Aspirin, acid $pK_a = 3.0$
4. A drug is excreted most rapidly if it is
   A. concentrated in the bile and returned to the intestinal tract.
   B. highly bound to plasma protein.
   C. filtered and secreted by the kidney.
   D. distributed to the extracellular fluid only.
   E. filtered and reabsorbed by the kidney.

A = 1,2,3; B = 1,3; C = 2,4; D = 4; E = All

5. The apparent volume of distribution of a drug
   1. relates the total amount of drug in the body to the plasma concentration.

2. is one of the essential facts required for estimating a drug's half-life.
3. serves to relate the cellular drug level to the extracellular concentration.
4. relates the plasma level of drug to the fraction of drug bound to the plasma proteins.

6. A lipid-soluble, unionized drug would be expected to be
   1. well absorbed orally.
   2. excreted rapidly.
   3. concentrated in the brain.
   4. rapidly metabolized by the liver.

7. The greater the binding of a drug to plasma proteins,
   1. the smaller its apparent volume of distribution.
   2. the longer its half-life.
   3. the greater its required dose.
   4. the greater the concentration of "active" drug in the cerebrospinal fluid.

8. Drugs that have a renal clearance rate of about 700 ml/min
   1. may be highly bound to the plasma proteins.
   2. are secreted by the kidney tubules.
   3. are generally highly ionized at plasma *p*H.
   4. readily cross the blood–brain barrier.

4

JEREMY H. THOMPSON

Drug Metabolism

Drug metabolism refers to the processes by which drugs are modified by the organism. Metabolites are chemically distinct from the parent drug and usually more polar. Thus they diffuse through cellular membranes less readily than the original drug and have a reduced renal tubular reabsorption. These properties limit pharmacologic activity, so metabolism usually converts a drug to a less active compound. This is not always the case, however, and pharmacologically active or even toxic metabolites are known. Therefore, drug metabolism and the enzymes responsible are important considerations in the evaluation of drug actions.

Although drug metabolism is presented in terms of individual reactions, like other biochemical reactions, it can occur as a series of interdependent reactions, with the product of one reaction becoming the substrate for another. The major drug metabolism reactions are *hydrolytic*, *oxidative*, and *conjugative*. Conjugative reactions are the result of a synthetic reaction whereby the drug or drug metabolite is coupled to an endogenous substance such as glucuronic acid or glutathione to form a molecule with markedly different chemical and physical properties.

DRUG METABOLISM REACTIONS

HYDROLYTIC REACTIONS

Plasma "pseudocholinesterase" hydrolyzes various choline or aminoethanol esters (*see* Chap. 15). The drugs succinylcholine and procaine are substrates for this enzyme, and the duration of their pharmacologic activity is dependent on enzymatic hydrolysis. Both compounds have very short half-lives, and succinylcholine must be continuously infused to maintain effective plasma levels (*see* Chap. 19). When infusion stops, the effects rapidly disappear, so the drug is well suited for use as a muscle relaxant in surgical procedures. There are individual differences in the activities of the esterase (*see* Chap. 6).

Carboxyesterase activity in the liver catalyzes the hydrolysis of procaine and other exogenous esters.

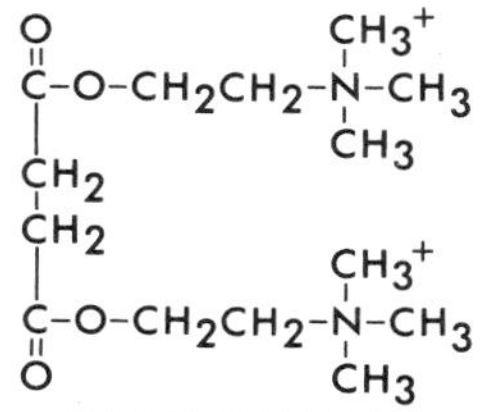

SUCCINYLCHOLINE

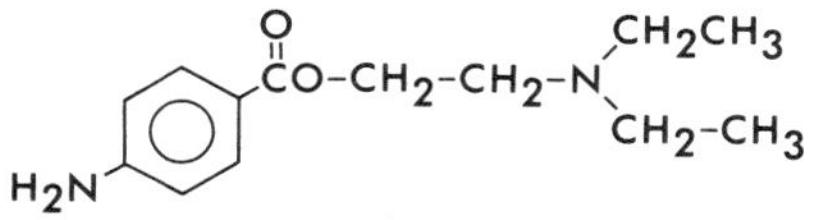

PROCAINE

Amides are also hydrolytically cleaved, but more slowly. An example of the differential susceptibilities of esters and amides of biochemical hydrolysis is provided by procaine (an ester) and its corresponding amide, procainamide. Procaine has a short duration of action (*see* Chap. 20) because it is readily hydrolyzed; procainamide has the same antiarrhythmic properties as procaine but has a longer duration of action because of slower hydrolysis. Lidocaine is another local anesthetic used as an antiarrhythmic agent. Its metabolism is summarized at the end of this chapter to provide an example of the multiple pathways of drug metabolism.

Epoxide hydrase converts epoxides to their corresponding diols, an important step in the "detoxification" of carcinogenic polynuclear aromatic hydrocarbons.

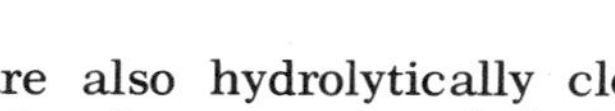

EPOXIDE DIHYDRODIOL

Epoxide hydrase is found in endoplasmic reticulum closely associated with cytochrome P-450 oxidase (*see* below), which oxidizes carcinogenic polynuclear aromatic hydrocarbons to their corresponding epoxides. Epoxides are highly reactive chemical species able to form covalent bonds with nucleophilic functional groups of nucleic acids, proteins, or other biological macromolecules producing mutagenesis or carcinogenesis. Epoxide hydrase hydrolyzes the reactive species to the corresponding diol, which is unreactive and readily eliminated from the cell.

OXIDATIVE REACTIONS

Biochemical oxidation of foreign chemicals is achieved either by the removal of hydrogen (dehydrogenation) or the addition of oxygen (oxygenation). There are a number of dehydrogenases, two of which are involved in the metabolism of ethyl alcohol. *Alcohol dehydrogenase* is a liver enzyme that catalyzes the following reaction.

$$NAD + CH_3CH_2{-}OH \xrightarrow[\text{dehydrogenase}]{\text{Alcohol}} CH_3{-}CHO + 2NAD{\cdot}H$$

The cofactor for this enzyme is nicotinamide adenine dinucleotide (NAD) which is reduced as ethanol is oxidized. There is also an *aldehyde dehydrogenase*, which converts the acetaldehyde to acetic acid. The kinetics of ethanol metabolism are different from those of most other foreign compounds because the dehydrogenase becomes saturated with respect to alcohol at "pharmacologically" effective doses. Then, the rate of metabolism becomes dependent only on the availability of NAD. Thus, the rate of alcohol metabolism is independent of the quantity ingested (*see* Chap. 27). For example, if metabolism will take 1 hour to lower body alcohol concentration from 200 to 100 mg/kg, it will take 3 hours to reduce the concentration from 400 to 100 mg/kg. In contrast, if the metabolism of alcohol followed first-order kinetics (*see* Chap. 3) with a half-life of 1 hour, body alcohol reduction by metabolism from 400 to 100 mg/kg would take only 2 "half-lives," or 2 hours (1 hour for reduction from 400 to 200 mg/kg and 1 hour further for reduction from 200 to 100 mg/kg). The oxidation of acetaldehyde to acetic acid can be inhibited by disulfiram, a drug used to treat alcoholism (*see* Chap. 27).

Monoamine oxidase (MAO), a mitochondrial enzyme found in liver, kidney, and neuronal tissue, metabolizes the neurotransmitters norepinephrine, epinephrine, and 5-hydroxytryptamine and other amines to their corresponding aldehydes plus ammonia.

$$R - CH_2 - NH_2 + H_2O + O_2 \rightarrow R - CH_2 - CHO + NH_3 + H_2O_2$$

MAO is of particular importance in the oxidative deamination of tryamine (*see* Chap. 8), an indirectly acting sympathomimetic amine found in high concentrations in fermented foodstuffs (*see* Table 8-8).

Dopamine β-hydroxylase is an enzyme in the biosynthesis of norepinephrine and epinephrine. It also effects the hydroxylation of compounds related to dopamine, the normal norepinephrine precursor, to form metabolites that

(*Text continues on p. 41*)

(A) Degradative or oxidative pathways of drug metabolism

Pathway	Enzyme (source)	Substrate	Metabolite	Other examples
Dehydrogenation	Alcohol dehydrogenase (brain, liver, etc)	CH_3CH_2OH ETHANOL	$CH_3C(H){=}O$	
Deamination	Monoamine oxidase (liver, nervous tissue)	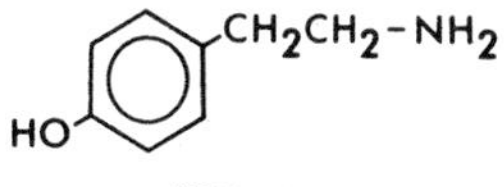 TYRAMINE	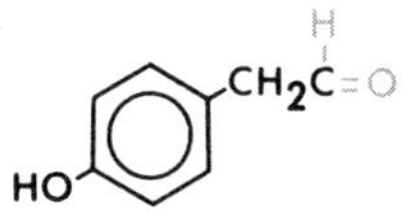	Phenylethylamine
Hydrolysis	Liver esterase (plasma pseudocholinesterase)	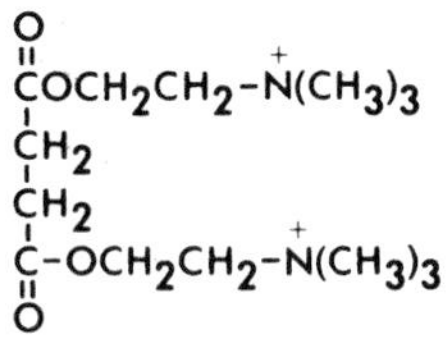 SUCCINYL CHOLINE	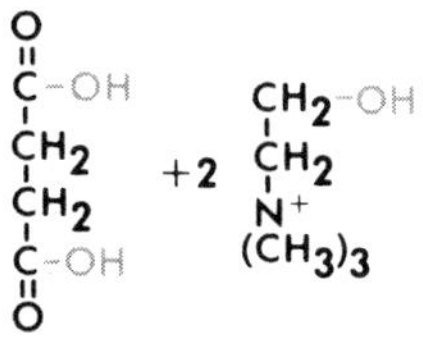	Procaine and other ester types of local anesthetics
Aromatic C hydroxylation	Mixed function oxidase (liver)	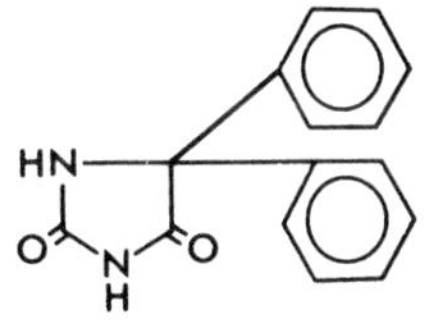 PHENYTOIN	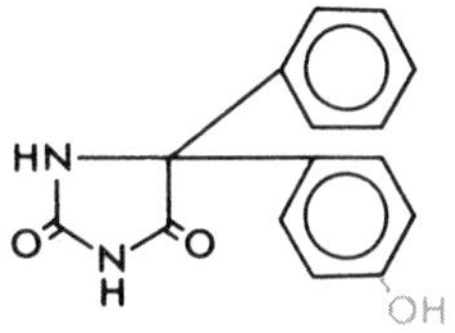	Amphetamine, phenobarbital, phenylbutazone, propranolol

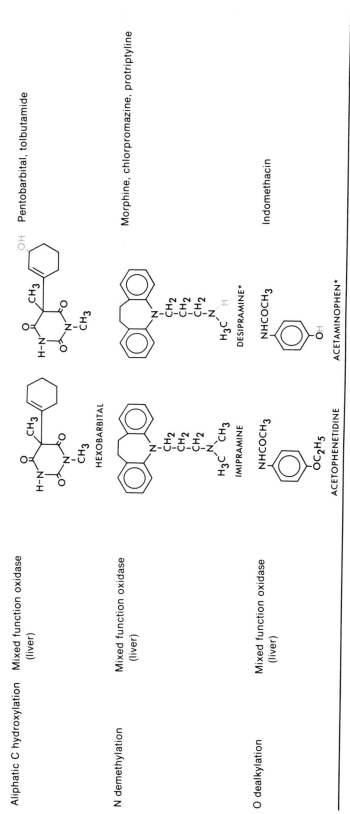

Aliphatic C hydroxylation	Mixed function oxidase (liver)	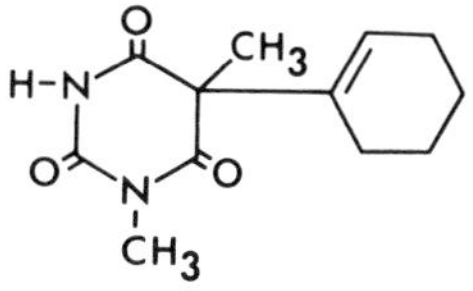 HEXOBARBITAL	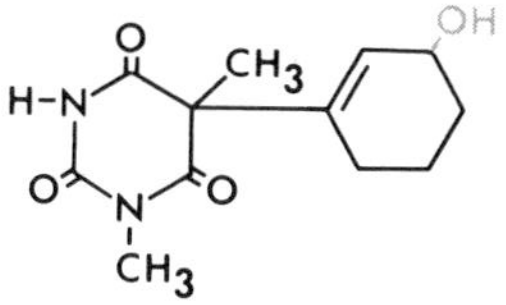	Pentobarbital, tolbutamide
N demethylation	Mixed function oxidase (liver)	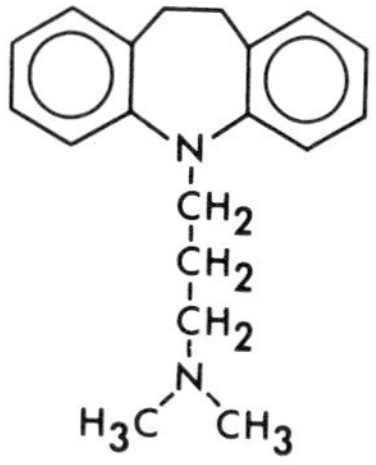 IMIPRAMINE	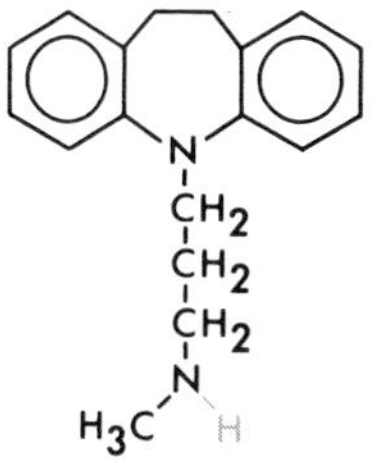 DESIPRAMINE*	Morphine, chlorpromazine, protriptyline
O dealkylation	Mixed function oxidase (liver)	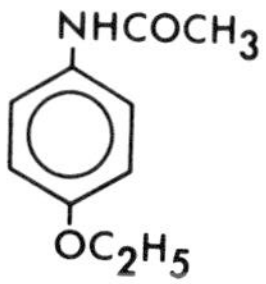 ACETOPHENETIDINE	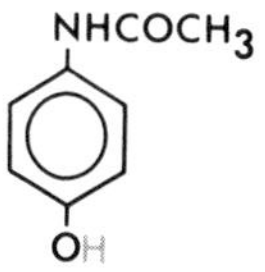 ACETAMINOPHEN*	Indomethacin

FIG. 4-1. Chemical structures of drugs and their metabolites. Changes in structure that result from metabolism are shaded. Pharmacologically active metabolites administered directly are indicated by asterisks.

(continued)

(B) Conjugative pathways of drug metabolism

Pathway	Enzyme (source)	Substrate	Metabolite	Other examples
Glucuronylation	Glucuronyltransferase (liver)	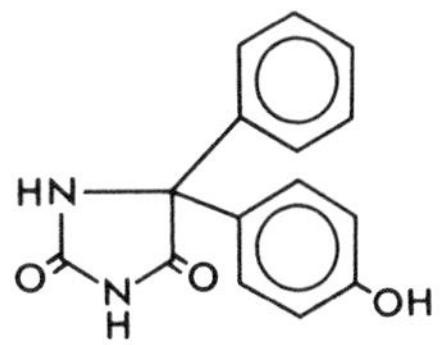 4-OH-PHENYTOIN (METABOLITE)	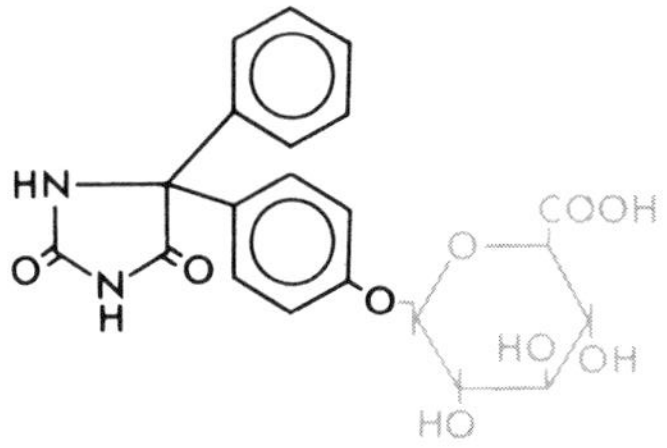	Morphine
Sulfonation	Sulfokinase (liver, kidney)	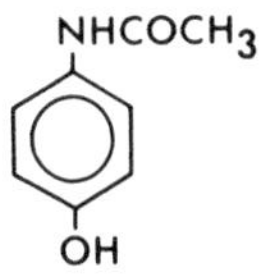 ACETAMINOPHEN	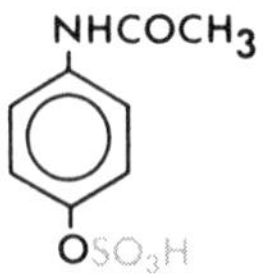	Steroids
Amino acid conjugation	Transacetylase (liver)	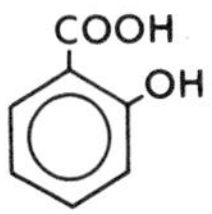 SALICYLIC ACID	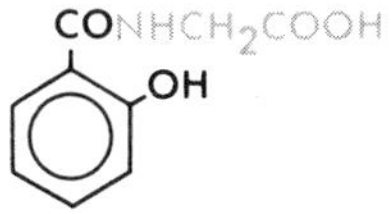	Benzoic acid
Mercapturic acid	Aryltransferase (liver, kidney)	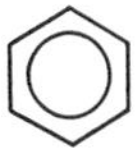 BENZENE	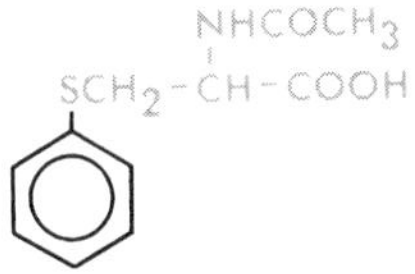	Aromatic hydrocarbons and halocarbons
N-Acetylation	Acetyltransferase (liver)	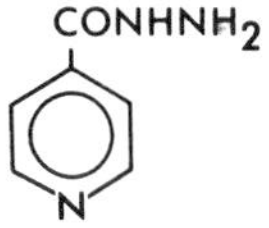 ISONIAZID (INH)	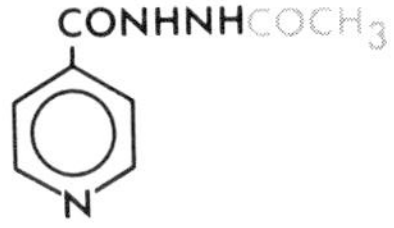	p-Aminosalicylic acid, sulfanilamide

have pharmacologic effects. These compounds, called false transmitters (*see* Chap. 13), are involved in the actions of several adrenergic agents.

Cytochrome P-450 Monooxygenase

The most important oxidative enzyme system for drug metabolism is the so-called cytochrome P-450 monooxygenase of the endoplasmic reticulum. This system effects a multitude of chemical reactions (Fig. 4-1), all involving the insertion of one atom of atmospheric oxygen into an organic substrate and the reduction of the other atom to water.

$$RH + O_2 + NADPH \rightarrow ROH + H_2O + NADPH$$

The system consists of a heme protein called *cytochrome P-450,* a flavin enzyme called *cytochrome P-450 reductase,* and a *phospholipid such as phosphotidyl choline.* Although there is only one molecular form of cytochrome P-450 reductase, there are many forms of cytochrome P-450, which presumably are responsible for the wide substrate specificity and the individual and species differences in activities. Enzyme activity can be increased or decreased by exposure of the organism to other foreign substances ("inducers" or "inhibitors"), so the past chemical environment of the organism can affect drug metabolism (*see* Chap. 8).

Substrates for cytochrome P-450 vary widely in structure, but all are highly lipid soluble. The enzyme is thus valuable in the initial conversion of lipophilic drugs and foreign compounds to more polar compounds that can be eliminated either directly or after conjugation (*see* below). The elimination of tranquilizers, antidepressants, anticonvulsants, and antihistamines, for example, is dependent on their metabolism by this enzyme system.

The heme protein component of cytochrome P-450 is specifically inhibited by compounds such as carbon monoxide, piperonylbutoxide (an insecticide synergist), and isoniazid. The interaction with carbon monoxide results in a characteristic absorption band in the region of 450 nm, which is the basis for the name of the enzyme. Functionally the heme protein binds both substrate and oxygen in a complex that allows the reduction of oxygen and the oxidation of the substrate. Although the system often is regarded as being nonspecific, there is increasing evidence that it is genetically controlled and that different hemes oxidize various molecular species. Attempts to characterize specific hemes or groups of hemes have used selected drug substrates. For example, debrisoquin (*see* Chap. 36) is dependent on aromatic ring hydroxylation for elimination. A study conducted in the United Kingdom showed that about 5% of British white persons were phenotypically poor "hydroxylators" of debrisoquin. These same subjects were later shown to have reduced ability to metabolize acetophenetidine by deethylation (Table 4-1), so the ability to metabolize both substances may be genetically related. These differences in metabolism result in a slower rate of drug removal and thus a longer duration of drug action in the poor hydroxylators.

Some drugs (*see* Table 8-5) increase the synthesis of cytochrome P-450 monooxygenase. Especially important are phenobarbital and the carcinogenic hydrocarbon 3-methylcholanthrene, whose biochemical actions have been extensively investigated. Both substances stimulate an increase in total cytochrome P-450 protein; but the molecules induced are chemically and enzymatically distinct, so the resultant increase in metabolic activity is not the same for all substrates. Clinically important enzyme inducers are alcohol (consumed chronically) and phenytoin. Enzyme inducers

TABLE 4-1. Species Variation in the Metabolism of Lidocaine*

	Percentage of Dose Recovered in Urine			
Compound	*Rat*	*Guinea Pig*	*Dog*	*Man*
Lidocaine	0.2	0.5	2.0	2.8
Monoethylglycinexylidide	0.7	14.9	2.3	3.7
Glycinexylidide	2.1	3.3	12.6	2.3
3-Hydroxylidocaine	31.2	0.5	6.7	1.1
3-Hydroxymonoethylglycine xylidide	36.9	2.0	3.1	0.3
2,6-Xylidine	1.5	16.2	1.6	1.0
4-Hydroxy-2,6-dimethylaniline	12.4	16.4	35.2	72.6
Total recovered	85.0	53.8	63.5	83.8

* Structures of the metabolites are shown in Figure 4-2. The animals were administered lidocaine and their urine collected for 24 hours. The quantities of metabolites indicated were measured and are expressed as the percentage of the original dose. The data are taken from Keenaghan JB, Boyes RN: The tissue distribution, metabolism and excretion of lidocaine in rats, guinea pigs, dogs, and man. J Pharmacol Exp Ther 180:454, 1972.

may be involved in significant drug interactions (*see* Chap. 8).

The inhibition of the P-450 system by drugs (*see* Table 8-6) is also documented. Usually enzyme inhibition results from two substrates successfully competing for a common enzyme and inhibiting the metabolism of each other. Examples of this type of interaction are those between dicumarol and tolbutamide, phenylbutazone and warfarin, and phenytoin and phenylbutazone.

The endoplasmic reticulum contains a toxicologically important flavin-dependent monooxygenase that oxidizes nitrogen and sulfur compounds. The enzyme converts some aromatic amines to their potentially carcinogenic *N*-hydroxy derivatives (*see* below).

REDUCTIVE REACTIONS

Compounds containing sites of unsaturation, such as carbonyl, azo, and nitro groups, are reduced by enzymes that oxidize other substrates. For example, liver alcohol dehydrogenase can reduce aldehyde and aliphatic ketones to the corresponding alcohols in the presence of NAD·H. Aromatic ketones are reduced by an NADP·H-dependent enzyme, aromatic aldehyde reductase. Both of these enzymes are found in the cytoplasm of the liver cell. The conversion of carbonyl groups to alcohols does not increase the polarity of the compound significantly, but the alcohol function can be readily converted to a highly polar conjugate (*see* below) that is rapidly excreted.

Azo and nitro functions are reduced by the liver mixed-functional oxidase under certain conditions. Nitro compounds, such as chloramphenicol, are reduced to the corresponding amines in the presence of NADP·H under anaerobic conditions. This nitro reductase activity is inhibited by carbon monoxide *in vitro* and is induced by phenobarbital, supporting the view that the cytochrome P-450 oxidase is involved. Prontosil, an azo compound, is reduced in the liver to form sulfanilamide:

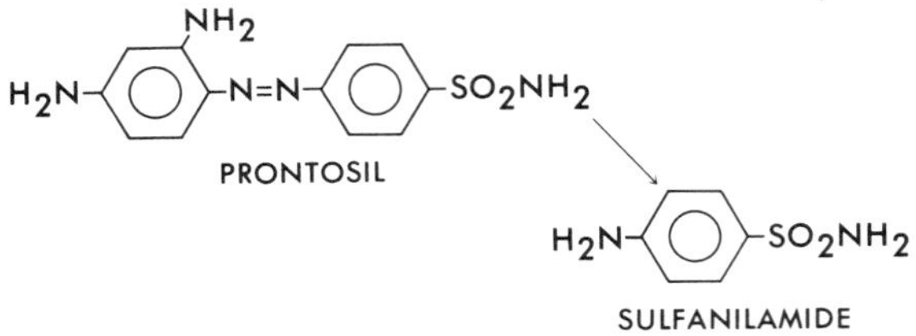

This reaction is an example of the metabolic activation of a drug (*see* Chap. 64). The azo group is also present in food dyes, many of which are metabolized by this route.

CONJUGATIVE REACTIONS

There are a number of different conjugative reactions (Fig. 4-1) in which the foreign compound or its metabolite is coupled to an endogenous compound. Hepatic conjugative enzymes are the most important. The conjugated product is considerably more polar than the parent drug, since the endogenous compound to which it is attached is highly polar and usually charged.

The most common conjugative reaction is *glucuronide formation,* occurring with different functional groups. In Fig. 4-1 a phenolic hydroxyl is shown as the functional group participating in this reaction, but aliphatic hydroxyl, hydroxylamine, amine, carboxyl, and thiol groups are also substrates. Glucuronyl transferase, the enzyme catalyzing this reaction, is found in the endoplasmic reticulum and is induced with drugs such as phenobarbital. Glucuronidation involves the reaction of a nucleotide derivative of the endogenous substrate (uridine phosphate glucuronic acid) with the drug substrate, as with phenol:

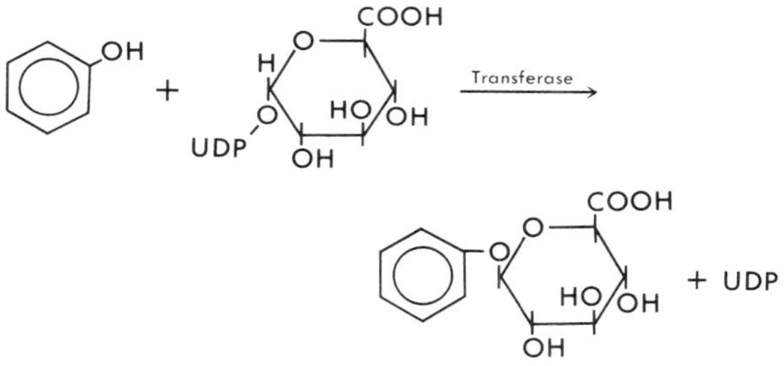

Several endogenous compounds, such as steroids, thyroxine, and bilirubin, are eliminated as glucuronides, and disease or toxicity may develop when the system is immature (*see* Chaps. 7, 11, 61.

In other conjugation reactions such as *N*-acetylation and amino acid conjugation, a coenzyme A-derivative of the endogenous substrate reacts with the drug or drug metabolite. The formation of mercapturic acids is a more complex reaction involving the reaction of glutathione (GSH) with an active organic substrate. In this reaction, the —SH group of glutathione (glutamyl-cysteinyl-glycine) acts as a nucleophilic reagent and reacts with a center such as an epoxide, e.g.:

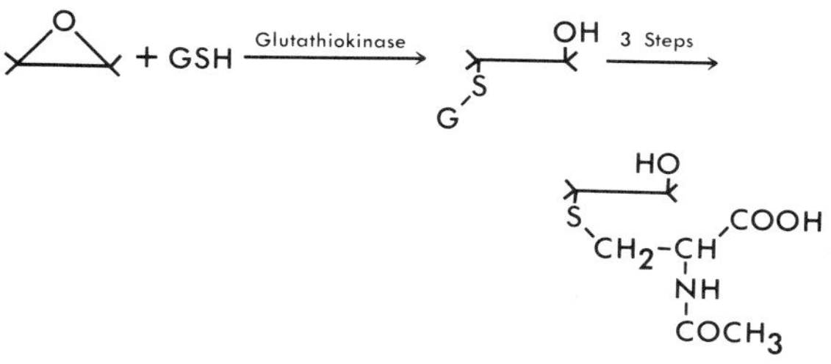

The resulting glutathione conjugate successively loses glutamate and glycine, and is then *N*-acetylated to form the mercapturic acid derivative. The reaction of —SH groups with epoxides and certain alkyl halides also readily occurs nonenzymatically and has been demonstrated with *N*-acetylcysteine. The products of *N*-acetylcysteine and reactive metabolites have been isolated after administration of epoxide-forming hydrocarbons and cysteine to experimental animals. The significance of this —SH conjugation is that compounds that undergo this reaction also react with essential cellular macromolecules to form covalent bonds resulting in cell damage or carcinogenesis.

CONSEQUENCES OF DRUG METABOLISM

TERMINATION OF DRUG ACTION

The most common result of oxidative or hydrolytic transformations is generation of a substance that is more readily eliminated from the body either directly or by subsequent conjugation. The addition of an OH group or the generation of an N—H function by hydroxylation makes the metabolite more polar. Polar groups reduce renal tubular reabsorption of the metabolite and enhance its excretion. The active hydrogen also can be replaced by one of the conjugative groups described above to generate an even more polar metabolite that is rapidly excreted. Moreover, conjugation with glycine, glucuronate, and sulfate generates an anionic function that can be eliminated by the tubular anion transport system.

The pharmacologic activity of drug metabolites is usually, but not always, lower than that of the parent drug, in part because of the increased polarity of the metabolite. Most drugs whose duration of action is metabolism-dependent are lipid-soluble nonpolar compounds such as central nervous system (CNS) drugs. When the polarity is increased, membrane penetration ability is reduced and a smaller fraction gains access to the intracellular space. Therefore, even though the potency of the metabolite at the receptor may not be altered, the reduced distribution of the metabolite diminishes its access to receptors.

TOXICOLOGIC CONSEQUENCES

Since the chemical properties of drug metabolites are determined by the structure of the drug and its interaction with relatively nonspecific enzymes, metabolites with deleterious effects can form also. This possibility has long been recognized, and several examples of the conversion of a drug to a toxic metabolite are known.

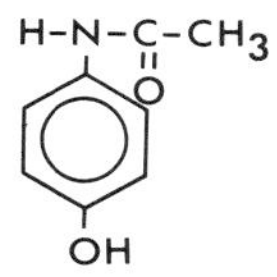

ACETAMINOPHEN

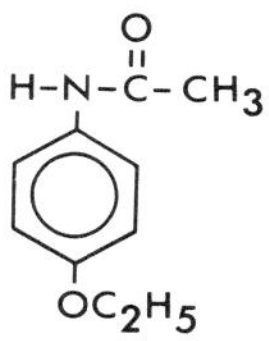

PHENACETIN

For example, acetaminophen, an analgesic, is considered to be the active metabolite of phenacetin, another analgesic. When these two substances are ingested in extremely high doses (20 to 50 times the therapeutic dose), the toxic effects are quite different. Phenacetin causes CNS toxicity—respiratory depression and cyanosis—while acetaminophen causes hepatic necrosis. The CNS toxicity of phenacetin is due to the unchanged drug, but the hepatotoxicity of acetaminophen is due to a reactive metabolite. This metabolite, generated by the cytochrome P-450 monooxygenase, is believed to covalently bind with vital cellular functional groups. Although the metabolite has not been identified, it has properties similar to those of the epoxide described above in that it reacts with nucleophiles, such as —SH groups. Thus a promising approach to the treatment of acetaminophen overdose is to administer large doses (140 mg/kg by mouth) of *N*-acetylcysteine, which will react rapidly with the metabolite (*see* Chap. 72) and convert it to a mercapturic acid derivative. This latter derivative is chemically unreactive and highly polar and hence is rapidly eliminated without generating toxicity. In essence, *N*-acetylcysteine is used to

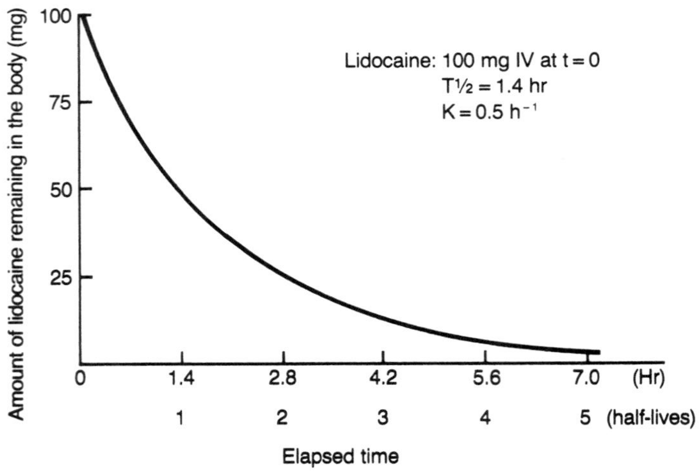

FIG. 4-2. The breakdown of lidocaine in the body.

supplement endogenous glutathione stores. Other toxic reactions due to reactive chemical species (such as those occurring with alkylating anticancer drugs) may be minimized by the selective use of *N*-acetylcysteine.

CARCINOGENICITY

Chemical carcinogenesis is an important example of metabolically induced toxicity. Chemical carcinogens, such as 2-aminofluorene and 3,4-benzpyrene, are by themselves relatively unreactive and will not form covalent bonds

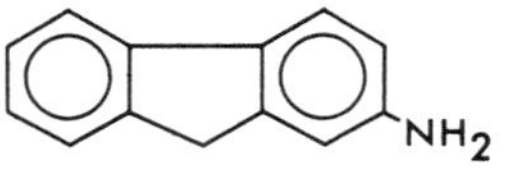

2-AMINOFLUORENE

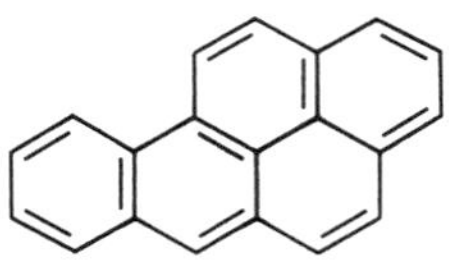

3,4-BENZPYRENE

with any tissue functional groups. However, both of these substances and some of their chemical congeners are metabolically activated to reactive intermediates that bind to macromolecules such as DNA to cause mutations, some of which are presumed to result in cancer. The "activation" reaction of 2-aminofluorene is believed to involve conversion to the *N*-hydroxy derivative by either the cytochrome P-450 monooxygenase or the flavin oxygenase (*see* above). The activation of the aromatic hydrocarbon 3,4-benzpyrene occurs via the epoxide and cytochrome P-450 (*see* above).

CONCLUSION

The breakdown of lidocaine (Fig. 4-2) is a useful illustration of the interplay of various enzymatic pathways of drug metabolism. Lidocaine is metabolized initially by an *N*-dealkylation reaction [A], an aromatic ring hydroxylation reaction [B], and a hydrolytic reaction [C]. The initial metabolites can undergo further degradative reactions or they can form conjugates such as the glucuronides of the ring-hydroxylated metabolites. Thus after an initial hydrolysis or oxidation, lidocaine is converted to metabolites containing polar functional groups suitable for conjugation.

Species differences in metabolism of lidocaine are summarized in Table 4-1, and although the same metabolites are formed, the relative amounts of each metabolite differ substantially between species. Despite numerous attempts, very little information of predictive value has been accumulated on species differences in drug metabolism. Therefore, most

LUDWIG REHN, 1849–1930. German surgeon. In 1895, some 35 years after the development of the synthetic dye industry, Rehn reported several cases of bladder cancer among workers involved in the preparation of fuchsin. Soon other similar cases came to light that revealed the delayed carcinogenic effects of the aromatic amines.

PERCIVALL POTT, 1714–1788. English physician. In 1775 Pott published a paper on scrotal cancer in chimney sweeps, the first description of an occupational cancer and probably the first paper on the carcinogenicity of benzpyrene, a common ingredient of soot. Pott is also remembered for Pott's disease, tuberculosis of the spine, and Pott's fracture of the ankle.

metabolic studies of new drugs involve studying many species to determine structures of different metabolites, with the understanding that the proportions in which they are found may vary between species (*see* Chap. 10). A problem arises when a metabolite or its precursor is potentially toxic, and species differences in drug metabolism prevent quantitative prediction of the formation such a compound in humans.

FURTHER READING

1. Welch RM: Toxicological implications of drug metabolism. Pharmacol Rev 30:457–476, 1978
2. Gorrod JW, Beckett AH: Drug Metabolism of Man. London, Taylor and Francis, 1978
3. Gillette JR, Mitchell JR (eds): Handbook of Experimental Pharmacology: Volume 28. Concepts of Biochemical Pharmacology, Part 3. Berlin, Springer-Verlag, 1975

CHAPTER 4 QUESTIONS

(See P. 7 for Full Instructions)

Select the One Best Answer

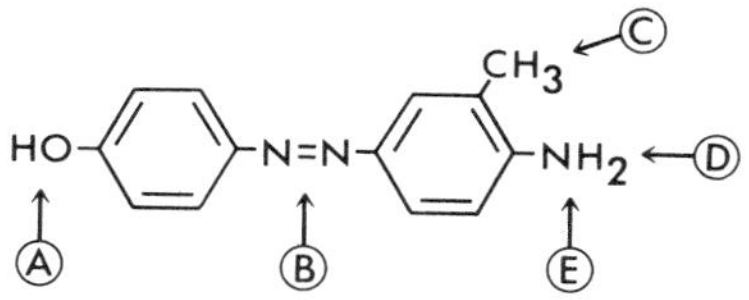

1. In the above chemical structure, each of the following is the characteristic metabolic transformation at the site indicated EXCEPT
   A. conjugation.
   B. reduction.
   C. acetylation.
   D. oxidation.

2. Because barbiturates stimulate liver microsomal enzymes, their use is absolutely contraindicated in
   A. chronic alcoholism.
   B. acute gout.
   C. kernicterus.
   D. hemolytic anemia.
   E. acute intermittent porphyria.

3. The duration of action of drug A is almost completely determined by its rate of metabolism by liver microsomal enzymes. When administered daily for 4 to 5 days, its duration of action decreases to about 25% of the duration of the initial dose. Drug B has a completely different spectrum of activity, but its administration increases the effect of subsequent doses of drug A. The best explanation for all these observations is that
   A. drug B is synergistic with drug A.
   B. drug A and B compete for plasma protein binding sites.
   C. drug A is a partial agonist.
   D. drug A is an inducer and drug B an inhibitor of drug metabolizing enzymes.
   E. drug A exhibits the phenomenon of tachyphylaxis.

A = 1,2,3; B = 1,3; C = 2,4; D = 4; E = All

4. Hepatic microsomal enzyme induction
   1. may be involved in the production of tolerance to some drugs.
   2. may involve "synthesizing" (conjugating) enzymes.
   3. may be used to therapeutic advantage in the treatment of neonatal hyperbilirubinemia.
   4. is an irreversible process.

5. The effects of barbiturates on liver microsomal enzyme systems have been implicated in
   1. precipitation of attacks of acute intermittent porphyria.
   2. diminution of bis-hydroxycoumarin effectiveness during chronic phenobarbital treatment.
   3. tolerance to barbiturates.
   4. potentiation of alcohol effects by barbiturates.

6. Drugs that have pharmacologically active metabolites include
   1. chloral hydrate.
   2. primidone.
   3. codeine.
   4. barbital.

7. Which of the following statements are true regarding drug metabolism?
   1. Drug metabolites usually are more easily excreted than are the parent drugs.
   2. Some drugs are metabolized to more active agents.
   3. Most drug metabolism occurs in the liver.
   4. Drugs must be metabolized before they can be excreted by the kidney.

5

DON H. CATLIN

Pharmacokinetics

Pharmacokinetics is the study of the time-course of absorption, distribution, metabolism, and excretion of drugs and their metabolites in body tissues and fluids. The study of pharmacokinetics begins with measurements of drug concentration in plasma at various times after its administration. Equations (or models) are then developed that describe or fit these data. The models define pharmacokinetic terms such as half-life, volume of distribution, and clearance (*see* Glossary). The final step is applying these models to clinical problems. Thus pharmacokinetics is used to make quantitative statements about the drug relative to the body, for example, kinetic principles are used to answer questions such as how much drug is in the body 1 hour after its administration; what is the drug concentration in plasma at a given time; how fast is a drug excreted by the kidney; and for how long must a drug be administered before steady-state is achieved. Comprehension of pharmacokinetic principles is essential for prescribing drugs safely because they are the basis of all dosage regimens. That is one reason why the kinetics of a new drug must be studied before it is released (*see* Chap. 10). Many diseases alter the pharmacokinetics of drugs; therefore some dosage regimens may need to be altered in proportion to the seriousness of a disease. An understanding of how diseases alter pharmacokinetic variables enables the physician to optimize therapy. *Pharmacodynamics* refers to the time-course of drug effects. One fundamental determinate of pharmacodynamics is the amount of drug at receptor sites. Although this amount cannot be directly measured, it relates to the drug concentration in plasma. Pharmacokinetic principles can be used to describe this latter relationship and thus to understand and to predict pharmacodynamics.

TERMINOLOGY

FIRST ORDER

First order refers to rates that are proportional to the amount present. If a drug is eliminated by a first-order process, the rate of elimination is proportional to the total amount of drug present in the system. Immediately after administering a drug, the amount present is large and the rate of elimination high; later when the amount is small, the rate of elimination is low. First order can describe other processes such as metabolism and absorption. The term is particularly fundamental to pharmacology because the kinetics of most drugs are first order.

RATE CONSTANT (K_e)

Rate constant describes the rate of a first-order process. The units of a rate constant are fractional change per unit of time (*e.g.*, $time^{-1}$ or 0.5/hr; 10%/hr = 0.1 hr^{-1}). If the rate constant that describes the elimination of a drug from the body is 0.3 hr^{-1}, the fractional rate of elimination is 30% of the drug/hr.

ZERO ORDER

Zero order refers to a constant or fixed rate. In contrast to a first-order process, a zero-order process is independent of the dose or amount of drug present. Processes such as drug administration, absorption, or metabolism may be characterized by zero-order kinetics. A zero-order infusion, for example, delivers a fixed amount of drug each minute. A good example of a drug with zero-order kinetics of metabolism is ethyl alcohol.

PHARMACOKINETIC MODELS

Pharmacokinetic models are abstractions that represent the body as one or more compartments. The volume of the compartments represent the volume of the body, and the amount of drug in the compartments equals the amount of drug in the body. Pharmacokinetic models have no physical meaning but can be described schematically (Fig. 5-1) or mathematically. To define a model completely, a series of assumptions that describe the operation of the model are needed. If all assumptions are true in humans, the model will provide an accurate description of the kinetics of a drug. Because humans obviously are much more complex than a simple model, often some discrepancy between the assumptions and the behavior of drugs in the body will occur. Nevertheless the models presented here provide a good description of data collected in humans. Models are used to define pharmacokinetic variables, devise dosage regimens, and predict the time-course of drug responses in humans.

ONE-COMPARTMENT MODEL

The most elementary model represents the body as a single compartment with a volume (V) and a concentration (C) (Fig. 5-1 inset). The assumptions of the model are that drug is rapidly distributed in the compartment and elimination is first order. If a drug is rapidly introduced into a single compartment and its concentration is determined at various times, a semilogarithmic plot of concentration (logarithmic) verses time (arithmetic) will be linear (Fig. 5-1). The slope of the line is $-K_e/2.3$, where K_e is the overall elimination rate constant and t is time. The concentration of drug at t = 0 is denoted C_0.*

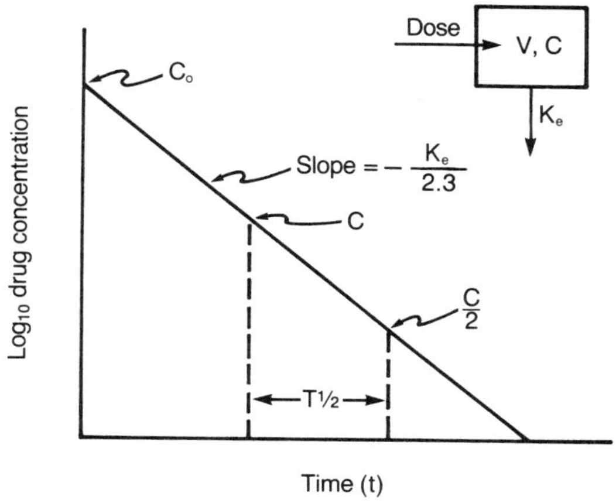

FIG. 5-1. Schematic representation of the one-compartment model (*inset*) and the concentration of drug in the compartment at various times (*t*) after the drug has been introduced into the compartment. C_o is the concentration of drug in the compartment at t=0; K_e is the elimination rate constant; and T½ is the half-life of the drug.

* Those with a working knowledge of calculus will recognize that the one-compartment model can be described as

$$\frac{dC}{dt} = -KeC, \qquad \text{A}$$

where dC/dt is the rate of change of concentration (C) with time, it is the time after drug administration, C is the concentration of drug at time t, and K_e is the elimination rate constant. After integrating equation A,

$$C = C_0 e^{-K_e t}. \qquad \text{B}$$

After converting equation B to logarithms,

$$\ln C = \ln C_0 - K_e t, \qquad \text{C}$$

and since

$$\ln x = 2.3 \log x, \qquad \text{D}$$

then

$$\log C = \log C_0 - K_e t/2.3. \qquad \text{E}$$

Thus a plot of log C versus t is a straight line with a slope $-K_e/2.3$.

The one-compartment model seemingly is not very useful because it vastly oversimplifies many complex processes. Moreover two of the model's assumptions cannot be completely true in humans: an i.v. injection of a drug cannot be given instantaneously and drugs do not distribute instantaneously throughout the body (compartment). Despite these imperfections, the model provides a reasonably accurate description of the plasma concentration time-plot of many drugs. The model is also important because it is used to define pharmacokinetic variables such as half-life and volume of distribution.

Half-Life ($T^1/_2$)

The *half-time* of a first-order process is the time required for one half of the process to be completed. In pharmacokinetics the analagous term is *half-life* ($T^1/_2$), which is used in different contexts. In this chapter, $T^1/_2$ refers to the half-life of a drug or drug metabolite in plasma unless otherwise designated. For a drug that conforms to first-order kinetics, the $T^1/_2$ is simply the time required for the concentration to decrease by one half (Fig. 5-1). The $T^1/_2$ of a drug in humans is determined experimentally by administering the drug intravenously, collecting blood at various times, and measuring the concentration of drug in plasma. The data are plotted on semilogarithmic coordinates to assess the linearity or "goodness of fit" of the data to the one-compartment model. The $T^1/_2$ may be determined graphically after visually fitting a straight line to the point, or more accurately by a least squares linear regression procedure. The relation between $T^1/_2$ and K_e is

$$T^1/_2 = \frac{0.693}{K_e} \approx \frac{0.7}{K_e}. \qquad 1$$

Equation 1 is obtained from equation D in the footnote on page 47 by noting that when $t = T^1/_2$, $C = {}^1/_2C_0$; thus $\log 0.5 = -K_eT^1/_2/2.3$, which simplifies to equation 1.

It is important to distinguish $T^1/_2$, K_e, and the rate of elimination. K_e is an elimination rate constant and describes the fraction of the total amount of drug present that is removed per unit of time. Elimination is not equivalent to excretion; it includes excretion by the liver, kidney, and other organs but also includes elimination by metabolism. K_e does not indicate the actual amount of drug eliminated per unit of time. That amount is given by

$$\text{Rate of elimination} = A_TK_e, \qquad 2$$

where A_T is the total amount of drug in the body. Thus both A_T and K_e determine the actual rate of elimination. If the amount present changes, the rate of elimination will also change, whereas the rate constant does not change. For example, if 100 mg of lidocaine ($T^1/_2 = 1.4$ hr, $k = 0.5$ hr^{-1}) is administered intravenously at $t = 0$ and the amount of lidocaine that remains in the body is plotted against elapsed time, the amount of lidocaine remaining will decrease by 50% every 1.4 hr (Fig. 5-2). During the first $T^1/_2$ (0–1.4 hr), the rate of elimination is 35.7 mg/hr (50 mg/1.4 hr) and the amount remaining at 1.4 hr is 50 mg. During the next $T^1/_2$ (1.4–2.8 hr), 25 mg is eliminated (50% of 50 mg), and the rate of elimination is only 17.8 mg/hr. By the time five half-lives elapse about 97% has been eliminated, and the rate is less than 3 mg/hr. Half-life is an exceedingly important pharmacokinetic parameter because a substantial portion of the individual variability in response to drugs is due to differences in $T^1/_2$. Some variables that influence $T^1/_2$ are state of induction or inhibition of drug-metabolizing enzymes (*see* Chap. 8), hepatic and renal function (*see* Chap. 11), age (*see* Chaps. 7, 11), diet (*see* Chaps. 8, 11), and genetic factors (*see* Chap. 6).

Volume of Distribution (V_d)

A proportionality constant, *volume of distribution* relates the total amount of drug in the body to the concentration of drug in plasma. The units of V_d are volume or volume/kg (*e.g.*, ml, liter, or liter/kg). If V_d and plasma concentration (C_p) are known, the total amount of drug in the body is

$$A_T = V_d \cdot C_p. \qquad 3$$

FIG. 5-2. The amount of lidocaine remaining in the body as a function of the number of hours and half-lives that have elapsed since drug administration.

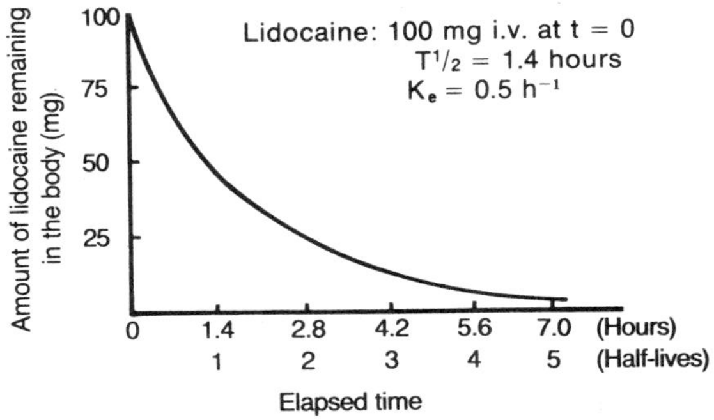

The V_d is analogous to the V of the one-compartment model. The volume of the compartment can be calculated if the total dose administered is known and the concentration of drug in the compartment is measured before any elimination takes place (i.e., at C_0, Fig. 5-1):

$$V = \frac{\text{dose}}{C_0}. \quad 4$$

The V_d of a drug in humans is determined experimentally from the plasma concentration versus time curve (Fig. 5-3). Because drugs do not distribute instantaneously in humans, C_0 cannot be measured directly. It can be estimated, however, by extrapolating the plasma disappearance curve to time zero as illustrated in Figure 5-3. Thus

$$V_d = \frac{\text{dose}}{C_0}. \quad 5$$

Another way to determine V_d is the relationship

FIG. 5-3. The use of a one-compartment model to determine the V_d, K_e, and T½ of antipyrine. Ten milligrams antipyrine was administered intravenously at t=0, and the plasma concentration was determined at various times. C_0 was obtained by extrapolating the curve to T=0. (Data adapted from Soberman et al: J Biol Chem 179:31–42, 1949)

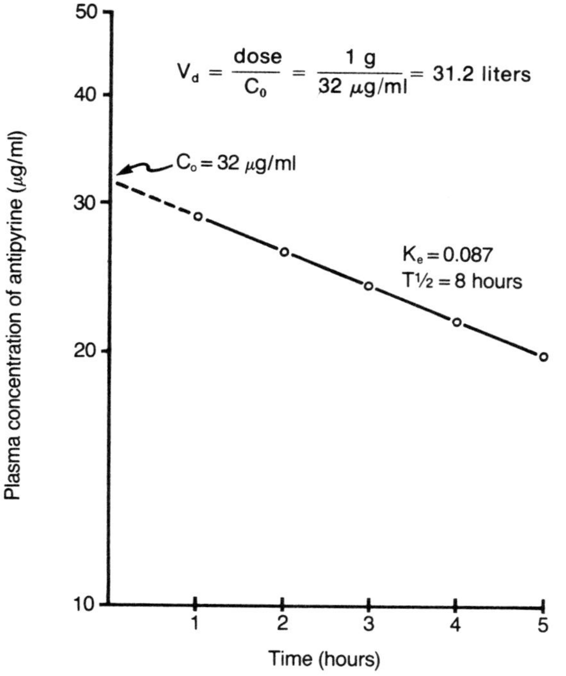

$$V_d = \frac{\text{dose}}{\text{AUC} \cdot K_e}, \quad 6$$

where AUC is the area under the plasma concentration versus time curve.

The V_d does not correspond to any anatomical space. It is a theoretical rather than a real volume. Nevertheless V_d is useful because it describes the distribution of a drug. A drug with a high V_d (*e.g.*, 20 liters/kg), for example, is present in high concentrations in tissues relative to plasma, whereas a low V_d (0.1 liter/kg) describes a drug that is concentrated in plasma relative to other tissues. Since the volume of plasma in a 70-kg man is about 2.1 liters, the total amount of drug in plasma (A_p) is $Cp \cdot 2.1$. Thus the fraction of A_T in the plasma space is A_p/A_T. The V_d of various drugs is listed in Table 2-2.

Drug distribution is determined by factors inherent in both the drug and the body. Thus distribution is affected by drug characteristics such as pK_a, lipid solubility, structure and molecular weight (*see* Chap. 2), and characteristics of the body and its tissues such as *p*H, blood flow, permeability, and tissue composition.

Clearance

Clearance of a drug from plasma (Cl) is the total volume of plasma from which drug is completely removed per unit of time (units = ml/min). Cl may be viewed as a proportionality constant that relates the rate of elimination to C_p:

$$\text{Rate of elimination} = \text{Cl} \cdot C_p \quad 7$$

Thus a drug with a very high clearance (1500 ml/min) may have a slower rate of elimination than a drug cleared at 100 ml/min (Table 5-1).

I have explained in previous sections how to

TABLE 5-1. Relation Between Clearance and Rate of Elimination*

	Drug	
Variable	***A***	***B***
Clearance, *ml/min*	1500	100
Rate of elimination, *μg/min*	15	500
Volume of distribution, *liter*	20	0.7
Plasma concentration, *mg/liter*	0.01	5

* This table shows that a rapidly cleared drug (A) can be eliminated slowly if the C_p is low. Drug B is rapidly eliminated even though the clearance is low because the V_d is small and the C_p correspondingly high.

determine V_d, K_e, and AUC from experimental data. Clearance is estimated from these variables by recognizing that

$$Cl = V_d \cdot K_e \quad \text{and} \qquad 8$$

$$Cl = \text{dose/AUC}. \qquad 9$$

These two equations were obtained by rearranging equation 7 and substituting from equations 1 and 2.

Clearance is a determinant of $T^1/_2$:

$$T^1/_2 = \frac{0.7\ V_d}{Cl}. \qquad 10$$

This relationship is important because it emphasizes that $T^1/_2$ is determined by both V_d and Cl. A decrease in Cl owing to hepatic or renal disease will increase $T^1/_2$ if V_d is unaffected. If both V_d and Cl change in the same direction, $T^1/_2$ may not change. Cl refers to clearance of the drug from plasma by organs (*e.g.*, hepatic clearance, Cl_H) by processes (*e.g.*, metabolic clearance), or it may denote clearance of a metabolite.

Clearances may be added. The Cl of a drug that is both metabolized by the liver and excreted by the kidney is represented by

$$C1 = Cl_H + Cl_R. \qquad 11$$

This relationship is particularly useful for devising dosage regimens in the presence of organ failure.

TWO-COMPARTMENT MODEL

The one-compartment model was discussed first because it is the least complicated model and it introduces several important pharmacokinetic variables. The two-compartment model accounts for its discrepancies and introduces the concept of a distribution phase followed by an elimination phase.

One type of two-compartment model is shown in Figure 5-4. Drug is either injected directly into the central compartment (i.v.) or reaches the central compartment after absorption. The drug may be eliminated directly from the central compartment or transferred to, then from, the peripheral compartment. All kinetics are assumed to be first order.

The plasma concentration time-curves plotted on arithmetic and semilog coordinates for a typical two-compartment drug are shown in

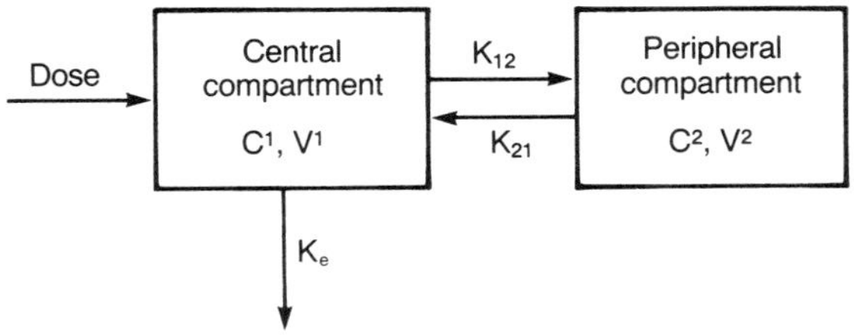

FIG. 5-4. A schematic of the two-compartment model. Drug administered to the central compartment distributes to the peripheral compartment and is eliminated (K_e) from the central compartment. C^1 and C^2 are the concentrations of drug and V^1 and V^2 the volumes of distribution of the two compartments, respectively. K_{12} and K_{21} are transfer rate constants between the two compartments.

Figures 5-5A and 5-5B, respectively. The typical characteristics of a drug in a two-compartment model are the sharp bend in the curve, as shown best in Figure 5-5A, and the linear terminal segment (Fig. 5-5B). During the initial phase, the plasma concentration falls rapidly as the drug is being distributed. Elimination also occurs, but the distribution process is relatively more important. During the later phase, distribution is essentially complete and elimination processes exert a greater influence on the shape of the curve. Whether the distribution phase is detected experimentally depends on its duration and on the frequency of sampling; for example, when the phase is long (hours), it is readily detected, but if it lasts only a few minutes it may not be detected unless sampling is early and frequent. In the latter case, the one-compartment model will usually provide a better fit to the data. It is not possible to allocate all organs and tissues to one or the other compartment, but as a first approximation the plasma, liver, kidney, and other organs with high blood flow are considered to be in the central compartment. Adipose tissue, muscle, and other poorly perfused tissues are in the peripheral compartment. Organs characterized by specialized membranes that may limit the distribution of a drug (*e.g.*, the brain) may be either in central or in peripheral compartments depending on the characteristics of the drug and the presence of specialized transport mechanisms.

Figure 5-5B shows that the plasma disappearance curve can be represented as the sum of two linear segments. Mathematically, the curve is defined as the sum of two exponential terms:

$$C_p = Ae^{-\alpha t} + Be^{-\beta t}, \qquad 12$$

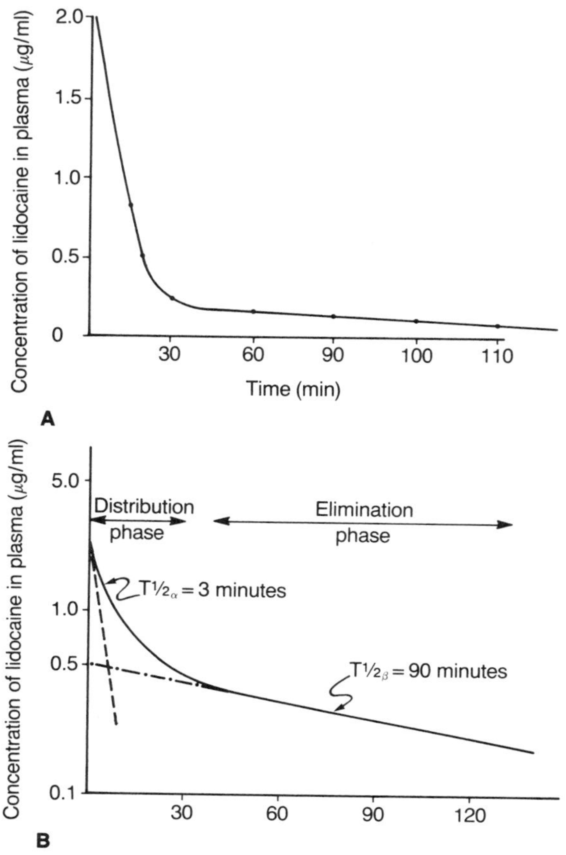

FIG. 5-5. A plot of the plasma concentration versus time data (___) for an intraveneously administered drug with kinetics that fit a two-compartment model. The coordinates in the left panel (*A*) are arithmetic; thus the curve rapidly falls, bends sharply, then slowly approaches the baseline. The same data plotted on semilogarithmetic coordinates (*B*) illustrate that the curve can be separated into two linear segments: (----α phase) and (---β phase). $T^1/_{2\alpha}$ = 0.693/3 min and $T^1/_{2\beta}$ = 0.693/60 min.

where A and B are proportionality constants and α and β are rate constants. A and B are analogous to C_0 in the one-compartment model, and α and β are similar to $T^1/_2$. In the two-compartment model V_d is the sum of V_c and V_p. $T^1/_{2\alpha}$, which is equal to $0.7/\alpha$, is referred to as the half-life of the α phase, and $T^1/_{2\beta}$ ($0.7/\beta$) is the half-life of the β phase. Thus the α phase principally represents distribution and the β-phase elimination. $T^1/_{2\alpha}$ is always shorter than $T^1/_{2\beta}$. Although $T^1/_{2\beta}$ and $T^1/_2$ (as defined for the one-compartment model) are not mathematically equivalent, they are essentially interchangeable in the equations above and below.

The parameters of the two-compartment model are determined by fitting experimental data to equation 12. Figure 5-6 shows the concentration of the drug in the two compartments. This information can be used to deduce the location of the receptors mediating the effects of the drug. If the onset of drug action is delayed and gradually reaches a peak, for example, one assumes that the receptors are in the peripheral compartment, whereas if the actions are immediate and decay rapidly, the receptors are probably located in the central compartment. A bolus injection often results in extremely high concentrations of drug in the central compartment. Hence if receptors that mediate toxicity are in the same compartment, toxicity will also occur almost immediately. Extremely high concentrations in the central compartment are readily avoided by administering the drug over a few minutes rather than as a bolus. Other dosage regimens that limit the concentration of a drug in the central compartment during the distribution phase are discussed later.

FIG. 5-6. Semilogarithmic plot of the amount of drug in the central and peripheral compartments of the two-compartment model at various times after i.v. administration. The configuration and relative positions of the curves depend on the model parameters. The curves may be markedly different if other parameters are used.

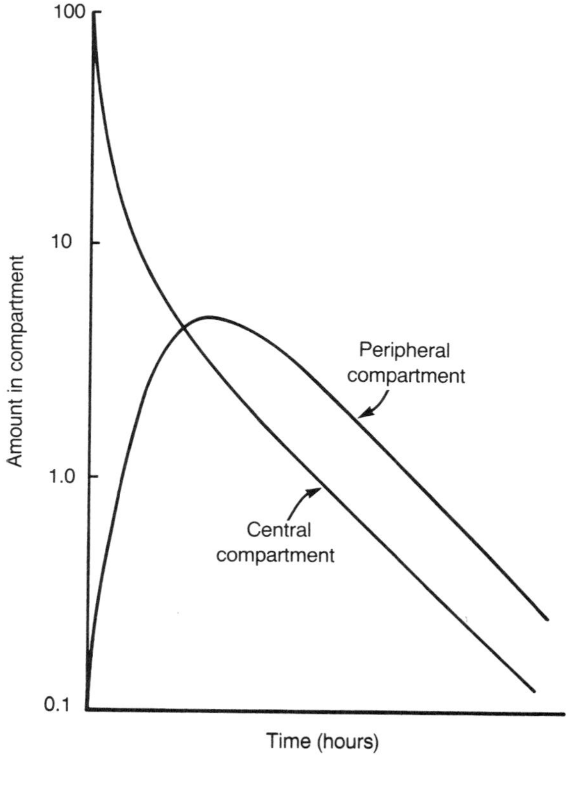

STEADY-STATE CONCENTRATION OF FIRST-ORDER DRUGS

PLATEAU PRINCIPLE

When a drug is administered intravenously at a constant rate, the amount of drug in the body will accumulate if the rate of administration exceeds the rate of elimination. The plasma concentration of a drug will increase until the rate of elimination and administration are equal (Fig. 5-7). At that point, the plasma drug concentration will plateau and remain constant until there is a change in the dosage regimen or kinetics. The plateau concentration or steady-state concentration (C_{ss}) is defined as

$$C_{ss} = \frac{\text{rate of administration}}{\text{clearance}} \qquad 13$$

Equation 13 is sometimes referred to as the plateau principle. A more convenient rearrangement of equation 13 is

$$C_{ss} = \frac{1.44\ T^{1}/_{2}\ D}{V_d\ \Delta T}, \qquad 14$$

where $D/\Delta T$ is the dosage regimen (dose/dosing interval) and the other terms are from equations 1 and 5 by rearrangement and substitution. The steady-state concentration is directly proportional to $T^{1}/_{2}$ and inversely proportional to V_d.

Time to the Plateau

The maximum effects of a drug will usually not be exerted until the C_{ss} is attained; it is thus important to know how long it will take to reach the C_{ss}. Equations 13 and 14 define the concentration of drug at steady-state but do not indicate the time to reach that state. It may seem paradoxical, but the only immediate determinant of the time to achieve the C_{ss} is the $T^{1}/_{2}$ (or K_e). The time to C_{ss} is completely independent of the dosage regimen. This is true *only* for first-order drugs administered at a fixed rate. If the dose is increased before the C_{ss} is achieved, the initial C_{ss} will be approached more rapidly, but the time to achieve the final C_{ss} still depends only on the $T^{1}/_{2}$. Because $T^{1}/_{2}$ is determined by V_d and Cl (Equation 5), a change in V_d or Cl will alter the time to attain C_{ss}.

The quantitative relation between $T^{1}/_{2}$ and C_{ss} is summarized in Table 5-2 and illustrated in Figure 5-7. After drug has been administered for one $T^{1}/_{2}$, the plasma concentration is 50% of the C_{ss}; after two half-lives elapse, the concentration is 75% of C_{ss}; after three half-lives 87%, and so forth.* An i.v. infusion of penicillin ($T^{1}/_{2}$ = 0.5 hr), for example, will take only 1.5 hr to reach 87% of the C_{ss}, whereas a drug with a $T^{1}/_{2}$ of 9 hours (*e.g.*, theophylline) will take more than 1 day to reach the same percentage of C_{ss}. In many clinical situations it is important to attain the C_{ss} as rapidly as possible by administering a single priming dose. When a drug has a low therapeutic index, however, a single priming dose is not usually safe. In this case, the priming is achieved with multiple closely spaced doses.

Because the effects of a drug are related to the C_p, another consequence of the plateau principle is that the maximum therapeutic

* In mathematical terms, the concentration of drug in plasma at any given time is

$$C_t = C_{ss}(1 - e^{-Ket}). \qquad E$$

When t = 1 $T^{1}/_{2}$, 2 $T^{1}/_{2}$, 3 $T^{1}/_{2}$, and so forth, the value of $1 - e^{-Ket}$ is 0.5, 0.75, 0.875, and so forth.

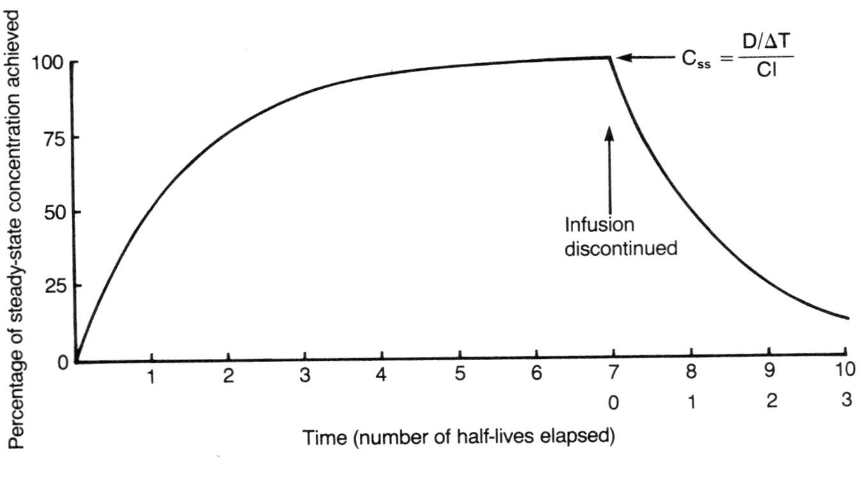

FIG. 5-7. Zero-order infusion of a first-order drug. Plasma concentrations are expressed as a percentage of C_{ss} and time as the number of half-lives elapsed. At the plateau, the rates of administration and elimination are equal. After discontinuation of the infusion, the rate of change in C_p is identical to that at the onset of the infusion.

TABLE 5-2. Quantitative Relation Between Time Expressed as the Number of Half-lives Elapsed and the Percentage of C_{ss} Achieved

Elapsed Half-lives	C_{ss} Achieved
no.	%
1	50.0
2	75.0
3	87.5
4	93.7
5	96.9
6	98.4
10	99.9

benefit usually will not be obtained until C_{ss} is achieved; however, it is not possible to distinguish clinically between the effects at C_{ss} = 90% and C_{ss} = 99% or greater. In terms of practical therapeutics, therefore, the full therapeutic benefit is essentially complete after 3.4 half-lives have elapsed. Another important consequence of the plateau principle is that diseases that prolong the $T^1/_2$ of a drug will prolong the time required to reach C_{ss}, resulting in an increase in the C_{ss} itself. Conversely, processes that decrease the $T^1/_2$ (*e.g.*, enzyme induction) will decrease C_{ss} and the time to C_{ss}.

ZERO ORDER VERSUS FIRST ORDER

An important difference between a first-order and a zero-order drug is that the relation between dose and C_{ss} is linear in arithmetic coordinates in first-order and nonlinear in zero-order drugs. As shown in Figure 5-8, when the dose of the first-order drug is increased, the C_{ss} increases proportionally, whereas an increased dose of a zero-order drug may result in a disproportionately greater increase in C_{ss}. At low doses, the dose versus C_{ss} relation is linear (pseudo-first order) for a zero-order drug, but at progressively higher doses the nonlinearity becomes apparent. Two commonly prescribed drugs that behave in this way are aspirin and phenytoin. Other drugs classified as first order may exhibit zero-order kinetics at very high doses.

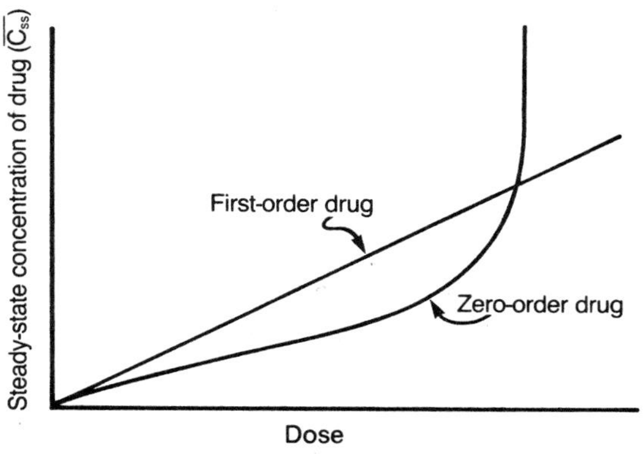

FIG. 5-8. Relation between the dose and $\overline{C_{ss}}$ of a zero-order and first-order drug. At high doses an increment in the dose of a zero-order drug results in a disproportionate increase in $\overline{C_{ss}}$, whereas the relation is linear at all doses for the first-order drug.

FIXED RATE MULTIPLE DOSE REGIMENS

INTRAVENOUS ROUTE OF ADMINISTRATION

When a single dose of drug is repeatedly administered at constant intervals, the C_p will fluctuate during the dosing interval. If the second dose is given before the first dose has been eliminated, the amount of drug in the body will accumulate until the steady-state is achieved. Equation 10 or 11 is still applied in this case, but the computed value represents the mean concentration ($\overline{C_{ss}}$) of drug during the dosing interval:

$$\overline{C_{ss}} = \frac{1.44\ T^1/_2\ D}{V_d\ \Delta T}. \qquad 15$$

ORAL ROUTE OF ADMINISTRATION

Bioavailability is that fraction (F) of the administered dose that reaches the central circulation. The fraction equals 1.0 for a drug completely absorbed and not metabolized by any tissues before it reaches the central circulation. The bioavailability of a drug may be determined from the ratio of the AUC after an oral dose (AUC_{oral}) to the AUC after an i.v. bolus of the same dose:

$$F = \frac{AUC_{oral}}{AUC_{i.v.}}. \qquad 16$$

Factors that result in bioavailability fractions of less than 1.0 are related to drug formulation (disintegration rates, solubility, excipients), gastrointestinal function (*p*H, motility, blood flow, disease), and metabolism (by bacteria, gastrointestinal tissue, and liver) (*see* Chaps. 2, 8, 11). Some commonly prescribed drugs that have low oral bioavailability are nitroglycerin, morphine, and lidocaine. The bioavailability of nitroglycerin is high when it is absorbed from the oral mucosa, but if nitroglycerin is swallowed the bioavailable fraction is about 0.1. A few drugs have low values of F, even if they are administered parenterally. Phenytoin is usually not completely bioavailable intramuscularly because it precipitates in the tissues. Different lots of drug, even if prepared by the same manufacturer, may differ in their bioavailability.

The formula for C_{ss} that takes the absorbed dose ($F \cdot D$) into account is

$$C_{ss} = \frac{1.44\ T^{1}/_{2}\ FD}{V_d\ \Delta T}. \qquad 17$$

PREDICTING THE STEADY-STATE CONCENTRATION

The normal values of $T^{1}/_{2}$, V_d, or their equivalents are reasonably well established for most commonly prescribed drugs. Usually the values have been determined in healthy, nonobese adults and therefore may not apply to patients with serious cardiac, renal, or hepatic disease or to pediatric (*see* Chap. 4) or geriatric populations. For some drugs, estimates of the parameters are available for these groups.

Sometimes it is useful to compare the predicted C_{ss} with the measured C_{ss} determined by analysis of plasma drawn from a patient in the steady-state. If the predicted C_{ss} and the actual C_{ss} do not agree, then the laboratory value was in error, the patient was not in the steady-state, or the predicted value of $T^{1}/_{2}$ or V_d was in error. Assuming the laboratory analysis was correct and the patient was in a steady-state, the estimates of V_d and $T^{1}/_{2}$ were incorrect. Often the clinical circumstances will suggest which variable was incorrect. Thus one can use the predicted versus the actual C_{ss} to estimate how the pharmacokinetics of a drug are altered in a given individual. In turn, this information is used to devise a new dosage regimen that will bring the measured and predicted C_{ss} into agreement.

ABSORPTION

FIRST ORDER

Generally a drug must be absorbed from the site of administration before it exerts effects (*see* Chap. 2). Most drugs are absorbed by a first-order process; the rate of absorption therefore depends on the total amount of drug remaining to be absorbed (A_{ab}). The rate constant for absorption (K_a) describes the fraction of A_{ab} absorbed per unit of time. Absorption processes are analogous to elimination processes. The half-life of absorption ($T^{1}/_{2a}$) is

$$T^{1}/_{2a} = \frac{0.7}{K_a}, \qquad 18$$

and the instantaneous rate of absorption is

$$\text{rate of absorption} = K_a\ A_{ab}. \qquad 19$$

Compared to the i.v. and intra-arterial routes, absorption from other sites results in a lower peak concentration of drug in plasma and a delay between drug administration and the peak. Consequently, absorption markedly influences the intensity and time-course of drug effects. The magnitude of the peak and the time to attain the peak depends on the rate of absorption relative to the rate of elimination. This relation may be expressed as the ratio of $T^{1}/_{2a}/T^{1}/_{2}$ or K_a/K_e.

Figures 5-9A and 5-9B illustrate the plasma concentration time curve for different $T^{1}/_{2a}/T^{1}/_{2}$ ratios. If absorption is rapid relative to elimination (*e.g.*, $T^{1}/_{2a} < T^{1}/_{2}$), absorption processes will predominate. In this case absorption will be nearly complete by the time the peak concentration is attained, and the curve will rapidly rise to a peak. Conversely, if $T^{1}/_{2a}$ is relatively slow, peak absorption will be lower and delayed.

The rate of drug absorption depends largely on the site of administration. Generally, the i.m. route results in a higher and earlier peak compared to the s.c. route. The configuration of the curve after oral administration is quite variable (*see* Chap. 2). An oral solution of a drug absorbed from the stomach, for example, will produce an early and high peak in contrast to a drug that must dissolve and pass into the small intestine before it is absorbed.

MULTIPLE DOSES

The rate of absorption influences the fluctuations in plasma concentration within the dosing interval (ΔT). As with a single dose, the height and timing of peak plasma drug concentration after multiple doses depend on the $T^{1}/_{2a}/T^{1}/_{2}$ ratio. This is illustrated in Figure 5-9B where the dosing regimen is the same in both curves but the $T^{1}/_{2a}/T^{1}/_{2}$ ratio is 3 for the solid curve and 1 for the dashed curve.

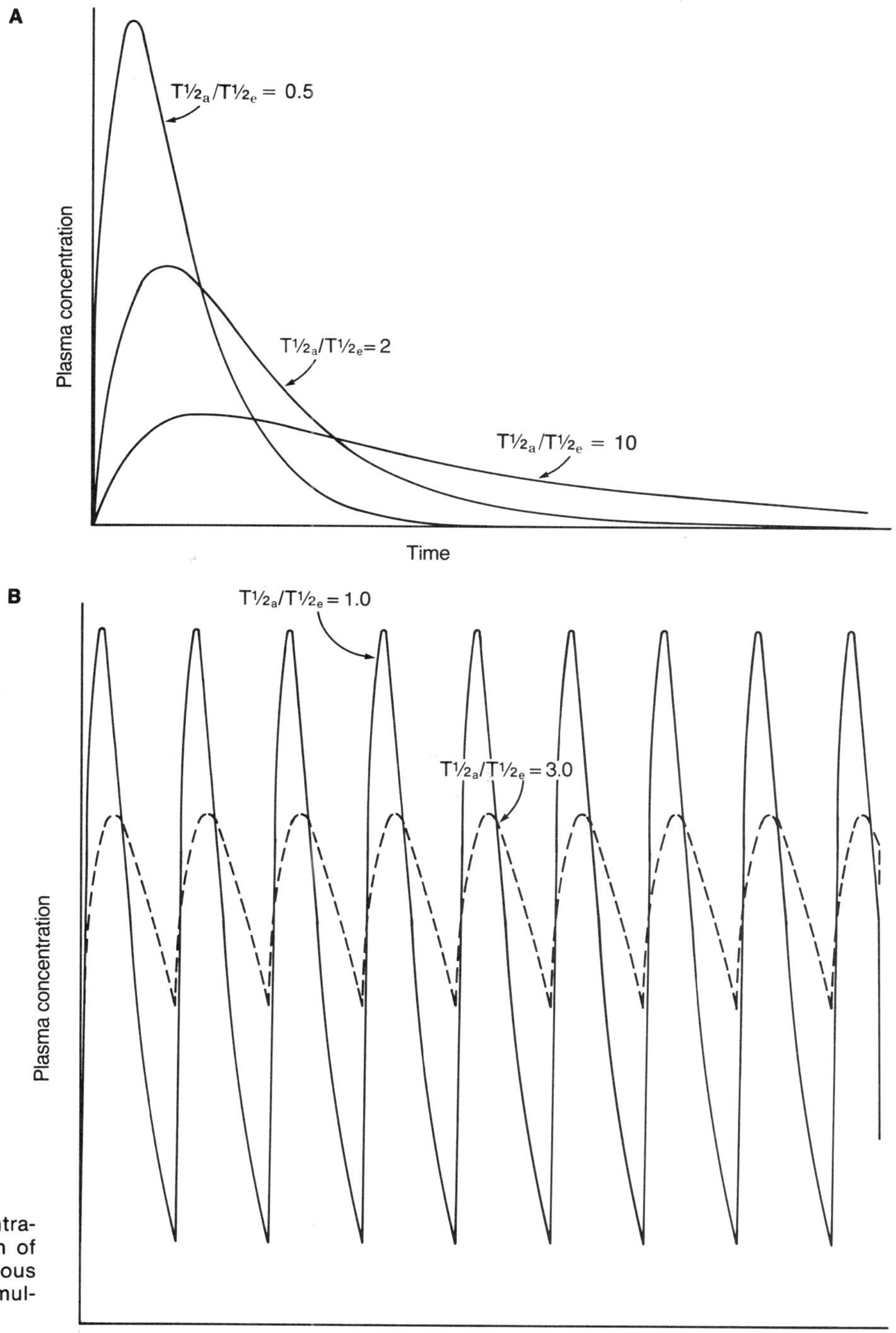

FIG. 5-9. Plasma concentration of drug as a function of the $T½_a/T½_e$ ratio at various times after single (*A*) and multiple (*B*) doses (*see* text).

ZERO ORDER

Some drugs are formulated to release their active principle slowly. The absorption of many of these sustained release preparations approximates zero-order kinetics. In reality, drug absorption is usually first order, but the active principle is released so slowly relative to the rate of absorption that the plasma concentration time-curve simulates zero-order absorption. The actual rate of release from these formulations may vary over a substantial range owing to a number of complex factors. Consequently the onset and intensity of drug effect may be quite variable.

INDIVIDUAL VARIATION IN PHARMACOKINETIC PARAMETERS

The response to a drug is determined by the amount of drug that reaches the receptors and the intrinsic activity of the drug/receptor complex. This chapter discusses some of the factors that affect the amount of drug that reaches its receptors—factors that determine or alter the pharmacokinetics of a drug. A few of the most important sources of variability that influence pharmacokinetic parameters are drug metabolism, genetics, age, sex, and drug interactions (*see* Chaps. 3, 6, 7, 8, 11).

Disease has a variable effect on pharmacokinetic variables. Thus a person with severe pneumonia or acute hepatitis may have pharmacokinetic variables indistinguishable from those of persons with no disease. In contrast, chronic hepatic or renal failure may produce a tenfold change in variables.

The organs that most commonly affect pharmacokinetic variables when diseased are the liver, kidney, and heart. The influence of renal disease is the best understood and the most predictable. The principles for alterating dosage regimens are independent of the disease; thus if the principles are understood for renal disease, they may be applied to patients with other diseases.

DOSAGE REGIMENS IN RENAL FAILURE

Renal insufficiency may alter the $T^1/_2$, V_d, Cl, F, or other pharmacokinetic characteristics of a drug. The most common alteration is diminished Cl and an increased $T^1/_2$. These changes result in increased C_{ss}; therefore, the maintenance dose must be decreased or administered less frequently. The V_d of some drugs decreases in renal failure, particularly if accompanied by cardiac failure. Completely metabolized drugs are not necessarily safe in renal failure. Normeperidine, for example, an active metabolite of meperidine, is rapidly eliminated by a normal kidney, but in renal failure normeperidine accumulates and causes CNS irritability. The effect of an abrupt decrease in renal function on the plasma concentration time-curve is shown in Figure 5-10.

One of the most common problems in therapeutics is adjusting the dosage regimen in patients with renal failure. The decision to alter the normal regimen depends on the fraction of the total clearance due to renal mechanisms; the degree of renal impairment; and the drug's therapeutic index. The fractional renal clearance (FCl_R) is

$$FCl_R = \frac{Cl_R}{Cl}. \qquad 20$$

The value of FCl_R for many of the most important drugs can be found in reference tables. Renal impairment is estimated from the serum creatinine or more precisely from the creatinine clearance (Cl_{cr}). The fractional degree of impairment may be estimated from

$$FCl_{cr\cdot rf} = \frac{Cl_{cr\cdot rf}}{Cl_{cr}}, \qquad 21$$

where Cl_{cr} is determined from tables of normal values or estimated at 100 to 120 ml/min. The $Cl_{cr\cdot rf}$ is the clearance of creatinine in the patient with renal failure. Ideally, $Cl_{cr\cdot rf}$ is calculated from recent measurements of the patients' serum and urine creatinine. If these values are not available, $Cl_{cr\cdot rf}$ must be estimated. One formula for estimating the maintenance dose in renal failure (D_{rf}) is

$$D_{rf} = (D)(FCl_R)(FCl_{cr\cdot rf}) + (D)(1\text{-}FCl_R), \qquad 22$$

where D is the maintenance dose in the absence of renal failure. Thus if D is 100 mg, the D_{rf} of a drug 90% eliminated by the kidney that is administered to a patient with a 50% reduction in Cl_{cr} will be 55 mg: {(100)(0.9)(0.5) + (100)(1 − 0.9)}. This approach does not consider the kinetics and toxicity of metabolites and assumes that nonrenal clearance is unchanged in renal failure. These assumptions are not valid for some drugs.

The D_{rf} may be administered at the (ΔT) ordinarily used in a normal person. Alternatively it may be more practical to increase ΔT and increase D_{rf} while still preserving the overall rate of administration. If the regimen for a patient with normal renal function is 100 mg every 8 hours and D_{rf} is 33 mg, three hypothetical regimens are (A) 33 mg every 8 hours; (B) 50 mg every 12 hours; and (C) 100 mg every 24 hours. The plasma concentration associated with these regimens are shown in Figure 5-11. Regimen A is similar to the normal regimen except that time to $\overline{C_{ss}}$ 90% is increased and the in-between-dose fluctuations are smaller. An impor-

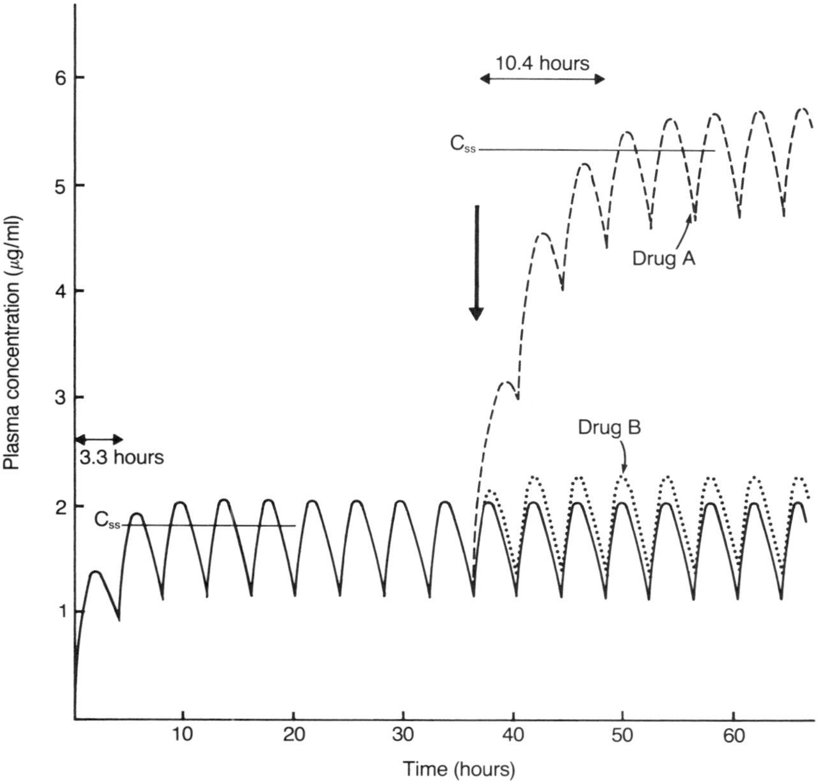

FIG. 5-10. The effect of a 70% reduction (↓) in renal function on the plasma-concentration-time curve of two drugs. Drug A and B have the same T½, V_d, and dosage regimen, but renal clearance (Cl_R) accounts for 90% of the total Cl of drug A and only 20% of the Cl of drug B. Since their pharmacokinetic parameters and dosage regimen are the same, their plasma-concentration-time curves are identical (___) in the absence of renal failure. The $\overline{C_{ss}}$ is 1.8 μg/ml, and the time to 90% of the $\overline{C_{ss}}$ is 3.3 hours. A 70% reduction in Cl_R has little effect on the $\overline{C_{ss}}$ and the time to 90% of $\overline{C_{ss}}$ for drug B (......). In contrast, both parameters are markedly increased for drug A (----). The $\overline{C_{ss}}$ and time to 90% of $\overline{C_{ss}}$ increase by a factor of about 3 to 5.7 μg/ml and 10.4 hours. This simulation assumed that V_d was not altered by renal failure. If there were a simultaneous decrease in V_d, the $\overline{C_{ss}}$ would be even higher.

tant advantage of regimen C is that the patient only requires one dose per day, but the fluctuations are large. Regimen B is a reasonable compromise because it closely simulates the normal regimen and requires fewer doses. In clinical practice, the choice of ΔT is a compromise between minimizing the interdose fluctuations in plasma concentration and the inconvenience of frequent drug administration. Because renal failure increases the T½, a priming dose may be needed.

Another commonly used technique for determining the maintenance dose in renal failure is a nomogram. The typical *nomogram* comprises three scales arranged on a planer surface. One scale represents the change of renal function (*e.g.*, $Cl_{cr \cdot rf}$), another scale the contribution of renal elimination to overall elimination (FCl_R), and the third scale, which is interposed between the other two, represents a pharmacokinetic variable such as Cl or T½. By connecting the two outer scales with a straight line, the value of the pharmacokinetic variable in renal failure is read off the center scale. The value of the variables is then used in one of the formulae relating dose to C_{SS} (*e.g.*, Equation 14).

Nomograms are based on a mathematical model. Although convenient to use, they are based on assumptions and population variables. The degree to which the assumptions and variables reflect the clinical state of renal failure determines the usefulness of the nomogram. Nomograms based on high-quality clinical data are very helpful in providing a reasonably accurate estimate of D_{rf}. Nomograms that do not account for all pertinent variables may be grossly inaccurate and should not be used.

Another means of devising a dosage regimen in renal failure is to consult the manufacturer's drug package insert. In most cases, the inserts that specifically address the problem of dosing in renal failure are accurate and reliable.

MONITORING PLASMA CONCENTRATION OF DRUGS

One of the most challenging aspects of therapeutics is individualization of the dosage regimen, which is easy in some drugs because clinical signs are readily observed or biochemical

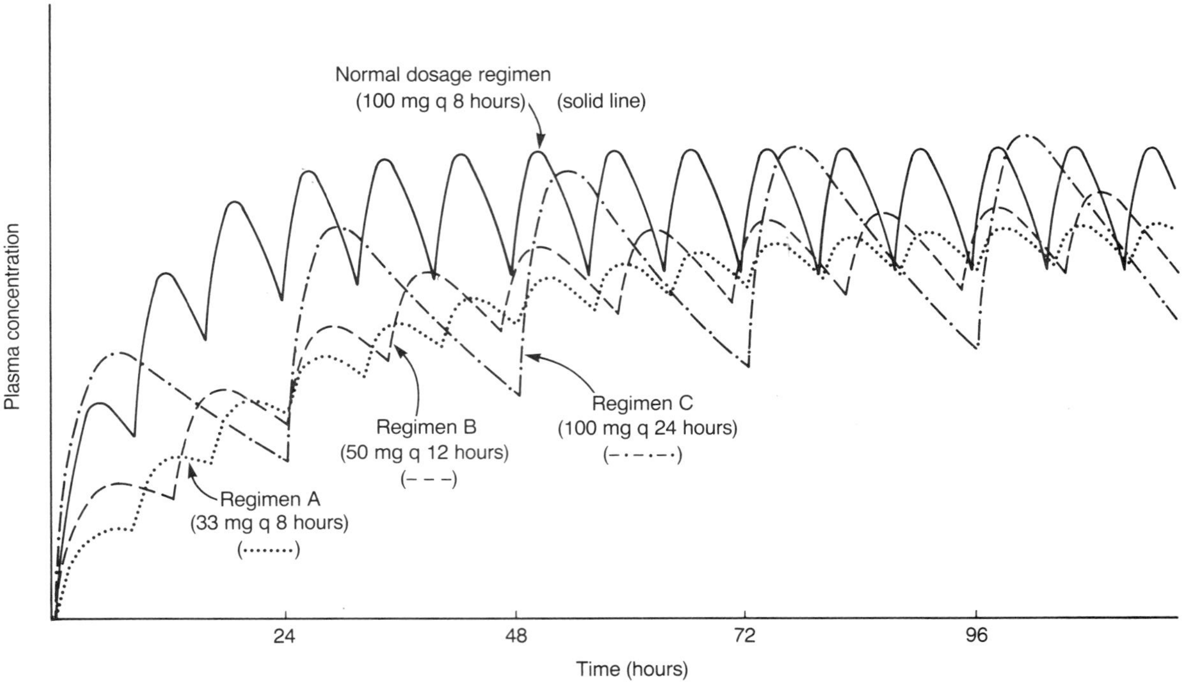

FIG. 5-11. A comparison of plasma concentration time curves in the absence (___) and presence (·····, -----, -·-·-·-) of renal failure. Dosage regimens A, B, and C produce the same $\overline{C_{ss}}$ but differing interdose fluctuations in plasma concentration (*see* text).

measurements indicate the desired or toxic responses. In these cases, it is relatively simple to titrate the dose to the person's response. Other drugs are more difficult to individualize because they do not exert actions readily measured or quantitated by clinical or biochemical means. In this circumstance, it is often useful to measure the concentration of drug in plasma and adjust dosage to provide levels known to produce the desired response in most patients. To use this approach—referred to as drug monitoring—one must understand the relationships of dose, plasma concentration, and desired response.

A particular dosage regimen administered to a large number of patients will result in a wide range of responses and steady-state concentrations (Fig. 5-12). The same regimen will produce a high C_{ss} (or C_{ss}) and toxicity in one patient and a low C_{ss} and insufficient response in another. The variability in the dose–effect relationship is largely due to individual differences in the C_{ss} established by the particular regimen. The highest concentration is commonly ten times greater than the lowest, and with some drugs the range may be fifty-fold. The relatively poor correlation between dose and C_{ss} is partly due to individual differences in absorption, distribution, metabolism, and elimination. The correlation between a given C_{ss} and intensity of drug action is quite good. Thus knowledge of the C_{ss} allows more accurate

FIG. 5-12. Frequency distribution resulting from administration of a standard dosage regimen to a large number of patients. Plasma concentrations that fall within the therapeutic window produce the desired response in most patients. High concentrations may be ineffective.

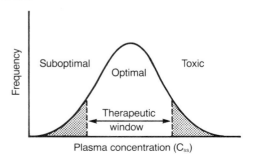

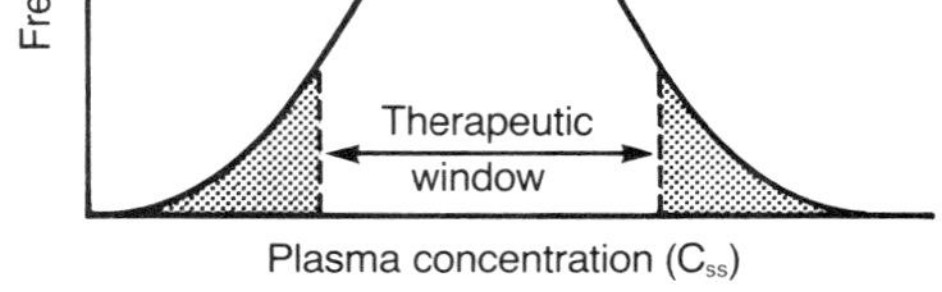

TABLE 5-3. Usual Therapeutic Ranges of Plasma Drug Concentration

Drug	Therapeutic Range
	μg/ml
Digitoxin	0.013–0.025
Digoxin	0.0005–0.002
Gentamicin	8–12
Lidocaine	2–5
Lithium	0.16–1.2 mEq/liter
Nortriptyline	0.05–0.08
Phenobarbital	10–30
Phenytoin	10–25
Primidone	5–10
Procainamide	4–8
Propranolol	0.03–0.15
Quinidine	3–7
Salicylates	150–300
Theophylline	5–20

individualization than does knowledge of the dose.

The process of adjusting the dosage regimen in accordance with the plasma concentration of drug is widely used to individualize and to optimize therapy. The therapeutic range or window is established by clinical studies and includes concentrations at which most patients experience the desired effects. Table 5-3 lists the therapeutic range of some frequently prescribed drugs that are commonly monitored. Usually it is not necessary or useful to monitor other drugs, and monitoring is not helpful if a drug forms covalent bonds, acts longer than it is present in plasma, or results in tolerance at its receptor sites. The drugs in Table 5-3 are characterized by a low therapeutic index, they do not produce readily quantitated clinical or biochemical responses, and they act reversibly over a short period. Monitoring is particularly helpful when a therapeutic failure is being evaluated, particularly if noncompliance and altered pharmacokinetics are likely possibilities, and when a toxic response is being evaluated. Careful clinical monitoring is usually the most reliable means of achieving accuracy while minimizing toxicity. Monitoring plasma drug concentrations is a useful adjunct but should not be used as a substitute for clinical observations and judgment.

GLOSSARY

Abbreviation:	*Meaning*	*Commonly Used Units*
D:	Dose	g, mg
D_{rf}:	Maintenance dose in renal failure	g, mg
t:	Time after drug administration	hr, min, days
ΔT:	Dosage interval	hr, min, days
$D/\Delta T$:	Fixed rate dosage regimen	mg/hr, g/day
A_T:	Total amount of drug in the body	g, mg
A_P:	Total amount of drug in plasma	g, mg
A_{ab}:	Total amount of drug remaining to be absorbed	g, mg
C:	Concentration of unchanged drug in plasma, serum, and whole blood	mg/ml
C_p:	Concentration of unchanged drug in plasma	mg/ml
C^1:	Concentration of unchanged drug in the central compartment of a two-compartment model	mg/ml
C^2:	Concentration of unchanged drug in the peripheral compartment of a two-compartment model	mg/ml
V:	Volume of a compartment	liter, ml or liter/kg, ml/kg
V_d:	Volume of distribution	
V^1:	Volume of the central compartment of a two-compartment model	
V^2:	Volume of the peripheral compartment of a two-compartment model	
K_e:	Elimination rate constant	hr^{-1}, min^{-1}
K_a:	Absorption rate constant	hr^{-1}, min^{-1}
k_{12}:	Transfer rate constant from the central to peripheral compartment	hr^{-1}, min^{-1}
k_{21}:	Transfer rate constant from the peripheral to central compartment	hr^{-1}, min^{-1}
Cl:	Clearance from plasma	ml/min or liters/hr
Cl_H:	Clearance by the liver	
Cl_R:	Clearance by the kidney	
Cl_{rf}:	Clearance by the kidney in renal failure	
Cl_{cr}:	Clearance of creatinine by the kidney	
FCL_R:	Fractional renal clearance	
$Cl_{cr\text{-}rf}$:	Clearance of creatinine in renal failure	

$T^{1}/_{2}$:	Half-life of elimination	min, hr
$T^{1}/_{2a}$:	Half-life of absorption	min, hr
$T^{1}/_{2\alpha}$:	Half-life of the alpha phase of a two-compartment model	min, hr
$T^{1}/_{2\beta}$:	Half-life of the beta phase of a two-compartment model	min, hr
AUC:	Area under the curve	mg/ml/min
AUC_0:	Area under the curve after oral administration	mg/ml/min
$AUC_{i.v.}$:	Area under the curve after i.v. administration	mg/ml/min
C_{ss}:	Steady-state concentration of drug in plasma resulting from a constant rate infusion	mg/ml, μg/ml
$\overline{C_{ss}}$:	Mean steady-state concentration of drug in plasma resulting from intermittent dosing	mg/ml, μg/ml

FURTHER READING

1. Sjöqvist F, Borgå O, Orme ML'E: Fundamentals of clinical pharmacology. In Avery GS (ed): Drug Treatment, pp 1–61. New York, Adis Press, 1980
2. Gibaldi M, Perrier D: Pharmacokinetics. New York, Marcel Dekker, 1975 (This book is part of a series of textbooks and monographs, Drugs and the Pharmaceutical Sciences, edited by James Swarbrick.)
3. Rowland M: Drug administration and regimens. In Melmon KL, Morrelli HF (eds): Clinical Pharmacology, pp 25–70. New York, Macmillan, 1978
4. Rowland M, Tozer TN: Clinical Pharmacokinetics: Concepts and Applications. Philadelphia, Lea & Febiger, 1980

CHAPTER 5 QUESTIONS

(*See* P. 7 for Full Instructions)

Select the One Best Answer

1. The bioavailability of a drug may be estimated most accurately by measuring
   - *A.* serum concentrations of the unaltered drug.
   - *B.* the intensity of a distinct therapeutic response.
   - *C.* urinary concentrations of the unaltered drug and its metabolites.
   - *D.* tissue concentrations of the drug.
   - *E.* the intensity of the adverse effects produced by the drug.

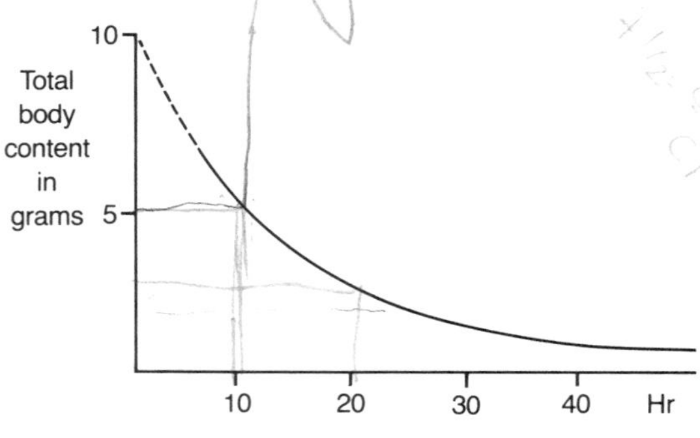

2. From the above graph, each of the following can be concluded to be correct EXCEPT
   - *A.* doses must be given every 10 hours to maintain an average content of 10 g.
   - *B.* the half-life is about 10 hours.
   - *C.* if the same dose is administered every 10 hours, the total body content will approach 20 g.
   - *D.* the elimination of the drug follows first-order kinetics.
   - *E.* a body content of 15 g will be reduced to less than 5 g in 30 hours.

3. A 25 mg/ml solution of drug X is available for intravenous injection. What volume is needed to give a dose of 8 mg/kg to a teenager weighing 50 kg?
   - *A.* 1.0 ml
   - *B.* 1.6 ml
   - *C.* 2.5 ml
   - *D.* 10 ml
   - *E.* 16 ml

4. The biological half-life of a drug in the body may be increased by each of the following EXCEPT
   - *A.* changes in urinary *p*H
   - *B.* the presence of another drug that competes for active renal tubular secretion.
   - *C.* decreased renal function.
   - *D.* another drug that induces microsomal enzymes.
   - *E.* a large increase in adipose tissue.

A = 1,2,3; B = 1,3; C = 2,4; D = 4; E = All

5. A long plasma half-life of a drug may be associated with
   - *1.* a high degree of binding of the drug by plasma proteins.
   - *2.* an apparent volume of distribution of > 1000 liters.
   - *3.* a specialized form of the drug that is slowly absorbed.
   - *4.* decreased renal function that serves to retard excretion of the drug.

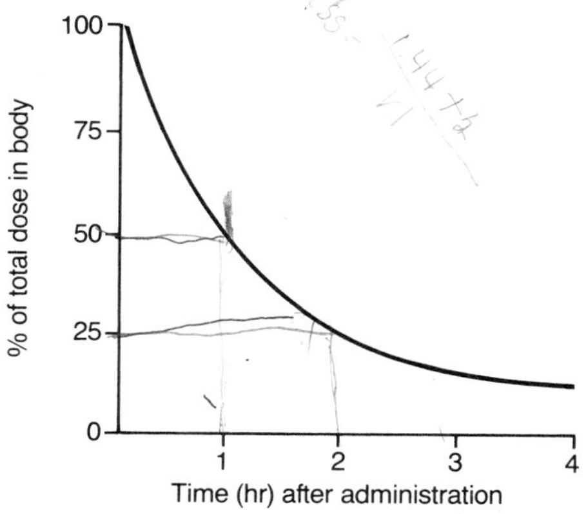

6. If a drug given in a single dose of 4 mg is eliminated according to the above graph, then
   1. the half-life of the drug is about 1 hour.
   2. the drug is eliminated according to zero order kinetics (dc/dt = k).
   3. with repeated administration at intervals of 1 hour, the maximum amount that can be accumulated in the body is about 8 mg.
   4. with repeated administration at intervals of 2 hours, the maximum amount that can be accumulated in the body is about 4 mg.

7. If a drug is metabolized according to first-order kinetics,
   1. its rate of metabolism would increase in proportion to its plasma level.
   2. its duration of action is doubled by the administration of twice the dose.
   3. a drop to half the initial blood level would occur in the same time-interval after a small or a large therapeutic dose.
   4. a constant rate of metabolism or excretion occurs.

8. A normal human volunteer is injected intravenously with drug X (a weak base, pK_a 7.4). Assume that the drug has reached steady state conditions with all body tissues, including the blood. Which of the following conditions would tend to lower the plasma concentration of the drug?
   1. The *p*H of the gastric content is raised to 7.4.
   2. A second drug is given that depresses respiration, resulting in decreased plasma *p*H.
   3. A second drug is given that competes with drug X for binding sites on serum albumin.
   4. The *p*H of the urine is decreased from 7.4 to 6.4.

9. An adequate blood level of a drug may be difficult to achieve by oral administration if the drug is
   1. a quaternary ammonium compound.
   2. rapidly metabolized by the liver.
   3. maximally secreted by the kidneys.
   4. a polypeptide.

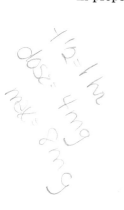

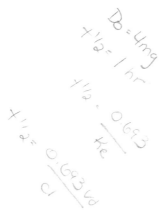

6

BERT N. LA DU, Jr.

Pharmacogenetics

Although it has been recognized for many years that genetic differences in people can modify their response to drugs, only during the past 20 years have systematic studies been conducted to evaluate the importance of genetic traits in drug effectiveness and adverse drug reactions. The scientific study of genetically determined individual variability in drug metabolism and unusual drug reactions is called *pharmacogenetics*. This relatively new field of pharmacologic investigation seeks answers to some important questions: How do genetic differences in people account for individual variability in the transformation, detoxification, and excretion of drugs? Do genetic factors explain clinical observations that some patients, given the recommended amounts of appropriate drugs, develop unexpected or adverse drug reactions? Certain human genetic traits are associated with unusual drug effects, and definite relations exist between genetic factors and drug disposition and metabolism.

DETECTION AND ANALYSIS OF PHARMACOGENETIC CONDITIONS

The observation that a patient has shown an exaggerated drug response or developed an unexpected drug reaction has been the starting point for many pharmacogenetic studies. Careful investigation of an individual patient's symptoms, however, is not enough to decide whether genetic or environmental factors are responsible, and a genetic approach, or a genetic analysis of the condition, is required. Whether the unusual drug response is familial (runs in certain families) and, if so, whether it occurs among selected members of the family pedigree in a pattern that agrees with expectation for an inherited trait must be ascertained. For example, a recessively inherited trait should occur, on the average, in one fourth of

---

ARNO GUNTHER MOTULSKY, 1923– . German-born American physician and geneticist. Has worked on the role of genetic variation in various diseases and in drug reactions.

FRIEDRICK VOGEL, 1925– . German geneticist. Has done extensive research on human genetics, including studies on genetic traits that account for different electroencephalographic patterns. Was the first to use the term *pharmacogenetics* in 1959.

the sibs (brothers and sisters) of the index patients. Other patterns of drug-sensitive family members would, of course, be expected for dominant traits, or for sex-linked hereditary conditions. If the unusual drug reaction is closely associated with a specific biochemical "marker," such as the deficiency of a particular enzyme, or the presence of an abnormal drug metabolite in the urine or blood, more conclusive genetic evidence can be obtained. These biochemical and genetic steps are rather easily followed for pharmacogenetic conditions that are inherited as simple mendelian dominant or recessive traits. The investigation becomes much more complicated, however, if several different genes are involved, and a particular combination of these genes must be inherited for patients to show the unusual drug reaction.

One general method that has been used in pharmacogenetic studies is to measure the relative contributions of genetic and environmental influences using identical and fraternal twins. The advantage of this method is that important information about the relative genetic contribution can be obtained from only a few test subjects, even though it does not indicate how many genes are involved or how the genetic factors operate. Basically, the twin study method is a comparison of variability of some pharmacologic measurement between pairs of identical (monozygotic) twins and pairs of fraternal (dizygotic) twins. Because monozygotic twins have the same genetic constitution, their variability is much less than the intrapair variability of fraternal twins for genetically determined traits.

A comparison of the percentage of a test dose of isoniazid excreted as acetylisoniazid in 24 hours (Table 6-1) by identical and fraternal twins shows this metabolic (conjugation) pathway for isoniazid to be determined primarily by genetic factors. Twin studies with several other drugs (phenylbutazone, antipyrine, bishydroxycoumarin, and ethanol) have led to similar results. These last-mentioned drugs are all handled mainly by biotransformation rather than by excretion into the urine as unchanged drug, and the rate of decline of the drug concentration in plasma was used as a measure of the rate of elimination. Close agreement in biological half-times was found within identical twin pairs; much wider variation occurred in pairs of fraternal twins. From all of these results, I conclude that genetic factors primarily determine the rate of metabolism of most drugs and chemicals in humans.

Pharmacogenetic conditions can also be investigated through population surveys by making some pharmacologic measurement in many people to see if the collected responses follow a unimodal, bimodal, or multimodal distribution. Bimodality suggests that there may be two distinct subpopulations but does not prove that there must be a genetic basis for the two groups. Testing can be done, on that premise, to find out if a genetic hypothesis is supported. Blood concentrations of isoniazid, for example, 6 hours after an oral dose of the drug show bimodality (Fig. 6-1). Further work has established that the rate of disappearance of the drug (rapid or slow) depends on the rate of isoniazid acetylation, and the latter is proportional to the level of the enzyme *N*-acetyl transferase in the liver. Slow acetylators of isoniazid have appreciably less *N*-acetyl transferase in their liver than do rapid acetylators. Family

TABLE 6-1. Excretion of Isoniazid by Identical and Fraternal Twins*

Identical Twins			Fraternal Twins		
Twin Pair Number	*Sex*	*Isoniazid Excreted in 24 hr (% of dose)*	*Twin Pair Number*	*Sex*	*Isoniazid Excreted in 24 hr (% of dose)*
1	M	8.8	6	F	12.1
	M	8.3		F	13.7
2	F	26.0	7	F	10.9
	F	25.2		F	4.6
3	M	11.8	8	M	11.0
	M	12.4		M	8.5
4	F	12.2	9	F	3.9
	F	11.5		F	15.2
5	F	4.1	10	M	10.5
	F	4.4		M	15.6

* (Bonicke R, Lisboa BP: Uber die Erbbedingtheit der intraindividnellen Konstanz der Isoniazidausscheidung beim Menschen. Naturwissenschaften 44:314, 1957)

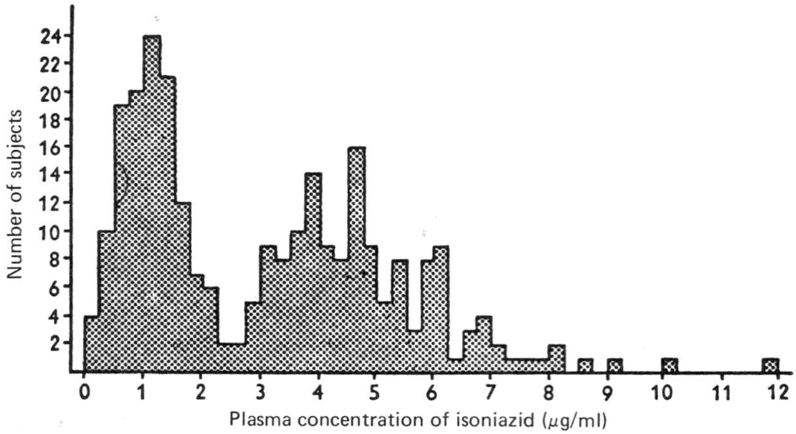

FIG. 6-1. Plasma concentrations of isoniazid 6 hours after oral administration to 267 members of 53 families. (Evans DA, Manley KA, McKusick VA: Genetic control of isoniazid metabolism in man. Br Med J 2:485, 1960)

studies and other genetic tests have led to the conclusion that two allelic genes (R = rapid acetylation; r = slow acetylation) at one locus control the rate of isoniazid metabolism. Thus there are three possible genotypic combinations (RR, Rr, and rr) and two phenotypes: rapid (RR or Rr) and slow (rr). Slow acetylators are homozygous for a recessive gene, but since about one half of the United States population has slow acetylators, the recessive gene is far from rare. The respective gene frequencies are r = 0.723 and R = 0.277. The relative gene frequencies differ in other geographic areas according to the particular ethnic groups and their genetic history. Asiatic groups are generally much higher in rapid acetylators, and Middle Eastern groups are higher in slow acetylators than are European and American populations.

OBJECTIVES OF PHARMACOGENETIC STUDIES

Whatever approaches are used in pharmacogenetic investigations, the objectives are the same: 1) to evaluate how genetics contributes to the condition; 2) to determine the inheritance pattern (dominant, recessive; sex-linked, autosomal); 3) to measure the frequency of the genes involved in the general population and different ethnic groups; 4) to find the biochemical basis for the variation; and 5) to establish the clinical importance of the condition.

PHARMACOGENETICS AND ECOGENETICS

Individual differences in response to drugs extend to the disposition of nontherapeutic, environmental chemicals, a concept that has been designated *ecogenetics*. Certain genetic traits modify the rate of biotransformation and the pattern of metabolites derived from environmental chemicals, and these may affect the degree of individual susceptibility of resistance to the agents. The pronounced polymorphic differences in human serum paraoxonase activity, for example, might confer greater protection to those with higher activity when exposed to parathion. Genetic differences have also been reported in the degree of inducibility of arylhydrocarbon hydroxylase activity of human lymphocytes after preincubation *in vitro* with 3-methylcholanthrene.

Since the same biochemical systems participate in the disposition of drugs and environmental agents, genetic traits identified by the unusual handling or response to any foreign chemical will probably affect additional compounds of both types. Pharmacogenetics and studies on genetic traits affecting the toxicity of environmental pollutants and carcinogens thus have common methods and objectives.

VARIATIONS IN DRUG METABOLISM

SERUM CHOLINESTERASE VARIANTS AND SUCCINYLCHOLINE SENSITIVITY

Several genetic variants of serum cholinesterase have been detected that are less effective in hydrolyzing the muscle relaxant drug succinylcholine than the common form of the esterase most people have in their blood. Succinylcholine, a dicholine ester of succinic acid, is inactivated by cleavage of one of the ester groups. After succinylcholine is given, an appreciable portion of the drug is hydrolyzed as it circulates through the blood and distributes to the tissues. Part of the drug reaches the tissues and binds to the myoneural junction sites (Ch. 19). The enzyme is probably less important in destroying receptor-bound drug than while it is being distributed through the blood and tissues. Persons with deficient serum cholinesterase have exaggerated responses to standard doses of the drug because more drug escapes hydrolysis and reaches the tissues. They develop muscular paralysis, particularly the respiratory muscles, which may last for several hours. Artificial respiration must be given during this period until the drug effects disappear, but patients properly oxygenated and cared for should completely recover. Presumably many other esterases in the body could also act on succinylcholine and compensate for a deficiency of serum cholinesterase, but clinical experience shows this not to be so. Serum cholinesterase is the principal enzyme responsible for succinylcholine hydrolysis in humans.

After succinylcholine was introduced into general use in the 1950s, occasional patients had prolonged and exaggerated responses, and a deficiency (reduced amount) of serum cholinesterase was suspected. It was found, however, that the serum esterase from sensitive patients was not reduced in quantity but modified, probably in its structure, to give it different qualitative properties. The atypical cholinesterase from these patients had a lower affinity for choline ester substrates, and it was a less efficient catalyst by far than the usual esterase for succinylcholine hydrolysis. It was also less susceptible to dibucaine inhibition and various other inhibitors. A simple inhibition test with dibucaine was developed to measure cholinesterase activity (with and without the inhibitor) to classify the type of esterase present. The inhibition by dibucaine, or *dibucaine number*, for the usual cholinesterase is about 80%; atypical cholinesterase has a dibucaine number of about 20%, and heterozygous carriers with serum cholinesterase of mixed or intermediate quality have dibucaine numbers of about 60%. The dibucaine inhibition test is useful in family studies, since both homozygous atypical (AA) persons and heterozygous (UA) can be distinguished from homozygous usual (UU) persons by analyzing serum samples; drug administration is not necessary to determine each individual's genotype. Family pedigree studies established that the subjects with atypical cholinesterase inherited a rare gene (A) from both parents and that all people with atypical esterase would be sensitive to succinylcholine if they were ever given the drug. In the general Canadian population, and probably in the United States, about 3.8% are heterozygous carriers of the atypical gene and 1:2820 are homozygous for the atypical gene (AA). Unless serum cholinesterase activity is greatly reduced, heterozygous carriers of the atypical gene (AU) are not unusually sensitive to succinylcholine. Clinically, then, sensitivity to succinylcholine is inherited as an autosomal, mendelian recessive trait.

Finding one genetic variant of an enzyme often leads to the discovery of others. Further variants of cholinesterase are known that also affect the response to succinylcholine. A fluoride resistant variant, detected by its greater resistance to fluoride inhibition than the usual cholinesterase, also has a lower affinity for choline ester substrates. Fluoride inhibition tests give "fluoride numbers" that can be used to distinguish whether persons have inherited a single or a double dose of the fluoride-resistant cholinesterase gene. Family studies in selected families carrying both the atypical (dibucaine resistant) and fluoride-resistant genes showed that these genes segregate as allelic genes at the same genetic locus, rather than as genes determined at different loci.

This evidence, and the fact that genes (A and F) produce active esterases with reduced affinities for substrates and inhibitors, suggest that they are both structural gene mutations in which the cholinesterases differ very slightly, perhaps only by single amino acids, from the amino acid sequence in the usual serum cholinesterase.

Another rare serum cholinesterase variant is determined by the "silent" gene. Persons homozygous for this gene have essentially no detectable cholinesterase activity, no signs or symptoms from this enzymatic deficiency, and no disturbance in their normal intermediary metabolic reactions. The only expression of the hereditary enzymatic defect is an exaggerated response to succinylcholine if these persons should receive the drug.

Additional rare variants of serum cholinesterase could be cited, but those given above illustrate some general pharmacogenetic principles worth noting again. The enzyme affecting succinylcholine hydrolysis does not participate in the metabolism of endogenous or dietary esters, and the enzymatic deficiency is apparent only when succinylcholine is given. The unusual drug reaction can be clearly associated with the altered quantity or quality of the specific enzyme protein. Susceptible patients can be detected and predicted by a simple blood test, and the same test can be used in families and sample populations to determine the frequency of the rare genes concerned with the drug reaction.

OTHER EXAMPLES OF HEREDITARY VARIATIONS IN DRUG METABOLISM

Isoniazid

Slow acetylators of isoniazid are more likely to accumulate the drug with repeated doses and to develop a peripheral neuritis (*see* Chap. 65). It is believed that isoniazid inhibits the enzyme that catalyzes the conversion of pyridoxine to pyridoxal phosphate, the coenzyme form of the vitamin. This complication can be prevented by giving extra pyridoxine, since the vitamin does not interfere with the antitubercular activity of isoniazid.

Phenytoin

Families are known with members who metabolize (*p*-hydroxylation) phenytoin much more slowly than expected. They are likely to develop symptoms of toxicity, nystagmus, ataxia, and drowsiness if given usual doses of the drug (*see* Chap. 29).

Acetophenetidin

Rarely, patients have been reported to develop hemolysis and methemoglobinemia after small doses of acetophenetidin. Such persons may have an inherited inability to metabolize the drug by the usual pathway (*O*-dealkylation and sulfate or glucuronide conjugation) and transform the drug through deacetylation and *p*-phenetidin to hydroxyphenetidin derivatives, which are toxic metabolites (*see* Chap. 31).

HEREDITARY METABOLIC DISORDERS OF PHARMACOGENETIC INTEREST

RED-CELL DEFICIENCIES

Some inherited traits not directly concerned with drug metabolism can change the cellular environment in such a way as to make cells vulnerable to adverse drug effects. A number of inherited enzymatic deficiencies of red blood cells, for example, will result in hemolysis if primaquine and certain other drugs are taken. Best known are the deficiencies of glucose-6-phosphate dehydrogenase (G6PD). At least 80 distinct variants of the enzyme have been identified, but not all of these are associated with drug-induced hemolysis. Generally, those variants with activity reduced to less than 30% of the normal are regularly associated with hemolytic reactions. It is not known exactly why a reduction in G6PD activity lead to hemolysis. G6PD is recognized as an important means of supplying NADPH, the cofactor for glutathione reductase, and glutathione appears to be essential for maintaining red-cell membrane functions. This explanation may not be entirely correct, but clearly the glutathione concentration falls in erythrocytes deficient in G6PD if they are incubated with acetylphenylhydrazine. This simple *in vitro* test has been used to identify persons who would be susceptible to drug-induced hemolysis.

Since the gene determining the characteristics of G6PD is carried on the X chromosome, G6PD deficiencies are inherited as sex-linked traits. Males are more likely to show drug-related hemolysis than are females. A survey of American blacks (Table 6-2) indicated that 15% of the males and 1.6% of the females were classified as "reactors" by the glutathione stability test. Although the test does not discriminate well between intermediate and normal responses, the figures establish the inheritance to be sex-linked, without dominance. Females are classified as reactors, intermediate or normal, depending on whether both, one, or neither of the X chromosomes carry the defective gene; males, having one X chromosome, are either reactors or normal.

TABLE 6-2. Glutathione Stability in Erythrocytes from American Blacks

	Genotype*	Expected Frequency†	Observed Frequency‡
Females (184 subjects)			
Normal	AA	0.742	0.935
Intermediate	Aa	0.239	0.049
Reactor	aa	0.019	0.016
Males (144 subjects)			
Normal	AY	0.864	0.833
Intermediate	—	0	0.021
Reactor	aY	0.136	0.146

* A = normal X chromosome; a = X chromosome with gene causing primaquine sensitivity.

† Calculated on the assumption of sex-linked inheritance without dominance, frequency of 0.136 for the reactor gene and frequency of 0.864 for the normal gene. (After Childs B et al: A genetic study of a defect in glutathione metabolism of the erythrocyte. Bull Johns Hopkins Hosp 102:21, 1958)

‡ The glutathione stability test does not discriminate well between normals and intermediates.

In addition to red-blood-cell enzymatic defects, abnormal forms of hemoglobin predispose the patient to hemolysis when sulfonamides and antimalarial drugs are given. Hemoglobin H and hemoglobin Zurich are hemoglobins of this type.

CONJUGATION DEFECTS

Several inherited defiencies in glucuronide conjugation are known characterized by hyperbilirubinemia and jaundice. Not only is the conjugation of bilirubin affected, but also the glucuronide formation may be reduced in such drugs and foreign chemicals as salicylates, menthol, and tetrahydrocortisone. Because these inherited disorders vary considerably in severity and in the specific molecular deficiency from family to family, the degree of drug conjugation impairment will also be variable.

VITAMIN RESPONSIVE CONDITIONS

Some persons have greatly increased above-average requirements for particular vitamins and may show symptoms of a vitamin deficiency unless the vitamin intake is increased manyfold over the usual daily requirement. Specific examples are known to defective conversion of vitamin B_{12} to cofactor forms of the vitamin. Some respond only to very high B_{12} administration. The therapeutic use of vitamins to treat hereditary disorders of this type illustrates the need to individualize therapy for each patient's particular genetic constitution.

INHERITED RESISTANCE TO COUMARIN ANTICOAGULANT DRUGS

It is unusual to find a true difference in responsiveness to drugs at the tissue level; most of the genetic differences in "response" can be explained by alterations in pharmacokinetics. The local dose-response relations rarely change. One exception is the hereditary resistance to coumarin anticoagulants. Such patients require nearly 20 times as much drug to produce the expected increase in prothrombin time, an amount that would cause a fatal hemorrhage in the usual patient (see Chap. 42). The first patient happened to be an identical twin, and his brother also required anticoagulant treatment and showed the same remarkable resistance to coumarin drugs. Their entire family, and one other large pedigree, has been tested for this genetic trait. Coumarin resistance is inherited as an autosomal-dominant trait. Resistant persons show another unusual feature: They are about 20 times more sensitive than usual to the antidotal effects of vitamin K. Since metabolism of the anticoagulant drugs is not unusual in these people, the most reasonable explanation for their resistance is a genetically altered tissue protein that regulates the synthesis of the blood clotting factors II, VII, IX, and X in the liver.

Surprisingly, there seems to be a natural animal model for this human pharmacogenetic condition. Warfarin is used as a rat poison, but natural resistance to this agent has been noted in rat populations after repeated use. Studies on some of the resistant rats have indicated that rare genes for resistance are selected out, and the rats have the same mechanism of resistance as found in human variants.

SOME MISCELLANEOUS HEREDITARY CONDITIONS THAT MODIFY DRUG EFFECTS

Drugs may produce undesirable effects in certain other patients with hereditary conditions or traits. A few are noted briefly in Table 6-3.

Malignant hyperthermia with muscular rigidity is a rare but serious complication associated with anesthesia. The condition is familial and appears to be inherited as an autosomal-dominant trait. Because hyperthermia may occur with or without muscle rigidity, probably more than one genetic disorder is represented. Patients are often young, healthy persons who unexpectedly develop these symptoms during surgery using halothane and succinylcholine. It can also occur with other anesthetic agents. Succinylcholine is not specifically associated with hyperthermia, but this combination is most frequently noted in the cases reported to date. About one half of the patients who develop hyperthermia and rigidity do not survive. Muscle biopsies from survivors respond abnormally to caffeine, and it has been suggested that the intracellular distribution of calcium is disturbed. The exact cause of this hereditary disorder is, however, still unknown.

I have intentionally closed with an example of a pharmacogenetic condition whose investigation is still in progress and unsolved because there are many such problems awaiting study and solution.

Aside from using specific examples of pharmacogenetic conditions above, I hope that those using drugs will appreciate that genetic differences must be considered in selecting the

TABLE 6-3. Some Hereditary Conditions That Modify Drug Effects

Conditions	Drugs	Pharmacologic Effects
Malignant hyperthermia	General anesthetics	Hyperthermia and rigidity
Angle closure glaucoma	Atropine	Intraocular pressure increased
Chronic, simple glaucoma	Dexamethasone	Intraocular pressure increased
Porphyria (hepatic)	Barbiturates	Porphyrin synthesis increased
Idiopathic hypertrophic subaortic stenosis	Digitalis	May not increase cardiac output
Mongolism	Atropine	Response increased
Familial dysautonomia	Norepinephrine	Increased pressor response

best drugs and the doses most appropriate for each patient. Further, when unexpected drug reactions do occur, an inherited drug anomaly ought to be considered, and at least a family history should be taken. Even in experimental pharmacology, genetics should be considered more, and unusual drug responses in animals should not be ignored. Studies over the years on hereditary metabolic diseases in humans have given us valuable insight into normal metabolism and the role of specific proteins. The same rewards can be expected if animal pharmacogenetic models are properly used.

FURTHER READING

1. Kalow W: Pharmacogenetics, Heredity and the Response to Drugs. Philadelphia, WB Saunders, 1962
2. La Du BN: Pharmacogenetics: Defective enzymes in relation to reactions to drugs. Annu Rev Med 23:453, 1972
3. La Du BN, Kalow W (eds): Pharmacogenetics. Ann NY Acad Sci 151:691, 1968
4. Stanbury JB, Wyngaarden JB, Fredrickson DS: Metabolic Basis of Inherited Disease. New York, McGraw-Hill, 1972
5. Vesell ES: Advances in Pharmacogenetics. In Steinberg AG, Bearn AG (eds): Progr Med Genet IX:291, 1973
6. Vogel E, Motulsky AG: Human Genetics, Problems and Approaches. Berlin, Springer-Verlag, 1979

CHAPTER 6 QUESTIONS

(See P. 7 for Full Instructions)

Select The One Best Answer

1. Pharmacogenetic mechanisms have been proposed to explain both the lack of sensitivity to, and the abnormal prolongation of, the response to
   - *A.* barbiturates.
   - *B.* phenytoin.
   - *C.* succinylcholine.
   - *D.* primaquine.
   - *E.* isoniazid.
2. An agent effective in the treatment of tuberculosis, whose rate of metabolism may be altered in patients with a specific pharmacogenetic abnormality, is
   - *A.* rifampin.
   - *B.* isoniazid.
   - *C.* nitrofurantoin.
   - *D.* ethambutol.
   - *E.* neomycin.
3. A patient with acute intermittent porphyria who needs treatment for anxiety might be prescribed
   - *A.* phenobarbital.
   - *B.* diazepam.
   - *C.* methaqualone.
   - *D.* chlorpromazine.
   - *E.* lithium carbonate.
4. Each of the following represents a drug and an idiosyncrasy established as a pharmacogenetic defect EXCEPT
   - *A.* succinylcholine–prolonged apnea.
   - *B.* sodium salicylate–tinnitus.
   - *C.* primaquine–hemolysis.
   - *D.* vitamin D-resistant rickets.
   - *E.* pentobarbital–porphyria.

A = 1,2,3; B = 1,3; C = 2,4; D = 4; E = All

5. Genetic abnormalities have been implicated in unusual responses to
   - *1.* primaquine.
   - *2.* phenytoin.
   - *3.* dicumarol.
   - *4.* phenobarbital.

BENJAMIN M. KAGAN

7 Pediatric Pharmacology

DIFFERENCES BETWEEN PEDIATRIC AND ADULT PHARMACOLOGY

An important difference between pediatric and adult patients is size. In addition, the growth and development of the infant and child are continually changing. In contrast, in the normal adult a relative plateau of maturation has been achieved, after which change proceeds in the opposite direction with aging and deterioration. The rate of change of different organ-systems varies throughout life. It follows, therefore, that the pharmacology of different drugs varies at different stages of life, particularly during the actively growing and developing period of infancy and childhood. In this chapter, pharmacology from the time of birth, whether low, normal, or above normal birth weight, premature, full term, or postmature, through adolescence (set arbitrarily through the 16th year of life) will be considered. A related and important subject, that of the effect of maternal drugs on the fetus, and consequently upon the infant, will also be discussed.

VEHICLES AND ROUTES

For older children who can swallow pills or capsules, vehicles are generally not a serious problem. For younger ones, however, the palatability of a suspension or a solution may make the difference between their receiving or not receiving the drug. An extreme example is the odor of the indanyl ester of carbenicillin in suspension that makes it impossible to administer. On the other hand, candylike chewable medications are hazardous because toddlers may eat them like candy. Jam, jelly, honey, applesauce, or sauce can be used to make some oral preparations more palatable.

Some drug forms—those in solution and suspension, for example—are less stable than others and have a shorter "shelf life." This is important to remember to avoid the use of preparations that may be ineffective or, worse yet, toxic—for example, prematurely degraded tetracycline antibiotics (*see* Chaps. 11 and 59).

For safety, the oral route is generally preferred because it tends to minimize "psychic" trauma and to preserve rapport for future visits to the physician's office or hospital. However, the tendency to vomit and the potential for aspiration when a child or infant is forced to take medication may create obvious problems. Aspiration of oily or chemically irritating substances may lead to a lipoid or chemical pneumonia.

When the oral route is not practical, the rectum can be used for some drugs. Other drugs, however, are not absorbed by this route, and diarrhea (sometimes even resulting from this procedure) can make this route impractical. Drugs can be suspended in 1 oz or 2 oz of water or in a starch solution and introduced rectally by way of a catheter or bulb syringe. The buttocks should be held or taped together to prevent loss.

When necessary, the i.v., i.m., intrathecal, or even intraventricular route is used. Each drug must be considered separately. One cannot assume that because any one of these routes is safe and effective, another will also be. For example, chloramphenicol can be given intravenously but not intramuscularly to attain predictable blood levels (*see* Chap. 59).

ABSORPTION

Because some intestinal transport mechanisms are underdeveloped in the neonate, some drugs, although eventually completely absorbed, are absorbed very slowly. Under such circumstances, these drugs must be administered less frequently in the pediatric patient than in the adult. Riboflavin is a good example of such a substance: In the older infant and adult, it is absorbed in as little as 3 to 4 hours, whereas in the newborn its absorption is only complete after 16 hours because it is absorbed almost exclusively by passive diffusion over a long segment of the intestinal tract.

Some orally administered antibacterial agents, such as triple sulfonamides, chloramphenicol, erythromycin, and the tetracyclines, are absorbed much more slowly in prematurely born than in full-term infants.

DISTRIBUTION AND METABOLISM

Distribution of a drug depends in part on whether it is water or fat soluble (Ch. 3). The process of growing older is a process of drying out. The egg has the highest percentage of water; as the fetus, the infant, and the child grow, the percentage of water decreases. The newborn for example, may be 70% water, and the premature baby as much as 80%. The extracellular water volume in the newborn is much greater than that in the adult. On the other hand, the fat content of the prematurely born may be only 1%, whereas the normal full-term infant has an average of 16% fat.

Drug distribution also depends on plasma protein binding (*see* Chap. 3). Thus phenytoin, when given to a mother about to deliver, is found in unbound form in twice the concentration in the cord blood of the infant as it is in the mother's blood. If hyperbilirubinemia develops, the unbound fraction may be three times that found in the mother.

Many drugs are metabolically transformed before excretion. The liver microsomal enzymes are primarily involved in these transformations. Generally, these systems function less well in the neonate than in older persons and reach a mature status at varying times after birth.

Giving several drugs at the same time may modify drug metabolism by affecting enzyme sites, as is the case with barbiturates that induce liver enzyme activity (*see* Chap. 8). Barbiturates have been shown to increase liver weight and also the size of the microsomal portion. Because of this effect, administration of phenobarbital to newborns significantly reduces blood bilirubin levels. This effect is of interest as an example of such activity but is not used clinically because it takes too long to achieve maximum effect and other methiods achieve reduction of serum bilirubin levels without the possible undesirable effects of the barbiturates in these infants.

During infancy and childhood, marked differences in other detoxification mechanisms are seen. An example is the relative inability of the neonate liver to inactivate or to conjugate drugs. The normal adult excretes 40% to 50% of an oral dose of salicylamide as the glucuronide. However, glucuronide excretion by full-term infants in the 5th day of life was found to vary 8% to 45%. Thus, there is considerable variation in response to drugs detoxified through this pathway—for example, sulfonamides (*see* Chap. 64) and chloramphenicol (*see* Chap. 59). On the other hand, some metabolic pathways, such as sulfation, appear to be as active in the neonate as in the adult.

EXCRETION

The ability of the liver and the kidney to excrete some drugs is incompletely developed in the full-term infant and even more so in the premature infant. Some antibacterial agents, for example, penicillin G, are excreted primarily by way of the kidney without previous metabolism. Renal function is, therefore, very important in determining dosage and the time-interval between doses. The kidneys are the most important route for excretion of most drugs. However, glomerular filtration rates and renal plasma flows in the newborn are only 30% to 40% of that in the adult. Excretion of hydrogen ion depends largely on tubular function, and the infant cannot excrete as much hydrogen ion as can an older child.

Ampicillin is excreted almost entirely by the kidney. The serum half-life of ampicillin is quite long during the first 2 weeks of life and declines over the next 2 to 3 weeks to a mature rate at about 1 month of age. The situation is similar for other penicillins such as carbenicillin, and for kanamycin, neomycin and streptomycin. However, no rule can be applied to all antibacterial agents, for example, the half-life of colistin is not prolonged in the neonate.

TOLERANCE AND TOXICITY

The pediatric patient is subject to the same drug idiosyncrasies or allergic reactions as is the adult (Ch. 11). These are usually drug dependent rather than dose dependent. The incidence may vary from that in the adult: With probenecid, for example, there are more reactions in children than in adults. With other drugs, such as the penicillins, the reverse is true.

The process of development may be responsible for some untoward results. For example, tetracyclines cause change in tooth texture and brown discoloration of the teeth (*see* Chap. 59).

Some drugs have greater toxicity in newborns than in persons of other ages. When chloramphenicol was widely used, the mortality rate among newborns actually rose. The "gray syndrome" largely responsible for this increase in mortality rate (*see* Chap. 59) developed as a result of high blood levels of this drug. These in turn were a consequence of poor glucuronide conjugation, competition for the carrier by serum albumin or other compounds such as bilirubin, and relatively poor renal excretion.

Both infants and young children tend to have problems with drugs that disturb acid–base balance. Thus overdosage with salicylates leads rather easily to metabolic acidosis, which is rarely seen in adults even with the same blood levels of salicylate. Likewise, when diuretics are given, serious depletion of sodium or potassium is more likely to occur in children than in adults.

The central nervous system of a developing neonate is peculiarly susceptible to toxicity. For example, when given to a neonate, a dose of morphine equivalent (based on surface area) to that given to an adult may produce severe respiratory depression. Yet the same is not true of meperidine hydrochloride. It is not uncommon in children for doses of salicylate, antihistamines, amphetamines, aminophyllin, or atropine to produce delirium or convulsions, whereas equivalent amounts tend not to do so in adults. On the other hand, whereas premature infants may have a diminished tolerance to digitalis, full-term and older infants and children are more resistant to the therapeutic effects of digitalis and related glycosides than are adults.

Small infants develop methemoglobinemia when exposed to water that contains high concentrations of nitrates or when their skin comes in contact with aniline dyes from freshly stamped diapers or clothes or even from some compounds formerly used in laundries. Methemoglobinemia may also result from the use of bismuth subnitrate, some local anesthetic ointments or suppositories, sulfonamides, or phenacetin.

During any growth period, the use of cortisone or related compounds may result in slowing of growth or osseous development. Usually "catch-up growth" occurs when these drugs are withdrawn. Conversely, androgens, such as testosterone, stimulate the rate of growth but also the rate of closure of epiphyses so that ultimate height is reduced.

SELECTION

Drug selection in infants and children is based on similar basic principles as those for adults. The etiology of disease and clinical symptoms and signs, however, tend to be very different. Generally, delays in starting therapy can be more devastating than can similar delays with adults. Early clinical diagnosis with an awareness of etiologic possibilities and a good knowledge of pediatric pharmacologic principles becomes paramount for the best care of pediatric patients.

DOSAGE

Relating the dose given to infants and children to a percentage of that given to an adult has been found to be unreliable, at times ineffective, and sometimes dangerous. Too much of the metabolic effect and the difference in binding, absorption, and excretion depends on the state of growth and development of the particular organ-system involved. The development of the various systems does not correspond uniformly to differences in weight, surface area, age, or other simple variable. Generally, each drug must be considered on its own. Many "rules" have been promoted to relate adult dosage to pediatric use. These rules or methods have been known under the names of Gaubius, Brunton, Cowling, Dilling, Starkenstein, Young, Fried, Clark, Augsburger, Cullis, among others. None of these, however, has been shown to be scientifically sound. Clearly there is a relationship between surface area and many physiologic functions, such as heat production, extracellular body water, plasma volume, cardiac output, glomerular filtration rate, organ size, oxygen consumption and also nitrogen, caloric, water and electrolyte requirements. Thus body surface measurements relate fairly well to dosage, but they are still imperfect since they do not take into account important variations such as those related to gestational age, age itself, variations in drugs unrelated to variations in body surface, and individual variations between patients of the same surface area and differential development of different organ systems. In the absence of better guidelines, however, the surface area relationships may be used as a preliminary estimate of drug dosage (Table 7-1). For some drugs in pediatrics, such as morphine, pentobarbital, atropine and scopolamine, this must be considered as especially crude.

While body surface is the most reliable single guide to dosage, no method provides for individual variations in response or for the need of careful consideration of many factors in each individual patient as well as of each individual drug and route of administration. Since there is so much to be considered which can make for large differences in the safe and effective use of drugs in pediatrics, frequent reference to the "package insert" is recommended (*see* Chap. 10), especially when drugs are being used with which the physician is not very familiar.

Tables 7-2 and 7-3 list common and emergency drugs, respectively, used in pediatrics.

TABLE 7-1. Determination of Children's Doses from Adult Doses on the Basis of Body Surface Area

	Weight *kg*	Weight *lb*	Surface Area* m^2	Fraction of Adult Dose†
	2.0	4.4	0.15	0.09
Birth	3.4	7.4	0.21	0.12
3 wk	4.0	8.8	0.25	0.14
3 mo	5.7	12.5	0.29	0.17
6 mo	7.4	16	0.36	0.21
9 mo	9.1	20	0.44	0.25
1 yr	10	22	0.46	0.27
1-½ yr	11	25	0.50	0.29
2 yr	12	27	0.54	0.31
3 yr	14	31	0.60	0.35
4 yr	16	36	0.68	0.39
5 yr	19	41	0.73	0.42
6 yr	21	47	0.82	0.47
7 yr	24	53	0.90	0.52
8 yr	27	59	0.97	0.56
9 yr	29	65	1.05	0.61
10 yr	32	71	1.12	0.65
11 yr	36	78	1.20	0.70
12 yr	39	86	1.26	0.74

* Approximate average for age.
† Based on adult surface area of 1.73 m^2.

MATERNAL DRUGS: EFFECTS ON FETUS AND CONSEQUENTLY ON THE INFANT

Few women go through pregnancy without taking some drugs. During embryogenesis, that is, especially during the first 3 months of pregnancy, the effects of drugs on the fetus can be significant and even devastating, causing disorganization of the developing process or even death of the fetus (*see* Chap. 11). Some severe malformations are clearly related to drugs taken by the mother in the first trimester. In the second trimester, or even the third, the result may be a malfunction of specific organ-systems. Toxic effects tend to be more acute and serious when the rate of growth and develop-

THOMAS YOUNG, 1773–1829. English physician, physicist, and Egyptologist. Has been called the founder of physiological optics, discovering accommodation, describing the cause of astigmatism, and developing a theory of color vision. He is also remembered for Young's modulus, for his contributions to the decipherment of the Rosetta stone, and for Young's Rule governing the amount of medicine to give a child.

ALFRED JOSEPH CLARK, 1885–1941. British physician and pharmacologist. Wrote on physiology as well as pharmacology, and the specifics of the mode of action of drugs. Was influential in showing the need for new legislation to control the marketing of patent medicines in Britain.

TABLE 7-2. Commonly Used Drugs in Pediatrics

Generic Name	Trade Name	Dose	Route*	How Supplied
Acetaminophen	Tempra, Tylenol, Liquiprin	10–15 mg/kg/dose q 4 hr	p.o., p.r.	Drops: 60 mg/0.6 ml Syrup: 120 mg/5 ml Chewable: 80 mg/tablet Suppository: 125, 300, and 600 mg
Aluminum hydroxide gel	Amphojel	15–30 ml q 4 hr	p.o. (gavage)	Suspension: 320 mg/5 ml
Aluminum hydroxide gel, magnesium hydroxide, and simethicone	Maalox	15–30 ml q 4 hr	p.o. (gavage)	Suspension: 2.5 mg/5 ml
Antibiotics		See Chapters 56–70		
Aspirin		10–15 mg/kg/dose q 4 hr		Drops: 60 mg/0.6 ml Syrup: 120 mg/5 ml Suppository: 120, 300, and 600 mg
Calcium gluconate		50–100 mg/kg/dose	i.v.	Ampule: 10 ml, 10%
Carbamazepine	Tegretol	10–20 mg/kg/24 hr in 3 divided doses	p.o.	Tablet: 200 mg
Chlorpromazine hydrochloride	Thorazine	0.5–1.0 mg/kg/dose	i.v.	Ampule: 1 or 2 ml; 25 mg/ml Vial: 10 ml; 25 mg/ml
Codeine		0.5–1.0 mg/kg	i.m., p.o.	Vial: 1 ml; 30 mg/ml Tablet: 15, 30, and 60 mg
Digoxin		See Chapter 33		
Dioctyl sodium sulfosuccinate	Colace	5 mg/kg/day	p.o. (gavage)	Capsule: 50 and 100 mg Liquid: 10 mg/ml Syrup: 20 mg/5 ml
Diphenhydramine hydrochloride	Benadryl	0.5–1.5 mg/kg/dose in 4 divided doses (maximum daily dose, 5 mg/kg)	p.o., i.v.	Capsule: 25 and 50 mg Ampule: 1 ml; 50 mg/ml Vial: 10 and 30 ml; 10 mg/ml
Emergency drugs		See Table 7-3		
Epinephrine, racemic	Vaponefrin	See Chapter 17		
Furosemide	Lasix	1 mg/kg/dose	i.v., i.m., p.o.	Tablet: 20 and 40 mg Ampule: 2 and 10 ml; 10 mg/ml
Hydralazine hydrochloride	Apresoline	0.2–0.5 mg/kg/dose q 4 hr	p.o., i.m., i.v.	Tablet: 10 and 50 mg Ampule: 1 ml; 20 mg/ml
Insulin		See Chapter 46		
Magnesia, milk of	Milk of Magnesia	15–30 ml q 1–2 h	p.o. (gavage)	
Mannitol		0.5–1.0 g/kg over 30 min q 4–6 hr	i.v.	Ampule: 50 ml, 25% (12.5 g/50 ml)
Meperidine hydrochloride	Demerol	1–2 mg/kg q 4 hr	i.m., p.o.	Ampule: 0.5, 1, 1.5, and 2 ml; 50, 75, and 100 mg/ml Syrup: 50 mg/5 ml Tablet: 50 and 100 mg
Methyldopa	Aldomet	10–50 mg/kg/day in 2 divided doses	i.v., p.o.	Vial: 5 ml; 250 mg/5 ml Tablet: 125, 250, and 500 mg
Morphine sulfate		0.1 mg/kg/dose q 4 h	i.m., i.v.	Ampule: 1 ml; 8, 10, and 15 mg/ml Vial: 20 ml; 15 mg/ml
Neomycin sulfate		100 mg/kg	p.o. (gavage)	Tablet: 500 mg
Pancuronium	Pavulon	0.1 mg/kg/dose	i.v.	Ampule: 2 and 5 ml; 2 mg/ml Vial: 10 ml; 1 mg/ml

(*continued*)

TABLE 7-2. *(Continued)*

Generic Name	Trade Name	Dose	Route*	How Supplied
Paraldehyde	Paral	0.3 ml/kg/dose	p.r.	Ampule: 5 ml
Phenobarbital	Luminal	Loading, 10 mg/kg Maintenance, 5 mg/kg/day in 2 divided doses	i.v. i.v., p.o.	Vial: 1 ml; 65 mg/ml Powder: dilute with 1 ml; 130 mg/ml Suspension: 20 mg/5 ml Tablet: 15, 30, 60, and 100 mg
Phenytoin	Dilantin	Loading, 10 mg/kg Maintenance, 5 mg/kg/day	i.v., p.o.	Suspension: 30 and 125 mg/5 ml Capsule: 30 and 100 mg Ampule: 2 and 5 ml; 50 mg/ml
Promethazine hydrochloride	Phenergan	0.5 mg/kg	i.m., i.v.	Ampule: 1 ml; 25 mg/ml
Propranolol hydrochloride	Inderal	0.5–2.0 mg/kg/day in 3 divided doses (slower than 1 mg/kg/min)	i.v., p.o.	Ampule: 1 ml; 1 mg/ml Tablet: 10, 40, and 80 mg
Sodium polystyrene sulfonate	Kayexalate	1 g/kg	p.o. (gavage), p.r.	Jar: 453.6 g
Spironolactone	Aldactone	3.3 mg/kg/day in 2 divided doses	p.o.	Tablet: 25 mg (must be made into suspension)
Succinylcholine chloride	Anectine	1.0–2.0 mg/kg/dose	i.v.	Vial: 10 ml; 20 mg/ml
Thiopental sodium	Pentothal	2–4 mg/kg/dose	i.v.	
Vasopressin	Pitressin	15–60 mU/hr	i.v.	20 units/ml
Vitamin K, phytonadione	Aquamephyton	1–5 mg	i.m., i.v.	Ampule: 1 and 2.5 ml; 10 mg/ml *or* 5 and 0.5 ml; 1 mg/ml

* p.o. = by mouth; p.r. = by rectum; i.m. = intramuscular; i.v. = intravenous.

ment is more rapid. Even during labor, drugs may change placental perfusion and thus affect transfer of other drugs to the fetus. Additionally, drugs during labor may lead to hypotension—and consequently poor perfusion of the placenta—to respiratory depression, to changes in the Apgar score of the newborn, and to alterations of the electroencephalogram or of neurologic signs. Sulfonamides are a good example; when one is given to the mother at a time close to delivery, it is transferred to the infant and thus potentiates the danger of hyperbilirubinemia and kernicterus. Sulfonamide competes with bilirubin for the limited glucuronide pathway for conjugation in the liver (*see* Chap. 63), after which it is readily excreted by the kidney. The sulfonamide also competes with bilirubin for albumin binding, resulting in more "free" bilirubin. Because of these factors, higher blood levels of free bilirubin develop, and the bilirubin enters and permanently damages brain tissue, resulting in kernicterus. This process is further aggravated by the fact that the normal newborn, especially the prematurely born infant, has less circulating albumin available for binding than do older infants or adults.

In addition to the sulfonamides, the following drugs have been found to displace bilirubin from protein binding: caffeine and sodium benzoate, salicylates, and probably also indomethacin, lanatoside C, menadiol, lobelin, ouabain, tolbutamide, polymyxin, sodium glucuronide, acetazolamide, epinephrine, penicillin, erythromycin, prednisolone, and the phenothiazines.

Other drugs increase the potential for kernicterus by increasing the rate of hemolysis of red cells. These include the sulfonamides, the nitrofurans, naphthyl and quinone derivatives, some antimalarials, perhaps some antibiotics, and large doses of vitamin K analogues. Because of the latter, the dosage of vitamin K in the newborn must be limited to a parenteral dose of 0.5 to 1.0 mg or an oral dose of 1 to 2 mg.

Nursing mothers may also pass drugs to their infants through their own breast milk in concentrations sufficient to have an effect on the suckling infant (*see* Table 81-26).

TABLE 7-3. Emergency Drugs in Pediatrics

Generic Name	Trade Name	Dose	Route*	How Supplied
Aminophylline		4–5 mg/kg/dose q 6 hr	i.v.	Ampule: 10 ml; 25 mg/ml
Atropine sulfate		0.01 mg/kg/dose	i.v., i.m.	Ampule: 1 ml; 1 mg/ml
Calcium chloride (10%)		0.25 ml/kg/dose (25 mg/kg/dose)	i.v.	Ampule: 10 ml; 10% calcium
Curare Tubocurarine chloride	Tubocurarine	0.5 mg/kg/dose	i.v.	Vial: 10 ml; 3 mg/ml
Dextrose (25%)		2 ml/kg (0.5 g/kg)	i.v.	Vial: 50 ml, 50% dextrose
Diazepam	Valium	For seizures, 0.3 mg/kg/dose	i.v.	Ampule: 2 ml; 5 mg/ml
Diazoxide	Hyperstat	5 mg/kg fast i.v. push	i.v.	Ampule: 20 ml; 15 mg/ml
Epinephrine hydrochloride (1:10,000 bolus)	Adrenalin	Bolus, 0.1 ml/kg/dose (10 μg/kg/dose)	i.v., i.c.	Ampule: 1 ml 1:1000 (1 mg)
Epinephrine hydrochloride infusion	Adrenalin	0.1–1.0 μg/kg/min	i.v.	Ampule: 1 ml 1:1000 (1 mg)
Isoproterenol hydrochloride	Isuprel	0.1–1,0 μg/kg/min	i.v.	Ampule: 1 and 5 ml; 1 mg/5 ml
Lidocaine	Xylocaine	1 mg/kg/dose	i.v.	Vial: 20 ml; 1%, 10 mg/ml
Methylprednisolone sodium succinate	Solu-Medrol	For shock, 30 mg/kg/dose	i.v.	Vial: 2 ml; 67.5 mg/ml
Naloxone hydrochloride	Narcan	0.01 mg/kg/dose	i.v.	Ampule: 1 ml; 0.4 mg/ml
Norepinephrine bitartrate	Levophed	0.1–1.0 μg/kg/min	i.v.	Ampule: 4 ml; 1 mg/ml
Phenobarbital sodium		10 mg/kg/loading dose	i.v.	Vial: 1 ml; 65 mg/ml
Salt-poor albumin (25%)	Albumisol	1 g/kg	i.v.	Vial: 50 ml; 25%, 1 g/4 ml
Sodium bicarbonate (0.9%)		1 mEq/kg; may repeat 3–5 times (or 0.3 × kg × base deficit)	i.v., i.c.	Vial: 50 ml; 1 mEq/ml

* i.v. = intravenous; i.m. = intramuscular; i.c. = intracardiac.

In summary, the infant and the child are by no means merely small editions of the adult. The choice of pharmacologic agents, their doses, and the routes of their administration must take into account the very important role of growth and development. Growth and development affect applied pharmacology through their influence on the manifestations and the etiology of various diseases, and also on the absorption, metabolism, excretion, and tolerance of drugs. Finally, drugs given to the mother may affect the fetus and newly born by means of the placenta and the infant through the breast milk.

FURTHER READING

1. Csay TZ: Cutting's Handbook on Pharmacology, 6th ed. New York, Appleton-Century-Croft, 1979
2. Gellis SS, Kagan BM: Current Pediatric Therapy, 10th ed. Philadelphia, WB Saunders, 1982
3. Kagan BM (ed): Antimicrobial Therapy, 3rd ed. Philadelphia, WB Saunders, 1980
4. Leach RH, Wood BSB: Drug dosage for children. Lancet 2:1350, 1967
5. Levin DL, Morriss FC, Moore GC (ed): A Practical Guide to Pediatric Intensive Care. Saint Louis, CV Mosby, 1979
6. Valman HB (ed): Paediatric Therapeutics. Saint Louis, CV Mosby, 1979
7. Wilson JT: Developmental pharmacology: A review of its application to clinical and basic science. Annu Rev Pharmacol 12:423–450, 1972
8. Yaffe SF (ed): Pediatric Pharmacology. New York, Grune & Stratton, 1980

CHAPTER 7 QUESTIONS

(See P. 7 for Full Instructions)

Select the One Best Answer

1. A pregnant woman has been receiving antihypertensive medication during the gestation period. On delivery the neonate has marked nasal congestion accompanied by mental depression. The offending drug most likely is
   A. hydrochlorthiazide.
   B. propanolol.
   C. reserpine.
   D. hydralazine.
   E. guanethidine.

A = 1, 2, 3; B = 1, 3; C = 2, 4; D = 4; E = All

2. With reference to the fetus *in utero* or the neonate, which of the following are true?
   1. Few drugs gain access because of the placental barrier.
   2. Hazard from teratogenic agents is greatest during the first 8 weeks of gestation.
   3. Permeability of the blood–brain barrier to gentamicin is the same as in the adult.
   4. Phenobarbital may lower the plasma bilirubin.

3. Kernicterus is more likely to occur in neonates given
   1. gentamicin.
   2. phenobarbital.
   3. sulfonamides.
   4. protamine sulfate.

JEREMY H. THOMPSON

8

Sites and Mechanisms of Drug Interactions

In most therapeutic situations, there is no major problem with drugs interacting with each other or with foods. As the number of "drugs" used together increases, however, the potential for interactions increases geometrically. A *drug interaction* occurs whenever the prophylactic, therapeutic, or diagnostic action of a drug is altered in or on the body by a second chemical administered previously, concurrently, or in close sequence. The second substance (interactant) may be another drug, an excipient, ethanol, a component of tobacco smoke, a food, or a dietary or environmental chemical or contaminant. The frequency of significant deleterious drug interactions is not known, and their importance has probably been exaggerated. Undoubtedly, a bewildering number have been described, but most have been poorly documented or studied. Additionally, the frequency of serious drug interactions is probably diminishing because of a greater awareness of potential problems.

Clinically significant drug interactions have been observed mainly with those drugs that have a *steep dose-response curve*, a *low therapeutic ratio*, a *dose-dependent rate of drug metabolism*, and a *measurable end-point of effect*, such as nonhormonal hypoglycemic agents, anticoagulants, hypotensives, cardiac glycosides, antiarrhythmics, and antiepileptic agents. Drug interactions will tend to have the greatest clinical significance if they take place at the rate-limiting step governing a drug's access to, or removal from, its receptor site. Significant effects, however, will be produced only if other sites or compartments (plasma protein, cell, or acceptor binding, or metabolism, and excretion) are unable to compensate for the rapid increase or decrease in free-drug levels. Prediction of a patient's response to multiple drug therapy is difficult because drugs may act at more than one site or by more than one mechanism. They do not necessarily occur in all patients given the same drug combination because many responses depend on other variables, that is, altered rates of drug metabolism (*e.g.*, isonicotinic acid hydrazide [INAH]-induced inhibition of phenytoin metabolism in slow acetylators, Chs. 6 and 65), drug response (monoamineoxidase inhibitors [MAOI] and foods, *see* below and Ch. 36), or disease-state (qualitative or quantitative differences in plasma proteins or renal or hepatic function, Ch. 5). Further, because of often subtle chemical differences, one cannot extrapolate with certainty from one drug combination to a second of chemically similar drugs, and species variation makes animal data unreliable for predicting human response. When evaluating potential drug interactions, one must remember that in cases of joint physician management, patients may be referred with a "drug legacy"; many physicians are unaware of the components of what they prescribe; patients with psychiatric illnesses may be so secretive with respect to antipsychotic or other drug ingestion that they deny the exposure; patients in a hospital environment may be brought surreptitiously "drugs of recreation" or other drugs by visitors; and substances such as tonics, antacids, laxatives, vitamins, over-the-counter preparations, oral contraceptives, tobacco, ethanol and dimethylsulfoxide (DMSO), occasionally responsible for initiating an important interaction, may be overlooked by the physician or patient.

When an interaction occurs, the action of either or both interactants may be increased, decreased, altered, or may show no change. Thus a patient may experience a therapeutic failure, an adverse drug reaction, or a potentiated therapeutic effect. Rarely does an interaction result in no obvious alteration in the expected response to individual agents.

DRUG INTERACTIONS: CLASSIFICATION AND CATEGORIES

A drug is usually administered to influence a specific target tissue. To do so, the agent must disintegrate and dissolve from its formulation, be absorbed and possibly metabolized, and be transported to its site of action. Subsequently, the drug may be metabolized further to more or less active products before its excretion. *Thus at numerous sites a second "drug" may act to alter the level of a primary drug (or its active metabolite) at receptor sites or to modify its pharmacologic action.*

Classically, sites of drug interactions are grouped as being pharmaceutic (Ch. 80), pharmacokinetic, and pharmacodynamic. *Pharmacokinetic interactions* are ones where the second drug may produce an alteration in the pharmacokinetics (Chs. 3, 4, and 5) of the primary agent, and *pharmacodynamic interactions* are ones where one drug may modify the action of a second agent at its receptor site. Clinically, however, overlap is considerable within these categories with more than one mechanism being involved, for example, the antacids (Table 38-2). Thus, such a classification is somewhat simplistic and artificial, serving primarily to emphasize and describe potential mechanisms of interactions.

It is impossible to memorize all known interactions. However, knowledge of potential mechanisms often enables the physician to minimize and to treat toxicity more adequately with minimum interference with therapy. Often unwanted drug interactions may be reduced by selecting an alternative agent; by altering the dose, time, or route of drug administration; or by retaining a stable drug and dietary regimen. Drug interactions *per se* may or may not be dangerous. Ignorance or failure to recognize that interactions may develop, however, can be dangerous. On occasion, beneficial interactions may be generated, for example, additive or potentiated responses with the use of two or more drugs in treating infections (Ch. 56), hypertension (Ch. 36), and malignant disease (Ch. 71). *In vitro* interference with, or direct *in vivo*, drug-induced alterations in clinical laboratory determinations are discussed elsewhere (Ch. 79).

Sites and mechanisms of drug interactions and some pertinent examples are given here. Numerous other interactions are described throughout the book and in Chapters 79 and 80.

PHARMACOKINETIC INTERACTIONS

DRUG INTERACTIONS DURING ABSORPTION

Drug interactions may develop after administration by any route, but those associated with oral administration are probably the most important. Certainly they have been subjected to more thorough study (Table 8-1).

Oral Administration

Interactions that produce reduced peak absorption of the primary drug (with the total quantity absorbed being relatively unchanged) must be distinguished from those that reduce the total quantity absorbed. Thus if a drug with a high first-pass metabolism (Chs. 3 and 4) or a short $T^1/_2$ (for example, procainamide) is absorbed at a reduced rate, therapeutic plasma levels may not develop. On the other hand, a diminution in the total quantity of drug absorbed (reduced bioavailability, Ch. 3) could be critical if the agent has a long $T^1/_2$, for example, anticoagulants, digitoxin, and phenytoin.

Hydrogen Ion Concentration. Alteration of the normal *p*H gastrointestinal gradients (*e.g.*,

TABLE 8-1. Potential Sites and Mechanisms of Drug Interactions

Classification	General Mechanisms	Examples
I. *Pharmaceutical interactions*	Chemical incompatibility	Acid-labile penicillins break down in acid solutions, that is, some D5W or normal saline solutions
		All penicillins break down in the presence of sugar at an alkaline *p*H
		Carbenicillin/gentamicin inactivate each other
	Physical incompatibility	Insulin binds to glass and Viaflex tubing
		Amphotericin B, sodium nitroprusside, and phenothiazines are light sensitive
II. *Pharmacokinetic interactions*		
Absorption, oral		
	1. *p*H: tablet disintegration/dissolution	Antacids reduce the disintegration and dissolution of digitalis and tetracycline preparations
	*p*H: drug stability/lability	Acid-labile penicillins variably destroyed in acid medium, but an acid *p*H facilitates iron absorption
	*p*H: degree of ionization	Absorption of weak acids (*e.g.,* aspirin) and weak bases (*e.g.,* H_1-blockers) altered by antacids or cimetidine
	*p*H: rate of gastric emptying	Atropine and propantheline delay gastric emptying
		Cimetidine and antacids may accelerate gastric emptying
	2. Rate of gastric emptying	*See* above. Opioids and tricyclic antidepressants delay gastric emptying. Metoclopramide and some laxatives accelerate gastric emptying
	3. Rate of intestinal motility	Metoclopramide and laxatives accelerate gastrointestinal motility
	4. Chelate formation	Tetracyclines and digoxin chelate to antacids. Tetracyclines chelate to zinc. Bishydroxycoumarin chelates with magnesium hydroxide, and the chelate may be more effectively absorbed
	5. Competition/interference with transport mechanisms	Levodopa absorption depends on quantity of dietary protein, and dietary purines and pyrimidines may depress the absorption of anti-cancer purines and pyrimidines
		Cimetidine inhibits intrinsic factor secretion
		Phenytoin and oral contraceptives depress mucosal conjugase, reducing the absorption of folic acid
	6. Toxic effects on intestinal mucosa	Neomycin, PAS, α-methyldopa, and phenolphthalein may produce a malabsorption syndrome

(*continued*)

TABLE 8-1. (*Continued*)

Classification	General Mechanisms	Examples
II. *Pharmacokinetic interactions* Absorption, oral (cont.)		
	7. Drug metabolism by intestinal microflora or mucosa	Broad-spectrum antibiotics potentiate coumarin-type anticoagulants by reducing vitamin-K-synthesizing bacteria Monoamineoxidase inhibitors may potentiate directly and indirectly acting sympathomimetic amines
	8. Miscellaneous	Castor oil sequesters fat-soluble vitamins
	9. Altered bioavailability	Reduced or increased bioavailability has been described for several drugs, especially digitalis, tetracyclines, chloramphenicol, and aspirin preparations
Absorption, parenteral		Reduced or increased bioavailability has been described for a few drugs, such as with benzodiazepines
Absorption, topical		Soaps may interfere with topical polymyxin B
Distribution	1. Plasma protein binding	Aspirin may displace sulfonylureas, coumarin anticoagulants, or indomethacin
	2. Blood flow	Sympathomimetic amines retard the absorption of local anesthetics. *Use of cocaine plus sympathomimetic amines systemically may result in significant sympathomimetic effects.*
	3. Transport across membranes	Tricyclic antidepressants block neuronal uptake of guanethidine, bethanidine, and debrisoquine into the nerve terminal. They also potentiate epinephrine and norepinephrine by blocking their reuptake into nerve terminals
Metabolism	1. Microsomal enzymes: induction	Common important inducers are phenobarbital, chronic ethanol ingestion, tobacco smoking, DDT, and rifampin. *See* also Table 8-5.
	Inhibition	Common important inhibitors are acute ethanol ingestion, oral contraceptives, and MAOI. *See* also Table 8-6.
	2. Nonmicrosomal metabolism	Allopurinol retards the metabolism of 6-mercaptopurine; PAS retards the metabolism of INAH
Excretion	1. Biliary excretion and the enterohepatic circulation	Broad-spectrum antibiotics potentiate methotrexate toxicity
	2. Renal: *p*H effects	*p*H effects on drug solubility, *e.g.*, crystallization of sulfonamides in acid urine (cranberry juice, vitamin C) *p*H effects on drug ionization, *e.g.*, loss of weak acids in alkaline urine, or reabsorption in acid urine. Opposite for weak bases

(*continued*)

TABLE 8-1. (*Continued*)

Classification	General Mechanisms	Examples
II. *Pharmacokinetic interactions* Excretion (cont.)		
	Renal: tubular mechanisms	Probenecid reduces tubular secretion of penicillins and cephalosporins (other than cephaloridine)
		Aspirin reduces tubular loss of methotrexate
III. *Pharmacodynamic interactions*	*Receptors*	
	1. Competitive/noncompetitive effects	Numerous examples in adrenergic, cholinergic, histaminergic fields, among others
	2. Physiologic antagonism	Epinephrine to reverse endogenous histamine effects in anaphylactic shock
	3. Physiologic synergism	Aspirin-induced bleeding with coumarin therapy or gastroduodenal ulceration with cortisone therapy
		H_1-blockers potentiate other CNS depressants (*e.g.*, ethanol, diazepam, chlordiazepoxide)
		Tricyclic antidepressants potentiate atropine (xerostomia, glaucoma, urinary retention, among others)
	4. Antibiotic interactions	Tetracyclines may reduce the effectiveness of penicillins
		Clindamycin may reduce the effectiveness of erythromycin
		Carbenicillin may reduce the effectiveness of gentamicin, and *vice versa*
		Penicillin and streptomycin may exhibit synergism
	5. Fluid and electrolyte interactions	Digitalis toxicity augmented by hypokalemia
IV. *Laboratory test interactions*		
In vitro interference	Various	*See* Chap. 79
In vivo drug toxicity	Various	*See* Chap. 79

with H_2-receptor antagonists, antacids, or anticholinergic agents) may significantly modify drug ionization, solubility (tablet disintegration/dissolution), or stability or the rate of gastric emptying (Ch. 3). Thus lowering or raising the intraluminal *p*H profoundly influences the rate and extent of absorption of weak electrolytes (Chs. 3 and 4); for example, peak absorption of nalidixic acid, salicylates, oral anticoagulants, nitrofurantoin, probenecid, and phenylbutazone (all weakly acidic drugs) is depressed with elevation of *p*H, and peak absorption of amphetamines, quinine, and ephedrine (all basic drugs) is depressed with lowering of *p*H.

Disintegration and dissolution of most oral formulations (other than enteric-coated drugs) depends on an acid milieu. Elevation of the gastric *p*H may thus reduce the release of certain active agents (*e.g.*, tetracycline hydrochloride and digoxin) from their complex formulations. The stability of many drugs depends on *p*H; for example, the acid-labile penicillins are variably destroyed in an acid environment

(Ch. 59), whereas an acid medium is optimal for iron absorption (Ch. 41). Alterations in the gastric hydrogen ion concentration influence the rate of gastric emptying (*see* below).

Rate of Gastric Emptying/Intestinal Motility. Drugs that alter the rate of gastric emptying or bowel motility (Table 8-2) may produce significant drug interactions by altering the rate of tablet disintegration/dissolution and by altering contact time with absorptive surfaces. Atropine and other anticholinergic drugs, or fatty drugs (*e.g.*, castor oil), delay gastric emptying, increasing or decreasing absorption of the second drug, depending on whether it is predominantly absorbed in the stomach or small intestine, respectively. Parasympathomimetic agents will have the opposite effect, as has been shown for ethanol, acetaminophen, diazepam, propranolol, and lithium. Levodopa (Ch. 30) is an interesting example; if it is retained in the stomach, mucosal metabolism reduces the amount available for small bowel absorption.

Increased peristalsis produced by laxatives and other drugs may reduce the time for tablet dissolution or absorption from enteric-coated or "slow release" tablets (Ch. 78).

Chelate Formation. Various components of foods, drugs, or their excipients may actively chelate or adsorb drugs intraluminally, reducing their absorption; for example, tetracycline antibiotics chelate to heavy metals (Ch. 61) and charcoal or cholestyramine chelate acidic drugs (warfarin, thyroxine, digitoxin, and digoxin). Additionally, kaolin and aluminum antacids depress the absorption of digitalis preparations and bentonite an excipient in some early formulations of para-aminosalicylic acid (PAS) bound rifampin (Ch. 65). Rarely does the chelate appear more readily absorbed than when the agents are given apart, for example, magnesium hydroxide may augment the absorption of coumarins, and caffeine may augment the bioavailability of ergotamine.

TABLE 8-2. Some Therapeutic Agents That Might Alter the Rate of Gastric Emptying or Affect Intestinal Motility

Antacids	Laxatives
Anticholinesterases	Metoclopramide
Antihypertensives	Narcotic analgesics
Antiparkinsonian drugs	Nitrites
Atropine and anticholinergics	Phenothiazines
Caffeine	Prostaglandins
H_1- and H_2-blockers	Sympathomimetic amines
Iproniazid	Tricyclic antidepressants

Transport Mechanisms. Alteration of gastrointestinal active and passive transport mechanisms (Ch. 3) may strongly influence drug absorption; *p*H effects on passive diffusion have been discussed above. Drugs related to normal dietary ingredients such as sugars, aminoacids, purines, and pyrimidines may have their absorption reduced by direct competition. Primary phenolic amino acids, for example, compete for the same transport mechanism as that absorbing α-methyldopa, and naturally occurring purines and pyrimidines may interfere with the absorption of purine and pyrimidine antimetabolites (Ch. 71). Additionally, barbiturates, phenytoin, nitrofurantoin, glutethimide, and oral contraceptives prevent ileal mucosal folate conjugase from splitting off monoglutamate from polyglutamates (Ch. 73), and tyramine in food may not be completely destroyed on absorption in patients taking monoamine oxidase inhibitors, possibly producing a hypertensive crisis (*see* below and Ch. 36). Levodopa absorption is reduced if the diet contains greater than 2.0 g/kg of protein, and possibly increased with dietary protein levels of less than 0.5 g/kg.

Physiochemical Interactions. Osmotically active agents (*e.g.*, saline cathartics; *see* Ch. 38) may alter absorption of other drugs. Salts may be formed that are more or less stable, soluble, or absorbable than the original agents. Fat-soluble agents (*e.g.*, vitamins A, D, E, and K) may be sequestered in fatty drugs, such as castor oil or mineral oil. Surface-active agents (*e.g.*, dioctyl sodium sulfosuccinate) may increase the absorption of poorly absorbed drugs by lowering surface tension or by facilitating intralumenal mixing and drug/mucosa contact.

Toxic Effects on Intestinal Mucosa. Neomycin, PAS, α-methyldopa, phenolphthalein, colchicine, mefenamic acid, and phenformin may produce varying degrees of villus atrophy, leading to malabsorption of both dietary constituents and drugs. A few drugs, however, (fusidic acid, propranolol, and trimethoprim) may be more rapidly and completely absorbed in states of malabsorption. Additionally, excessively rapid drug absorption may be seen if the intestinal villi have been partially destroyed by toxic agents such as tannic acid.

Drug Metabolism by Intestinal Microflora or Mucosa. Modification or elimination of the host microflora can substantially alter the susceptibility of patients to some drugs. For example, broad-spectrum antibiotics, by destroying vitamin K-synthesizing flora, may potentiate oral anticoagulants (Ch. 73). Similarly, methotrexate, which undergoes an enterohepatic circulation, is markedly more toxic if the microflora is depressed, since it normally is biotransformed by intestinal organisms to a nontoxic metabolite (Ch. 71). Drug effects on ileal folate conjugase and the potential consequences of monoamine oxidase inhibition are discussed above.

Disruption of Lipid Micelles. Drugs that alter the formation of lipid micelles may interfere with the absorption of fat-soluble drugs and fatty substances. Neomycin (Ch. 60), for example, reduces the absorption of vitamin A and cholesterol independent of any evidence of villus atrophy (*see* above).

Parenteral Administration

Little definitive information exists on potential drug interactions following routes of administration other than oral. Two examples, however, can be cited: Epinephrine retards the absorption of local anesthetics (Ch. 20), and subcutaneous (s.c.) hyaluronidase injected with a primary drug may increase the rate of its absorption. Pharmaceutical interactions developing on i.v. administration are discussed in Ch. 80. Little is known about the effects of formulation factors, excipients, or blood flow on drug absorption after i.m. or s.c. administration.

Topical and Intradermal Administration

Drugs administered systemically and topically may interact. Systemic glucocorticosteroids and H_1-blockers, for example, may modify the response to intradermal skin test antigens, and topically administered cholinesterase inhibitors in the eye (*e.g.*, echothiopate) may be absorbed sufficiently to potentiate systemically administered muscle relaxants. Some drugs applied topically interact with one another; for example, soaps can depress the antibacterial properties of polymyxin B (Ch. 62).

DRUG INTERACTIONS ALTERING DISTRIBUTION

Important interactions may alter drug distribution and the concentration of free (unbound) drug at receptor sites by affecting drug plasma binding, blood flow to organs of biotransformation, or drug transport across membranes.

Plasma Protein Binding

Proteins, and other components of blood including cellular elements, carry various endogenous substances (*e.g.*, hormones) as well as drugs and their metabolites. Binding depends on the number of binding sites available, the affinity of the drug for loci (of which there are several types; Chs. 3, 5), and the drug concentration. Bound drug is considered "inactive" pharmacologically but is in reversible equilibrium with the free (unbound) active fraction (Chs. 3, 5). Binding to plasma albumin has been studied most frequently.

One drug may displace another if the affinity of the displacing agent for the attachment sites is greater than that of the bound drug. When a drug is displaced, the increase in its free fraction may be associated with an immediate increase in activity and, paradoxically, with a temporarily accelerated half-life, since the displaced drug is susceptible to redistribution (governed by its physiochemical properties), metabolism, and excretion. Usually within 1 hour a new equilibrium (steady-state) between the bound and free fractions of the displaced drug develops with restabilization of response. If drug dosage is not altered after displacement, the new steady-state is characterized by a lower total blood drug level but the same unbound drug level and intensity of action before displacement. Obviously, all other factors being equal, a 2% displacement of a drug bound 98% is of far greater importance than a similar displacement of a drug bound 20%. In practice, the pharmacokinetic time-course of displacement interactions is highly complex. The development and extent of any interaction are influenced by many variables, including, for the displacing agent, its rate of administration or absorption, its volume of distribution, and its rate of metabolism and excretion. In general, where clinically significant "displacement" interactions have been proved to occur, an additional mechanism, such as altered metabolism, has been identified; for example, phenylbutazone displaces protein-bound warfarin and inhibits the rate of metabolism of the S isomer while stimulating the rate of metabolism of the R isomer (Ch. 42). The S isomer is about five times more potent an anticoagulant than is the R isomer, and numerous deaths caused by hemorrhage were reported before recognition of this interaction. Similarly, sulfaphenazole, in addition to displacing tolbutamide from binding sites, reduces the rate of its metabolism, and various acidic drugs may displace methotrexate, dramatically increasing its toxicity.

Usually highly acidic drugs bind to plasma proteins (Table 8-3). Unfortunately, however, many studies of pure displacing interactions were conducted before the complexity of the problem was recognized. Thus, how many of these agents produce clinically significant displacement is uncertain. Acidic drugs with the particular properties of high protein binding, a long $T^1/_2$, a small V_d, and dependence on hepatic metabolism or renal excretion should be highly suspect as potential displacers (Chs. 3, 4, 5). Withdrawal of the displacing agent theoretically should result in a reduced response to the displaced drug because of its increased binding. This is not commonly observed, however, presumably because of the gradual elimination and redistribution of the displacing and displaced drugs, respectively. Hypoalbuminemia and renal failure (with its variable alteration in drug binding to plasma proteins; Ch. 5) compound the evaluation of displacement interactions. Displacement interactions have not been described for basic drugs presumably [1] because they bind to different loci than do acidic drugs and [2] because of their large volume of distribution the plasma concentration is only a very small fraction of the drug concentration within the body.

Blood Flow

Epinephrine/local anesthetic interactions have been mentioned above. Since most nonpolar drugs are metabolized in the liver, concomitantly administered drugs that influence hepatic blood flow, or liver disease, may alter the response of agents such as propranolol, INAH, or lidocaine that are measurably cleared by "first-pass" effect (Chs. 3, 4, 5).

TABLE 8-3. Some Drugs That Displace Other Drugs from Plasma Protein-Binding Sites

Acetaminophen	Mefenamic acid
p-Aminobenzoic acid (PABA)	Methotrexate
Barbiturates	Nalidixic acid
Chloral hydrate*	Oxyphenbutazone
Chlorpropamide	Penicillins
Clofibrate	Probenecid
Cyclosphosphamide	Salicylates
Diazoxide	Sulfinpyrazone
Phenytoin	Sulfonamides
Ethacrynic acid	Thiazide diuretics
Ethyl biscoumacetate	Tolbutamide
Flufenamic acid	Tranquilizers
Furosemide	Triiodothyronine
Halofenate	Valproic acid
Indomethacin	Warfarin

* A metabolite, trichloracetic acid, is probably the displacing agent.

Transport Across Membranes

Most drugs have to cross various membrane barriers to reach their receptor (Chs. 3, 5); other drugs may alter such passage. The antihypertensive agents guanethidine, bethanidine, and debrisoquine, for example, are taken into the adrenergic nerve terminal by the norepinephrine pump (Ch. 36). Tricyclic antidepressants, phenothiazines, sympathomimetic amines, and some antihistamines, by blocking the norepinephrine pump, can reverse the action of the antihypertensive agent.

DRUG INTERACTIONS ASSOCIATED WITH METABOLISM

The intensity and the duration of the pharmacologic effect of many drugs depend on their rate of metabolism by specific enzyme systems or by "microsomal" enzymes, particularly those of the liver, kidney, and gastrointestinal mucosa (Ch. 4). Both specific enzyme systems and microsomal enzymes may be influenced by various drugs. Drug interactions in this general area are probably the *most common* and the *most important* in clinical practice.

Microsomal Enzymes

Through direct or indirect actions on tissue microsomal enzymes, lipid-soluble drugs or drug metabolites may accelerate (enzyme induction) or reduce (enzyme inhibition) the rate of metabolism of themselves or other related or unrelated drugs or physiological compounds. There is no simple chemical relation between inducers and inhibitors and the drugs that are affected in either category. Further, some drugs may have a biphasic effect. Because the metabolite(s) may be relatively more or less pharmacologically active or toxic than the parent drug (Table 8-4), the end result and clinical response are often complex. Thus when two inducers, both of which produce sedation (*e.g.*, a barbiturate and an H_1-blocker), are given together clinically, it is impossible to predict the clinical outcome with regard to the net effect of potentiation of sedation versus induction. In general, the microsomal enzymes in induction and inhibition are those mediating dealkylation, aromatic hydroxylation, side-chain oxidation, deamination, sulfoxidation, azolink reduction, and glucuronidation (Ch. 4).

Depending on the drug and dose, enzyme induction or inhibition usually takes about 1 to 3 weeks to become apparent after the offending stimulus has been introduced. Similarly, it usually takes 1 to 3 weeks for the effects of in-

TABLE 8-4. Possible Effect of Drug-Metabolism Inducers and Inhibitors on Pharmacologic Activity

Metabolism Situation	Inducer	Inhibitor	Examples
Drug → more active metabolite	Response enhanced	Response diminished	Chloral hydrate Cyclophosphamide Phenacetin
Drug → inactive metabolite	Response diminished	Response enhanced	Barbiturates Phenytoin Tolbutamide Warfarin
Drug 1 → drug 2	Effects of drug 2 increased	Effects of drug 1 increased	Imipramine (desmethylimipramine) Phenylbutazone (oxyphenbutazone)

duction or inhibition to revert to normal after withdrawal of the stimulus. However, with agents such as the chlorinated insecticides, which are highly lipid soluble, profound effects may persist for months after cessation of exposure owing to slow release of the inducer from adipose tissue stores and slow rates of excretion. Similarly, the inducing effect of tobacco smoke may take several months to return to normal. Because of the slow development of enzyme induction under certain circumstances, the phenomenon may be very difficult to detect. Enzyme induction may have a greater effect on drugs exhibiting a high "first-pass" metabolism (Ch. 3).

Microsomal Enzyme Induction

An increase in the quantity of drug-metabolizing enzymes usually arises through augmented synthesis of microsomal protein; reduced catabolism of enzyme protein may rarely be involved. In the liver, enzyme induction is associated with an increase in liver weight, an increase in production of cytochrome P_{450}, and changes in the smooth membrane of the endoplasmic reticulum; enzyme induction is prevented by inhibitors of RNA synthesis, such as actinomycin-D (Chs. 4, 71).

Several hundred drugs are known to produce enzyme induction in laboratory animals, but only a few have been proved to do so in humans (Table 8-5). Generally, a compound is likely to cause enzyme induction if it is lipid soluble at physiologic *p*H, not rapidly metabolized and moderately bound to plasma proteins. Phenobarbital appears to be a universal inducer because it increases the metabolism of more than 60 different agents, including itself, phenytoin, griseofulvin, digitalis, cortisol, and oral anticoagulants. Enzyme-inducing agents frequently act to displace drugs from plasma-binding sites. Other important inducing

TABLE 8-5. Some Drug-Metabolizing Enzyme Inducers

Alcohol (ethanol)	Chlorcyclizine	Hexachlorocyclohexane	Phenaglycodol
Aldrin	Chlorobutanol	Hexobarbital*	Phenobarbital*
Aminopyrine*	Chlordane	Imipramine*	Phenylbutazone*
Amobarbital*	Chlordiazepoxide	Insecticides, halogenated	Phenytoin*
Androstenedione	Chlorinated hydrocarbons	Lindane	Prednisolone
Antihistamines	Chlorinated insecticides	Meprobamate*	Prednisone*
Barbiturates*	Chlorpromazine*	Methoxyflurane*	Probenecid*
Bemegride	Cortisone	Methylphenylethylhydantoin	Promazine
Benzene*	Cotinine	Methyprylon	Pyridione
3,4-Benzpyrene (charcoal broiled meats, cigarette smoke)*	o,p-DDD	Nicotine (tobacco smoking)	Secobarbital*
	Dieldrin	Nikethamide	Stilbestrol*
Butabarbital	Diphenhydramine	Nitrous oxide	Testosterone and its derivatives
Carbromal	Ethchlorvynol	Norethynodrel	
Carbutamide	Glutethimide*	Orphenadrine*	Tolbutamide*
Carcinogens (polycyclic aromatic hydrocarbons)	Griseofulvin	Paramethadione	Trifluperidol
	Haloperidol	Pentobarbital*	Triflupromazine
Chloral betaine	Heptabarbital	Pesticides	Urethane
Chloral hydrate	Heptachlorepoxide	Phenacetin	

* These drugs stimulate their own metabolism either in test animals or in humans during chronic administration.

"agents" are chronic ethanol administration, tobacco smoking, and chlorinated hydrocarbons.

The interaction between phenobarbital and bishydroxycoumarin serves to illustrate the clinical importance of enzyme induction. If a patient's prothrombin time is well controlled on a daily dosage of bishydroxycoumarin, the introduction of phenobarbital (which increases the rate of metabolism of the anticoagulant) will be associated with the risk of thrombosis. On the other hand, if the patient is concomitantly taking phenobarbital while the dose of bishydroxycoumarin is being adjusted, fatal hemorrhage may develop 1 to 3 weeks after the phenobarbital has been withdrawn if the dose of bishydroxycoumarin is not adjusted downward. Other pertinent clinically important examples are rifampin-induced metabolism of methadone leading to withdrawal symptoms; induction of oral contraceptive metabolism resulting in pregnancy; tobacco smoking induction of theophylline and phenacetin metabolism; and accelerated metabolism of cortisone resulting in transplant rejection.

Stopping sedative or hypnotic therapy on leaving the hospital is frequently an important cause of morbidity. Because diazepam and chlordiazepoxide do not cause enzyme induction in humans, they are usually preferred to barbiturates as "sedatives" where induction may be a problem. Enzyme induction may be responsible for the development of tolerance to such drugs as barbiturates, glutethimide, and meprobamate because these drugs stimulate their own metabolism. The ability of drugs to increase the rate of metabolism of themselves or of other drugs often confuses the results of new drug studies.

The phenomenon of enzyme induction may also be used in the treatment of disease. Phenobarbital, phenytoin, o, p'DDD, and phenylbutazone enhance, for example, hepatic hydroxylase activity and are associated with an accelerated metabolism of cortisol to the inactive 6-β-hydroxycortisol. This therapeutic approach has been used in treating Cushing's syndrome in certain patients. Similarly, inducers have been used to treat neonatal hyperbilirubinemia and patients with familial unconjugated hyperbilirubinemia.

Enzyme induction is not rapid enough to be of value in treating overdosage with drugs such as phenobarbital. It may, however, alter the results of clinical laboratory test values (phenobarbital and phenytoin increase the metabolism of cortisol, estrogens, progesterones, and androgens) and be responsible for disease. (Griseofulvin, by inducing δ-amino levulinic acid synthetase, may precipitate acute intermittent porphyria.)

Microsomal Enzyme Inhibition

Drug metabolism by microsomal enzymes can be reduced by other drugs or drug metabolites (Table 8-6). No single mechanism has been identified, and competitive inhibition, interference with drug transport, and induction of functional impairment (direct toxicity or depletion of glycogen stores) have been identified. Generally, the net effects are opposite to those seen with enzyme induction (*see* above). Bishydroxycoumarin, phenyramidol, phenylbutazone and some sulfonamides, for example, inhibit the metabolism of tolbutamide to carboxymethyl- and hydroxymethyl-tolbutamide, thus potentiating the hypoglycemic effect of the sulfonylurea (Ch. 46). Phenylbutazone and the sulfonamides have an additional potentiating effect in that they displace tolbutamide from plasma protein-binding sites. Phenindione is a useful anticoagulant in diabetic persons because it does not alter drug metabolism. Enzyme inhibition may be stereospecific, as illustrated by metronidazole and phenylbutazone inhibiting the metabolism of S-warfarin but having little or no activity against the less potent R-isomer.

Enzyme inhibition is associated with drug cumulation, a prolonged action, and, if the parent drug is toxic, toxicity. On the other hand, therapeutic failure may result if the inhibited drug's metabolite is the active agent; for example, PAS, isoniazid, bishydroxycoumarin, disulfiram, methylphenidate, phenyramidol, and sulfonamides depress the hepatic metabolism of phenytoin. Thus if a patient is stabilized (with respect to control of seizure activity) on phenytoin therapy and if an inhibitor is introduced, anticonvulsant toxicity may develop rapidly (Ch. 29). On the other hand, if the patient is initially stabilized on phenytoin therapy and an inhibitor, seizures may redevelop if the inhibitor is withdrawn.

Enzyme inhibition can also be associated with altering the results of clinical laboratory tests. Glutethimide, for example, inhibits the biosynthesis of cortisol by depressing the 2-α-hydroxylation of cholesterol. Several examples of drug toxicity due to enzyme inhibition are given in Table 8-7.

DRUG INTERACTIONS DURING EXCRETION

Drugs are excreted by numerous routes (Ch. 3), but drug interactions that involve the urinary

TABLE 8-6. Some Drug-Metabolizing Enzyme Inhibitors

Acetohexamide	Clofibrate	Metronidazole	Procarbazine
Allopurinol	Coumarins	Mushrooms (*Coprinus atramentarius*)	Prochlorperazine
Anabolic steroids	Disulfiram	Nialamide	Quinacrine
Androgens	Estrogens	Nitrofurantoin	SKF-525A
Anticholinesterases	Furazolidone	Norethandrolone	Sulfonylureas
Bishydroxycoumarin	Insecticides	Oral contraceptives	Sulfaphenazole
Calcium carbimide	Iproniazid	Paraaminosalicylic acid	D-Thyroxine
Carbon disulfide	Isocarboxazid	Pargyline	Tolbutamide
Chloramphenicol	Isoniazid	Phenelzine	Tranylcypromine
Chlordiazepoxide	MAO inhibitors	Phenyramidol	Triparanol
Chlorpromazine	Methandrostenolone	Prednisolone	Warfarin
Chlorpropamide	Methylphenidate		

tract and bile are the only ones clinically important.

Biliary Excretion

Water-soluble drugs are excreted in the bile either unchanged or after conjugation, usually as glucuronides. Drugs or their metabolites may produce significant alterations in therapy by interfering with conjugation (for example, acetaminophen metabolites and BSP), or biliary excretion (for example, probenecid blocks rifampin excretion). Drug conjugates may be hydrolyzed in the intestinal lumen with subsequent reabsorption of the active agent. Foods and antibiotics, especially broad-spectrum antibiotics, by altering the intralumenal flora, may affect the hydrolyzation of conjugates.

Renal Excretion

Drug interactions may alter the urinary excretion of other drugs by increasing or decreasing glomerular filtration, tubular secretion, or active or passive tubular reabsorption. The most important mechanisms involved in these inter-

TABLE 8-7. Examples of Drug Toxicity Produced by Inhibition of Drug Metabolism

Drug Producing Toxicity	Enzyme-Inhibiting Drug	Toxicity
Azathioprine, or 6-mercaptopurine (6-MP)	Allopurinol	Bone marrow toxicity (Chap. 71)
Isoniazid	Paraaminosalicylic acid (PAS)	Peripheral neuropathy (Chap. 65)
Suxamethonium	Propranidid	Prolongation of muscle paralysis (Chap. 19)
Warfarin	Dextropropoxyphene, disulfiram, phenylbutazone	Bleeding (Chap. 42)
Ethanol	Disulfiram, metronidazole	Antabuse or antabuse-like reaction, respectively (Chap. 27)
Phenytoin	Dicoumarol, disulfiram, chloramphenicol, chlordiazepoxide, diazepam, phenylbutazone	Phenytoin intoxication (Chap. 29)
Tolbutamide	Dicoumarol, chloramphenicol, phenylbutazone	Hypoglycemia (Chap. 46)
Foods containing dopamine or tyramine (Table 8-8), or directly (epinephrine) or indirectly (amphetamine) acting sympathomimetic amines	Monoamine oxidase inhibitors (MAOI)	Hypertension, heart failure, cerebrovascular accidents (Chap. 36)

TABLE 8-8. Foods Containing Tyramine/Dopamine

Dairy Products	Alcoholic Beverages	Meats	Vegetables	Others
Yogurt	Beer and ale	Dried fish Herring Cod Caplin	Italian broad beans with pods (fava beans)	Chocolate
Aged cheeses Brie Camembert Cheddar Emmentaler Gouda Gruyere Mozzarella Parmesan Provolone Romano Roquefort Stilton	Wine Chianti Riesling Sauterne Sherry	Game		Soya sauce
		Liver		Vanilla
		Pickled herring		Yeast and yeast extracts

actions are changes in osmotic or pH gradients within the tubules or competition for tubular transport systems.

***p*H Effects.** The effects of pH are clinically important if the pK_a of the "affected" drug or active metabolite is in the range of 3.0 to 7.5 for weak organic acids and 7.5 to 10.0 for weak organic bases and if a significant proportion of the drug or active metabolite is normally excreted in the urine. (Strong acids and bases, by their almost complete ionization at physiologic pH, are unaffected by alterations of urinary pH.) Thus urinary alkalinizers (thiazide diuretics, acetazolamide, potassium citrate, sodium bicarbonate, citrate, or lactate) will favor the ionization of weak acidic drugs and augment their excretion but will favor nonionization of weak basic drugs and allow their reabsorption. Urinary acidifiers (ammonium chloride, vitamin C, cranberry juice) will have the opposite effect. Control of urinary pH is of some importance in treating overdosage with certain drugs, such as the barbiturates, aspirin, and amphetamines (Ch. 72).

The urinary solubility of many drugs depends on pH. For example, sulfonamides readily precipitate out in acid urine (Ch. 64), and some antibiotics (particularly the aminoglycosides and tetracyclines) may be more active in an acid urine.

Tubular Mechanisms. Many weak acidic drugs (and their weakly acidic metabolites), such as aspirin, sulfonamides, sulfonylureas, methotrexate, acetazolamide, thiazide diuretics, probenecid, phenylbutazone, diazoxide, dicoumarol, indomethacin, and the penicillins, are actively secreted by the same transport system in the proximal renal tubules. Drug interactions may therefore arise through competition for these sites of transport. Probenecid, for example, blocks the secretion of penicillins, all cephalosporins except cephaloridine (Ch. 59), and indomethacin, and the hypoglycemic effect of acetohexamide is enhanced by phenylbutazone, which inhibits the tubular secretion of hydroxyhexamide, an active metabolite. Additionally, the excretion of penicillin is reduced by phenylbutazone, indomethacin, aspirin, and sulphinpyrazone. Aspirin, by blocking the secretion of methotrexate, can rapidly produce serious toxicity (Ch. 71). Many of the aforementioned agents may also be involved in displacement interactions.

PHARMACODYNAMIC INTERACTIONS

DRUG INTERACTIONS AT RECEPTOR AND ACCEPTOR SITES

Drug interactions at the level of receptors are invariably complex. The following mechanisms can be identified and are illustrated with some pertinent examples: [1] alteration in the release of an endogenously stored compound (tyramine and amphetamine potentiate each other in the release of epinephrine); [2] alteration in the concentration of an endogenous compound at the receptor (desmethylimipramine and cocaine block the uptake of norepinephrine); [3] alteration in the sensitivity of a receptor for a drug (thyroxine increases the sensitivity of hepatic receptors to coumarins); [4] an additive effect on the same receptor (lithium and haloperidol, or lithium and α-methyldopa, may produce dementia and extrapyramidal symptoms); and [5] drugs can interact at the same receptors. The actions of particular agonists can be antagonized by specific antagonists. Thus one of the two agents may have a greater affinity for a receptor, as with atropine and curare reducing the access of acetylcholine (Ch. 14), naloxone competing with narcotic analgesics (Ch. 31), H_1-, and H_2-receptor antagonists blocking histamine (Ch. 51), and vitamin K antagonizing coumarin anticoagulants (Ch. 42). Many other examples occur among the drugs that act on the nervous system (Chs. 22–30). Such receptor interactions are governed by strict physiochemical laws (Ch. 2). Thus, for example, the use of neostigmine (a cholinesterase inhibitor) will reverse the action of curare (Ch. 15).

Drugs that have a similar mode of action or physiological response may interact. Thus CNS depression is frequently produced with the concomitant use of any two or more of the following: ethanol, barbiturates or other hypnotics, tranquilizers, opioids, H_1-blockers, and antiepileptic agents. Similarly, in the treatment of hypertension, hypotension may be produced with two or more of the following: antihypertensive agents, diuretics, ethanol, β-blockers, MAOI, general anesthetics, and CNS depressants (Ch. 36). Drug interactions at acceptor sites (other than plasma binding sites) are difficult to quantitate. However, quinacrine may displace the 8-aminoquinolines, thus potentiating their toxicity (Ch. 67).

ANTIBIOTIC INTERACTIONS

Several interactions that involve antimicrobial and antiinfective agents are discussed here because they are difficult to classify elsewhere and because they may involve an action on "receptors" in bacteria. Theoretically, a bacteriostatic agent should not be combined with a bactericidal drug (Ch. 56). However, a mixture of penicillin (bactericidal) and streptomycin (bacteriostatic), and numerous other pairs (methicillin/kanamycin, carbenicillin/gentamicin) exhibit a potentiated antibacterial effect under certain circumstances *in vivo*. Despite producing a potentiated effect *in vivo*, carbenicillin and gentamicin should not be mixed in the same syringe or infusion bottle or injected into the same muscle site because they chemically inactive each other. A similar problem may rarely be observed in tissue fluids in the presence of renal failure. An additive or a potentiated antimicrobial response is observed in the treatment of tuberculosis with two or more agents (Ch. 60), with cotrimoxazole) where the components act at sequential steps in folic acid synthesis (Ch. 64)), and in treatment of typhoid fever with ampicillin (bactericidal) plus chloramphenicol (bacteriostatic). Amphotericin B and miconazole are antagonistic (Ch. 69; *see* also Ch. 56).

DRUG INTERACTIONS WITH FLUID AND ELECTROLYTES

A few pertinent examples of such drug interactions are cited. Pyrazolone derivatives (Ch. 31), by causing fluid retention, may reduce the effectiveness of diuretics in the treatment of hypertension. Since lithium ions act by replacing sodium (Ch. 22), severe fluctuations in serum lithium levels are possible when the sodium content of the diet is altered drastically, or if sodium loss by the kidneys or intestine is augmented through the concomitant use of diuretics. Hypokalemia, induced by diet or drugs (diuretics, laxatives, carbenoxolone sodium, carbenicillin), will profoundly affect digitalis toxicity (Ch. 33), the effectiveness of certain antidysrrhythmic agents (lidocaine, quinidine, and phenytoin), and certain nondepolarizing muscle relaxants (Ch. 19). Significant hyperkalemia may be induced by excesses of diet, or by the ingestion of potassium supplements concomitantly with spironolactone and other "potassium-sparing" diuretics. Hyperkalemia may in turn potentiate skeletal muscle disorders and antidysrrhythmic drug myocardial toxicity (Ch. 34).

FURTHER READINGS

1. Corrigan L: Evaluations of Drug Interactions, 2nd ed. Washington DC, American Pharmaceutical Manufacturers Association, 1976
2. Hansten PD: Drug Interactions, 4th ed. Philadelphia, Lea & Febiger, 1979
3. Hurwitz A: Antacid therapy and drug kinetics. Clin Pharmacokinet 2:269–280, 1977
4. Martin EW: Hazards of Medication, 2nd ed. Philadelphia, JB Lippincott, 1978
5. Roe DA: Interactions between drugs and nutrients. Med Clin North Am 63:985–1007, 1979

CHAPTER 8 QUESTIONS

(See P. 7 for Full Instructions)

Select the One Best Answer

1. In which of the following pairs of drugs does the first agent decrease the therapeutic effectiveness of the second?
   A. Propranolol–guanethidine (Ismelin).
   B. Phenobarbital–prednisone.
   C. Probenecid–ampicillin.
   D. Allopurinol–6-mercaptopurine.
   E. Carbidopa (α-methyldopa-hydrazine)–levodopa.

2. In which one of the following pairs of drugs does pretreatment with the first drug *reduce* the pharmacologic effect of the second drug?
   A. paragyline–levodopa
   B. ethyl alcohol–chlorpropamide
   C. streptomycin–tubocurarine
   D. bis-hydroxycoumarin–phenytoin
   E. protamine–heparin

3. Antacids may retard the gastrointestinal absorption of a weak acid such as aspirin because
   A. they increase intragastric destruction of aspirin.
   B. they interfere with aspirin's ionization.
   C. they form an insoluble chelate with aspirin.
   D. they increase prostaglandin formation.
   E. they inhibit gastric pepsin activity.

A = 1,2,3; B = 1,3; C = 2,4; D = 4; E = All

4. Which of the following correctly describes the action of the first drug on the second drug by the mechanism cited?
   1. Phenobarbital will reduce the activity of warfarin by increasing its rate of metabolism.
   2. Pyridoxine (vitamin B_6) will increase the beneficial effect of *l*-dopa (levodopa) by decreasing its peripheral decarboxylation.
   3. Desipramine (desmethylimipramine) will reduce the antihypertensive action of guanethidine by inhibiting its uptake by sympathetic nerve endings.
   4. Probenecid will reduce the action of penicillin by increasing its rate of renal excretion.

5. Which of the following correctly associates a drug with a mechanism by which that drug is known to alter the effect of the second drug?
   1. phenobarbital—enzyme induction—dicoumarol.
   2. sulfonamides—displacement from binding site—tolbutamide.
   3. probenecid—inhibition of active transport—penicillin.
   4. hydrochlorothiazide—increased potassium excretion—digoxin.

6. Both coumarin anticoagulants and methotrexate
   1. undergo significant enterohepatic circulation.
   2. effects are increased by treatment with broad-spectrum antibiotics.
   3. actions are immediately reversed by protamine sulfate.
   4. actions are potentiated by aspirin.

7. Both aluminum hydroxide and magnesium hydroxide
   1. may significantly change urinary *p*H.
   2. may delay gastric emptying.
   3. may chelate drugs, reducing their absorption after oral administration.
   4. may cause laxation.

8. Both mineral oil and neomycin
   1. may cause a malabsorption syndrome with steatorrhea and structural alteration of intestinal villi.
   2. may adsorb vitamin A, reducing its gastrointestinal absorption.
   3. potentiate drug-induced ototoxicity after oral administration.
   4. use may be associated with diarrhea.

DONALD J. JENDEN

9 Biologic Variation and the Principles of Bioassay

The assay of drugs serves many purposes. Accurate estimation of potency is essential in the development and evaluation of new compounds for therapeutic purposes and in their isolation if derived from natural sources. Some compounds, such as insulin, vitamin B_{12}, and many antibiotics, must be assayed biologically for purposes of formulation and dispensing. The concentration of drugs and their metabolites in plasma, urine, and other biologic fluids is frequently measured as part of a research protocol and increasingly for purposes of therapeutic monitoring.

Most drugs are pure chemical compounds of known structure. Quantities suitable for therapeutic use may be dispensed by weighing or by chemical estimation. Many agents commonly used in therapeutics, particularly extracts of plants or animal tissues, are not pure, and the chemical structure of the active principle is not always known. In these cases the quantity must be determined by observing the biologic responses to the drug. The estimation of drug potency by the reactions of living organisms or their components is known as *bioassay*. The principles of bioassay are important not only because some of the most valuable drugs currently in use must be subjected to bioassay to determine the activity of each batch, but also because the same basic principles are applicable to all comparisons of drug effectiveness, including clinical trials of new drugs and their continuing practical evaluation.

Bioassay is frequently used for estimating drug concentrations and endogeneous compounds in biologic fluids. Its sensitivity frequently exceeds that of the most refined physicochemical methods, and in principle a bioassay method can be developed for any compound with a well-defined pharmacologic activity by using the biologic response as an endpoint in a suitably controlled experimental design.

Bioassays are sometimes very specific, but, more often, related compounds share a similar effect, and a single bioassay therefore cannot discriminate between them. This limitation can sometimes be overcome by using more than one bioassay, based on different types of pharmacologic response. This technique is

---

JOHN WILLIAM TREVAN, 1887–1956. English physician and pharmacologist. Pioneered the development of standards and assays for drugs.

called *parallel bioassay*. If the sample has the same activity relative to the standard reference compound in several different assays, this provides evidence that the activity in the sample is due to the same compound. The specificity of bioassays can also be enhanced by preliminary partial purification of the sample by chemical means, such as solvent extraction or chromatography.

Another disadvantage of bioassay is interference by other drugs or endogenous compounds in the sample, particularly in investigative work in which agents other than the one to be assayed must be in the sample because of the purpose of the experiment (*e.g.*, in studies of the effect of neurotransmitter analogues on evoked release of neurotransmitters).

Finally, the precision of bioassays is considerably less than that of physical or chemical assays. The error associated with physical or chemical assays is usually less than 1% to 5%, whereas bioassay error is generally 5% to 50%. Bioassay error is basically the result of biologic variation, and the principles of bioassay design are derived from the need to reduce the sources and effects of biologic variation.

During the past decade, a number of assay methods have been developed that can be regarded as hybrids of bioassay and chemical assay in that they use biologic components such as enzymes, receptors, or antibodies to confer specificity on the assay but depend on a physical measurement such as fluorescence or radioisotope counting for quantitation. These assays include radioimmunoassay, receptor binding assays, and enzymatic derivative methods, which frequently yield an excellent compromise between the conflicting demands of sensitivity, specificity, and simplicity.

NATURE AND SOURCES OF BIOLOGIC VARIATION

The net effect produced by a drug is the result of a number of interacting factors. In addition to the basic propensity of a compound to react with and alter a normal physiologic or biochemical function, the observed response depends on the rate at which the drug is absorbed and excreted; its ability to bind with, and hence to be removed by, nonspecific tissue acceptors; reversible binding to plasma proteins; its rate of metabolism in the organism as a whole and sometimes in the tissues that it affects; its distribution throughout the body; and the efficiency of normal compensatory and adaptive mechanisms of the organism. All these factors not only vary from animal to animal but also change in a single animal in response to alterations in the internal and external environment. Not surprisingly the quantity of drug needed to produce a given effect may vary widely in different experiments. The principal objective of bioassay design is to minimize this inherent variability.

DOSE-RESPONSE CURVES

A graphic picture of biologic variation may be obtained by plotting the percentage of a large group of animals that respond to a drug in a specific way against the dose of the drug (Fig. 9-1). A sigmoid curve is generally obtained that is roughly symmetrical if the dose axis is logarithmic. The steepest part is approximately in the middle of the curve. Because a given change in dose corresponds to the greatest change in response where the curve is steepest, the dose required to produce a given effect can be most accurately estimated at the 50% point. This dose is conventionally referred to as the ED_{50} (effective dose for 50%), or *median effect dose*. If the "effect" is a lethal response, the dose is called the LD_{50} or *medial lethal dose*. The ratio of the LD_{50} to the ED_{50} for a desired effect is a measure of the safety margin of a drug and is sometimes known as the *therapeutic index*. The term therapeutic index is sometimes used more generally to refer to the ratio of ED_{50} for a toxic and desired therapeutic effect. A symmetric curve such as that in Fig. 9-1 is usually not obtained unless the dose is plotted logarithmically on the abscissa. Partly because of the greater ease with which a symmetric curve can be analyzed, bioassay data are usually collected with logarithmically spaced doses.

A curve of similar shape is usually obtained if a continuous measure of mean drug response (*e.g.*, contraction of a smooth muscle strip or elevation in blood pressure) is plotted on the ordinate instead of the percentage that shows a specific threshold response. In this case, however, the ordinate frequently has no definable limit. For this reason and because the response measure is usually continuous rather than quantal, a different type of statistical analysis must be used. When two different drugs are being compared in this way, they often differ not only in their potency (the dose required to produce 50% of their maximum effect) but also in the maximum effect they can exert. Figure

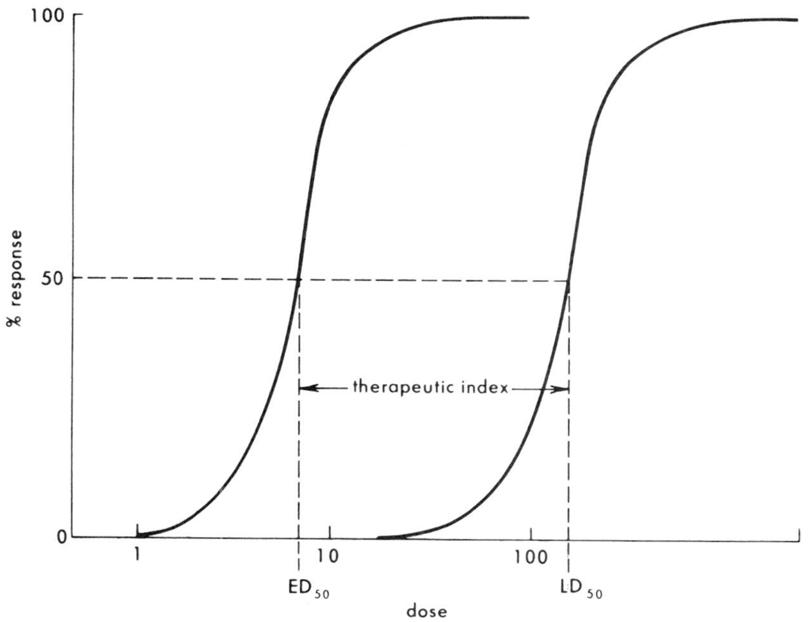

FIG. 9-1. Typical cumulative dose-response curve.

9-2 illustrates schematically an example of this in which the analgesic effects of morphine and codeine are compared. The curves for morphine and codeine differ in two respects: The entire morphine curve is located to the left of the codeine line, indicating that morphine is more potent than codeine regardless of the response level at which they are compared; and the codeine curve shows a ceiling, indicating that the drug cannot produce more than a certain degree of analgesia whatever the dose. In contrast, morphine produces an increasing analgesic effect over the entire practical dose range. The relative potency of these two drugs is not a fixed number but a function of the degree of analgesia (*i.e.*, response) at which they are compared. A nonparallel shift in the dose-response curve is also produced by a noncompetitive antagonist, in contrast to a competitive antagonist, which causes a shift to the right of an agonist's dose-response curve without changing the slope.

FIG. 9-2. Schematic representation of dose-response curves for analgesic action of morphine and codeine. Morphine is more potent in the sense that the required dose is lower and it can produce more profound analgesia than any dose of codeine.

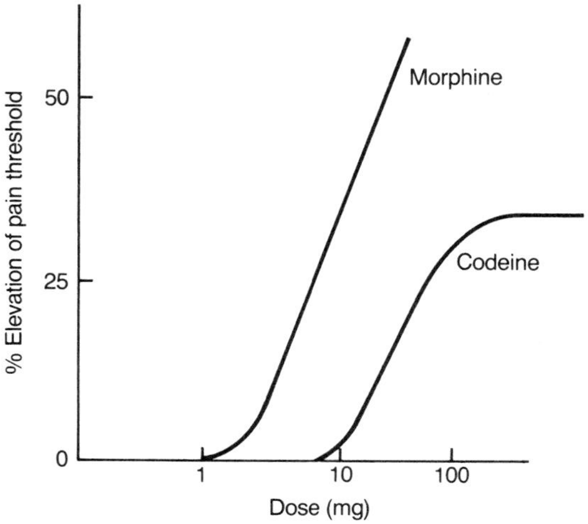

Because of the greater ease with which straight lines may be fitted to data both visually and statistically, an empirical or semiempirical transformation is usually applied to the response measurement so that a straight line relation is obtained. There are both theoretical and empirical reasons to believe that many quantal responses, like that represented in Fig. 9-1, follow a normal, or Gaussian, probability distribution. In this case the cumulative dose-response curve can be transformed into a straight line if the number of standard deviations above the mean is plotted as the ordinate instead of the percentage that corresponds to it. This basic procedure is used in probit analysis. Because of the exaggeration of random error at extreme values of the ordinate, an iterative weighted regression procedure must be used for statistical analysis of the results and not a simple linear regression.

DESIGN OF BIOASSAYS

THE REFERENCE STANDARD

At one time the biologic activity of some drugs was expressed directly in terms of a simple pharmacologic response. For example, the quantity of digitalis extract required to kill a frog was defined as a "frog unit." Because frogs differ greatly in their sensitivity, depending on season, species, and weight, among other factors, this kind of definition did not provide a basis for an accurate and reproducible assay. These units have been replaced by absolute reference standards, and therefore the role of the biologic test is to provide end-points (responses) to allow the standard and the unknown to be quantitatively compared. Reference standards for therapeutic agents that must be bioassayed are maintained in the United States by the Board of Trustees of the United States Pharmacopeial Convention and other agencies and are distributed to pharmaceutical manufacturers for standardization of their products. A specific quantity of the standard is defined as having one unit of activity, and pharmaceuticals that require biologic standardization must be labeled according to the number of units of activity per gram or milliliter. The use of reference standards in pharmaceutical standardization is analogous to the internationally accepted definitions of length and weight and has been the single most important factor in establishing confidence in, and reliability of, bioassay. In clinical drug evaluation or trial, inclusion of one or more established drugs is important to serve as a standard with which to compare a new agent.

MINIMIZATION OF BIOLOGIC VARIATION

To minimize the effects of biologic variation, the responses to standard and unknown samples should be observed in animals that are as similar as possible. Factors such as age, sex, genetic strain, weight and environment can exert a major influence on the sensitivity to drugs, and unless they are carefully controlled the precision of the assay will be reduced and the result biased. Individual animals should then be assigned to receive standard or unknown preparations on an objectively random basis, such as the throwing of dice or the use of a table of random numbers. Ideally a cross-over design should be used in which the assay is repeated with standard and unknown preparations administered to the opposite groups of subjects, so that standard and unknown are compared independently in each animal. When more than two drugs are being compared or more than one dose level of each is being tested, a more complicated balanced experimental design, such as a Latin square, should be used in which the same principle is observed. This is not always possible because observation of the response may involve sacrifice of the animal. Some of the most accurate bioassays are made on a single piece of isolated tissue, such as a strip of rat uterus or guinea pig ileum, thus eliminating most of the factors that contribute to variability of response between animals. Whatever the experimental format, both the selection of animals and the procedure itself must be rigorously controlled and precisely reproduced.

OBJECTIVE EVALUATION

Wherever possible, the biologic response should be measured objectively. When different drugs are being compared or a galenical product (*i.e.*, a mixture of potentially active components) is being assayed, a response should be selected that is as closely related as possible to the intended therapeutic effect. Sometimes, particularly in clinical trials, no relevant objective criterion of response is available, and assessment of efficacy depends primarily on subjective evaluation by the patient or the physician. In this case, subjective bias should be minimized by use of a double-blind system in which neither the patient nor the observing physician knows to which group the patient has been assigned. Unfortunately it is not always possible to keep a study double-blind because both the patient and the physician can sometimes easily recognize either the therapeutic or adverse effects of a drug and thus distinguish it from a placebo.

Bioassays may be classified in various ways depending on the quantal or continuous nature of the reponse, the empirical relation between dose and response, and the system used for assignment of subjects to different groups, among other considerations. The most important distinction is between assays using a single predetermined end-point (direct assays) and those that establish a dose-response relation (indirect assays).

DIRECT ASSAY

The classic head-drop assay for *d*-tubocurarine is an example of a direct assay. The end-point response is head drop in rabbits, which results from neuromuscular paralysis. A sample of the drug is injected intravenously in small aliquots at constant time-intervals until head drop is observed, and this is repeated with a series of 12 to 16 animals, half of which receive the reference standard and the other half the unknown. From the relative mean amounts of standard and unknown needed to produce head drop, the relative activity can be estimated. The reliability of the assay is estimated from the variability of the results by standard statistical procedures and is expressed in terms of 95% confidence limits for the activity of the unknown preparation.

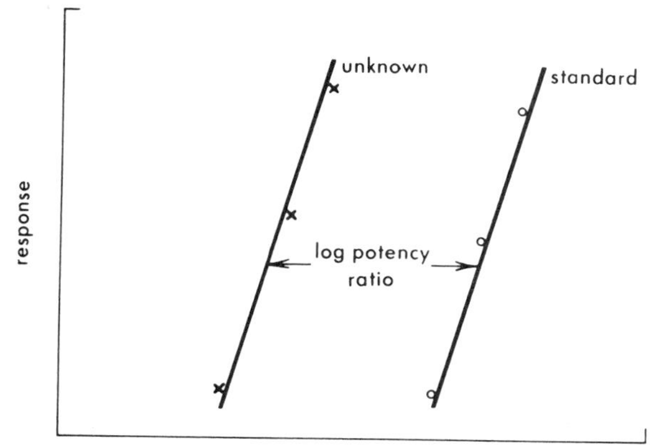

FIG. 9-3. Typical indirect bioassay in which the log dose-response curves are parallel. The unknown preparation is less active than the reference standard by a factor given by the antilogarithm of the horizontal distance between the lines. Confidence limits can be calculated from the scatter of the experimental points about the fitted parallel lines.

INDIRECT ASSAY

Direct assay is the simplest type of bioassay in which an end-point response is predetermined and the dose needed to produce it is measured. Such an end-point cannot always be established, and an indirect assay must be done. Here two or more fixed doses of both standard and unknown are used and the responses to each measured. From the results, log dose-response curves are constructed (Fig. 9-3), and the potency of the unknown sample relative to the reference standard is estimated by fitting parallel lines to the data statistically and by calculating the horizontal distance between the two lines. This gives the logarithm of the relative potency.

The statistical calculations needed to determine this ratio and its confidence limits are more complex than those for a direct assay. They yield an additional piece of information, however, that may be important when the sample contains a mixture of pharmacologically active components, namely, an assessment of whether the log dose-response curves are parallel. When only a single active substance is present, the standard and the unknown differ only in dilution, and this difference should be the same no matter how it is measured or what the end-point is. If more than one active component is present in the preparation, the standard and the unknown may differ in their dose-response curves, and the relative activity of the standard and the unknown may depend on the response level chosen for the comparison, that is, the log dose-response curves may not be parallel (Fig. 9-4). A direct assay uses only one end-point response and cannot detect this lack of parallelism. Since nonparallelism indicates that the potency ratio is not constant, the active components are probably not present in the

FIG. 9-4 Schematic representation of an indirect assay in which the log dose-response curves are not parallel. The activity of the unknown increases relative to the standard as the response level chosen for comparison increases.

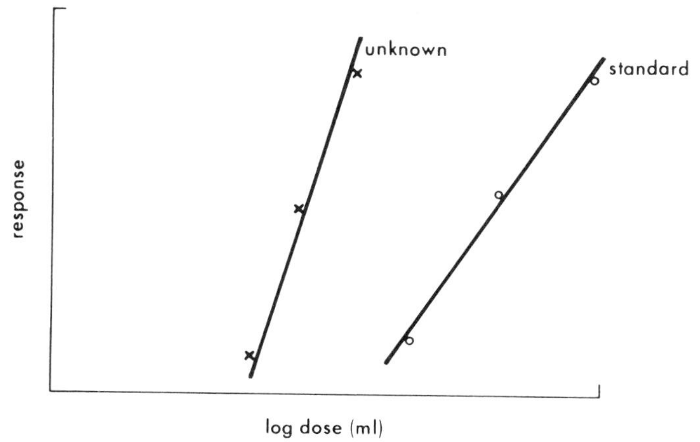

same proportions in the standard and the unknown preparations, and projection of the results to clinical use may involve serious errors. A statistical test for parallelism is therefore included in the routine analysis and may lead to rejection of the assay or of the drug preparation.

CLINICAL TRIALS

A clinical trial is basically a bioassay in which the response to a drug is assessed in human subjects. Ethical considerations place limitations on the design of the assay.

The principles underlying a clinical trial are the same as those governing any other type of assay, but they are more difficult to implement. A new drug should not be assessed alone but must always be compared with a placebo and one or more accepted agents (analogous to the reference standard). Each drug should be tested using at least two dose levels to establish meaningful estimates of relative potency. The subjects involved in the trial should be divided into groups that are balanced to every possible extent. Obviously, although animals of inbred strains can be grouped rather simply, the number of variables in a clinical trial is much greater: Sex, race, weight, and age can easily be balanced if the groups are sufficiently large, but when pathologic states are superimposed it may be possible to balance the groups only approximately.

Whereas in a conventional bioassay a single simple objective measurement generally provides the information from which drug potency is estimated, usually no such simple measurement can be made clinically. Judgment of efficacy in disease-states is usually based not only on several objective tests, but also on subjective evaluation by both the patient and the physician. Clearly, objective measurements are preferable to subjective judgments, but a relevant subjective judgment is better than the most precise measurement of a variable that gives no direct information about the drug effect sought. The format and basis of the evaluation must be determined completely before the trial, and, to avoid bias, both the physician and the patient should be ignorant of which drug any person is receiving (double-blind format).

FURTHER READING

1. Bliss CI: Statistics of Bioassay. New York, Academic Press, 1957
2. Finney DJ: Statistical Method in Biological Assay. New York, Hafner, 1952
3. Gaddum JH: Bioassays and mathematics. Pharmacol Rev 5:87, 1953
4. Biological Tests and Assays, In U.S. Pharmacopeia, 15th ed, pp 882–905.

CHAPTER 9 QUESTIONS

(*See* P. 7 for Full Instructions)

A=1,2,3; B=1,3; C=2,4; D=4; E=All

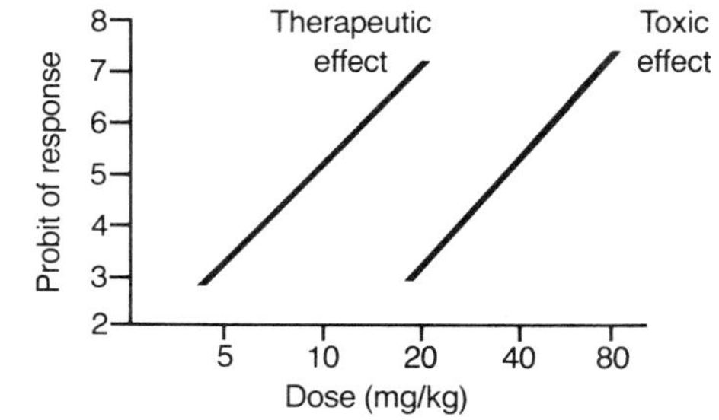

1. If the above graph depicts the dose-response curves for a therapeutic effect and a toxic effect of drug X in a group of patients, then
   1. the ED_{50} is about 20 mg/kg.
   2. all patients will show the therapeutic effect before showing the toxic effect.
   3. the TD_{50} is about 80 mg/kg.
   4. the therapeutic index is about 4.

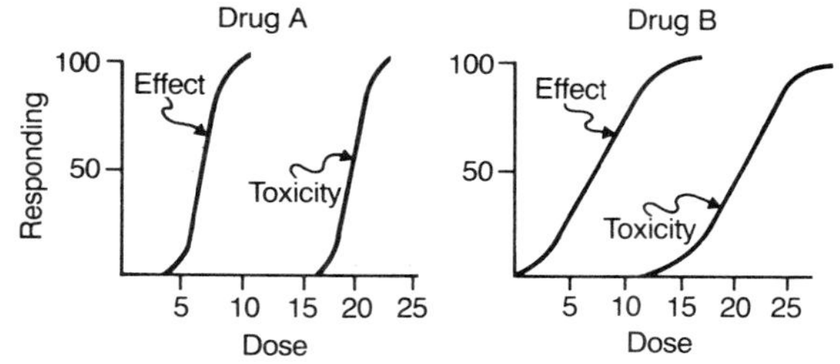

2. Graphs A and B represent the effects of two drugs that produce the same qualitative therapeutic effect. From these data, one can conclude that
   1. administration of ED_{99} doses of each agent would be expected to produce a similar incidence of toxic effects.
   2. the two drugs are equally safe.
   3. the therapeutic index for drug A approximates 0.3.
   4. the therapeutic indices for the two drugs are the same.

3. Placebos are used in medicine because
   1. in double-blind drug studies they allow

for evaluation of the psychological factors involved.
2. they show less variability in response than do active drugs.
3. they may be as effective as drugs in some persons.
4. they do not produce gastrointestinal symptoms.

4. The "therapeutic index" (LD_{50}/ED_{50}) of a drug
1. gives the best indication of the safety of the drug.
2. is independent of the slopes of the dose-response curves.
3. must be greater than 2 if the drug is to be used in human therapy.
4. requires the determination of two dose-response curves to obtain data for its calculation.

10

HAROLD E. PAULUS

Development of New Drugs

Perhaps the single most significant occurrence in the 20th century has been the remarkable increase in the average life expectancy of human populations; substantial changes in the organization and goals of society are occurring in response to the increased numbers and longevity of its members. Although improvements in public health engineering, sanitation, insect control, and agricultural productivity have been vital prerequisites to increased life expectancy, the development and dissemination of new drugs and vaccines have contributed substantially to the elimination of many scourges that previously held human populations in check. The development of new methods of birth control soon may provide a more acceptable method of population limitation. The rate of introduction of drugs with significant new actions has accelerated greatly, and, to a considerable extent, the methods involved in the development of new drugs have become codified and organized into the pharmaceutical industry and are regulated by governmental agencies. The goal of this collaboration between government, industry, academicians, and practicing physicians is the safe and orderly evaluation and introduction of new drugs in such a way that the risk-to-benefit ratio is favorable at all stages of the process.

FINDING A POTENTIAL NEW DRUG

New drug candidates may be found in a number of ways.

SERENDIPITY

The astute appreciation and the exploitation of an unanticipated effect have resulted in many important classes of drugs being introduced, starting with the prehistoric tribal medicine man who observed reduced fever when he chewed on (salicylate-containing) willow bark, or relief of pain on ingesting the sap of the opium poppy. Other important drugs in this category include colchicine (autumn crocus), digitalis (foxglove), atropine (belladonna plant), quinine (cinchona tree bark) and penicillin (*Penicillium* mold).

NEW USES FOR OLD DRUGS

An unanticipated drug effect may be noted and exploited when a drug is used for a known indication or when a drug is given for a nonstandard indication. These new applications tend to be developed by physicians using the drugs rather than by scientists introducing them. The use of the local anesthetic lidocaine and the anticonvulsive phenytoin to control cardiac arrhythmias; amphetamines to control hyperkinetic behavior in children; the anticancer agent methotrexate to control severe psoriasis, and the anticancer drugs cyclophosphamide and azathioprine as immunosuppressive agents to prevent rejection of kidney transplants and to treat autoimmune diseases are examples of new uses developed by physicians.

EXTRACTION OF A NATURAL REGULATOR FROM AN ANIMAL PRODUCT

Insulin from the pancreas, heparin from mast cells, adrenocorticotropin from the pituitary, thyroid extract from the thyroid, and estrogens from the urine of pregnant mares are natural regulators extracted from an animal product. These drugs are usually obtained as byproducts of the processing of domesticated meat-producing animals such as hogs and cattle. The deliberate hyperimmunization of animals to certain antigens has used the animal as a factory to produce drugs (antisera) effective against various bacteria and toxins, for example, tetanus and diphtheria antitoxin and type-specific pneumococcal and rabies antisera.

EMPIRICAL SCREENING OF CHEMICALS FOR A DESIRED EFFECT

This time-honored method, perfected by the pharmaceutical industry, requires a relatively easy and inexpensive method for detecting the desired effect. *In vitro* examples include the use of bacterial cultures to detect the antibacterial effects of antibiotics and the use of tissue cultures of tumor cell lines to detect the effects of potential antitumor agents. Small animals may be used to screen for hypnotic, sedative, and anesthetic effects, whereas the injection of irritating substances into small animals may be used to screen for antiinflammatory activity. When a reproducible routine test system has been standardized, the number of chemicals that can be processed is limitless. The rapid proliferation of antibiotic compounds is a tribute to the effective application of this approach.

DELIBERATE CHEMICAL MODIFICATION OF A KNOWN ACTIVE AGENT TO ENHANCE AN EFFECT (OR A SIDE-EFFECT)

Having found and characterized the effects and side-effects of a drug, pharmaceutical chemists can synthesize a myriad of cogeners of its basic chemical structure. By careful correlation of the changes in drug effect that occur with changes in structure, it is sometimes possible to develop rational structure-effect relationships to maximize the desired effects and to minimize the undesired effects of a particular family of chemicals. Examples are modification of antihistamines to produce the phenothiazine tranquilizers, of the steroid molecule to enhance the potency of corticosteroids, and of the basic structure of sulfa compounds to enhance hypoglycemic or diuretic effects.

LOGICAL FORMULATION OF A NEW CHEMICAL TO PRODUCE A DESIRED EFFECT

Based on a detailed knowledge of physiologic chemistry in the normal and diseased state, it should be possible to formulate specifically new drugs to correct a defect or to modify an undesired manifestation of disease. Detailed structural characterization of a physiologic mediator may permit the development of an analogue to block its effects. An example is allopurinol, an analogue of xanthine, which blocks the enzyme xanthine oxidase, thus preventing the production of uric acid. Use of this drug results in decreased concentrations of uric acid in the blood and benefits patients with gout. Although few currently available drugs have been discovered in this way, the increasing knowledge of molecular biology should make this an important source of new drugs. For example, cimetidine was specifically developed to inhibit competitively the action of histamine at the histamine H_2 receptor sites of acid-producing gastric parietal cells.

PRECLINICAL EVALUATION OF A CANDIDATE COMPOUND

The purposes of preclinical drug evaluation are to document reasonably that the drug may be tested safely in humans and to obtain some indication that it may be effective in certain human disease-states. Thus the two major areas of preclinical evaluation are *efficacy evaluation* and *toxicity screening*. The major effort in these areas is expended by the pharmaceutical industry and is conducted by the experimental pharmacologist. Specialization may limit the role of an individual pharmacologist to the evaluation of a particular class of drug actions or to toxicology. At this stage there are many candidate drugs, but the investment in each is relatively small. Because the cost of drug development increases exponentially as the drug progresses through preclinical and clinical evaluation, the emphasis at this stage is the elimination of compounds that may later prove to be unacceptable.

SCREENING FOR EFFICACY

Several approaches may be taken. Many compounds may be screened for a specific effect, and those with the desired effect may then be evaluated more extensively for the presence of other (side) effects. Another approach is to screen all new compounds in a standard set of test systems to evaluate efficacy in various organ-systems. *In vitro* assays are used when appropriate, particularly when searching for antibacterial properties or for effects on cell metabolism that can be elicited in tissue culture systems. Sometimes drug effects can be studied in an isolated organ-system; examples include the evaluation of ion transport across the excised toad bladder; the transmission of nerve impulses through the squid axon; and the effects of various substances on the contractility of isolated segments of guinea pig intestine, rat uterus, or other muscle preparations. More frequently, however, drug effects are evaluated in intact animals. Cardiorespiratory, renal, endocrine, and CNS effects may be studied in normal animals. A useful technique for evaluation of drug effects on gastric acid secretion and transport across the gastric mucosa is the preparation of an isolated gastric pouch that allows one to quantitate these factors in a normal unanesthetized animal.

Generally drug actions intended to modify normal physiologic response patterns can be studied in normal animals. For the evaluation of drug activity against specific disease processes, diseases or models of disease may be induced in the animal, or inbred animal strains may be selected for the natural occurrence of certain diseases. The NZB mouse and certain inbred dog strains that develop an autoimmune illness similar to systemic lupus erythematosus can be used to evaluate immunosuppressive therapy. Antitumor drugs may be studied in strains of mice that either develop specific tumors or accept transplanted tumors. Specific infections or hypertension may be induced and treated with candidate compounds. Drug effects on hyperuricemia and gouty nephropathy may be evaluated in rodents fed oxonic acid (an inhibitor of uricase) and uric acid. Mice, rats, guinea pigs, and dogs are the most frequently used experimental animals, but various monkey species are also used for some studies.

Activity of a drug in preclinical tests of efficacy does not necessarily mean that the drug will be active or useful in human disease-states. The reliability with which *in vitro* and animal models can select drugs that will be effective in human diseases is constantly being reevaluated against the performance of new compounds. Results tend to be better when the pathophysiology of the human disease process is clearly understood.

Metabolic Studies

If a compound appears to be promising, its absorption and metabolism are generally studied in several species of animals, usually rats, dogs, and sometimes monkeys. These metabolic studies should establish the relative bioavailability of the compound when administered orally and parenterally, should determine the rate at which it is metabolized and excreted, and should characterize its metabolic products. Usually the administration of radioisotope-tagged compounds is followed by timed collections of serum, urine, stool, and sometimes bile for quantitative analysis. In addition, relative drug concentrations in various tissues and organs may be determined after acute or chronic administration of the drug. The metabolites themselves should be evaluated for efficacy because active compounds frequently have pharmacologically active metabolic products. The rate of excretion can be expressed as a half-life, that is, the time required for one half of the drug to be excreted (*see* Chap. 3). This information is useful in estimating optimal dosage intervals, but information obtained in animals can be applied to humans only in a general way.

EVALUATION FOR DRUG TOXICITY

If given in sufficient dosage, all pharmacologically active drugs produce toxic effects. Those candidate compounds that, on the basis of their preclinical efficacy, are considered worthy of evaluation in humans are subjected to rigorous preclinical toxicity evaluation. Preclinical toxicity screening has been substantially standardized and in the United States is regulated by the Food and Drug Administration (FDA). Its purpose is to characterize the toxic effects and to determine the relative margin of safety, that is, the difference between the median lethal dose (LD_{50}) and the median effective dose (ED_{50}) (*see* Chap. 9). This margin of safety, or therapeutic index, cannot be precisely defined for a compound because it may vary with the conditions of administration and the drug effect being observed.

Initially a wide range of single doses are given to mice or rats to determine the minimum lethal dose and to estimate the biologic activity of the drug. Based on the results of acute toxicity studies, the range of doses and routes of administration are determined for subsequent subacute toxicity studies. The drug is evaluated in several species of animals by repeated administration at a number of dose levels ranging from median effective levels to levels that are lethal after only a few doses. Chronic toxicity studies require continued drug administration for up to 2 years in several dosage ranges, at least one of which must be high enough to produce substantial toxicity. Generally three species of animals are studied, frequently the rat, the dog, and the monkey. Additional studies are done to determine the effects of the compound on fertility and pregnancy. Decreased fertility, increased fetal wastage, and fetal malformations are sought. Mutagenicity is evaluated by quantitating the development of adaptive mutations in bacterial cultures exposed to the drug (and its metabolites) under specific adverse culture conditions (Ame's test). Carcinogenicity is evaluated as part of the chronic toxicity studies.

At the end of the preclinical evaluations, one should be confident that the candidate compound is safe for initial introduction into human subjects and reasonably certain that it may be therapeutically effective. Only a small percentage of the originally synthesized candidate compounds are selected for clinical evaluation. At this point the sponsor is required to submit the results of the preclinical investigations to the FDA, along with proposals for initial clinical evaluations. If the FDA is satisfied that the compound is reasonably safe, permission is given to begin initial clinical trials in humans.

CLINICAL EVALUATION OF THE NEW DRUG

Having survived the rigors of preclinical efficacy and toxicity evaluation, the candidate compound, which may now be called a new drug, must be evaluated in the human subjects for whom it is intended. The purpose of clinical evaluation is to determine whether a new drug is effective for its projected therapeutic indications and to characterize its toxicity in order to define the conditions under which it may be ultimately prescribed for general use. The standards and conditions for clinical evaluation of new drugs are specifically regulated by the FDA, and drugs cannot be released for general use in the United States without its approval. In 1938, the FDA was made legally responsible for determining the safety of new drugs before their release. Until 1962, however, it was not necessary to prove that a new drug was therapeutically effective. Stimulated by the thalidomide tragedy in 1962 (*see* Chap. 11), the FDA was directed to require proof of effectiveness as well as safety. This new requirement substantially increased the complexity of the clinical evaluation of new drugs and slowed the flood of new preparations into the pharmacy.

To carry out its responsibility, the FDA requires complete information about the methods and quality controls used for the synthesis and manufacture of the compound, in addition to complete records of all preclinical studies. For each clinical study, both the protocol and the clinical investigators must be approved by the FDA; upon its completion, detailed case reports of each subject must be submitted, along with general summaries of the conclusions drawn from the trials. This carefully regulated procedure for the development and evaluation of new drugs is called the investigational new drug (IND) process. When the sponsor feels that sufficient information has been gathered to justify approval for marketing, a new drug application (NDA) is submitted to the FDA. After careful review of the NDA, the package insert is written and the drug may be approved for general prescription.

THE CONTROLLED CLINICAL TRIAL

The crucial element in the clinical evaluation of a new drug is the controlled clinical trial,

1962—Thalidomide tragedy stimulated Kefauver hearings, resulting in the current FDA regulations that require proof of efficacy as well as safety.

which in essence is the application of the scientific method of clinical investigation to prove or disprove a prestated hypothesis. Controlled clinical trials compare a treated group with an untreated, or control, group. This comparison is necessary because of the complexity of human subjects and the multitude of uncontrollable or unknown variables that may affect the results of the trial. A prerequisite of any clinical trial is the informed consent of its participants. Each subject must understand the general structure of the trial, the therapeutic agents he may be exposed to, and all possible risks of the trial, whether from treatment, lack of treatment, or diagnostic maneuver. Alternative treatment methods must be explained, and the patient's privacy must be protected. An institutional review committee is required to determine that the rights and welfare of all subjects affected are adequately protected; the methods used to obtain informed consent are appropriate; and the risks to the subject are outweighed by the potential benefit to him, to knowledge, or to humanity. The time used to explain carefully a proposed clinical trial to its subjects is amply repaid because the subjects then become active, cooperating participants in the trial rather than passive subjects upon whom observations are made.

The elements of a controlled clinical trial collectively may be referred to as the design of the trial.

1. A clearly defined therapeutic objective (hypothesis)
2. A quantitative scale of accomplishment (to indicate attainment of the objective)
3. Representative subjects
4. Unbiased subject assignment to treatment or control groups
5. Control of bias (of investigator and subject)
6. Equal distribution of uncontrollable environmental and genetic factors
7. Statistical methods to determine the significance of differences between study groups

The therapeutic objective, or hypothesis, must be clearly stated and answerable. The methods by which attainment of the objective will be recognized must be defined and should be quantitated by an appropriate scale. The scale may be based on the patient's report, for example, severe, moderate, mild, or none with respect to pain, or on a laboratory observation, for example, blood sugar or serum drug concentration. The study subjects must be representative of the population to whom the hypothesis is to be applied. The results of a study of normal subjects cannot be indiscriminately applied to patients with a disease, and the findings of a study of subjects with minimal disease manifestations may not be applicable to those with severe disease manifestations.

The subjects must be assigned to the treatment or control group in an unbiased manner, generally by *random assignment*, using a list of randomly generated numbers to determine the sequence in which subjects are assigned to the study groups. In the case of a *cross-over trial*, each subject receives both the investigative and the control treatment, but the order in which they are given is randomly predetermined. The cross-over trial has an additional advantage in that uncontrollable environmental and genetic factors tend to remain more or less constant within the subject, who acts as his own control. However, either spontaneous or treatment-induced changes in the subject during the course of the study, and carryover effects of one drug on the subsequent treatment may confound the investigation. These problems are avoided in a *parallel study* design in which each subject receives only one treatment, but larger numbers of subjects must be studied to distribute uncontrollable factors by randomization equally. The unavoidable bias of both the investigator and the subjects is frequently controlled by using a *double-blind* study design; here neither the investigator nor the subject knows which of the possible therapies is being given. Blindness is ensured by preparing the various treatments in identical dosage forms: identical capsules, tablets, and injections, for example. A code that indicates the patient's actual treatment is readily available if this information should be needed. During a double-blind trial, the investigator or the subject frequently thinks that he can recognize the treatment by its characteristic side-effects or in some other way, but his lack of insight is usually evident when the code is broken at the end of the study. As long as some element of uncertainty is present, the double-blind design has attained its objective. At the conclusion of the clinical trial the treatment codes are broken, the data are tabulated and then subjected to statistical analysis to determine the significance of observed differences between the study groups. Various statistical methods may be applied, but they should be preselected to avoid bias. Mathematically massaging the data until the desired result is obtained is not a legitimate application of statistical methods to controlled clinical trials.

Placebos are frequently used as the control therapy in double-blind trials. A *placebo* is a substance, for example, lactose capsules or saline injections, thought to be pharmacologically inert. The use of placebos is particularly helpful in controlled trials because it helps quantitate the degree to which subject responses are due to the study situation, the mere ingestion of capsules, or other uncontrollable variables. Subject response to the administration of a placebo is called *placebo effect* and, when specifically studied, has been seen in about one third of subjects. Placebo effects are more likely to be seen when the pertinent effect is subjectively reported by the patient rather than when it is objectively measured by the investigator or by his laboratory. To some extent, the placebo effect is due to the suggestibility of the subject. It may be either positive or negative and applies not only to therapeutic effects but also to side-effects of the treatment.

PHASES OF CLINICAL EVALUATION

Evaluation of a new drug in humans follows a logical pattern and is usually subdivided into distinct stages referred to as phases. The purpose of phase I—the initial exploratory introduction of the drug to human subjects—is to determine that the drug is not generally toxic and to accumulate information that will be helpful in establishing dosage and dosage intervals for subsequent studies. A single tiny dose is usually given to the first subject; if well tolerated, single doses of increasing size are then given to a series of subjects until a dose in the anticipated therapeutic range is reached, or until some side-effects are observed. Clinical laboratory evaluations are done in all subjects to detect possible adverse effects on the blood, liver, kidneys, or gastrointestinal tract, and the subjects are carefully observed for subjective or objective evidence of drug effects. The choice of the initial dose and the maximum dose to be used in a phase I trial is difficult to decide; the doses chosen depend to a greater extent on the "gut reaction" of the clinical pharmacologist conducting the trial than on any scientific formula. As part of the single dose trials, a metabolic study is usually done to determine that the drug can be found in the plasma (is bioavailable) and to determine the rate at which it disappears from the plasma. In addition, the rate and character of urinary excretion products may also be ascertained. The rate at which a drug disappears from plasma, or its half-life, is important in estimating the frequency with which doses should be administered in subsequent multiple-dose trials. A rapidly metabolized drug must be given frequently to maintain plasma concentrations, whereas a slowly metabolized drug must be given less frequently to avoid accumulation. If no problems develop during single-dose studies, multiple-dose trials are begun. Again, a small number of subjects are given small doses of the drug in trials of 4 to 6 weeks' duration. If no problems are encountered, other subjects are given larger doses; thus the dose and duration of treatment are gradually increased, always with the knowledge that the previous dosage level was safe. Metabolic studies should be done during the multiple-dose studies to ascertain the plateau concentrations developing during clinical therapy. Phase I studies generally use healthy normal volunteer subjects, although sometimes patients for whom the drug might reasonably be used as treatment are allowed to volunteer. In either case, the subjects must understand that there is no likelihood they will benefit personally from phase I drug administration. If the drug has an action that can be measured in normal subjects, this can be studied during phase I; for example, the effects of a diuretic or an antihypertensive agent could be evaluated. However, evaluation of safety is the prime concern. Phase I studies are almost always undertaken by experienced clinical pharmacologists. Double-blind, placebo controlled studies are not always necessary, but this design is useful because it establishes a reference group against which incidental or minimal abnormalities can be judged.

Phase II is divided into early and late stages and comprises the initial introduction of the drug into patients who have the disease or condition that the drug is intended to treat. Early phase II studies should establish that the drug is as safe in patients as it was in the normal volunteers studied in phase I. Small numbers of patients are intensively studied to assess the potential usefulness and dosage range of the drug. Increasing doses of the drug may be given in an open or blind fashion by an experienced investigator. In addition to routine monitoring of safety, the beneficial effects of the drug are evaluated intensely. If the new drug is promising therapeutically and has not shown excessive toxicity, extensive and expensive clinical and preclinical studies are initiated. These comprise long-term chronic toxicity studies and evaluations of drug effects on reproduction and fertility in animals and the entire spectrum of clinical studies leading to eventual approval of the drug for general distribution. Because the investment in these subsequent studies is great, a drug that has modest toxicity or uncertain efficacy is likely to be dropped at the end of the early phase II studies.

Assuming that the drug appears safe and that therapeutic effects were shown at some dosage level in the early phase II studies, late phase II studies are begun. Late phase II studies represent a substantial commitment to the drug and are intended to provide statistical proof that the drug is therapeutically beneficial in the dosage to be ultimately recommended. Larger numbers of patients are studied in tightly controlled double-blind trials in which the drug is compared to placebo and to standard forms of therapy. At the end of phase II, one should be convinced that the drug is therapeutically useful and that it is generally safe for its proposed indication, and one should know the therapeutic dose range. Late phase II studies tend to merge into phase III studies in which the role of the drug in clinical practice is ascertained. A large number of patients are studied by various investigators, and the drug is given in situations similar to those of actual clinical practice. The duration of administration should approach that anticipated in subsequent clinical practice. A sufficient number of subjects should be studied to uncover the possibility of rare but serious toxicity. Special aspects of safety and metabolism are evaluated, for example, drug dosage in patients with hepatic or renal insufficiency, interactions with other drugs, drug concentrations in milk, and transmission across the placental barrier. If it is anticipated that the drug may be used during pregnancy or in children, studies in the appropriate subjects are done late in phase III. Although many phase III studies are more valid if they are carried out in a double-blind controlled manner, unblinded administration of the drug in a clinical setting is also useful, if drug effect and side-effects are carefully documented.

At the end of phase III, both the sponsor and the FDA must be satisfied that the drug is both safe and effective for its proposed uses, even when prescribed by busy physicians to sometimes forgetful patients. At this time, the "package insert" is written by the sponsor under the watchful eye of the FDA. This important document, inserted in every package of the drug and quoted in the Physician's Desk Reference (PDR), summarizes everything that is known about the drug and specifies the conditions under which it should be used, dosage information, possible side-effects, precautions, and any other significant factors known about the drug. Whenever one uses an unfamiliar drug, the package insert should be carefully and completely read rather than being hastily discarded, for it contains the most authoritative current statement available about that drug.

The evaluation of a new drug does not stop when it has been released for general prescription. Drug evaluation is then referred to as phase IV and comprises continued surveillance during general clinical use. Unusual types of toxic reactions are often noted during phase IV, sometimes many years after the drug was introduced to medicine. Examples include bone marrow suppression by chloramphenicol and by phenylbutazone, hepatitis induced by isoniazid, hepatic fibrosis induced by methotrexate, and the drug-induced lupus syndrome caused by various agents. An aspirin-induced hepatitis was only recently recognized, even though this ubiquitous drug has been used for more than 75 years. Thus phase IV evaluation continues as long as the drug is used. In addition to observations on toxicity, further refinement of dosage schedules, metabolism, interactions with other drugs, effects of various disease-states on the drug and its metabolism, and additional clinical indications for use of the drug frequently develop during phase IV, which is monitored by the FDA.

SCIENTIFIC PERSONNEL INVOLVED IN NEW DRUG DEVELOPMENT

In addition to those persons needed for the commercial aspects of the pharmaceutical industry, a number of distinct scientific roles are involved in new drug development. The *pharmaceutical chemist* must be well versed in both synthetic biochemistry and pharmacology in order to synthesize the compounds that may become new drugs. He must be able to isolate, identify, and then synthesize the active principle of a naturally occurring herb or other product with medicinal properties. The *experimental pharmacologist* searches for evidence of drug activity in experimental animal and *in vitro* models of physiologic processes or diseases. Although he may evaluate the whole spectrum of drug activity, a person may limit his work to a specific organ-system or type of drug action. *Toxicologists* are experimental pharmacologists who specialize in the preclinical assessment of drug toxicity and are generally distinct from persons who evaluate the drugs for preclinical efficacy. Sometimes *veterinarians* supervise the care of the large variety of experimental animals used in preclinical studies; their knowledge of the naturally occurring incidence of certain abnormalities or diseases in these animal populations is particularly important. Early human studies are usually undertaken by *clinical pharmacologists*, that is, physicians especially trained in the design, conduct, and evaluation of studies of drug effects in humans. Later trials in patients are conducted by *clinical investigators* with experience and expertise in the treatment of patients with diseases for which the drug is indicated. These studies are monitored by other physicians who attempt to assure that the study protocol is properly adhered to and finally are evaluated by physicians or pharmacologists employed by the FDA. Of great importance in the evaluation of both preclinical and clinical studies is the *biostatistician*, who is frequently assisted by specialists in computerized data storage, retrieval and processing.

Thus the development of a new drug requires the diligent application of skills drawn from a number of disciplines. The long and torturous path involved in the development of a successful new drug is frustrating because so few candidate drugs complete it, but the satisfactions gained from the introduction of a substantial therapeutic advance make the effort worthwhile.

FURTHER READING

1. Feinstein AR: Clinical Judgement. Baltimore, Williams & Wilkins, 1967
2. Harris EL, Fitzgerald JD (eds): The Principles and Practice of Clinical Trials. Edinburgh, E and S Livingstone, 1970
3. Melmon KL, Morrelli HF (eds): Clinical Pharmacology. Basic Principles in Therapeutics, 2nd ed. New York, Macmillan, 1978

11

JEREMY H. THOMPSON

Adverse Drug Reactions

Drugs are powerful chemicals that unfortunately may produce effects other than those sought by the prescriber. Such unsolicited effects may be harmful or harmless; if harmful, they are called *adverse drug reactions*. Adverse drug reactions are consequently one facet of *iatrogenic disease,* which encompasses the spectrum of adverse effects produced unintentionally by physicians while caring for their patients. Iatrogenic disease includes not only the direct injuries that may result from drugs or from diagnostic or therapeutic procedures, but also the states that may arise from personality conflicts between the physician and the patient. This chapter is concerned only with adverse effects produced by drugs.

Although the laity expect drugs to cure most disease and suffering without danger or undesirable effects, the use of any drug inevitably entails some risk. No drug is so specific that it produces only desired effects in all patients. No clinically useful drug (not even a placebo) is entirely devoid of toxicity. Both the patient and the doctor should recognize and accept these facts. The physician should neither become a therapeutic nihilist for fear of adverse drug reactions nor prescribe indiscriminately. Before administering a drug, he or she should carefully consider its possible adverse effects versus the potential therapeutic benefits.

DIAGNOSIS AND FREQUENCY OF ADVERSE DRUG REACTIONS

The frequency of adverse drug reactions is difficult to determine (*see* below) since the same response may be either beneficial or adverse depending on the clinical situation. For example, sedation with an H_1-antagonist (*see* Chap. 51) is generally undesirable when it occurs during the day, but will be desirable when the drug is used as a hypnotic; moreover, H_1-blocker-induced sedation may be desirable in treating a patient with a severe pruritic drug reaction. Thus "adverse" is one of many qualifying adjectives applied to drug effects. The tendency in the past to classify all unwanted drug effects as adverse has led to some confusion. Because of these and other difficulties in definition, data on the frequency of occurrence of adverse drug reactions should be interpreted carefully. Most drugs are relatively safe, but some have so low a therapeutic ratio that there is little difference between the effective dose and the toxic dose.

Adverse drug reactions have accounted for 3% to 20% of hospital admissions, and 5% to 40% of patients in hospitals experience an adverse drug reaction. Also, 30% of patients admitted for a drug reaction have a further reaction while in the hospital, and the average length of hospital stay is doubled for patients who experience a reaction.

The "incidence" of adverse drug reactions has increased in recent years. This increase may be a result of more people taking more drugs, often for longer periods; more drugs being used concomitantly without a parallel increase in our knowledge of their pharmacokinetics and the diseases for which they are being given; a changing pattern of diseases being treated, with a greater percentage of older patients or those receiving chronic immunosuppressive therapy, for example; and greater exposure to environmental agents that may alter the response to drugs. Potent drugs with a potential for life-threatening reactions, such as chloramphenicol, should not be used for trivial illnesses.

VARIABLES IN ASSESSING THE INCIDENCE OF ADVERSE DRUG REACTIONS

Several variables influence the frequency of adverse drug reactions. Diagnosis may be difficult, or debatable, as with H_1-antagonist-induced sedation (*see* above) or atropine-induced xerostomia; some physicians view the latter effect as an adverse reaction, whereas others consider it to be merely a useful indicator in determining the optimum dose. Similarly, reaction rates differ widely depending on whether they were obtained prospectively or retrospectively or on how the reactions were defined, that is, by such means as clinical impression, biochemical or immunologic test, or drug rechallenge.

Only rarely (*e.g.*, with a new drug under trial or with Schedule II drugs; *see* Chap. 12) are accurate records available on the number of prescriptions written or on the use of prescription and nonprescription (over-the-counter) drugs. If such figures are not known, no true incidence rates of adverse reactions can be calculated, and assessing the benefit-risk ratio of any agent for any patient is virtually impossible. This problem is compounded by nursing errors in drug administration and patient noncompliance. Time is also an important variable. Thus adverse effects of some therapies (*e.g.*, x-irradiation, teratogens, gold salts) may not appear for months or years after the patient has been at risk, and with other drugs (*e.g.*, chloroquine), damage may be seen only after chronic administration if cumulation develops.

Errors in prescription filling and in drug administration are surprisingly common. It is essential to establish whether a patient suspected of suffering an adverse drug reaction has actually received the drug in question. Moreover, in this lawsuit-conscious age, many physicians fail to report adverse reactions for fear of legal complications.

There is often failure to recognize that a new "symptom" developing under therapy is in fact a drug reaction rather than some manifestation of the underlying disease. This is particularly likely if the reaction is either very common or highly unusual.

The patient who receives only a single drug is rare. Thus, if a reaction develops during multiple drug administration, it may be impossible to decide which agent, if any, was responsible. Symptoms often listed as being caused by drugs are common. A survey of 414 healthy university students and hospital staff who were not taking medications indicated that 81% of the subjects had experienced a variety of symptoms in the preceding 72 hours (Table 11-1). The median number of symptoms experienced was two per person, and 10% of the subjects experienced six or more!

TIME OF ONSET OF DRUG REACTIONS

Depending on its pathogenesis, a reaction may appear within seconds (*e.g.*, anaphylactic shock, Table 59-1) to years (*e.g.*, chloroquine-induced retinopathy) after drug administration. Most reactions, however, develop within 7 to 10 days of the start of therapy. Some reactions may persist after the offending drug has been excreted, such as catecholamine sensitivity after monoamine oxidase inhibitors (*see* Chap. 8), where the enzyme has been irreversibly inactivated.

REPORTING OF REACTIONS

Deciding what is or is not appropriate to tell a patient about the drugs he or she is taking is sometimes difficult. In general, however, patients should be fully informed, particularly on what side-effects to expect and how they can be

TABLE 11-1. Percentage of Subjects Reporting Each Symptom

Symptom	Medical Group	Nonmedical Group
Skin rash	8	3
Urticaria	5	1
Bad dreams	8	3
Excessive sleepiness	23	23
Fatigue	41	37
Inability to concentrate	25	27
Irritability	20	17
Insomnia	7	10
Loss of appetite	3	6
Dry mouth	5	3
Nausea	3	2
Vomiting	0	0
Diarrhea	5	2
Constipation	4	3
Palpitations	3	3
Giddiness or weakness	2	3
Faintness or dizziness on first standing up	5	5
Headaches	15	13
Fever	3	1
Pain in joints	9	5
Pain in muscles	10	11
Nasal congestion	31	13
Bleeding or bruising	3	3
Bleeding from gums after brushing teeth	21	20
Excessive bleeding from gums after brushing teeth	1	1

(Reidenberg MM, Lowenthal DT: Adverse, non-drug reactions. N. Engl J Med 279:678–679, 1968)

minimized with least interference in therapy. Such candor fosters a better doctor-patient relationship and also aids compliance. Patients also should be instructed to report certain warning symptoms so that a drug can be discontinued promptly in an attempt to minimize progression to more serious disease, as with sore throat subsequent to drug-induced neutropenia (*see* Chap. 64). Physicians should not be reticent about reporting known serious reactions or potential new reactions to the proper authorities.

FACTORS PREDISPOSING TO ADVERSE DRUG REACTIONS

Although deriving accurate figures on the incidence of adverse drug reactions is impossible, many of the variables that influence their development are known. Predicting which patients are most likely to suffer adverse reactions to drugs, however, is still generally impossible. In the discussion that follows, the considerable overlap between individual categories will become evident.

PREDISPOSING DRUG FACTORS

Chemical Characteristics

Polarity and pK$_a$. Highly polar (water soluble) drugs (*see* Chap. 3) (*e.g.*, aminoglycoside antibiotics, thiazide diuretics) primarily are excreted by the kidney unchanged and are thus likely to accumulate in patients with renal insufficiency. Conversely, nonpolar (fat-soluble) drugs (*see* Chap. 3) (*e.g.*, phenothiazines, barbiturates) require metabolic conversion to polar metabolites for their excretion. They also tend to be highly plasma protein bound and to cause enzyme induction or inhibition (*see* Chaps. 3, 4, 8). Thus knowledge of the chemical characteristics that determine a drug's polarity may facilitate prediction of adverse drug reactions in patients with disease of excretory organs and prediction of drug interactions at the level of plasma protein binding and hepatic metabolism (*see* Chap. 8). Similarly, appreciation of a drug's pK$_a$ (*see* Chap. 3) will facilitate prediction of certain drug interactions since the pharmacokinetics of weak electrolytes are dramatically modified by altering the pH of the bowel lumen and the urine.

Chemical Similarities

Certain chemical groupings predictably yield adverse reactions, although they may occur in drugs with totally different pharmacologic properties. For example, hepatic damage induced by one "hydrazine" will almost invariably develop with another agent containing that grouping, and aniline-like drugs may produce hemolysis in subjects with glucose-6-phosphate dehydrogenase deficiency (*see* Table 81-23).

Similarly, in persons hypersensitive to certain chemical groups, related drugs usually produce symptoms of allergy. A patient hypersensitive to a specific sulfonamide will usually show a similar response to all other antimicrobial sulfonamides and sulfones and to the chemically related but nonantibacterial sulfonylureas, thiazide diuretics and acetazolamide.

Bioavailability

A drug is formulated (manufactured, compounded) with a variety of additional agents (excipients) such as buffers, and flavoring agents (Table 11-2). Since the specific drug salt, the formulation process, and the number, type, and concentration of excipients are patentable, it is not surprising that the bioavailability of the active ingredient in similar drugs from different manufacturers may vary (*see* Chaps. 3, 8). Although the degree of bioavailability is important for most therapeutic agents, it is of critical importance with antiepileptic drugs, anticoagulants, digitalis, and endocrine agents. For example, switching to the same antiepileptic chemical supplied by a second manufacturer may lead to redevelopment of seizure activity if the bioavailability of the new formulation does not equal that of the initial preparation. In contrast, if the bioavailability of the second agent is greater than that of the initial preparation, an exaggerated therapeutic response or toxicity may ensue.

Drug Degradation

Potentially unstable drugs are formulated with various excipient buffers and stabilizers. Such formulations are given an expiration date indicating the time period for which a manufacturer guarantees the product against decomposition under normal storage conditions. Owing to adverse storage conditions (particularly extremes of temperature and humidity) some drugs may degrade prematurely; out-of-date drugs are not necessarily degraded, but they should not be used. If a drug degrades, the patient is deprived of the active ingredient, and the degradation product may produce toxicity (*e.g.*, the Fanconi-like syndrome with tetracyclines*; *see* Chap. 61); if either of these occurs, the physician and the pharmacist are open to litigation.

Drug Purity

It is rare that the active (drug) ingredient of any preparation is not what the manufacturer states it is, but mistakes do occur. In the United States, for example, some early preparations of digitalis glycosides were accidently contaminated by estrogens that caused puzzling gynecomastia in several patients, and a minor epidemic of precocious puberty in young girls taking isoniazid was traced to contamination of the drug by female sex hormones in an improperly cleaned tablet-making machine. Impure drugs rarely reach the United States market today. A tourist or alien, however, may bring in a drug purchased abroad that, because of less stringent controls in its country of manufacture, contains contaminants.

* See footnote in Chapter 61 (protein synthesis inhibitors II).

TABLE 11-2. Some of the Factors That May Alter Drug Bioavailability

Formulation and manufactoring factors		
Additives (adjuncts)	Excipients	Preservatives
Adjuvants	Flavors	Pressure of tablet punches
Binders	Formulation	Purity
Buffers	Friability	Solubility (of adjuncts)
Chelators	Granulators	Solubility (of drug)
Coating composition	Hardness	Solvation
Coating thickness	Hydration, degree of	Stereoisomeric stability
Coloring agents	Impurities	Stereoisomerism
Compactness of fill	Incompatibilities	Surface activity
Complexation	Lubricants	Surface area
Crystal structure	Packaging materials	Surfactants
Deaggregation rate	Particle size	Suspending agents
Diluents	pH	Uniformity of composition
Disintegrators	Porosity	Vehicles
Dissolution rate	Potency	Wettability
Emulsifying agents		
Distribution Factors		
Age of drug product	Moisture, atmospheric	Stability of ingredients
Deterioration	Oxidation	Stereoisomeric shifts
Epimerization	Packaging	Storage conditions
Humidity	Radiation	Temperature of environment
Inertness of atmosphere	Reduction	Transportation stress

(Modified from Martin EW: Hazards of Medication, 2nd ed. Philadelphia, J B Lippincott, 1978)

More commonly, questions arise on the safety or dangers of contaminants or excipients. For example, the sodium content of antacids may pose a significant hazard to patients with compromised cardiovascular function, and drug solutions may become contaminated by bacteria. In recent years considerable publicity has been directed toward the potential dangers of particulate matter (fibers) in solutions (large-volume parenterals) for intravenous (i.v.) administration. Specific excipients may cause toxicity (*e.g.*, yellow dye-induced photodermatitis) or drug interactions (*e.g.*, bentonite in some early preparations of para-aminosalicylic acid (PAS) chelating rifampin; *see* Chap. 8).

Route of Drug Administration

Generally speaking, serious adverse reactions are more common after parenteral administration, particularly by the i.v. route, compared with oral or topical administration. The topical application of some drugs, however—for example, the penicillins—is followed more frequently by sensitivity reactions than is parenteral administration. "Nonabsorbable" drugs given for an effect in the bowel lumen, such as group 4 sulfonamides (*see* Chap. 64), magnesium and aluminum antacids (*see* Chap. 38), and aminoglycoside antibiotics (*see* Chap. 60), are absorbed to a slight degree. Under normal circumstances such absorption is harmless, but with hypersensitivity to the compound or compromised excretory organ function, toxicity may readily develop. Localized toxicity is also common when specific routes of drug administration are used, for example, thrombophlebitis when too concentrated a drug solution is infused intravenously, or chemical meningitis, and neuropathies, after poorly controlled intrathecal drug administration.

Too large a volume should not be injected intramuscularly since necrosis may result. Similarly, drugs intended for subcutaneous (s.c.) or intramuscular (i.m.) injection may be dangerous when accidentally administered intravascularly, and drugs formulated for i.v. injection may cause intense spasm of local arterioles if injected intraarterially.

Number of Drugs Administered

In one detailed epidemiologic study of medical patients, the number of adverse drug reactions was reported to increase exponentially with the number of drugs given (Fig. 11-1). The types of medication given to patients receiving many drugs and those receiving fewer drugs were similar. Furthermore, although patients who received more drugs had a higher mortality and a longer hospital stay than those who received fewer drugs, the types of illnesses in the two groups were not different. Considerable sophistication is required to evaluate the multipotential for drug interactions when many drugs are given together (*see* Chap. 8). The *benefit-risk ratio for each drug usually decreases when multiple drugs are given.*

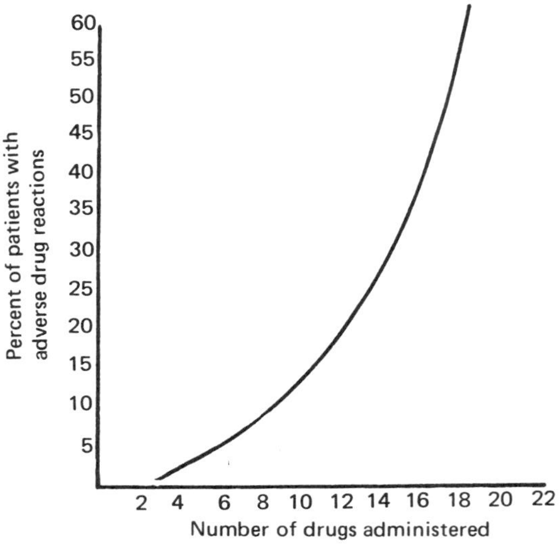

FIG. 11-1. The relationship of rate of adverse drug reactions to number of drugs administered. (Smith JW, Seidl LG, Cluff LE: Studies on the epidemiology of adverse drug reactions: V. Clinical factors influencing susceptibility. Ann Intern Med 65:629–640, 1966)

Drug Dosage and Duration of Treatment

In general, the longer the duration of treatment and the higher the dosage, the greater is the chance of development of adverse drug reactions. Interrupted short courses of some drugs, however, can be just as dangerous, as with antibiotics (*see* Chap. 56).

Most responses to drugs are dose dependent, but drugs may have more than one effect, each with a different dose response, such as sedation, antihistaminic actions, and anticholinergic effects with the H_1-blockers (*see* Chap. 51). Nevertheless, only minute quantities of a drug can generate severe anaphylactic shock in subjects hypersensitive to that agent. Drug dosage must be individually tailored so that the optimally effective dose yielding the fewest side-effects is given.

Addition or Antagonism of Pharmacologic Effects

If the pharmacologic effects of two drugs are additive, adverse drug reactions may develop. A patient taking PAS, for example, may develop salicylism on taking small doses of aspirin (*see* Chap. 31), or *vice versa*. Similarly, atropinism may readily develop if an H_1-blocker and a phenothiazine are combined, since both drugs possess some parasympatholytic activity (*see* Chap. 51). Various additive and antagonistic drug effects may be observed with mixtures of antibiotics (*see* Chap. 56). *Alcohol and H_1-blockers are the most common potentiators of central nervous system depressants, such as diazepam and barbiturates* (*see* Chap. 51).

Combination of Drugs and Adjuvants

Excipients used as repository vehicles for drugs given parenterally may increase their sensitizing potential. Examples are the inclusion of procaine or benzathine in penicillin preparations (*see* Chap. 8) or the use of heparin in oil.

Drug Cost

The high cost of some drugs may increase the rate of patient noncompliance or encourage the patient to "shop around" in an attempt to buy a generically prescribed drug (with possibly altered bioavailability characteristics) more cheaply.

PREDISPOSING PATIENT (HOST) FACTORS: INTRINSIC

Patient variables may alter the pharmacodynamics or pharmacokinetics of drugs, producing adverse effects. Computer-based data-gathering programs, such as the Boston Collaborative Drug Surveillance Program (*see* Chap. 82), will undoubtedly identify numerous other important factors.

Age

At the extremes of life, the functions of absorption, metabolism, and excretion may be imperfectly developed, as in the newborn (particularly the premature infant), or diminished, as in the elderly subject (*see* Chaps. 7, 11). Furthermore, the responsiveness of certain tissues and homeostatic mechanisms may be different from those in the healthy adult, and the ability of the body to oppose drug effects may be altered. Thus therapy based on pharmacokinetic data derived from adults may lead to unexpected toxicity or failure of therapy. The developing fetus is particularly susceptible to drug effects (*see* below).

Pediatric Age Group. Compared with adults, children have a more rapid gastrointestinal transit time, a higher body water content (70% to 75% compared to 60%), a relatively smaller body surface area, differences in tissue distribution of drugs (*e.g.*, the relative permeability of the blood brain barrier), a relatively low glomerular filtration rate and renal plasma flow, plasma proteins that do not bind drugs as well, and difficulty (and therefore unreliability) with oral therapy. These factors may influence the development of adverse drug reactions (*see* also Chap. 7).

Geriatric Age Group. In 60- to 70-year-old persons the risk of an adverse drug reaction is about double that in a young adult. This risk results predominantly from a diminution in the function of the organs of metabolism and excretion due to age or associated disease. For example, symptom-free patients of 65 years of age may have lost as much as 50% of their renal glomerular and tubular functions. Diminished renal function is accentuated by such states as dehydration, congestive heart failure, urinary retention, and electrolyte abnormalities. Thus, drugs excreted by the kidney may rapidly achieve high plasma levels in geriatric patients if dosage is not adjusted downwards.

Geriatric patients may have reduced sensitivity (responsiveness) to some drugs compared with adults. Therefore, a gradual loss in sensitivity of autonomic reflexes in the cardiovascular system may influence the response of patients to drugs such as guanethidine (*see* Chap. 36). Similarly, phenothiazines are more prone to produce Parkinson's disease in the elderly. Emotional problems and cerebral arteriosclerosis can contribute to unintentional drug abuse, imperfect compliance (*see* below), or an irrational attitude toward a drug reaction.

Weight and Body Composition

Body weight, composition (especially fat content), and degree of physical fitness may be important. For example, phenobarbital (a nonpolar drug) rapidly accumulates in adipose tissue, from where it is slowly released to act on the central nervous system (*see* Chaps. 3, 25, 28). Thus the pattern and deviation of pharmacologic effects of this agent will vary with the amount of body fat. In general, drugs should be given in doses based on *ideal* rather than *actual* body weight.

Sex

Although various sex differences in drug distribution, response, and metabolism have been described in animals, these are not (excluding those associated with pregnancy and lactation; *see* below) of major importance in humans. Epidemiologic studies have shown that drug reactions are two to three times more common in women than in men. For example, blood dyscrasias with phenylbutazone, aminopyrine, and chloramphenicol have an unexplained 3:1 preponderance in women. The reason for the preponderance of reactions in women is not known, but women may have a greater tendency to seek care or report reactions. Moreover, many reactions may be due specifically to treatment of obstetric or gynecologic conditions. For example, oral contraceptive steroids retard drug metabolism, whereas androgens are enzyme inducers and the half-lives of some drugs vary with the menstrual cycle.

Sex differences influence the severity of some diseases in humans, for example, essential hypertension. Since hypertension is usually associated with greater end-organ damage in men than women, more potent drugs tend to be used in men. Finally, sex-linked genetic factors may be important, such as glucose-6-phosphate dehydrogenase (*see* Chap. 6).

Race and Heredity

Pharmacogenetics. Genetic polymorphisms of drug metabolism can be responsible for the production of adverse drug reactions (*see* Chap. 6).

Blood Group

Associations between blood group and secretor status and various disease states, although unexplained, have been recognized for many years. For example, women of blood group A recently have been found to be nearly three times more likely to develop vascular complications while receiving oral contraceptive steroids than are women of blood group O.

Temperament

Emotional, sensitive, frail, asthenic, high strung, hypochondriacal subjects report more adverse drug reactions and tend to be greater placebo responders (*see* Chap. 10) than more stable, stoic persons. Geriatric patients may have wide swings of mood owing to cerebral arteriosclerosis and other factors and thus suffer more "subjective" drug reactions.

Skin Color

Melanin in the skin protects against injury by external agents, such as radiant energy. Thus photodermatitis (*see* below) is very rare in black subjects, not uncommon in white persons, and frequent in albinos of any race.

History of Drug Reaction

Patients with previous drug reactions are at greater risk of experiencing second reactions (Table 11-3).

TABLE 11-3. Incidence of Adverse Drug Reactions in Relation to History of Drug Reactions and to Drug Allergy

	Reaction Rate	
History	*United States**	*United Kingdom†*
	%	
No previous reaction	9	9
Previous reaction	14	28
No history of allergy	11	9
Previous allergies	13	28

* (Smith JW, Seidl LG, Cluff LE: Studies on the Epidemiology of Adverse Drug Reactions. Ann Intern Med 65:629, 1966)

† (Hurwitz N: Predisposing factors in adverse reactions to drugs. Br Med J 1:536, 1969)

Allergic Diathesis

Drug allergy is more likely to develop in patients with an "allergic diathesis" (eczema, hay fever, asthma, hives, urticaria, angioedema) than in nonhypersensitive persons (Table 11-3). In patients with ulcerative gastrointestinal disease, drug allergy to orally administered drugs may be more likely to develop than in other persons. A patient known to have suffered an allergic drug reaction should not be exposed again to the offending agent or to related chemicals without full consideration of the risk of inducing fatal anaphylaxis. In one study, the penicillins, streptomycin, barbiturates, meprobamate, codeine, and the thiazide diuretics were responsible for 70% of the allergic reactions encountered. Penicillin allergy is covered more fully in Chapter 59; little is known about allergies to other drugs.

Concomitant Disease

Specific disease-states may predispose to adverse drug reactions in several ways. For example, *multiple drug therapy* is often required (*e.g.*, in infections, edema, heart failure, hypertension), a situation predisposing to adverse drug reactions (*see* above).

Disease of the organs of drug absorption, metabolism, and excretion; congenital anomalies; or other drugs may significantly alter drug pharmacodynamics and or pharmacokinetics. Numerous examples are given throughout the text and in Chapters 5, 6, and 8.

Little is known about the way disease states may alter drug handling or tissue sensitivity. Many diseases are associated with hypoproteinemia or hyperproteinemia, but whether plasma protein binding of drugs is significantly altered in these situations is not clear. Certainly, low serum albumin levels have been associated with increased phenytoin and prednisone toxicity; reduced protein binding of many drugs, for example, the sulfonamides, occurs in uremia.

Drugs may exaggerate overt disease, or they may precipitate latent disease. For example, hyperuricemia may be produced directly (ethionamide, pyrazinamide, and thiazide diuretics) or indirectly (methotrexate), precipitating gout; glucocorticosteroids can "induce" diabetes mellitus (*see* Chap. 47); barbiturates and griseofulvin, by inducing the synthesis of δ aminolevulinic acid, may precipitate acute hepatic porphyria; neuromuscular blockade in patients with myasthenia gravis is accentuated by aminoglycoside antibiotics and various antimalarial agents; patients with the Crigler-Najjar syndrome develop jaundice with drugs that are cleared via glucuronidation, since glucuronyl transferase is poorly developed in such patients, and the drugs compete successfully with bilirubin for the enzyme. Numerous other examples are given throughout the text.

Drug reactions are more likely to develop in patients with infections. The reason is unclear, but experimentally the central nervous system toxicity of some drugs is increased in the presence of fever.

Physiological Status

Pregnancy. Major alterations in body function develop during pregnancy. It has been suggested, for example, that the increased demand for protein anabolism makes the liver more susceptible to drugs like the tetracyclines, which depress this function (*see* Chap. 61). Moreover, during pregnancy the metabolism of some drugs (*e.g.*, succinylcholine) is delayed, and transport processes that clear drugs (*e.g.*, sulfobromophthalein) through the liver cell are depressed. Changes in hemodynamics and renal function may alter drug clearance and response. The fetus may suffer adverse drug reactions (*see* below).

Lactation. Many drugs are excreted in breast milk (*see* Table 81-26) and thus can produce adverse effects in breast-fed infants.

Circadian and Other Physiological Variations. Many physiological variations occur in the body during the day, and these functions may alter if a patient is placed on a regimen of complete bed rest. Moreover, prolonged bed rest is associated with a reduced plasma volume and depressed cardiovascular function. Stresses of heat, exercise, and fluid deprivation may alter the rate of drug metabolism, and circadian effects with regard to drug absorption, metabolism, and excretion are only now being identified (*see* Chaps. 47, 51). Daily fluctuations in urinary *p*H occur, particularly in relation to meals, and this may alter the excretion of weak electrolytes (*see* Chap. 8).

The normal human organism is populated by several hundred different microorganisms, particularly in the gastrointestinal tract. That this microflora is important in drug metabolism is just being realized (*see* Chap. 4): For example, patients stabilized on anticoagulants usually need their dose adjusted downward if broad-spectrum antibiotics are added to the drug regimen (*see* Chap. 8).

Social Awareness

A patient's expectations and perspectives about drug reactions and effects often vary depending on how they are viewed in the community. Thus, for example, American women complained more of the adverse effects of oral contraceptives than did women of a non-American social environment, even though the groups experienced similar drug effects.

Patient Noncompliance and Errors of Drug Administration

Patients may interfere with therapy either by not following directions or by self-medication. The patient who does not comply with drug therapy is usually poorly compliant with other aspects of management, such as dietary restrictions, termination of tobacco smoking, and exercise regimens. Patients may take either more or less than the prescribed dose; both usually result in suboptimal therapy. The common (and fallacious) rationale for taking more than the prescribed dose is "if three of these pills a day are making me better, six of them a day will make me better twice as quickly." However, taking drugs irregularly is far more common than overmedication. A careful study of 40 patients receiving a total of 143 different drugs in a medical clinic indicated that only 10% were taking their drugs as prescribed. Noncompliance rates of 20% to 80% have been reported in studies involving antibiotics, antacids, antidepressants, and antimalarials. Noncompliance may be serious; for example, in a

---

JOHN F. CRIGLER, JR., 1919– . American pediatrician. In 1950, reported Crigler–Najjar syndrome, a form of congenital hyperbilirubinemia with brain damage. Special interest in pediatric endocrinology.

VICTOR ASSAD NAJJAR, 1914– . Lebanese-born pediatrician, came to the United States in 1938. Co-reporter of Crigler–Najjar syndrome. Special interest in vitamin metabolism, immunochemistry, and enzyme chemistry.

study of patients with congestive heart failure, 92% continued to take their digitalis as prescribed, whereas 83% took their thiazide diuretic and only 60% continued to take potassium supplements, thus encouraging digitalis toxicity (*see* Chap. 33).

Noncompliance is more difficult to predict than to detect since the causes are poorly understood, but correlations between noncompliance and various factors have been determined (Table 11-4). Two important points are clear: Noncompliance increases with increasing dose (increasing number of tablets) and the number of different drugs prescribed, and *in many instances, failure to comply results from failure of the physician to fully inform the patient about the drug, its purpose, and its dosage schedule.*

Consequences of Noncompliance. The consequences of noncompliance are either adverse drug reactions or apparent therapeutic failure. Failure to take an antibiotic regularly often leads to relapse of the original infection, emergence of resistant organisms, or suprainfection (*see* Chap. 56). On occasion, however, no real disadvantage can be observed. For example, in a study of antacid therapy in the treatment of peptic ulcer disease, noncompliance was not associated with increased morbidity, suggesting that antacids may have a minimal role, if any, in therapy!

Since noncompliance rates are high, noncompliance should be suspected in every patient. Many techniques for measuring the degree of noncompliance have been tried but they are rarely foolproof. Direct measurements of the concentration of a drug or its metabolite in urine or feces or tests for the presence of an inert marker (*e.g.*, riboflavin-produced fluorescence) are more satisfactory than pill counting, special drug dispensers, or quantitation of a measurable side effect (such as dry mouth with atropine). Tests that can directly measure drug effect (such as prothrombin time) are most valuable.

TABLE 11-4. Patients Likely to be Noncompliant or factors contributing to, or associated with, patient noncompliance

Children, particularly when poorly supervised
Geriatric subjects
Disadvantaged subjects
Patients living alone
Single or divorced patients
Low socioeconomic status
Psychiatric disease or other personality disorder
Occurrence of an adverse drug reaction
Unfamiliar or uncommunicative physicians
Unhelpful or uncommunicative pharmacists
Drug administration more frequent than once per day
Chronic illness with chronic therapy
Increasing the number of drugs

The best treatment for noncompliance is prophylaxis. Physicians should thoroughly explain drug therapy to the patient, giving the drug name, its purpose, and how it should be taken. In addition, any prescription drugs, over-the-counter drugs, or foods that might interfere with the agent should be identified.

Self-Medication

Self-medication with drugs remaining from previous prescriptions or with over-the-counter preparations (tonics, vitamins, aspirin, iron tablets, laxatives, dimethyl sulfoxide) is not unusual and may lead to drug interactions (*see* Chap. 8). Similarly, care must be taken with regard to drugs the patient may be taking concomitantly that were prescribed by another physician. One of the most important parts of history taking is a thorough inquiry into the nature and dosage of all drugs taken in the immediate past.

PREDISPOSING PATIENT (HOST) FACTORS: EXTRINSIC

Diet, Environment, and Climate

Foods may alter the rate or degree of drug absorption, and tobacco smoking and ethanol are potent enzyme inducers (*see* Chap. 8). For example, tobacco smoking increases the activity of benzpyrene reductase and hepatic oxidases, and heavy cigarette smokers are less likely than nonsmokers to suffer excessive sedation from benzodiazepines. Exposure to DDT and other insecticides is unavoidable for almost everybody in the United States, and some foodstuffs contain up to 5 ppm of DDT, a concentration that causes enzyme induction in animals. Many other common substances produce enzyme induction (*see* Table 8-5), and some industrial solvents can produce hepatic or renal damage. Extreme heat or cold is associated with hypovolemia or hypervolemia, respectively, with concomitant development of changes in pH and electrolytes in tissue fluids. Hypoxia (living at high altitude) is a stimulus to enzyme induction. Picas, such as clay or starch eating, can be associated with drug interactions. Undoubtedly many other environmental and dietary factors are unknown.

PERSONNEL FACTORS

Influence of the Physician

Physicians may be tempted to use drugs when little or no clinical benefit can be expected, for example, the unwise prophylactic use of antibiotics, or the use of digitalis glycosides in subjects with heart failure secondary to aortic stenosis or mitral insufficiency, when clinical benefits are typically minimal. Under such circumstances, digitalis may be "pushed" to toxic levels in an attempt to produce some clinical improvement.

Influence of the Nurse

Some degree of error is inevitable in all human performance, but studies have indicated that in some hospitals (where the quality of drug therapy should be at the highest level), between 10% and 20% of all doses of medication were incorrect. A careful study of nine nurses in a teaching hospital indicated that there was one error in every six drug doses ordered. Statistically, 40% were omission of a dose, 20% were the administration of a drug not ordered, and 40% were drugs administered at the wrong time, in the wrong dosage form, in an extra dose, or in under- or overdosage. It is hoped that the fraction of errors in this example is extreme, but nursing medication mistakes increase logarithmically with the number of drugs prescribed.

Influence of the Pharmacist

The pharmacist is an integral cog in the health care team and not only may affect patient compliance significantly, but also may contribute to the development of adverse drug reactions through errors in prescription, labeling, or other aspects.

CLASSIFICATION OF ADVERSE DRUG REACTIONS

Adverse drug reactions are difficult to classify because of the many variables or "risk" factors that may influence their development and because the definition of such a reaction is often not clear-cut. A simple classification based primarily on pathogenic mechanisms is given here that, although by no means comprehensive, should clarify this heterogeneous and complex subject; many categories overlap. Specific reactions and the drugs that may cause them are tabulated in Chapter 81.

REACTIONS ASSOCIATED WITH THERAPEUTIC EFFECTS OF DRUGS

Many adverse reactions are produced through an extension of a therapeutic effect. *Overdosage* is seen when too large a dose of an agent is given, for example, respiratory depression and coma with the barbiturates or hemorrhage with the anticoagulants. Overdosage may also occur with standard therapeutic doses owing to failure of drug metabolism or excretion, such as antibiotic toxicity in the presence of renal failure, the gray baby syndrome with chloramphenicol (*see* Chap. 61), or succinylcholine sensitivity (*see* Chap. 6).

A therapeutically useful action of a drug may be harmful when it involves a tissue other than the target organ, for example, with autonomic or anticancer agents (*see* Chaps. 15, 16, 71).

Depression of host "resistance" is a direct extension of the mode of action of many drugs that interfere with leukocyte function, lysosomal activity, and immune mechanisms. Examples occur with glucocorticosteroids (*see* Chap. 47), immunosuppressants (*see* Table 56-1), and anticancer drugs (*see* Chap. 71).

Depression of the inflammatory and repair processes is the basis of the use of glucocorticosteroids and immunosuppressive agents in autoimmune and some chronic inflammatory diseases and in suppression of graft-versus-host reactions. However, in some situations (*e.g.*, peptic ulcer disease, postoperative wound healing), such effects may be dangerous.

Interference with the normal body flora may lead to suprainfections (*see* Chap. 56) and often poses a therapeutic problem. For example, antibiotic suppression of the normal bacterial flora in the bowel may lead to symptoms of vitamin B deficiency or to an altered responsiveness to anticoagulants (*see* Chap. 8) or methotrexate (*see* Chap. 71).

REACTIONS ASSOCIATED WITH NONTHERAPEUTIC EFFECTS OF DRUGS

Direct pharmacologic effects are very common. Drowsiness from the H_1-blockers or morphine-induced constipation are typical examples. Reactions associated with the intensification of concurrent disease are an exceedingly important category. Thus a patient with peptic ulcer may have a relapse if treated with certain drugs (*see* Table 38-4). Similarly, hepatic coma may follow administration of morphine, ammonium chloride, or thiazide diuretics in patients with cirrhosis.

Many drugs cause local tissue irritation. Upper gastrointestinal symptoms (nausea, vomiting, dyspepsia, heartburn) are common after oral administration of many drugs, especially antibiotics, iron preparations, and aspirin. These are mild adverse effects, and slight reduction in dosage or proper spacing of the drug in relation to meals usually reduces symptoms. Similarly, hypertonic or hypotonic parenteral injections may cause considerable local edema or pain. Occasionally a sterile abscess develops after a large parenteral injection or repeated injections to the same muscle of, for example, an iron-dextran complex. Tetracycline antibiotics are notoriously prone to produce thrombophlebitis (due to endothelial irritation) after i.v. administration.

Tissue deposition of drug crystals may develop in the urinary tract, as in sulfonamide crystalluria (*see* Chap. 64). Some drugs can produce blockade of nutrient absorption. For example, several agents produce malabsorption (*see* Table 81-27). Similarly, barbiturates and phenytoin may block the absorption of folic acid, resulting in megaloblastic anemia.

Delayed adverse effects may be seen after the use of radioactive drugs. Thorium dioxide (Thorotrast), for example, used for many years as a radio-opaque dye in arteriography, is stored in the reticuloendothelial system and has been incriminated, after a latency of up to 20 years, in producing generalized atrophy, fibrosis, and malignant degeneration, especially in the liver. Similarly, the use of radioactive iodine (^{131}I) in the treatment of hyperthyroidism has been linked with the subsequent development of thyroid carcinoma and leukemia.

Effects due to drug degradation have been discussed above.

REACTIONS ASSOCIATED WITH ALLERGY

Hypersensitivity (allergic) reactions represent the largest single group of adverse drug reactions. While most drugs are capable of producing an allergic response, penicillin, streptomycin, the sulfonamides, and quinidine are notorious offenders. To give rise to an allergic reaction, the drug, drug metabolite(s) (haptene), or drug contaminants must combine strongly with a tissue or plasma protein. This complex is processed by the reticuloendothelial system, with the ultimate production of specific antibody. Antibodies can react with both the complex and the haptene, but our knowledge of their production is far from clear. Antibodies against the offending drug or its metabolites cannot be demonstrated in every case of suspected drug allergy, and reexposure of the patient to the original drug may not elicit an allergic reaction.

There are four main categories of allergic drug reactions: type I (anaphylaxis), type II (cytotoxic), type III (immune complex-mediated), and type IV (delayed hypersensitivity).

REACTIONS ASSOCIATED WITH SUNLIGHT

By far the most important precipitating exogenous factor is sunlight, and reactions are either phototoxic or photoallergic (Table 11-5). In addition, drug photosensitivity has been documented in at least three diseases: porphyria, lupus erythematosus, and pellagra. Phototoxic reactions occur when a nontoxic substance is converted into a toxic one in the patient's skin by the absorption of photoenergy. Photoallergic reactions occur when the absorption of photo energy by a chemical converts it into a metabolite that may then sensitize the patient. Photosensitization may also arise after topical exposure of various compounds, particularly antiseptics and antibiotics in soaps, hair rinses, shampoos, perfumes, and antiseptic creams (Table 81-8). Drugs that produce photoallergies absorb light in the ultraviolet and near-ultraviolet range. Thus blue discoloration after exposure to ultraviolet light occurs only in those phenothiazine derivatives that are able to induce photoallergy, not in other representatives of this class. Similar changes have been noted with the tetracyclines and the sulfonamides. Photoallergic rashes may persist for long periods after termination of drug exposure. The patient may remain permanently sensitized to the offending drug, even in the absence of sunlight.

REACTIONS ASSOCIATED WITH PREGNANCY AND FETAL DEVELOPMENT

Effects on Reproduction

Parasympatholytic drugs (*see* Chap. 16) may produce impotence. Thorazine and related psychopharmacologic agents have been shown to interfere with ejaculation without affecting orgasm.

PHILIP GEORGE HOUTHEN GELL, 1914– . British pathologist and immunologist.

TABLE 11-5. Characteristics of Drug-Induced Photosensitivity

Reaction	Phototoxic	Photoallergic
Reaction possible on first exposure	Yes	No
Incubation period necessary after first exposure	No	Yes
Chemical alteration of photosensitizer	No	Yes
Covalent binding with carrier	No	Yes
Clinical changes	Usually like sunburn	Varied morphology
"Flares" at distant previously involved sites possible	No	Yes
Can persistent light reaction develop	No	Yes
Cross-reactions to structurally related agents	Infrequent	Frequent
Broadening of cross-reactions following repeated photo-patch testing	No	Possible
Concentration of drug necessary for reaction	High	Low
Incidence	Usually relatively high (theoretically 100%)	Usually very low (but theoretically could reach 100%)
Action spectrum	Usually similar to absorption spectrum	Usually higher wavelength than absorption spectrum
Passive transfer	No	Possible
Lymphocyte stimulation test	No	Possible
Macrophage migration inhibition test	No	Possible

(Baer RL, Harber LC: Reactions to light, heat, and trauma. In Swater M (ed): Immunologic Diseases, Volume II. Boston, Little, Brown & Co, 1971)

Effects During Intrauterine Development

Adverse drug effects are nowhere more dramatically evident than in the fetus and neonate. Most drugs with a molecular weight of 1000 or less can easily cross the placental barrier (*see* Table 81-25). The effects of rubella virus (German measles) during the first trimester of pregnancy are well known. Of more importance and not generally recognized is that many drugs can cause similar effects. The effect of a drug given early in pregnancy may be fetal death. During organogenesis, in the first trimester, malformations may be produced. Later in pregnancy or during labor, drugs may cause fetal morbidity or death. Morbidity in the perinatal period is more common in premature infants.

Drug exposure during pregnancy is unfortunately commonplace. Studies have reported that 82% to 92% of women were given at least one drug during pregnancy, with four being the average number of drugs prescribed; 4% of patients were given ten drugs or more.

Teratogenesis. The thalidomide disaster focused attention on the potential danger of administering drugs during pregnancy. Although thalidomide is no longer available, a brief discussion of the incident is instructive.

A German pharmaceutical firm in the late 1950s developed thalidomide, a drug that induced sleep without residual hangover. Subsequently, because of its apparently minimal side effects, thalidomide was manufactured and sold in many countries, often combined with analgesics, hypnotics, and antiinflammatory drugs. Some 90 different brand names under which thalidomide was sold have been identified. The first cases of phocomelia, or seal limbs (Figs. 11-2 and 11-3), were detected in Germany in September 1960, and since then, according to the German minister of health, approximately 6000 cases have been reported in that country alone. Of these patients, about half have died. Besides phocomelia, malformations of the gastrointestinal tract, ears, and heart were seen. Facial hemangiomas were fairly common, but the babies were usually normal mentally. Parenthetically, it should be stressed that the only notable adverse effect in adults taking thalidomide is peripheral neuritis.

The critical time during organogenesis for an individual tissue to be affected by teratogenic agents is usually considered to be the time that coincides with the greatest mitotic activity in that organ. For example, the limb buds exhibit maximal susceptibility between 18 and 28 days of gestation, or, in other words, 38 to 48 days after the first day of the last menstrual period. This indicates the importance of not exposing women of childbearing age to un-

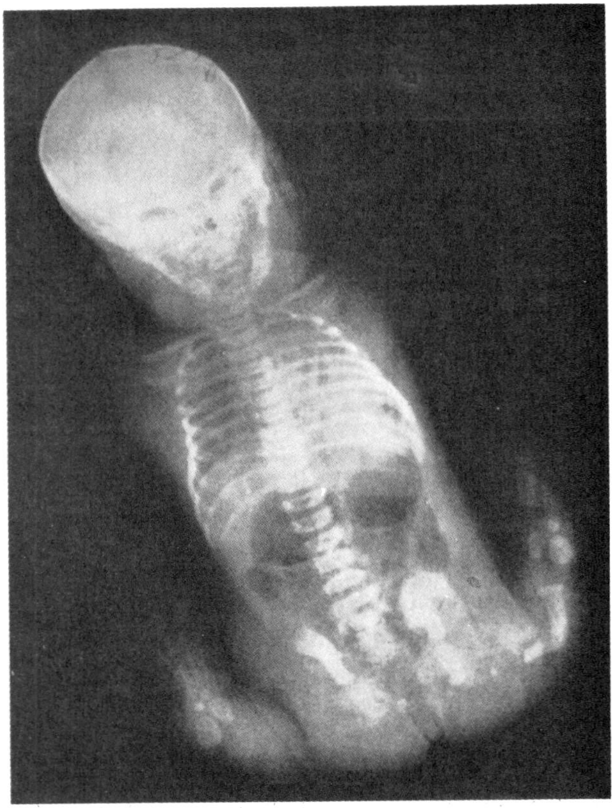

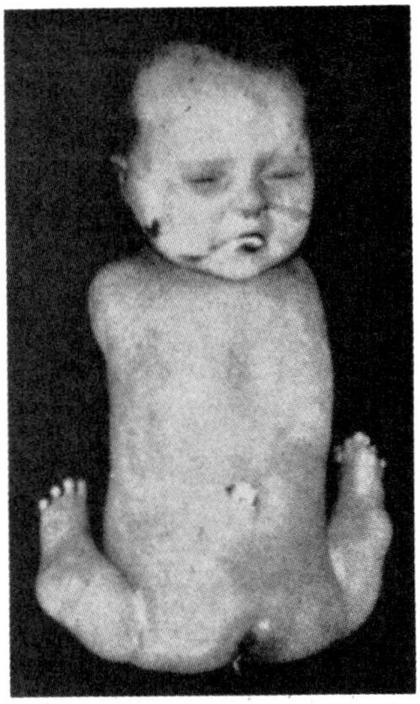

FIG. 11-2. Female infant who died 24 hours after birth. (Ward, Shirley P: Br Med J 8: 646, 1962. Reprinted from the *British Medical Journal* by permission of the author, editor, and publishers, B.M.A. House, Tavistock Square, London, W.C. 1)

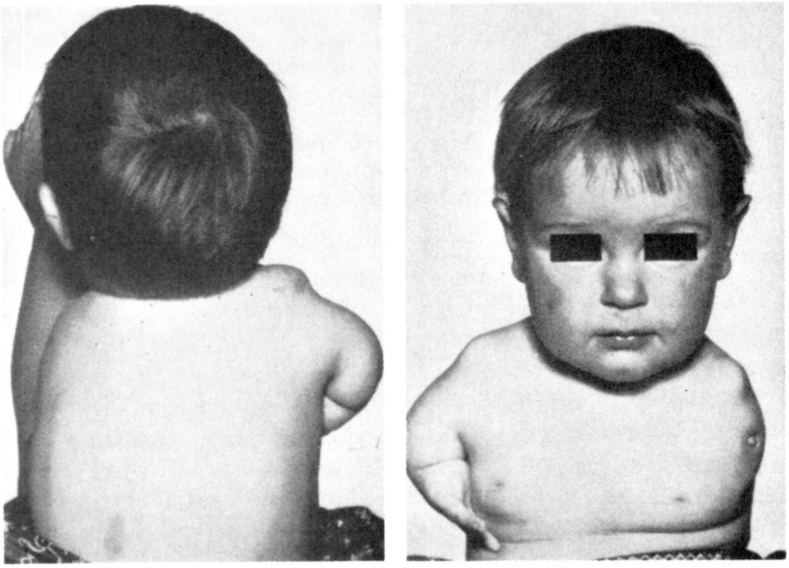

FIG. 11-3. Boy, aged 18 months, whose mother had taken thalidomide during early pregnancy. Note saddle nose and hemangioma situated on the right cheek. The left upper limb is absent; on the right side there is a rudimentary humerus, no radius, and two rudimentary digits. (Gillis L: Br Med J, September 8, 1962. Reprinted from the *British Medical Journal* by permission of the author, editor, and publishers, B.M.A. House, Tavistock Square, London, W.C. 1)

necessary medication, as teratogenic effects may be produced before pregnancy is diagnosed or even suspected.

Many experiments have been undertaken in animals in an attempt to demonstrate thalidomide teratogenicity. Most have been unsuccessful. This poses the question of how accurate and useful are animal experiments in predicting the potential toxicity of new drugs to humans (*see* Chap. 10).

Several other potent pharmacologic agents, including anticancer drugs, sulfonylureas, and corticosteroids, are suspected of being teratogenic.

Masculinization of the Female Fetus. Before embryonic sexual structures differentiate, they are susceptible to the influence of exogenous endocrine agents. Female pseudohermaphroditism, for example, has been produced by testosterone (given for hyperemesis gravidarum) and by a variety of synthetic progestational agents commonly used in the treatment of habitual or threatened abortion.

Perinatal Effects

Drugs given to the mother before or during labor may cross the placenta, and the baby may be born still under their influence (*see* Table 81-25). In most instances, the drug is an anesthetic, analgesic, tranquilizer, antidiabetogenic agent, antibiotic, or antihypertensive. Side-effects of simple overdose tend to result, similar to those seen in adults. Paralytic ileus from antihypertensive drugs and ventilatory depression after reserpine, hypnotics, and narcotics are not unusual. Occasionally, barbiturates induce hemorrhagic disease of the newborn owing to depression of the Stuart–Prower factor.

Neonatal Effects

The neonate is not just a miniature young adult. This point is discussed above under Age Factors and in Chapter 7.

MISCELLANEOUS REACTIONS

Effects After Use of Placebos

The basic emotional pattern of a patient may influence his or her response to drugs. This is particularly true of drugs affecting the central nervous system and of placebos. Many physicians have observed mild adverse reactions to placebos, such as depression, sleepiness, sleeplessness, anorexia, nausea, tremulousness, dizziness, palpitations, and lassitude. Some puzzling severe reactions to placebos have been reported, such as fixed drug eruptions, anaphylactic shock, and even death. Many "reactions" to placebos are in reality an expression of "adverse" nondrug reactions (Table 11-1).

A placebo is by definition innocuous. It is a pharmacologically inert agent, or a food substance (iron capsule, bread pill, sugar pill, vitamin C tablet). No substance should be used as a placebo if there is even remote danger of a harmful effect. Thus aspirin should not be used, especially in children. Similarly, the ever-present danger of serum hepatitis makes it impossible to guarantee the harmlessness of parenteral injections of normal saline, a common placebo. On the other hand, failing to recognize the need for precise treatment and substituting a placebo for necessary drug (or psychiatric) therapy is also a danger. Megadoses of many vitamins are potentially toxic (*see* Chaps. 8, 73).

Drug Interactions

Adverse drug reactions may develop through drug interactions (*see* Chap. 8).

Effects on Laboratory and Diagnostic Procedures

It is now recognized that many commonly prescribed drugs can invalidate diagnostic tests (*see* Chap. 79). Furthermore, drugs may produce pathologic changes in tissue; for example, a megaloblastic bone marrow may be associated with ingestion of barbiturates, and lymph node changes suggestive of sarcoidosis or lymphoma may attend phenytoin administration.

Effects Owing to Failure to Institute Correct Therapy

Frequently drugs are prescribed because the patient expects a pill. In these instances (by giving a potentially harmful agent without a true indication for its use), the physician can be criticized justifiably. For example, the administration of antibiotics to patients with uncomplicated coryza is therapeutically unsound. On the other hand, indirect harm can be caused by postponing correct therapy.

A related topic of particular importance in the United States is the long time lag in Food and Drug Administration approval of new drugs developed overseas (*see* Chap. 10).

FURTHER READING

1. Forfar JO, Nelson MM: Epidemiology of drugs taken by pregnant women: Drugs that may affect the fetus adversely. Clin Pharmacol Ther 14:632–642, 1974

The Stuart–Prower blood clotting factor, later identified with the previously described Factor X, was named for the first two patients studied, in 1956 and 1957.

2. Harber LC, Baer RL: Pathogenic mechanisms of drug-induced photosensitivity. J Invest Dermatol 58:327–342, 1972
3. Hurtwitz N: Predisposing factors in adverse reactions to drugs. Br Med J 1:536, 1969
4. Martin EW: Hazards of Medication, 2nd ed. Philadelphia, JB Lippincott, 1978
5. Smith JW, Seidl LG, Cluff LE: Studies on the epidemiology of adverse drug reactions. Ann Intern Med 65:629, 1966
6. Smithells RW: Drugs and human malformations. Adv Teratol 1:251, 1966
7. Zbiden G: Experimental and clinical aspects of drug toxicity. Adv Pharmacol 2:1, 1963

CHAPTER 11 QUESTIONS

(*See* P. 7 for Full Instructions)

Select the One Best Answer

1. In each of the following a skin eruption is paired with an agent that characteristically produces the eruption EXCEPT
   A. erythema multiforme—penicillin G.
   B. fixed eruption—phenolphthalein.
   C. photosensitization—tetracycline HCl.
   D. erythema nodosum—mineral oil.
   E. acneiform eruption—bromide.

2. Which of the following substances would be the most likely causative agent for the agranulocytosis that develops in a house painter?
   A. Lead
   B. Mineral spirits
   C. Turpentine
   D. Benzene
   E. Titanium dioxide

3. Each of the following drugs is properly paired with its characteristic effect on blood cells EXCEPT
   A. lead—Heinz bodies.
   B. quinine—thrombocytopenia.
   C. trimethadione—hemolytic anemia.
   D. chloramphenicol—aplastic anemia.
   E. phenylbutazone—agranulocytosis.

4. An adverse effect that chlorpromazine, phenytoin, and methyltestosterone have in common is
   A. gum hyperplasia.
   B. extrapyramidal reactions.
   C. jaundice.
   D. excessive body hair.
   E. induction of lactation.

5. Phenytoin, methotrexate, and pyrimethamine can cause symptoms of deficiency of
   A. folic acid.
   B. vitamin B_{12}.
   C. thiamine.
   D. riboflavin.
   E. nicotinic acid.

A = 1,2,3; B = 1,3; C = 2,4; D = 4; E = All

6. Systemic anaphylacticlike reactions can be produced by the parenteral administration of
   1. iron dextran.
   2. iodinated organic contrast materials.
   3. morphine.
   4. procaine.

7. Aplastic anemia has been associated with exposure to
   1. phenacemide.
   2. tolbutamide.
   3. benzene.
   4. trimethadione.

8. Severe hepatic damage may occur
   1. in tuberculous patients treated with isoniazid.
   2. commonly after anesthesia with ether.
   3. after attempted suicide with acetaminophen.
   4. in most chronic abusers of phenobarbital.

9. The use of iodides in treating bronchial asthma can lead to
   1. pain and swelling of the parotid gland.
   2. hypothyroidism.
   3. acneiform eruptions of the skin.
   4. rhinorrhea.

10. Deafness may be a side-effect of
   1. furosemide.
   2. streptomycin.
   3. ethacrynic acid.
   4. tetracycline hydrochloride.

Prescription Writing

12

DIANE ZALBA, MERCEDES TOKORCHECK

The prescription has come to represent more than written instructions by a physician to a pharmacist for the preparation of a medication. It is a summary of the physician's diagnosis and proposed drug treatment and a method of instructing the patient on the proper method of taking the prescribed medication. Thus the prescription is the instrument by which the science of pharmacology is applied to the practice of medicine.

One of the earliest records of prescription writing is contained in the Ebers Papyrus, an Egyptian medical compendium dating back to about 1700 B.C. The importance of drug therapy in Egyptian medicine is demonstrated by the fact that the largest portion of the compendium is devoted to pharmaceutical prescriptions. These prescriptions or recipes resemble modern prescriptions in that they consist of a title, the disease for which the recipe was to be used, a list of the name and amount of each ingredient, compounding instructions, and directions for the patient.

LAWS REGULATING THE PRESCRIBING AND DISPENSING OF DRUGS

The practice of ordering medication for a particular patient, or "prescribing," is closely governed by a number of federal and state regulations.

FEDERAL REGULATIONS

Federal regulations classify drugs into two categories. An *over-the-counter* (OTC) drug is a "drug preparation which may be safely employed in self-treatment and which is properly labeled with directions for use." Such drugs may be obtained without a prescription.

Prescription or *legend* drugs are those limited to dispensing by, or upon an order from a legally authorized practitioner (physician, dentist, veterinarian, podiatrist) because they have been determined to be habit forming, toxic, or have the potential for harm.

The two major laws that affect the handling of drugs from their manufacture, distribution, and sale to their disposition to the patient are the *Federal Food, Drug and Cosmetic Act* of 1938 and the *Federal Comprehensive Drug Abuse Prevention and Control Act* of 1970.

The Federal Food, Drug and Cosmetic Act of 1938

Enacted to assure the quality and purity of drugs by requiring accurate labeling, this act's enforcement is entrusted to the Food and Drug Administration (FDA). The Drug Amendment Act of 1962 expanded the responsibility of the FDA to include an evaluation of the efficacy and safety of new drugs as well as those drugs already in general use.

In the last 12 years, the FDA has begun to issue a number of regulations aimed at increasing patient awareness of possible drug side-effects. For example, in 1970, a regulation was issued that required a summary of potential benefits and risks associated with the use of oral contraceptives be included in each package of the drug given to a patient. In 1980, the FDA published regulations in an attempt to initiate procedures for the preparation and distribution of patient package inserts (PPIs) for ten classes of drugs (ampicillin, benzodiazepines, cimetidine, clofibrate, digoxin, methoxsalen, thiazides, phenytoin, propoxyphene, and warfarin). Such PPIs would contain a summary of the potential risks and benefits associated with each drug, directions for use, and information on proper storage and handling. These PPIs are intended to be given to each patient to whom the drug is initially dispensed.

The Federal Comprehensive Drug Abuse Prevention and Control Act of 1970

This 1970 federal act regulates the manufacture, distribution, and sale (dispensing/administration) of certain chemicals identified as "controlled substances," which are drugs subject to or having a potential for abuse or physical and/or psychological dependence. Enforcement of this act is entrusted to the Drug Enforcement Administration (DEA).

Owing to the potential for abuse, all persons involved with controlled substances, from procurement to distribution or dispensing, must be federally registered. Thus medical practitioners who wish to prescribe controlled substances must obtain authorization from the state in which they are licensed to prescribe as well as registering with the DEA. Only under special circumstances (*i.e.*, federal and state government practice settings such as the Veteran Administration Hospitals) may a practitioner be considered exempt from registration.

Under the act, controlled substances are classified into five schedules (*see* Table 12-1). The requirements placed on the medical practitioner when writing a prescription for a controlled substances may vary according to the drug's schedule. However, each prescription for a controlled substances must include the practitioner's DEA registration number.

The Poison Prevention Act of 1970

Another federal regulation that affects the handling of drugs, the Poison Prevention Act requires that certain household substances (*e.g.*, aspirin) and all oral legend drugs with the exception of sublingual nitroglycerin preparations and the 2.5-mg and 5-mg dosages of the sublingual and chewable isosorbide dinitrate preparations be packaged in "special containers." The special containers are designed so that they would be extremely difficult for a child under the age of 5 years to open but not difficult for healthy adults. The use of these "childproof" containers was instituted to ensure maximum protection against accidental poisoning of children. Because this type of container frequently poses a problem for the elderly or those with arthritis of the hands, the medical practitioner may indicate on the prescription that a "non-childproof" container be used.

STATE REGULATIONS

A number of states have individually enacted laws that affect the manner in which drugs are handled within that state. Federal laws may differ in some instances from state laws, but the *more stringent law or regulation is to be followed in all cases.*

COMPOSITION OF THE PRESCRIPTION

No matter how carefully thought out the prescription order, it may be therapeutically useless unless clearly communicated to the pharmacist. Because many drug names look alike when written, or sound alike when spoken, the importance of legibly indicating the drug name on a written prescription and speaking slowly and distinctly when giving a verbal prescription cannot be overemphasized.

The completed prescription must adequately instruct the patient on how to use the medica-

TABLE 12-1. Controlled Substance Schedules

Schedule	Definition	Prescription Requirements	Examples
I	Drugs that have no accepted medical use in the U.S. and that have a high potential for abuse	All nonresearch use is forbidden	Heroin, marijuana, peyote, mescaline, psilocybin
II	Drugs that have a high potential for abuse with severe psychic or physical dependence liability	DEA registration number Date of issuance Written in ink or indelible pencil Signature of physician (last name in full) with ink or indelible pencil Not refillable	Morphine, codeine, hydromorphone, methadone, meperidine, oxycodone, dextroamphetamine, methylphenidate
III	Drugs that have an abuse potential less than that of schedule I or II drugs. Abuse may lead to moderate or low physical dependence or high psychological dependence	DEA registration number Date of issuance Prescription must be rewritten after five refills or 6 months (cannot be filled or refilled more than 6 months after date of issuance)	Acetaminophen with codeine, aspirin with codeine, glutethimide, methyprylon
IV	Drugs that have an abuse potential less than drugs in schedule III	DEA registration number Date of issuance Prescription must be rewritten after five refills or 6 months (cannot be filled or refilled more than 6 months after date of issuance)	Chlordiazepoxide, diazepam, flurazepam, meprobamate, propoxyphene, phenobarbital
V	Drugs that have an abuse potential less than drugs listed in schedule IV. Comprises preparations containing moderate quantities of certain opioid drugs, generally for antidiarrheal or antitussive purposes	May be dispensed without a prescription provided 1. such distribution is made only by the pharmacist. 2. not more than 240 ml of any schedule V substance containing opium, or more than 120 ml or more than 24 solid dosage units of any other controlled substance, is sold to the consumer in any given 48-hour period without a valid prescription order. 3. the purchaser at retail is at least 18 years of age. 4. the pharmacist obtains suitable identification. 5. a record book is maintained that contains the name and address of the purchaser, name and quantity of controlled substance purchased, date of sale, and initials of pharmacist. 6. other federal, state, or local law *does not* require a prescription order.	Promethazine expectorant with codeine syrup, loperamide, diphenoxylate, kaolin-pectin with paregoric, terpin hydrate with codeine elixir

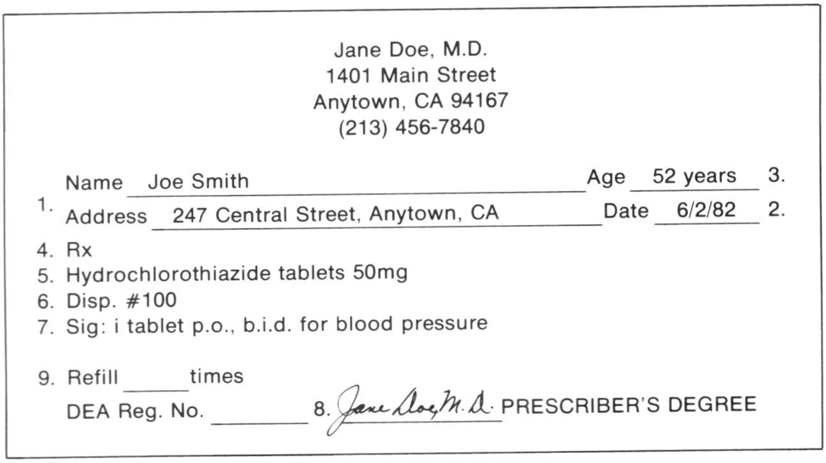

Jane Doe, M.D.
1401 Main Street
Anytown, CA 94167
(213) 456-7840

1. Name Joe Smith — Age 52 years 3.
Address 247 Central Street, Anytown, CA — Date 6/2/82 2.

4. Rx
5. Hydrochlorothiazide tablets 50mg
6. Disp. #100
7. Sig: i tablet p.o., b.i.d. for blood pressure

9. Refill _____ times
DEA Reg. No. _______ 8. Jane Doe, M.D. PRESCRIBER'S DEGREE

FIG. 12-1.

tion. The practitioner must discuss with the patient the nature and prognosis of his illness, including the role of the prescribed medication. In this manner, the practitioner should be able to minimize potential problems with patient noncompliance (*see* Chap. 11).

THE PRESCRIPTION

A legally authorized practitioner may prescribe a medication (depending on the specific setting) by [a] an entry in the patient's hospital chart; [b] a verbal order to a health professional authorized to receive such an order, for example, a pharmacist; or [c] a written prescription for use by an outpatient.

The basic composition of the prescription may be viewed according to its components (Fig. 12-1).

1. The *name and address* of the patient should be as complete as possible to avoid confusion with medications intended for someone else.
2. The *date* the prescription is written should be clearly indicated. Federal law requires that all schedule II, III, and IV prescription orders be dated (Table 12-1).
3. The *age* of the patient should be indicated. This allows the pharmacist to determine accurate dosing of various drugs (*see* Chaps. 7–11).
4. The *superscription* consists of the symbol Rx (Table 12-2). It functions as a directive to the pharmacist to prepare the medication as specified.
5. The *inscription* constitutes the principal part of the prescription and contains the name, dosage form, and strength of the medication to be dispensed. Drugs can be prescribed by the manufacturer's proprietary (trade) name or by the nonproprietary (generic) name. When the proprietary name is used, the pharmacist filling the prescription order must dispense the drug of the indicated manufacturer. If the generic name of the drug is used, the pharmacist may dispense any manufacturer's generically equivalent preparation. Because most drugs are available in various dosage forms, strengths, and formulations, the information present in the prescription should be as specific as possible to prevent potential errors.
6. The *subscription* historically has contained compounding directions. This section is now limited to the number of doses or quantity of medication to be dispensed (*see* Drug Measurement).
7. The *signatura*, usually abbreviated as sig. (Table 12-2), gives the necessary directions for use of the medication. These instructions are usually written in a mixture of Latin and English. The use of Latin is limited to specific key words and phrases (Table 12-2).

The pharmacist translates these directions for the patient, providing the information on the label attached to the medication container. The prescriber's instructions should be clear and concise so that the patient understands the proper use of the medication. The use of the phrase "as directed" should be avoided whenever possible because misunderstandings or patient forget-

---

Rx symbol is believed to have originated from the sign of Jupiter, used in ancient times to request aid in healing. It is now generally understood to be a contraction of the Latin verb "recipe," meaning take thou.

TABLE 12-2. Some Latin Words, Phrases, and Numbers used in Prescription Writing

Abbreviation	Latin	English Meaning
a	ante	before
aa, $\overline{aa}$	ana	of each
a.c.	ante cibum	before meals
ad	ad	to, up to
ad lib.	ad libitum	at pleasure (as desired)
aur.	auris	ear
b.i.d.	bis in die	twice a day
bis	bis	twice
c, $\bar{c}$	cum	with
cap.	capsula	capsule
d.	dexter	right
d.	dies	day
disp.	dispensa	dispense
d.t.d.	dentur tales doses	give such doses
et	et	and
f., ft.	fac, fiat	make
gm., Gm.*, g.	gramma	gram
gr	grana	grain
gtt.	gutta	drop
h.	hora	hour
h.s.	hora somni	at bedtime
m.	misce	mix
mixt.	mixtura	mixture
no.	numerus	number
noct.	nocte	at night
non rep.	non repetatur	do not repeat
o.d.	oculus dexter	right eye
o.h.	omni hora	every hour
o.s.	oculus sinister	left eye
o.u.	oculus uterque	each eye
p.o.	per os	by mouth
p.c.	post cibum	after meals
placebo	placebo	I please
p.r.n.	pro re nata	as needed
pulv.	pulvis	powder
q.	quaque	each, every
q.h.	quaque hora	every hour
q.i.d.	quater in die	four times a day
q.s.	quantum sufficit	as much as suffices
Rx	recipe	take thou
s	sine	without
s.	sinistro	left
sig.	signa	label, let be written
sol.	solutio	solution
s.s., $\overline{s.s.}$	semi	one-half
stat.	statim	at once, immediately
syr.	syrupus	syrup
tab.	tabella	tablet
t.i.d.	ter in die	three times a day
tinct., tr.	tinctura	tincture
ung.	unguentum	ointment
ut dict.	ut dictum	as directed
unus,-a,-um	i, I	1
duo, duae, duo	ii, II	2
tres, tria	iii, III	3
quattuor	iv, IV	4
quinque	v, V	5
sex	vi, VI	6
septem	vii, VII	7
octo	viii, VIII	8
novem	ix, IX	9
decem	x, X	10
viginti	xx, XX	20
trigenta	xxx, XXX	30
quadraginta	xl, XL	40
quinquaginta	l, L	50
sexaginta	lx, LX	60
septuaginta	lxx, LXX	70
octoginta	lxxx, LXXX	80
nonaginta	xc, XC	90
centum	C	100

* The abbreviation Gm is preferred to minimize confusion with other symbols.

fulness may lead to errors. The directions should include such phrases as "for relief of pain," "for itching," and so forth to remind the patient of the intended purpose of the medication. The prescriber should not hesitate to provide the patient with a separate sheet of instructions for his own use, especially when directions are complex.

8. The *signature of the prescriber* is placed at the bottom of the prescription and must include the degree (*e.g.*, M.D.). If the information is not preprinted on the prescription blank, it is advisable to include the printed or stamped name of the prescriber. This facilitates identification of the practitioner in those instances that involve signatures which are difficult to read. The address and telephone number of the prescriber should also be indicated.
9. *Auxiliary information* may vary according to the specific needs of the patient. Since legend drugs may not be refilled without the consent of the prescriber, instructions on refilling the prescription should always be included. Statements such as "refill p.r.n." or "refill ad lib" are not appropriate. The prescriber may also wish to indicate that a nonchildproof container be used.

DRUG MEASUREMENT

Specifying the amount of medication prescribed may involve either or both of two systems of measurement. The older apothecary system is based on unrelated units of measurement such as scruples and grains, ounces and pints. In contrast, the newer metric, or decimal system, based on mathematically related units such as milligrams and grams, milliliters and liters, provides for easier calculations and greater accuracy and flexibility. Although *use of the metric system in prescription writing is preferable,* practitioners should still retain familiarity with both systems, since the transition from use of the apothecary to the metric system has been a gradual process. For example, apothecary system is still used with some of the older drugs such as nitroglycerin, which is often specified in fractional grain dosages (gr 1:150) or 0.4 mg metric equivalent dose).

For practical purposes, translation between the apothecary and metric systems may be accomplished by remembering the following basic conversions.

Apothecary System	Metric System
1 grain (gr)	= 0.065 gram (g) (60 mg for the usual approximation)
15 gr	= 1 gram (g)
1 ounce (oz)	= 0.03 liters (30 ml)

For further information, Table 12-3 provides a summary of approximate and exact equivalents.

TABLE 12-3. Apothecary/Metric Dose Equivalents*

Approximate Equivalents	
Liquids	
1 gallon = 3800 ml	8 fluid ounces = 240 ml
1 quart = 950 ml	1 fluid ounce = 30 ml
1 pint = 475 ml	10 minims = 0.6 ml
1 teaspoonful = 5 ml	1 tablespoonful = 15 ml
Solids	
1 ounce = 30 g	1/8 grain = 8 mg
15 grains = 1 g	1/12 grain = 5 mg
10 grains = 600 mg	1/100 grain = 0.6 mg
7.5 grains = 500 mg	1/150 grain = 0.4 mg
5 grain = 300 mg	1/200 grain = 0.3 mg
1.5 grain = 100 mg	1/250 grain = 0.25 mg
1 grain = 60 mg	1/300 grain = 0.2 mg
Exact Equivalents	
1 pint = 473.17 ml	1 kg = 2.2 pounds
1 fluid ounce = 29.57 ml	1 ounce = 28.35 g
16.23 minims = 1 ml	1 grain = 64.8 mg

* Use exact equivalents for compounding and calculations that require a high degree of accuracy.

INPATIENT MEDICATION ORDERS

Essentially, with the exception of possible hospital-mandated regulations, each order written for a patient is assumed to be *current therapy* unless changed or discontinued by the prescriber. Failure to realize this circumstance and develop appropriate inpatient prescribing patterns has been the pitfall of many practitioners. For this reason, the practitioner is advised to develop a few basic prescribing habits.

1. When considering the addition of a new medication order, review the patient's current therapy and other information, such as disease state, laboratory test values, and potential drug interactions, before prescribing.
2. Each medication order should begin with the date and time that the order is being written and should end with the prescriber's signature.
3. For any change in a medication order, designate clearly the status of the previous order. Any possible misinterpretation or confusion regarding the prescriber's wishes may then be minimized.
4. *Never* cross out any notation that is part of a medication order. This practice has frequently led to errors in medication dosing because the order may already have been noted and recorded by hospital personnel. Once these latter steps have occurred, the intended deletion may not be noted, and the original order will remain current. Any medication or dosing change may be indicated immediately and appropriately by means of a new order.
5. Review the patient's drug regimen on a regular basis, preferably daily. This provides for review of "p.r.n." medication orders which should be reviewed, orders requiring discontinuation, and a host of other considerations involving drug therapy. Routine medication review also allows the prescriber to assess as a whole the scope and appropriateness of therapy.
6. Review periodically the nursing notes on medication charting. Valuable information pertaining to use of "p.r.n." medications, refused doses, or medication orders entirely missed by the nursing staff may be determined.

TWO

Systematic Pharmacology

DRUGS ACTING PREDOMINANTLY ON THE PERIPHERAL NERVOUS SYSTEM

13 Introduction

JOHN A. BEVAN

The peripheral nervous system comprises the afferent and efferent neurons of the autonomic and somatic nervous system. All drugs of clinical importance that act on the peripheral nervous system, except local anesthetics (*see* Chap. 20) and veratrum alkaloids (*see* Chap. 36), do so by modifying the transmission of excitation between two serial neurons or between the junction of neurons with effector cells (glands or muscle). The region of contact between two nerve cells or between a nerve and an effector cell used for the transference of excitation or inhibition is termed a *synapse*. The synapse between a motor neuron and an effector cell is also known as a *neuroeffector junction*.

The peripheral junctional sites are models of synapses in the central nervous system. Consequently the mode of action of drugs on the brain is frequently inferred from a study of their peripheral effects, although direct studies on central synapses are becoming increasingly common.

A knowledge of the anatomy, physiology, and biochemistry of the peripheral nervous system, particularly in its junctional sites, is essential to understanding its pharmacology. Drugs that modify the neuroeffector mechanism at the synapse between motor nerves and voluntary muscle, the *neuromuscular junction*, are discussed in Chapter 19.

ANATOMY OF THE AUTONOMIC NERVOUS SYSTEM

The autonomic (visceral, vegetative, automatic) nervous system innervates almost all tissues of the body; the notable exception is voluntary muscle. *Visceral afferent or sensory fibers* are more numerous than autonomic motor fibers (Fig. 13-1). They pass via either somatic nerves or the various ramifications of the autonomic nervous system into the cerebrospinal axis. Such fibers carry general visceral sensation and information from the specialized reflexogenic areas of the cardiovascular, ventilatory, and other systems.

Integration of autonomic activity occurs at all levels of the cerebrospinal axis. A study of patients with high spinal cord lesions shows that a number of reflex changes are mediated at the spinal or segmental level. The medulla and pons contain the "vital" centers important in controlling the ventilatory and cardiovascular systems. The principal site of organization

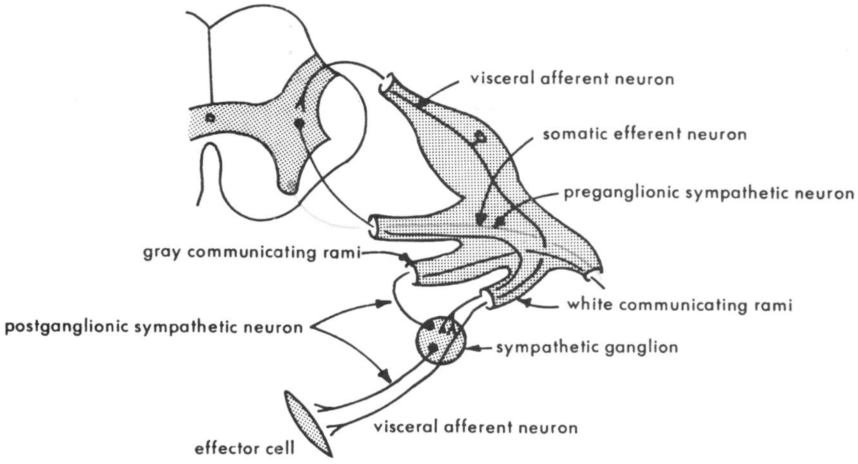

FIG. 13-1. Neuronal arrangement of the afferent and efferent neurons of the peripheral autonomic nervous system.

and coordination of the autonomic nervous system is the hypothalamus. Sympathetic functions are controlled by the posterior nuclei and parasympathetic by the middle and some anterior nuclei. The supraoptic and paraventricular nuclei are anatomically and functionally associated with the posterior lobe of the pituitary. Integration of autonomic with somatic motor and sensory function, as in fainting at the sight of blood, must occur in higher centers.

Although the pharmacology of these integrative centers will not be described systemically, many drugs owe some of their important effects to actions upon them, including reserpine (*see* Chap. 36), barbiturates (*see* Chap. 25), morphine (*see* Chap. 32), and digitalis (*see* Chap. 33).

Visceral efferent fibers are divided among the two divisions of the autonomic nervous system. These divisions are distinguished anatomically (Fig. 13-2) and functionally. The fibers of the *sympathetic division* emerge from the

FIG. 13-2. Autonomic efferent outflow.

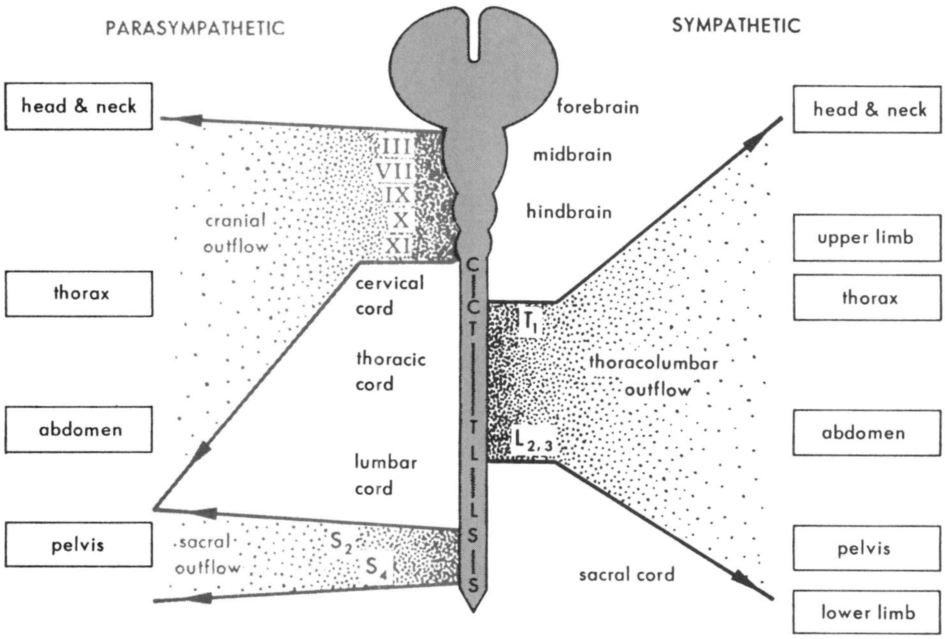

thoracolumbar levels of the spinal cord and those of the *parasympathetic division* from the sacral part of the spinal cord and in association with certain cranial nerves. Both divisions can be represented schematically as two serial neurons (Figs. 13-1, 13-3). The proximal (preganglionic) neurons originate in the parasympathetic components of the nuclei of some cranial nerves and from the interomediolateral gray column of the spinal cord and synapse with distal (postganglionic) neurons in ganglia.

The sympathetic or thoracolumbar division arises from segmental levels T_1 to L_2 or L_3 of the spinal cord (Fig. 13-2). Fibers pass via white communicating rami (myelinated fibers) and by nerves to ganglia, most of which are found in the sympathetic chains and paravertebral ganglia (Figs. 13-1, 13-2). Postganglionic fibers are distributed to visceral structures by way of terminal plexuses and by specific autonomic nerves and to somatic tissues by the gray communicating rami (nonmyelinated fibers) and the spinal nerves. The cells of the adrenal medulla are homologous to sympathetic postganglionic neurons and are innervated by preganglionic fibers that pass in the splanchnic nerves. They form an integral part of the sympathetic autonomic division.

Sympathetic postganglionic fibers are subdivided into "long" fibers that innervate the heart, blood vessels, smooth muscle, glands, and intramural ganglia and "short" fibers to the vas deferens, uterus, and urinary bladder. The neuronal organization of the long fibers of the sympathetic nervous system is designed to ensure a generalized influence on the innervated viscera. One preganglionic fiber influences a large number of postganglionic neurons, and any one ganglion contains neurons that are distributed to a number of organs. Furthermore, the adrenal medulla, an integral part of this division, on activation releases epinephrine and norepinephrine into the circulation, which potentially can influence all cells of the body.

The parasympathetic or craniosacral division emerges in association with cranial nerves III, VII, IX, X, and XI and at segmental levels S_2 to S_4 of the spinal cord (Fig. 13-2). The cranial outflow of this division carries fibers to most structures in the head, neck, thorax, and abdomen. The left half of the transverse colon,

FIG. 13-3. Anatomic, physiologic, and pharmacologic classification of efferent neurons and junctional sites of the peripheral nervous system. Ach = acetylcholine; Norepi = norepinephrine; Epi = epinephrine.

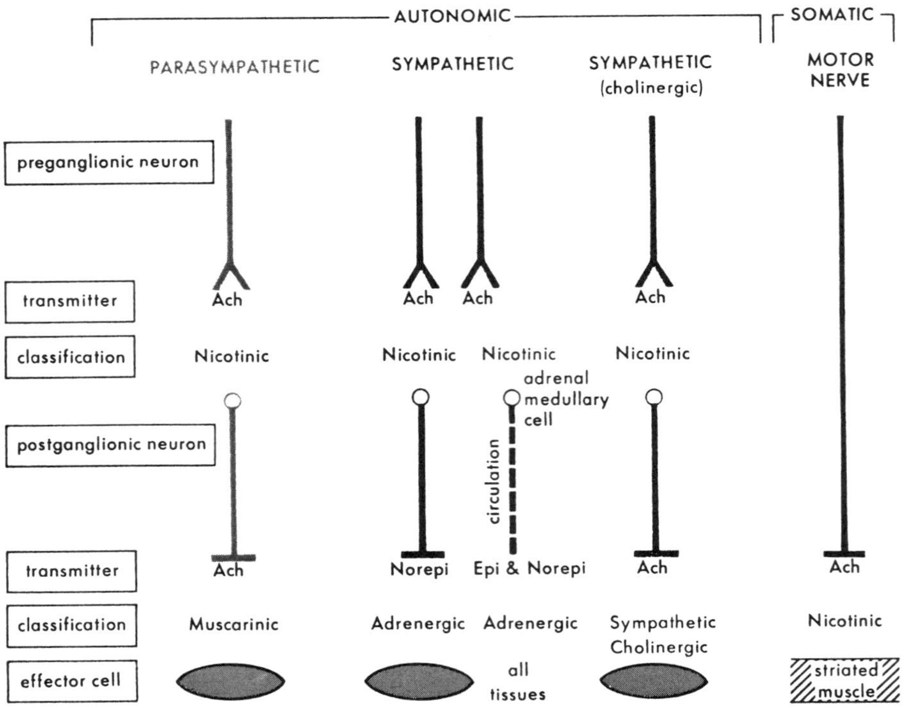

the descending colon, and the pelvic viscera are supplied by the sacral outflow (pelvic nerve). Parasympathetic ganglia are small and situated either close to, or buried within, the structures they innervate.

In contrast to the sympathetic division, the neural arrangement of the parasympathetic efferent limb is consistent with discrete, limited, localized effects. A typical parasympathetic preganglionic neuron synapses with only a few postganglionic neurons. Juxtaposition of parasympathetic ganglia to the viscera is consistent with a limited distribution of postganglionic fibers. The main exception to this generalization is Auerbach's plexus.

PHYSIOLOGY OF THE AUTONOMIC NERVOUS SYSTEM

Many tissues are innervated by both divisions of the autonomic nervous system. Although the actions of the two divisions are supplementary in some tissues (*e.g.*, the salivary gland), generally activities of the two divisions produce opposite effects (as in the bladder, bronchi, gastrointestinal tract, heart, and pupil). *In vivo*, however, these two parts of the autonomic nervous system act synergistically and tend to be complementary. Denervation studies show that many autonomically innervated structures possess intrinsic activity that is modified by autonomic activity. A few tissues, including most blood vessels, sweat glands, and spleen, are innervated by only one division (Table 13-1).

The autonomic nervous system acts to regulate and to maintain the constancy of the internal environment of the body despite many influences that threaten to alter it, such as temperature change, alteration in posture, exercise, food ingestion, and anger. The responses of the various organs to autonomic activity and, where known, the dominant regulating division are summarized in Table 13-1. Because the sympathetic system discharges diffusely in response to fear or anger, causing the physiological changes appropriate to fight or flight, these at first seemingly unrelated effects appear to have cohesion and purpose and are more readily understood and remembered. They are similar to the effects of epinephrine described in Chapter 17.

Sympathetic activity causes an elevation of cardiac output due to an increased heart rate, stroke volume, and total peripheral resistance. Generalized venous constriction occurs. These changes, along with the contraction of the spleen that occurs in some species, are responsible for the rise in arterial pressure. Cardiac output is redistributed among the various regions of the body. As a result of active vasoconstriction it is shifted away from the skin, gastrointestinal tract, glands, and, to a lesser extent, the kidney to organs of more immediate biologic importance: the heart, voluntary muscle, brain, and lungs. Glandular secretions dry up, sphincters of the gastrointestinal tract and urinary system contract, peristalsis is inhibited, and the tone in the wall of these organs is reduced. Pupils and bronchi dilate. Erector pili and sweat glands are activated. Glycogenolysis is initiated. Blood levels of free fatty acids rise. Transient elevation and depression of blood potassium and inorganic phosphate, respectively, occur.

In contrast, the parasympathetic nervous system is designed for conservative and discrete action. It can effect changes in a single organ; for example, vagal bradycardia can occur without concomitant salivary secretion or a change in gastric tone. Only the parasympathetic nervous system of the two divisions is essential for life.

NEUROHUMORAL TRANSMISSION

Transmission of excitation across junctional regions of the peripheral nervous system in mammals occurs through the mediation of liberated chemical substances. Of the many experimental studies that led to the establishment of this theory, those of Otto Loewi, in 1921, are the most simple and convincing. Loewi perfused two frog hearts (Fig. 13-4): He stimulated the vagus of one (A) and then transferred the fluid from that heart to the second one (B). The second heart slowed. When the sympathetic supply was stimulated, the trans-

CLAUDE BERNARD, 1813–1878. French physiologist. Founder of the experimental method in physiology. Originated the idea of "internal secretions" from work on the functions of the pancreas and developed the concept of a constant *milieu intérieur*. First French scientist honored with a state funeral.

OTTO LOEWI, 1873–1961. German physician and pharmacologist, came to United States in 1940. Demonstrated in 1921 that nervous stimulation of the heart was chemically mediated. Won Nobel prize in 1936 with Henry Dale for work on nervous transmission.

TABLE 13-1. Effector Responses to Autonomic Nervous Activity

Effector System	Predominant Division*	Response	Receptor Type	Response to Other Division	Receptor Type
Iris					
Dilator pupillae	Symp.	Contraction (mydriasis)	α	–	–
Sphincter pupillae	Parasymp.	Contraction (miosis)	Chol.	–	–
Ciliary Muscle	Parasymp.	Contraction (near vision)	Chol.	Opposite (weak)	β
Bronchi and Bronchioles	Parasymp.	Contraction	Chol.	Relaxation	β_2
Heart	*See* Chap. 33				
SA node	Parasymp.	Slowing	Chol.	Opposite	β_1
Atria	Parasymp.	Increased conduction velocity, shortened refractory period	Chol.	Mixed; increased conduction velocity; increased contractility	β_1
A-V node and bundle	Parasymp.	Decreased conduction velocity, lengthened refractory period	Chol.	Opposite	β_1
Ventricles	Symp.	Increased conduction velocity, increased contractility, increased automaticity	β_1	–	–
Blood Vessels					
Abdominal viscera	Symp.	Constriction > dilation	α,β_2	–	–
Coronary	Symp.	Dilation > constriction	α,β_2	?Dilation	Chol.
Glands	Parasymp.	Complex dilation	Chol.	Opposite	α
Pulmonary	Symp.	Constriction > dilation	α,β_2	?Opposite	?Chol.
Skeletal muscle	Symp.	Complex dilation	β_2 Chol.	–	–
Skin, mucosa	Symp.	Constriction	α	–	–
Veins	Symp.	Constriction > dilation	α,β_2	–	–
Gastrointestinal Tract					
Liver	Symp.	Glycogenolysis, lipolysis	α,β_2	Same	Chol.
Muscle wall	Parasymp.	Increased tone and motility	Chol.	Opposite	α_2,β_2
Sphincters	Parasymp.	Relaxation	Chol.	Opposite	α
Glands					
Gastrointestinal	Parasymp.	Secretion	Chol.	–	–
Lacrimal	Parasymp.	Secretion	Chol.	–	–
Nasopharyngeal	Parasymp.	Secretion	Chol.	–	–
Respiratory	Parasymp.	Secretion	Chol.	?Opposite	α
Salivary	Parasymp.	Thin secretion	Chol.	Same, thick secretion	α
Skin					
Pilomotor	Symp.	Piloerection	α		–
Sweat glands	Symp.	Secretion	Chol.	Symp. similar in special areas	α
Urinary Bladder					
Detrusor	Parasymp.	Contraction	Chol.	Opposite	β
Sphincter and trigone	Parasymp.	Relaxation	Chol.	Opposite	α
Sex Organs	Parasymp.	Erection	Chol.	Ejaculation	?α

* During rest and normal physiologic function.

Parasymp. = parasympathetic; Symp. = sympathetic; Chol. = cholinergic; α = alpha adrenergic receptor; β = beta adrenergic receptor.

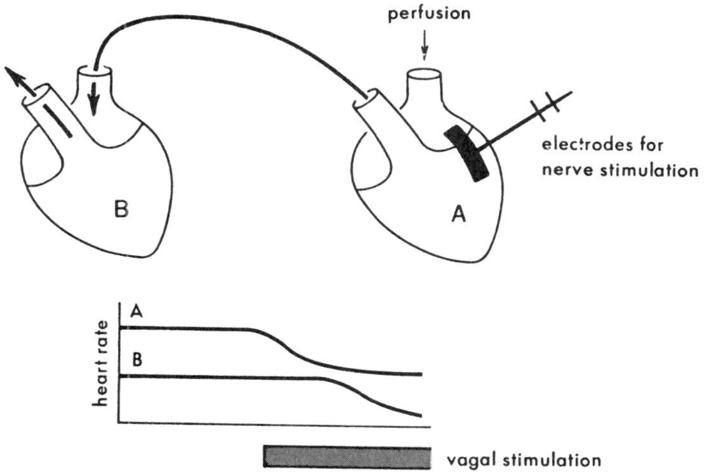

FIG. 13-4. Loewi's experiment. The perfusion fluid flows from frog heart *A* to heart *B*. Stimulation of the autonomic innervation of heart *A* causes changes first in *A* and then in *B*.

ferred fluid accelerated the second heart. Loewi argued that the autonomic nervous activity influenced the myocardium through the liberation of specific chemical substances. Such a substance was contained in the fluid transferred from heart A to heart B.

The supporting evidence for the theory of neurohumoral transmission is now overwhelming. The minimum criteria necessary to establish a substance as a neurohumoral transmitter are as follows.

1. Demonstration of liberation of the active substance from junctional sites during presynaptic nervous activity.
2. Identification by chemical or biologic methods of the liberated substance.
3. Identity of the response to nerve stimulation and local injection of liberated substance.
4. Similar modification of responses to nerve stimulation and the local injection of transmitter substance by drugs and other procedures.
5. Demonstration of synthetic mechanisms for the disposition of the proposed transmitter in the region of the junction.

Acetylcholine mediates transmission between the preganglionic and postganglionic neurons of both parasympathetic and sympathetic divisions (ganglionic transmission). Acetylcholine is also the chemical transmitter between postganglionic parasympathetic neurons and their effector cells and between the motor nerves of the somatic nervous system and voluntary muscle. The transmitter released at the postganglionic sympathetic nerve ending is almost exclusively *l*-norepinephrine and from the adrenal medulla, a mixture of *l*-norepinephrine and *l*-epinephrine. In Figure 13-3, the efferent neurons and the principal neurohumoral transmitters of the peripheral nervous system are represented schematically. There is one notable exception: Fibers to sweat glands and to certain blood vessels (*e.g.*, in skeletal muscle) liberate acetylcholine, although they are anatomically part of the sympathetic nervous system. Other exceptions to this seemingly simple arrangement are under experimental investigation. Other possible transmitters include histamine, serotonin, γ-aminobutyric acid, purines, and possibly some amino acids and polypeptides. A role of some of these substances in modulating transmission has been proposed.

PRINCIPAL EVENTS IN TRANSMISSION

Vesicles (secretory granules) are aggregated in neuronal terminations or in periodic swellings in the plexi formed by their terminations. These are storage sites for the transmitter. During nervous activity, the vesicles appear to migrate toward the neurilemma and release their contents into the extracellular space probably by exocytosis. The released transmitter diffuses across the synaptic or junctional cleft, which is generally around 200 to 400 Å in width but sometimes may, in some blood vessels, be as great as 10,000 Å. There it combines with specific receptors probably found in the axonal membrane of the postganglionic neuron or the cell membrane of the effector cell. In some cells, such as skeletal muscle, the postjunctional membrane is specialized into a receptor-containing area or end plate. In other cells such as vascular muscle, the receptors are probably distributed more widely over the cell surface, and there is no postsynaptic specialization. The precise nature of the reaction of the transmitter with its receptors and the subsequent events that lead to excitation or inhibition vary widely in different tissues.

Vesicles are manufactured in the cell body and pass along the axon to its terminal areas. At each junctional site, special mechanisms exist for the synthesis, release, and disposition of the transmitters. A number of feedback systems regulate each of these processes and contribute to the precise control of response. Three disposition mechanisms (Fig. 13-5) are possible: diffusion from the junctional cleft; destruction by enzymatic activity; or reuptake of the transmitter into the nerve endings. The relative importance of these pathways varies from one junction to another.

Cholinergic Transmission

In the nerve ending acetylation of choline transported into the neuroplasm is catalyzed by choline acetyltransferase. The acetylcholine formed is stored within the synaptic vesicles. The rate of synthesis of neuronal acetylcholine is linked to the level of neuronal activity. Within a few milliseconds of its release from the nerve ending into the synaptic cleft probably by exocytosis, and its subsequent reaction with cholinergic receptors, the transmitter is hydrolyzed by acetylcholinesterase found at the neuromuscular junction. At cholinergic sites, transmitter inactivation by metabolism is the dominant mechanism. Acetylcholine often causes a local depolarization or hyperpolarization of the postsynaptic membrane (*see* Chap. 14), for example, in skeletal muscle at the end plate, the released acetylcholine causes a local depolarization, an end plate potential (*see* Chap. 19). If this is of sufficient magnitude, it gives rise to a regenerative or action potential.

Adrenergic Transmission

Although *l*-norepinephrine is present in the synaptic vesicles that pass from the cell body to neuronal sites of release, the main site of amine formation is in or near the nerve endings. Phenylalanine or tyrosine is taken up by an active transport mechanism into the axoplasm of the nerve terminal and there synthesized into either *l*-norepinephrine or epinephrine. The pathways and the enzymes that regulate these processes are shown in Figure 13-6. The initial steps in this process that lead to the synthesis of dopamine are carried out in the cytoplasm from where the amine must enter a synaptic vesicle before finally being converted into norepinephrine by dopamine β-hydroxylase. The rate-limiting step in biosynthesis is the conversion of *l*-tyrosine to *l*-dopa. The rate of synthesis of transmitter mainly depends on the level of autonomic activity and is regulated by several mechanisms, including the regulation of tyrosine hydroxylase activity by the local cytosol concentration of norepinephrine.

FIG. 13-5. Stages of neurohumoral transmission and sites of pharmacologic modification. (*See* text discussion under Classification by Mode of Action.) T = transmitter.

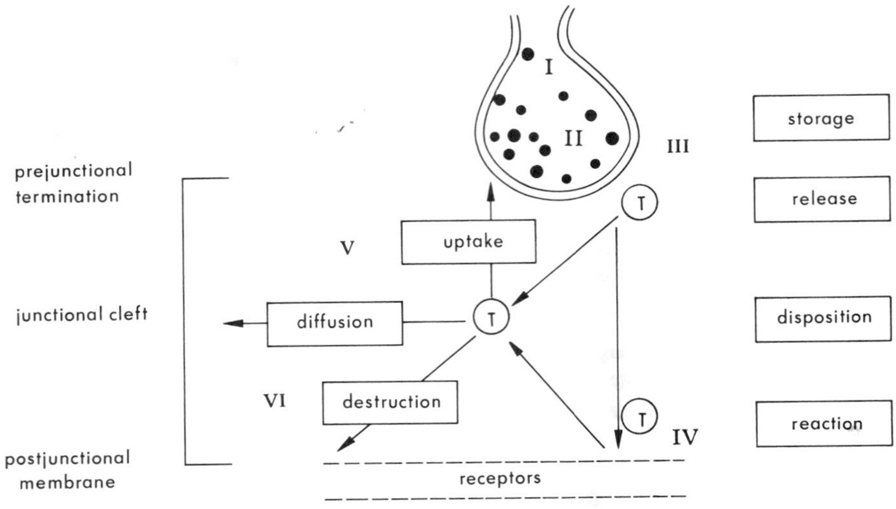

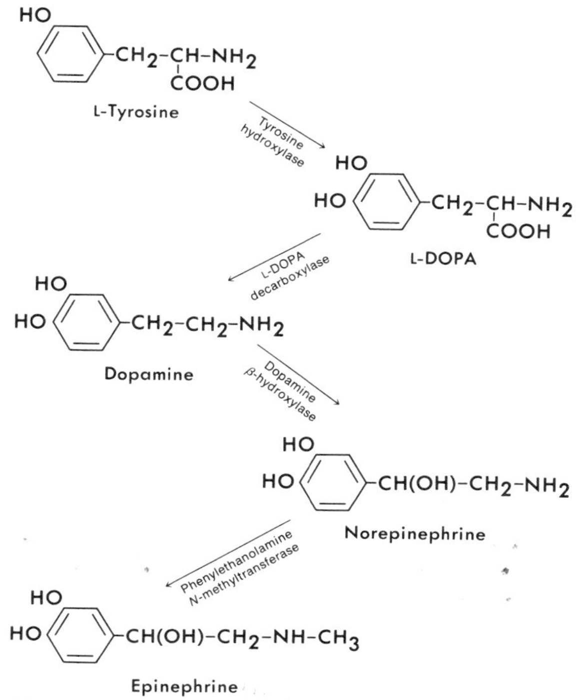

FIG. 13-6. Synthetic pathway of sympathetic transmitters.

The *l*-norepinephrine released from the terminal plexus by neuronal activity is derived from that taken up into the terminal from the extracellular space (*see* below) and from that locally synthesized. Transmitter release from the varicosity as a result of neuronal function is intimately regulated by local norepinephrine concentrations. Although a number of presynaptic mechanisms influence or modulate transmitter release, that mediated through presynaptic α receptors is of greatest physiological importance. This is a negative feed-back system. The form of the presynaptic and postsynaptic receptors is different (*see* Chap. 18): They are referred to as α_2 and α_1 adrenoceptors, respectively.

The released amine is disposed of mainly by reuptake into the nerve terminals. Small amounts of endogenous catecholamines are taken up and subsequently metabolized in nonneuronal tissues. A variable proportion diffuses into the extracellular space. The biologic activity of the transmitter on the effector cells of a number of tissues is terminated almost entirely by reuptake. In others, these additional mechanisms are relatively important. The two enzymes that catalyze the degradation of norepinephrine and epinephrine are monamine oxidase and catechol-O-methyltransferase. These enzymes influence predominantly presynaptic and postsynaptic intracellular catecholamine concentrations, respectively, and play a relatively minor role in terminating transmitter action, at least in peripheral tissues. Circulating catecholamines, on the other hand, are metabolized rapidly mainly by catechol-O-methyltransferase present in the liver through a complex degradative pathway.

PHARMACOLOGY

The drugs that modify the activity of the peripheral nervous system are described in succeeding chapters. These agents are classified according to their site of action (Fig. 13-3) and the mechanism whereby they exert their principal effects.

CLASSIFICATION BY SITE OF ACTION

Drugs that act in the region of the postganglionic sympathetic nerve ending are commonly known as *adrenergic drugs*. *Sympathomimetic drugs* mimic at least some of the actions of the sympathetic nervous system (*mimetic* means simulating or imitating); *sympatholytic drugs* (*lysis* means dissolution) block sympathetic activity. Drugs that act in the region of the postganglionic parasympathetic nerve endings are *cholinergic*. The terms *parasympathomimetic* and *parasympatholytic* are self-explanatory. Because sympathetic and parasympathetic ganglia are pharmacologically identical, the simple terms *ganglionic stimulating* or *ganglionic blocking* are applied to drugs that act at these sites.

Since acetylcholine is the mediator at autonomic ganglia, postganglionic parasympathetic endings, and the neuromuscular junction, and since drugs with actions specific to each site are known, distinguishing names are necessary. Early pharmacologists were aware that muscarine, derived from the poisonous mushroom *Amanita muscaria*, stimulated specifically cholinergic receptors at the postganglionic parasympathetic junctions. Consequently, these sites are commonly referred to as *muscarinic* receptors or sites. Since small doses of nicotine act on cholinergic receptors in the ganglia and the neuromuscular junction, these sites are often referred to as *nicotinic;* it is better that the term be restricted to ganglionic sites.

CLASSIFICATION BY MODE OF ACTION

Autonomic drugs exert their effects by modifying one or more of the steps or stages of neurohumoral transmission and may be classified on this basis (Fig. 13-5; *see* Chap. 21 where a similar classification is extended to CNS synapses).

I. *Interference with transmitter biosynthesis.* No drug of therapeutic value causes its effects exclusively by interfering with transmitter biosynthesis. α-Methyl-p-tyrosine and hemicholinium are experimentally used drugs that interfere with adrenergic and cholinergic transmission, respectively.

α-Methyldopa is metabolized in the adrenergic transmitter pathway to α-methylnorepinephrine, which displaces norepinephrine and is released in its place as a false transmitter.

II. *Interference with transmitter storage.* Certain sympathomimetic amines, such as amphetamine, ephedrine, and tyramine, act in part by displacing and thus releasing endogenous transmitter. The released transmitter in turn reacts with the receptor in the normal way causing sympathomimetic effects (*see* Chap. 36). Reserpine prevents the entry of norepinephrine into storage granules and possibly interferes with storage itself. Thus, after norepinephrine is released, its uptake is prevented, making it susceptible to neuronal monoamine oxidase. The end-result is norepinephrine depletion.

III. *Interference with transmitter release.* The only drug of therapeutic value in this category, bretylium acts by interfering with the link between the action potential and the mechanism of release in the postganglionic sympathetic neuron (*see* Chap. 36). Botulinus toxin prevents the release of acetylcholine by an unknown mechanism.

Clonidine is an α_2-adrenoceptor agonist that reinforces the physiological negative feed-back system modulating norepinephrine release (*see* above and Chap. 18). This results in a reduction of the average amount of transmitter that leaves the nerve terminal.

IV. *Stimulation of postjunctional receptors.* Many drugs mimic autonomic activity by reacting with the same receptors on postjunctional membranes as the physiologic transmitters. They are frequently related chemically to the transmitter. Muscarine, nicotine in small doses, and the choline esters react with cholinergic receptors (*see* Chap. 14). Certain sympathomimetic amines—norepinephrine, epinephrine, isopropylnorepinephrine, and phenylephrine—are agonists at adrenergic receptors (*see* Chap. 17).

Interference with the action of endogenous transmitter at postjunctional receptors. Certain drugs, by reacting with the receptors of the effector cells, prevent or block the normal effects of the transmitter. These are commonly referred to as blocking agents and are classified according to their site of action as neuromuscular (*see* Chap. 19), adrenergic (*see* Chap. 17), ganglionic (*see* Chap. 36), or muscarinic (*see* Chap. 16) blocking agents.

V. *Interference with the reuptake of transmitters.* Drugs such as cocaine and imipramine act by inhibiting the reuptake of the adrenergic transmitter. Thus they prolong its local effect within the synapse (*see* Chaps. 20, 22).

VI. *Interference with transmitter metabolism.* Anticholinesterases act by inhibiting the hydrolytic action of acetylcholine esterases. The result is an increased local concentration of acetylcholine in the synaptic cleft and an increased effector response (*see* Chap. 5). Inhibitors of monoamine oxidase and catechol-O-methyl transferase effect adrenergic transmission in peripheral synapses to a variable and relatively minor degree.

FURTHER READING

1. Bevan JA, Bevan RD, Duckles SP: Adrenergic regulation of vascular smooth muscle. In Bohr DF, Somlyo AP, Sparks HV (eds): Handbook of Physiology, Section 2. The Cardiovascular System, Volume 2: Vascular Smooth Muscle, pp 515–566. Baltimore, American Physiological Society, 1980
2. Burnstock G, Costa M: Adrenergic Neurons. London, Chapman and Hall, 1975
3. Koelle GB: Microanatomy and pharmacology of cholinergic synapses. In Tower DB (ed): The Nervous System, Volume 1, pp 363–371. New York, Raven Press, 1975
4. Triggle DJ, Triggle CR: Chemical Pharmacology of the Synapse. New York, Academic Press, 1972
5. Westfall TC: Local regulation of adrenergic neurotransmission. Physiol Rev 57:659–728, 1977

CHAPTER 13 QUESTIONS

The Student May Need to Read Other Chapters in This Section Before Answering These Questions

Select the One Best Answer

(See P. 7 for Full Instructions)

1. Ganglionic blocking drugs produce all of the following effects EXCEPT
   A. postural hypotension.
   B. blurred vision.
   C. dry mouth.
   D. atrioventricular block.
   E. constipation.

2. Difficulty in focusing for near vision might be expected after the oral administration of
   A. ephedrine.
   B. bethanecol.
   C. propantheline.
   D. propranolol.
   E. guanethidine.

3. A large dose of acetylcholine would be expected to cause a rise in blood pressure after fully effective treatment with which of the following agents?
   A. atropine.
   B. chlorisondamine.
   C. reserpine.
   D. neostigmine.
   E. propranolol.

4. The intravenous administration of drug X results in hypotension, increased intestinal motility, miosis, salivation, and bradycardia. The class of drugs to which drug X belongs is
   A. β-adrenergic stimulants.
   B. ganglionic blocking agents.
   C. ganglionic stimulating agents.
   D. muscarinic agents.
   E. antihistaminic agents.

5. Drug X produces vasoconstriction (not blocked by phentolamine) and bradycardia (blocked by atropine or chlorisondamine). Drug X could be
   A. norepinephrine.
   B. angiotensin.
   C. nicotine.
   D. phenylephrine.
   E. tyramine.

A = 1,2,3; B = 1,3; C = 2,4; D = 4; E = All

6. Nicotine
   1. is readily absorbed through the skin.
   2. produces only depression in the central nervous system.
   3. may cause severe nausea.
   4. acts directly on receptors in smooth muscle of the gut.

7. The administration of a ganglionic stimulating agent to an animal previously treated with propranolol (Inderal) will cause a decrease in heart rate. This response is abolished by
   1. atropine.
   2. section of the vagus nerves.
   3. hexamethonium.
   4. reserpine.

8. Neurotransmitter responses are usually terminated by
   1. destruction of the neurohormone in the parasympathetic system.
   2. diffusion of the neurotransmitter at the motor end-plate.
   3. neurotransmitter reuptake into the nerve terminal in the sympathetic system.
   4. binding of neurotransmitter to "spare" receptors in the gut.

9. The diagram below represents mean blood pressure responses to drug A before and after treatment with a fully effective dose of atropine.

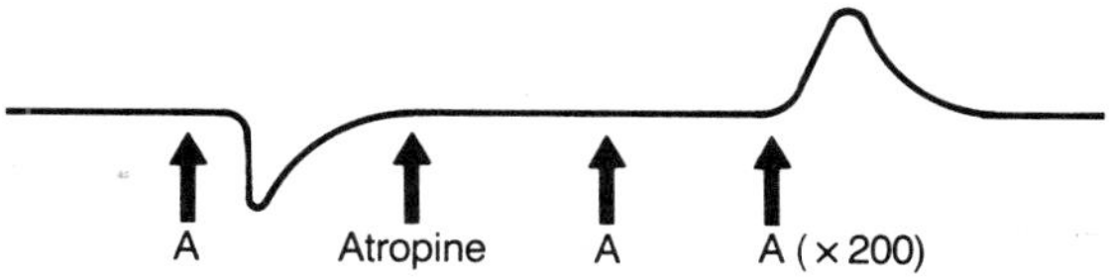

The response to the high dose of drug A would be antagonized by pretreatment with
   1. chlorisondamine.
   2. reserpine.
   3. phentolamine.
   4. neostigmine.

14

THOMAS C. WESTFALL

Muscarinic Agents

The primary action of muscarinic agents is at cholinergic receptors located at parasympathetic postganglionic junctions (smooth muscle, cardiac muscle, and various glands). Interaction with these receptors results in activation or inhibition of the various effector systems. Parasympathetic innervation of a particular organ is not, however, a prerequisite for the presence of muscarinic receptors. Other names given to muscarinic agents are parasympathomimetics or cholinomimetics (*see* Chap. 13). Additional actions may also be produced by means of muscarinic receptors located on autonomic ganglia and in the central nervous system. The prototype drug of this group is acetylcholine, which serves as the transmitter at the postganglionic parasympathetic junction. Various muscarinic drugs differ from acetylcholine in being more resistant to inactivation by cholinesterase and therefore in having more prolonged and useful action. These drugs are primarily directly acting agents, which implies that they combine directly with muscarinic receptors on the effector cells, in contrast to cholinesterase inhibitors (*see* Chap. 15), which act indirectly and, in addition to their muscarinic action, have prominent effects at other sites. Muscarinic agonists are of two types: synthetic choline esters, including bethanechol, carbachol, methacholine, and furtrethonium; and naturally occurring alkaloids, such as pilocarpine.

Most evidence indicates that the muscarinic receptor on various effector cells is homogeneous; however, recent binding studies with newer muscarinic antagonists suggest that the homogeneity of muscarinic receptors may be an oversimplification and that subclasses may exist. This could conceivably set the stage for more selective muscarinic and antimuscarinic action by drugs.

ACETYLCHOLINE

Acetylcholine is not important therapeutically because of its diffuse action on cholinergic

---

Walter Ernest Dixon, 1870–1931. Cambridge, England, pharmacologist. One of the founders of experimental pharmacology. In 1907 showed similarity between nerve stimulation of the heart and the effects of certain drugs; he suggested that neural effect was due to chemical substance release. Verified later by others.

sites throughout the body and its susceptibility to hydrolysis by acetylcholinesterases. A knowledge of its pharmacologic actions forms the basis for our understanding of the pharmacology, toxicology, and therapeutic usefulness of muscarinic agents, and for this reason it is the prototype drug.

CHEMISTRY

Acetylcholine is a quaternary ammonium compound (Fig. 14-1) that contains three spatially separated centers of importance for its biologic activity: the positively charged nitrogen, the carboxyl oxygen carrying a relatively negative charge, and the relatively electron-poor esteratic oxygen. Although acetylcholine has three reactive sites, only two are necessary for the various actions of the compound. The quaternary nitrogen is necessary for the activation of all acetylcholine receptors but must be coupled with either the positive or the negative oxygen.

For muscarinic activity, the combination of the quaternary nitrogen and the positive oxygen separated by a particular distance predicted by molecular orbital studies is necessary. This type of binding and spatial orientation is present in the alkaloid muscarine (*see* Chap. 14) whose effects were originally used to distinguish the various actions of acetylcholine. Another combination of sites is found in nicotine. When acetylcholine is in this spatial configuration, it can activate nicotinic receptors (autonomic ganglia and skeletal-neuromuscular junctions; *see* Chaps. 13, 19).

FIG. 14-1. Principal muscarinic agents.

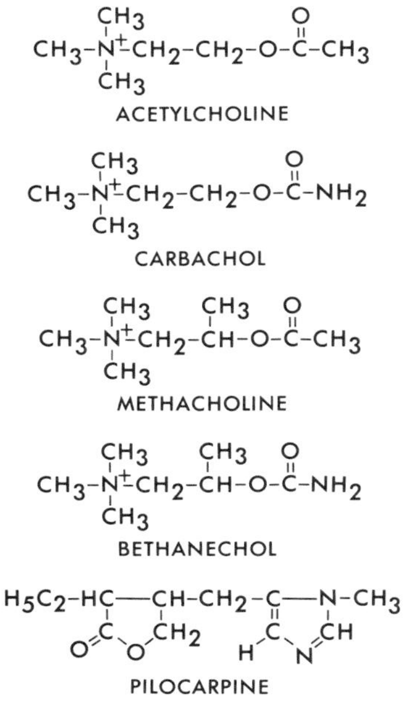

PHARMACOLOGIC ACTIONS

The pharmacologic effects produced by acetylcholine and other muscarinic agents can, to a considerable extent, be deduced from a knowledge of the physiology of the autonomic nervous system. A brief discussion follows.

Cardiovascular System

Acetylcholine lowers arterial pressure as a result of vasodilation of vascular smooth muscle and decreased cardiac function. This response is potentiated by a cholinesterase inhibitor and blocked by atropine. In the presence of both drugs, acetylcholine may raise arterial pressure by stimulating sympathetic ganglia (nicotinic effect) and releasing catecholamines from the adrenal medulla.

Acetylcholine seems to have a greater effect on small resistance vessels, arteries, and arterioles than it has on larger vessels and veins. Acetylcholine appears to produce dilation of essentially all vascular beds after its administration probably by releasing dilator material from the tunica intima. However, the lack of parasympathetic innervation to certain vascular beds suggests that these responses are not of primary physiological importance. In addition, activation of muscarinic receptors on peripheral sympathetic nerve terminals leads to a decrease in the release of norepinephine, thus reducing sympathetic vascular tone.

In the heart, cholinergic parasympathetic fibers are distributed extensively to the sinoatrial and atrioventricular nodes and the atrial muscle. Cholinergic innervation of the ventricular myocardium is sparse, and the axons terminate predominately on specialized conduction tissue such as the Purkinje fibers. Acetylcholine resembles vagal stimulation in producing bradycardia, prolongation of atrioventricular conduction, and a negative inotropic effect on the atria and ventricle. The bradycardia is primarily the result of the action

---

ADOLF JOHANN FRIEDRICH WILHELM VON BAEYER, 1835–1917. Munich chemist. Discovered barbituric acid (1863); did much work on organic dyes, discovering the molecular structure of indigo; developed tests for glucose and acetone; and, in 1870, distinguished the dark and light reactions of photosynthesis. Won the Nobel prize for chemistry in 1905.

of acetylcholine at the sinoatrial node, where it decreases the rate of spontaneous diastolic depolarization. This decreases the time for reaching the threshold potential and the subsequent events in the cardiac cycle. The drug shortens the atrial action potential, and conduction velocity may actually increase. This combination of factors is the basis for the perpetuation or exacerbation by vagal impulses of atrial flutter or fibrillation arising at an ectopi foci (*see* Chaps. 34, 35). Mechanistically acetylcholine increases the permeability of cardiac fibers to potassium. This increase, relative to the change in permeability to sodium, decreases the rate of discharge of sinoatrial pacemaker fibers. Decreased conduction velocity and an increased refractory period occur in the atrioventricular node. High concentrations of drug produce complete heart block. Acetylcholine decreases the slope of the diastolic prepotential.

In addition to direct effects of acetylcholine on the vascular system, indirect reflex effects are produced. The fall in arterial pressure produced by acetylcholine reflexly activates sympathetic activity through pressor receptive mechanisms, resulting in an increased heart rate.

Smooth Muscle

Smooth muscles of the gastrointestinal urogenital and respiratory tracts, as well as the eye, are stimulated by acetylcholine. In the gastrointestinal tract there is increased tone and motility. With high concentrations, spasm and tetanus can occur. The motility of the gall bladder and bile ducts is also increased. The smooth muscles of the ureters and urinary bladder are contracted and their sphincters relaxed, leading to voiding of urine. The physiology of these systems is, however, rather complex. For instance, studies have shown that it is extremely difficult to isolate and differentiate the sympathetic from the parasympathetic system in the lower urinary tract because both appear to work as a single unit. Noradrenergic sympathetic fibers, for example, influence the action of parasympathetic fibers, and parasympathetic stimuli regulate the activity of the sympathetic fibers. Moreover, the traditional concept that the pudendal nerve (somatic) is the only outlet for the external sphincter musculature is incorrect because there is autonomic as well as somatic innervation to the external sphincter.

Cross-talk between cholinergic and adrenergic fibers in the gastrointestinal tract also appears to exist. In the bronchial smooth muscle, contraction by acetylcholine results in bronchospasm. In the eye, acetylcholine produces pupillary constriction (miosis), spasm of accommodation, and a transitory rise in intraocular pressure, followed by a more persistent fall.

At all these sites acetylcholine produces increased permeability of the muscle cell to all ions with a resultant depolarization of the cell membrane. In addition to this partial depolarization, acetylcholine increases the frequency of the spontaneous action potentials presumably by increasing pacemaker activity.

Glands

Acetylcholine causes increased secretions from lacrimal, salivary (profuse and watery), nasopharyngeal, bronchial, gastric, intestinal, pancreatic, and sweat glands. At these sites acetylcholine causes an increased permeability, leading to an inward flux of calcium which, in turn, activates the specific cellular function. Acetylcholine also increases the release of catecholamines from the adrenal medulla by activation of either nicotinic or muscarinic receptors.

MECHANISM OF ACTION

Acetylcholine and other muscarinic agents exert their principal action at the cell membrane by combining with specific receptors. This action results in alterations in membrane permeability. In the presence of the drug the membrane becomes more permeable to one or more various ions (*e.g.*, potassium, sodium, and calcium). The pre-existent flux equilibrium is disturbed and the membrane potential altered. The direction of the change depends on the magnitude of the membrane potential and on the ratio between the increased sodium and potassium conductance. Under the influence of acetylcholine the membrane permeabilities for potassium and sodium increase unequally, so that the ratio of permeability for potassium to that of sodium may either increase, resulting in hyperpolarization, or decrease, leading to depolarization. The final result can be either depo-

---

REID HUNT, 1870–1948. American pharmacologist. In 1906 reported the hypotensive effect of acetylcholine and in 1911 showed physostigmine pretreatment to increase sensitivity to acetylcholine. First to show thyroid hormone in human blood and to correlate the activity of the thyroid with its iodine content.

MORRIS ZIFF, 1913– . American physician and chemist. Special interest in biochemistry and immunology of rheumatoid arthritis and related diseases.

larization (as in smooth muscle cells) or hyperpolarization (as in myocardial pacemaker cells).

BETHANECHOL (URECHOLINE)

The most widely used muscarinic agent in urology, bethanechol has structural features common to both methacholine and carbachol (Fig. 14-1). It is not hydrolyzed by acetylcholinesterase or butyrocholinesterase and thus has a longer duration of action. Bethanechol's major pharmacologic effects result from interaction with muscarinic receptors with minor nicotinic effects in normal persons.

The activity of bethanechol is largely confined to the urinary bladder and gastrointestinal tract, and bethanechol is preferred to other cholinergic drugs for stimulation of these systems. Its important pharmacologic actions on the urinary bladder include a decreased bladder capacity, increased tone of the detrusor muscle, and increased maximum voluntary voiding. When the bladder is empty, bethanechol does not initiate a desire to urinate. When used to treat patients with hypotonicity of the detrusor (atonic bladder), bethanechol results in a consistently elevated intravesical pressure, decreased capacity, increased detrusor tone, increased maximum voluntary voiding pressure, and decreased residual volume. It has been reported that a combination of bethanechol and the α-adrenoceptor antagonist phenoxybenzamine may result in effective voiding in patients with atonic bladder and functional outflow obstruction when they are not responsive to bethanechol itself.

Bethanechol is also used to restore normal micturition in selected patients with acute urinary retention related to surgery and parturition. The drug is administered orally and subcutaneously but never by the intramuscular or intravenous route. Although the effect on organ-systems other than the urinary bladder and gastrointestinal tract are minimal, side-effects include lacrimation, flushing, sweating, gastrointestinal disturbances, abdominal cramps, difficulty in visual accommodation, and headache. These side-effects are less pronounced after oral administration compared to after subcutaneous administration.

METHACHOLINE (MECHOLYL)

Methacholine differs from acetylcholine only by the addition of a methyl group to the β-methyl position of choline (Fig. 14-1). It is hydrolyzed by acetylcholinesterase but not by butyrocholinesterase (*see* Chap. 15). Because its rate of hydrolysis is considerably slower than that of acetylcholine, methacholine's actions are more persistent. Methacholine acts principally on muscarinic receptors and is essentially devoid of nicotinic effects; its muscarinic actions are qualitatively the same as those of acetylcholine. The drug is administered orally but is poorly and irregularly absorbed from the gastrointestinal tract. Methacholine is partly destroyed by gastric secretions. It differs from bethanechol by eliciting gastrointestinal and detrusor effects only after doses that also induce relatively prominent cardiovascular effects that limit its clinical usefulness. The drug is still useful, however, in ophthalmology.

CARBACHOL

Carbachol is one of the most powerful of the choline esters (Fig. 14-1). Its acid component is carbamic rather than acetic, and the carbamic ester linkage is not readily susceptible to hydrolysis by acetylcholinesterase or butyrocholinesterase. Carbachol has both muscarinic and nicotinic actions, but muscarinic actions predominate. Its pharmacologic actions are similar to those of acetylcholine. Carbachol is not as useful in treating gastrointestinal and urinary tract atony because of its considerable stimulation of ganglionic nicotinic receptors.

FURTRETHONIUM

The most potent cholinergic drug acting on the bladder, furtrethonium is seldom used clinically. In normal persons it causes a sharp rise in intravesical pressure with decreased capacity and an earlier desire to void.

PILOCARPINE

In contrast to the above drugs, pilocarpine is not a choline ester but is a naturally occurring muscarinic alkaloid with additional nicotinic actions. This agent is obtained from the leaves of tropical American shrubs belonging to the genus *Pilocarpus*. The hydrochloride salt is hygroscopic and is inactivated by light. The nitrate salt is not hygroscopic and therefore offers some advantages.

Pilocarpine has a direct effect on muscarinic effector cells and stimulates autonomic ganglia. It very markedly stimulates the secretion of sweat and saliva. As much as 2 to 3 liters of sweat and 350 ml of saliva can be secreted in a few hours. Pilocarpine produces effects on smooth muscle and glands similar to those of acetylcholine. On the cardiovascular system, however, hypertension and tachycardia may result from its nicotinic actions on the sympathetic ganglia and the adrenal medulla. Despite this, pilocarpine has been the mainstay of therapy in primary open-angle and most other chronic glaucomas for more than 100 years and is still the standard drug used in treating various forms of this disease.

The major action of pilocarpine in the treatment of various forms of glaucomas is to increase aqueous outflow through the trabecular network and Schlemm's canal. Its effects on aqueous humor dynamics are complex, and despite extensive research, still not completely known. Pilocarpine produces contraction of the ciliary muscle and contraction of the circular muscle of the iris, producing pupillary constriction and causing a mechanical change in the configuration of the meshwork, increasing its fluid conductance. In addition, pilocarpine may also act directly on the meshwork or the canal. It appears to dilate the trabecular network and veins leading away from Schlemm's canal, resulting in increased outflow. Pilocarpine also appears to affect aqueous humor formation and composition of unknown mechanisms. The importance of these actions and the precise mechanism by which they are produced in explaining the therapeutic efficacy and toxicity of pilocarpine in primary open-angle and other chronic glaucomas still await definition.

In contrast, the primary beneficial effects of pilocarpine and other miotics in angle-closure glaucoma result in its above-mentioned constriction of the pupil, which pulls the iris away from the trabeculum. Pilocarpine penetrates the eye well and induces miosis 15 to 30 minutes after topical application. Its duration of action after this type of application is 2 to 4 hours. Pilocarpine is tolerated better than most other miotics; however, ciliary spasm and miosis may be troublesome. Systemic side-effects and allergic reactions are uncommon.

Various routes for the delivery of pilocarpine have been developed in addition to traditional eye drops: soft contact lens reservoirs; membrane controlled delivery system; high viscosity gels; and polymer emulsions. If the patient can tolerate these forms of the drug, administration is better in maintaining around the clock intraocular pressure control than it is with pilocarpine eye drops.

If refractoriness to pilocarpine develops during long-term treatment, responsiveness can often be restored by withdrawing pilocarpine and substituting another miotic, such as carbachol, for a short time.

THERAPEUTIC USES

Gastrointestinal and Urologic Disorders

Muscarinic agents, in particular bethanechol, are used to treat nonobstructive urinary retention and gastrointestinal atony by virtue of their ability to stimulate the smooth muscles of the gastrointestinal and urinary tracts. These agents are used to restore normal micturition in patients with urinary retention related to surgery, parturition, trauma, or psychic factors. They are also useful in treating postoperative gastrointestinal atony, including postvagotomy atony and adynamic ileus secondary to trauma, infection, or neurogenic disorders.

Ophthalmologic Disorders

Muscarinic agents are used as miotics in the treatment of glaucoma but have also been applied in accommodative estropia or convergent strabismus. When applied directly to the eye, these drugs cause miosis, spasm of accommodation, and a persistent fall in intraocular pressure that may be preceded by a transitory rise. *Glaucoma* is traditionally defined as an ocular disease characterized by an elevated intraocular pressure sufficient to interfere with vision. The elevation of pressure can be sufficient to impair retinal and optic nerve circulation with possible irreversible visual loss. It is responsible for 10% to 20% of the cases of blindness in the United States. The primary goal of treatment is to prevent damage to the optic nerve fibers by lowering the elevated intraocular pressure.

Primary Open-angle (Chronic Simple) Glaucoma. In primary open-angle glaucoma, the most common form, increased intraocular pressure is the result of an unknown abnormality that involves the trabecular network, causing interference with the outflow of aqueous humor to Schlemm's canal. This decreased outflow occurs in the presence of a normal angle. Pilocarpine is the drug of choice for initial and maintenance therapy, and this or other muscarinic drugs may have to be given indefinitely. As discussed above, the mechanism of the lowering of intraocular pressure by miotics in this form of glaucoma is not known. It appears that they facilitate the filtering of aqueous humor from the anterior chamber through the trabecular network. They appear to dilate the trabecular network and veins leading away from Schlemm's canal, resulting in increased outflow. Contraction of the ciliary body caused by these drugs may also help open the trabecular network. Miotics are generally not used to treat secondary glaucomas.

Primary Angle-closure (Acute Congestive or Narrow Angle) Glaucoma. Far less common and in contrast to open-angle glaucoma, the angle-closure form has a normal filtration mechanism and normal intraocular pressure, as long as aqueous humor can gain access to the filtration angle. The iris, however, bows forward and makes contact with the corneal endothelium, and the anterior chamber becomes shallow. Where access to the filtration angle is eliminated, the pressure rises suddenly and dramatically. Treatment comprises reversing the relative pupillary block and allowing the aqueous humor to gain access to the filtration angle and is carried out by surgical intervention. An iridectomy, using surgery or a laser beam, provides an opening through the peripheral iris between the anterior and posterior chambers. Before surgery can be undertaken, the pressure must be controlled. Pilocarpine or other miotics are used to constrict the pupil and break the pupillary block, along with osmotic agents and carbonic anhydrase inhibitors. This is a medical emergency, and drugs must be used as soon as possible because a prolonged attack can result in permanent adhesions between the peripheral part of the iris and the corneal endothelium.

ADVERSE EFFECTS AND CONTRAINDICATIONS

Since muscarinic agents produce ubiquitous effects on numerous organ-systems, all effects except the desired one can be considered adverse. These are likely to be particularly serious if the drug is given intravenously, and consequently this route should never be used. The more common adverse effects include severe gastrointestinal cramping, profuse sweating, generalized or localized paresthesia, shock, bladder pain, salivation, and diarrhea. When used in ophthalmology as miotics, these drugs may produce ciliary spasm, browache, headache, false myopia, and undesirable rises in intraocular pressure. In addition, patients may become hypersensitive or refractory to the effects of the drug.

Muscarinic agents are contraindicated in any condition in which one or more of their actions is likely to be particularly dangerous, including in patients with myasthenia gravis who are receiving neostigmine in those with progressive muscular atrophy, or in those with bulbar palsy. These drugs are contraindicated in patients with bronchial asthma because of the possibility of inducing bronchospasm. Hyperthyroidism is another contraindication due to possible production of atrial fibrillation. Because of their effects in increasing gastrointestinal motility, muscarinic agonists such as bethanechol or pilocarpine should not be given to patients with peptic ulcers or other gastrointestinal lesions. Likewise, they are contraindicated in the presence of organic urinary tract or gastrointestinal obstruction. Because muscarinic agonists may lower blood pressure, they should be used cautiously in patients with hypotension.

FURTHER READING

1. Carrier O Jr: Pharmacology of the Peripheral Autonomic System. Chicago, Year Book Publishers, 1972
2. Durkee DP, Bryant BG: Drug therapy reviews: Drug therapy of glaucoma. Am J Hosp Pharm. 35:682–690, 1978
3. Finkbeiner AE, Bissada NK, Welch LT: Uropharmacology: Choline esters and other parasympathomimetic drugs. Urology 10:83–89, 1977
4. Levy NN: Parasympathetic control of the heart. In Randall WC (ed): Neural Regulation of the Heart, pp 97–129. New York, Oxford University Press, 1977
5. Raz S: Pharmacological treatment of lower urinary tract dysfunction. Urol Clin North Am 5: 323–334, 1978
6. Snyder SH, Chang KJ, Kuhar MJ et al: Biochemical identification of the mammalian muscarinic cholinergic receptor. *Fed Proc* 34:1915–1921, 1974

CHAPTER 14 QUESTIONS

(See P. 7 for Full Instructions)

Select the One Best Answer

1. An effect produced by intravenous injection of methacholine but not by stimulating the parasympathetic nervous system is

A. bradycardia.
B. peripheral vasodilation.
C. contraction of the circular muscle of the iris.
D. increased gastrointestinal activity.
E. increased salivation.

2. Which of the following will occur in poisoning caused by the mushroom *Amanita muscaria* (muscarine)?
A. Bronchodilation, lacrimation, and hypotension
B. Dry mouth, miosis, and intestinal colic
C. Salivation, miosis, and bronchiolar spasm
D. Spasm of the ciliary muscle, decreased intestinal motility, and bradycardia
E. Sweating, cycloplegia, and colic

3. The intravenous administration of drug X results in hypotension, increased intestinal motility, miosis, salivation, and bradycardia. The class of drugs to which drug X belongs is
A. β-adrenergic stimulants.
B. ganglionic blocking agents.
C. ganglionic stimulating agents.
D. muscarinic agents.
E. antihistaminic agents.

A = 1,2,3; B = 1,3; C = 2,4; D = 4; E = All

4. Side-effects that may accompany the topical use of pilocarpine in the treatment of glaucoma include
1. spasm of accommodation.
2. dry mouth.
3. induction of extreme miosis and an immobile pupil that curtails night vision.
4. twitching of the striated muscle of the eyelids.

5. Agents used in the treatment of chronic open-angle glaucoma include
1. pilocarpine.
2. *l*-epinephrine (Epitrate).
3. acetazolamide (Diamox).
4. echothiophate (Phospholine).

6. Which of the following effects of methacholine (Mecholyl) limit its clinical usefulness?
1. Excessive salivation
2. Marked hypotension
3. Bronchiolar constriction
4. Skeletal muscle fasciculations

7. Methacholine
1. prolongs the refractory period of atrial muscle.
2. prolongs the refractory period of the A-V node.
3. increases the rate of firing of latent pacemaker tissue.
4. decreases the slope of slow diastolic depolarization (phase 4 of the action potential).

8. Both carbachol and bethanecol (Urecholine) are
1. adequately absorbed after oral administration.
2. metabolized by cholinesterases.
3. active on the muscarinic receptors of the gastrointestinal tract.
4. effective therapy for myasthenia gravis.

THOMAS C. WESTFALL

15

Cholinesterase Inhibitors

Cholinesterase inhibitors represent a second major group of drugs that produce effects similar to acetylcholine. These actions are the result of inhibition of the enzymes (acetylcholinesterase and butyrocholinesterase) involved in the hydrolysis of acetylcholine. Acetylcholinesterase (specific cholinesterase, true cholinesterase) is the enzyme that destroys the acetylcholine involved in synaptic transmission. This represents the principal mechanism for the disposition of the transmitter after its liberation from nerve terminals. Pharmacologic evidence indicates that acetylcholinesterase is also active presynaptically and plays a role in regulating acetylcholine levels in cholinergic nerve terminals. The enzyme is found in high concentrations at all sites at which acetylcholine serves as a transmitter, including the skeletal-neuromuscular junction, autonomic ganglia, postganglionic parasympathetic neuroeffector sites, and at certain synapses in the central nervous system (CNS). Butyrocholinesterase (nonspecific cholinesterase, pseudocholinesterase, plasma cholinesterase) is a related enzyme with less substrate specificity found in plasma, intestine, glial cells, and other organs. The function of this enzyme is less clear.

The pharmacologic effects of cholinesterase inhibitors are principally due to their action on acetylcholinesterase, whose inhibition results in the accumulation of excessive amounts of the acetylcholine transmitter in the synaptic region. The action of acetylcholine released from nerve terminals is potentiated and prolonged, resulting in increased skeletal muscle contraction, increased activity of organs and tissues receiving postganglionic parasympathetic innervation (glands, smooth muscle, heart), increased ganglionic transmission, and cholinergic effects in the CNS. In addition, some of these drugs have a direct cholinomimetic action by directly stimulating cholinergic receptors.

Cholinesterase inhibitors are useful in the treatment of myasthenia gravis, in the management of glaucoma, and in atony of the gastrointestinal and urinary tracts. They are active ingredients of many potent insecticides and thus of toxicologic importance. They are extensively used as investigative tools. Finally, cholinesterase inhibitors represent a potential hazard as chemical warfare agents.

CHEMISTRY AND MECHANISM OF ACTION

A great deal of information on the structure and activity of acetylcholinesterase exists. The enzyme is a tetramer made up of four equal subunits (80,000 molecular weight) each of which has an active center. Acetylcholine attaches to the active center of acetylcholinesterase at two sites, one specific for the quaternary ammonium moiety of acetylcholine—the anionic site—and the other for its esteratic site where nucleophilic attack occurs on the acyl carbon of the substrate. The anionic site is negatively charged, is stereospecific, and is a carboxyl group of a decarboxylic amino acid such as glutamic acid. This site attracts the positively charged nitrogen atom of acetylcholine and binds the attached methyl groups by Van der Waal's forces. The esteratic site of the enzyme where nucleophilic attack occurs on the acyl carbon of the substrate comprises two basic groups: serine and histadine and one acid group, the hydroxyl of tyrosine. The esteratic site combines with the carbonyl carbon atoms of the acetyl group and forms a covalent bond with the enzyme, resulting in the acetylation of the enzyme, rupture of the ester linkage, and elimination of choline.

The hydrolysis of acetylcholine, or any other substrate, takes place in three steps, presented schematically in Figure 15-1. The first step consists of the reversible formation of a complex between acetylcholine and the enzyme in which the principal bonds are formed with the cationic site of acetylcholine and the carbonyl atom of the ester group. The second step results in an acyl transfer through nucleophilic attack on the ester carbonyl by a serine residue in the enzyme, releasing choline and forming an acyl-enzyme intermediate. In the third step hydrolysis of the acylenzyme (rate limiting step) occurs, yielding acetate and hydrogen ions and regenerating the enzyme.

The hydrolysis of acetylcholine occurs extremely fast. Each active site in a purified sample of ox red blood cell acetylcholinesterase can hydrolyze 3×10^5 molecules of acetylcholine per minute, equivalent to a turnover time of 150 microseconds.

Cholinesterase inhibitors prevent the above reactions by forming inhibitor-enzyme complexes in competition with acetylcholine. Although these drugs react with the enzyme in essentially the same manner as acetylcholine, these complexes are more stable (covalent) than is the acetylcholine enzyme complex; they therefore delay the hydrolysis of acetylcholine. The most convenient way of classifying the cholinesterase inhibitors is based on quantitative temporal differences. Drugs are classified as reversible or nonreversible cholinesterase inhibitors. Reversible cholinesterase inhibitors delay the hydrolysis of acetylcholine from 1 to 8 hours. The breakdown of the inhibitor-enzyme complex in the case of nonreversible agents is much slower.

REVERSIBLE INHIBITORS

Reversible cholinesterase inhibitors can interact with acetylcholinesterase in two ways. First, a reversible complex between the enzyme and the inhibitor is formed (step I), but steps analogous to steps II and III do not occur. Edrophonium (Fig. 15-2), an example of this type of inhibition, binds only with the anionic site of acetylcholine to form a rapidly reversible enzyme-substrate complex.

Second, a reversible complex between the inhibitor is formed, and steps analogous to II and III occur very slowly. Physostigmine and neostigmine (Fig. 15-2) are examples of this type of inhibitor. Both are substituted carbamate esters, and the enzyme-inhibitor complex decomposes to yield the corresponding alcohol and carbamylated enzyme. Unlike the acetylated enzyme, the carbamylated enzyme is relatively stable, and free enzyme is slowly regenerated by hydrolysis.

In addition, both edrophonium and neostigmine have a direct stimulating action at cholinergic sites.

NONREVERSIBLE CHOLINESTERASE INHIBITORS

Nonreversible cholinesterase inhibitors are mostly organophosphate compounds widely used as the active ingredients of many insecticides and war gases (Fig. 15-2). With the organophosphate cholinesterase inhibitors, steps corresponding to I and II are very rapid, but step III does not occur at any appreciable rate. These agents form a stable phosphorylated enzyme intermediate resulting from nucleophilic displacement by the enzyme at its esteratic site.

Nonreversible cholinesterase inhibitors produce an essentially permanent inactivation of the enzyme because the organically substituted phosphoryl enzyme formed is extremely

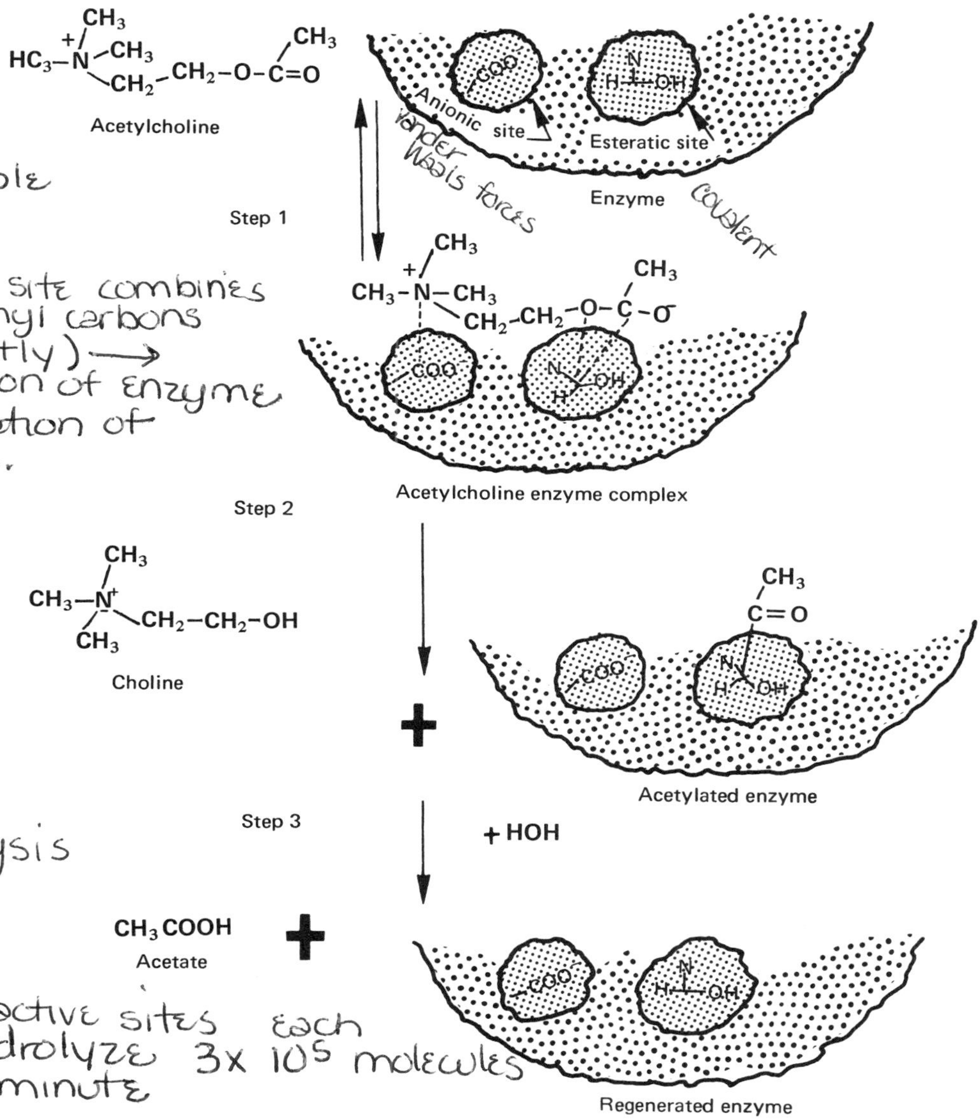

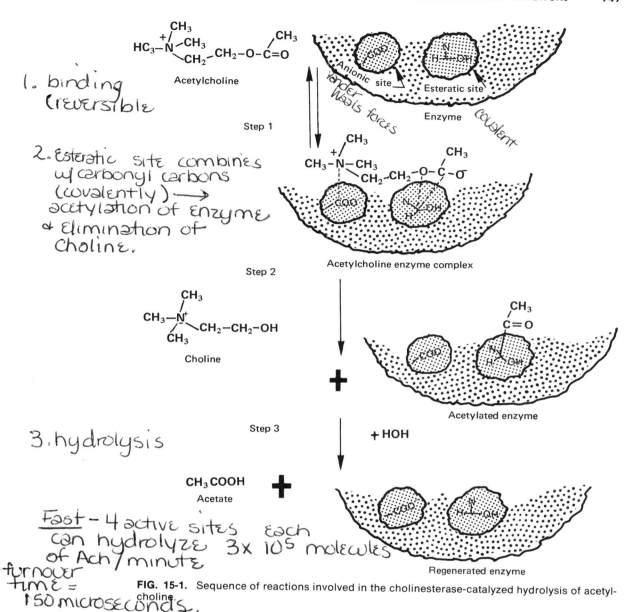

1. binding (reversible

2. Esteratic site combines w/ carbonyl carbons (covalently) → acetylation of enzyme & elimination of choline.

3. hydrolysis

Fast - 4 active sites each can hydrolyze 3x 10^5 molecules of Ach/minute
turnover time = 150 microseconds.

FIG. 15-1. Sequence of reactions involved in the cholinesterase-catalyzed hydrolysis of acetylcholine.

resistant to attack by water. The phosphorylated enzyme cannot hydrolyze acetylcholine and thus is inhibited. Eventually hydrolysis of the ester bond by water occurs, but this hydrolytic step is extremely slow, and for some agents the reaction is not measurable. Most members of this class lack a cationic group and thus attack only the esteratic site of the enzyme. Both types of cholinesterase are inactivated. Some drugs, such as *echothiophate*, are quaternary compounds that contain a cationic group and appear to be potent and selective inhibitors of acetylcholinesterase. They interact with both the esteratic and anionic sites in the active center to produce a stable complex. Their duration of action is longer than that of cholinesterase inhibitors that contain no cationic group and is determined principally by the rate of synthesis of new enzyme. (It may be several weeks.)

PHARMACOLOGIC ACTIONS

The administration of cholinesterase inhibitors results in generalized cholinergic responses. The most prominent effects are those that originate from the parasympathetic postganglionic

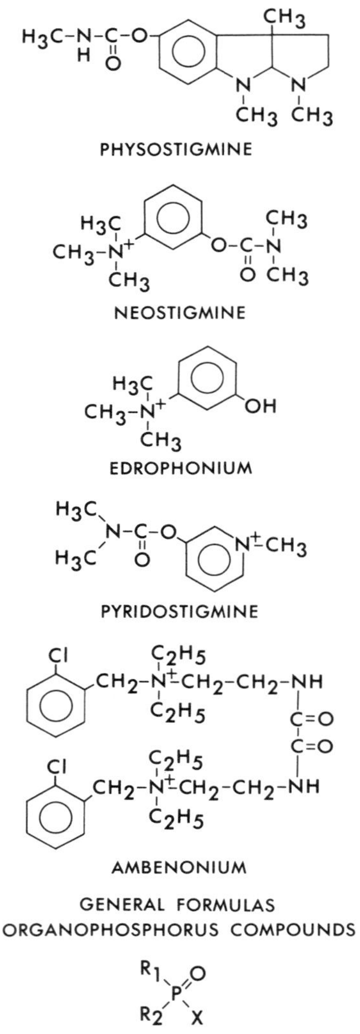

FIG. 15-2. Principal cholinesterase inhibitors.

nerve terminals due to activation of muscarinic receptors, including a decreased heart rate; vasodilation with resultant decreased arterial pressure; increased skin temperature; increased gastrointestinal activity; bronchial constriction and spasm; pupillary constriction; and increased secretions of salivary, sweat, gastric, and mucosal glands. A local action restricted to the eye may be achieved by conjunctival instillation, results in miosis, conjunctival hyperemia, spasm of the ciliary muscle that may be painful, and accommodation for near vision.

In low doses, cholinesterase inhibitors have little effect at the skeletal neuromuscular junction. At higher doses, however, muscle fasciculations associated with augmentation of miniature end-plate and excitatory postsynaptic potentials, conversion of twitch to tetanus, and ultimately depolarizing block may be seen. If neuromuscular transmission has been impaired by antidepolarizing blocking agents such as *d*-tubocurarine, protection of the liberated acetylcholine against destruction of cholinesterase may cause a significant improvement (*see* Chap. 19). A similar improvement may be seen in myasthenia gravis, a disease in which local or general muscular weakness is produced by a disorder in neuromuscular transmission (*see* below). Inhibition of acetylcholinesterase and accumulation of acetylcholine can lead to repetitive antidromic firing.

Ganglionic stimulant and subsequent blocking effects can be seen only after high doses of cholinesterase inhibitors, and for the most part these effects are of no practical import. A considerable proportion of the acetylcholinesterase in autonomic ganglia seems to be excessive. In the superior cervical ganglion of the cat, for instance, at least 50% of the acetylcholinesterase must be inhibited before a potentiation of the effects of preganglionic stimulation can be demonstrated. An effect on the nerve plexus of the gastrointestinal tract may play a part in the increased gastrointestinal motility seen after cholinesterase inhibitors.

Various central effects may be produced after high doses of those cholinesterase inhibitors that cross the blood–brain barrier. These include drugs that contain a tertiary nitrogen such as physostigmine, but not a quaternary nitrogen, such as neostigmine. These effects are characterized by stimulation followed by depression and include disturbances of sleep, tremor and ataxia, hallucinations, and desynchronization of the electroencephalogram. Death from cholinesterase inhibitors is usually due to respiratory paralysis secondary to depression of the respiratory centers.

REVERSIBLE CHOLINESTERASE INHIBITORS

Physostigmine (Eserine)

Physostigmine was the first specific cholinesterase inhibitor. Its discovery is important for two reasons: First, it was the first instance in which the mechanism of action of a drug was defined in relatively simple chemical terms. Physostigmine is the active ingredient of the

ROBERT CHRISTISON, 1797–1882. Scottish physician and toxicologist. As well as extensive drug studies, worked on renal pathology and medical jurisprudence. Developed generally accepted cadaver examination methods for legal purposes. Early description of the ordeal or calabar bean.

calabar bean (the nut of Etu Esére), extracts of which were used in the trial by ordeal of Nigerian women suspected of witchcraft. If the accused could save her life by vomiting the poison, she was deemed innocent of the charge brought against her. The properties of this drug were studied as early as 1855. Second, it proved to be an important tool with which evidence was secured to support the theory of chemical neurotransmission.

The drug is a tertiary ammonium alkaloid (Fig. 15-2) that is well absorbed from the gastrointestinal tract and enters the CNS. Physostigmine appears about equally effective against acetylcholinesterase and butyrocholinesterase. Physostigmine is the drug of choice for reversing the signs and symptoms of anticholinergic poisoning and is particularly effective in antagonizing the central actions of drugs with anticholinergic activity. Although not popular as a primary miotic agent, physostigmine is occasionally used to treat angle-closure glaucoma and accommodative estropia (overconvergence caused by excessive accommodation). Miosis occurs in about 30 minutes and may last 12 to 36 hours. Physostigmine can cause hyperemia of the conjunctiva and iris and is rarely tolerated for prolonged periods because of conjunctivitis and allergic reactions. Physostigmine has been replaced in the treatment of myasthenia gravis by quaternary amines that do not significantly penetrate the CNS.

The principal use of this drug is as a miotic and thus is used to treat narrow angle glaucoma and to reverse the mydriasis caused by atropine. It is also the antidote of choice to treat atropine poisoning.

NEOSTIGMINE (PROSTIGMINE)

A synthetic, reversible quaternary (Fig. 15-2) cholinesterase inhibitor, neostigmine differs from physostigmine in that, because it is a quaternary ammonium nitrogen compound and is poorly and irregularly absorbed from the gastrointestinal tract, it does not cross the blood–brain barrier (*see* Chap. 3). This irregular absorption produces some problems in therapy but minimizes CNS toxicity. The presence of the quaternary nitrogen enables the drug to have a direct action on both nicotinic and muscarinic receptors, which makes it particularly useful for its effect at the neuromuscular junction.

Neostigmine has a very powerful anticurare action: It increases the amount of acetylcholine liberated from nerve terminals, preserves the liberated acetylcholine by blocking acetylcholinesterase, and has a direct action on the skeletal-neuromuscular end-plate. The neuromuscular action of the neostigmine has made it beneficial in the management and diagnosis of myasthenia gravis. It has also been used as a miotic and in treating postoperative atony of the intestine and urinary bladder.

Adverse side-effects occur more frequently with neostigmine than with pyridostigmine or ambenonium.

Pyridostigmine Bromide (Mestinon)

Pyridostigmine is a reversible cholinesterase inhibitor with pharmacologic properties and a therapeutic response similar to those seen with neostigmine. It has several advantages over neostigmine, however, that contribute to its being the most widely used oral cholinesterase inhibitor for the treatment of myasthenia gravis: its more predictable oral absorption; its slightly longer duration of action; and its less frequent adverse effects after oral administration.

Nevertheless, individual dosage and intervals of administration must be carefully determined because of wide fluctuations among patients in absorption, metabolism, and excretion to avoid fluctuations in strength and to anticipate periods of greatest need. A relatively simple method for determining blood levels of pyridostigmine by gas chromatography now exists. Sustained release preparations are available that can be used at bedtime to maintain the patient's strength at night or in the early morning.

Ambenonium (Mytelase Chloride)

Ambenonium is a bis-quaternary compound with anticholinesterase activity about six times greater than that of neostigmine. It facilitates transmission at the neuromuscular junction, has anticurare actions, and at high doses exhibits neuromuscular blocking activity. The drug is generally given orally when treating myasthenia gravis and has fewer side-effects and a longer duration of action than does neostigmine. Ambenonium is used less commonly

---

THOMAS RICHARD FRASER, 1841–1920. Scottish pharmacologist. With Alexander Crum Brown, was the first to study the relation between a drug's chemical structure and its action. Developed an antisnake venom (1895) and characterized physostigmine and strophanthus (an African arrow poison).

GEORGE BARGER, 1878–1939. English chemist. Isolated ergotoxine from ergot in 1906 and histamine in 1910–1911 with Henry Dale. Synthesized thyroxine in 1927.

than pyridostigmine or neostigmine but is very useful in treating patients who cannot tolerate neostigmine bromide or pyridostigmine bromide because of sensitivity to bromide ion. Overdosage can result in all of the typical cholinergic effects.

Edrophonium (Tensilon)

A synthetic cholinesterase inhibitor, edrophonium is unique in having a much shorter onset and duration of action than neostigmine. The absence of the carbamate group results in a marked reduction in its ability to inhibit acetylcholinesterase. It acts only at the anionic site to form a rapidly reversible enzyme substrate complex and has a direct stimulant action on the motor-end plate and probably stimulates the skeletal-neuromuscular junction by this direct action. This agent is more effective at the skeletal neuromuscular junction than at postganglionic parasympathetic neuroeffector sites.

Edrophonium is important in establishing the diagnosis of myasthenia gravis and in differentiating between "myasthenia weakness or crises" and "cholinergic crises." To diagnose myasthenia gravis, small amounts of edrophonium are injected intravenously in divided doses. An improvement in muscle strength within 1 to 3 minutes is diagnostic in myasthenic patients. A smaller i.v. dose will produce a brief remission of symptoms if they are caused by inadequate anticholinesterase therapy ("myasthenia crisis") but will further weaken patients suffering from an overdose of medication ("cholinergic crisis").

Edrophonium has a very powerful anticurare action and is used to reverse curare paralysis of skeletal muscle. This action does not appear to be due to a cholinesterase inhibitor action but rather to a facilitation of transmitter release and a direct displacement of curare from the motor end-plate. This action of edrophonium is prolonged.

Because the drug has a short duration of action, side-effects are not as severe as with other cholinesterase inhibitors. Most muscarinic symptoms can be seen after i.v. administration and are readily reversed with atropine.

THERAPEUTIC USE OF CHOLINESTERASE INHIBITORS

MYASTHENIA GRAVIS

One of the principal uses of the reversible cholinesterase inhibitors is in the diagnosis and treatment of myasthenia gravis. This disease is characterized by the weakness and rapid fatigability of skeletal muscle. The pattern of the disease is variable and may be diffused or limited to specific muscles. Often muscle weakness is severe and widespread and during an exacerbation typically begins in the face and neck and then spreads progressively to involve the upper limbs, the abdomen, and muscles of respiration.

The nature of neuromuscular defects in myasthenia gravis has been more clearly defined recently. The defect in neuromuscular transmission has been localized to the skeletal muscle motor end-plate, which possesses morphological, electrophysiological, and biochemical abnormalities. The disorder is caused by an autoimmune reaction that reduces the number of available acetylcholine nicotinic receptors on postjunctional membranes of the neuromuscular junction. The number of interactions between the acetylcholine released by nerve stimulation and the receptors is decreased, resulting in a reduction of muscle strength or progressive failure of contractions from repeated nerve stimulation. There are anatomical changes in the neuromuscular junction of the myasthenic patient: fewer junctional folds and wider synaptic clefts on the postjunctional side of the synapse. Circulating antibodies to acetylcholine receptors have been seen in about 90% of patients with myasthenia gravis. In fact, this may be an important new diagnostic tool because these antibodies are not found in patients with other autoimmune diseases. Moreover, IgG immune complexes can be demonstrated electromicrographically.

The severity of the disease does not seem to correlate with the antibody titer, although the severity of clinical signs increases with an increased proportion of receptors bound by antibody. Although the source of the immune stimulation of the antibody synthesis in myasthenia gravis is unknown, the disease may be initiated in a genetically susceptible person by an alteration of thymic cell function. There are decreased antibody titers after a thymectomy, a procedure known to benefit myasthenic patients. The precise role that the thymus plays in myasthenia gravis still awaits definition.

Reversible cholinesterase inhibitors are used for both diagnosis and treatment of myasthenia gravis. For diagnosis, edrophonium and neostigmine are used. In most cases, dramatic improvement in muscle strength can be observed shortly after the administration of either of these two drugs. Physostigmine, the first cholinesterase inhibitor used to treat myasthenia gravis, has now been replaced by the more effective quaternary ammonium compounds neostigmine, ambenonium, and pyridostigmine. These drugs are given orally, with pyridostigmine being the most widely used. In severe cases, neostigmine can be given parenterally. The maximal muscle strength attained after optimal doses of these agents is about the same, but the effectiveness of therapy varies among patients. In addition, there are differences in onset and duration of action. Major problems occur in regulating the dosage to maintain a uniform level of strength throughout the day and yet minimize the production of side-effects. With insufficient drug a "myasthenia crisis," an exacerbation of the disease, results and can be precipitated by infection, surgery, pregnancy, emotional upset, or some undetermined cause. If there is too much drug a "cholinergic crisis" may be precipitated, which for muscle strength resembles a myasthenic crisis. In addition, there may be muscarinic side-effects, the most common being excessive salivation, perspiration, abdominal distress, nausea, and vomiting.

Not all patients are helped by the use of cholinesterase treatment. In addition, the sensitivity to these drugs may decrease in chronic treatment. The lack of an effect of cholinesterase inhibitor in the initial treatment of myasthenia gravis can be explained in several ways, based on our current understanding of the pathophysiology of the disease. For instance, postjunctional acetylcholine receptors may be completely absent; therefore increased acetylcholine in the neuromuscular junction would not be expected to improve muscle contraction. Another explanation is based on the observation of the markedly altered anatomy of the neuromuscular junction. The wider subsynaptic gap may allow increased acetylcholine to diffuse away before it can act on the available acetylcholine receptors. The loss of sensitivity to cholinesterase inhibition after chronic treatment could be due to a progression of the disease to where the two explanations above apply. Additionally, the cholinesterase inhibitors themselves may be responsible in the refractoriness by causing a continual increase in acetylcholine levels at the neuromuscular junction. Such a build-up may result in a decreased concentration of acetylcholine receptors at the motor end-plate. Such a loss of receptors has been demonstrated in experimental animals and is consistent with the observation that taking patients off cholinesterase inhibitor therapy results in a beneficial effect perhaps by their reacquiring acetylcholine receptors.

In addition to cholinesterase inhibitors additional therapeutic measures include thymectomy, adrenal corticosteroids, and other immunosuppressants, such as azathioprine and plasmapheresis (removing all the patient's plasma and replacing it with an artificial substitute).

Drugs Contraindicated in Myasthenic Patients

Certain drugs are contraindicated in patients suffering from myasthenia gravis. Curare and other nondepolarizing muscle relaxants, for instance, are 10 to 100 times more potent in these patients. Moreover, sedatives, hypnotics, and narcotics should be used cautiously as should antibiotics that have neuromuscular blocking properties.

More than 30 drugs are in current clinical use, besides those used in anesthesia, that may interfere with neuromuscular transmission. These drugs can produce postoperative respiratory depression, aggravate or unmask myasthenia gravis, or induce a myasthenic syndrome. Included in this grouping are antibiotics, cardiovascular drugs, psychotropic drugs, antiepileptics, hormonal agents, and antirheumatic drugs, as well as some miscellaneous agents.

OPHTHALMOLOGIC DISORDERS

Cholinesterase inhibitors may be used with, or in place of, directly acting muscarinic agents (*see* Chap. 14) to treat glaucoma and other ophthalmologic indications. These agents are applied directly to the eye and produce conjunctival hyperemia, miosis, spasm of accommodation, and reduced intraocular pressure. When administered locally, systemic adsorption is minimal but can take place with high doses of the drugs.

Short-acting agents such as physostigmine or neostigmine are occasionally used in the emergency treatment of primary angle-closure glaucoma, usually with pilocarpine. They are also sometimes used in treating primary open-angle glaucoma but are not usually as well tolerated as pilocarpine and may cause local irritation or allergic reactions.

Long-lasting cholinesterase inhibitors such as demecarium (Humorsol) and the organophosphate compounds isoflurophate (Floropryl) and echothiophate (Phospholine) are used to treat primary open-angle glaucoma. Because of their much longer duration of action, these drugs have a clear advantage when long-continued medication is needed. Owing to their toxicity, they are generally reserved for use when shorter-acting miotics have failed. In such situations, these long-lasting cholinesterase inhibitor drugs should be used because the risk of visual loss owing to uncontrolled open-angle glaucoma is greater than the potential toxicity of the compounds. Because of the possibility of precipitating an attack, these long-acting inhibitors are not advocated before iridectomy in angle-closure glaucoma; however, they may be used after iridectomy.

GASTROINTESTINAL AND UROLOGIC DISORDERS

Quaternary cholinesterase inhibitors such as neostigmine may be used to treat postoperative abdominal distention or urinary retention because of their ability to stimulate the smooth muscle. They may also be used to counteract the constipating effect of morphine. Quaternary cholinesterase inhibitors should not be used in the presence of mechanical obstruction.

ORGANOPHOSPHATE ANTICHOLINESTERASE POISONING

As mentioned above, organophosphate cholinesterase inhibitors such as isoflurophate (DFP), echothiophate (Phospholine), and parathion (Tables 15-1, 15-2) are highly toxic compounds that produce nonreversible inhibition of acetylcholinesterase and butyrocholinesterase. These drugs were developed as potential chemical warfare agents because of their extreme toxicity and free absorption through the intact skin. Although they have some therapeutic application, their principal interest is toxicologic because a number of organophosphate anticholinesterases are widely used as agricultural insecticides and because of their potential as warfare agents (Table 15-2). For these reasons, the diagnosis and treatment of poisoning by organophosphate anticholinesterases are of considerable practical import.

When these agents are administered, the clinical picture is a combination of peripheral cholinergic and CNS effects. The most pronounced systemic effects are profuse salivation, sweating, diarrhea, muscular weakness and fasciculations, mental confusion and ataxia, and disturbances of ventilation, culminating in respiratory paralysis and death.

At least four contributing causes lead to respiratory failure: excessive secretions from the salivary and bronchial glands, leading to obstruction of the airway; bronchoconstriction and laryngospasm; neuromuscular blockade of the respiratory muscles; and central respiratory failure. Severe dehydration may also develop. Depending on the route of administration, various local effects may also be observed: bronchoconstriction and increased bronchial secretion are prominent after inhalation, whereas nausea, vomiting, and intestinal cramps occur earliest after ingestion.

If the outcome is not immediately fatal, the effects may persist for several days or weeks. The rate of recovery depends on the rate of synthesis of new cholinesterase.

Delayed neurotoxic effects may begin 3 months or more after exposure to certain organophosphate agents, including the triaryl phosphates, which may be metabolized to form cholinesterase inhibitors. The latter are extensively used commercially as hydraulic fluids and gasoline additives. Symptoms include polyneuritis with flaccid paralysis of the upper and lower extremities and degeneration of myelin sheaths and axons in the spinal cord sciatic nerve and medulla. The mechanism is not understood.

TREATMENT

Atropine provides a specific and effective antidote to the muscarinic effects of cholinesterase inhibitors and to some degree is also active against the CNS effects. It must be given in large and repeated doses until the muscarinic effects are controlled. Supportive measures, including artificial ventilation, if necessary, must also be applied. Atropine antagonizes the effects of cholinesterase inactivation and does not restore the cholinesterase. Because of the prolonged inactivation of cholinesterase, atropine treatment may have to be continued for several days or weeks.

Although attack by the organophosphate cholinesterase inhibitors on the enzyme yields a phosphorylated enzyme resistant to attack by water, spontaneous hydrolysis of phosphorylated acetylcholinesterase and butyrocholines-

---

LUDWIG LAQUEUR, 1839–1909. German ophthalmologist. Introduced the use of physostigmine for glaucoma treatment in 1876.

TABLE 15-1. Principal Cholinesterase Inhibitors Used Therapeutically

Drug	Trade Name	Source	Type of Inhibition*	Dose	Route of Administration	Duration of Action	Major Therapeutic Indications
Ambenonium	Mytelase	Synthetic	2	10–30 mg	Oral	4 hr	Myasthenia gravis
Demecarium	Humorsol	Synthetic	2	0.2–0.5%	Conjunctival	3–5 days	Glaucoma
Echothiophate	Phospholine	Synthetic	3	0.25%	Conjunctival	3–7 days	Glaucoma
Edrophonium	Tensilon	Synthetic	1	2–8 mg	i.v.	1–2 hr	Diagnosis of myasthenia gravis; *d*-tubocurarine overdose
Neostigmine	Prostigmine	Synthetic	2	0.022 mg/kg (for diagnosis)	i.m.		Diagnosis and management of myasthenia gravis
				0.5–2 mg	i.m.	3–6 hr	
				30 mg	Oral	2–4 hr	
Pyridostigmine	Mestinon	Synthetic	2	60–300 mg	Oral	4 hr	Myasthenia gravis
Physostigmine	Eserine	Calabar bean (Physostima *venenosum*)	2	0.2–1%	Conjunctival	6–12 hr	Ophthalmologic applications

* The numbers 1, 2, and 3 refer to the types of cholinesterase inhibition discussed in the text under "Chemistry and Mechanism of Action."

TABLE 15-2. Representative Organophosphate Cholinesterase Inhibitors

Drug	Use	Comment
Diisopropyl fluorophosphonate (isoflurophate, DFP)	Investigative, medical	First organophosphate cholinesterase inhibitor discovered. Rarely used therapeutically. Water soluble
Malathion	Insecticide	Relatively safe to mammals because of rapid metabolism in liver
Parathion	Insecticide	Highly toxic to higher animals. Frequent cause of accidental poisoning
Sarin (GB)	Chemical warfare	Extremely toxic. No commercial use
Tabun	Chemical warfare	Extremely toxic. No commercial use

terase is accelerated by nucleophilic reactivators such as hydoxamic acids and oximes that can displace the phosphoryl group and reactivate the enzyme. Inclusion of a quaternary ammonium group in the reactivator may greatly increase its potency, although diminishing its ability to penetrate into the CNS.

The most commonly used reactivator is pralidoxime (pyridine-2-aldoxime-methiodide; PAM), which is effective principally at the neuromuscular junction and to some extent at muscarinic sites but is ineffective in the CNS. Pralidoxime must be administered parenterally, usually by i.v. infusion. The agent has some depolarizing effect of its own in addition to enzyme reactivation. As a supplement to atropine and general supportive therapy, pralidoxime is valuable in the treatment of poisoning by both organophosphate and carbonyl ester cholinesterase inhibitors. Sometimes the aging process renders the phosphorylated enzyme refractory to reactivation by agents like pralidoxime, presumably because the anionic site of acetylcholinesterase is occupied. In this case, treatment is restricted to general supportive measures and atropine.

Side-effects of pralidoxime are surprisingly mild if the drug is given in the dosage suggested.

FURTHER READING

1. Aquilonius SM: Physostigmine in the treatment of drug overdose. In Jenden DJ (ed): Cholinergic Mechanisms and Psychopharmacology 24, pp 817–825. New York, Plenum Press, 1977
2. Brimblecombe RW: Drugs acting on central cholinergic mechanisms and affecting respiration. Pharmacol Ther B 3:65–74, 1977
3. Carrier O Jr: Pharmacology of the Peripheral Autonomic System. Chicago, Year Book Publishers, 1972
4. Drachman DB: Myasthenia gravis. N Engl J Med 298:136–142, 186–193, 1978
5. Havener WH: Ocular Pharmacology, 4th ed, pp 318–335. Saint Louis, CV Mosby, 1978

CHAPTER 15 QUESTIONS

(See P. 7 for Full Instructions)

Select the One Best Answer

1. After the administration of a cholinesterase inhibitor to a normal person, one would expect each of the following EXCEPT
   A. accommodation for near vision.
   B. increased sweating.
   C. increased muscle strength.
   D. increased adrenalin secretion.
   E. increased lacrimation.
2. Clinical conditions for which *both* muscarinic agents and cholinesterase inhibitors are effective include each of the following EXCEPT
   A. acute narrow angle glaucoma.
   B. paralytic ileus.
   C. congenital megacolon.
   D. chronic wide-angle glaucoma.
   E. postoperative urinary retention.
3. Edrophonium
   A. produces mydriasis.
   B. is useful in the differentiation of cholinergic crisis from myasthenic crisis.
   C. inhibits plasma cholinesterases but not tissue cholinesterases.
   D. reduces the bradycardia induced by the Valsalva maneuver.
   E. potentiates the effects of carbachol.

A = 1,2,3; B = 1,3; C = 2,4; D = 4; E = All

4. Irreversible cholinesterase inhibitors include
   1. echothiophate.
   2. isoflurophate.
   3. malathion.
   4. physostigmine.
5. Treatment for poisoning with parathion may include
   1. pralidoxime.

2. atropine in large doses.
3. artificial respiration.
4. pilocarpine.

6. Neostigmine is
   1. a competitive antagonist of pseudo- (plasma) and true (cell) cholinesterase.
   2. beneficial in the treatment of myasthenia gravis.
   3. effective in the treatment of narrow-angle glaucoma.
   4. highly toxic when the usual oral dose is administered parenterally.

7. Physostigmine and neostigmine differ in that
   1. only neostigmine penetrates the CNS readily.
   2. only physostigmine produces miosis in the denervated eye.
   3. only neostigmine is useful in treating glaucoma.
   4. only neostigmine stimulates denervated skeletal muscle.

8. Neostigmine may prolong the half-life of
   1. methacholine.
   2. succinylcholine.
   3. procaine.
   4. bethanechol.

16

THOMAS C. WESTFALL

Antimuscarinic Agents

Antimuscarinic agents antagonize the muscarinic actions of acetylcholine and related compounds. They act at the receptors of organs innervated by cholinergic postganglionic autonomic nerves by blocking the effects of liberated acetylcholine. Like acetylcholine, these drugs possess a high affinity for these receptors, but unlike acetylcholine they have no intrinsic activity or ability to stimulate or inhibit the tissue through these receptors. Generally the doses required to block the effects of nerve stimulation are greater than those that block the effects of injected acetylcholine or choline esters. The terms *cholinolytic*, *anticholinergic*, or *cholinergic blocking* have often been applied to this group of drugs. Because they imply antagonism of the effects of acetylcholine at all sites, they are imprecise and broad.

The principal actions of these drugs include inhibition of secretions from lacrimal, salivary, nasopharyngeal, bronchial, gastric, intestinal and sweat glands, and the pancreas; increase in heart rate, depression of the tone and motility of the stomach and intestines, and relaxation of bronchial and tracheal smooth muscle; and dilation of the pupil (mydriasis) and paralysis of accommodation (cycloplegia). All postganglionic autonomic neuroeffector junctions are not equally sensitive to antimuscarinic agents, although the order of sensitivity of various organs to blockade by these agents varies little.

In higher doses antimuscarinic agents have antinicotinic actions, blocking cholinergic transmission at motor nerve endings and ganglionic synapses. Muscarinic actions on autonomic ganglia are also antagonized. Several drugs in this group have important actions on the CNS resulting in part from actions on cholinergic synapses that are pharmacologically similar to the postganglionic cholinergic junction. In addition, these drugs have central actions apparently unrelated to their antimuscarinic properties.

The most important and best known of the antimuscarinic drugs are atropine (*dl*-hyoscyamine) and scopolamine (*l*-hyoscine). For this

---

George Gabriel Sigmond, 1794–   . English physician. Lectured in London on Materia Medica and medical jurisprudence. Wrote on the medical and moral effects of tea and the curative properties of mercury and the early materia medica of anti-muscarinic drugs.

reason this group of drugs is often referred to as atropinic (Fig. 16-1). Atropine and scopolamine have widespread actions and have been used in the treatment of a large number of clinical conditions. In attempts to obtain atropine-like drugs with a greater selectivity, with a different duration of action, or with fewer side-effects, a large number of related synthetic or semisynthetic drugs have been introduced. Because the actions and effects of the antimuscarinic agents differ only quantitatively from those of atropine or scopolamine, these two drugs will be discussed as prototypes and their properties considered in detail. Differences between these and other agents are discussed subsequently.

SOURCE AND CHEMISTRY

Atropine (*dl*-hyoscyamine) and scopolamine (*l*-hyoscine) are found in a number of plants belonging to the potato family, the order Solanacea. These include *Atropa belladonna* (deadly night shade), *Hyoscyamus niger* (black henbane), and *Datura stramonium* (thorn apple, Jamestown weed, or Jimson weed). The major active ingredient in these plants is *l*-hyoscyamine, with smaller quantities of *l*-scopolamine (hyoscine). Atropine is a mixture of equal parts of *dl*-hyoscyamine. It may be prepared by racemization of the L-rotatory hyoscyamine after extraction from plants, or it may be manufactured synthetically. The *l*-isomer is more potent both peripherally and centrally than is the D-form, which is almost inert, but the racemic form is preferred because it is more stable chemically. *l*-Hyoscine is more active peripherally than *d*-hyoscine, but the actions of the isomers on the CNS are similar.

Atropine, scopolamine, and most synthetic antimuscarinic agents are esters of complex organic bases with tropic acid. Atropine is *dl*-tropyl tropine and is an ester of tropic acid and the organic base tropine. Scopolamine is *l*-tropyl-α-scopine and is an ester of tropic acid and the organic base scopine. These two drugs differ only by the presence of an epoxide bridge on the amino acid moiety of scopolamine. Many synthetic antimuscarinic agents are quaternary ammonium compounds, which are generally more potent than corresponding tertiary amines and which have some ganglionic blocking activity but lack effects on the CNS. They are also less well absorbed after oral administration and tend to have a shorter duration of action.

MECHANISM OF ACTION

Atropine, scopolamine, and most synthetic antimuscarinic agents are competitive or surmountable antagonists of acetylcholine at muscarinic receptor sites in smooth muscle, cardiac muscle, exocrine glands, and the CNS. Their blocking action can be overcome by increasing the local contraction of acetylcholine or choline ester. They do not react chemically with acetylcholine, nor do they affect the release or rate of hydrolysis of acetylcholine. The effectiveness of antimuscarinic agents is

FIG. 16-1. Some representative antimuscarinic compounds. Shaded C indicates an asymmetric carbon atom responsible for natural isomers of belladonna alkaloids.

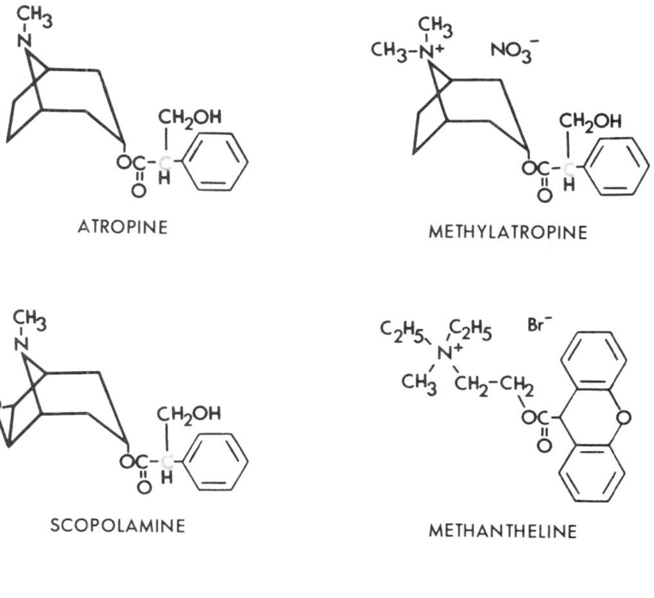

greater against the muscarinic effects of injected cholinergic drugs than for the stimulation of cholinergic postganglionic nerves. This difference in sensitivity is most likely due to release of the chemical mediator in an area in which it has much greater proximity to the receptor, and is therefore present in higher concentration than is capable by exogenous administration. With some drugs the antagonism of muscarinic receptors is preceded by a brief agonist action. The sensitivity of the various effector cells to the effects of atropine and scopolamine is different. For instance, low doses may be sufficient to inhibit salivation and sweating, whereas larger doses are needed for action on the cardiac vagus and smooth muscle of the gastrointestinal tract.

Atropine and similar drugs produce a highly selective antagonism of muscarinic receptors so selective that atropine blockade of a drug's actions has been taken as evidence that the drug is acting on muscarinic receptors. The selectivity for muscarinic receptors is not absolute, however, and in very large doses and with intraarterial administration these drugs can antagonize ganglionic as well as neuromuscular transmission. In addition, in a concentration about 1000 times the muscarinic blocking dose, atropine also antagonizes 5-hydroxytryptamine (serotonin), histamine, and norepinephrine receptors.

Atropine, scopolamine, and similar drugs may form a three-point attachment to the receptors: on the onium nitrogen, on the tropyl hydroxyl group, and on the benzene ring. Structure activity studies support this concept.

PHARMACOLOGIC ACTIONS

CARDIOVASCULAR EFFECTS

The administration of atropine produces complex effects on the human heart rate. Soon after its administration, atropine produces a transient slowing of the heart. This bradycardia is due to the stimulation of the medullary cardioinhibitory center. The main effect of atropine, however, particularly with larger doses (1–2 mg), is to produce an increase in heart rate from blockade of the normal action of the vagus nerve at the postganglionic neuroeffector junction. Vagal tone, hence the cardioaccelerator effect of atropine, varies considerably. In humans this tone is most marked in the trained athlete and in the young adult, whereas in children and old persons it is slight. Tachycardia produced by atropine is fairly marked in the former but quite small in the latter group. Atropine and similar drugs can reverse all the cardiac effects of acetylcholine and vagal stimulation; therefore, it reverses the shortening of the refractory period, the prolongation of the P-R interval, the decreased conduction, and the decreased cardiac output and oxygen consumption (*see* Chap. 14). The effect on cardiac output is generally slight because of compensatory circulatory mechanisms. Atropine also reduces or abolishes cardioinhibitory reflexes produced as a result of irritant vapors, stimulation of the carotid sinus, pressure on the eyeballs, pulling of extraocular muscles, or peritoneal stimulation, although some cardiac slowing can occur owing to reduction of sympathetic tone. Atropine will frequently stop atrial fibrillation induced by acetylcholine during vagal stimulation. In addition, it has a quinidine-like action on the equivalent to one half the activity of procaine (*see* Chap. 20). This is seen only at doses greatly in excess of those required to block muscarinic receptors. With such doses, atropine can prevent cardiac arrhythmias produced by epinephrine in the presence of cyclopropane anesthesia (*see* Chap. 28). Arrhythmias such as atrio-ventricular (A-V) nodal dissociation, A-V block nodal rhythm, and ventricular extrasystoles have been reported after atropine administration. These arrhythmias may be more frequent during anesthesia and are dependent on the anesthetic agent used. Cardiac contractility is generally unaffected by atropine except at high doses where it produces depression. Because acetylcholine can decrease the release of norepinephrine after nerve stimulation by means of an action on prejunctional receptors, atropine may potentiate effects of sympathetic nerve stimulation in the myocardium.

PEPTIC ULCER

The antimuscarinic drugs are obsolete when used alone since they have been replaced by more selective agents, particularly the H_2-antagonists (*see* Chap. 51). Theoretically atropine and related drugs could benefit patients with peptic ulcer by reducing the vagal stimuli of

---

VELYIEN EWART HENDERSON, 1877–1945. Canadian pharmacologist. In 1929, he and G. H. W. Lucas reported the experimental use of cyclopropane gas as a general anesthetic. Also worked in aviation medicine. He first described the effect of muscarinic drugs on gastric secretion.

acid/pepsin secretion, and by prolonging the action of antacids through delaying gastric emptying. However, significant gastric effects are produced only in the face of systemic signs and symptoms of parasympathetic blockade. These effects are usually intolerable and often dangerous (*see* Chap. 38).

Because antimuscarinic drugs augment the acid-inhibiting properties of H_2-antagonists, they may occasionally be combined with cimetidine particularly to control nocturnal hypersecretion, "escape" from control in the Zollinger–Ellison syndrome, or rarely in chronic gastric ulcer disease. Little is known with respect to the effects of such combination treatment on ulcer healing or relapse.

Because few blood vessels receive cholinergic innervation, the effect of atropine on arterial pressure in humans is small. At higher doses a slightly decreased systolic arterial pressure may be seen and may be due to reduced filling of the heart during tachycardia. Atropine can block the muscarinic receptors on blood vessels and thereby block the depressor response to acetylcholine and other muscarinic agents.

Large doses of atropine cause vasodilation of cutaneous blood vessels, unrelated to its muscarinic blocking properties. This is due to a direct action on blood vessels or to local histamine release. Flushing of the skin, the result of this vasodilation, may be very noticeable after moderately high doses of atropine. In addition, in warm environments atropine may cause cutaneous vasodilation secondary to blockage of the sweat glands, resulting in a rise in body temperature.

OCULAR EFFECTS

When atropine or related drugs are administered systemically or locally into the conjunctival sac of the eye, they produce dilation of the pupil (mydriasis), paralysis of accommodation of the lens (cycloplegia), and increased intraocular pressure. All these effects can be deduced from an understanding of the autonomic innervation of the eye. The circular smooth muscle of the iris and the ciliary muscles are innervated by parasympathetic neurones in the third cranial (oculomotor) nerve. The radial muscles of the iris are innervated by sympathetic adrenergic fibers that originate from the superior cervical ganglion. Under normal circumstances, the parasympathetic system is tonically active. Atropine causes pupillary dilation by blocking the effects of tonic vagal activity on the muscarinic receptors in the circular muscle and by leaving unopposed the influence of the sympathetic dilator fibers. An atropinized pupil does not respond to light.

Accommodation for near vision depends on the contraction of the ciliary muscles, which slackens the suspensory ligament, reducing tension on the lens and allowing it to become more convex. Atropine prevents contraction of the ciliary muscle, paralyzing accommodation (cycloplegia). Distant vision remains good, but near vision is indistinct.

The effects of antimuscarinic agents differ from those of sympathomimetic amines in that the latter have no effect on the ciliary muscle and cause mydriasis by stimulation of the radial muscle of the iris. Accommodation, therefore, is not lost, and the pupillary responses to light and accommodation are retained.

Atropine also increases intraocular pressure. This is a purely mechanical effect resulting from pupillary dilation, which causes thickening of the peripheral part of the iris with a consequent narrowing of the iridocorneal angle. This restricts the drainage of aqueous humor, which is normally continuously secreted by the ciliary processes. The rise in intraocular pressure rarely does harm in the normal eye of young adults. However, when the intraocular pressure is raised, particularly in people over 40, an attack of glaucoma may be precipitated. This constitutes a serious hazard. Scopolamine appears more potent than does atropine in producing the various ocular effects.

GASTROINTESTINAL, BILIARY, AND GENITOURINARY TRACTS

Atropine, scopolamine, and related drugs antagonize the increase in smooth muscle tone and activity that follows activation of cholinergic nerves and muscarinic drugs in the gastrointestinal, biliary, and urinary tracts. Generally they decrease tone and the amplitude and frequency of peristalsis of all segments of the intestinal tract. The degree of inhibition depends on the level of the existing cholinergic (vagal) nerve activity, since intestinal movements and tone of intestinal muscle are under predominantly parasympathetic control.

The bladder has a very complex innervation, but detrusor muscle undoubtedly is primarily innervated by parasympathetic nerves. Stimulation of muscarinic receptors in the detrusor muscle leads to a forceful contraction. Generally, atropine and other anticholinergics will release the tone and spontaneous activity of the fundus and contraction of the sphincter, thus favoring urinary retention.

The bile ducts and gall bladder are slightly relaxed by atropine. The parasympathetic nerves appear to be unimportant in the control of the uterus, and consequently atropine has little effect.

RESPIRATORY SYSTEM

Bronchial smooth muscle is predominantly under parasympathetic control. Following the administration of atropinic drugs, bronchial and tracheal smooth muscles relax, particularly when parasympathetic tone is high or muscle tone has been increased by muscarinic agents. The bronchodilation produced by atropine results in a larger vital capacity and decreased bronchial resistance. These drugs also inhibit secretions from bronchial glands, and decreased frequency of cough and laryngospasm results at the induction of anesthesia after their administration. Some evidence suggests that antimuscarinic drugs will also cause increased mucous viscosity and decreased mucociliary clearance in the tracheobronchial tree.

GLANDS

Atropine and related drugs reduce or abolish secretions from glands that receive cholinergic innervation. This includes tears, sweat, saliva, mucus, and digestive juices. The flow of saliva and mucus from the glands that line the respiratory tract is reduced, and drying of the mucous membranes of the mouth, nose, and bronchi occurs. Complaints of a dry mouth (xerostomia) and difficulty in swallowing are common. Eccrine sweat gland activity that depends on cholinergic sympathetic nerve fibers is suppressed, and the skin becomes hot and dry. After large doses of atropine, the body temperature rises. The apocrine sweat glands found in the axilla and around the nipples, labia majora, and mons pubis are not blocked. Both thermal and emotional sweating is reduced by atropinic drugs. The secretions of the stomach, the actions of the hormone gastrin, and the exocrine secretion of the pancreas are at least partly blocked by atropine (*see* Chap. 38). There is no inhibition of the secretion of milk, urine, or bile.

Suppression of the secretion of tears by atropine results in drying of the conjunctiva and exposes the eye to a greater risk of superficial injuries from dust and other particles in the atmosphere.

CENTRAL NERVOUS SYSTEM

The principal difference between atropine and scopolamine is in their central action. In doses usually used in humans, atropine mildly stimulates the CNS. This is generally seen as a slight bradycardia that results from stimulation of medullary centers with increased vagal outflow. With higher doses, the central effects are more pronounced, and restlessness, irritability, disorientation, hallucinations, and delirium can occur. If the dose is further increased, stimulation is followed by depression, then respiratory paralysis, causing death. Scopolamine has a more pronounced central effect and at therapeutic levels causes drowsiness, euphoria, amnesia, fatigue, and sleep. Restlessness and other signs of central stimulation occur only after high doses of the drug. Scopolamine has been found to have a central potency 8 to 9 times that of atropine. Physostigmine (*see* Chap. 15) is highly effective in reversing these central effects. Other central effects of these prototype and similar acting drugs are used to treat motion sickness and Parkinson's disease (*see* Chap. 31). Atropine and scopolamine are well absorbed from the gastrointestinal tract and from other mucosal membranes but only to a limited extent from the eye or intact skin. Quaternary derivatives are poorly adsorbed from all routes but are still effective as cycloplegics or mydriatics. Distribution occurs throughout the body and across the placenta. About 85% to 90% is excreted in the urine within 24 hours. Metabolism is still incompletely understood, but about half of the drug is excreted unchanged and the rest as tropic acid esters or tropine. Enzymatic hydrolysis and conjugation take place in the liver.

THERAPEUTIC USES

Because of the multitudinous pharmacologic effects of the belladonna alkaloids, they have been used in many therapeutic applications. Regardless of the particular effect sought therapeutically, however, side-effects invari-

---

HENRY CHARLES STOLL, 1922– . American pathologist. Most of his work has been in oncology, especially of the head and neck. Described the pharmacodynamics of atropine and related compounds.

ably occur. Whether an effect of the drug is termed adverse or therapeutic depends on the reason for drug administration. More than 600 pharmaceutical preparations and combinations containing atropine or scopolamine are available, as are more than 60 atropine-like synthetic substitutes. These have been introduced in an attempt to achieve greater specificity and hence fewer side-effects. Despite aggressive advertising claims that particular drugs are selective for various organ-systems, all these drugs produce dose-dependent muscarinic blockade identical to that produced by atropine or scopolamine. The two naturally occurring alkaloids are still the drugs of choice and the most commonly used for therapeutic measures calling for an antimuscarinic agent.

CENTRAL NERVOUS SYSTEM DISORDERS

Vestibular Disturbances

Anticholinergic agents are effective in treating the nausea and vomiting resulting from vestibular disturbances, such as motion sickness and vertigo. Motion sickness is a functional disorder caused by repetitive angular, linear, or vertical motion. Vertigo refers to a feeling of whirling or rotation accompanied by nonvoluntary swaying, weakness, and lightheadedness. The mechanism of action of these drugs in vertigo and motion sickness has not been precisely defined. Anticholinergic drugs might be acting on at least two levels: in the central nervous system, and in the periphery. Acetylcholine, histamine, and norepinephrine have all been implicated as transmitters in transferring information from receptors located in the vestibular center, the eight cranial nerves, the retina, and the proprioreceptors of the joints and muscles to the midbrain and cerebellum for integration of normal body posture. Moreover, increasing the activity of cholinergic or histaminergic or decreasing the activity of noradrenergic nerves appears to increase vertigo and motion sickness. Antimuscarinic, antihistaminic, or adrenergic agents may be effective by decreasing or increasing the appropriate neurotransmitter system. Anticholinergic drugs may also act by blocking vagalmediated effects peripherally. Scopolamine appears to be the most effective anticholinergic drug.

Parkinson's Disease

Belladonna alkaloids have long been used and are beneficial in treating Parkinson's disease. The principal drugs are trihexyphenidyl and benztropine, both used as adjuncts in the treatment of parkinsonism and in the prophylaxis and control of extrapyramidal symptoms secondary to the use of phenothiazines (*see* Chap. 30 for more complete details).

Ophthalmologic Use

Although only a brief duration of action is required when these agents are used for most diagnostic purposes, prolonged mydriasis is required in the treatment if iritis and certain other conditions. The principal antimuscarinic agents used to produce mydriasis and cycloplegia are listed in Table 16-1 and include atropine, scopolamine, homatropine, cyclopentolate, tropicamide, and eucatropine.

Antimuscarinic drugs are applied topically to the eye to produce paralysis of accommodation (cycloplegia) and pupillary dilation (mydriasis). These effects are produced by blocking muscarinic receptors located in the ciliary muscle and iris, which are both under predominant cholinergic tone. They are used primarily as an aid in measuring refractive errors and for other diagnostic purposes, preoperatively and postoperatively in intraocular surgery and in the treatment of anterior uveitis and some secondary glaucomas.

Both the cycloplegic and mydriatic actions of the antimuscarinic drugs are useful in estimating errors of refraction. Paralysis of accommodation reveals latent refractive errors, and dilation of the pupil facilitates estimation of the refractive error. Short-acting drugs are used to dilate the pupil for examination of the intraocular structures and are also used as a provocative test for angle-closure glaucomas. In the latter situation a positive result is said to occur when intraocular pressure rises 8 mm Hg within 1 (one) hour of installation of an agent

TABLE 16-1. Antimuscarinic Agents Commonly Used in Ophthalmology

Drug	Concentration	Duration of Action	Cycloplegia
	%		
Atropine sulfate	1–4	6–12 days	+++
Cyclopentolate hydrochloride	1–2	12–24 hr	++
Eucatropine hydrochloride	5–10	2–4 hr	–
Homatropine hydrobromide	2	12–48 hr	+
Scopolamine hydrobromide	0.25	1–3 days	+++
Tropicamide	0.5–1	1–2 hr	++

like eucatropine. These drugs are used to produce maximal mydriasis during intraocular surgery and in the nonspecific treatment of anterior uveitis and glaucoma secondary to ocular inflammation. Although the precise mechanisms for the beneficial effects in the latter situations are not known, three beneficial actions seem to exist: they relax intraocular pressure, which seems to relieve pain and photophobia; they reduce abnormal vascular permeability, which allows an outpouring of protein and inflammatory cells into the anterior chamber that may clog the angle and promote the development of adhesions that seal the iris to the trabecular network; and they dilate the pupil, which prevents the formation of posterior synechiae and may aid in breaking these adhesions once they have formed.

Cyclopentolate, homatropine, eucatropine, or tropicamide are generally used in diagnostic work because they produce the same effects as atropine but for a much shorter period. The effects of one or two drops of atropine, for instance, may persist for a week or more. Short-acting antimuscarinic agents are often combined with a sympathomimetic amine such as phenylephrine or hydroxyamphetamine to ensure a more rapid effect and faster recovery with minimal cycloplegia.

Muscarinic agents such as pilocarpine or physostigmine are frequently used by topical application to terminate the mydriatic and cycloplegic effects of antimuscarinic agents more rapidly. Although these agents are applied topically in the form of eyedrops and their systemic absorption is minimal, antimuscarinic eyedrops are important household poisons. Accidental ingestion of very small quantities can produce a severe atropine psychosis and is particularly dangerous in children (*see* Chap. 7).

Gastrointestinal Tract

Because antimuscarinic drugs reduce the tone and motility of smooth muscle, naturally occurring belladonna alkaloids, their derivatives, and numerous synthetic substitutes have been widely promoted as antispasmodics (for details, (*see* Chap. 38). Atropine and related drugs reduce both the peristaltic and secretory activity of the entire gastrointestinal system, reduce the tone of the ureter and urinary bladder, and have a slight inhibitory action on the bile ducts and gallbladder. Adequate doses of antimuscarinic antispasmodics apparently relieve pain by inhibiting both motility and secretions, and some of these agents may have a local anesthetic action. Table 16-2 lists some commonly used antimuscarinic antispasmodics.

The synthetic anticholinergics are substituted quaternary ammonium compounds,

TABLE 16-2. Antimuscarinic Agents Used as Antispasmodics or to Treat Peptic Ulcer

Drug	Trade Name	Dose	Duration
		mg	*hr*
Belladonna alkaloids			
Atropine sulfate	—	1	6
Hyoscyamine hydrobromide	—	0.25	6
Quaternary ammonium derivatives of belladonna alkaloid			
Homatropine methylbromide	(Many trade names)	6	6
Methscopolamine bromide	Pamine	5	6
Methylatropine nitrate	Metropine	2	6
Synthetic substitutes			
Anisotropine methylbromide	Valpin	10	6
Diphemanil methylsulfate	Prantal	100	6–8
Glycopyrrolate	Robinul	2	8
Hexocyclium methylsulfate	Tral	25	6
Isopropamide iodide	Darbid	5	12
Mepenzolate bromide	Cantil	25	6
Methantheline bromide	Banthine	50	6
Oxyphencyclimide hydrochloride	Daricon	10	12
Oxyphenonium bromide	Antrenyl bromide	10	6
Pentapiperium methylsulfate	Quilene	10–20	8
Pipenzolate bromide	Piptal	5	6
Poldine methylsulfate	Nacton	4	8
Propantheline bromide	Pro-Banthine	15	8
Tridihexethyl chloride	Pathilon	25	8

with the exception of oxyphencyclimine, a tertiary amine. Quarternary ammonium compounds are less readily absorbed than are tertiary amines when given orally, and individual variability in response is considerable. These drugs rarely exert effects on the CNS because they do not readily cross the blood–brain barrier.

Antispasmodics. Many of these drugs are packaged in pharmaceutical preparations which also contain antianxiety agents or antacids in addition. The routine use of such mixtures is generally frowned upon because of the problem of regulating the dosage of each component of the mixture.

Preanesthetic Medication. The administration of an antimuscarinic agent as a preanesthetic medication is a time honored and universally accepted procedure. Its use originated because some inhalation anesthetics stimulate bronchial secretions, and this effect can be prevented by atropine or scopolamine. An additional reason for their use is to afford protection against vagal reflexes. The sedative action of scopolamine is also useful in calming patients before surgery. The routine use of antimuscarinic agents preoperatively is now questionable, since newer anesthetic gases are far less irritating to the bronchial mucosa. In addition, noninhalation anesthesia has become more common. Limiting preoperative antimuscarinic medication to patients who have a specific indication is wise. Specific indications include repeat administration of suxamethonium, bradycardia during an operation, administration of an ether anesthetic, intravenous or intramuscular ketamine with neostigmine at the time of reversal of nondepolarizing neuromuscular block, if awake tracheal intubation is anticipated in an outpatient especially an infant and if a peroral endoscopic procedure is to be performed.

Cardiac Disease

Atropine is beneficial in treating patients with severe bradycardia complicated by excessive hypotension or excessive ventricular activity that develops in the first few hours after acute myocardial infarction. Such treatment can restore adequate ventricular rates and cardiac output while reducing ectopic activity. This often obliterates the need for adrenergic agents, external pacing, or antiarrhythmics. Therefore, although the use of atropine for this indication, particularly in the setting of the coronary care unit, appears well founded, the potential benefit of its routine use in patients with acute myocardial infarction remains controversial. In fact evidence suggests that the administration of atropine increases the heart rate and may actually increase the incidence of arrhythmias. The criteria for using atropine as well as the appropriate dose and route of administration of the drug in the therapy of bradycardia are under active debate and investigation. It is current practice not to treat patients who have asymptomatic sinus bradycardia. Atropine may enhance A-V conduction in Wenckebach type I second-degree A-V block, but A-V block may be observed in some patients. This paradoxical effect may occur because small doses of atropine have little direct effect on the A-V node but nevertheless increase the sinus rate.

Atropine is the drug of choice in treating heart block due to digitalis toxicity.

Anticholinesterase and Muscarine Poisoning

Anticholinesterases are the active ingredients of many insecticides commonly used by the agricultural industry (*see* Chap. 15). Poisoning by these substances produces cholinergic hyperactivity, including bradycardia, sialorrhea, bronchospasm, and depolarizing neuromuscular block. The muscarinic effects of these indirectly acting cholinergic toxins can be promptly antagonized by atropine. The neuromuscular paralysis is treated with cholinesterase reactivators such as prolidoxime. Recovery from anticholinesterase intoxication is enhanced if the antidotes are given soon after exposure to the toxin. Atropine-like drugs are routinely administered concomitantly with neostigmine at the time of reversal of nondepolarizing block to counteract muscarinic side-effects.

A second use of antimuscarinic agents is in treating intoxication by mushrooms (*Amanita muscaria*) that contain muscarine (*see* Chap. 14). Poisoning by these mushrooms is likewise manifested by signs and symptoms of cholinergic hyperactivity, which can be successfully neutralized by the administration of atropine or similar compounds.

Miscellaneous Uses

The antisecretory effect of belladonna alkaloids is used in numerous combinations with antihistamines and sympathomimetics and widely promoted as proprietary (over the counter) cold remedies. These should be used with caution in patients with asthma or respiratory tract infection. The principal side-effect is dry mouth.

Scopolamine has been used in many sleep-inducing proprietary preparations and is frequently used in combination with a sedative antihistamine. The hypnotic efficacy of these preparations is questionable.

MEDICATIONS WITH ANTIMUSCARINIC PROPERTIES OR SIDE-EFFECTS

In addition to the standard atropine-like drugs and antihistamines, a broad range of drugs exhibit antimuscarinic properties. The drug classes are listed in Table 16-3; nearly all currently marketed psychiatric medications are included. Most authorities consider the antimuscarinic actions of these compounds as side-effects rather than as therapeutic effects. However, in some cases this property might well contribute to the mechanism of their therapeutic effect. These drugs have the potential to produce the whole range of antimuscarinic effects, and additivity can be produced if more than one agent is administered.

ADVERSE EFFECTS

The principal adverse effects of antimuscarinic agents may be deduced from a consideration of their total pharmacologic properties in relation to the therapeutically desirable effect. As mentioned earlier, the use of these drugs is coupled with widespread side-effects, and whether these effects are termed adverse or therapeutic depends on the reason for drug administration. The most common troublesome effects are dry mouth, blurred vision, tachycardia, constipation, and urinary hesitancy and are not really adverse effects but reflect the primary pharmacologic action of antimuscarinic drugs. Tolerance is lower in subjects with glaucoma or prostatic hypertrophy. The danger of precipitating acute glaucoma in susceptible persons by conjunctival application and the danger of hyperthermia in hot climates as a result of inhibition of sweating have already been mentioned. Central nervous effects of these drugs are much less tolerable, less predictable, and more variable. Up to 20% of patients receiving antimuscarinic drugs for Parkinson's disease experience CNS toxicity.

Recently there have been several reports of abuse of centrally acting antimuscarinic drugs, especially the antiparkinson drugs trihexyphenidyl and benztropine. Some authorities believe that this is a common problem and that antiparkinson antimuscarinic drugs are gaining increasing popularity as street drugs.

TABLE 16-3. Medications with Anticholinergic Properties or Side-Effects

Atropine products
Antihistamines
Antipsychotics
Tricyclic antidepressants
Monoamine oxidase inhibitors
Lithium
Antiparkinson agents

POISONING BY BELLADONNA ALKALOIDS

Acute poisoning by belladonna alkaloids may result from the accidental ingestion of berries or seeds, from dosage errors, and occasionally from systemic absorption of a drug applied to the conjunctiva after it has transversed the nasolacrimal duct. Although an alarming reaction may occur, a fatal outcome is uncommon, for atropine has one of the widest safety margins of all commonly used drugs. Patients have survived the ingestion of 1 g of atropine. Patients poisoned with atropine or scopolamine rapidly develop these symptoms: dryness of the mouth; blurred vision and photophobia; hot, dry skin; fever in about one fourth of patients, which may reach dangerously high levels; weak but rapid pulse; and increased arterial pressure.

Central nervous system effects include hallucinations, disorientation, delirium, hyperactivity, and seizures. Mental state is abnormal, fluctuating unpredictably from unresponsiveness and coma to an agitated, confused, combative, delirious, or psychotic state.

Dry mucous membranes, widely dilated unresponsive pupils, tachycardia, hot skin, and fever should produce immediate suspicion of atropine toxicity. The diagnosis of antimuscarinic poisoning may be confirmed by administration of a dose of 10 to 30 mg of methacholine given parenterally. Failure to elicit bradycardia, rhinorrhea, salivation, sweating, and

WILLIAM DAMESHEK, 1900–1969. Russian-born American physician. Worked chiefly in hematology, the hemolytic disorders, anemias, leukemias, and agranulocytosis. Was the first editor of the journal *Blood* and remained its editor-in-chief until his death. He suggested that mecholyl be used as a diagnostic test for atropine poisoning.

abdominal distress unequivocally indicates that an atropine-like substance is involved.

Intoxication is usually of short duration and relatively benign, but recovery may take a week or more and is usually followed by amnesia. Diazepam or chlordiazepoxide is often used to treat the psychotic effects if reassurance alone is ineffective. Phenothiazines are contraindicated because of their anticholinergic properties. Physostigmine, a nonquaternary cholinesterase inhibitor (*see* Chap. 15), is the specific antidote reversal of delirium and hyperpyrexia. Treatment with physostigmine should be guarded, however, because it can lead to severe cardiac and respiratory complications. Other cholinesterase inhibitors such as neostigmine do not cross the blood–brain barrier and are ineffective. Except for counteracting the central effects of atropine poisoning, cholinesterase inhibitors are of doubtful value, and treatment is mainly supportive.

FURTHER READING

1. Brimblecombe RW: Drug Actions on Cholinergic Systems. Baltimore, University Park Press, 1974
2. Finkbeiner AE, Bissada NK, Welch LT: Uropharmacology: VI. Parasympathetic depressants. Urology 5:503–510, 1977
3. Greenblatt DC, Shader RI: Anticholinergics. N Engl J Med 288:1215, 1973
4. Mirakhur RK: Anticholinergic drugs. Br J Anaesth 51:671–679, 1979
5. Rumack BH: Anticholinergic poisoning: treatment with physostigmine. Pediatrics 52:449, 1973

CHAPTER 16 QUESTIONS

(*See* P. 7 for Full Instructions)

Select the One Best Answer

1. The changes in the near-point brought about by homatropine are due to
   - *A.* contraction of the radial fibers of the iris.
   - *B.* contraction of the ciliary muscle.
   - *C.* contraction of the sphincter fibers of the iris.
   - *D.* relaxation of the sphincter fibers of the iris.
   - *E.* relaxation of the ciliary muscle.
2. Atropine
   - *A.* penetrates the blood–brain barrier poorly.
   - *B.* is the drug of choice in bronchial asthma.
   - *C.* will antagonize acetylcholine stimulation of the adrenal medulla.
   - *D.* will reduce the bradycardia in response to phenylephrine.
   - *E.* increases cholinesterase activity.
3. Difficulty in focusing for near vision might be expected after the administration of
   - *A.* ephedrine.
   - *B.* bethanecol.
   - *C.* propantheline.
   - *D.* propranolol.
   - *E.* guanethidine.
4. Atropine can produce each of the following EXCEPT
   - *A.* cycloplegia.
   - *B.* flushing.
   - *C.* bradycardia.
   - *D.* hyperthermia.
   - *E.* parkinsonism.

A = 1,2,3; B = 1,3; C = 2,4; D = 4; E = All

5. Antimuscarinic agents may
   - *1.* reduce gastric secretions.
   - *2.* cause urinary retention.
   - *3.* precipitate glaucoma.
   - *4.* be effective in treating all mushroom poisonings.
6. Propantheline
   - *1.* inhibits nocturnal HCl secretion.
   - *2.* produces sedation.
   - *3.* blocks muscarinic receptors.
   - *4.* increases blood pressure.
7. Both atropine and epinephrine
   - *1.* produce mydriasis.
   - *2.* are useful in terminating an attack of bronchial asthma when given alone.
   - *3.* may produce a positive chronotropic effect.
   - *4.* are effective orally.
8. The usefulness of propantheline in the treatment of acid-peptic disease is based on its ability to
   - *1.* reduce significantly basal or nocturnal acid secretion.
   - *2.* prolong the action of antacids by delaying gastric emptying.
   - *3.* reduce motility and hence inhibit production of pain.
   - *4.* produce sedation similar to that of scopolamine.

17

JOHN A. BEVAN

Sympathomimetic Drugs

The term *sympathomimetic*, if used strictly, should be reserved for drugs that mimic the peripheral effects of sympathetic nervous activity whose activity can be looked upon as preparing the body for muscular activity (Cannon 1928). By general assent, however, this term is applied to all drugs that, whether or not chemically related to the sympathetic transmitter *l*-norepinephrine, act on the peripheral nervous system and its effector organs to cause at least some effects similar to activation of the sympathetic nervous system via an action on the peripheral adrenergic apparatus. Many of these drugs do not produce identical peripheral responses, as do norepinephrine and epinephrine, and some have additional actions on the central nervous system that are more prominent than their peripheral actions. Thus the term has become somewhat loose.

The sympathetic nervous system orchestrates a large number of body responses to stress, either physical, psychological, or generated as a result of disease. Generally they represent the mobilization of the organism—of the cardiovascular, respiratory, muscular, metabolic, and other systems in response to stress. Specificity of effect from among this range of possibilities is a desirable attribute of a drug.

Although dozens of sympathomimetic amines exist, and many are used clinically, only the prototype epinephrine and four others —norepinephrine, isopropylnorepinephrine (isoproterenol), ephedrine, and amphetamine (Fig. 17-1)—will be described in detail. All sympathomimetic amines may be described in terms of these five classic compounds. Agents in this class are useful clinically because they can treat signs and symptoms of various diseases. Some other newer therapeutically advantageous derivatives of clinical significance will be detailed.

Some aspects of the physiologic role and pharmacologic effects of dopamine will be discussed. Dopamine is not, strictly, a sympathomimetic amine, but because, in addition to an action on a specific dopamine receptor, it has some major effects mediated through the sym-

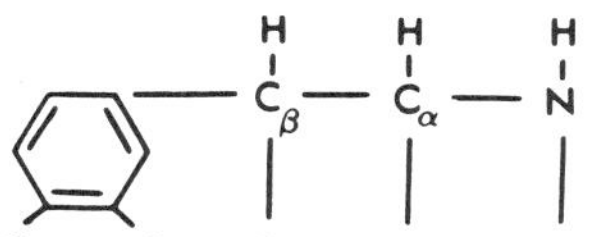

EPINEPHRINE	HO	HO	OH	H	CH_3
NOREPINEPHRINE	HO	HO	OH	H	H
ISOPROPYLNOREPINEPHRINE	HO	HO	OH	H	$CH(CH_3)_2$
EPHEDRINE	H	H	OH	CH_3	CH_3
AMPHETAMINE	H	H	H	CH_3	H
DOPAMINE	OH	OH	H	H	H

FIG. 17-1. Sympathomimetic drugs and dopamine.

pathetic nervous system and is chemically related to catacholomines, it is included in this chapter.

MECHANISMS OF ACTION

Epinephrine, norepinephrine, and isopropylnorepinephrine differ chemically only in the group substituted on the amine N atom (Fig. 17-1). Because they combine directly with postjunctional adrenergic receptors of effector cells to cause their pharmacologic effects, they are known as *directly acting amines* (*see* Chap. 13). This terminology, although usually used in relation to their postsynaptic effects mediated through receptors on effector cell membranes, also pertains to their action on transmitter release mediated through presynaptic adrenergic receptors, which are found on the neurilemma of the terminal adrenergic plexus (*see* below and Fig. 17-2).

In contrast, ephedrine and amphetamine are described as indirectly acting amines because they cause most of their pharmacologic effect by releasing the sympathetic transmitter from the terminations of the postganglionic sympathetic neurons and the adrenal medullary cells. This distinction between directly and indirectly acting amines is not absolute. Most amines act predominantly by one mechanism or the other and are sometimes referred to as *mixed action sympathomimetic amines*. However, phenylephrine is almost exclusively directly acting, and small doses of tyramine are indirectly acting. There are a number of consequences of this difference in mechanism of action: Drugs that block norepinephrine reuptake and those that deplete stored norepinephrine (*see* Chaps. 13, 36) will tend to inhibit effects of indirect, but not direct, sympathomimetic action. Blockade of neuronal and other cellular uptake disposition routes will actually potentiate the action of many directly acting amines by increasing local concentrations of norepinephrine, for example, at receptor sites.

ADRENERGIC RECEPTORS

To many, the present classification of adrenergic receptors is confusing. Indications are that considerable modification will take place in the next few years. It does, however, still represent a system of considerable pharmacologic and therapeutic value, which can be best appreciated from its historical perspective.

Postjunctional adrenergic receptors have been classified as α and β on the basis of a pharmacologic study by Ahlquist (1948), who

RAYMOND PERRY AHLQUIST, 1914– . American pharmacologist. Described mechanism of action of adrenaline and related compounds, classified α and β adrenergic receptors, developed β-adrenergic blocking agents. (Ahlquist RP: Study of adrenotropic receptors. Am J Physiol 153:586–600, 1948)

FIG. 17-2. Presynaptic and postsynaptic α and β adrenoceptors and their involvement in adrenergic transmitter release and action of sympathominetic amines.

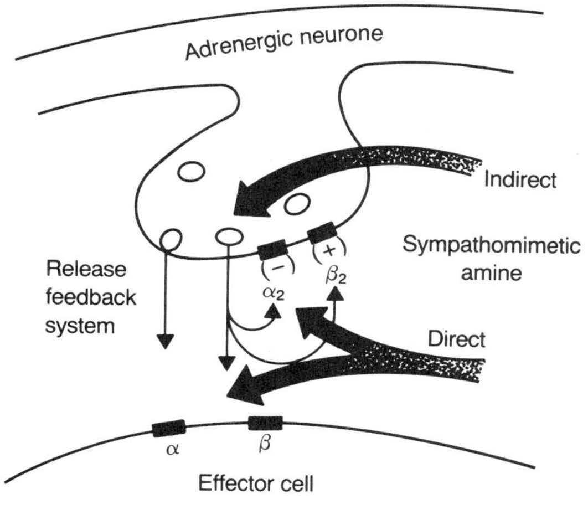

found that the potency order of a small series of closely related catecholamines on various organs fell into two groups. Generally binding to α adrenoceptors leads to excitation or elevation of basal tissue activity and binding to β receptors to the inhibition or depression of intrinsic or ongoing function. Because the change in an organ with stress can be inferred from the "fight or flight" response pattern, the dominant receptor type can often be logically derived. There are a number of important exceptions to this generalization. Amine occupation of myocardial adrenoceptors, while pharmacologically exhibiting β receptor attributes, results in excitation. However, as the classification is primarily a pharmacologic one, these are designated β adrenoceptors. The nature of the elicited change is secondary from the point of view of receptor classification. Further, inhibition of gastrointestinal mobility is mediated by both α and β adrenoceptors. This apparent discrepancy has been explained: The α adrenoceptors are at presynaptic sites on terminal cholinergic excitatory neurons of Auerbach's plexus. In this case, an α-adrenoceptor effect eventually results in an inhibition of the effector cell and gut smooth muscle function. Other exceptions include certain central nervous system and metabolic effects. Multiple types of receptors mediate the latter changes and vary considerably between species.

In the last decade the problem of receptor classification has become more complex and generalization more tenuous. Most cells contain both types of adrenergic receptors; the relative proportion differs even in different representations of the same cell type in different parts of the body. The dominant receptor seems to dictate the response. In general inhibitory β adrenoceptors have a lower drug threshold than do excitatory α adrenoceptors (*see* "Epinephrine" below). Both α_1 and α_2 adrenoceptors have now been identified and refer to the most common post- and pre-alphalike adrenergic synaptic receptors, respectively. In some effector tissues, however, α_1 and α_2 are both found. Binding to presynaptic α_2 adrenoceptors invariably leads to inhibition of norepinephrine release: Binding to postsynaptic α_1 receptors commonly but not invariably leads to excitation. Potency ranking for the three basic types of amines are epinephrine (EPI) $\geq$, norepinephrine (NE) $>>$ isoproterenol (ISO) for α_1, and EPI $\geq\leq$ NE $>>>$ ISO for α_2. Clonidine and α-methylnorepinephrine are more effective on α_2 than on α_1: Phenylephrine and methoxamine favor the α_1 adrenoceptor. Prazosin and yohimbine are relatively specific blockers of α_1 and α_2 adrenoceptors, respectively (*see* Table 17-1).

The β adrenoceptors have also been divided into two groups: β_1 predominates in the heart and β_2, in effector cells in blood vessels, bronchi, and glands. As with the α receptors, the distinction is not absolute. Some blood vessels contain β_1 receptors, others β_2 (the most common), whereas some blood vessels contain both. The tissue response to β_2 activation wherever this occurs is almost invariably inhibition, whereas those responses that arise through β_1 occupation in the heart and, rarely, β_2 in the pancreas result in tissue excitation. Potency rankings for β_1 and β_2 adrenoceptors are ISO $>>$ EPI $\geq$ NE and ISO $\geq$ EPI $>>>$ NE, respectively. There are various relatively selective drugs for the two types of receptors: for β_2 receptors, agonists include metaproterenol and albuterol (Salbutamol); and for β_1 receptors, antagonists such as metoprolol.

The events that follow receptor occupation are extremely complex and vary from one effector cell to another (*see* Chaps. 2, 50). Excitation and inhibition both probably involve an al-

TABLE 17-1. Pharmacologic Characteristics of Adrenergic Receptors

Receptor Type	Amine Potency Ratios*	"Specific" Agonist	"Specific" Antagonist
α_1	E $\geq$ NE $\gg$ ISO	Phenylephrine Methoxamine	Prazosin
α_2	E $\geq\leq$ NE $\ggg$ ISO	Clonidine α-Methylnorepinephrine	Yohimbine
β_1	ISO $\gg$ EPI $\geq$ NE		Metoprolol
β_2	ISO $\geq$ EPI $\ggg$ NE	Terbutaline Albuterol	

* E = epinephrine; NE = norepinephrine; ISO = isopropylnorepinephrine.

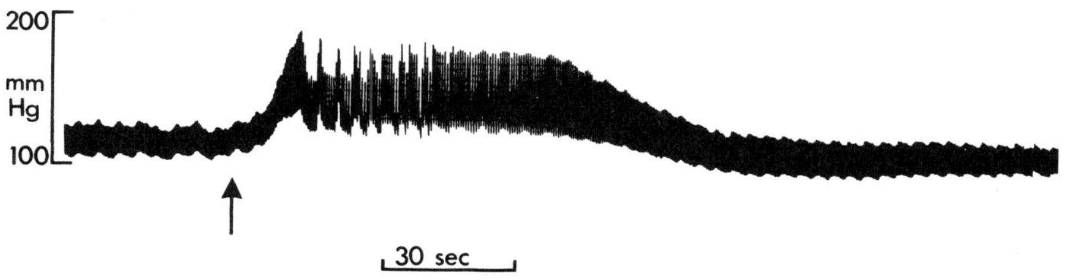

FIG. 17-3. Arterial pressure response to i.v. injection of epinephrine in an experimental animal.

teration in the calcium economy of the cell. The increase in intracellular calcium associated with excitation may involve electrical events that in turn alter ion exchange across the cell membrane. The additional ion species involved also varies from one tissue to another. Some of the changes that follow receptor occupancy are part of the long series of events that lead to change in cellular function and are discussed in Chapters 2 and 50.

EPINEPHRINE

The naturally occurring *l*-isomer of epinephrine, also known by its official British name adrenaline, is as much as 50 times more active pharmacologically than is the *d*-isomer. It was first proposed as the sympathetic transmitter by Elliott in 1904.

Epinephrine is found in nervous tissue, in the adrenal medulla, and scattered throughout the body in chromaffin cells. Activation of the adrenal medulla leads to the secretion of varying proportions of epinephrine and norepinephrine. The importance or significance of the "extraneuronal" epinephrine in the chromaffin cells is unknown. Its blood levels are increased in some pathologic states, for example, in pheochromocytoma.

ACTIONS

Although epinephrine is considered to have both α and β stimulating properties, in small doses it causes a predominantly β effect, since these receptors are more sensitive to epinephrine than are α receptors. The effect of higher doses depends on the relative importance of α- and β-adrenoceptor-mediated response in any one organ. Responses of different organs can be inferred from Table 13-1. In comparison to the fairly rapid tachyphylaxis seen to "indirectly acting" sympathomimetic amines, responses to an average dose of epinephrine tend not to diminish with repetition.

The effects described below are those that result from an intravenous (i.v.) injection of epinephrine into an experimental animal. The words *experimental animal* are italicized to emphasize (*see* below) that because of potential adverse effects such injections of epinephrine are given in humans only as heroic treatment. The effects are listed because they best illustrate the pharmacologic action of the drug.

Cardiovascular Effects

After the i.v. injection of epinephrine into an experimental animal (Fig. 17-3), a rise in arterial pressure is followed by a moderate fall before levels become normal again.

Hypertension

Increased systolic and diastolic arterial pressures and pulse pressure occur. The causes are cardiac and vascular. Cardiac output increases owing to an increased heart rate (β_1 effect) and stroke volume (β_1 effect), the result of direct myocardial stimulation. At the same time the myocardium becomes more susceptible to arrhythmias (β_1 effect) (*see* Chap. 35). Total peripheral resistance is increased. Epinephrine constricts resistance and capacitance vessels in the skin, mucosa, splanchnic organs, and kidney because α effects predominate over β effects in these regions. It dilates vessels in the coronary and skeletal muscle beds (β_2 effect). In some species splenic constriction (α effect) increases the circulating blood volume. Probably the direct action of epinephrine on the coronary and skeletal muscle vessels is small compared with the increased flow in these beds secondary to the rise in systemic arterial pressure and metabolic changes. Alterations in the cerebral, renal, and pulmonary beds are ini-

---

THOMAS RENTON ELLIOTT, 1877–1961. London physician. Proposed in 1904 that sympathetic nerves release adrenaline at smooth muscle. In 1914 suggested treatment of pulmonary collapse by artificial pneumothorax.

tially passive following the arterial pressure, but flow tends to return to control levels as a result of local autoregulatory mechanisms. Veins are constricted (α effect), decreasing venous volume and increasing venous return and, as a result, cardiac output.

These direct effects of the drug are modified by compensatory mechanisms in the circulation. Homeostatic pressoreceptor reflexes tend to reduce the drug-induced hypertension by reflex bradycardia and (possibly β_2) vasodilation as evidenced by an early hypotensive "notch" in the arterial pressure record. These cardiac effects are atropine sensitive (*see* Chap. 16). If these homeostatic reflexes were abolished, the hypertensive and hypotensive response to the drug (*see* below) would be considerably greater and more prolonged.

In summary, after epinephrine administration, blood circulates faster and is redistributed to the vital organs. It is diverted away from the skin and splanchnic regions to the heart, skeletal muscles, brain, and lungs.

Hypotension

As the plasma concentration of the intravenously administered dose of epinephrine falls, both β_1 and β_2 effects predominate. The decrease in peripheral resistance, however, outweighs the cardiac excitatory effects of epinephrine, and arterial pressure in particular, and diastolic pressure falls. This resembles the effect produced in humans by a slow i.v. infusion or subcutaneous injection of epinephrine (Fig. 17-4). Under these circumstances, the tachycardia and small rise in systolic pressure are the consequence of cardiac stimulation (β_1 effect). The fall in diastolic pressure is the result of a decreased peripheral resistance due to the effect, predominantly β_2, of small doses of epinephrine on blood vessels, particularly those in skeletal muscle. Small doses of epinephrine in animals produce similar pictures.

Effects on the Bronchi

Bronchial muscle is relaxed (β_2 effect), and the microcirculation in the bronchial mucosa is constricted (α_1 effect). All changes contribute to a decreased bronchial resistance. Owing to a CNS effect, ventilatory stimulation is preceded by transient apnea in humans and some animals.

Other Effects

Eyes. Provided the dose is sufficient, the radial muscles of the iris contract, resulting in mydriasis (α effect).

Gastrointestinal Tract. Tone, frequency, and amplitude of peristalsis are reduced (α_2 and β_2 effects). Sphincters are constricted (α effect).

Glands. Saliva becomes sparse, thick, and mucoid; other secretions are inhibited (α effect). Although sweat glands receive a cholinergic innervation, they are stimulated by epinephrine (α, β).

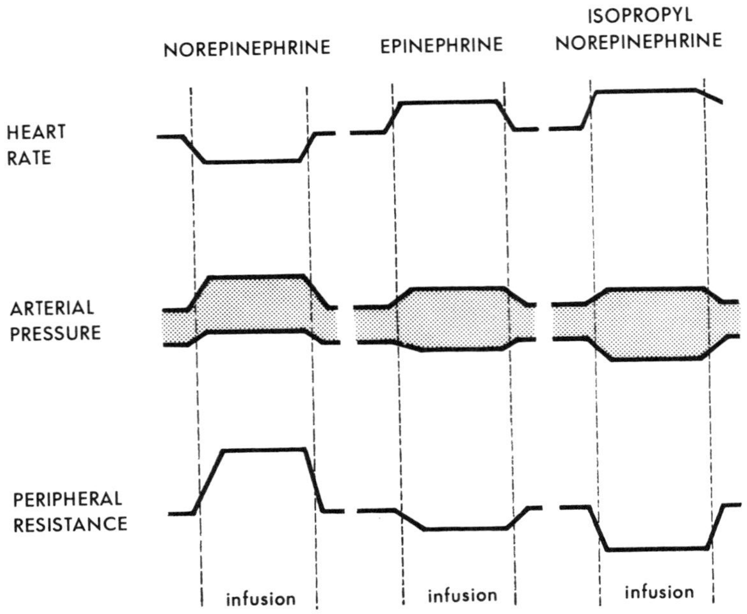

FIG. 17-4. Cardiovascular effects of infusions of norepinephrine, epinephrine, and isopropyl norepinephrine in humans. (Allwood MJ, Cobbold AF, Ginsberg J: Peripheral vascular effects of noradrenaline, isopropylnoradrenaline, and dopamine. Br Med Bull 19:132, 1963)

Urinary Tract. The detrusor muscle is relaxed (β effect); the trigone and sphincters are constricted (α effect).

Uterus. Effect varies with dose, species, pregnancy, and stage of estrous cycle. The pregnant human uterus contracts (α effect); however, the β_2-adrenoceptor-mediated inhibition of tonic contractions of the pregnant uterus is clinically important (*see* below).

Central Nervous System. Feelings of anxiety, apprehension, restlessness, and sometimes tremor and weakness are experienced.

Metabolic Effects

Glycogenolysis in the liver and skeletal muscle (α_1, β_2 effects) leads to hyperglycemia. Oxygen consumption may increase up to 25%. Lipolysis in adipose tissue (commonly α and β_1 effects) results in lipemia. An increase in basal metabolic rate and the cardiovascular effects cause a rise in body temperature (calorigenic effect).

Uses

Allergic Disorders. Epinephrine is the drug of choice in acute moderate to severe bronchial asthma. The symptoms and signs of this condition are the result of increased bronchial resistance. Epinephrine causes bronchodilation (reduces bronchial resistance) by relaxing bronchial muscle (β_2 effect), constricting or shrinking the bronchial mucosa (α effect), and inhibiting mucoid secretions. Other potentially serious manifestations of acute allergic reactions, including those to drugs (*e.g.*, including anaphylaxis, urticaria and angioneurotic edema) and hypotension may be treated similarly. (In these conditions epinephrine is eliciting a physiological antagonism. The substances responsible for the changes are not specifically antagonized. Epinephrine not only reduces the changes that occur in anaphylaxis but also often reverses them.) Epinephrine given orally as droplets or by aerosol may not always reach its site of action; however, when given parenterally it invariably does. The use of epinephrine in allergy is discussed in Chapter 51.

Local Anesthetics. The vasoconstrictor action of epinephrine is used to decrease the absorption of local anesthetics from their injection sites, which prolongs their local action, limits their spread, minimizes their absorption and, therefore, their systemic toxicity (*see* Chap. 20).

Control of Bleeding. Local arteriolar constriction caused by epinephrine-soaked packs or sprays is sometimes used to control superficial hemorrhage from small blood vessels of the skin and mucous membranes.

Cardiac Arrest. In cardiac arrest after external physical methods have failed and before manual cardiac massage is attempted, cardiac puncture with or without an intracardiac injection of epinephrine may be performed, followed by an intravenous infusion, although cardiac arrhythmias, including ventricular fibrillation, are definite and serious dangers. If induced, ventricular fibrillation may be controlled by electrical defibrillation. Pharmacologic procedures are only temporarily effective, and usually an artificial pacemaker must be applied.

Preparations and Dosage

Because epinephrine is destroyed in the gastrointestinal tract and that which is absorbed is detoxified in the liver, it is ineffective by mouth and must be administered parenterally, as a nebula, or applied locally. Many preparations are available. Epinephrine injection, U.S.P., B.P., is a 1:1000 solution of epinephrine base. The dose is 0.1 to 0.5 ml by s.c. injection. The i.v. or intracardiac (i.c.) route is used only in extreme conditions. During routine use the needle must *not* be in a vein; an i.v. injection must not be given in error.

Epinephrine inhalation, U.S.P., is a nonsterile 1:100 solution of epinephrine base, for oral inhalation from a nebulizer.

Great care must be used in distinguishing the two preparations. The parenteral use of the inhalation concentration is an established cause of accidental death.

Adverse Effects

Adverse effects occur most frequently in the very young and very old, in patients who because of hyperthyroidism or hypertension are hypersensitive, and after inadvertent i.v. injection or overdosage. They also result when used in patients receiving monoamine oxidase inhibitors and tricyclic antidepressants (*see* Chap. 22).

Central Nervous System. The effects of even therapeutic doses can sometimes be very disturbing and cause considerable alarm, but they are generally not dangerous. The effects include a sense of uneasiness, anxiety, tension, and sometimes tremor.

Cardiovascular System. An excessive rise in arterial pressure may result in cerebral or subarachnoid hemorrhage and myocardial infarction. The concomitant increase in cardiac work may lead to coronary insufficiency and angina pectoris. The increased myocardial contractility and irritability may lead to palpitations and atrial, and possibly ventricular, arrhythmias. Inhalation anesthesia using cyclopropane or the halogenated hydrocarbon anesthetics appears to sensitize the heart to this effect (*see* Chap. 28).

LEVARTERENOL (NOREPINEPHRINE)

Nor is derived from the German N(itrogen) O(hne) R(adikal)—nitrogen without radical. Levarterenol differs chemically from epinephrine in that "nitrogen is without" the methyl substitution (Fig. 17-1). The *l*-isomer is the neurohumoral transmitter at the postganglionic sympathetic nerve ending. Some evidence suggests that there may be an alteration in norepinephrine metabolism or release in essential hypertension.

ACTIONS

Norepinephrine has a predominant action on α adrenergic receptors. Its potency related to epinephrine is described above.

Cardiovascular

Norepinephrine causes a rise in both systolic and diastolic pressures due to an increase in total peripheral resistance, which is independent of dose. Cardiac output is either unchanged or reduced. The β_1 stimulating effect of the drug on the heart is antagonized by reflex cardiac inhibitory changes via the aortic and carotid pressoreceptors secondary to the hypertension. The bradycardia seen in Figure 17-4 is secondary to the hypertension.

Other Effects

Specific cardiovascular actions and other effects in humans in doses used clinically are minimal and unimportant. They may be accurately forecast by reference to Table 13-1.

USES

Shock

Shock is a condition of acute peripheral vascular failure when there is inadequate tissue perfusion. Its treatment is mainly determined by its cause, the intent being to restore tissue perfusion. In addition to vascular fluid replacement and improvement in oxygenation, peripheral vasoconstrictors, including norepinephrine, may be helpful.

Norepinephrine raises arterial pressure almost exclusively by increasing peripheral resistance. This, it has been argued, would be advantageous in cardiogenic shock secondary, for example, to myocardial infarction. Unfortunately, however, even though the damaged myocardium is not stimulated pharmacologically, the increased peripheral resistance inevitably increases the work load on the heart. Because of the pharmacologic vasoconstriction, neither coronary blood flow nor that to other important areas such as the brain and kidney necessarily increases with pressure rise. Particularly when blood loss has occurred, the opposite is often the case. Restoration of arterial pressure with a vasopressor agent is therefore not always the best procedure, although it may be useful in an emergency. The important consideration under these circumstances—apart from the heart—is not the absolute level of arterial pressure but the adequacy of local blood flow. As can be inferred from this discussion, there is a debate on the usefulness of vasoconstrictor therapy by this or any other agent in this type of condition.

PREPARATIONS AND DOSAGE

Levarterenol bitartrate injection, U.S.P., is a 1:1000 solution of norepinephrine base. It is administered by i.v. infusion (4 mg/1000 ml of solution), the rate being adjusted to maintain the desired level of arterial pressure. Ascorbic acid (0.5 g/liter) is added to prevent breakdown of the amine in the infusion system.

ADVERSE EFFECTS AND TOXICITY

If an excessive rise in arterial pressure is allowed, cardiovascular effects similar to those described for epinephrine occur.

Extravasation produces intense cutaneous vasoconstriction, which may lead to necrosis and sloughing. The local infiltration of an α-adrenergic blocking agent or its inclusion in the infusion medium is prophylactic, although this latter technique is rarely used. Because it stimulates the gravid uterus, epinephrine should not be administered to pregnant women.

ISOPROTERENOL (ISOPROPYLNOREPINEPHRINE)

ACTIONS

Isopropylnorepinephrine (Fig. 17-1) acts almost exclusively on β-adrenergic receptors.

Cardiovascular Effects

The change in arterial pressure is the net result of the drug's positive inotropic and chronotropic cardiac actions (β_1) and its vasodilator effects (β_2) mainly in skeletal muscle and, to a lesser extent, in renal and mesenteric beds, which tend to increase and decrease arterial pressure, respectively. The doses commonly used in humans usually cause a slight drop in mean arterial pressure (Fig. 17-4). Generally an increased pulse pressure, a rise in systolic pressure, and a fall in diastolic pressure occur. Higher doses cause a more dramatic fall in mean arterial pressure.

Bronchial Effects

Bronchial muscle contains a predominance of β_2 receptors; isopropylnorepinephrine decreases muscle tone. Unlike epinephrine, isopropylnorepinephrine does not constrict the mucosal circulation (α effect).

Other Effects

Other effects in doses commonly used clinically are not important but may be predicted by reference to Table 13-1.

USES

Bronchial Asthma

Isopropylnorepinephrine is sometimes effective in moderate to severe bronchial asthma in patients resistant to epinephrine. It may be administered sublingually or by oral inhalation, which is the preferred route because the incidence of palpitations is lower.

Heart Block

Isopropylnorepinephrine, the most potent cardiac stimulant in the pharmacopeia, is useful in the *immediate* treatment of heart block. Heart rate is increased, and the incidence and severity of syncopal seizures (Stokes–Adams syndrome) are reduced. Usually a cardiac pacemaker is implanted.

Preparations and Dosage

Isoproterenol hydrochloride inhalation (Isuprel), U.S.P., is a 1:100 solution of the amine base. Other concentrations are dispensed: Sublingual tablets of 10 and 15 mg are available in sustained action form. Isoproterenol is ineffective by mouth.

Adverse Effects and Toxicity

Isoproterenol causes flushing, headache, and tremor. Direct myocardial stimulation (β_1) and vasodilation (β_2) produce tachycardia and palpitations, which often limit its usefulness. These effects are smaller after inhalation compared to after sublingual administration.

Increased mortality among asthmatic patients has been associated with excessive use of β-adrenoceptor agonist therapy (*see* below).

SELECTIVE β_2 ADRENERGIC AGONISTS

The frequency of dangerous side-effects of isoproterenol that limit the dose that can be used in the treatment of bronchial asthma, even when administered by inhalation, has led to a search for more specific agonists. A number of drugs are now available with varying degrees of β_2-adrenoceptor agonist specificity. These drugs cause relaxation of bronchial, some vascular (especially in blood vessels to voluntary muscle), and also uterine smooth muscle but are devoid of a stimulant action on the heart. Selectivity, however, is relative, and, although this class of compounds has considerable β_2-adrenoceptor specificity, it is not absolute.

All these new agents are effective by mouth, but their selectivity of action on the bronchi is enhanced if they are given by inhalation ensuring a high concentration in the respiratory tract. These compounds, unlike isoproterenol, are not taken into effector cells and thus act longer. On i.v. infusion they all inhibit premature uterine contractions, thus delaying labor (*see* Chap. 39).

ALBUTEROL

The first β-receptor agonist for which some modest selectivity was claimed was metaproterenol, which is chemically related to isoproterenol. This has been superceded by albuterol (Salbutamol), which shows significant selectivity for β_2 adrenoceptors and is equipotent with isoproterenol on bronchial smooth muscle. Tachyphylaxis is not an important consideration. Because of initial concern over the reported induction of myomas in rats, it has only recently been released in the United States in inhalation form.

TERBUTALINE

Terbutaline is similar in many respects to albuterol. It lasts 4 to 6 hours after s.c. injection and several hours longer after oral ingestion. Its selectivity is enhanced by oral inhalation. Side-effects are usually mild and diminish with continuing administration.

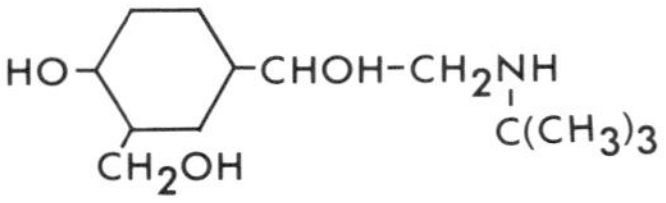

ALBUTEROL

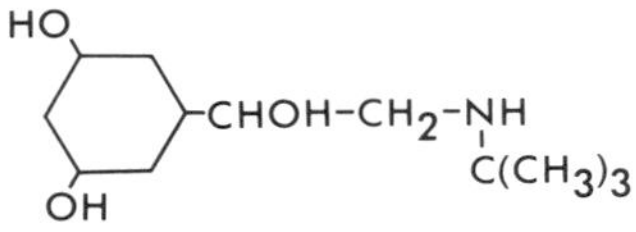

TERBUTALINE

There have been an increasing number of reports of death associated with the use, and particularly the misuse, of sympathomimetic drugs in bronchial asthma. This may result from a progressive desensitization of bronchial muscle β adrenoceptors. Patients often experience a waning in the effectiveness of bronchial dilator therapy with the frequent use of β-receptor agonists in high concentration. Their response to this, since medication is usually self-administered, is to increase the dose. Drug effectiveness is usually restored when therapy is withheld for a few days. The nature of the desensitization process is not known but may involve a diminution in the number of β adrenoceptors, a blunting of the coupling between receptors and adenylate cyclase (*see* Chap. 50), or possibly an imbalance of α and β adrenoceptors. Some of these changes may be prevented by glucocorticosteroids.

DOPAMINE

Dopamine (*see* Fig. 17-1), an endogenously occurring catecholamine, is a precursor of norepinephrine (*see* Chap. 13) and a transmitter in the CNS and possibly in some peripheral vascular sites, such as the kidney. Alteration in dopaminergic neuronal mechanisms in the substantia nigra is linked with parkinsonism (*see* Chap. 30).

Dopamine receptors, distinct from α- and β-adrenergic receptors, occur in peripheral organs and are blocked by haloperidol, among other drugs. Small doses of dopamine dilate mesenteric and renal vascular beds through these specific receptors. In addition, dopamine exerts a positive inotropic effect by means of myocardial β_2 adrenoceptors. Larger doses of dopamine have additional effects attributable to the two mechanisms of a "mixed action" sympathomimetic amine (*see* above).

The hemodynamic response to an average infusion of dopamine is different from that of any other amine: Cardiac output is increased, but mean arterial pressure and heart rate are unaltered. Cardiac output increases, primarily by the positive inotropic effect. Systolic, but not diastolic, pressure rises, as the renal dilation balances the vasoconstriction in other beds. When relatively higher doses are used, significant and potentially dangerous rises in arterial pressure occur along with vascular constriction. (These effects are the result of the indirect sympathomimetic property of the drug.)

Since dopamine is a substrate for monoamine oxidase and catechol-o-methyl transferase, it is ineffective orally and does not pass the blood–brain barrier.

USES

Dopamine is useful in congestive heart failure especially when associated with poor renal perfusion and diminished renal function. The increased cardiac output is associated advantageously with renal and mesenteric arterial dilation. Thus it has been used in the management of liver and renal failure and in the treatment of chronic refractory congestive heart failure.

PREPARATION AND DOSAGE

Dopamine hydrochloride is administered by i.v. infusion in a concentration of 400 or 800 μg/ml, beginning at a rate of 5 μg/kg/min. Cardiovascular status must be monitored with particular attention to arterial pressure and cardiac rhythm.

ADVERSE EFFECTS AND TOXICITY

Adverse effects are the consequence of the indirect and direct sympathomimetic actions of dopamine and are qualitatively, but not quantitatively, equivalent to those seen with epinephrine and norepinephrine. Excessive responses, if the immediate stoppage of infusion is insufficient, may be controlled with an α-adrenoceptor blocking agent (*see* Chap. 18).

DOLBUTAMINE

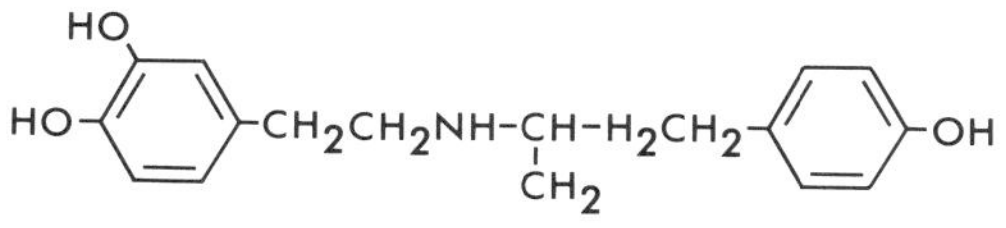

DOLBUTAMINE

Although chemically related to dopamine, the synthetic drug dolbutamine has a different spectrum of autonomic effects. It stimulates cardiac β_1 adrenoceptors preferentially, producing inotropic rather than chronotropic effects, particularly in the ventricle. It enhances cardiac automaticity but to a lesser degree than does isoproterenol and weakly stimulates peripheral α adrenoceptors. Unlike dopamine, dolbutamine has only weak indirect action. Thus cardiac output is raised primarily by a cardiac action in which diastolic time, and thus coronary flow, is well maintained and oxygen consumption only minimally raised. A modest renal vasoconstriction occurs.

USES

Like dopamine and isoproterenol, dolbutamine is useful in the treatment of heart failure superimposed on myocardial infarction or resulting from cardiopulmonary bypass. Oxygen demands seem to be elevated minimally, and improvement in urinary function is secondary to the rise in perfusion pressure. Reduction in tissue blood flow is less than that with norepinephrine, and the liability for arrhythmias is less than that with isoproterenol.

PREPARATION AND DOSAGE

Dolbutamine is administered 2.5 to 10 μg/kg/min by i.v. infusion. As its half-life in plasma is only several minutes, regulation of its infusion rate will control the extent of its pharmacologic effects.

ADVERSE EFFECTS

At high dosage, tachycardia or a raised systolic pressure and a lowering of peripheral resistance are encountered. However, reduction in dosage rapidly reverses the effects. Nausea, headache, anginal pain, palpitations, and shortness of breath occur in 1% to 3% of patients.

EPHEDRINE AND AMPHETAMINE

Ephedrine and amphetamine are typical members of two classes of therapeutically valuable amines. Although these drugs are classified as sympathomimetic amines, in contrast to the preceding agents, they are orally active, relatively stable in the body, and therefore of longer duration of action (measured in hours rather than minutes) and of lower absolute potency. They are mixed-action sympathomimetic amines with a predominant indirect effect (*see* above); in addition, they stimulate the cerebrospinal axis.

Tachyphylaxis results with continuing therapy, probably from transmitter depletion, since the mechanims of transmitter synthesis do not keep pace with its loss through release.

EPHEDRINE

For many centuries ephedrine extracted from various plant sources has been used medicinally. It is now obtained entirely by chemical synthesis. As both the α and β carbon atoms are asymmetric (Fig. 17-1), six isomers exist. Although subtle differences of action between these isomers have been described, their pharmacologic properties are practically identical.

Actions of Ephedrine

Cardiovascular. Ephedrine causes typical adrenergic or sympathomimetic changes. In comparison with epinephrine, the changes are slow in onset and persist longer. Ephedrine-induced hypertension in humans is principally due to an increased cardiac output rather than to an increased peripheral resistance.

Bronchial. Bronchodilation is weaker, slower in onset, but more persistent than that of epinephrine.

Ocular. On instillation of ephedrine into the conjunctival sac, the pupil dilates (mydriasis) but is not paralyzed. Accommodation and intraocular pressure are unaffected. The drug is relatively inactive in heavily pigmented irises.

Central Nervous System. The central stimulant effects of ephedrine are similar to, but less marked than those of amphetamine. Doses that have appreciable central effects also cause peripheral changes of significance. In therapeutic doses, ephedrine causes insomnia, restlessness, tremor, alertness, and feelings of tension, anxiety, and agitation. It is a weak analeptic.

Uses

Allergic Disorders. Ephedrine is the preferred prophylactic and is also used therapeutically in mild or moderate bronchial asthma. It is limited by its slow rate of onset, modest potency, tachyphylaxis, and CNS effects. It has the advantage of a long duration of action. Ephedrine is commonly used to relieve nasal congestion of allergic origin (hay fever) and after viral or bacterial infections of the upper respiratory tract and to prevent barotrauma. The small vessels in the mucous membranes are constricted and mucous secretions inhibited, providing not only subjective relief by allowing nasal breathing but better drainage of sinuses and eustachian passages.

Nasal decongestants, as a class, should in effective dosage cause only minimal local and systemic side-effects. They should be nonirritant and not induce secondary or rebound congestion of the mucosa. Spray application is usually preferred to drops. Ephedrine is effective at first, but when tachyphylaxis occurs its value diminishes; central stimulant effects occur, especially in babies, owing to systemic absorption. Medication should therefore be avoided late in the evening if a night's sleep is to be achieved. Transitory stinging and burning of the mucosa is sometimes experienced, but in comparison with some other amines ephedrine is relatively nonirritant; even so, it often causes sufficient rebound congestion secondary to the irritation and necessitates repetition of use. This unfortunate circle can lead to increased dependence on the decongestant. Rebound congestion may partly result from tissue anoxia or ischemia after intense vasoconstriction. Because of these disadvantages, nose drops and sprays are now less popular and have been somewhat superceded by oral vasoconstrictors, sometimes combined with an antihistamine and often dispensed in a prolonged action form.

Heart Block. More reliable and effective electric pacemakers are replacing long-term ephedrine therapy in the treatment of Stokes–Adams syndrome.

Other. Ephedrine is used to produce mydriasis not accompanied by cycloplegia, in the treatment of enuresis in children, as a mild central stimulant in narcolepsy and as a pressor agent during spinal anesthesia. In general, however, other drugs have replaced ephedrine in these conditions.

Preparations and Dosage

L-Ephedrine sulfate, U.S.P., and L-ephedrine-hydrochloride, N.F., are available in various forms and dilutions for oral administration, as nose drops and as sprays. The oral dose varies between 15 and 50 mg. Ephedrine sulfate (and hydrochloride) injection, rarely used, contains 20 to 50 mg/ml.

Adverse Effects and Toxicity

Apart from its adverse cardiovascular effects, which are essentially the same as those described for epinephrine, ephedrine produces CNS stimulation. The drug does not cause addiction. It may cause urinary retention in elderly men and glycogenolysis in diabetics. Children are particularly susceptible to general sympathomimetic effects. Tachyphylaxis disappears if the drug is withdrawn for 3 or 4 days.

AMPHETAMINE

Amphetamine (Benzedrine) is a powerful cerebrospinal stimulant. In therapeutic doses this action overshadows its peripheral sympathomimetic effects. The term *amphetamine* refers to the racemic form of the drug and *dextroamphetamine* (Dexedrine), to the *d*-isomer. Both amphetamine and dextroamphetamine are of synthetic origin. On the CNS the *d*-isomer is the more potent, whereas the *l*-isomer is more active at peripheral sites.

Actions and Uses

Peripheral Nervous System. Generally, the peripheral effects of amphetamine are similar to those of ephedrine.

Central Nervous System. The central stimulant effects of amphetamine are dramatic and best described in terms of its clinical uses. Amphetamine causes a general euphoria, producing a sense of well-being, confidence, self-satisfaction, and self-esteem. These actions underlie its previous use in some psychoses and neuropsychoses (*see* Chaps. 22–24). Amphetamine is usually valuable in reducing the incidence of narcoleptic attacks.

The performance of dull, repetitive tasks is temporarily improved by amphetamine. Physical fatigue is allayed. Both effects have led to abuse by students and athletes. In contrast, intellectual effort or creativity, although subjectively improved, objective assessment shows deterioration. Errors are more common and self-criticism less censorious, especially if the subject is mentally fatigued. These apparently beneficial effects are lost after higher doses or after repeated use and are replaced by depression, apprehension, agitation, and panic. Amphetamines are sometimes used as an aid in the management of minimal brain dysfunction in children, for example, hyperkinetic behavior disorders.

A piperidine derivative of amphetamine, methyl phenidate (Ritalin) is a mild central stimulant that is probably superior to amphetamine in the management of minimal brain dysfunction. Reports of improvement in behavior and learning must be balanced against the possibility of growth suppression and unpleasant mental experiences.

Obesity. Because amphetamine is an anorexiant (anoretic) that reduces the desire for food and diminishes the hunger drive, it has been considered a useful adjunct in the treatment of obesity. The small increase in basal metabolic rate induced by the drug is not responsible for this effect. Unfortunately tolerance develops, and because of its addictive properties its use is not without danger (*see* Chap. 26).

Amphetamine is a Schedule II drug. Because of its abuse potential and because drugs prescribed for weight control are a major source of abuse, this prescribing indication will probably be removed. Other amines have been claimed to be more specific and less addicting than amphetamine, such as phenmetrazine, and are listed in Table 17-2.

Other. Amphetamine has been used to counteract some undesirable sedative side-effects of other medication such as antiepileptic agents (*see* Chap. 29).

Preparations and Dosage

Amphetamine sulfate, *N.F.*, amphetamine phosphate, *N.F.*, and dextroamphetamine sulfate, *U.S.P.*, are available in many forms. Tablets usually contain 5 or 10 mg. The usual initial oral dose is 2.5 to 5.0 mg.

Adverse Effects and Toxicity

Amphetamine addiction is discussed in Chapter 26. Adult patients taking amphetamine for legitimate purposes should be warned to guard against the morbid curiosity of adolescents. Doctors should never prescribe the drug for themselves. In certain personalities, amphetamine precipitates acute psychotic episodes during which suicide may be attempted. Its continuous use over time may mask an underlying progressive chronic fatigue, and severe depression may follow withdrawal of the drug.

High doses of amphetamine produce typical peripheral sympathomimetic effects, mainly cardiovascular, along with signs of exag-

(*Text continues on p. 179*)

TABLE 17-2. Drug Interactions

Sympathomimetic Amine	Interacting Drugs	Mechanism of Interaction
Indirectly acting sympathomimetic amines: (tyramine, ephedrine, amphetamine)	Norepinephrine (NE) Neurone uptake inhibitors cocaine, tricyclic antidepressants	Prevent entry of indirectly acting amines into nerve terminals
Indirectly acting sympathomimetic amines: (tyramine, ephedrine, amphetamine)	Norepinephrine depleters (reserpine, guanethidine)	Loss of NE stores on which the indirectly acting sympathomimetic amines depend for their effect
Dopamine	Tricyclic antidepressants	Prevent the indirect action of dopamine
Tyramine and tyramine-containing foods (ephedrine, amphetamine, and Dopamine)	Monoamine oxidase inhibitors	By preventing intraneuronal degradation of drugs or intraneuronally released NE, they sensitize to their effects

TABLE 17-3. Sympathomimetic Amines (Those Not Discussed in Text)

Drug	Trade Name	Dose	Comment
Compounds resembling l-norepinephrine (predominantly α stimulating; causing minimal central stimulation)			
Metaraminol bitartrate	Aramine bitartrate	5–10 mg i.m.	Orally active, less potent, longer acting vasopressor agent. May be given intravenously. Has little action on the heart
Methoxamine hydrochloride	Vasoxyl hydrochloride	10–20 mg i.m.	Longer-acting vasopressor agent. Can be used to inhibit cardiac irregularities by reflex increase in vagal tone. Nasal decongestant
Phenylephrine hydrochloride	Neo-Synephrine	0.25–10% topically; 5 mg i.m.	Orally active, less potent, longer-acting vasopressor. May be given intravenously. By local application, nasal decongestant and mydriatic
Mephentermine sulfate	Wyamine sulfate	0.5% topically; 10–30 mg i.m.	Long-duration vasopressor agent. Nasal decongestant
Compound resembling l-epinephrine			
Nordefrin hydrochloride	Cobefrin hydrochloride	1:10,000 solution	Used with local anesthetics
Compounds resembling isopropylnorepinephrine (predominantly β stimulating; causing minimal central effects)			
Isoxsuprine hydrochloride	Vasodilan hydrochloride	5–10 mg p.o.	Orally active, long-duration vasodilator, especially in skeletal muscle. Myocardial stimulant
Nylidrin hydrochloride	Arlidin hydrochloride	6 mg p.o.	Orally active, long-duration vasodilator, especially in skeletal muscle. Myocardial stimulant
Protokylol hydrochloride	Caytine	1% inhalant; 2–4 mg p.o.	Orally active, persistent bronchodilator
Compounds resembling ephedrine (causing peripheral sympathomimetic and central stimulation)			
Hydroxyamphetamine hydrochloride	Paredrine hydrochloride	1–3% topically; 20–60 mg p.o.	Similar to ephedrine in uses but with less central stimulant action
Phenylpropanolamine hydrochloride	Propadrine	25 mg p.o.	Similar to ephedrine in uses but with less central stimulant action
Compound resembling amphetamine (causing predominantly central stimulation)			
Methamphetamine hydrochloride	Methedrine hydrochloride	2.5–5.0 mg p.o.	Probably more pronounced central stimulant action. Vasopressor agent
Miscellaneous anoretic drugs			
Benzphetamine	Didrex		
Chlorphentermine	Pre-Sate		
Diethylpropion	Tenuate, Tepanil		
Fenfluramine	Pondimin		
Phenmetrazine	Preludin		
Phentermine hydrochloride	Wilpo		
Phentermine resin	Ionamin		
Miscellaneous bronchodilator drugs			
Ethylephedrine	Nethamine		
Methoxyphenamine	Orthoxine		
Pseudoephedrine	Sudafed		
Racemic ephedrine	Racephrine		
Miscellaneous nasal decongestants			
Cyclopentamine hydrochloride	Clopane		

(*continued*)

TABLE 17-3. (*Continued*)

Drug	Trade Name	Dose	Comment
Miscellaneous nasal decongestants (continued)			
2-Methylaminoheptane	Oenethyl		
Methylhexaneamine	Forthane		
Phenylpropanolamine hydrochloride	Propadrine hydrochloride		
Phenylpropylmethylamine hydrochloride	Vonedrine hydrochloride		
Propylhexedrine	Benzedrex		
Tetrahydrozoline hydrochloride	Tyzine		Volatile for inhalation
Tuaminoheptane sulfate	Tuamine		

gerated central stimulation: insomnia, confusion, hallucinations, panic, tremor, and even syncope and collapse.

OTHER SYMPATHOMIMETIC AMINES

Other clinically useful sympathomimetic amines are described briefly in Table 17-3 in terms of the compound discussed above that they most resemble pharmacologically, not chemically. Brevity of description does not imply clinical or therapeutic inferiority. Reference sources should be consulted when further details are required.

FURTHER READING

1. Avado DM Jr: Cardiovascular effects on some commonly used pressor amines. Anesthesiology 20:71–97, 1959
2. Conolly M: Sympathomimetic amines, beta receptors and bronchial asthma. In Weiner N, Trendelenberg U (eds): Catecholamines. II Berlin, Springer–Verlag (in press)
3. Cotton M de V, Moran NC: Cardiovascular pharmacology. Annu Rev Pharmacol 1:261–285, 1961
4. Furchgott RF: The classification of adrenoceptors (adrenergic receptors); an evaluation for the standpoint of receptor theory. In Blaschko H, Muscholl E (eds): Catecholamines, Handbuch der Experimentellen Pharmakologie. Berlin, Springer–Verlag, 33:283–335, 1972
5. Goldberg LI: Cardiovascular and renal actions of dopamine: Potential clinical applications. Pharmacol Rev 24:1–29, 1972
6. Sutherland EW, Rall TW: The relation of adenosine 3′, 5′-phosphate and phosphorylase to the action of catecholamines and other hormones. Pharmacol Rev 12:265–300, 1960
7. Westfall TC: Local regulation of adrenergic neurotransmission. Physiol Rev 57:659–728, 1977

CHAPTER 17 QUESTIONS

(*See* P. 7 for Full Instructions)

Select the One Best Answer

1. Because of its action on β-adrenergic receptors, epinephrine is used to
   - A. relieve nasal stuffiness.
   - B. alleviate bronchial asthma
   - C. treat cardiac arrest and heart block associated with syncope.
   - D. reduce absorption of local anesthetics.
   - E. control hemorrhage from small blood vessels.

2. The vasopressor effect of tyramine is likely to be enhanced after pretreatment with
   - A. chlorpromazine.
   - B. cocaine.
   - C. a monoamine oxidase inhibitor such as phenelzine.
   - D. reserpine.
   - E. imipramine (Tofranil).

3. Each of the following statements is correct for ephedrine EXCEPT that
   - A. its effects are reduced in a patient under treatment with tricyclic antidepressants.
   - B. it is effective both when administered orally and systemically.
   - C. it reduces the rate of spontaneous firing of the sinoatrial node.
   - D. it enters into the adrenergic nerve varicosity by way of the same transport mechanism as norepinephrine.
   - E. tachyphylaxis occurs to its hypertensive effect.

4. Dopamine
   - A. has essentially the same actions as dobutamine but is short acting.
   - B. is a general circulatory vasodilator.

C. is a breakdown product of catecholamine.
D. can increase renal blood flow during congestive heart failure.
E. is rapidly effective after oral administration.

A = 1,2,3; B = 1,3; C = 2,4; D = 4; E = All

5. Norepinephrine infusion is sometimes found to slow the human pulse rate because it
   1. stimulates β_2-adrenoceptors.
   2. causes increased acetylcholine release by means of a presynaptic receptor.
   3. decreases venous return by causing venous pooling.
   4. has an action that activates the baroreceptor reflex.

6. Agonist action on β-adrenoceptors is associated with
   1. relaxation of bronchial smooth muscle.
   2. dilation of arterioles in blood supply to gracilis muscle.
   3. binding to a receptor that is antagonized by propranolol.
   4. feedback inhibition of adrenergic transmitter release.

7. Isoproterenol is a drug of choice in treating complete heart block because it
   1. increases the rate of firing of the sinoatrial node.
   2. shortens the refractory period of the atrioventricular node.
   3. has a positive inotropic action.
   4. increases the slope of phase 4 depolarization of specialized myocardial conduction tissue.

8. Amphetamine and related drugs
   1. are used in the treatment of the hyperkinetic syndrome in children.
   2. do not usually cross the blood–brain barrier.
   3. in therapeutic dose cause an elevation in diastolic blood pressure.
   4. produce an anorectic effect to which tolerance rapidly develops, limiting their usefulness.

JOHN A. BEVAN

18

Adrenergic Receptor Blocking Drugs

Adrenergic receptor blocking agents antagonize the effect of endogenously released norepinephrine and epinephrine and also exogenous sympathomimetic amines on α- and β-adrenergic receptors (*see* Fig. 17-2).

The consequences of agonist action on the postsynaptic α and β adrenoceptors at various sites are summarized in Table 13-1. If the tonic discharge of the sympathetic nervous system or the effects of a sympathomimetic amine on an effector cell are mediated by either an α or β adrenoceptor or both, then an appropriate receptor blocking agent would diminish or antagonize that influence. In many cells adrenoceptors are not innervated, that is, are not exposed to amine released by local tonic sympathetic discharge. Occupation of such receptors by blocking agents would have functional consequence only if they are influenced by circulating amines. In many healthy mammals at rest there is little or no tonic sympathetic influence on the myocardium by β adrenoceptors. Sympathetic activation has been shown to occur during stress, exercise, or disease, as in heart failure. Blockade of myocardial β adrenoceptors thus would have consequence only in a disease state. On the other hand exogenous agonists do not depend for their action on tonic sympathetic influence; all their actions would usually be expected to be antagonized by the appropriate receptor blocking drugs.

Adrenergic receptors are also located at presynaptic sites. Although both α- and β-receptor-mediated presynaptic effects that lead to inhibition and augmentation of transmitter release, respectively, are present in most adrenergic synapses, only the α-adrenoceptor negative feed-back system is commonly and significantly involved in physiological regulation. Thus presynaptic α-adrenoceptor blockade usually leads to increased transmitter release owing to inhibition of this tonically active system (Fig. 17-2). In most synapses, presynaptic β-adrenoceptor blockade has no effect on transmitter function. Blockade of either receptor would prevent this presynaptic influence when it is functional and also the presynaptic effects of exogenous sympathetic agonists.

Because of the diverse structure of adrenoceptor antagonists, some specificity of action on presynaptic (α_2) versus postsynaptic (α_1) receptors and on β_1 and β_2 adrenoceptors is found among this group of agents (*see* Table 18-1). This specificity can be used to clinical advantage to increase the selectivity of effect of this group of drugs that potentially have extremely widespread and diverse effects, since these types of receptors are found on most effector cells and relate to so many responses.

Adrenergic receptor blocking agents must be distinguished from *adrenergic neurone blocking agents* such as guanethidine (*see* Chap. 36). This latter class of drugs exerts a primarily presynaptic effect (at the termination of the postganglionic adrenergic neuron), preventing transmitter release. Drugs of this class prevent both the α- and β-adrenoceptor-mediated effector cell consequences of tonic sympathetic neural activity. They do not interfere with the postsynaptic actions of endogenous and exogenous α- and β-adrenoceptor agonists. In addition, by virtue of their prevention of transmitter release, they block drug actions dependent on occupation of presynaptic receptors. Adrenergic neurone blocking agents do not prevent the actions of indirectly acting sympathomimetic amines (*see* Chap. 36) provided that transmitter stores are intact and these amines have access to them. On the other hand, the indirect effects of these amines are susceptible to direct receptor blockade.

A detailed description of the effects of receptor blocking drugs will not be given here because this can usually be worked out; for example, if the predominant adrenergic receptor and the influence of tonic sympathetic activity on the various organs are known, the pharmacologic actions of receptor blocking drugs may be easily deduced (*see* Table 13-1).

ALPHA-ADRENERGIC RECEPTOR BLOCKING AGENTS

There are two groups of this class of drugs: irreversible and reversible. After an interim period during which blockade is reversible, phenoxybenzamine and related compounds bind covalently to the α adrenoceptor, resulting in an irreversible block—one that cannot be overcome or surmounted by high agonist concentrations and one that persists for a number of days. The reversible group of α-adrenoceptor blocking agents are of diverse chemical structure and form a competitive or surmountable blockade. They are relatively nonspecific.

IRREVERSIBLE BLOCKING AGENTS

Phenoxybenzamine is a haloalkylamine that exhibits considerable specificity in its reaction with postsynaptic α_1 adrenoceptors. It inhibits postsynaptic-mediated actions of α agonists in doses lower than those that increase transmitter release by a presynaptic effect. Higher concentrations prevent neuronal uptake of sympathomimetic amines and also bind at nonadrenergic sites, including serotonin, acetylcholine, and histamine receptors. Many tissues contain an excess of adrenergic receptors—more than are necessary to mediate the maximum response of the tissue. As the concentration of phenoxybenzamine is increased, the agonist dose-response curve of such tissues is shifted to the right without a change in its maximum or slope, as long as there are sufficient receptors remaining to mediate a maximum response. When the number of available receptors—those not irreversibly inactivated by the drug—falls below this level, the maximum response to the agonist and the slope of the dose-response curve is reduced (*see* Chap. 2).

Phenoxybenzamine hydrochloride, USP (Dibenzyline), is irregularly absorbed after oral ingestion, and thus its i.v. injection is often preferred when it is given well diluted. Phenoxybenzamine is very fat soluble, and details of its distribution and subsequent fate have been poorly studied. Evidence suggests that a small percentage remains in the body for some weeks.

The adverse effects of phenoxybenzamine are mainly the result of undesirable α-adrenoceptor blockade. Inhibition of compensatory circulatory reflexes results in postural hypotension. The associated fall in blood pressure is accompanied by tachycardia. There is an exaggerated response to other cardiovascular drugs, in particular vasodilators and antihypertensives. Other effects include nasal stuffiness, miosis, failure to ejaculate, and local consequences of the drug's irritative properties (it is chemically related to the nitrogen mustards), which vary with the administration route.

REVERSIBLE BLOCKING AGENTS

Although many types of compounds have been introduced over the course of the last half century, including some early agents by Bovet,

---

DANIEL BOVET, 1907– . Swiss-born pharmacologist working in France and Italy, often with his wife Filomena Bovet-Nitti. Codiscoverer of antibacterial action of sulfanilamides. Worked on relation between structure and activity of pharmacologicals. Won Nobel prize 1957.

only a few are in vogue currently. Phentolamine (Regitine) shows modest selectivity and prazosin, a relatively new agent, high selectivity for α_1 postsynaptic adrenoceptors. Yohimbine, a drug with little clinical value, favors the α_2 receptor. Other agents in this general class include some ergot alkaloids and their derivatives, tolazoline (Priscoline)—similar to phentolamine but less selective—and azapetine (Ilidar). Except for prazosin, these agents are not highly specific and exert a host of other effects at doses that cause α adrenoceptor blockade.

Phentolamine

Only doses of this drug that produce a modest or incomplete level of α adrenoceptor blockade can be tolerated clinically. This lack of specificity is associated with a paradoxical sympathomimetic effect particularly on the heart, probably owing to blockade of presynaptic α_2 receptors and a parasympathomimetic effect manifested mainly on the gastrointestinal tract. Higher doses of phentolamine will release histamine, block serotonin receptors, and cause peripheral vasodilation by direct action on vascular smooth muscle. There are many less common adverse effects.

Phentolamine mesylate, USP (Regitine mesylate), is available for oral or parenteral use. After an initial trial dose, the standard intravenous dose when testing for pheochromocytoma is 5 mg. Phentolamine hydrochloride is available in 5-mg tablets.

Prazosin

Prazosin is a specific postsynaptic α_1 adrenoceptor antagonist that has been introduced as an antihypertensive agent (*see* Chap. 36). Its lack of affinity for α_2 adrenoceptors probably explains the modest tachycardia and low level of renin release that occurs with its use. Other actions attributed to prazosin—phosphodiesterase and dopamine-β-hydroxylase inhibition, a central action, and augmentation of baroreceptor sensitivity—are probably of little consequence in causing its clinically useful effects.

In addition to its uses shared with other α-adrenoceptor blocking agents (*see* below), prazosin is valuable as an antihypertensive. It has been used to treat severe congestive heart failure. Its salutary effects are attributable to peripheral vasodilation of both arterial and venous beds, resulting in a reduction in cardiac preload and afterload (*see* Vasodilators in Heart Failure, Chap. 35).

Adverse effects of prazosin are fairly mild. Problems are often encountered with the first dose administered that seem to be due to an exaggerated postural hypotensive response. After more prolonged administration, many undesirable effects can be related to α adrenoceptor blockade. Headache, nausea, drowsiness, depression, fluid retention, urinary incontinence, and polyarthralgia have been reported.

GENERAL USES OF ALPHA-ADRENOCEPTOR BLOCKING AGENTS

With the exception of the ergot alkaloids, α-adrenergic blocking agents have been used to treat peripheral vascular spastic disease for such conditions as thromboangiitis obliterans (Buerger's disease) and Raynaud's syndrome. Sympathetic hyperactivity probably contributes in part to these conditions, this component is eliminated by α receptor blockade (*see* Chap. 35). Because the vessel wall is often rigid and narrowed by pathologic change, this precludes a satisfactory dilator response. Further, the fall in perfusion pressure caused by the general vascular effect of these agents often offsets their therapeutic value. Obviously they are of less use in vascular beds dominated by autoregulatory or β-adrenergic receptor dilator mechanisms. These actions are augmented by the direct smooth muscle relaxant properties of the drugs.

Alpha receptor blocking agents have a rational place in the control of pheochromocytoma. Adrenoceptor blocking agents may protect against the high concentration of catecholamines released into the circulation after histamine challenge (*see* Chap. 51) Phenoxybenzamine particularly can be used profitably in preoperative management, protecting against the surge of vasoactive substances often released during surgical manipulation. Because of its specificity and prolonged blockade, this drug can be used advantageously to control the circulatory and other manifestations of inoperable tumors.

In certain types of shock, when reflex neurogenic vasoconstriction owing to the hyperactivity of compensatory mechanisms is a prominent feature, the judicial use of α-receptor blocking agents can increase blood perfusion of important areas.

ERGOT ALKALOIDS

Although traditionally the ergot alkaloids are classified as α-adrenergic receptor blocking agents and they were the first of this type of

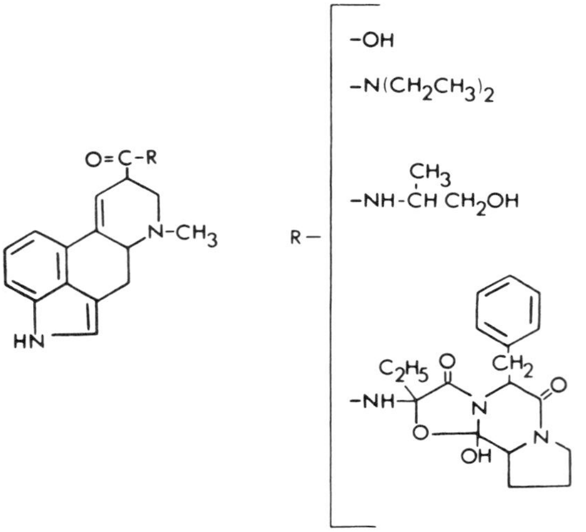

FIG. 18-1. Some derivatives of lysergic acid.

drug to be described by Dale, their present clinical uses depend on other pharmacologic properties.

SOURCE AND CHEMISTRY

Ergot alkaloids along with many other substances are extracted from a fungus (*Claviceps purpurea*) parasitic to rye and other grains. Even today in the United States, infected rye is fairly common. The substances derived from ergot that are commonly used in medicine are all related to lysergic acid (Fig. 18-1). The most important are ergotamine and ergonovine. Hydrogenation of one of the double bonds in the lysergic acid nucleus enhances the adrenergic blocking properties of these compounds and reduces their other actions. Lysergic acid diethylamide (LSD) is an easily prepared congener (*see* Chap. 26).

ACTIONS

In addition to their α-adrenoceptor blocking activity, ergot alkaloids constrict smooth muscle, particularly vascular and uterine, and cause endothelial damage in the small peripheral blood vessels. The increase in smooth muscle tone is due to a direct action of the drug on the muscle cells independent of adrenergic mechanisms. In addition, by an action on the cardiovascular centers in the medulla, mild hypotension and depression of reflex compensatory mechanisms occur.

Henry Hallett Dale, 1875–1968. London physiologist. Demonstrated the inhibitory action of acetylcholine on the heart in 1914, isolated it from spleen in 1929, and showed its release at the neuromuscular junction in 1936. Won Nobel prize, with O. Loewi, in 1936 for work on neural transmission. Isolated ergotoxine and worked on histamine and histamine shock.

USES AND EFFECTIVENESS

Migraine Headaches

The pain of migraine headaches is associated with vasodilation, edema, and sometimes visible pulsation of extracranial blood vessels. This is possibly associated with the local release of serotonin (*see* Chap. 52) in periarterial tissues. The prodromal symptoms or aura that precedes the headache, on the other hand, is associated with excessive constriction of the same vessels. The ergot alkaloids are effective in migraine headache because of their vasoconstrictor, or smooth muscle stimulant, properties. However, their specificity for migraine headache and not other types of headaches suggests that this explanation may not be entirely correct. They should not be administered more than once a week, avoided during pregnancy, and used with care in patients with peripheral vascular disease.

Ergotamine is effective in almost 90% of migraine attacks if given early, preferably during the prodromal phase. In nonmigraine headaches, only 15% of patients claim relief. They are ineffective if given during an attack.

Dihydroergotamine, a weaker vasoconstrictor but a more potent adrenergic blocking agent, is generally less effective than ergotamine in the treatment of migraine headache, although preferred by some patients. In contrast to other vascular beds, where it causes vasodilation, caffeine constricts cerebral blood vessels. Thus it enhances the therapeutic effectiveness of the ergot alkaloids, presumably by adding to the direct vasoconstriction action of ergotamine.

Methysergide (Sansert) (*see* Chap. 52), a congenor of ergonovine and a potent serotonin antagonist, is effective prophylactically only after a latency of several days. Protection persists for some time after its withdrawal. Unfortunately in about 20% of patients the frequency of adverse effects limits its use (*see* Chap. 52).

Propranolol is also beneficial in preventing migraine attacks (*see* below).

For ergotamine's use as an oxytocic, *see* Chapter 39.

PREPARATIONS AND DOSAGE

Ergotamine tartrate, *U.S.P.* (Gynergen), is available in sublingual tablets. The dose is 3 to 4 mg stat, then 0.5 to 1.0 mg hourly to a total of 10 mg. The course is not to be repeated within a week. Dose by injection is 0.25 to 0.5 mg stat, intramuscularly, or subcutaneously, to be repeated once if ineffective. It is also effective in an inhaled form.

Ergotamine tartrate (1 mg) plus caffeine (100 mg) (Cafergot) is a commonly used mixture. The dosage is as above.

Ergonovine maleate, *U.S.P.* (Ergometrine maleate, *B.P.*), may be given intramuscularly, orally or sublingually. The dose for injection is 0.2 mg. The oral or sublingual dose is 0.5 mg.

ADVERSE EFFECTS

Acute effects such as headache, nausea, vomiting, diarrhea, extreme thirst, weakness, muscle pain, confusion, depression, convulsions, and various neurologic symptoms and cutaneous manifestations—itching, numbness, and tingling—are experienced by about 15% of patients. Other symptoms, such as hypertension, especially in patients with toxemia of pregnancy and angina, are probably the result of direct vasoconstriction. Many of these effects may be minimized by symptomatic treatment with other agents (vasodilators, antiemetics), allowing the continued use of the drug in migraine headache.

The dramatic chronic effects of ergot ingestion, sometimes of epidemic proportions, witnessed in the past from eating bread prepared from infected rye are seldom seen today. This condition in its extreme is characterized by convulsions, abortion, and peripheral vascular stasis and gangrene, the result of the intense vasoconstriction and toxicologic damage to the vascular endothelium of the small peripheral blood vessels. Sporadic reports of these effects still appear, presumably owing to accidental overdosage or to an increased sensitivity to the drug, probably associated with hepatic disease or pre-existing vascular disease.

BETA-ADRENERGIC RECEPTOR BLOCKING AGENTS

All β-adrenergic receptor blocking agents are synthetic. The dichloro derivative of isoproterenol, dichloroisoproterenol, was the first effective drug of this class (Fig. 18-2). Unfortunately, in addition to its β-receptor blocking action, it exhibited β-receptor stimulating activity and thus is a partial agonist. Recently pronethalol (Nethalide) and subsequently propranolol (Inderal), both related to isoproterenol, were developed. Pronethalol was found to produce lymphosarcoma in mice, and its use has been discontinued. Propranolol appears to be without this undesirable property and, as can be seen from its inclusion in a number of chapters, is proving to be quite valuable clinically.

Propranolol, however, is a nonselective β-adrenoceptor blocking agent. Its actions are valuable in the treatment of diseases of the heart and circulation. In addition to these clinically advantageous effects, however, it antagonizes the actions of the sympathetic nervous

FIG. 18-2. The β-adrenoceptor stimulating agent (isoproterenol) and the β-adrenoceptor blocking agent (propranolol).

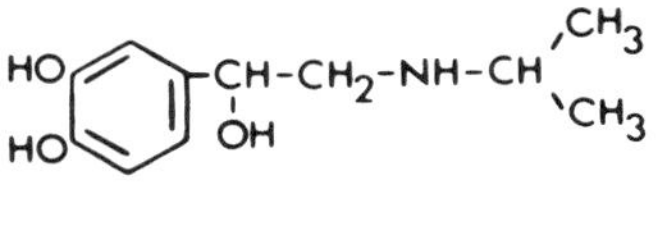

ISOPROTERENOL

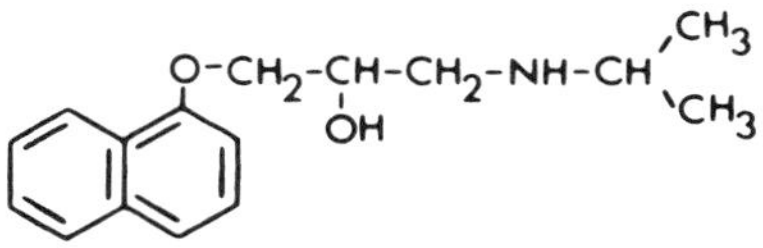

PROPRANOLOL

system on the bronchi, often leading to bronchial constriction. It also interferes with glycogenolysis, a physiological response to hypoglycemia. These disadvantages have prompted the search for cardioselective β_1 receptor antagonists. *Practolol*, the first drug of this type, caused major toxic changes in some epithelial structures such as the lens, but more recently recognized agents do not show this toxicity (*see* below).

In this chapter propranolol will be discussed in some detail and compared with other β adrenoceptor agents in Table 18-1. The relative advantages and disadvantages of these various agents are not sufficiently well established to justify their separate description.

PROPRANOLOL

Propranolol is a reversible, competitive antagonist of sympathomimetic amines at β_1 and β_2 adrenergic receptors. Its effects can be deduced from a knowledge of those physiological consequences of sympathetic tone mediated through the β adrenergic receptor. For example, the sympathetic nervous system to some degree at rest, and particularly during stress, exerts a positive inotropic and chronotropic effect on the myocardium. Thus the administration of propranolol has little effect at rest but a marked negative inotropic and chronotropic action during heart failure, for example, when sympathetic tone is elevated.

Propranolol has little action on the vasculature since the sympathetic drive to this system is mediated predominantly through α adrenoceptors. It has little of the intrinsic sympathomimetic activity prominent in other agents in this class (Table 18-1), which offset some of the consequences of blockade itself. The total effects of propranolol on the heart are the result not only of β adrenoceptor blockade but an additional quinidinelike action (*see* Chap. 34).

Propranolol lowers arterial pressure, probably by reduction in cardiac output, by blockade of renin release mediated by β_2 receptors on the juxtaglomerular apparatus, and by an as yet undefined central mechanism (*see* Chap. 35).

Administration and Excretion

Propranolol is rapidly and completely absorbed from the gastrointestinal tract. Individual variation is remarkable in the dose needed to cause the same effect, which can be determined only by trial and error. Ninety percent to 95% of the drug in the plasma is bound to protein, which is probably responsible for the variability of dose and lack of predictability of effect based on total plasma values. Maximum effects are realized within 90 minutes. Its halftime in the plasma is 2.5 to 3.0 hours. Propranolol is completely metabolized to a variety of products, including many glycuronide conjugates. At least one of these metabolites has a similar pharmacologic effect to the parent compound.

Preparations and Dose

Propranolol hydrochloride, USP (Inderal), is usually administered orally but can be given intravenously for the rapid control of serious arrhythmias (*see* Chap. 34 for details of dosage).

Uses and Effectiveness

Propranolol is being found to be useful in diverse conditions. Only some of these uses can be associated with its β-adrenoceptor blocking propensity.

Angina Pectoris. Propranolol and other β-adrenergic blocking agents are effective in reduc-

TABLE 18-1. Some Characteristics of β-Adrenergic Receptor Blocking Drugs

	Receptors Blocked	Intrinsic Sympathomimetic Activity	Local Anesthetic Activity
Propanolol (Inderal)	β_1 β_2	±	+++
Oxprenolol (Trasicor)	β_1 β_2	++	++
Alprenolol (Aptin)	β_1 β_2	++	+
Pindolol (Viskin)	β_1 β_2	++	+/−
Sotalol (Betacardone)	β_1 β_2	−	+/−
Timolol (Blocadren)	β_1 β_2	±	±
Alebutolol (Sectral)	β_1	+	++
Atenolol (Tenormin)	β_1	−	−
Metoprolol (Betaloc, Lopressor)	β_1	−	±

ing the incidence and severity of attacks in some patients by depressing the sympathetic drive to the heart (*see* Chap. 35).

Propranolol may also be responsible for redistribution of intramyocardial blood flow. The cardiac response to exercise is blunted (*see* Chap. 35).

Cardiac Arrhythmias. Propranolol is used to treat arrhythmias, including those that result from digitalis toxicity. Presumably because of its antiarrhythmic properties, propranolol reduces the mortality associated with myocardial infarction.

Hypertension. Propranolol is widely used in the treatment of essential hypertension (*see* Chap. 36).

Pheochromocytoma. Propranolol is sometimes combined with an α-adrenergic receptor blocking agent in the pharmacologic premedication of the patient before surgery for pheochromocytoma.

Hyperthyroidism. Many features of hyperthyroidism are similar to increased sympathetic activity. Whether owing to altered effector sensitivity associated with changes in β adrenoceptor and/or their coupling, to increased sympathetic adrenergic tone, or to raised catecholamine levels in the region of the adrenergic receptors has not been resolved. Propranolol and related drugs do offer some relief, especially in thyrotoxic crises. Clearly those drugs with intrinsic sympathomimetic activities should be avoided (Table 18-1). The use of β-adrenoceptor blockers is not considered a long-term substitute for the specific therapy of the thyroid abnormality.

Hypertropic Cardiomyopathy. β-adrenoceptor blocking drugs reduce the intraventricular pressure gradient and probably the impaired ventricular compliance seen in hypertropic cardiomyopathy. There is often considerable associated symptomatic relief.

Migraine Prophylaxis. Many patients show singular decreases in numbers and severity of migraine attacks. The required dose of ergot alkaloids (*see* above), if still needed, is reduced, with obvious advantage.

Anxiety. Although not established by appropriate controlled trial, propranolol may lower the systemic manifestations of anxiety, especially in temporary and periodic circumstanes. Propranolol does reduce action tremors.

Open-Angle Glaucoma. Timolol is probably the best specific β-adrenoceptor blocking drug for open-angle glaucoma. It decreases intraocular pressure when applied topically.

Central Disorders. Propranolol has been used in the management of acute psychotic states and in the withdrawal of abused drugs. Adequate assessment of its usefulness in central disorders is awaited.

Diabetes. Propranolol potentiates the effect of insulin by reducing the response of the sympathetic nervous system to hypoglycemia. It interferes with the usual warning symptoms of palpitations, tachycardia, and sweating that alert patients to diabetes. If possible, propranolol should be avoided in the diabetic patient. Because it interferes with the physiological response to hypoglycemia, propranolol use during general anesthesia and major surgery puts patients at increased risk.

Adverse Reactions

General symptoms include nausea, vomiting, mild diarrhea; skin changes such as reversible alopecia, agranulocytosis, and purpura; lightheadedness, depression, hallucinations, visual disturbances, short-term memory loss, insomnia and various psychologic disturbances have been reported.

More serious effects are associated with blockade of sympathetic β-receptor-mediated drive. Heart failure may develop slowly, especially in those with a compromised myocardium. Existing heart failure may be exacerbated by blocking compensatory and supportive sympathetic hyperactivity. High doses of propranolol directly depress the heart. Concomitant administration of digitalis, can often minimize this problem, although both depress atrioventricular conduction. Propranolol is contraindicated in patients with asthma. Even cardioselective β_1-adrenergic receptor blockers are not sufficiently discriminating to be used with impunity in asthma.

The higher the dose of the so-called cardioselective blockers, the less selective they are. A blocker with intrinsic sympathomimetic action may have some advantages under some circumstances; however, its use can result in bronchial spasm.

Abrupt withdrawal of propranolol after chronic therapy often leads to a sudden exacerbation of sympathomimetic effects with potentially serious consequences. This "rebound" effect may be due to compensatory changes in receptor number that have occurred during its use. Therapy should be reduced over a number of days.

Some characteristics of newer nonselective and selective β-adrenergic receptor blocking drugs are summarized in Table 18-1.

FURTHER READING

1. Barger G: Ergot and Ergotism. London, Gurney, 1931
2. Conolly ME, Kerstung F, Dollery CT: The clinical pharmacology of β-adrenoceptor-blocking drugs. Prog Cardiovasc Dis 19:203–234, 1976
3. Epstein SE, Braunwald E: Beta adrenergic receptor blocking drugs. N Engl J Med 275:1106, 1966
4. Frishman W, Silverman R: Clinical pharmacology of the new beta-adrenergic blocking drugs: Part 3. Comparative clinical experience and new therapeutic applications. Am Heart J 98:119–131, 1979
5. Graham RM, Pettinger WA: Prazosin. N Engl J Med 300:232–236, 1979
6. Nickerson M: The pharmacology of adrenergic blockade. Pharmacol Rev 1:27–101, 1949
7. Wolff HG: Headache and Other Head Pains. London, Oxford University Press, 1948

CHAPTER 18 QUESTIONS

(*See* P. 7 for Full Instructions)

Select the One Best Answer

1. Phentolamine (Regitine) will reduce each of the following responses to sympathetic activity EXCEPT
   A. arteriolar constriction.
   B. increased venomotor tone.
   C. muscle glycogenolysis.
   D. one type of sweating.
   E. mydriasis.

2. Phenoxybenzamine (Dibenzyline) causes all of the following effects EXCEPT
   A. a marked drop in blood pressure when administered alone in the presence of hypovolemic shock.
   B. inhibition of tachycardia produced by epinephrine.
   C. inhibition of the bradycardia produced by norepinephrine.
   D. potentiation of the depressor response to epinephrine.
   E. reduction of the pressor response to bilateral carotid occlusion.

3. Which of the following bronchodilators would be expected to be clinically most effective in the presence of propranolol (Inderal)?
   A. Isoproterenol
   B. Aminophylline
   C. Epinephrine
   D. Ephedrine
   E. Terbutaline

A = 1,2,3; B = 1,3; C = 2,4; D = 4; E = All

4. Dihydroergotamine
   1. competitively antagonizes the action of epinephrine on bronchial smooth muscle.
   2. is contraindicated in pregnancy.
   3. is useful in the treatment of peripheral vascular disease.
   4. has an action on blood vessels augmented by caffeine.

5. β-Adrenoceptor blocking drugs should be given very cautiously or not at all when which of the following conditions exists?
   1. Peripheral vascular insufficiency
   2. Increased airway resistance
   3. Depression of atrioventricular conduction rate with partial heart block
   4. Anxiety

6. Propranolol
   1. will reduce the pulmonary edema associated with idiopathic hypertrophic subaortic stenosis.
   2. antagonizes digitalis induced ventricular arrhythmias.
   3. in most patients acutely increases diastolic blood pressure.
   4. reduces catecholamine-induced renin release from the juxtaglomerular apparatus.

7. Reversal of the vasomotor effects of a hypertensive dose of epinephrine by α-adrenoceptor blocking drugs is due to one or more of the following factors:
   1. Drug-induced overaction of homeostatic circulatory reflexes.
   2. Metabolic conversion of epinephrine to a dilator congener by the liver and/or lung.
   3. Unmasking of the venodilator effect of epinephrine by the predominantly arteriolar site of action of the blocking drugs.
   4. Unmasking of concomitant vasodilator effects of the amine.

8. The action of phenoxybenzamine or phentolamine at presynaptic receptors on sympathetic neurones
   1. augments their postsynaptic effect.
   2. can be surmounted by exogenous α-adrenoceptor agonists.
   3. shows that presynaptic and postsynaptic α-adrenoceptors are identical in their chemical structure.
   4. are opposite to those of clonidine.

GENERAL QUESTIONS ON AUTONOMIC DRUGS

The following questions span the knowledge encompassed in several of the chapters in this section and may provide useful review.

Select the One Best Answer

1. Administration of methoxamine, a peripheral sympathomimetic drug with primarily alpha-adrenoceptor agonist properties, causes a reflex change in heart rate. This is antagonized by
   A. methysergide.
   B. neostigmine.
   C. atropine.
   D. cimetidine.
   E. captopril.
2. The increase in arterial pressure after the intravenous injection of tyramine into anesthetized animals would be expected to be smaller if there had been previous administration of each of the following EXCEPT
   A. guanethidine.
   B. desmethylimipramine.
   C. reserpine.
   D. phenoxybenzamine.
   E. pentolinium, a ganglionic blocking agent.
3. When surgical removal of a pheochromocytoma is in progress, which drug regimen from among the following would be most clinically useful in the control of typical signs and symptoms?
   A. Propranolol
   B. Prazosin
   C. Propranolol + prazosin
   D. Neither propranolol nor prazosin
   E. Phentolamine + prazosin
4. Ganglionic blocking drugs (agents that block both parasympathetic and sympathetic ganglia) would be expected to produce all of the following effects EXCEPT
   A. postural hypotension.
   B. blurred vision.
   C. dry mouth.
   D. atrioventricular block.
   E. constipation.
5. Difficulty in focusing on near objects might be expected after the oral administration of
   A. ephedrine.
   B. bethanecol.
   C. scopolamine, an antimuscarinic drug.
   D. propranolol.
   E. guanethidine.
6. A large dose of acetylcholine would be expected to cause an increase in blood pressure after fully effective pretreatment with which of the following agents?
   A. Atropine
   B. Chlorisondamine, a ganglionic blocking agent
   C. Reserpine
   D. Neostigmine
   E. Propranolol
7. The intravenous administration of drug X results in hypotension, increased intestinal motility, miosis, salivation, and bradycardia. The class of drugs to which drug X belongs is
   A. beta-adrenergic stimulants.
   B. ganglionic blocking agents
   C. ganglionic stimulating agents.
   D. muscarinic agents.
   E. antihistaminic agents.
8. Drug X produces vasoconstriction (not blocked by phentolamine) and bradycardia (blocked by atropine or chlorisondamine, a ganglionic blocking drug). Drug X could be
   A. norepinephrine.
   B. angiotension.
   C. dopamine.
   D. phenylephrine.
   E. tyramine.

A = 1,2,3; B = 1,3; C = 2,4; D = 4; E = All

9. The administration of a ganglionic stimulating agent to an animal previously treated with propranolol will cause a decreased heart rate. This response is abolished by
   1. atropine.
   2. section of the vagus nerves.
   3. hexamethonium, a ganglionic blocking drug.
   4. reserpine.
10. In many peripheral synapses, neurotransmitter responses are often terminated predominantly by
    1. destruction of the neurohormone in the synapse between the parasympathetic nerve terminal and effector cells.
    2. diffusion of the neurotransmitter away from the motor end-plate.
    3. neurotransmitter reuptake into the nerve terminal of postganglionic sympathetic neurons.

4. binding of neurotransmitter to "spare" receptors as in the gut.

11. Nicotine in small doses stimulates ganglia and increases heart rate and blood pressure. Which of its following actions could contribute to this effect?
    1. Parasympathetic ganglionic cell stimulation
    2. Stimulation of carotid chemoreceptors
    3. Blockade of sympathetic ganglionic transmission
    4. Liberation of adrenal medullary catecholamine

NICHOLAS N. DURANT,
RONALD L. KATZ

19

Muscle Relaxants: Peripheral and Central

This chapter deals with three types of clinically useful skeletal muscle relaxants: the *neuromuscular blocking agents* (nondepolarizing and depolarizing); *dantrolene sodium,* which acts on the contractile mechanism of skeletal muscle fibers; and the *centrally acting* muscle relaxants. The neuromuscular blocking agents are used primarily during anesthesia whereas the others are used mainly to treat muscle spasticity.

PHYSIOLOGY OF THE NEUROMUSCULAR JUNCTION

Skeletal muscles receive somatic efferent innervation from fast-conducting group A axons, which have their cell bodies in the midbrain or in the anterior horns of the spinal gray matter. These lower motor neurons are divided repeatedly at the nodes of Ranvier as they approach the muscle, the degree of this division depending on the function of the muscle: The larger muscles of the limbs are supplied with neurons having fewer divisions than those muscles whose function is dependent on fine control. There are two types of innervation to skeletal muscle in mammals: *Focal innervation,* the most common, is characterized by each muscle fiber having one point or focus (or at most three in long muscle fibers) of innervation; much less common is *multiple innervation,* in which each muscle fiber is innervated by several nerves. Terminally, in close proximity to the muscle fiber, the axon loses its myelin sheath and forms multiprocessed endings that lie in grooves in the muscle cell membrane to form the *neuromuscular junction* (Fig. 19-1). The surface of the muscle fiber opposite the nerve terminal is a specialized postjunctional membrane known as *the motor end-plate,* this region consists of folds that increase its surface area, and is the site of acetylcholine (ACh) receptors and acetylcholinesterase (AChE). The prejunctional and postjunctional membranes of the neuromuscular junction are about 50 nm apart and form the junctional (synaptic) cleft. Other characteristics of the junctional

Louis Antoine Ranvier, 1835–1922. French histologist. In 1871 discovered the nodes of myelinated nerves that bear his name, but also developed many new histologic methods, including the picrocarmin stain in 1868. Often described as the founder of experimental histology.

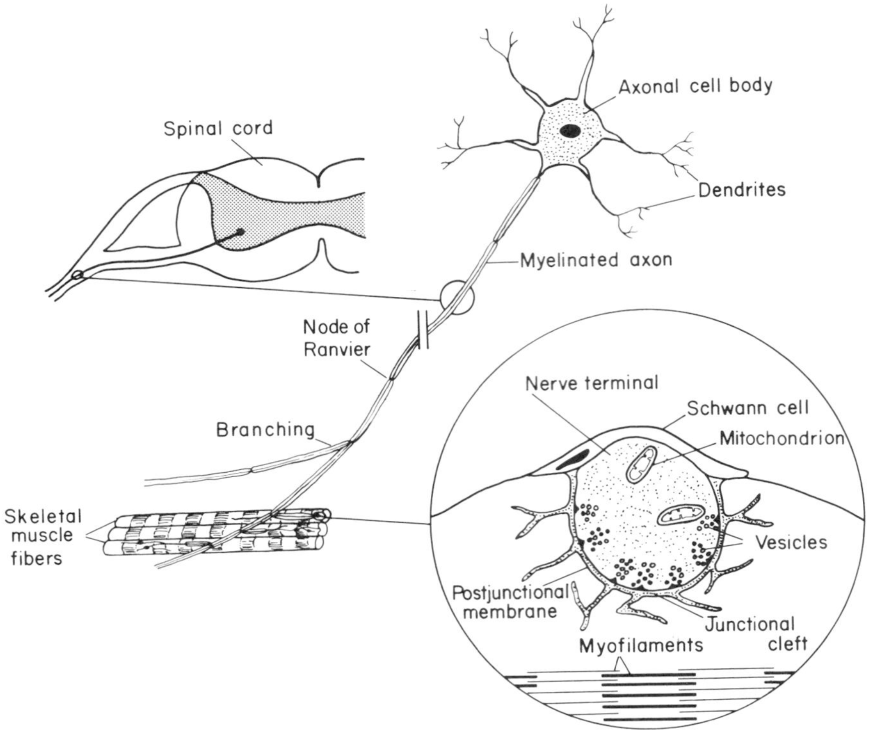

FIG. 19-1. Diagrammatic representation of a motor unit that comprises the lower motor neuron (*left, middle*) and the neuromuscular junction (*right*).

area are the axonal Schwann cells, which enclose the neuromuscular junction, and the nerve terminal, which serves to synthesize, store, and release ACh. ACh is stored in vesicles that congregate opposite the postjunctional membrane. Between the nerve impulse and excitation-contraction (E-C) coupling there are several steps as follows:

Step 1 2 3 4
Nerve impulse → Acetylcholine →

5 6 7
Muscle action potential → E-C coupling,

where step 2 is the release of ACh, step 4 is its interaction with the receptors, and step 6 is the release of calcium from the sarcoplasmic reticulum of the muscle fiber and the calcium influx into the muscle fiber. The peripherally acting muscle relaxants (the neuromuscular blocking agents) block step 4, whereas dantrolene sodium interferes only with step 6. The centrally acting muscle relaxants only decrease the traffic of nerve impulses, and some drugs and ions interfere with step 2 (see below).

THEODOR SCHWANN, 1810–1882. German anatomist and physiologist. Demonstrated the fundamental concept of the cellular structure of animals in 1839, but also discovered pepsin (1835), demonstrated respiration in the chick embryo (1834), and showed bile to be essential to digestion (1844). Also remembered for the Schwann cells of the myelin sheath.

NEUROMUSCULAR TRANSMISSION

Neurohumoral transmission is outlined in Chapter 13, but the distinctive characteristics of ACh transmission at the neuromuscular junction are described below.

ACETYLCHOLINE SYNTHESIS, STORAGE, AND RELEASE

ACh is synthesized in the nerve terminal from choline and acetylcoenzyme A by choline-O-acetyltransferase. Choline is originally synthesized in the liver and partially supplemented by dietary choline and to some extent (about 50%) by reuptake into the nerve terminal (Fig. 19-2). Choline uptake can be weakly inhibited by some drugs (*d*-tubocurarine, decamethonium, physostigmine, neostigmine, atropine, and hexamethonium) whose main action is

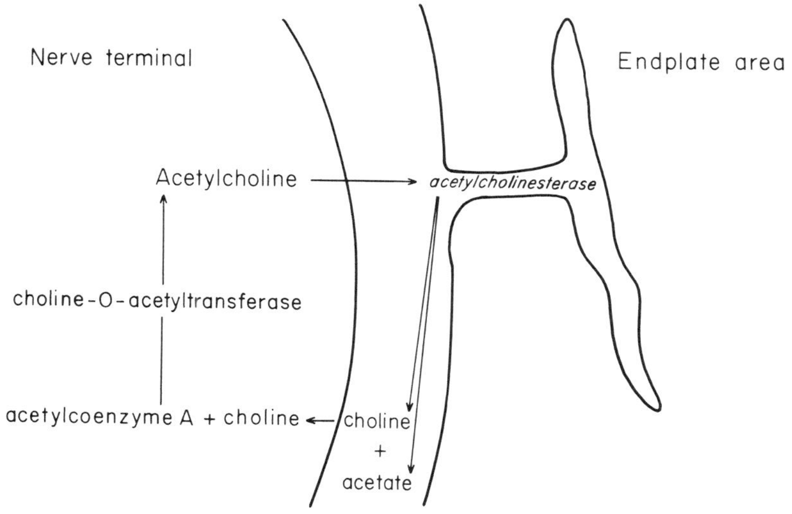

FIG. 19-2. Schematic representation of the synthesis and destruction of acetylcholine at the neuromuscular junction.

elsewhere. Normally this inhibition is unimportant but should be considered if unusual effects occur after prolonged drug administration.

Storage vesicles contain approximately 10,000 to 30,000 molecules of ACh. When triggered by a nerve action potential, about 200 to 350 vesicles simultaneously fuse with the nerve terminal membrane and release their ACh by exocytosis; vesicles can subsequently reform and be reused several times. Calcium ions are vital to exocytosis, whereas magnesium ions are antagonistic and at high concentrations (*i.e.*, plasma concentrations greater than 4 mEq/liter) will cause neuromuscular block. Procaine, aminoglycoside antibiotics (*see* Chap. 60), and botulinum and tetanus toxins may produce an effect similar to that produced by magnesium ions.

INTERACTION OF ACETYLCHOLINE WITH POSTJUNCTIONAL RECEPTORS

The motor end-plate is normally the only region of focally innervated muscle with ACh receptors. ACh-receptor interaction generates an *end-plate potential* (depolarization from the normal resting potential of about −80 mV to a threshold potential of about −60 mV; Fig. 19-3) owing to the rapid influx of sodium ions and an efflux of potassium ions through end-plate ionic channels. Normally the end-plate potential triggers a *muscle action potential* that reaches a level of ±10 mV and is propagated both ways along the muscle fiber.

The two ionic channels involved in the generation of muscle action potentials are selective for sodium and potassium ions, respectively, and are also voltage dependent and, as such, distinct from those channels involved in the generation of the end-plate potential that are not selective for either sodium or potassium ions nor voltage dependent. The muscle action potential initiates excitation-contraction coupling, which results in muscle contraction. The entire process from arrival of the nerve impulse to genesis of the muscle action potential takes

FIG. 19-3. A drawing taken from an oscilloscope tracing of the voltage changes recorded at the neuromuscular junction during a muscle action potential. The point at which the end-plate potential triggers the action potential is indicated by an arrow.

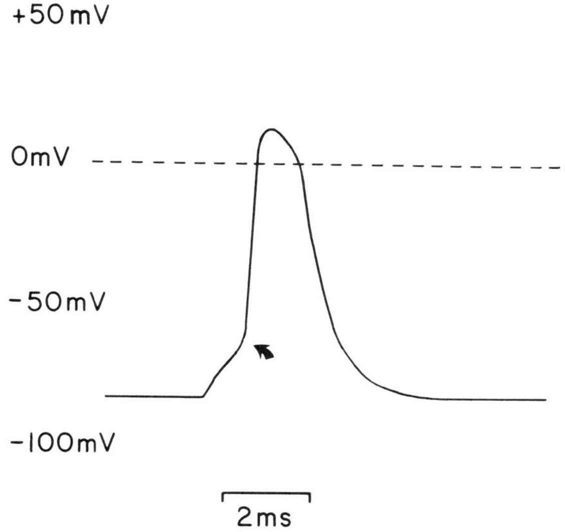

about 2 to 3 msec, and when repeated many times per second produces a sustained muscle contracture; for example, inspiration involves bursts of nerve impulses at a frequency of about 30 Hz (Hertz).

TERMINATION OF THE ACTION OF ACETYLCHOLINE

After depolarizing the end-plate, ACh is promptly degraded to choline and acetate by AChE located in the postjunctional folds (Fig. 19-2).

NONDEPOLARIZING NEUROMUSCULAR BLOCKING AGENTS

HISTORY

d-Tubocurarine was long recognized by South American Indians as an extremely useful arrow poison but remained unknown to Europeans until 1516, when the first account of the poison appeared in a Latin book called *De Orbo Nova* (The New World), written by Pieter Matyr d'Anglera. Much mystery and confusion surrounded the arrow poisons for the next 300 years, mainly because alkaloids such as strychnine were also present. The main source of *d*-tubocurarine was then and is now the bark of the creepers *Chondodendron tomentosum Ruiz* and *Pavon* native to the forest of South America and in particular Peru. The disappearance of the creepers has in recent years led to shortages of *d*-tubocurarine.

Brodie established that death due to *d*-tubocurarine could be prevented by artificial respiration, and in 1856 Claude Bernard found that *d*-tubocurarine administration resulted in paralysis of all muscles of a pithed frog except those deprived of arterial circulation. Furthermore Bernard found that although the paralyzed muscles did not respond to nerve stimulation, they did respond to direct electrical stimulation. Bernard concluded that *d*-tubocurarine acted independently of the central nervous system, not affecting nerves or muscles directly but blocking neuromuscular transmission.

The first commercial preparation of *d*-tubocurarine (Intocostrin, Squibb Laboratories) was hailed as "a milestone in anesthesia" when introduced clinically in 1942.

The nondepolarizing muscle relaxants have greatly increased the safety of anesthesia (since far less anesthetic is required to achieve muscle relaxation) and have facilitated and made possible new surgical and clinical techniques. The four main agents are indicated in Fig. 19-4.

MODE OF ACTION

These drugs have a common mode of action in that they prevent the interaction of ACh with its postjunctional receptor such that the end-plate potential is reduced in amplitude or even abolished. Thus, the trigger threshold for the muscle action potential is not reached; these drugs also may have presynaptic effects that contribute to the block. All the nondepolarizing agents have at least one quaternary nitrogen in their molecular structure (Fig. 19-4), which is responsible for receptor-binding and the lack of lipid solubility preventing access to the brain (*see* Chap. 3).

DURATION OF ACTION

The duration of action of the nondepolarizing neuromuscular blocking agents is determined primarily by three factors: first, the association and dissociation of the drug with its receptor, second, the redistribution of the drug to nonactive sites, and third, the rate of elimination via the liver and kidneys.

The effects of low doses of all these agents can be reversed by anticholinesterase agents such as neostigmine or pyridostigmine (*see* Chap. 15), which indirectly cause an increase in drug-receptor complex dissociation; the anticholinesterases also may act presynaptically to increase transmitter release. The redistribution of a drug to nonactive sites together with cumulation is responsible for less intense neuromuscular block and duration of

---

HEINRICH RUDOLF HERTZ, 1857–1894. German physicist. Worked on electrical discharge in gases and the electromagnetic theory of light. Around 1886 observed electromagnetic (Hertzian) waves for the first time and showed that radio waves had similar physical properties to those of light.

De Orbo Nova was translated into English in 1555 and contains stories, many of which are fanciful, relating to the explorers who visited the New World not long after Columbus.

BENJAMIN BRODIE, an Englishman, used samples of curare obtained by the explorer Charles Waterton to show that it caused death by respiratory paralysis. He reported his findings to the Royal Society in 1811 and 1812.

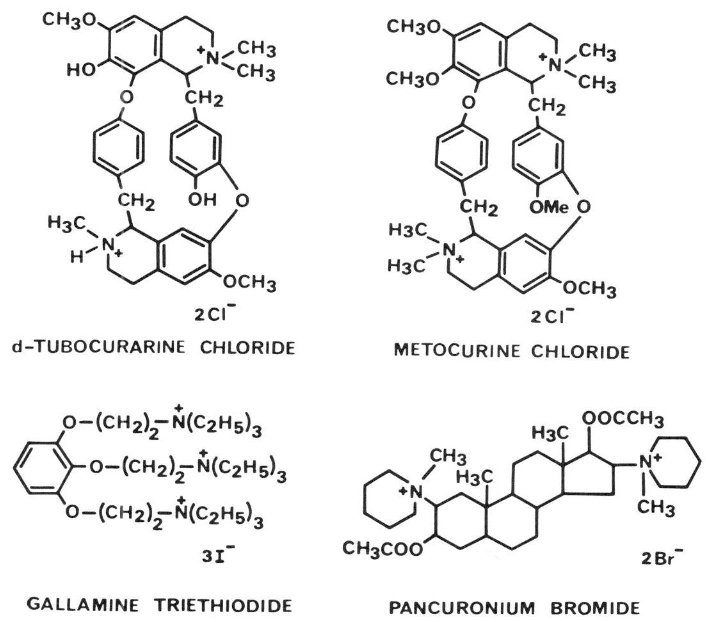

FIG. 19-4. Chemical structures of the four most commonly used nondepolarizing muscle relaxants.

effect of the first administration compared with subsequent administrations. *d*-Tubocurarine is excreted primarily via the biliary route, while pancuronium is primarily dependent on renal elimination. In cases of renal or biliary insufficiency, the duration of action of these agents may be prolonged. Thus, in the selection of muscle relaxants, the route of elimination should be considered.

ADVERSE EFFECTS

Blockade of Cardiac Vagus Neuroeffector Transmission

Since neuromuscular blocking agents inhibit the action of ACh at the neuromuscular junction, it is not surprising that some of them block other cholinergic synapses. Gallamine and pancuronium block the cardiac vagus neuroeffector junction, producing a cardioselective atropine-like action (Table 19-1). Several novel nondepolarizing muscle relaxants (*e.g.*, vecuronium, atracurium) lacking this and other undesirable side effects are under current investigation with a view to entering clinical use in the next few years.

Autonomic Ganglion Block

Occurring primarily with *d*-tubocurarine, ganglion block contributes to the hypotension and tachycardia often observed in patients and results from nonselective interaction with cholinergic nicotinic receptors.

Histamine Release

Histamine release is important with *d*-tubocurarine and is partly responsible (together with ganglion blockade) for the hypotensive response that this agent produces at neuromuscular blocking doses.

DOSAGE

d-Tubocurarine, for many years the most widely used agent, now has been superseded by pancuronium. The dosage and side effects of these drugs are given in Table 19-1.

Clinically, an initial test dose is given, followed by supplemental doses as required (*see* Table 19-1). The dose-response curves for pancuronium and *d*-tubocurarine are not parallel, with pancuronium being five times more potent at the lower end and seven times more potent at the upper end of the dose-response curve. Pancuronium is also shorter acting than *d*-tubocurarine and lacks most of its side-effects.

MONITORING OF NEUROMUSCULAR TRANSMISSION

The most satisfactory method of monitoring the dose of muscle relaxants is to use a peripheral nerve stimulator and either observe or record the twitch response of the thumb adductor pollicis muscle. A peripheral nerve stimulator supplies a stimulus, the variables of which

TABLE 19-1. Summary of Dose, Time-Course, and Side-Effects of More Commonly Used Nondepolarizing Muscle Relaxants*

Drug	Test Dose	Intubation Dose	Duration of Action	Initial Dose After Intubation	Supplemental Dose	Comments
	mg/kg		*min*	*mg/kg*		
d-Tubocurarine	0.1	0.6–0.7	25–90	0.1–0.2	0.05–0.1	Histamine release, ganglion blockade
Metocurine	0.05	0.3–0.4	25–90	0.05–0.1	0.025–0.05	Histamine release, ganglion blockade (but not as marked as with *d*-tubocurarine)
Pancuronium	0.02	0.05–0.1	30–60	0.02–0.04	0.01–0.02	Tachycardia (less than with gallamine)
Gallamine	0.7	3.0–4.0	25–90	0.7–1.5	0.35–0.7	Tachycardia, hypertension

* The intubation dose includes the test dose in the total; the initial dose is used when intubation is carried out with the aid of succinylcholine but the relaxation has worn off. The supplemental dose is used when either the intubation or the initial dose of the same relaxant has worn off. Metocurine is the trimethylated derivative of *d*-tubocurarine and is otherwise known as d-0,0,*N*-trimethyltubocurarine, or commonly misnamed as dimethyltubocurarine.

(pulse width, voltage, and frequency) can be controlled. A square wave of 0.1 msec duration, 0.1 Hz frequency, and supramaximal voltage is usually used and applied to the ulnar nerve via two-surface or subcutaneous electrodes. As the neuromuscular blockade becomes more intense, the elicited twitch tension decreases.

DEPOLARIZING NEUROMUSCULAR BLOCKING AGENTS

HISTORY

The depolarizing neuromuscular blocking agents were introduced as synthetic alternatives to *d*-tubocurarine. *Decamethonium* is one of a series of methonium drugs that were found to be most active when 10 carbon atoms separated the quaternary nitrogen groups (n = 10 in Fig. 19-5). Succinylcholine (suxamethonium), the equivalent of two acetylcholine molecules joined back to back (Fig. 19-5), was soon recognized to have an extremely rapid onset and a short duration of action and thus gained clinical acceptance for use when rapid endotracheal intubation was required. Today succinylcholine is still the shortest-acting muscle relaxant and is in widespread use, whereas decamethonium is virtually obsolete.

MODE OF ACTION

Succinylcholine is bisquaternary and resembles ACh in molecular structure, mimicking its action at the motor end-plate. Succinylcholine initially depolarizes the end-plate (phase I block) such that further depolarization by endogenous ACh is impossible. Pseudocholinesterase (plasma cholinesterase) hydrolyzes succinylcholine to choline and succinylmono-

FIG. 19-5. Chemical structures of the methonium series and succinylcholine chloride.

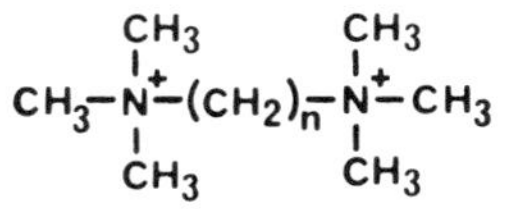

THE METHONIUM SERIES

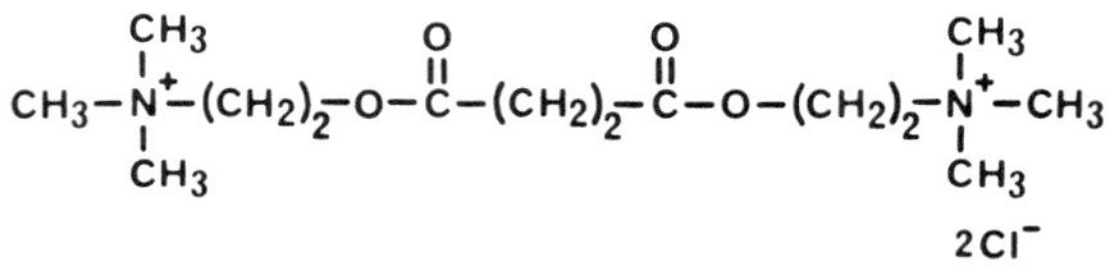

SUCCINYLCHOLINE CHLORIDE

choline, which is then further hydrolyzed (at about one seventh the rate) to choline and succinic acid. The first hydrolysis by pseudocholinesterase confers a duration of action on succinylcholine that is far shorter than that of *d*-tubocurarine; however, the depolarization that succinylcholine produces at the endplate is far longer than that produced by ACh released from the nerve terminal.

Phase I block can progress with increasing dosage and time to the development of phase II block with characteristics of block similar to that produced by the nondepolarizing neuromuscular blockers.

Phase I blockade is characterized by muscle fasciculations at the onset, absence of fade of tetanic tension in response to an indirect stimulus at a frequency of 50 Hz, and little or no post-tetanic twitch facilitation. In contrast, phase II blockade is characterized by tetanic fade and post-tetanic facilitation and often occurs during prolonged or repeated administrations of succinylcholine; the mechanisms involved in phase II block are still a matter of controversy.

DURATION OF ACTION

Succinylcholine is destroyed by plasma cholinesterase (pseudocholinesterase) with a half-life of about 1 to 3 minutes, and genetic variants with coding are known that result in atypical enzyme levels (*see* Chap. 6). Approximately one person in 2800 has abnormal genes for pseudocholinesterase and thus metabolizes the drug very slowly. In homozygotes (with two genes for atypical pseudocholinesterase) the effective dose of succinylcholine for endotracheal intubation may be as low as 0.05 mg/kg of body weight, while in normal persons 1.0 mg/kg is commonly used. Approximately 4% of patients are heterozygous (with one normal and one abnormal gene), some responding normally but others having a prolonged response to succinylcholine. If a peripheral nerve stimulator is used to monitor the effects of succinylcholine, patients with one or even two abnormal genes present no problem. Family members should be informed and if possible tested to see if they have inherited this abnormality.

ADVERSE EFFECTS

Succinylcholine has more side-effects than the nondepolarizing neuromuscular blocking agents, but its main advantage of brevity of action often outweighs its disadvantages. *Muscle fasciculation* at the onset of neuromuscular block, characterized by intense contraction of neck muscles, grimacing, clenching of the fist, and waves of transiently increased muscle tone are common. *Muscle aches* and *pain* usually occurring the first day or so after surgery may also follow administration of the drug. Although the fasciculations and muscle pain are suspected to be related, this has been never clearly proved. Diazepam (0.05 mg/kg intravenously) decreases muscle pain and fasciculations and appears to have an advantage over pretreatment with a small dose of nondepolarizing agent.

Hyperkalemia may occur. In normal patients the potassium level may increase from 3.5 mEq/liter before to 4 mEq/liter after administration of succinylcholine, but in patients with burns, upper or lower motor neuron disease, and other conditions, a rise from 3.5 to 13.5 mEq/liter may occur and can cause severe cardiac arrhythmias or arrest.

A rise in *intraocular pressure* may develop owing to contraction of the extraocular muscles, which, unlike most other muscles in mammals, are multiply innervated (*see* above) and respond to succinylcholine by contracture rather than by depolarization. Thus if the eye is injured the increase in intraocular pressure may extrude vitreous humor and result in permanent loss of vision.

Tachycardia or *bradycardia* may develop when succinylcholine is given to an adult. Bradycardia also may be seen with the first dose in a child and on the second dose in an adult if the two doses are given 5 to 15 minutes apart. Other complications that may be encountered with succinylcholine include *raised intragastric pressure, malignant hyperthermia, myotonia, and myoglobinuria.* Despite these side-effects and complications, however, succinylcholine is in widespread use because of its short duration of action. A short-acting nondepolarizing neuromuscular blocking agent without the side effects of succinylcholine is needed, and in some cases the new nondepolarizing agents vecuronium or atracurium may be appropriate.

CLINICAL PHARMACOLOGY OF NEUROMUSCULAR BLOCKING AGENTS

Use of the peripherally acting muscle relaxants is confined almost entirely to the operating room for facilitating intubation and providing general muscle relaxation during surgery. These drugs also are used occasionally to prevent tetanic muscle contraction during electroconvulsive therapy, and in patients with tetanus or in intensive care units. When they are used, facilities for ventilatory assistance must be available.

CHOICE OF A MUSCLE RELAXANT

For endotracheal intubation, the most common choice is a single i.v. dose of succinylcholine. For maintained muscle relaxation during surgery, an infusion of succinylcholine can be used, but a continuous infusion should be limited to 60 minutes since recovery may be prolonged with longer use. More commonly used is the technique of intubation with the aid of succinylcholine followed by change to a nondepolarizing agent such as pancuronium or *d*-tubocurarine (*see* Table 19-1). The proper doses of muscle relaxants can be determined easily by the use of a peripheral nerve stimulator. A common practice is to use repeated small doses of muscle relaxant as long as relaxation is required.

FACTORS AFFECTING SENSITIVITY TO THE NEUROMUSCULAR BLOCKING AGENTS

Inhalation anesthetics (halothane, methoxyflurane, isoflurane, diethyl ether, cyclopropane, and enflurane) all increase a patient's sensitivity to neuromuscular blocking agents, but nitrous oxide/narcotic anesthesia does not produce such noticeable potentiation.

Other factors that may be associated with an altered sensitivity to *d*-tubocurarine and pancuronium are acidosis; a decrease in body temperature; concomitant medication with aminoglycoside antibiotics, local anesthetics, and lithium carbonate; and hypokalemia. Renal and hepatic insufficiency should be expected to prolong the effect of muscle relaxants, especially with repeated administrations. Patients with myasthenia gravis or the Eaton–Lambert syndrome are exquisitely sensitive to nondepolarizing neuromuscular blocking agents. The potential problems of altered sensitivity can be minimized by using a small test dose and assessing the degree of block with the aid of a nerve stimulator.

REVERSAL OF NEUROMUSCULAR BLOCKADE

The anticholinesterases (*see* Chap. 15) are the only clinically available antagonists of nondepolarizing neuromuscular block, and they usually will restore adequate muscle power within 10 minutes or less provided a twitch response to nerve stimulation can be seen before the anticholinesterase is administered. The anticholinesterases have also been used successfully to counteract the desensitization (phase II or dual) block produced with succinylcholine, but this should be done only by an expert and with great caution since any remaining phase I block will be potentiated.

SAFETY DURING USE OF NEUROMUSCULAR BLOCKING AGENTS

Neuromuscular blocking agents can be used safely and effectively if the following points are appreciated: *Ventilatory assistance* should always be immediately available; the *first dose should be the minimum dose required;* and the effect of each dose should be *adequately monitored,* preferably with the aid of a peripheral nerve stimulator.

DANTROLENE SODIUM: A DIRECTLY ACTING MUSCLE RELAXANT

The only clinically available muscle relaxant that acts directly on the contractile mechanism of skeletal muscle is Dantrolene sodium (Fig. 19-6). This agent blocks excitation-contraction coupling by preventing calcium release from the sarcoplasmic reticulum and also by preventing calcium influx. It has not been shown to have any clinically significant effect on neuromuscular transmission. Dantrolene sodium

FIG. 19-6. Chemical structure of the directly acting muscle relaxant dantrolene sodium.

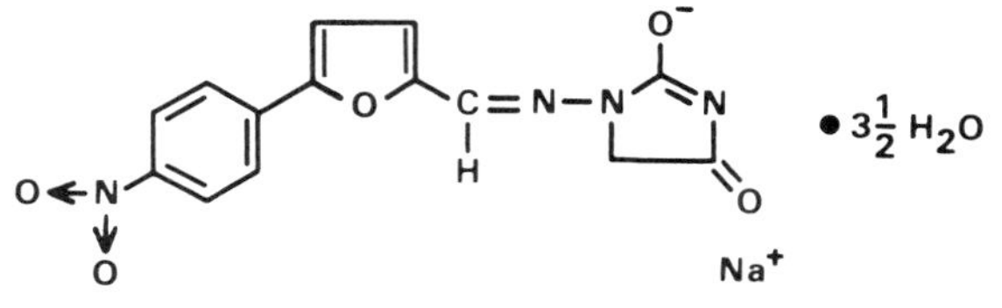

DANTROLENE SODIUM

is not used as an adjunct to anesthesia because of its slow onset of action, long duration of blockade, and lack of a suitable antagonist; however, it has the advantages of being active orally, being unable to totally block skeletal muscle activity, and having little effect on sustained tetanic muscle contractions such as breathing.

INDICATIONS

Dantrolene sodium is indicated for chronic disorders characterized by skeletal muscle spasticity, such as spinal cord injury, stroke, cerebral palsy, and multiple sclerosis: given i.v. it is indicated in the treatment of malignant hyperthermia (*see* Chap. 6). Malignant hyperthermia can be triggered by halothane (or other potent halogenated anesthetics) and/or succinylcholine, and may be seen during anesthesia and surgery or postoperatively after all anesthetic agents have been discontinued. One feature of malignant hyperthermia is a sudden rise of the calcium ion concentration within muscle fibers; this can be beneficially antagonized by dantrolene sodium. The agent may be effective prophylactically in patients at risk of developing malignant hyperthermia. Of course, all triggering agents such as halothane and succinylcholine should be avoided in susceptible patients.

METABOLISM AND EXCRETION

Dantrolene sodium has a half-life of between 7 and 9 hours and is metabolized predominantly by the liver and excreted in the urine; only 1% to 4% of the orally administered dose remains unchanged in the urine. The principal metabolite, 5-hydroxydantrolene sodium, is considerably less active as a muscle relaxant than dantrolene sodium itself.

ADVERSE REACTIONS

Commonly reported side effects, particularly at the start of therapy, are transient drowsiness, general malaise, and diarrhea. The drug is also known to impair hepatic function in about 0.1% to 1% of patients; this should be monitored during long-term treatment. Less commonly, dantrolene sodium causes dermatoses, enuresis, visual disturbances, dizziness, and hallucinations. Nondepolarizing muscle relaxants have an additive action with dantrolene sodium, and therefore the dose of such agents used in patients already receiving dantrolene sodium should be reduced accordingly.

DOSAGE

The usual oral dose of dantrolene sodium for control of muscle spasticity is 12 to 25 mg once daily, increased at 4- to 7-day intervals to the minimum dosage that produces the maximum benefit (up to a maximum total dose of 100 mg every 6 hours). When used for prophylaxis of malignant hyperthermia the drug should be given in doses of 4 to 5 mg/kg of body weight, for 1 to 3 days; for acute treatment an initial dose of 1 mg/kg intravenously is recommended. Usually control can be achieved with 3 to 4 mg/kg, with 10 to 15 mg/kg considered the upper limit. The doses described for the treatment of hyperthermia are tentative since this application of the drug is fairly new.

CENTRALLY ACTING MUSCLE RELAXANTS

HISTORY

Centrally induced muscle relaxation without loss of conciousness was first shown in 1910 in animals using phenoxypropanediol (autodyne). In 1946 a phenoxypropanediol-related compound, *mephenesin*, also was found to produce muscle relaxation. Mephenesin, although no longer widely used, is regarded as the prototype of the centrally acting muscle relaxants since it produces muscle relaxation by means of a central action with minimal sedation. The structures of some of the centrally acting muscle relaxants are shown in Fig. 19-7.

MODE OF ACTION

The precise mode of action of these agents is not known, although some reflexes involving interneurons are suppressed, especially in the brain stem, thalamus, and basal ganglia. The centrally acting muscle relaxants have no significant effect on the neuromuscular junction or on neuronal conduction. The classification is

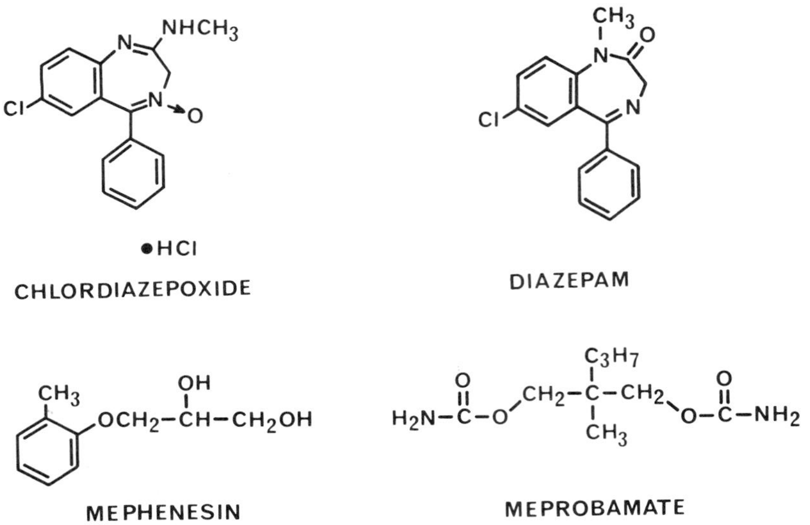

FIG. 19-7. Chemical structures of some of the centrally acting muscle relaxants.

somewhat confusing, however, since some of these agents, such as diazepam, are also central depressants while some, such as mephenesin, do not possess this property.

Centrally acting muscle relaxants are never used to produce muscle relaxation for surgery but may be used for premedication or as an adjunct for the induction of anesthesia. Diazepam and lorazepam are two commonly used premedicants in the United States. For muscle relaxation and amnesia, diazepam has been determined to be more effective intravenously than either intramuscularly or orally; however, the reason for this has not been clearly determined.

Baclofen, an analogue of the central transmitter gamma-aminobutyric acid (GABA), may inhibit monosynaptic and polysynaptic spinal reflexes, although its precise mechanism of action is not fully understood.

INDICATIONS

Centrally acting muscle relaxants are used to treat muscle tension and pains associated with stress and anxiety and muscle spasms due to inflammation and trauma. Diazepam is also of value in the treatment of tetanus, and baclofen is used for treating spasticity due to spinal cord injury and multiple sclerosis.

ADVERSE EFFECTS

Large doses of drugs of this group are likely to result in prolonged flaccid paralysis with attendant respiratory depression. These agents (other than mephenesin) commonly cause drowsiness and sedation. General weakness, blurred vision, dizziness, and headache with gastrointestinal upsets occur commonly with oral therapy.

DOSAGE

Diazepam has been used clinically in individual doses of up to 10 mg intravenously for the treatment of tetanus, although very much larger cumulative doses have been used for this purpose. Chlordiazepoxide usually is used in the dose range of 50 to 100 mg intravenously or intramuscularly. Baclofen is administered orally, starting with a low dose (15 mg/kg) and building up by 0.6 to 1.0 mg/kg per day. Mephenesin is given orally at a dose of about 1.2 g/day and meprobamate also orally at a dose of 1.2 to 1.6 g/day.

FURTHER READING

1. Bowman WC: Pharmacology of Neuromuscular Function. Bristol, Wright, 1980
2. Cheymol J (ed): Neuromuscular Blocking and Stimulating Agents, Oxford, Pergamon Press, 1972
3. Cookson JC, Paton WDM: Mechanisms of neuromuscular block. Anesthesia 24:395, 1969
4. Durant NN, Bowman WC, Marshall IG: A comparison of the neuromuscular and autonomic blocking activities of (+)-tubocurarine and its N-methyl and O,O,N-trimethyl analogues. Eur J Pharmacol 46:297, 1977
5. Durant NN, Katz RL: Suxamethonium. Br J Anaes 54:195, 1982

6. Foldes FF (ed): Muscle relaxants. Philadelphia, FA Davis, 1966
7. Greenblatt DJ, Shader RI: Benzodiazepines in clinical practice. New York, Raven, 1975
8. Katz RL (ed): Muscle Relaxants, Volume 3. Monographs in Anesthesiology, Amsterdam, North-Holland, 1975
9. Pinder RM, Brogden RN, Speight TM, Avery GS: Dantrolene sodium: A review of its pharmacological properties and therapeutic efficacy is spasticity. Drugs 13:3, 1977

CHAPTER 19 QUESTIONS

(See P. 7 for Further Instructions)

Select the One Best Answer

1. Both *d*-tubocurarine and succinylcholine (Anectine)
   - A. produce hyperkalemia.
   - B. are used as diagnostic agents in myasthenia gravis.
   - C. stimulate the spinal cord.
   - D. are inactivated by pseudocholinesterase.
   - E. depress respiration.

2. Muscle fasciculation might be expected after the intravenous injection of each of the following drugs or drug combinations EXCEPT
   - A. succinylcholine.
   - B. nicotine.
   - C. atropine followed by neostigmine
   - D. atropine followed by hexamethonium.
   - E. neostigmine alone.

3. Muscle relaxation by diazepam (Valium) is attributed to
   - A. decreased acetylcholine synthesis.
   - B. increased metabolism of acetylcholine.
   - C. depressed polyneuronal reflexes.
   - D. decreased acetylcholine release by the nerve action potential.
   - E. blockade of acetylcholine receptors at the neuromuscular junction.

4. The early phase of succinylcholine-induced neuromuscular blockade is not antagonized by neostigmine because
   - A. neostigmine acts only at cholinergic autonomic nerve endings.
   - B. succinylcholine is not hydrolyzed by plasma pseudocholinesterase.
   - C. an excess of acetylcholine produces the same effect on the motor endplate as does succinylcholine.
   - D. both act on the same receptors and succinylcholine has a greater affinity for the receptor.
   - E. neostigmine is rapidly hydrolyzed by cholinesterases.

5. Both pancuronium and tubocurarine
   - A. release histamine.
   - B. relax skeletal muscles at a dose of 0.02 mg/kg.
   - C. exert a cardioselective atropine-like action.
   - D. block ganglia at neuromuscular blocking doses.
   - E. have a longer duration of action than succinylcholine.

A = 1,2,3; B = 1,3; C = 2,4; D = 4; E = All

6. Tubocurarine
   1. may produce a fall in blood pressure that would be reduced by diphenhydramine.
   2. will reduce the effects of hexamethonium on ganglia.
   3. will antagonize the stimulating effect of neostigmine on skeletal muscle.
   4. will produce analgesia.

7. Succinylcholine
   1. may produce muscle fasciculations during administration.
   2. -induced paralysis is accentuated by neostigmine.
   3. may acutely elevate plasma K^+.
   4. is hydrolyzed by plasma cholinesterase.

8. Succinylcholine chloride
   1. is useful for preventing harmful muscle contractions in electroconvulsive shock.
   2. may increase intraocular pressure.
   3. bradycardia is prevented by atropine.
   4. produces flaccid paralysis

9. Patients with myasthenia gravis have an increased sensitivity to the paralyzing effects of
   1. gentamycin.
   2. *d*-tubocurarine.
   3. pancuronium.
   4. succinylcholine.

10. Dantrolene sodium is indicated for
    1. relaxation of muscle before surgery.
    2. treatment of muscle spasticity associated with multiple sclerosis.
    3. decreasing skeletal muscle activity during electroconvulsive therapy.
    4. acute treatment of malignant hyperthermia.

20

PETER LOMAX

Local Anesthetics

Local anesthetics are drugs that block conduction in nerve tissue when applied in appropriate concentrations. Many compounds have this property but often cause permanent neural damage or else are too toxic following systemic absorption from their site of application. With clinically useful local anesthetics, the blocking effect is completely reversible, no functional damage to the nerve occurs, and serious systemic effects are rare.

A good local anesthetic should be nonirritating to the tissues, cause no permanent damage, have a low systemic toxicity, be effective both topically and when injected, have a short latent period before onset and an adequate duration of action, be soluble in water and stable in solution, and be sterilizable without deterioration.

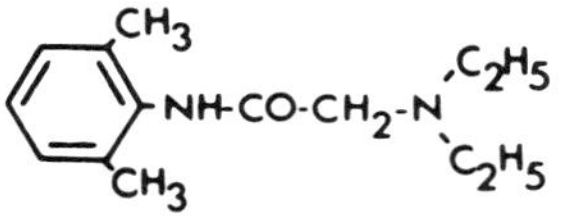

LIDOCAINE

The naturally occurring alkaloid cocaine was the first local anesthetic used clinically. A chemical search for substitutes led to the discovery of procaine in 1905. Subsequently an extremely large number of local anesthetics

---

ALBERT NIEMANN, German scientist. In 1860 published an account of the pure alkaloid he had extracted from coca leaves and named it "cocaine."

SIGMUND FREUD, 1856–1939. Austrian psychoanalyst. Best remembered for his revolutionary psychoanalytic techniques and psychological theory. Worked with cocaine in 1884 and suggested that it might be useful as a stimulant and in the cure of morphine addiction. Used it himself for 3 years.

CARL KOLLER, 1857–1944. Czechoslovakian-born American ophthalmologist. In 1884 introduced the use of cocaine as a local anesthetic for ocular surgery. At that time he was working in Vienna and was introduced to cocaine by Sigmund Freud.

KARL GUSTAV AUGUST BIER, 1861–1949. German surgeon. In 1899 introduced the use of cocaine as a spinal anesthetic. Also was the first to use artificial hyperemia in surgery in 1892. In 1904 he used it for acute infections.

WILLIAM STEWART HALSTED, 1852–1922. American surgeon. One of the first to use cocaine as a nerve blocking agent, he became addicted to it after using himself as an experimental subject in 1885. Halsted is remembered as a great, innovative surgeon and the first leading surgeon to use rubber gloves in the operating theater, in 1890.

ALFRED EINHORN, 1857–1917. German chemist. Published the synthesis of novocaine (procaine) in 1899.

has been synthesized. The local anesthetics in common use are described in Table 20-1.

CHEMISTRY

The useful local anesthetics are structurally similar and comprise a lipophilic aromatic group, an intermediate chain, and a hydrophilic amine group. The general formula is shown in Figure 20-1 with that of procaine. The amino group is always either a tertiary or a secondary amine. The link between the aromatic and the intermediate group is either an ester link —CO—OCH_2, as in procaine, or an amide link —NH—$COCH_2$, as in lidocaine (*see* Table 20-1).

Changes in any part of the molecule may alter the potency or toxicity of the drug. Increasing the length of the intermediate chain leads to greater potency and toxicity. A compound with an ethyl ester link, such as procaine, is usually the least toxic. The toxicity and potency of synthetic local anesthetics are always compared with procaine as the standard.

All local anesthetics are bases with a pK_a in the 7 to 9 range and are only sparingly soluble in water. These compounds form salts with strong acids and most often are supplied for clinical use as the hydrochlorides. The salts are freely soluble in water and give rise to solutions with a *p*H of 6 or less. When these salts are injected into the tissues (*p*H 7.4), the buffering effect of the tissue fluids leads to the release of free base (Fig. 20-2).

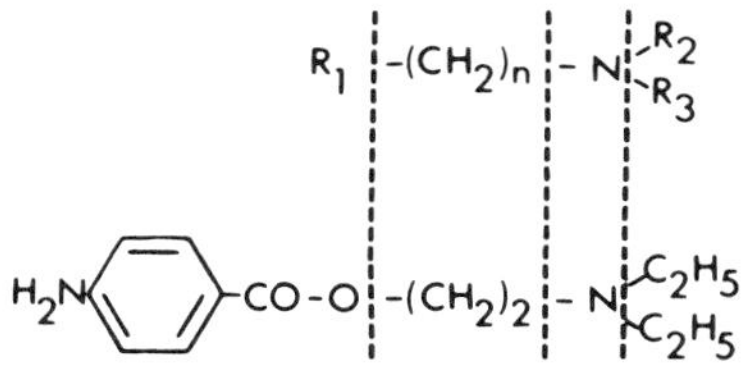

PROCAINE

FIG. 20-1. General structural formula of local anesthetics and procaine.

The products of infection in inflamed tissues tend to lower the *p*H, and if a local anesthetic is injected into such sites less base is liberated and consequently less effective anesthesia results.

MECHANISM OF ACTION

The sequence of changes in the nerve fiber after local application of an anesthetic agent can be followed by electrophysiological methods. Changes consist of an increase in the threshold for electric stimulation, slowing of

TABLE 20-1. Common Local Anesthetics

Drug	Trade Name	Concentration	Latency	Duration	Comment (Type)
		%	*min*	*hr*	
Dibucaine hydrochloride	Nupercaine	0.1	10	3	Fifteen times potency and toxicity of procaine (amide)
Lidocaine hydrochloride	Xylocaine	0.5–2.0	1	4–5	About equal toxicity to procaine. Best surface anesthetic. Effective without epinephrine in patients sensitive to epinephrine. So dissimilar to procaine that it can be used in patients sensitive to former. Causes sleepiness (amide)
Mepivacaine hydrochloride	Carbocaine	1–2			Similar to lidocaine with slightly faster onset and longer-duration (amide)
Procaine hydrochloride	Novocaine	1–2	2–5	1	(ester)
Tetracaine hydrochloride	Amethocaine, Pontocaine	0.25	5–10	2	Ten times potency and toxicity of procaine. Good surface anesthetic (ester)
Prilocaine hydrochloride	Citanast	4.0	2–5	5+	May cause cyanosis in large doses. 50% toxicity of lidocaine (amide)

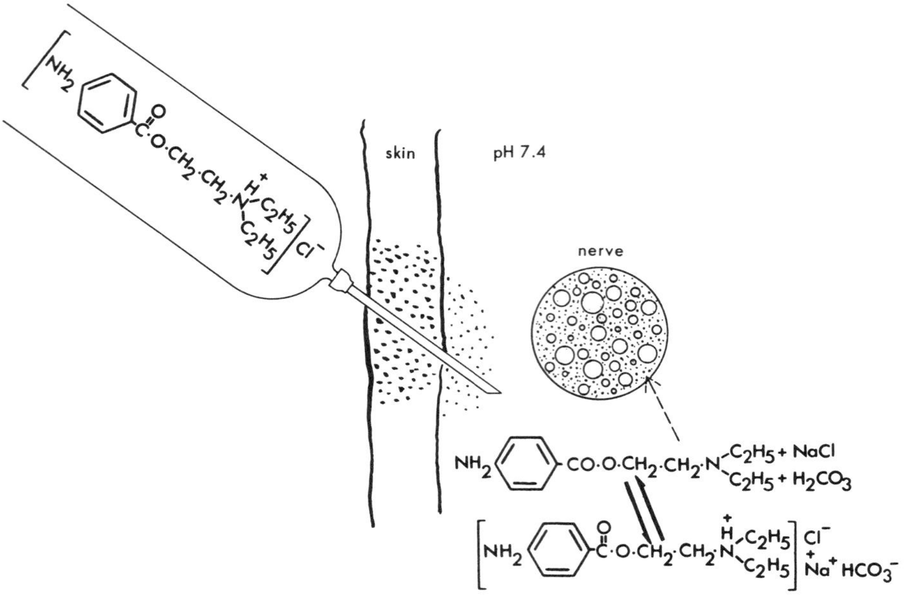

FIG. 20-2. Procaine injected subcutaneously as the chloride salt is buffered by the extracellular fluid and free procaine base is liberated and enters the nerves.

the rate of propagation of the impulse, reduction in the rate of rise of the action potential, and eventual complete block of conduction.

The fundamental process in nerve conduction is the large transient rise in sodium permeability of the neural membrane, which is triggered by a slight depolarization of the membrane. The changes enumerated above can be explained as the result of increasing blockade of this process. The end-effect of these changes is that the nerve membrane becomes stabilized and cannot be depolarized by the potentials reaching the blocked region. Thus conduction is blocked.

The local anesthetic must enter the nerve fiber to reach its site of action. The anesthetic crosses the nerve membrane in the uncharged form. Inside the fiber a large proportion returns to the charged form, and it may be this cationic state of the drug that is responsible for its action. Differences in *p*H on each side of the neural membrane may lead to a higher concentration of local anesthetic inside than outside the fiber (*see* Chap. 3). The intimate processes involved in the transient depolarization of the membrane are still poorly understood.

Local anesthetics interfere with the fundamental process that causes the voltage-dependent rise in membrane conductance. There are several sites in the neural membrane where sodium permeability may be affected by different classes of drugs, including

1. at the external opening of the sodium channel (site of action of tetrodotoxin);
2. at receptors at the inner opening of the sodium channel (some quaternary compounds perfused into the axoplasm block at this site);
3. Nonspecific hydrophobic regions along the channel that block sodium movement (alcohols and barbiturates attach to such regions).

Local anesthetics act by interfering with sodium conduction by a combination of effects at sites 2 and 3. Calcium binding to phospholipids is inhibited by local anesthetics, and calcium is displaced. The drugs may compete with calcium for a phospholipid receptor, and calcium displacement may be necessary for local anesthesia. However, inhibition of calcium binding is not thought to be involved in the mechanism of nerve blockade.

PHARMACOLOGIC ACTIONS AND THERAPEUTIC APPLICATIONS

Whatever the mechanism of action of local anesthetics, a critical concentration must be built up inside the nerve fiber to block conduction. To achieve this, the concentration around the nerve must be many times the level that would be toxic systemically. Thus local application is necessary.

One of the major factors governing the time taken to reach this particular axoplasmic concentration is the ratio of volume to surface area of the fiber. Small fibers tend to be blocked before large fibers. This sequence can sometimes be seen clinically when the small autonomic fibers are blocked before the larger diameter sensory or motor fibers to voluntary muscle.

Increasing the concentration of the local anesthetic injected increases the amount that enters the nerve fiber. This does not alter the degree of block in an individual fiber once the threshold level is reached, but since the time taken for the greater amount of anesthetic to diffuse from the nerve is longer, the duration of blockade will be increased. However, the higher the concentration, the greater the chance of systemic toxicity.

With topical application of local anesthetics to mucous membranes, there appears to be an optimal concentration. Further increases in concentration not only fail to prolong the duration of anesthesia but may even reduce it.

There is a latent period, which may amount to several minutes, between administration of the anesthetic and onset of blockade. The longer-acting local anesthetics have longer latent periods, for example, dibucaine > tetracaine > procaine (Table 20-1). Failure to allow for this latency, and the application of unnecessary further quantities of the drug to shorten it, can lead to severe or lethal toxic reactions.

All the local anesthetic is eventually absorbed into the blood stream, regardless of its site of administration. If this absorption is slow, then dilution, storage, and metabolism prevent toxic blood levels from occurring.

After perineural infiltration in quantities normally used, the concentration of the drug in blood is barely perceptible. Rapid absorption occurs from the mucous membranes after topical application, and the blood levels approach 50% of those found after rapid i.v. injection of the same dose. For anesthetizing mucous membranes, the dose should be divided into several fractions, and a few minutes should elapse between each application. The relative blood levels of a local anesthetic after various methods of administration are shown in Figure 20-3. Absorption from mucous membranes varies considerably: It is more rapid from the trachea than from the larynx and pharynx, and

FIG. 20-3. Relative blood levels of a local anesthetic following various methods of administration.

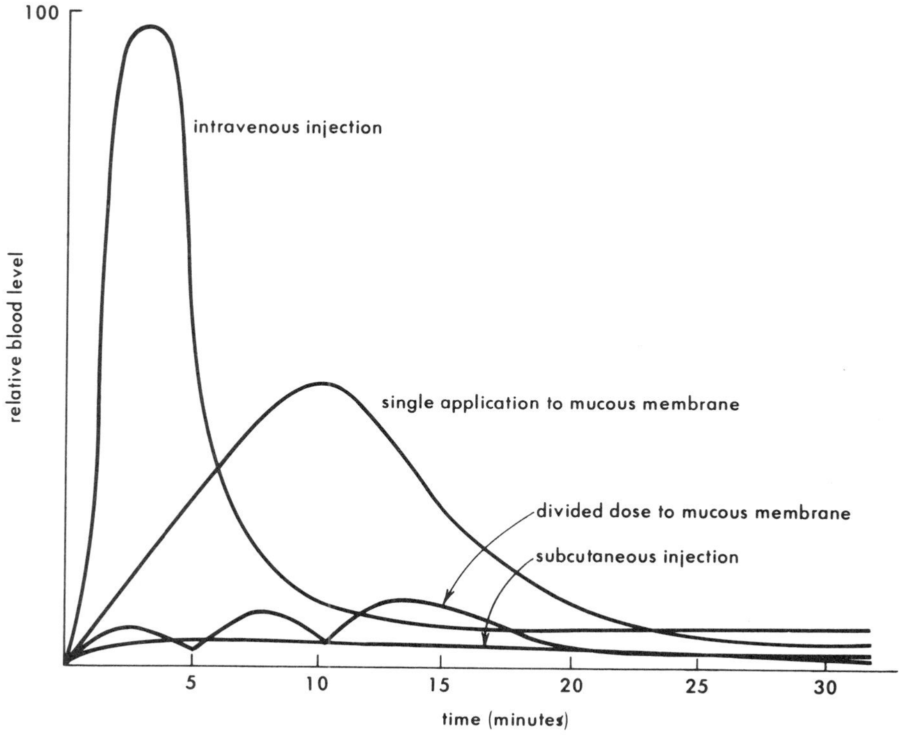

gravitation into the trachea can be avoided by anesthetizing the larynx with the patient in a head-down position. No appreciable absorption occurs from the stomach or from the bladder and urethra. Instrumental trauma at these latter sites, however, may allow absorption through the damaged epithelium. Local anesthetics are not absorbed through the unbroken skin or from the denuded areas of first- or second-degree burns.

To slow absorption and prolong the duration of action, vasoconstrictors are frequently added to local anesthetic solutions. Epinephrine is most effective. Norepinephrine may cause sloughing of the tissues. Vasoconstrictors can be used effectively when the anesthetic is infiltrated around nerve fibers or under the skin or used intrathecally for spinal anesthesia. However, vasoconstrictors do not alter the duration of action or rate of absorption of local anesthetics applied to mucous membranes.

Effective constriction of the vessels is achieved with a concentration of, for epinephrine, 1:200,000. Generally about twice this concentration is mixed with the anesthetic initially to allow for deterioration and losses during sterilization.

Most local anesthetics are vasodilators owing to direct paralysis of the muscle of the vessel wall. Cocaine is the only true vasoconstrictor: It blocks the uptake of catecholamines released from the vasoconstrictor nerve terminals and thus enhances the sympathetic effect (*see* Chap. 13). Owing to its high toxicity, cocaine is now little used except for shrinking the mucous membranes before antrostomy. This constrictive action of cocaine does not, however, retard its rate of absorption from the mucous membrane.

Norepinephrine may be responsible for delayed wound healing, because it not only reduces the blood supply but also increases tissue oxygen consumption. Trials have been initiated using vasopressin (*see* Chap. 42) or a synthetic analogue (fellypressin) as the vasoconstrictor since it does not have this metabolic effect.

ADVERSE EFFECTS

The ester and amide types of local anesthetics undergo hydrolytic cleavage, and the products are excreted in the urine. Detoxification takes place mainly in the liver, and little or no destruction of the drug occurs in the perineural tissues. Data on the metabolic fate in humans of many of the drugs are lacking. Cholinesterases are involved in the degradation of the ester-linked compounds. The rate of removal varies with the metabolic state of the patient, and esterase activity may be reduced in certain diseases such as toxic goiter, severe anemia, hepatic dysfunction, and any debilitating condition.

Paraminobenzoic acid is produced from metabolism of procaine and other anesthetics, and this may interfere with the action of sulfonamides. Amide-linked local anesthetics should not be used during sulfonamide therapy.

The value of a local anesthetic depends on its toxicity, although potency and duration, although not clearly related, are important. The type and severity of toxic reactions to local anesthetics depend on many factors, including the inherent toxicity of the drug, the susceptibility of the patient, and the blood level. The blood level depends on the rate of absorption from the injection site, the rate of diffusion through the tissues, and the rate of inactivation. Certain precautions can ensure that the concentration of the anesthetic in the blood is kept at a low level. The amount used should be kept to a minimum; the most dilute effective solution should be used; vasoconstrictors should be used whenever possible; and care should be taken to avoid intravascular injection.

Toxic reactions are referable to either CNS or the cardiovascular system. The onset of toxic effects is generally heralded by prodromal symptoms and signs. Epinephrine may cause tachycardia, palpitations, restlessness, and anxiety. Such symptoms and signs may be confused with toxic reactions to the anesthetic. Epinephrine should not be used in patients with thyrotoxicosis.

CENTRAL NERVOUS SYSTEM

Initially signs of central stimulation may be due to depression of inhibitory areas. Depression follows if the blood levels of the drug continue to increase. Prodromal signs are excitement, apprehension, disorientation, nausea, and vomiting. The condition may then progress to twitching, convulsions, and finally respiratory paralysis and circulatory failure. The convulsive phase is treated by giving an ultra-short-acting barbiturate, administering oxygen, and providing general supportive therapy. Pretreatment with a barbiturate has been recommended for procedures involving extensive nerve block in hospitalized patients.

CARDIOVASCULAR

The onset of toxic effects may be heralded by pallor, tachycardia, and syncope. The drug may have a toxic effect directly on the myocardium and circulation, and gradual or sudden general circulatory failure results. Drowsiness and coma can occur. Vasopressor agents such as ephedrine, methoxamine, or phenylephrine are used to treat the circulatory collapse. Oxygen, artificial respiration, and cardiac massage should be used without delay if needed.

Local anesthetics are frequently used preferentially in so-called poor-risk patients. These same patients, however, are also more likely to develop adverse reactions to local anesthetics.

Type I allergic reactions to local anesthetics occur rarely and appear to be confined to the ester-linked derivatives of p-aminobenzoic acid. The preservative methylparaben, used in certain preparations, may also be antigenic. Because many of the ester-linked local anesthetics exhibit cross-allergenicity, an amide-type compound should be used in patients claiming such sensitivity. Drug screening by sensitivity testing yields frequent false-positives and is not reliable.

TECHNIQUES FOR LOCAL ANESTHESIA

SURFACE

For application to wounds, ulcers, and burns, the local anesthetic bases can be dissolved in ointments. A 2% solution of lidocaine in carboxymethylcellulose can be used to anesthetize the mucous membranes of the mouth and pharynx, for example, before subcutaneous infiltration or the passage of gastric tubes. Solutions are usually sprayed onto the mucous membranes of the larynx and nasal passages. Many local anesthetics such as procaine are ineffective as surface anesthetics unless applied in extremely high concentrations; they are therefore not used in this manner.

INFILTRATION

The nerve endings in the infiltration area are blocked directly.

BLOCK

The main nerve trunks (*e.g.*, the occipital nerve) or a plexus (*e.g.*, brachial plexus) are infiltrated so that the field of distribution of the nerves is anesthetized.

SPINAL

The spinal nerve roots are anesthetized by injecting the local anesthetic into the subarachnoid space (into the cerebrospinal fluid). The injection is generally made into the fourth lumbar intravertebral space. The level of anesthesia attained depends on many factors, mainly the position of the patient and the specific gravity of the injected solution, which is adjusted by the addition of glucose.

EPIDURAL

The anesthetic is introduced into the epidural space below the second lumbar segment. The mixed nerves in the paravertebral space and nerve roots are blocked.

CAUDAL

The anesthetic is introduced into the epidural space of the sacral canal.

FURTHER READING

1. Adriani J: The clinical pharmacology of local anesthetics. Clin Pharmacol Ther 1:645, 1960
2. Adriani J: The Pharmacology of Anesthetic Drugs. Springfield, Illinois, Charles C Thomas, 1960
3. Adriani J, Naraghi M: The pharmacologic principles of regional pain relief. Annu Rev Pharmacol Toxicol 17:223, 1977
4. Ritchie JM, Greengard P: On the mode of action of local anesthetics. Annu Rev Pharmacol 6:405, 1966

CHAPTER 20 QUESTIONS

(See P. 7 for Full Instructions)

Select the One Best Answer

1. Lidocaine (Xylocaine) is characterized by all of the following EXCEPT that it
   A. decreases membrane responsiveness of the ventricle.

B. usually produces sedation with intravenous administration.
C. interferes with conduction of nerve impulses.
D. can produce complete A-V block.
E. can produce general anesthesia.

2. Which of the following is administered intravenously for its antiarrhythmic effect and administered by several routes for its local anesthetic effect?
A. Procainamide
B. Phenytoin
C. Lidocaine
D. Cocaine
E. Benzocaine

A = 1,2,3; B = 1,3; C = 2,4; D = 4; E = All

3. Procaine
1. can block conduction in both afferent and efferent nerves.
2. produces depolarization blockade.
3. in toxic doses produces convulsions.
4. produces local vasoconstriction.

4. Lidocaine has largely displaced procaine (Novocaine) in clinical practice because lidocaine
1. is less allergenic.
2. has less central depressant activity.
3. is better absorbed by mucous membranes.
4. is more readily hydrolyzed by plasma enzymes.

5. Lidocaine
1. is effective when given orally.
2. is effective in the treatment of most ventricular arrhythmias.
3. usually depresses A-V conduction.
4. produces paresthesias as an early manifestation of toxicity.

6. Lidocaine
1. is a vasoconstrictor.
2. causes sleep as an after effect.
3. can cause muscle relaxation.
4. interferes with rapid sodium influx in the nerve.

DRUGS ACTING PREDOMINANTLY ON THE CENTRAL NERVOUS SYSTEM

ISRAEL HANIN

Central Nervous System Neurotransmitter Mechanisms and Psychopharmacology

21

Many hypotheses that link mood disorders with alterations in endogenous neurotransmitter mechanisms have been suggested to date. These hypotheses have stemmed from parallel observations that certain psychopharmacologic agents can alleviate particular syndromes in humans and can actively impinge on, and influence, the function of certain neurotransmitters in brains of experimental animals. These two groups of phenomena may be interrelated, and thus these effects and hypotheses are the subject of intense investigation.

Before it can be stated with certainty that a particular neurotransmitter substance, or even a constellation of neurotransmitters, is involved in the etiology of a specific disease-state, a good understanding of a number of factors related to central neurotransmitter mechanisms is essential. Specifically it is important to identify the various neurotransmitter substances in brain; to understand which factors are important in regulating the synthesis, breakdown, and availability of these neurotransmitter substances; and to have a mechanism or technique whereby the availability and rate of use of these neurotransmitter substances can be studied and ascertained *in vivo*.

Identification of brain neurotransmitters is crucial. If a psychogenic illness is caused by an imbalance in one or more neurotransmitters in the brain, it is important to know about the existence and anatomical localization of these neurotransmitters before conducting studies that attempt to link neurotransmitter deficits to any type of centrally mediated abnormalities. Another important factor is the discernment of factors that affect, either in a facilitatory or inhibitory manner, the rate of metabolism and availability of the various neurotransmitter substances. If a psychotropic agent exerts its mode of action at some step in the transmitter synthetic process in the nerve terminal, the elucidation of the compound's precise site of action may ultimately serve to unravel the potential weak link in a person's central neurochemical organization, which may be an important contributing factor in the disease-state. Last, it is important to develop some tests with which central neurotransmitter function can be studied *in vivo*. Such tests can be applied to patients both before, and during, appropriate drug treatment and compared with similar tests conducted in control subjects. Findings from such an approach may begin to unravel some of the clues as to which neurotransmitter mechanism, if any, is involved in any particular disease-state.

Our current status of information in each of the above areas is growing but is by no means comprehensive. The various chapters that follow in this section will, in general terms, discuss our current knowledge in these categories and will attempt to provide an introductory basis for understanding neurotransmitter-related correlates of activity of the classes of compounds covered in the subsequent chapters. References provided in the reading list at the end of this chapter are primarily review articles and will equip the reader with a broader literature base from which to obtain more comprehensive coverage of available information.

NEUROTRANSMITTER CANDIDATES

The list of endogenous compounds believed to function as central nervous system neurotransmitters is quite extensive. Compounds that have been implicated as neurotransmitter substances to date are listed in Table 21-1. Of these, only a fraction are currently accepted as "neurotransmitters." The following arbitrary set of criteria have been established by investigators in the field and are used to qualify a compound for consideration as a *bona fide* central neurotransmitter agent.

1. The substance should exist as an endogenous compound in the brain.
2. The substance should be stored in the presynaptic neuron.
3. The substance should be released from the neuron upon nerve depolarization.
4. When applied postsynaptically, the agent should mimic the physiologic effects seen after depolarization of the neuron (excitation or inhibition).
5. Pharmacologic agents known to modify its action should exert the same effect whether the compound is applied postsynaptically or released after nerve depolarization.
6. The postsynaptic action of a potential neurotransmitter substance should be efficiently terminated by some specific endogenous mechanism.

To date, only acetylcholine (ACh) has fulfilled all the established criteria for a central transmitter. The weight of evidence that favors a central neurotransmitter role for dopamine (DA), epinephrine, gamma-aminobutyric acid (GABA), glycine, histamine, 5-hydroxytryptamine, and norepinephrine is, however, quite considerable. Some of the other compounds mentioned in Table 21-1 are referred to as "putative" neurotransmitters because only partial fulfillment of the above criteria has been demonstrated for these agents. Further supportive evidence favoring the role of these compounds as central neurotransmitter agents will certainly be forthcoming.

NEUROTRANSMITTER DISTRIBUTION AND FUNCTION

The distribution in the brain of the various neurotransmitter agents is predicated by the neuronal networks in the brain. Different nerve tracts connect various anatomical locations in the brain. Many have been identified; some have yet to be discovered. In general, nerves that contain a specific neurotransmitter substance will cluster in tracts. The area in which the tract terminates is rich in nerve terminals that contain the specific neurotransmit-

TABLE 21-1. Substances Implicated to Date as Potential Central Neurotransmitter Agents (in Alphabetical Order)

Acetylcholine	Angiotensin II	Aspartic acid
Bombesin	Carnosine	Cholecystokinin
Corticotropin	Dopamine	β-Endorphin
Epinephrine	Gamma-aminobutyric acid	Gastrin
Glutamic acid	Glycine	Histamine
5-Hydroxytryptamine	Insulin	Leu-enkephalin
Luteinizing hormone releasing hormone	Melanocyte stimulating hormone	Met-enkephalin
Neurotensin	Norepinephrine	Oxytocin
Prolactin	Proline	Somatostatin
Substance P	Taurine	Thyrotropin releasing hormone
Vasoactive intestinal peptide	Vasopressin	

ter substance, and consequently the measured concentration of the neurotransmitter is high. More than one nerve tract may innervate a particular brain area. Consequently more than one neurotransmitter substance can be identified and measured in this area. For example, DA-containing neurons have been shown to project from the substantia nigra to the caudate nucleus in brain. As would be predicted from this observation, the caudate nucleus contains high concentrations of the neurotransmitter DA. The caudate nucleus, however, is also rich in ACh. It is therefore evident that cholinergic nerve endings are concentrated in the caudate nucleus, as well as DA-ergic nerve endings. In fact, a major portion (although not all) of cholinergic neurons originates and terminates in the caudate nucleus; that is, cholinergic neurons exist primarily as interneurons. The tasks of identification, anatomical localization, and quantitation of the various neurotransmitter substances have been the subject of extensive investigation over the past two decades and have resulted in a number of excellent sources of reference information.

Intricate interactions exist between the various neuronal terminals found in brain areas. Nerve terminals that originate from one projection or tract are postulated to impinge on and influence the function of nerve terminals or dendrites from cell bodies of nerves from one or several other projections or tracts. This results in an interaction between the neurons involved. Consider the following simple hypothetical example of one neuronal tract impinging on another tract. Electrical stimulation of the first nerve tract results in mobilization and release of the neurotransmitter from its nerve terminals. The released neurotransmitter substance diffuses across the synaptic cleft between the originating nerve terminals and the so-called effector nerve terminals or dendrites of the second tract, which are influenced by the released transmitter. The sum total of this sequence is the transmission of information from one nerve tract to another as a combined result of electrical and neurochemical phenomena. The neurotransmitter's interactions with receptors result either in the activation or the inhibition of transmission of an impulse on the effector side. Whether activation or inhibition occurs, depends on a complex sequence of events related to the chemical nature of the neurotransmitter substance and the physiological properties of the effector neuron.

Such an interaction actually occurs between DA-containing nerve terminals within the caudate nucleus and the cholinergic interneurons within the same brain area. The DA-containing nerve terminals appear to impinge on dendrites of cell bodies of the cholinergic interneurons. Moreover, DA appears to exert a tonic inhibitory effect on the postsynaptic receptor site. Consequently, stimulation of the release of DA from these nerve terminals results in the reduction of activity of the ACh-containing neurons in the caudate nucleus.

Alternatively, if one diminishes the afferent influence of the DA-containing neurons in the caudate nucleus (*e.g.*, by blocking the postsynaptic DA-specific receptors with a pharmacologic "neuroleptic" agent), the tonic inhibitory influence of these neurons on the cholinergic interneurons is released. The end-result of this action is a reduction in DA activity and a concomitant increase in ACh activity within the caudate nucleus. The cholinergic interneurons, in turn, are known to impinge on other neurotransmitter systems (*e.g.*, GABA and substance P-containing neurons), which extend out of the caudate nucleus to other brain areas.

Thus a sequence of interacting mechanisms exists both intraneuronally and extraneuronally located in the brain, each subject to the specific characteristics of the neurotransmitter mechanisms involved. A disturbance of this sequence at any point triggers a chain reaction and attempts by the brain to restore normalcy.

The complexity of this picture is further compounded when the number of intertransmitter interactions that could, and do, exist *in vivo* are considered, as well as the number of brain areas involved in these interactions. Different brain areas control different functions in our bodies. Consequently a perturbation, whether endogenously or drug induced, even in a very specific brain area or a very specific group of nerve terminals, may result in a series of physiological as well as neurologic or mental aberrations. The nature and extent of such aberrations depends on the neuronal circuitry that connects the particular affected brain area with other parts of the brain; and the precise site of action of the endogenous, or the pharmacologically induced, perturbation that ultimately leads to the particular clinical imbalance.

How does one study the factors involved in the various complex sequelae of events listed above? Painstaking experiments are required at the neuronal as well as the integrative whole organ-system levels using a combination of approaches, including techniques in neurochemistry, pharmacology, histochemistry, behavior, and the development of appropriate animal models that attempt to simulate the disease-state under investigation.

STUDY OF CENTRAL NEUROTRANSMITTER MECHANISMS *IN VIVO*

The complexities involved in understanding the interaction of psychopharmacologic agents with central neurotransmitter mechanisms are enormous. Moreover, attempts at interpreting the nature of a suspected neurotransmitter-related imbalance in the central nervous system, based on the response of a patient to a specific psychopharmacologic agent with its known interactive effects on neurotransmitter mechanisms, must be tempered with considerable caution and restraint. Many laboratories are nevertheless currently involved in studies attempting to discover so-called biological markers in human subjects that would provide a reliable index of central neurotransmitter-related function *in vivo*. These studies, although elaborate and extensive, are in their infancy.

CONCLUSION

Increasing knowledge about the interaction of commonly used psychopharmacologic agents with central neurotransmitter systems has contributed to the development of various neurotransmitter-related hypotheses on the etiology of various psychogenic disease-states. Interpretation of clinical data obtained in this area of investigation depends on a broad base of information gleaned from studies in the sphere of basic animal research. The subject matter is complex, and many questions remain to be answered. However, herein lies the excitement in this field, which combines both clinical and basic research, encompasses diverse areas of investigation, and holds promise of many new findings in the immediate future.

FURTHER READING

1. Barchas JD, Berger PA, Ciaranello RD, Elliott GR: Psychopharmacology: From Theory to Practice. New York, Oxford University Press, 1977
2. Cooper JR, Bloom FE, Roth RH: The Biochemical Basis of Neuropharmacology, 3rd ed. New York, Oxford University Press, 1978
3. Hanin I, Usdin E: Animal Models in Psychiatry and Neurology. Oxford, Pergamon Press, 1977
4. Iversen SD, Iversen LL: Behavioral Pharmacology, 2nd ed. New York, Oxford University Press, 1981
5. Usdin E, Hanin I: Biological Markers in Psychiatry and Neurology. Oxford, Pergamon Press, 1982

CHAPTER 21 QUESTIONS

(*See* P. 7 for Full Instructions)

A = 1,2,3; B = 1,3; C = 2,4; D = 4; E = All

1. Both imipramine and chlorpromazine
   1. enhance amphetamine-induced CNS stimulation.
   2. prolong barbiturate sleeping-time.
   3. produce sedation in agitated psychotic states.
   4. sedate normal volunteers.

2. A neurotransmitter is a substance that transmits an impulse from
   1. a nerve to another nerve.
   2. a muscle to a nerve.
   3. a nerve to a muscle.
   4. the adrenal medulla to the liver.

3. When nerve stimulation causes release of a neurotransmitter, subsequent expected events include
   1. increased transmitter at the postsynaptic receptors.
   2. activation of postsynaptic mechanisms.
   3. counteraction of effect by reuptake or inactivation mechanisms.
   4. positive feedback promotion of further release of transmitter.

ALAN G. MALLINGER

22 Antidepressant Drugs

Depression is a clinical condition in which profound lowering of mood is the predominant symptom. Depressed persons often lose the capacity to experience pleasure, are overwhelmed by feelings of hopelessness, helplessness, and worthlessness or guilt, and experience disturbances of sleep, appetite, and sex drive. The social and personal consequences of depressive illness can be serious. Untreated, depression may lead to loss of employment, the destruction of interpersonal relationships, and, in a significant number of cases, suicide.

Two groups of drugs commonly are used to treat severe depression. The most widely used are referred to as *tricyclic antidepressants* because of their three-ring chemical structure. A less frequently used group, the *monoamine oxidase inhibitors,* are chemically heterogeneous, but have in common the ability to block the enzymatic breakdown of amine neurotransmitters.

TRICYCLIC ANTIDEPRESSANTS

HISTORY

Imipramine, the prototype drug for the tricyclic antidepressants, initially was synthesized and tested in the late 1940s for possible use as an antihistamine or sedative. Because of its structural similarity to the phenothiazines, imipramine was tested clinically for antipsychotic activity. Although imipramine was found to be ineffective for treating psychotic patients, Kuhn reported in 1958 that depressive symptoms improved markedly during treatment with this agent. Since that time, numerous clinical investigations have confirmed the effectiveness of imipramine for treating depression, and a number of chemically related compounds have been synthesized and found to be similarly effective.

CHEMISTRY

Imipramine has a three-ring chemical structure that differs from that of the phenothiazines

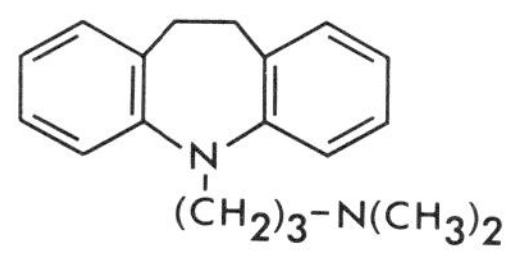

IMIPRAMINE

only by replacement of the sulfur atom in the central ring with an ethylene bridge. However, this causes the three-dimensional molecular conformation of imipramine to be very different from that of the phenothiazines, which probably accounts for the differences in their clinical actions. An aminopropyl side chain containing a nitrogen atom is attached to the central ring of the tricyclic nucleus of imipramine.

The tricyclic antidepressants are categorized as either tertiary or secondary amines. Tertiary amines have three organic groups (two methyl groups) attached to the nitrogen atom of the side-chain. Included among the tertiary amines are imipramine, amitriptyline, doxepin, and trimipramine. Secondary amines have only two organic groups (one methyl group) attached to the nitrogen atom of the side chain. This category of drugs includes desmethylimipramine or desipramine, nortriptyline, and protriptyline. Clinically and pharmacologically, there are characteristic differences between the tertiary and secondary amine compounds.

MECHANISMS OF ACTION

The pathophysiologic processes underlying depressive illness are incompletely understood, and therefore any proposed mechanism of action for antidepressant drugs must be speculative. Imipramine is known, however, to affect the metabolism of amine neurotransmitters at the neuronal level, and this effect is thought to be important in the therapeutic action of this drug.

At noradrenergic nerve terminals, norepinephrine is released into the synaptic cleft, where it can interact with postsynaptic receptors. This process is subsequently terminated, primarily by reuptake of norepinephrine into the presynaptic neuron. A similar sequence of events occurs at serotonergic nerve terminals. The predominant current view of the mode of action of imipramine is that it enhances the synaptic activity of norepinephrine, serotonin, or both by blocking their reuptake (*see* Chap. 13). In this way, imipramine is thought to enable the brain to compensate for a postulated deficiency of noradrenergic or serotonergic activity in depression.

The various tricyclic antidepressants differ in their abilities to block the reuptake of particular neurotransmitters. In general, tertiary amines tend to be more effective at blocking serotonin reuptake, whereas secondary amines tend to be more effective at blocking norepinephrine reuptake. These effects are relative, however, and depend to a large extent on the particular experimental system used for performing the studies.

Although it is generally accepted that tricyclic antidepressants block reuptake of amine neurotransmitters, the relationship of this effect to the antidepressant action of these drugs remains unproven for several reasons. First, although blockade of amine reuptake occurs rapidly, antidepressant effects are not seen clinically for several weeks. Second, some drugs that are structurally similar to imipramine are effective antidepressants but have no effect on norepinephrine or serotonin reuptake. An example is iprindole, which currently is unavailable in the United States. Finally, since the postulated deficiency of neurotransmitter activity in depressive illness never has been demonstrated conclusively, the clinical significance of the blockade of amine reuptake is speculative.

Other theories to explain the mechanism of action of imipramine and related tricyclic antidepressants have been proposed. Some investigators have suggested that the anticholinergic activity of these drugs may contribute to their antidepressant action. Other workers have noted that these drugs affect presynaptic alpha-adrenergic autoreceptors, as well as causing desensitization of beta-adrenergic systems. However, there is not sufficient evidence at present to support any of these proposed explanations.

EFFECTS

Central Nervous System

Although imipramine is an antidepressant, it does not typically produce euphoria. In a normal subject, the drug generally causes sedation, an unpleasant subjective effect, and difficulty with concentration. But when imipramine is given to a depressed patient, a reversal of the depressed mood occurs, with an accompanying improvement in thinking, decision making, and other goal-directed activities. In a simplistic way, this is analogous to the effect of aspirin on body temperature: Aspirin reduces fever, but not the temperature of a normal organism.

In certain cases, imipramine may precipitate manic excitement. This is seen most often in patients with a history of bipolar (manic-de-

---

Johannes Thiele, 1865–1918. German chemist. Worked especially with guanidine and tetrazol derivatives. In 1894 discovered semicarbazide.

pressive) illness, a condition that is discussed in greater detail in the chapter on antimanic agents. Such patients should be closely monitored for the appearance of manic symptoms during treatment with imipramine.

Sedation is a common central effect of imipramine. In general, tertiary amines such as imipramine tend to produce more sedation than secondary amine tricyclic antidepressants. In cases where depression is accompanied by agitation, patients may benefit from these sedative effects. Likewise, the sedative properties of imipramine may help to alleviate insomnia in depressed patients. Additionally, imipramine has specific effects on sleep that include a decrease in the total number of awakenings, an increase in the amount of stage four sleep, and a decrease in the amount of rapid-eye-movement sleep.

Imipramine and the other tricyclic antidepressants have central anticholinergic activity. Under some circumstances, this can give rise to confusional reactions or toxic delirium.

Autonomic Nervous System

The peripheral anticholinergic effects of imipramine include reduced visual accommodation, dry mouth, constipation, urinary retention, and tachycardia. These effects are additive with those of other anticholinergic drugs such as chlorpromazine, and can be antagonized by administration of neostigmine (an inhibitor of acetylcholinesterase). Imipramine enhances and prolongs the responses of the peripheral nervous system to injected norepinephrine by blocking the uptake of norepinephrine into sympathetic nerve terminals, which is a major route for inactivation of this substance. Imipramine also enhances and prolongs noradrenergic responses elicited by preganglionic or postganglionic sympathetic nerve stimulation, presumably because the reuptake of released endogenous norepinephrine is inhibited. However, imipramine also blocks the neuronal uptake of indirectly acting sympathomimetic amines and thereby reduces their effectiveness (*see* Chaps. 13, 17).

Cardiovascular System

The most common effect of imipramine on the cardiovascular system is orthostatic hypotension, which occurs frequently with therapeutic doses. Imipramine can also produce a variety of cardiac arrhythmias. Tachycardia can result from the anticholinergic effects of this drug. Slowing of conduction may be produced by a direct cardiotoxic effect. Other arrhythmias are thought to arise as a consequence of inhibited amine reuptake, which leads to elevated norepinephrine concentrations in cardiac tissue.

ABSORPTION, METABOLISM, AND EXCRETION

Absorption of imipramine from the gastrointestinal tract is rapid and nearly complete. The drug is extensively bound to plasma proteins, which limits its availability to tissues. The plasma half-life of imipramine is highly variable among individuals but is generally in the range of 9 to 24 hours. Because of this relatively large variability of the plasma half-life, persons on similar doses of this drug will have substantially different steady-state plasma imipramine levels. The relation of these plasma drug levels to therapeutic response is discussed in a later section of this chapter. Because imipramine is highly lipid soluble and binds extensively to tissue constituents as well as plasma proteins, its apparent volume of distribution is large and may exceed 20 liters/kg of body weight in some persons.

Imipramine is metabolized by two major routes. The first involves alteration of the side-chain, particularly by demethylation of the nitrogen atom. A single demethylation converts imipramine to desipramine, which is also marketed separately as an antidepressant. Thus both the parent drug and an active metabolite will be present in a patient treated with imipramine, and the demethylated metabolite may actually accumulate in concentrations exceeding those of the parent drug. Similarly, a single demethylation of amitriptyline produces nortriptyline, which also is available as a separate antidepresant. Further demethylation of desipramine and nortriptyline produces inactive metabolites. *N*-oxidation of imipramine also occurs, and this metabolite is excreted in the urine.

The second major metabolic route for imipramine is hydroxylation of the tricyclic nucleus, which can be followed by glucuronide formation. The metabolites are excreted primarily by the kidneys. Metabolites accounting for 70% of an administered dose of imipramine can be recovered from the urine within 72 hours.

Combinations of the metabolic steps described above can produce a variety of metabolites. Some have pharmacologic activity, but their clinical effects on the central nervous system are not known at present.

CLINICAL USE

The tricyclic antidepressants are the most effective medications available for treating depression. In general, between 65% and 70% of depressed patients will respond favorably to treatment with these drugs. Many depressed patients improve without treatment, however, because there is a high rate of spontaneous remission in depressive illness; it is therefore important to determine whether drug treatment is indicated for a particular patient. Several considerations are involved in making this decision.

First, the possibility of a medical or pharmacologic basis for the depressive symptoms must be ruled out. Depression can result from various medical conditions, including mononucleosis, hepatitis, viral pneumonia, carcinoma of the pancreas, epilepsy, and endocrine disorders such as Cushing's syndrome, Addison's disease, hyperthyroidism, hypothyroidism, and hyperparathyroidism. Moreover, a number of pharmacologic substances can induce depression, including antihypertensives (especially reserpine and methyldopa), corticosteroids, oral contraceptives, thyroid medication, antianxiety drugs, and sedative-hypnotics. Tricyclic antidepressants should not be used to treat depression that is secondary to medical or pharmacologic causes; instead, treatment should be aimed at correcting the underlying disorder.

The severity of depression must also be considered in determining the need for drug treatment. Most persons have intermittent variations of mood, and some sad days are a part of the human condition. In general, imipramine and similar drugs should not be used unless a patient's ability to function in interpersonal relationships or employment is impaired significantly by the illness.

Finally, the pattern of depressive symptoms is important to consider in selecting a therapeutic agent. For example, findings from clinical trials indicate that imipramine is most effective for treating endogenous depression characterized by disturbances of major bodily functions such as sleep, appetite, libido, and motor activity. However, depressed patients who have psychotic symptoms (such as delusions) may need to be treated with antipsychotic drugs, since imipramine has no inherent antipsychotic activity. Moreover, patients with bipolar (manic-depressive) illness may experience "mixed states," in which both manic and depressive symptoms occur. For such patients, a trial of treatment with lithium may be warranted.

DOSAGE

Treatment with imipramine should be initiated with a small daily dose, typically 50 mg administered at bedtime, to allow early recognition of adverse effects in patients who are particularly sensitive to the agent. If a patient tolerates the drug for 2 days, the dose can be increased gradually during a 2-week period. The usual adult daily dose ranges for drugs in this class are as follows: imipramine, amitriptyline, and trimipramine, 75 to 300 mg; desipramine and doxepin, 75 to 250 mg; nortriptyline, 50 to 100 mg; and protriptyline, 10 to 60 mg. These ranges are necessarily wide because the optimal drug dosage varies substantially among patients. In general, somewhat lower doses should be administered to elderly patients, who typically have reduced plasma protein binding and slower drug metabolism. Large doses should be reserved for severely ill hospitalized patients, who can be closely monitored.

The recent trend has been to give all or most of the daily dose at bedtime, which simplifies the dosage schedule and does not seem to increase the frequency of adverse effects. Further, the sedative effects of these drugs may help to relieve insomnia, which frequently occurs in depressed patients.

Clinical improvement may begin after 3 to 10 days of treatment with imipramine, but the full therapeutic effect may not be evident for 2 to 3 weeks. It is therefore important to perform an adequate therapeutic trial with this drug before concluding that it is ineffective in a particular patient. Of the tricyclic antidepressants currently available, none has been shown consistently to be more effective than the others. In the treatment of a particular patient, however, one drug is often found to be clinically superior. Thus, if a patient has responded to a particular tricyclic antidepressant during a previous depressive episode, the same agent should be tried in treating later episodes. In this regard, there has been interesting but unproven speculation that individual differences in drug response could reflect distinct pathophysiologic processes in depressed patients. For example, patients with an underlying disturbance of noradrenergic function might respond best to drugs that preferentially block norepinephrine reuptake, whereas patients with a disturbance of serotonergic function might respond to drugs that preferentially inhibit serotonin reuptake.

PLASMA DRUG LEVELS

Certain pharmacologic effects of the tricyclic antidepressants are related more closely to the plasma drug level than to the dose. For example, inhibition of the pressor response to indirectly acting sympathomimetic amines is correlated with the plasma level, but not with the dose, of nortriptyline. Plasma drug levels differ substantially among patients receiving similar doses of tricyclic antidepressants because the rates of drug elimination and metabolism vary greatly among individuals. The relation between such plasma drug levels and therapeutic response has been investigated, but the results have been controversial. In general, there appears to be a minimum level of drug that must be reached to attain a therapeutic effect. With nortriptyline, further increases in the plasma level apparently lead to a decline in therapeutic response, although with other tricyclic antidepressants this phenomenon has not been seen. As additional research is completed, plasma drug levels are likely to become clinically useful as a guide to dosage.

ADVERSE EFFECTS

The most frequently occurring adverse effects of imipramine are due to its anticholinergic properties. Specifically, this drug can cause loss of visual accommodation, dry mouth, constipation, and urinary hesitancy or retention. On rare occasions, narrow-angle glaucoma can be precipitated, but an underlying predisposition to this disorder must be present. Some degree of urinary retention is common in patients treated with imipramine because bladder sphincter tone is increased and more fluid is required to evoke detrusor contraction. This phenomenon generally does not become a clinically significant problem unless there is preexisting prostatic hypertrophy.

The most clinically important adverse effects of imipramine are cardiovascular. Orthostatic hypotension is very common and is especially problematic in the elderly. The anticholinergic properties of imipramine may produce tachycardia. The drug also causes widening of the QRS complex and can produce bundle branch block or even complete heart block. Other commonly occurring electrocardiographic changes are flattened T waves, prolonged QT intervals, and depressed ST segments. Imipramine and the other tricyclic antidepressants should be used with great caution in patients who have heart disease. These drugs have been implicated in the precipitation of congestive heart failure, myocardial infarction, and sudden death from ventricular arrhythmias.

Imipramine can produce a variety of adverse effects in the central nervous system, including drowsiness, tremor, headache, epileptiform seizures, confusional reactions, and manic excitement. The confusional reactions are believed to be due to central anticholinergic effects and are most common in patients over 40 years of age. Weight gain, a commonly reported adverse effect of imipramine, may be due to a drug-induced craving for sweets or carbohydrates. The weight gained during treatment tends to be lost when the drug is discontinued. Rare but serious adverse effects include cholestatic jaundice and agranulocytosis.

DRUG INTERACTIONS

Imipramine blocks the antihypertensive actions of guanethidine, bethanidine, and debrisoquine (*see* Chap. 36). The entry of these antihypertensive agents into noradrenergic nerve terminals via the amine uptake system is blocked by imipramine, so they are prevented from reaching their site of action. When imipramine treatment is initiated in patients being treated with these antihypertensives, loss of blood pressure control can occur within days. Doxepin is less likely to produce this effect because it is a relatively weak blocker of amine uptake. Imipramine also antagonizes the antihypertensive action of clonidine, although the mechanism of this effect is unknown.

Imipramine can potentiate the effects of central depressant drugs, such as alcohol or sedatives. In addition, imipramine augments the effects of directly acting sympathomimetic amines because inactivation of these substances by means of uptake into nerve terminals is blocked. However, the effects of indirectly acting sympathomimetic amines are inhibited by imipramine, which prevents these agents from reaching their intraneuronal site of action.

In some cases, the concomitant administration of tricyclic antidepressants and monoamine oxidase inhibitors can cause severe reactions characterized by hypertension, hyperpyrexia, coma, and seizures. Such reactions are relatively rare, however, and in a number of cases these two drug classes have been combined safely. Nevertheless, because of the potential seriousness of this drug interaction, these drugs should be used in combination only with great caution.

ACUTE OVERDOSAGE

Imipramine and the other tricyclic antidepressants are among the most toxic drugs in clinical use, and the depressed patients who take them are at high risk for attempted suicide. For this reason, the amount of drug prescribed should be kept small, and, when practical, treatment should be monitored by a family member.

Acute overdosage with imipramine is characterized by hyperpyrexia, respiratory depression, seizures, coma, and cardiac arrhythmias. Hypertension or hypotension may be present, and anticholinergic effects are prominent. The overall treatment approach in acute imipramine intoxication includes the physical maintenance of respiration and temperature, control of seizures, and administration of antiarrhythmic agents such as lidocaine when indicated. Because the cardiac arrhythmias that occur are potentially life threatening, patients must be monitored carefully.

MONOAMINE OXIDASE INHIBITORS

The monoamine oxidase (MAO) inhibitors are considered to be somewhat less generally effective than the tricyclic antidepressants. Nevertheless, they can often be useful for treating patients who are unresponsive to drugs such as imipramine. The main disadvantage to the use of MAO inhibitors is their potential for causing serious adverse effects and drug interactions.

HISTORY

In the early 1950s, isoniazid and its derivative, iproniazid, were developed for the treatment of tuberculosis. During clinical trials, it was noted that iproniazid had mood-elevating effects and could be used for treating depressed patients. This clinical observation was accompanied by the biochemical finding that iproniazid was an inhibitor of the enzyme MAO. These events subsequently had an important influence on the development of theories pertaining to the pathophysiology of depression.

After its initial clinical use, iproniazid was withdrawn from the market because of unacceptable hepatic toxicity. Several other MAO inhibitors that had been introduced were also withdrawn, and at present the only drugs of this category available for use in depression are phenelzine, tranylcypromine, and isocarboxazid. Because there is little clinical evidence to support the efficacy of isocarboxazid, it is seldom used and will not be discussed further in this chapter.

CHEMISTRY

The MAO inhibitors are a heterogeneous group of substances that have in common the ability to inhibit the enzyme that catalyzes oxidative deamination of monoamines (including norepinephrine and serotonin). MAO is distributed throughout the body, although the activity of this enzyme is especially high in blood, the liver, and the central and peripheral nervous systems.

Structurally, MAO inhibitors may be classified as hydrazines or nonhydrazine compounds. The hydrazines, for which phenelzine is the prototype,

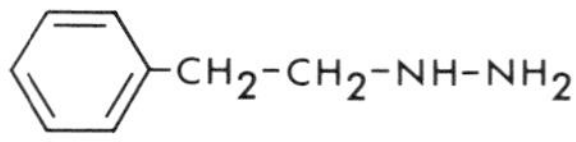

PHENELZINE

can react chemically with MAO. Phenelzine initially binds to MAO as if it were an ordinary substrate. The drug is then oxidized by MAO but subsequently forms a covalent bond with the enzyme. This process results in irreversible MAO inhibition.

Tranylcypromine is the prototype nonhydrazine MAO inhibitor.

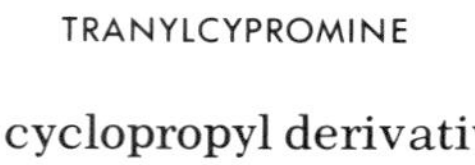

TRANYLCYPROMINE

This drug is a cyclopropyl derivative of amphetamine, in which the amphetamine side chain is closed to form a cyclopropyl ring. Although tranylcypromine does not react covalently with MAO, it is tightly bound to the enzyme, so that inhibition in this case is also functionally irreversible. The cyclopropyl ring apparently has a major role in the binding of tranylcypromine to

MAO, because neither amphetamine nor the cyclobutyl derivative of amphetamine is an irreversible inhibitor of this enzyme.

MECHANISMS OF ACTION

The drugs in this category can inhibit many enzymes other than MAO and have numerous direct effects on tissues unrelated to enzyme inhibition. The therapeutic action of these drugs, however, is believed to be a consequence of MAO inhibition.

The function of MAO in blood, liver, intestine, and other non-nervous tissues is to metabolize circulating monoamines. These amines, which may be produced endogenously or consumed with food or drugs, can have a variety of undesirable physiological effects (such as elevating blood pressure). Thus, the body must be able to inactivate these substances.

The role of MAO is more complex, however, in neurons that utilize monoamines as neurotransmitters. Monoamines that are synthesized in such neurons have two potential fates: They may be stored in synaptic vesicles for later release, or they may be metabolized by mitochondrial MAO. By means of this latter process, MAO may be involved in the regulation of intraneuronal amine levels. In addition, MAO can metabolize amines that enter the neuron via the reuptake system.

The neurotransmitters most commonly believed to be associated with the therapeutic action of MAO inhibitors are norepinephrine and serotonin. MAO has an important role in the metabolism of both of these substances. The initial step of norepinephrine metabolism may be performed by MAO or by catecholamine-O-methyltransferase (COMT) (*see* Chap. 13). In either case, oxidative deamination by MAO eventually occurs in the metabolic sequence, and an aldehyde is produced. In the central nervous system, such aldehydes can be metabolized further to form 3-methoxy-4-hydroxyphenglycol (MHPG).

Serotonin, in contrast to norepinephrine, cannot be metabolized by COMT. Serotonin is first deaminated by MAO and subsequently oxidized by aldehyde dehydrogenase. Inhibition of MAO can therefore lead to major changes in the metabolism of both norepinephrine and serotonin (*see* Chaps. 13, 52).

At least two forms of MAO exist, designated types A and B. Serotonin is metabolized almost exclusively by the type A enzyme. Norepinephrine is metabolized by MAO-A, and to some extent by MAO-B as well. Phenelzine and tranylcypromine inhibit both the A and B types of MAO, but there are investigational agents with more selective inhibitory properties. Clorgiline, for example, primarily inhibits MAO-A, whereas deprenyl is a relatively selective MAO-B inhibitor.

Inhibition of MAO leads to increased amine levels in the brain. The amounts of endogenous norepinephrine, dopamine, and serotonin can be increased by a single dose of an MAO inhibitor. The antidepressant action of these drugs is hypothesized to be due to increased availability of one or more of these amines, particularly norepinephrine or serotonin, in the nervous system. Like the tricyclic antidepressants, the MAO inhibitors are thus supposed to enable the brain to compensate for a presumed deficiency of noradrenergic or serotonergic activity in depression. As stated earlier, however, such a deficiency never has been demonstrated conclusively. Moreover, although MAO inhibitors increase norepinephrine and serotonin levels almost immediately, the clinical effects of these drugs are not evident for several days to weeks.

Both phenelzine and tranylcypromine can inhibit amine reuptake to some extent, but in this action they are less potent than the tricyclic antidepressants. Conversely, most tricyclic antidepressants have some MAO inhibitory activity, but this effect is generally weak and reversible and is of doubtful clinical significance.

EFFECTS

Central Nervous System

Depressed patients experience an elevation of mood when treated with MAO inhibitors. Unlike the tricyclic antidepressants, however, the MAO inhibitors are general psychomotor stimulants in both depressed and normal subjects. They produce psychological effects that include increased psychomotor speed, enhanced externally directed motivation, improved cognitive and perceptual test performance, and increased intensity and structural detail of visual imagery. The MAO inhibitors also can cause overstimulation, irritability, restlessness, and insomnia. The frequency of these latter effects is generally related to the dose of drug and to the duration of treatment. In some cases, mania or confusional behavior may be produced.

The MAO inhibitors, like the tricyclic antidepressants, decrease the amount of rapid-eye-movement sleep. Because of this effect, these drugs are sometimes used in the treatment of narcolepsy.

Cardiovascular System

The MAO inhibitors can cause hypotension, usually postural. This effect is thought to be due to a direct action of the drug on the vascular system rather than to inhibition of MAO. A possible mechanism for this hypotensive effect is sympathetic ganglionic blockade. The MAO inhibitors can also cause hypertensive reactions as a consequence of drug or food interactions.

ABSORPTION, METABOLISM, AND EXCRETION

Because these drugs produce more or less irreversible MAO inhibition, their clinical effects are not closely related to their pharmacokinetic profiles. They are absorbed readily from the gastrointestinal tract and produce maximal inhibition of MAO activity in biopsy samples within 5 to 10 days. Although these agents are probably in the body for a relatively short time, their effects are persistent because regeneration of the enzyme can take several weeks.

The hydrazine MAO inhibitors such as phenelzine are inactivated by acetylation. In the United States, about 50% of the population are "slow acetylators," who inactivate the drug less rapidly than other persons. Such persons may be at greater risk for adverse reactions to phenelzine because they have a greater total exposure to the drug.

CLINICAL USE

The MAO inhibitors are not usually drugs of first choice for the treatment of depression. Clinical trials generally have shown that the tricyclic antidepressants are more effective, and the MAO inhibitors have potentially serious adverse effects and drug interactions. Nevertheless, these drugs are often useful for treating patients who fail to respond to tricyclic antidepressants and also should be considered for patients who have responded to MAO inhibitors in the past.

There may be specific clinical indications for the use of MAO inhibitors, but this area is controversial at present. So-called atypical depressions may be particularly responsive to treatment with these drugs. Further, patients with hypersomnia and decreased psychomotor activity may benefit from the psychostimulant properties of MAO inhibitors.

DOSAGE

Treatment with MAO inhibitors should begin with a small dose, which gradually can be increased. Recommended therapeutic daily dose ranges are 15 to 75 mg of phenelzine and 20 to 40 mg of tranylcypromine. (This dose exceeds the Food and Drug Administration's recommended limits.) As with the tricyclic antidepressants, high doses should be reserved for hospitalized patients. Satisfactory clinical response is more likely when MAO activity, measured in blood platelets, is inhibited by at least 70%. This test, however, is generally available only in research settings.

Because they tend to produce insomnia, MAO inhibitors are not administered at bedtime. These drugs generally are given in divided doses before 3:00 p.m., with the larger part of the total dose being administered in the morning.

ADVERSE EFFECTS

The MAO inhibitors frequently act on the central nervous system to produce adverse effects that are consistent with their central stimulant properties. The most common effects include insomnia, irritability, motor restlessness, agitation, and tremor. Psychotoxic effects, such as manic excitement or confusional states, may also occur. These drugs may act on the autonomic nervous system to produce dry mouth, urinary hesitancy, constipation, delayed ejaculation, and orthostatic hypotension although such effects occur less frequently than with the tricyclic antidepressants. Peripheral neuropathy, which is occasionally caused by the hydrazine MAO inhibitors, may be related to pyridoxine deficiency.

The MAO inhibitors can cause serious hepatic toxicity, in which the clinical picture is similar to that of viral hepatitis. This toxic syndrome is characterized by jaundice, diffuse hepatocellular damage, and elevated serum liver enzyme levels. The emergence of this syndrome is not related to the dose of drug or the duration of treatment. Hepatic toxicity was more common with formerly marketed hydrazine MAO inhibitors; with the currently used drugs, this problem occurs infrequently.

DRUG INTERACTIONS

The MAO inhibitors induce major changes in the body's response to various pharmacologic agents. One category of such drug interactions occurs because MAO inhibitors decrease the activity of hepatic drug-metabolizing enzymes. Thus, the central nervous system depressant effects of alcohol, barbiturates, chloral hydrate, and benzodiazepines can be potentiated because the metabolic inactivation of these drugs is reduced. Similarly, the metabolism of anticholinergic agents is reduced and their effects therefore enhanced.

Adverse drug interactions can also result from the alterations of amine metabolism produced by MAO inhibitors. Monoamines that cannot be inactivated because of MAO inhibition may accumulate in the body and produce untoward physiologic responses to certain drugs. Thus, a serious hyperpyrexic reaction can occur when meperidine is administered to patients taking MAO inhibitors. This reaction appears to be mediated by the release of endogenous serotonin, and does not occur in animals when they have been pretreated with inhibitors of serotonin synthesis. A similar mechanism could be responsible for the severe reactions that can occur when tricyclic antidepressants and MAO inhibitors are administered concomitantly. Such reactions are characterized by hypertension, hyperpyrexia, coma, and seizures. Because of the irreversible nature of MAO inhibition, MAO inhibitors ordinarily should be discontinued for 10 days to 2 weeks before treatment with tricyclic antidepressants is initiated.

The administration of metabolic precursors of amine neurotransmitters may cause marked effects during MAO inhibitor treatment. Administration of DOPA or 5-hydroxytryptophan to animals treated with MAO inhibitors causes catecholamine and serotonin levels in the brain to increase and produces signs of central excitation. In patients receiving levodopa treatment for parkinsonism, administration of MAO inhibitors may produce hypertension and palpitations.

The MAO inhibitors can potentiate the pressor response to sympathomimetic amines (*see* Chap. 17). This potentiation is much more pronounced in the case of indirectly acting amines because levels of norepinephrine in the adrenergic neurons of patients taking MAO inhibitors are abnormally elevated. Thus, if an indirectly acting sympathomimetic drug is administered to such patients, the drug causes release of greater than usual amounts of norepinephrine, leading to excessive alpha-adrenergic stimulation and an exaggerated pressor response. Therefore, patients taking MAO inhibitors may have hypertensive reactions after receiving indirectly acting sympathomimetic amines, such as those commonly found in cold or hay fever remedies.

Tyramine is an indirectly acting sympathomimetic amine that is particularly important because large amounts may be present in cheese, beer, red wine, pickled herring, chicken liver, raw yeast preparations, canned figs, and other foods. The tyramine in food is ordinarily inactivated by MAO in the intestine and liver, but during MAO inhibitor treatment, tyramine can accumulate in the systemic circulation and cause excessive release of norepinephrine by the sympathetic nervous system. This process may lead to hypertensive crisis, a medical emergency characterized by severe blood pressure elevation that may be accompanied by headache or fever. The elevated blood pressure can lead to intracranial bleeding, and this complication has occasionally been fatal.

Hypertensive crisis may occur after the ingestion of foods that are high in tyramine or dopamine or after the administration of other sympathomimetic amines. Treatment consists of lowering the blood pressure, which usually can be accomplished by administration of an alpha-adrenergic blocking agent such as phentolamine. All patients being treated with MAO inhibitors should be given a list of foods and specific drugs to avoid, as well as a general warning to consult the prescribing physician before using any other medication.

ACUTE OVERDOSAGE

Acute overdosage with MAO inhibitors is manifested by agitation, hallucinations, hyperreflexia, hyperpyrexia, and seizures. The clinical picture may include either hypotension or hypertension. Treatment decisions should take into consideration the complex drug interactions of these agents. In general, treatment should be conservative and directed toward maintaining normal temperature, respiration, blood pressure, and fluid and electrolyte balance. Because of the irreversible nature of MAO inhibition, delayed toxic effects may appear; patients therefore should remain in the hospital for at least 1 week after an overdose with these drugs.

FURTHER READING

1. Hollister LE: Tricyclic antidepressants. N Engl J Med 299:1106–1109, 1168–1172, 1978
2. Kupfer DJ, Detre TP: Tricyclic and monoamine-oxidase-inhibitor antidepressants: Clinical use. In Iverson LL, Iverson SD, Snyder SH (eds): Handbook of Psychopharmacology, Volume 14: Affective Disorders: Drug Actions in Animals and Man, pp 199–232. New York, Plenum Press, 1978

3. Morris JB, Beck AT: The efficacy of antidepressant drugs. Arch Gen Psychiatry 30:667–674, 1974
4. Robinson DS, Nies A, Ravaris CL, Ives JO, Bartlett D: Clinical psychopharmacology of phenelzine. In Lipton MA, DiMascio A, Killam KF (eds): Psychopharmacology: A Generation of Progress, pp 961–973. New York, Raven Press, 1978

CHAPTER 22 QUESTIONS

(*See* P. 7 for Full Instructions)

Select the One Best Answer

1. Adverse effects common to both imipramine and tranylcypromine include
   A. insomnia.
   B. hypotension.
   C. heart block.
   D. hypertension.
   E. drowsiness.

2. Imipramine
   A. produces its maximum therapeutic effects within 24 hours.
   B. irreversibly inhibits monoamine oxidase.
   C. has anticholinergic effects like those of chlorpromazine.
   D. usually increases blood pressure.
   E. is contraindicated in depressed patients.

3. A patient presenting at the emergency room with severe headache and elevated blood pressure was recently released from a psychiatric hospital, but she cannot recall the name of the medication she has been taking. She also reports taking an over-the-counter decongestant for cold symptoms shortly before her headache began. One suspects that she has been treated with
   A. chlorpromazine.
   B. amitriptyline.
   C. diazepam.
   D. imipramine.
   E. tranylcypromine.

4. For treating severe mental depression characterized by agitation and insomnia, the agent of choice is
   A. tranylcypromine.
   B. imipramine.
   C. amphetamine.
   D. phenelzine.
   E. diazepam.

5. Imipramine may produce each of the following effects EXCEPT the
   A. reduction of the seizure threshold.
   B. depression of the T wave of the ECG.
   C. enhancement of the clinical effectiveness of guanethidine.
   D. inhibition of barbiturate metabolism.
   E. precipitation of psychotic behavior.

6. Tranylcypromine has each of the following characteristics EXCEPT that it
   A. is chemically very similar to amphetamine.
   B. can produce an increased concentration of norepinephrine in the brain.
   C. can produce an increased concentration of serotonin in the brain.
   D. can produce an increased concentration of acetylcholine in the brain.
   E. can produce an increased concentration of dopamine in the brain.

A = 1,2,3; B = 1,3; C = 2,4; D = 4; E = All

7. The side-effects most likely to be troublesome during therapy with imipramine are
   1. urinary retention.
   2. cardiac arrhythmias.
   3. blurred vision.
   4. physical dependence.

ALAN G. MALLINGER

23 Antimanic Drugs

Mania is a state of euphoria, inflated self-esteem, and excitement that is behaviorally the opposite of depression. The manic patient typically has increased physical activity, a decreased need for sleep, and a heightened sex drive. In addition, mental activity is characteristically increased in mania so that the patient has racing thoughts and pressured speech. The social activity of manic patients is also increased and often inappropriate. They may approach other persons with grandiose schemes, spend large amounts of money during buying sprees, or make foolhardy business investments. In extreme cases, the manic patient can lose touch with reality and may have delusions of grandeur when this occurs.

Hypomania is a less severe form of the same syndrome. Hypomanic persons have increased physical, mental, and social activity. In certain cases this less severe form of mood disturbance may actually be socially rewarding because such persons are typically energetic and ambitious. However, most patients with mania or hypomania also experience recurrent episodes of depression—hence the name manic-depressive or bipolar illness. Mania and hypomania can be treated with lithium salts or with antipsychotic drugs. A more detailed discussion of antipsychotic drugs is found in Chapter 24.

LITHIUM

HISTORY

Lithium was first used for the treatment of mania by Cade, who in 1949 reported that lithium treatment seemed to have a specific antimanic effect. In the late 1940s, lithium chloride was introduced in the United States as a substitute for table salt to be used by cardiac patients who needed to limit their sodium intake. This unsupervised use of lithium led to a number of severe intoxications and deaths.

JOHN F. J. CADE. Australian physician. Published his use of lithium for the treatment of mania in 1949, but it was little noticed at the time.

Consequently the need for careful monitoring of patients who received lithium treatment became widely recognized.

CHEMISTRY

As a drug, lithium is unusual (although not unique) because it is an inorganic element. Lithium is common in the earth's surface, where it frequently occurs as a lithium–aluminum–silicate ore known as spodumene. In nature, lithium is more abundant than tin, lead, silver, or gold.

Lithium is a group I alkali metal, like sodium and potassium, and in aqueous solutions has a single positive charge. Clinically it is administered as a salt. The most commonly used salt is lithium carbonate. A liquid dosage formulation that contains lithium citrate is also available. Sustained-release preparations of lithium carbonate allow less frequent administration of the drug.

MECHANISMS OF ACTION

Lithium has diverse effects on neurotransmitter systems, cyclic AMP-dependent systems, and membrane function. However, the basic mechanism for its antimanic action is not currently known.

Mania is thought by some investigators to be caused by excessive activity of amine neurotransmitters. For this reason, there has been much interest in lithium's effect on brain amine metabolism. When administered acutely, lithium inhibits the release and increases the reuptake of norepinephrine. This effect on amine reuptake is the opposite of that produced by tricyclic antidepressants. Currently the effects of lithium on serotonin metabolism are controversial and incompletely understood.

Lithium also affects various cyclic AMP-dependent systems (*see* Chap. 50). Adenyl cyclase is the enzyme that, when stimulated by a "first messenger" such as a hormone, converts ATP to cyclic AMP. The cyclic AMP produced then interacts with other cell components to regulate various physiological processes. In the brain, lithium can inhibit norepinephrine-stimulated adenyl cyclase, although relatively high concentrations of lithium may be needed to produce this effect. At therapeutic concentrations, lithium inhibits TSH-stimulated adenyl cyclase in the thyroid and ADH-stimulated adenyl cyclase in the kidney. The effects of lithium on these cyclic AMP-dependent systems are the basis for several significant adverse drug effects that will be discussed below.

Because of the physicochemical similarities between lithium and sodium ions, lithium can interact with certain sodium-dependent functions of the cell membrane. Sodium is ordinarily removed from cells by the sodium-pump so that extracellular concentrations of this ion are substantially higher than intracellular concentrations. During depolarization of a neuron or other excitable cell, sodium-channels in the membrane become more permeable to sodium, which diffuses inward. The membrane potential is thereby reversed. Lithium can substitute for sodium in this process. Thus, in perfused axon preparations, substitution of lithium for extracellular sodium will support nerve excitation, with lithium entering the cells by way of the sodium-channels during the action potential. However, lithium is not effectively removed from cells by the sodium-pump, which may result in altered intraneuronal ionic composition. In this regard, lithium has been referred to as an imperfect substitute for sodium in the neuron. Sodium is known to be importantly involved in several aspects of central nervous system physiology, including the cellular uptake of neurotransmitter precursors, the conduction of the action potential, the reuptake of neurotransmitters by presynaptic neurons, and the postsynaptic actions of certain neurotransmitters. Thus an interaction of lithium with these sodium-dependent processes could significantly affect neuronal function.

EFFECTS

Central Nervous System

When administered to manic patients, lithium reduces motor activity, diminishes euphoria, and relieves insomnia. When administered to psychiatrically normal subjects, however, its psychological effects are less pronounced than are those of the antipsychotic or antidepressant drugs. Lithium produces characteristic EEG changes, including generalized slowing with increased amplitude, decreased alpha activity, and increased delta and theta activity.

JOHAN AUGUST ARFVEDSON, 1792–1841. Swedish chemist. Prepared lithium sulfate in 1817 under the direction of J. J. Berzelius. (Sir Humphrey Davy isolated pure lithium in 1818.) Worked on mineral composition, including uranium ores, and prepared uranous oxide in 1823.

Water and Electrolyte Metabolism

Lithium has pronounced effects on water metabolism, with polyuria and polydipsia being frequent during lithium treatment. These effects apparently are due to inhibition of the antidiuretic action of ADH on the kidney. Antidiuretic hormone, secreted by the posterior pituitary, ordinarily causes the renal collecting ducts to become more permeable to water. When this occurs, water flows out of the collecting ducts into the hyperosmolar region of the kidney medulla, where it is reabsorbed, leading to the production of smaller volumes of more concentrated urine. In contrast, when ADH is absent or its action is inhibited, the collecting ducts become relatively impermeable to water, which therefore remains in the ducts and subsequently is excreted. This process results in polyuria and decreased urine osmolarity.

Intravenous infusion of lithium in animals inhibits the antidiuretic action of ADH, an effect very specific for the lithium ion and not seen during infusion of potassium, rubidium, magnesium, or calcium. The action of ADH on the kidney is mediated by cyclic AMP. However, the exact mechanism by which lithium inhibits this action is not known because lithium treatment not only diminishes the activity of ADH-stimulated adenyl cyclase, but also blocks the effect of exogenous cyclic AMP on urine osmolarity. Which of these effects is more important in the production of lithium-induced polyuria is not clear.

Thyroid

Lithium decreases the secretion of T_3 and T_4 from the thyroid. Reduced circulating levels of these thyroid hormones then stimulate TSH secretion by the pituitary. Thus elevated TSH levels are seen in about 30% of lithium-treated patients. In a smaller percentage of patients, goiter or clinical hypothyroidism may occur, although these are more common when there is pre-existing thyroid disease.

As in the case of the kidney, the effect of lithium on thyroid function is thought to involve cyclic AMP. Ordinarily TSH stimulates adenyl cyclase activity, and the cyclic AMP produced then promotes release of thyroid hormone. Lithium interferes with this process, but the exact mechanism is controversial. Lithium does strongly inhibit TSH-stimulated adenyl cyclase, but lithium can also block TSH secretion that is stimulated by exogenous cyclic AMP. Thus lithium can act on adenyl cyclase but can also act on a physiological process distal to this enzyme. This situation is similar to that already discussed for the kidney.

ABSORPTION, METABOLISM, AND EXCRETION

Absorption of lithium from the gastrointestinal tract is rapid, with peak plasma levels being reached within 1 to 3 hours after an oral dose of the drug. Nearly all of an administered dose is absorbed. Lithium is not bound to plasma proteins and distributes throughout the total body water. No metabolites of lithium are produced in the body. Lithium is eliminated primarily by the kidneys, which account for about 98% of the total drug excretion. Small amounts of lithium may also leave the body in the feces and sweat. Lithium is secreted into saliva and into breast milk.

In the kidneys, about 80% of the lithium originally present in the glomerular filtrate is reabsorbed. For this reason, factors that affect lithium reabsorption ultimately affect the renal excretion of this drug. Most of the filtered lithium is reabsorbed in the proximal tubule. In hyponatremic patients, proximal tubular reabsorption of both sodium and lithium increases, which can lead to significant lithium retention that may eventually precipitate lithium toxicity. Conversely, sodium loading produces a small enhancement of lithium excretion as a consequence of decreased renal reabsorption.

Renal lithium clearance varies considerably among different persons; it is thus necessary to measure serum lithium levels to determine the appropriate dose of this drug. Renal lithium clearance tends to increase during pregnancy and to decrease after delivery. Lithium clearance also tends to be lower in elderly patients, who ordinarily require a lower dose of this drug.

CLINICAL USE

Considerable evidence suggests that lithium is an effective antimanic agent. About 80% of manic patients respond favorably to treatment. Those patients with typical manic syndromes that include symptoms such as flight of ideas or grandiose delusions tend to respond best. Patients having atypical clinical features, such as mood-incongruent delusions or prolonged hallucinations, tend to respond less well. Unlike the antipsychotic drugs, lithium is generally ineffective for treating excited psychotic conditions other than mania.

Clinically, 6 to 10 days are needed for lithium to exert its full therapeutic effect. Because manic patients are often destructive and unmanageable, faster-acting or injectable antipsychotic drugs may be needed initially to control acute manic episodes. Patients can later be gradually switched to lithium treatment when they become more cooperative.

Lithium is also used for the prevention of both manic and depressive episodes in bipolar (manic-depressive) patients. Lithium maintenance treatment prevents the recurrence of manic episodes in about 85% of cases and appears to reduce the frequency, duration, and intensity of depressive episodes. (However, the Food and Drug Administration approves of lithium maintenance treatment only for the prevention of manic episodes.) Recent studies of patients with recurrent depression (unipolar patients) suggest that lithium treatment may also prevent affective episodes in this population. Such unipolar patients could alternatively receive maintenance treatment with imipramine or other tricyclic antidepressants. These drugs are, however, less useful for maintenance treatment of bipolar patients because they cannot prevent manic episodes. In fact, tricyclic antidepressants may actually precipitate such episodes in certain cases.

DOSAGE

Lithium dosage is routinely monitored by the measurement of serum lithium levels. In acute mania, the therapeutic range for these serum levels is generally considered to be between 0.8 and 1.5 mEq/liter. For maintenance treatment, the range is 0.6 to 1.2 mEq/liter. The dose of drug needed to produce serum levels in the desired range varies greatly among persons, depending on factors such as renal lithium clearance. In general, treatment should begin with 600 to 900 mg of lithium carbonate per day. This dose should be increased gradually using the serum lithium concentration as a guide. Generally, the serum level will equilibrate within 4 to 6 days after a change in lithium dose.

Serum lithium levels should be drawn frequently at first, until the optimum dosage can be determined. Blood for serum lithium measurements should be drawn 12 hours after the most recently administered dose because, for several hours after ingestion of lithium, the serum level fluctuates rapidly as a consequence of drug absorption and distribution. After 12 hours, the serum lithium level becomes more stable. Large single doses of lithium tend to produce high peak serum levels owing to rapid drug absorption. Because these high peak levels may be associated with transient adverse effects, lithium should always be administered in divided doses.

ADVERSE EFFECTS

Prominent adverse reactions to lithium may occur in the nervous and neuromuscular systems. Fine tremor is common, although this can be treated, if necessary, with low doses of propranolol. Other common adverse effects on the nervous and neuromuscular systems include muscular weakness, headache, twitches, incoordination, ataxia, impaired concentration, lethargy, somnolence, and slurred speech. Most of these effects can be minimized by lowering the dose of lithium.

Adverse effects of lithium on the gastrointestinal system include nausea, vomiting, and diarrhea. Such effects are most common when serum levels are rising rapidly during the initiation of lithium treatment. Lithium-induced diarrhea can have serious consequences because of the potential for sodium depletion. As the kidney attempts to compensate for gastrointestinal sodium losses by increased proximal tubular reabsorption of this ion, lithium reabsorption is concurrently increased. This process leads to lithium retention, which elevates the serum level further and can lead to a progressive cycle of gastrointestinal sodium loss followed by renal lithium retention. The same sequence of events, moreover, can occur as a consequence of diarrhea of any other etiology. Therefore the serum lithium level must be closely monitored in any patient taking lithium who develops severe diarrhea.

Renal effects of lithium include polyuria and polydipsia, nephrogenic diabetes insipidis, and possibly irreversible renal damage. Polyuria and polydipsia occur in 40% to 50% of lithium-treated patients. In about 10% of patients, this progresses to nephrogenic diabetes insipidis, with urine volumes greater than 3 liters per day. Thiazide diuretics may paradoxically decrease the urine volume in this condition.

Irreversible renal damage in biopsy specimens from lithium-treated patients has been

MOGENS ABELIN SCHOU, 1918–. Danish physician. First used lithium for maintenance treatment of manic-depressive psychoses in 1954.

reported. The observed lesions have included focal nephron atrophy and interstitial fibrosis. The clinical significance of these findings is controversial. Nevertheless, renal function should be evaluated at least semiannually in patients who receive long-term lithium treatment.

Lithium effects on the thyroid can lead to goiter, hypothyroidism, or abnormal thyroid function test findings. The incidence of lithium-induced goiter is low, and when this does occur it usually responds to thyroid hormone replacement or discontinuation of lithium treatment. Similarly hypothyroidism is rare. Lithium-induced hypothyroidism differs clinically from primary hypothyroidism in that radioactive iodine uptake is elevated. Changes in thyroid function test findings commonly produced by lithium include elevated TSH and reduced T_4 and T_3. Patients typically remain clinically euthyroid despite these changes.

Lithium can also produce leukocytosis, with white blood cell counts that range from 10,000 to 14,000. Neutrophils are the predominant cell type affected.

DRUG INTERACTIONS

Lithium interacts with several classes of diuretics. Osmotic diuretics generally increase renal lithium elimination because of their proximal tubular effects. Thiazide diuretics, in contrast, decrease renal lithium elimination. Thus if thiazides are administered to a patient being treated with lithium, the dose of lithium should be lowered.

Lithium potentiates the effects of neuromuscular blocking agents. This occurs with depolarizing agents such as succinylcholine, as well as with nondepolarizing agents such as curare.

ACUTE OVERDOSAGE

Lithium toxicity usually occurs at serum levels greater than 2 mEq/liter, although some patients will develop toxicity at lower levels. Except in cases of intentional overdose, the onset of symptoms is usually gradual. The prodromal symptoms are extensions of the common adverse effects of this drug and may include gastrointestinal distress, slugglishness, drowsiness, slurred speech, and ataxia. Patients should consult their physician when effects such as these occur. The most prominent manifestations of lithium toxicity occur in the nervous system and include confusion, hyperreflexia, coarse tremor, and nystagmus. Impaired consciousness, coma, or seizures may occur. Treatment is directed toward support of vital functions. Maintenance of electrolyte and fluid intake is essential, and if hyponatremia is present it must be corrected to allow maximum renal lithium elimination. Most patients who recover do so without sequelae, but some instances of irreversible brain damage leading to permanent ataxia, nystagmus, or choreoathetotic movements have occurred.

FURTHER READING

1. Amdisen A: Monitoring of lithium treatment through determination of lithium concentration. Dan Med Bull 22:277–291, 1975
2. Klerman, GL: Long-term treatment of affective disorders. In Lipton MA, DiMascio A, Killam KF (eds): Psychopharmacology: A Generation of Progress, pp. 1303–1311. New York, Raven Press, 1978
3. Prien RF, Caffey, EM: Long-term maintenance drug therapy in recurrent affective illness: Current status and issues. Dis Nerv Syst 38:981–992, 1977
4. Shopsin B, Gershon S: Lithium: Clinical considerations. In Iverson LL, Iverson SD, Snyder SH (eds): Handbook of Psychopharmacology, Volume 14, Affective Disorders: Drug Actions in Animals and Man, pp 275–325. New York, Plenum Press, 1978

CHAPTER 23 QUESTIONS

(See P. 7 for Full Instructions)

Select the One Best Answer

1. Lithium-induced polyuria
   - *A.* is due to inhibition of posterior pituitary release of ADH.
   - *B.* can be mimicked by the intravenous infusion of magnesium sulfate.
   - *C.* is due to the inhibition of the action of ADH on the renal tubules.
   - *D.* is a rarely encountered adverse drug effect.
   - *E.* commonly occurs at serum lithium concentrations below 1.0 mEq/liter.

A = 1,2,3; B = 1,3; C = 2,4; D = 4; E = All

2. Serum concentrations of lithium
   - *1.* should be determined using blood drawn within 2 hours after the last administered dose.

2. are affected by any large change in sodium ingestion.
3. usually reach a plateau on the third day of constant daily dosages.
4. are considered in the toxic range when they are above 1.5 mEq/liter.

3. Lithium carbonate
1. is safe for use as a salt substitute.
2. must be administered for several days to attain a full therapeutic effect.
3. toxicity is immediately reversed by giving large amounts of sodium.
4. produces little or no sedation in therapeutic doses.

4. Lithium carbonate
1. is effective in long-term control of manic cycles.
2. should never be coadministered with antipsychotic drugs.
3. may produce vomiting and diarrhea.
4. stimulates Na/K ATP-ase to exchange intracellular sodium for extracellular lithium.

ROBERT H. GERNER

24

Neuroleptic Drugs

The antipsychotic (or neuroleptic) drugs are a family of chemical compounds that have a wide range of use in psychiatric and neurologic disorders. The term *neuroleptic,* as opposed to *antipsychotic,* is generally favored because the drugs in this class have certain specific effects on the dopaminergic system and commonly produce extrapyramidal as well as antipsychotic effects. Further, many compounds that have antipsychotic effects (such as lithium) are clearly outside this class of agents.

The use of these compounds is the single most important reason for the abrupt reduction in the population of public mental hospitals in the United States, which up until 1955 had shown a gradual and seemingly inexorable increase. The widespread use of psychotropic agents effective in ameliorating psychoses resulted in the rapid decrease of the number of patients in hospitals by approximately 50%.

The immediate impetus for the development of neuroleptic drugs as we know them today was the search for a better sedative for use in potentiating general anesthetics. The first compound of this class, *chlorpromazine,* was synthesized in 1949 and used effectively in psychiatric patients by 1952. Subsequently, numerous other agents, both related to and different from chlorpromazine, have been marketed. Now over a dozen neuroleptics are available in the United States; yet more are prescribed in Europe.

CLASSES OF NEUROLEPTIC DRUGS

PHENOTHIAZINES

All of the *phenothiazines* are chemically related to chlorpromazine and are similar in having a tricyclic ring structure with a sulphur atom and a nitrogen atom connecting the two external rings. They differ in the substitutions at R-1 and R-2 (Fig. 24-1). Substitution at R-1 divides the phenothiazines into three major groups: Those with an aliphatic group include chlorpromazine and triflupromazine; a piperidine group, thioridazine and mesoridazine; or a piperazine group, prochlorperazine, trifluoperazine, perphenazine, fluphenazine, and

Pierre G. Deniker, 1917– . French psychopharmacologist and psychiatrist. Pioneered work in chemotherapy of psychiatric disorders.

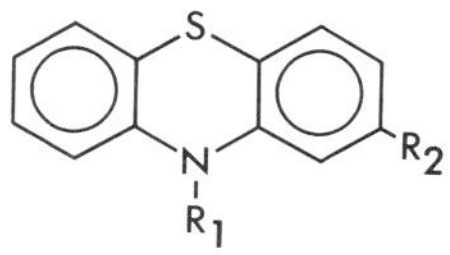

FIG. 24-1. Phenothiazine.

acetophenazine. The drugs in each group have different substitutions at R-2 that modify in a minor way the activity of the individual drugs. The aliphatic and piperidine substituted compounds are the least potent neuroleptics and have the greatest antimuscarinic activity. The piperizine side group confers high potency and low antimuscarinic activity. This inverse relationship between potency and antimuscarinic activity is generally true for all of the neuroleptics.

THIOXANTHENES

The *thioxanthenes* (Fig. 24-2) are similar to the phenothiazines in having a tricyclic ring, but a carbon instead of a nitrogen atom connects the two external rings. These compounds also have R-1 and R-2 substitutions. The two drugs in this class available in the United States are thiothixene and chlorprothixene, the former being a high-potency neuroleptic and the latter having moderate potency.

BUTYROPHENONES

Two members of the *butyrophenones* are available in this country: haloperidol and droperidol (Fig. 24-3). Both compounds are relatively potent; the latter is used mainly in anesthesia but also is given parenterally for acute psychiatric emergencies.

DIHYDROINDOLONES

The *dihydroindolones* are represented by only one drug, molindone, of moderate potency (Fig. 24-4).

FIG. 24-2. Thioxanthene.

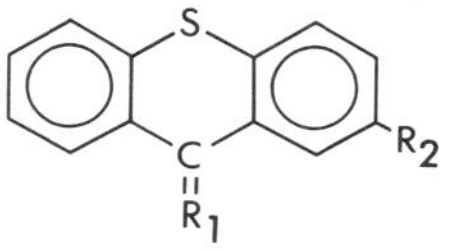

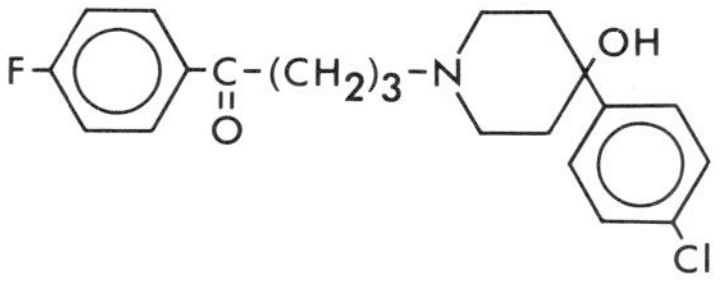

FIG. 24-3. Butyrophenone (haloperidol).

DIBENZOXAZEPINES

Loxapine, which is moderately potent, is the only congener of the *dibenzoxazepines* available for use (Fig. 24-5).

DIPHENYLBUTYLPIPERIDINES

The diphenylbutylpiperidines are represented by two drugs that may soon be available in the United States, penfluridol and pimozide (Fig. 24-6). These compounds are among the most potent known, and penfluridol is unique in its long action after oral administration.

Although historically used as antipsychotic agents, rauwolfia alkaloids (reserpine) are only rarely used to treat psychotic symptoms. The mechanism of action in treating psychosis is similar to that of their hypotensive action (*i.e.*, depletion of presynaptic catecholamines and thus decreased postsynaptic stimulation of receptors).

PHARMACOLOGIC EFFECTS

DOPAMINE RECEPTOR BLOCKADE

Although all of these compounds are chemically distinct, they have several pharmacologic similarities: part of their molecular structure is congruent with the structure of dopamine, which possibly plays a major role in mania, schizophrenia, and perhaps depression; presumably they all exert their therapeutic action by occupying dopamine receptors on postsynaptic neurones in the limbic system (Fig. 24-7), thus diminishing the effect of dopamine released from the presynaptic neuron. The pathophysiologic mechanisms for the antipsychotic

FIG. 24-4. Dihydroindolone (molindone).

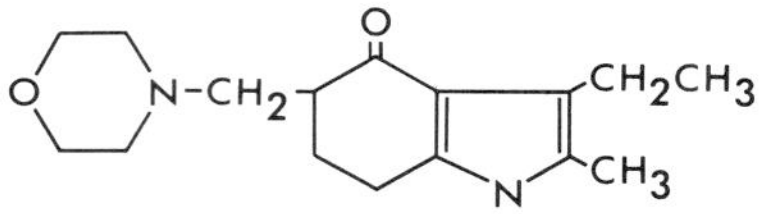

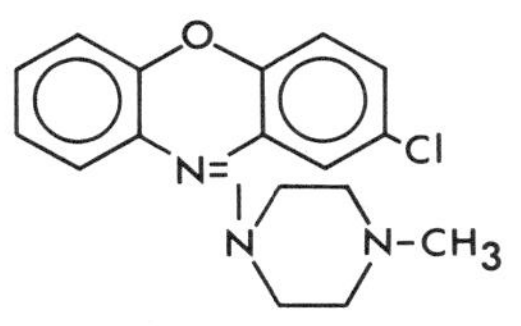

FIG. 24-5. Dibenzoxazepine (loxapine).

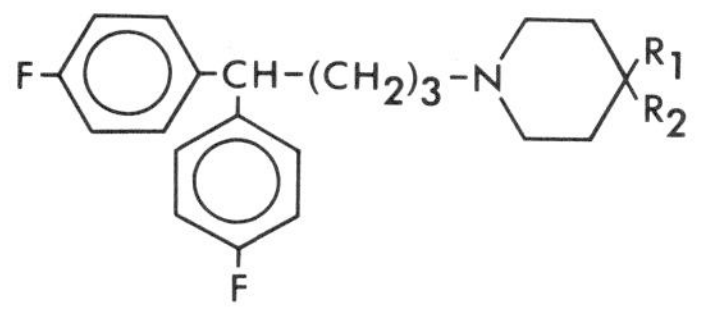

FIG. 24-6. Diphenylbutylpiperidine.

effect of neuroleptics are still being studied. In actuality, the blockade of dopamine receptors occurs within hours of administration, but their antipsychotic effect typically takes days to weeks to become manifest. Thus their antipsychotic effects may be mediated through indirect mechanisms (such as the brain adapting to the acute effects of the drugs) rather than by simple dopamine receptor blockade. All investigators do agree that their effectiveness can be related to dopamine receptor blockade. Many studies that use animal models and studies of dopamine receptor binding *in vitro* have shown a very high correlation of the average clinical dose of each agent and its ability to bind to dopamine receptors.

ALPHA-ADRENOCEPTOR BLOCKADE

All neuroleptics appear to compete with norepinephrine for binding at alpha-adrenergic receptor sites (*see* Chap. 18). The potency of this alpha-adrenergic antagonism varies considerably. It is not related to the therapeutic effect of the drugs. Rather, certain side-effects have been posited to be due to this, including hypotension, ejaculatory impairment, miosis, and dry mouth. The neuroleptics with the most potent alpha adrenoceptor antagonist action are, in descending order, droperidol, triflupromazine, chlorpromazine, and thioridazine; those with lesser effect range downward from fluphenazine, haloperidol, and trifluperazine to pimozide.

MUSCARINIC RECEPTOR BLOCKADE

Virtually all neuroleptics possess some antimuscarinic effects, including, but not limited to, central anticholinergic syndromes of confusion, delirium, and psychosis; tremors; decreased salivation; urinary hesitancy or urinary retention (especially in older males); constipation, decreased intestinal motility that may clinically result in constipation or adynamic ileus; and blurred vision and exacerbation of narrow-angle glaucoma. The most potent antimuscarinic agent in this group is thioridazine, then chlorpromazine. All potent neuroleptics have minimal anticholinergic side-effects at clinical doses. Sedation appears to parallel anticholinergic potency.

When considering potentiality for both alpha-adrenergic and muscarinic blockade effects, one must remember that clincal dosage is not based on potency for side-effects but on effectiveness in dopamine receptor blockade. Thus because of the high doses used, the low potency neuroleptics are usually those associated with clinically significant symptoms from alpha adrenoceptor and muscarinic receptor antagonism.

FIG. 24-7. Site of action of neuroleptics at the dopamine synapse.

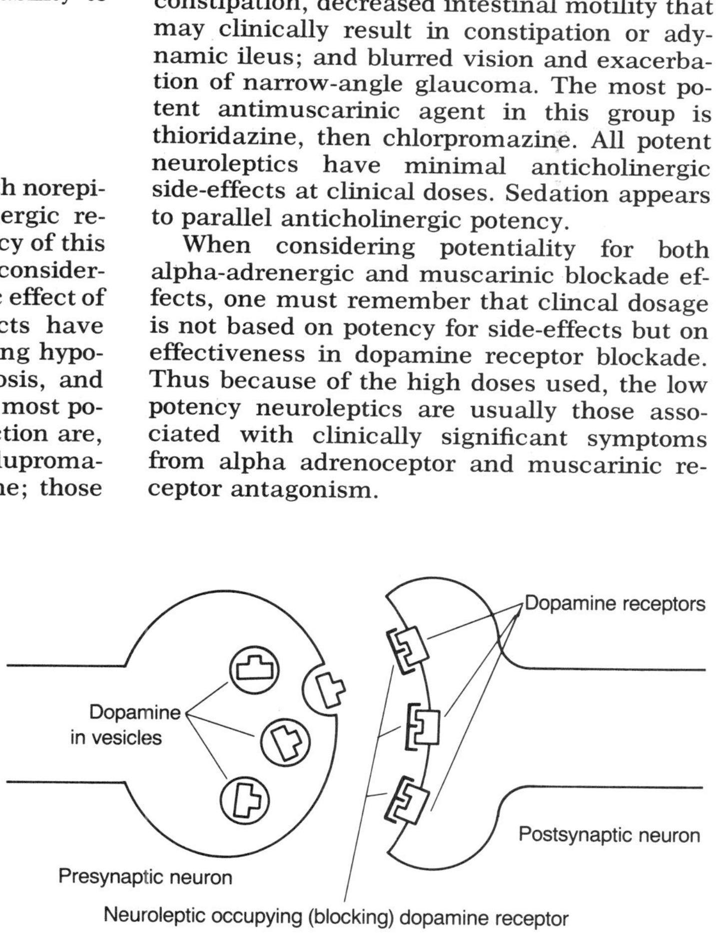

ABSORPTION

Neuroleptics are available in a wide range of preparations: tablet, liquid, rectal suppository, and parenteral preparations. Parenteral administration is generally 25% to 50% of the initial oral dose. Two long-acting parenteral forms of neuroleptics—*fluphenazine* esterified as a decanoate or enanthate—are slowly released after intramuscular injection.

Individual blood levels vary greatly after oral administration of any neuroleptic compound, perhaps reflecting genetic differences in their absorption and metabolism. The specific variables related to absorption are still being studied. The clinical import of these differences is that the optimal dosage range may vary many fold from one person to another. The wide interindividual range of absorption of neuroleptics is diminished considerably by the use of parenteral forms.

METABOLISM

Many neuroleptics have active metabolites, (chlorpromazine has more than 20), immensely complicating studies of their metabolism. Two major metabolic mechanisms for their metabolism exist: glucuronic conjugation and oxidation by hepatic microsomal enzymes. Induction of both hepatic metabolism and conjugation occurs with chlorpromazine and is probably a factor with other less potent neuroleptics. Thus blood levels and possibly clinical response may diminish over time owing to increased metabolism of the active compound.

Metabolism may be impaired with consequent increased drug levels in patients with liver disease, the elderly, children, and, of course, the fetus. The half-life of the neuroleptic drugs varies considerably as a function of the differences in metabolism between individuals. Commonly a figure of 12 to 24 hours is given for the elimination half-life (penfluridol and pimozide excepted); however, although the half-life is relatively long compared to that of many other compounds, the biologic effects of the neuroleptics tend to persist for a much longer time. Electroencephalographic changes in patients who have been maintained on neuroleptic therapy have been found up to 2 months after the drugs have been withdrawn, and active metabolites of some compounds are excreted for weeks after the drug has been withdrawn. Because of this prolonged biologic effect, the entire daily dose of any neuroleptic is commonly given at one time once the patient is on maintenance dosage. Sustained release preparations make little sense for drugs with such long half-lives. During the initial acute treatment phases, however, the dose is commonly divided several times during the day, minimizing the sedative side-effects and allowing for a more rapid increase in dosage. The depot injectable or long-acting oral forms of neuroleptic drugs are, however, extremely useful for many schizophrenic patients who, because of their illness, are not responsible enough to take medication reliably each day.

The large variation in individual metabolism of neuroleptic drugs necessarily results in a wide range of therapeutic doses. Generally there seems to be a tendency in the United States to use too high a regimen, especially on schizophrenic patients. Commonly used initial dosages are shown in Table 24-1.

CLINICAL PHARMACOLOGY

SCHIZOPHRENIA

Except for neuroleptic drugs used specifically to treat nausea, all compounds of this class have been shown to be an effective single main treatment for acute and chronic schizophrenia. Neuroleptic drugs are significantly more effective than placebos or purely sedative agents in treating this disease. There are no data showing that one neuroleptic is more effective than another or that a combination is more effective than a single neuroleptic drug given alone. The drugs normalize the patient's behavior and thinking. Thus, withdrawn and retarded, as well as agitated and hyperactive, schizophrenic patients tend to become normalized with any neuroleptic drug. Contrary to popular belief, the less sedating neuroleptics are just as effective as the more sedating ones for any of the behavioral subtypes of this disorder. The less potent neuroleptic drugs tend to be overused to "sedate" agitated or violent patients. If such behavior is secondary to a psychosis, it will respond favorably and as rapidly to any neuroleptic agent. Sedation *per se* can be better achieved with short-acting barbiturates, which will not cloud the diagnostic picture or produce side-effects common to neuroleptic drugs. Generally the acute symptoms respond most rapidly and substantially to neuroleptic drugs: hallucinations, delusions, poor sleep, fearfulness, combativeness, hyperactivity, and asocialization. Symptoms that have become chronic and those referable to insight, judgment, and affect are less likely to re-

TABLE 24-1. Neuroleptic Compounds

Form*	Drug†	Daily Oral Starting Dose‡		Antipsychotic Potency	Class
		Psychiatric	*Antiemetic*		
		mg			
Also R	Chlorpromazine	100–400	10–100	Low	Aliphatic
	Triflupromazine	50–200	20–30	Low	Phenothiazine
Not parenteral	Thioridazine	25–200		Low	Piperidine
	Mesoridazine	50–150		Moderate	Phenothiazine
Also R	Prochlorperazine		10–50		
	Perphenazine	16–64	8–16	Moderate	Piperazine
	Trifluoperazine	10–20		High	Phenothiazine
Also D	Fluphenazine	2.5–10 (depot 12.5–50 q 1–3 weeks)		High	
	Thiothixene	5–20		High	Thioxanthene
	Haloperidol	5–15		High	Butyrophenone
	Loxapine	20–50		Moderate	Dibenzoxazepine
Tablet only	Molindone	25–75		Moderate	Dihydroindolone
(Not yet available in USA)	Pimozide	1–5		High	Diphenylbutylpiperidine
	Penfluridol	20–80 (orally q week)		High	

* All are available as pills, liquid, and parenteral preparations except as indicated. R = rectal suppository, D = depot injectable. Parenteral dosage should be 30–50% of low oral dosage, particularly with low potency agents.

† Only the more common neuroleptics are listed.

‡ Dosage for outpatients, medically ill patients, and geriatric patients should be decreased by 50%, particularly with low potency agents. Initial daily dosage is usually divided into 2–4 increments.

spond to treatment. Improvement generally occurs within the first few days after starting neuroleptic agents and continues for about 6 weeks. Slower improvement then continues for several months, at which time the patient's behavior and social skills tend to plateau. Commonly, well-diagnosed schizophrenic patients are placed on maintenance neuroleptic medication to prevent relapse of psychosis. There is a consensus from several excellent, well-controlled studies that most schizophrenic persons will have severe repeated relapses unless they are maintained on neuroleptic medication. Most patients need not be maintained, however, on the high doses given during the acute treatment phase. It is clinically important to give the lowest effective dose to minimize the likelihood of developing severe extrapyramidal side-effects such as tardive dyskinesia.

MANIA

During the manic phase of bipolar disorder, treatment with lithium alone has not been found to be as rapidly effective as has a combination of lithium and a neuroleptic agent. As in schizophrenia, one neuroleptic drug is as effective as another. Common clinical experience suggests that very high doses of neuroleptic agents may be needed to control severe manic behavior. After the mania is under control, the neuroleptic drug should be slowly decreased over several weeks, after which the patient may be kept on lithium therapy alone (*see* Chap. 22).

DEPRESSION

Neuroleptic medications are not generally considered as effective as antidepressants or electroconvulsive therapy in the treatment of depression (*see* Chap. 22). When used for severe agitated and psychotic depression, however, they rapidly and effectively diminish the agitated and psychotic aspects of the episode. Commonly they are initially combined with standard antidepressants and then discontinued within several weeks, as the antidepressants alone are continued. The use of combination drugs that contain an antidepressant and neuroleptic agent for long-term treatment of patients with depression should be discouraged because of the likelihood of developing tardive dyskinesia.

OTHER PSYCHOSES

Patients who develop acute psychoses as an apparent reaction to life stresses, medical procedures, or drug abuse (*see* Chap. 26; LSD or amphetamines) respond rapidly to neuroleptic drugs. Treatment is usually discontinued a few days after clinical remission occurs.

NEUROSES

The risk of side-effects is such that neuroleptic drugs are rarely indicated for neuroses. Few, if any, neurotic disorders have been found to respond better to neuroleptic agents than to other compounds. Their use is temporarily indicated for mildly ill patients who may be threatened with emerging psychotic features.

CHRONIC BRAIN SYNDROMES

In organic mental syndromes with mild to severe psychotic features such as delusion, agitation, and disorientation, low doses of the potent neuroleptic drugs may diminish these symptoms so that the patient may be more confortable and managed in a more open setting.

GILLES DE LA TOURETTE SYNDROME AND TICS

Standard treatment is very careful and slow titration of either haloperidol or pimozide. Relief of tics usually occurs at relatively low doses of either compound, but patients may be sensitive to as little as a 0.25-mg difference in dosage a day.

NAUSEA AND EMESIS

All neuroleptic drugs except thioridazine are effective in suppressing nausea and emesis due to central dopaminergic stimulation of the chemoreceptor trigger zone. The antiemetic effect occurs rapidly and with doses far below those that are antipsychotic. The compounds most commonly used for antiemetic effect are chlorpromazine, prochlorperazine, promethazine, triflupromazine, and perphenazine. The side-effects from the neuroleptic agents used as antiemetics are the same as for those used specifically as antipsychotic agents. Subsequently treatment of side-effects is the same.

ADVERSE EFFECTS

Before using neuroleptic drugs in children, geriatric patients, and medically ill patients, one should remember side-effects, which are more likely to occur in these populations (in particular, cardiovascular side-effects), and that dosages should be decreased by about one half to two thirds. There are no specific clinical contraindications to using any neuroleptic drug in these subgroups, but clinical experience suggests that agents likely to cause hypotension or that possess marked antimuscarinic effects should be avoided when possible.

Neuroleptic drugs are contraindicated in patients with Parkinson's disease because the blockage of dopamine receptors will worsen the disorder. Although not specifically linked to teratogenic effects, neuroleptic drugs are relatively contraindicated in pregnant and nursing women because they rapidly cross the placental barrier and enter breast milk in meaningful quantities.

The adverse effects most specific to neuroleptic drugs are those related to the extrapyramidal system. These effects are due to dopamine receptor blockade in the basal ganglia and can be divided into four major categories.

1. *Parkinsonian* features of bradykinesia, rigidity, and tremor are more likely to occur with potent neuroleptic agents. The parkinsonian symptoms seen with neuroleptic drugs are virtually exact duplicates of those seen in idiopathic Parkinson's syndrome. These side-effects may diminish significantly after several weeks of neuroleptic treatment.
2. *Akathesia* is a very important but less common side-effect. This syndrome includes an inner sense of restlessness, which may mimic agitation or anxiety. The patient may progress to feeling compulsed to move his legs or his whole body, sometimes jumping out of the chair and rolling on the floor. The diagnosis of akathesia is extremely important lest it be thought that the patient's illness is worsening and his neuroleptic dosage be raised. This side-effect is more common with the potent neuroleptic agents.
3. Acute extrapyramidal effects include *dystonias,* which are spasms of muscle groups in the face, neck, back, or extremities. These usually occur within the first 2 weeks of treatment and are immediately reversed by anticholinergic agents.
4. *Tardive dyskinesia* usually does not occur until after the patient has been exposed to neuroleptic drugs for more than 12 months.

It may be found in as many as 35% of persons given prolonged maintenance treatment with neuroleptic agents. Older patients and women are more susceptible. Patients may develop tardive dyskinesia while they are taking neuroleptic drugs or, more commonly, when they are acutely withdrawn from such drugs. Contrary to common belief, if diagnosed early, tardive dyskinesia generally will gradually remit over 6 months to 1 year. Symptoms of tardive dyskinesia are rhythmic, involuntary, muscle movements occurring over the face, mouth, and tongue as well as in the extremities. Tardive dyskinesia may be due to development of supersensitivity of dopamine receptors after prolonged blockade.

TREATMENT OF ADVERSE EFFECTS

Extrapyramidal side-effects can be controlled by using anticholinergic drugs or amantadine, which are effective for most anticholinergic symptoms except tardive dyskinesia and, to a lesser extent, akathesia. These drugs are usually given in divided doses during the day with the dosage being titrated by the patient's clinical response. Care must be exercised with anticholinergic agents because they can cause confusion or psychosis, which may mimic the patient's illness and result in an unnecessary dosage increase of neuroleptic drug. Initiating prophylactic use of these agents at the same time that neuroleptic drug therapy is started is controversial. Compliance in some patients is increased if they do not experience any extrapyramidal effects. Their routine chronic use without consideration of the patient's pharmacologic and neurologic status is poor practice.

Compounds most commonly used are benztropine (0.5–10 mg daily); trihexyphenidyl (2–10 mg daily); biperiden (2–8 mg daily); procyclidine (5–20 mg daily); and amantadine (100–200 mg daily). Diphenhydramine, 50 mg parenterally, will acutely reverse most dystonias within 5 minutes of administration.

INTERACTION WITH OTHER DRUGS AND MEDICAL CONDITIONS

The more sedating neuroleptic agents potentiate the respiratory depression of anesthetic agents and opiates. Significant alpha-adrenoceptor blockade can unpredictably affect blood pressure in persons taking antihypertensive drugs. The effect of neuroleptic agents on cardiac function is probably insignificant for the very potent neuroleptics, but the anticholinergic actions of thioridazine and chlorpromazine may cause tachycardia. Thioridazine, in particular, has quinidine-like effects similar to the tricyclic antidepressants and can cause mild myocardial depression. Other less common clinical interactions reported in only a few patients taking chlorpromazine include increased cholesterol, impairment of glucose tolerance, photosensitivity, and a gray–blue skin pigmentation in exposed body areas. Pigmentary retinopathy has been reported only with thioridazine in doses greater than 1000 mg/day. Blood dyscrasias with neuroleptic drugs are rare. Patients who develop symptoms of respiratory infection, however, while taking neuroleptic agents, should be evaluated immediately and have a complete blood count and differential. The occurrence of an obstructive jaundice with high alkaline phosphatase and bilirubin levels is also rare, and most reports of this have been limited to the phenothiazine class of neuroleptic drugs. The jaundice clears over weeks to months following withdrawal. Since the etiology of the obstructive jaundice is thought to be an idiosyncratic hypersensitivity reaction, patients can be treated concomitantly with another class of neuroleptic drugs, while liver function tests are serially followed.

Other side-effects of neuroleptic drugs include drowsiness, which is usually accommodated within a week of treatment. Most patients who receive low potency neuroleptic agents experience drowsiness during the initial treatment phase, and they should be warned about it.

Weight gain is common with all neuroleptic agents except molindone. A gain of 10% to 20% of baseline body weight is fairly common, and some patients develop overt obesity. The relationship of weight gain to alteration of endocrine systems or glucose metabolism is controversial.

The less potent phenothiazines are associated with lowering of the seizure threshold. The neuroleptic drugs least likely to affect the seizure threshold are fluphenazine, thiothixene, and molindone. When given to epileptic patients, neuroleptic drug doses should be increased slowly and carefully. If seizures occur and the drug cannot be withdrawn for clincal reasons, the anticonvulsant dosage should be increased.

Normal people who ingest an antipsychotic dose of neuroleptic agents report feelings of unreality, inability to feel pleasure, and difficulty in initiating activities. This occurrence is a sign that the diagnosis should be reevaluated. Withdrawal symptoms *per se* do not occur with neuroleptic medications, although some patients who have neuroleptic drugs abruptly withdrawn will develop nonspecific gastrointestinal symptoms. Convulsions do not occur after neuroleptic withdrawal.

Numerous endocrinologic effects occur from the use of neuroleptic agents. Dopaminergic blockade particularly is associated with markedly increased prolactin levels. This is not known to have any clinical consequence other than breast engorgement and galactorrhea in some male, as well as female, patients. One should ask about this side-effect because commonly people are embarrassed to mention it. It is treated by reassurance. Normally patients with established breast carcinoma are not given neuroleptic drugs because of the predictable increase of prolactin. There is an unknown incidence of inhibition of the release of growth hormone (also due to dopaminergic blockade but of no clinical significance) and ammenorrhea with chlorpromazine.

POISONING

Although overdosage of neuroleptic agents is relatively common, death from these drugs is rare. Combined with other sedative agents, neuroleptics (especially the less potent ones) may additively increase respiratory depression. The other serious effects of overdosage is marked hypertension, which again is more common with the less potent agents. If necessary, the blood pressure can be raised using phenylephrine or metaraminol, which are alpha-adrenoceptor agonists. Compounds that stimulate both alpha and beta receptors, such as norepinephrine, may produce further decrease in the blood pressure due to beta-adrenoceptor stimulation. (The alpha receptors are blocked by the neuroleptic agent.) Arrhythmias have not been specifically linked to neuroleptic drugs, but the less potent agents do have a quinidine-like effect, and thus quinidine or digitalis preparations should be given cautiously. Very rarely patients may develop a hypothalamic syndrome, manifested by inability to control body temperature and accompanied by tachycardia, diaphoresis, and delerium. This may develop very rapidly over 1 to 2 hours; it is a medical emergency requiring immediate admission to an intensive care unit with constant monitoring and external support of cardiovascular functions and temperature. Anticholinergic psychosis is not uncommonly seen with overdosage of the less potent neuroleptic agents. A careful differential diagnosis is essential so that additional neuroleptic drugs are not given for anticholinergic delerium. Most people poisoned with neuroleptic agents will become stuporous for hours to days but will respond to supportive care in an intensive care unit, where vital signs and respiratory functions can be closely monitored. Renal dialysis, alkalization, and forced diuresis are not effective. The use of stimulant drugs should be avoided because they may cause hyperpyrexia and convulsions.

FURTHER READING

1. Appleton S: Fourth psychoactive drug usage guide. J Clin Psychiatry 43:12–27, 1982
2. Davis JM: Overview: Maintenance therapy in psychiatry: 1. Schizophrenia. Am J Psychiatry 132:1237–1245, 1975
3. Feinberg AP, Snyder H: Phenothiazine drugs: Structure–activity relationships explained by a conformation that mimics dopamine. Proc Nat Acad Sci USA 72:1899–1903, 1975

CHAPTER 24 QUESTIONS

(See P. 7 for Full Instructions)

Select the One Best Answer

1. Chlorpromazine and reserpine are similar in that both agents
   A. possess antiepileptic activity.
   B. produce alpha-adrenergic receptor blockade.
   C. are clinically effective antiemetics.
   D. reduce catecholamine activity in the brain.
   E. can produce orthostatic hypotension.

2. Chlorpromazine may produce all of the following EXCEPT
   A. anticonvulsant effects.
   B. delayed menstruation.
   C. photosensitivity reactions.
   D. gynecomastia in males.
   E. disturbances in temperature regulation.

3. In a patient with manifestations of schizophrenia with acutely agitated behavior, the treatment of choice would be
   A. chlorpromazine.
   B. imipramine.
   C. diazepam.
   D. lithium carbonate.
   E. phenobarbital.

4. Which of the following antiemetic compounds is most likely to produce jaundice and parkinsonism when used for prolonged periods?

A. Dimenhydrinate
B. Chlorpromazine
C. Scopolamine
D. Meclizine
E. Diphenidol

A = 1,2,3; B = 1,3; C = 2,4; D = 4; E = All

5. Trifluoperazine is more likely than chlorpromazine to produce
   1. oversedation.
   2. postural hypotension.
   3. allergic skin reactions.
   4. Parkinson's syndrome.

6. Chlorpromazine administered chronically in high therapeutic doses may produce
   1. lens opacities.
   2. skin pigmentation.
   3. obstructive jaundice.
   4. tardive dyskinesia.

7. Chlorpromazine is effective as an antiemetic when nausea and vomiting are the result of
   1. radiation sickness.
   2. motion sickness.
   3. morphine administration.
   4. local irritation of the gastric mucosa.

8. The interactions of chlorpromazine with other drugs is shown by the
   1. prolongation of barbiturate sleeping-time.
   2. antagonism of alcohol depression.
   3. increased meperidine-induced respiratory depression.
   4. decreased analgesic effect of morphine.

GENERAL QUESTIONS ON NEUROLEPTIC DRUGS

Select the One Best Answer

1. All of the neuroleptic drugs have antipsychotic efficacy by virtue of
   A. blockade of norepinephrene receptors.
   B. blocking dopamine receptor.
   C. A and B above.
   D. reducing cholinergic tone in the limbic system.
   E. sedating the psychosis.

2. The more potent neuroleptics are
   A. less likely to cause extrapyramidal side-effects.
   B. less likely to cause anticholinergic side-effects.
   C. less likely to cause hypotension.
   D. A and B above.
   E. B and C above.

3. The dosage of neuroleptic drugs is best determined by
   A. serum blood levels.
   B. standard treatment tables.
   C. the patient's clinical response.
   D. using higher doses, which is always better.

4. Of the different classes of neuroleptics, the most effective for treating schizophrenia is
   A. phenothiazines.
   B. thioxanthines.
   C. butyrophenone.
   D. diphenylbutylpiperidines.
   E. all of the above because they all have equivalent antipsychotic properties.

5. Choose the symptoms that would most likely be troublesome during therapy with thioridazine.
   A. Blurred vision, orthostatic hypotension, and urinary retention.
   B. Muscle stiffness, rigidity, and bradykinesia.
   C. Dependence and addiction.
   D. All of these are equally likely.
   E. None of these is likely.

6. The neuroleptic drugs are particularly indicated for the treatment of
   A. mania.
   B. depression.
   C. schizophrenia.
   D. anxiety.
   E. A and C.

7. Overdoses with the neuroleptic drugs are *usually* associated with
   A. death.
   B. prolonged sedation.
   C. heart block.
   D. respiratory apnea.
   E. hypothalamic syndrome.

8. A patient taking prochlorperazine for 2 days develops acute spasm of the right sternocleidomastoid that pulls the head into a fixed turn to the left, accompanied by severe agitation and the feeling that he is going to "jump out of his skin." The appropriate treatment would be to
   A. call for a psychiatric consult.
   B. administer 50 mg of diphenylhydramine intramuscularly.
   C. administer 1 mg of haloperidol intramuscularly.
   D. administer 50 mg of secobarbital.
   E. administer 10 mg of diazepam intravenously.

25

RICHARD W. JOHNSON
HENRY I. YAMAMURA

Sedative-Hypnotics and Antianxiety Agents

Among the most widely used drugs in the physician's neuropharmacologic armamentarium are those that produce sedative/hypnotic or anxiolytic effects. The term "sedative-hypnotic" is actually somewhat atavistic, dating from the days when the only drugs available to sedate "disturbed" patients such as psychotics were those that, at higher doses, caused progressive central nervous system (CNS) depression and were therefore often used as hypnotic agents as well. However, the introduction of the phenothiazines and subsequent neuroleptic derivatives, often called "major tranquilizers," largely supplanted CNS depressants in the treatment of such neuropsychiatric conditions. The term "sedative," then, often implied antianxiety efficacy. Recent developments in neurochemistry, however, suggest that the sedative properties of certain drugs are mechanistically distinct and separate from their anxiolytic effects. One often encounters references to "minor tranquilizers"; this term includes all clinically used antianxiety agents. The two remaining therapeutic applications of the drugs discussed herein are as *hypnotics* (in the treatment of insomnia) and as *anticonvulsants*.

Historically, the oldest sedative/hypnotic agents are *opiates* and *alcohol*. More recently, during the 19th century, the *bromides* were introduced into medicine. Toward the beginning of the 20th century, *chloral derivatives* and *barbiturates* were found to be somewhat more convenient and efficacious and are still used widely today. The most recent class of sedative/hypnotic agents are the *nonbarbiturate* drugs, which at times have little or no advantage over the barbiturates but include certain agents that are clearly safer than the earlier sedative/hypnotic drugs, and other drugs that display enhanced pharmacologic specificity as compared to barbiturates and similar agents.

Many drugs used to induce sleep also have antianxiety effects; the ratio of the former action to the latter effect constitutes an important clinical consideration for any agent used to treat anxiety. Until recently the only drugs available for treating anxiety were sedative/hypnotic agents, the most widely used being barbiturates and, more recently, certain carbamates. A major and ineluctable side-effect of antianxiety medication, then, has always been sedation. Within the last few years, however, novel anxiolytics have been developed that are reportedly devoid of sedative effects, indicating that these actions are mechanistically distinct pharmacologic effects.

Barbiturates are often used as prototypes of sedative/hypnotic agents. Therefore the overall pharmacologic profile of the barbiturates is worth considering because of their still widespread use and the many similarities that exist between these agents and other, newer sedative/hypnotic drugs. Further, the barbiturates illustrate the addiction liability and withdrawal syndrome that characterize many CNS depressants.

The first half of this chapter focuses on the use of CNS depressants as sedative/hypnotic agents and includes an extensive description of barbiturates. Newer sedative/hypnotic agents are then discussed with reference to these drugs. It will quickly become apparent that pharmacologic similarities between most sedative/hypnotic agents are quite extensive.

The second half of the chapter deals with anxiolytic pharmacotherapy, the prototypical drugs being the benzodiazepines; other CNS depressants still used as antianxiety agents are, however, also mentioned. Finally, the rationale for development of novel antianxiety drugs is discussed, along with the pharmacologic characteristics of such drugs known to science but yet to be introduced into clinical medicine.

Many of the drugs listed herein also have pronounced anticonvulsant activity and have been used in the acute control of certain types of convulsions. The suitability of a particular compound for long-term anticonvulsant therapy is, however, dictated not only by its anticonvulsant efficacy, but also by sedation and impaired judgment. The ideal anticonvulsant would have no appreciable sedative/hypnotic activity, although this cannot be said of any drug in this chapter. Certain drugs, however, have an acceptable balance for long-term use as anticonvulsants. Among the barbiturates, phenobarbital has the optimal anticonvulsant specificity and is thus widely used both acutely and chronically to treat certain types of epilepsy. Additionally, certain benzodiazepines are gaining popularity as anticonvulsants in certain conditions, including status epilepticus and petit mal seizures. The suitability of various agents for anticonvulsant pharmacotherapy is discussed as the drugs appear throughout this chapter.

SEDATIVE/HYPNOTIC AGENTS

The treatment of insomnia is a very frequently occurring problem for today's physician. Unfortunately, there is no panacea among the myriad sedative/hypnotic drugs available. Each has certain drawbacks, and some have associated problems that preclude their being used by an intelligent practitioner to treat a patient who has difficulty in sleeping.

Insomnia is a very real and often highly debilitating condition. Lack of sleep can quickly lead to a variety of serious neurotic and even psychotic phenomena, and therefore an efficacious treatment is important. Ultimately, the physician must compromise and accept certain liabilities in order to offer some form of drug treatment under these circumstances.

BARBITURATES

Chemistry

No pharmacology textbook would be complete without an account of Baeyer's original synthesis of barbituric acid from malonic acid and urea. Baeyer reportedly decided on the name "barbituric" for the resulting cyclic diureide while celebrating at a local pub with a group of artillery officers whose patron saint was St. Barbara, which amalgamated with "urea" formed the word "barbituric." All clinically used barbiturates are derivatives of barbituric acid, which is itself devoid of CNS depressant effects but is subject to modification by altering the nature of the substituents at four basic points, as summarized in Table 25-1. The pharmacologic profile of a particular barbiturate is a function of the exact combination of substituents composing that barbituric acid derivative.

The barbiturates are very weak acids that exhibit an interesting acid/base equilibrium. In most drug molecules, nitrogen-containing functions are, if anything, basic. However, the electron-withdrawing effect of the carbonyl moiety adjacent to the amide nitrogen at position #1 facilitates ionization of the amide hydrogen by stabilizing the resulting negative charge, which is actually borne by the carbonyl oxygen atom by means of keto-enol tautomerization (Fig. 25-1).

Because ionization of the barbiturates occurs only in highly alkaline solutions, the injectable barbiturate preparations are strongly basic and, as such, can cause extensive tissue necrosis if not carefully administered. At physiologic pH levels, however, barbiturates exist largely in their nonionized forms and are therefore highly lipid soluble.

The structure–activity relationships of the barbiturates have been extensively characterized and can be exploited by selecting a partic-

TABLE 25-1. Barbituric Acid Derivatives

Drug	Trade Name	Duration	R1	R2*	R3	R4
Phenobarbital	Luminal	Long	C_2H_5	C_6H_5	0	H
Mephobarbital	Mebaral	Long	C_2H_5	C_6H_5	0	CH_3
Metharbital	Gemonil	Long	C_2H_5	C_2H_5	0	CH_3
Amobarbital	Amytal	Intermediate	C_2H_5	1	0	H
Butabarbital	Butabon	Intermediate	C_2H_5	2	0	H
Pentobarbital	Nembutal	Short	C_2H_5	3	0	H
Secobarbital	Seconal	Short	$CH_2CH{=}CH_2$	3	0	H
Hexabarbital	Sombucaps	Ultrashort	CH_3	4	0	H
Thiamylal	Surital	Ultrashort	C_3H_5	3	S	H
Thiopental	Pentothal	Ultrashort	C_2H_5	3	S	H

* 1 = isopentyl; 2 = sec-butyl; 3 = 1-methylbutyl; 4 = 1-cyclohexen-1-yl.

ular derivative for a given clinical application. Phenobarbital, for example, is a barbituric acid derivative with an aromatic substituent at C5. This relatively minor structural feature confers a pronounced anticonvulsant action (*see* Chap. 29). Other structural variations may alter their effective durations of action. Overall trends in this regard, however, appear to involve the physicochemical properties of a particular derivative as opposed to the actual steric parameters that characterize a given combination of structural variables. Variations in the properties of various barbiturates consist mainly of differences in potency, rapidity of onset, and duration of action.

The most important physicochemical variable that can be related to the pharmacologic characteristics of barbituric acid derivatives is their lipid/water partition coefficients. There is a strong positive correlation between potency and lipophilicity; further, more hydrophobic barbiturates have a faster onset of action and, because of enhanced metabolic degradation, a shorter duration of action. Additionally, lipophilicity and the overall extent of metabolic biotransformation correlate strongly such that while the least hydrophobic barbiturates may be excreted unchanged in the urine, the fraction of a more hydrophobic derivative that may be excreted unchanged in the urine is negligible. The most highly lipophilic barbiturates, the thiobarbiturates, have a sulphur atom instead of an oxygen at C3 and are therefore more lipophilic than the corresponding oxybarbiturates. The thiobarbiturates have such a brief duration of action that they are not used as sedative/hypnotic or anxiolytic agents but in the induction of surgical anesthesia. A large bolus injection of thiopental, for example, results in loss of consciousness within several seconds. This effect, though, is extremely short-lived, owing to redistribution of the thiopental from the brain to less well-perfused tissues, not to rapid metabolic inactivation. The barbiturates themselves have no actual analgesic effect and are usually combined with a gaseous anesthetic agent for surgical anesthesia.

FIG. 25-1. Acid–base chemistry of barbituric acid derivatives.

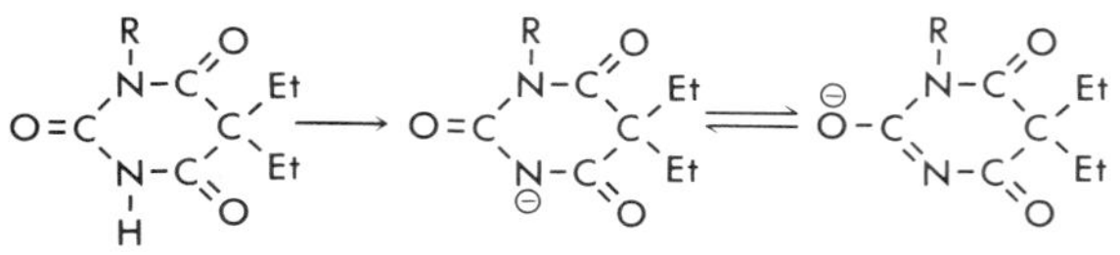

Absorption, Metabolism, and Excretion

Variations in the pharmacokinetic disposition of barbiturates depend largely on their lipophilicity. The following generalizations apply best to derivatives that have intermediate degrees of hydrophobicity.

Most barbiturates are well absorbed after oral administration and, when given as sedative/hypnotic agents, are administered almost exclusively by this route.

Metabolism of barbiturates yields hydrophilic derivatives that are more readily excretable. The half-life of certain barbiturates in the body, interestingly, would be decades rather than days or hours without metabolic biotransformation.

The most important metabolic reaction is oxidation of the substituents at C5. Generally the larger of the two side-chains at this point is converted to an oxygen-containing function that can either be excreted directly or first be conjugated with glucuronic acid. Other metabolic fates include N-dealkylation, ring cleavage, and, with the thiobarbiturates, replacement of the sulphur atom with oxygen. N-Demethylation can yield pharmacologically active products; for example, methabarbital is converted to barbital, and mephobarbital is transformed into phenobarbital by this enzymatic reaction.

Hydrophilic barbiturates are not extensively metabolized because they do not dissolve well in microsomal membranes and because they can be excreted in the urine without transformation into polar derivatives. Physical redistribution rather than metabolic inactivation is the primary mechanism for terminating the effects of the highly lipophilic, ultra-short-acting thiobarbiturates, although these drugs, too, are eventually metabolized and excreted.

Major Actions

Barbiturates are general depressants that inhibit various cellular functions in many different tissues. Their relevant actions stem from selective inhibition of neuronal activity at certain loci within the CNS. Barbiturates induce sleep similar to, with the exception of a certain degree of REM suppression, normal physiologic sleep.

When administered in increasing dosages, barbiturates produce progressive CNS depression ranging from mild sedation to hypnosis and eventually to coma and death. Although the exact molecular mechanism of action is incompletely understood, clinical levels appear to have a relatively selective effect on synaptic transmission in the reticular activating system. Depression of neural function at this locus can account for certain effects of barbiturates, including their hypnotic action. At progressively higher doses, though, barbiturates begin to inhibit neurons nonselectively in all brain areas. The anxiolytic action of these drugs may be mediated through some neuroanatomical locus besides the reticular activating system. Similarly the anticonvulsant effects of certain barbiturates appear to be mechanistically and anatomically distinct from their sedative/hypnotic actions.

Subsidiary Actions

The cardiovascular and respiratory depression accompanying barbiturate-induced sleep is similar to that characterizing physiologic sleep. At higher doses, however, barbiturates are respiratory depressants and progressively inhibit respiratory drive of neurogenic, chemical, and even hypoxic origin. Similarly, while hypnotic levels of barbiturates have no significant effect on the cardiovascular system other than a slightly decreased heart rate and blood pressure similar to that which accompanies ordinary sleep, extremely large doses of barbiturates may inhibit myocardial contractility. Although vascular smooth muscle is unaffected by hypnotic doses of barbiturates, high concentrations effect relaxation.

Metabolic biotransformation by the liver is the major route of termination of barbiturate activity. Barbiturates, in turn, exert two reciprocal effects on the P-450 system (*see* Chap. 4). Acutely, barbiturates, being substrates for the P-450 metabolic enzymes, competitively inhibit the metabolism of many other endogenous and exogenous substances whose biotransformation is catalyzed by these enzymes. Chronically, barbiturates rank at the top of a large number of drugs that induce this hepatic microsomal enzyme system. The resulting augmentation of enzyme activity results in an acceleration not only of the metabolism of barbiturates but also of a host of other exogenous and endogenous substances. This pharmacokinetic alteration by no means fully accounts for barbiturate tolerance that involves a very substantial pharmacodynamic component as well.

A very serious, albeit fairly infrequent, consequence of hepatic microsomal enzyme induction occurs in patients who suffer from *intermittent polyporphyria*, an aberration in heme metabolism characterized by the production, by the microsomal enzymes in the liver, of a very toxic metabolite. Induction of hepatic microsomal enzymes will result in production of extremely high levels of this toxic substance, thereby precipitating a crisis in patients who suffer from this condition. Obviously, then, barbiturates and other compounds that cause hepatic microsomal enzyme induction are strictly contraindicated in such patients. Unfortunately many other sedative/hypnotic agents mimic the barbiturates with respect to hepatic microsomal enzyme induction and are therefore also contraindicated.

Mechanism of Action

Barbiturates are CNS depressants and, at higher doses, are nonspecific inhibitors of cellular function throughout the body.

Although there is a plethora of information on the cellular and systemic effects of barbiturates, the exact molecular mechanism by which these agents produce such effects has yet to be defined precisely. The complexity of this issue is compounded when one considers that the different pharmacologic effects of barbiturates may involve distinct molecular mechanisms. Moreover, cause and effect relations between the biochemical effects produced by these drugs and their concomitant cellular and systemic effects are difficult to define.

The involvement of "barbiturate receptors" in the mechanism of action of barbiturates has recently been studied, although the use of the term "receptor" in this context may be somewhat misleading. Early theories on the mechanism of action of barbiturates implied, by analogy to the general (gaseous) anesthetics, that barbiturates, being highly lipophilic compounds, acted by dissolving in the lipid bilayer of the nerve membrane, rendering them less excitable. Stabilization of excitable membranes would presumably involve increasing resistance to sodium ion movement. This general hypothesis was supported by the strong correlation between potency and lipophilicity for a series of barbiturates. Clearly the concept of barbiturate receptors, even using the least strict definition of "receptor," has no place in such a mechanism.

Certain considerations, however, indicate that the mechanism of barbiturate action is somewhat more complex than is suggested by the foregoing model. Given the foregoing concept of "receptor," the macromolecule to which a barbiturate binds to produce a particular effect obviously must have some relatively important physiologic role such that this event results in an altered cellular function. With regard to the effects of barbiturates on nerve cells, ion channels are logical candidates as pharmacologically relevant barbiturate binding sites. Thus certain effects of barbiturates on neuronal conduction may involve sodium channels. These so-called local anesthetic effects, however, may not be relevant to the characteristic clinical effects of the drugs. More recently, barbiturates have been suggested to bind to chloride channels, which may also be linked to gamma-aminobutyric acid (GABA) receptors and benzodiazepine binding sites, possibly eliciting a conformational change in the proteinaceous ionophore that facilitates the flux of chloride ions across the nerve membrane and thereby causing hyperpolarization and stabilization of the membrane. Referring to sodium channels as "barbiturate receptors" does not imply that an endogenous ligand exists for these binding sites. Evidence suggests, however, that there may be an endogenous substance that binds to barbiturate receptors associated with the chloride channel/GABA receptor complex.

Certain effects of barbiturates can, insofar as they involve inhibition of neuronal activity, be explained by the foregoing mechanism. Other effects may well involve different mechanisms, for example, structure–activity considerations indicate that the anticonvulsant action of barbiturates may be mechanistically distinct from their sedative/hypnotic effects. If both of these processes are receptor mediated, as defined above, there would appear to be multiple, functionally distinct types of macromolecules to which the barbiturates may bind.

Adverse Effects

In addition to the suppression of REM sleep (*see* above), other minor adverse effects of barbiturates on the normal sleep-waking cycle include drowsiness and a "hangover" syndrome often experienced on the morning after use of these drugs as hypnotic agents. Short-acting compounds have a lower incidence of this effect and are preferred to longer-acting drugs in the treatment of insomnia.

Another common adverse effect is sometimes referred to as *paradoxic excitation*. At sedative/hypnotic doses, certain patients fail to exhibit the usual tranquil response to barbiturates and manifest restlessness, excitement, or even delirium. This response may relate to the release of inhibitions that accompanies mild barbiturate intoxication, which is quite similar to the effect of alcohol in some persons. The neurophysiological basis of this phenomenon may involve an effect known as "barbiturate activation," whereby neurons in certain brain areas may be stimulated instead of inhibited by moderate barbiturate concentrations.

Excitement and delirium are occasionally seen when these drugs are administered to patients experiencing pain. In some experimental animals, barbiturates have a pronounced hyperalgesic effect and may even antagonize the effects of analgesic agents. Obviously coadministration of a suitable analgesic with the barbiturate is advisable under these conditions.

Barbiturates are contraindicated in patients with intermittent polyporphyria and should be administered cautiously to patients who suffer from pulmonary or hepatic disease. Hypersensitivity occurs occasionally and may produce extensive damage to the liver, often accompanied by dermatitis and dysfunction of other parenchymous tissues. The most common and dangerous adverse effect associated with chronic use of barbiturates is addiction. Barbiturates are typical of many other CNS depressants in this regard. Abuse of barbiturates is often coupled with abuse of another highly addictive CNS depressant, alcohol. Ingested together, alcohol and barbiturates are *synergistic*, and combined abuse of barbiturates and alcohol is difficult to manage and constitutes a major health problem (*see* Chap. 27).

NONBARBITURATE SEDATIVE/HYPNOTIC AGENTS

In Table 25-2 are listed a number of commonly used nonbarbiturate sedative/hypnotic agents, along with their trade names, relative durations of action, and dosages. More complete descriptions of each drug are included below.

CHLORAL HYDRATE

Chloral hydrate, a white crystalline substance, has an aromatic odor and a bitter taste and is soluble in water and alcohol.

Major Actions

Along with other hydrate derivatives, chloral hydrate is a relatively safe and efficacious hypnotic agent that at one time was widely used. Although its use has waned appreciably during the last few decades, chloral hydrate has been used especially as a geriatric hypnotic during the last few years.

The overall effects of chloral hydrate are largely indistinguishable from the barbiturates. Moreover it shares the barbiturates' lack of analgesic activity. Like the barbiturates, chloral hydrate has some anticonvulsant activity, although the ratio of its anticonvulsant effects to its sedative/hypnotic effects renders it unsuitable for long-term anticonvulsant prophylaxis. Similarly, while complete anesthesia can be achieved with large doses of chloral hydrate, the long-lasting respiratory depression produced under these conditions limits its suitability for the induction of surgical anesthesia, which is much more efficiently achieved by the

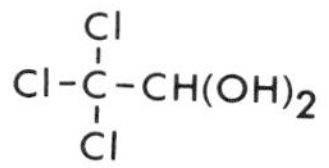

FIG. 25-2. Structure of chloralhydrate.

ultra-short-acting barbiturates. Thus chloral hydrate is largely limited to use as a sleep-inducing agent. At the usual dose of 0.5 to 1.0 g, chloral hydrate produces sedation within 15 minutes, usually followed by sleep within 1 hour and lasting from 5 to 8 hours.

An additional use of chloral hydrate at one time was in conjunction with alcohol as knockout drops, known commonly as a "Mickey Finn." Like other CNS depressants, chloral hydrate is synergistically potentiated by alcohol, and therefore such knockout drops mixed into a cocktail can produce a potent hypnotic effect.

Absorption, Metabolism, and Excretion

Chloral hydrate, on oral administration, is rapidly absorbed. Its characteristic pharmacologic effects appear to be produced largely by trichloroethanol, a metabolite of chloral hydrate that is itself a potent hypnotic. Chloral hydrate's action is terminated by metabolic biotransformation in the liver, where trichloroethanol is conjugated with glucuronic acid, forming a highly polar compound readily excreted in the urine and, to a small extent, in the bile.

Adverse Reactions

As with barbiturates and other CNS depressants, chronic intoxication with chloral hydrate can be accompanied by tolerance and physical dependence. The symptoms that accompany withdrawal of chloral hydrate from an addicted person are characteristically quite severe, often including delirium.

TABLE 25-2. Nonbarbiturate Sedative/Hypnotic Agents

Drug	Trade Name	Duration	Dose
Chloral hydrate	Noctec	Short	0.5–1.0 g
Paraldehyde		Short	5–10 ml
Ethchlorvynol	Placidyl	Short	500–700 mg
Ethinamate	Valmid	Short	0.5–1.0 g
Glutethimide	Doriden	Intermediate	250–500 mg
Methyprylon	Nodular	Intermediate	200–400 mg
Methaqualone	Quaalude	Intermediate	150–300 mg
Flurazepam	Dalmane	Intermediate	15–30 mg

PARALDEHYDE

Paraldehyde is an orally active hypnotic agent somewhat less potent than chloral hydrate. It is a colorless liquid with a characteristic odor and an unpleasant taste.

FIG. 25-3. Structure of paraldehyde.

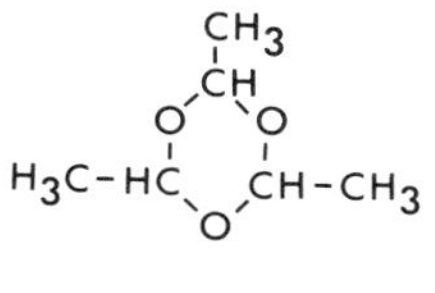

Major Actions

Paraldehyde, a relatively safe hypnotic, produces sleep accompanied by negligible alterations in respiration and circulation. Like the barbiturates, this sedative/hypnotic agent has no appreciable analgesic activity and can produce delirium in the presence of pain. It has marked anticonvulsant activity but is not used chronically to treat epilepsy, although it has been used in emergency treatment of certain convulsions. It is also used in the management of various abstinence syndromes and in certain types of anesthesia.

Absorption, Metabolism, and Excretion

After ingestion of the usual dose of 4 to 8 ml of paraldehyde, the patient falls asleep very rapidly, often within 10 to 15 minutes. Paraldehyde is rapidly metabolized by the liver, although a significant fraction of an oral dose is excreted by way of the lungs, imparting a characteristic unpleasant odor. Because of the odor, paraldehyde is not preferred by ambulatory patients and is therefore not usually subject to abuse. In fact, the reputation of paraldehyde as a relatively safe hypnotic may be partly due to its usual administration under controlled conditions by trained personnel. Chronic use of this drug is, however, accompanied by tolerance and physical dependence; as with other CNS depressants, withdrawal can be characterized by severe, highly unpleasant symptoms, sometimes including vivid hallucinations. In certain respects, paraldehyde addiction resembles addiction to alcohol, and the paraldehyde withdrawal syndrome may be accompanied by delirium tremens.

ETHCHLORVYNOL

Ethchlorvynol, a colorless or yellow liquid with a pungent odor, discolors on exposure to air and light.

Major Actions

This tertiary alcohol is an effective sedative/hypnotic agent with a rapid onset and a short duration of action. As with the drugs above, ethchlorvynol is pharmacologically similar to the barbiturates in several respects; for example, the EEG pattern that characterizes ethchlorvynol-induced sedation and sleep is similar to that after administration of barbiturates. Further, ethchlorvynol has anticonvulsant effects besides its sedative/hypnotic action.

The short duration of action of ethchlorvynol is in contrast to that of another related tertiary alcohol, meparfynol, whose long duration of action limits its clinical usefulness. The transient effects of ethchlorvynol render it suitable for treatment of insomnia when the patient has difficulty falling asleep as opposed to insomnia characterized by interrupted sleep.

Absorption, Metabolism, and Excretion

Ethchlorvynol is adequately absorbed after oral administration, producing CNS depression within 30 minutes and achieving maximal blood concentrations within 60 to 90 minutes. Ethchlorvynol is metabolized primarily in the liver but does not induce hepatic microsomal enzymes.

FIG. 25-4. Structure of ethchlorvynol.

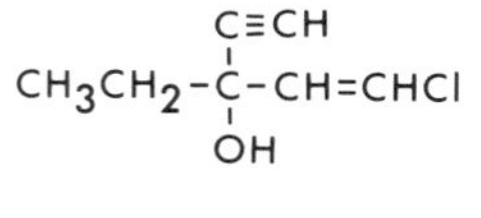

ETHINAMATE AND MEPROBAMATE

Chemistry

Esterification of monohydric alcohols with carbamic acid produces a class of compounds known as urethanes, which includes ethinamate. Meprobamate is a dicarbamate of a dihydric alcohol and has been thought to exhibit a somewhat wider spectrum of action than ethinamate.

Major Actions

Ethinamate is pharmacologically quite similar to the barbiturates: It has a rapid onset of action, and its sedative/hypnotic effects are relatively short lived. Thus, like ethchlorvynol, it is ideally suited to people who have trouble falling asleep but who, once asleep, remain so for the night.

Absorption, Metabolism, and Excretion

Ethinamate is adequately absorbed after oral administration. It is metabolized by the liver, first by hydroxylation, followed by conjugation of the resulting alcoholic function with glucuronic acid and excretion in the urine.

FIG. 25-5. Structure of ethinamate.

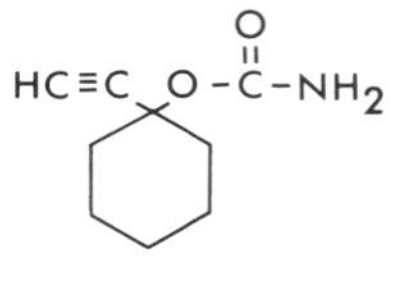

Adverse Effects

Prolonged administration of large doses of ethinamate may result in addiction, and the associated withdrawal syndrome is similar to that of barbiturates and other CNS depressants.

Nausea and, less frequently, vomiting are occasional side-effects of ethinamate administration. More infrequent side-effects include rash and, rarely, fever and thrombocytopenia.

Meprobamate is an effective sedative/hypnotic agent that is more often used as an anxiolytic (*see* below). As a sedative/hypnotic agent, meprobamate is similar to barbiturates and other CNS depressants.

Abuse of meprobamate is common, partly owing to its widespread use as a minor tranquilizer. Like all of the preceding examples, meprobamate is addictive and is characterized by an abstinence syndrome of the CNS depressant type.

GLUTETHIMIDE AND METHYPRYLON

Although glutethimide and methyprylon are both piperidinediones with many structural similarities, their pharmacologic characteristics differ markedly.

Glutethimide is a white powder that is practically insoluble in water. Thus it has a high lipid/water partition coefficient.

Glutethimide was introduced as a sedative/hypnotic agent in 1954 and was thought to be a nonbarbiturate drug devoid, according to popular sentiment at that time, of many of the problems associated with barbiturate use. As with many other drugs, however, the initial widespread use of glutethimide showed it to be much more dangerous than originally thought. In fact, the consensus today suggests that glutethimide is at least as addictive as the barbiturates and perhaps even more toxic while actually being therapeutically inferior in certain respects. Moreover, treatment of glutethimide overdoses is complicated by the highly lipophilic nature of the drug, which precludes elimination by dialysis.

FIG. 25-6. Structure of meprobamate.

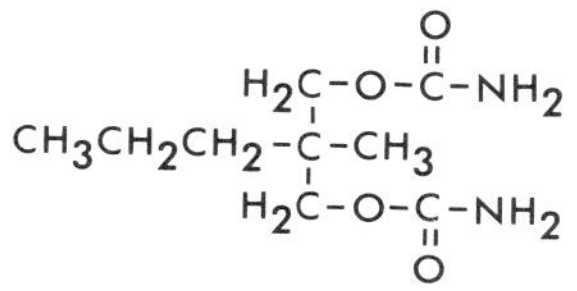

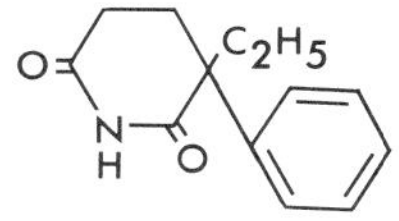

FIG. 25-7. Structure of glutethimide.

Major Actions

The general pharmacologic profile of glutethimide is similar to that of the barbiturates: It is an effective sedative/hypnotic agent with no analgesic activity. Unlike several drugs above, glutethimide does not have pronounced anticonvulsant effects.

Absorption, Metabolism, and Excretion

The absorption of glutethimide after oral administration is unpredictable, presumably owing to its unusually high degree of hydrophobicity. Thus after ingestion of a given dose of this drug, blood levels can vary by 50% to 100%.

Metabolism of glutethimide proceeds by means of hepatic hydroxylation and conjugation with glucuronic acid. The resulting glucuronides, however, are not readily excreted in the urine due to enterohepatic circulation. Ultimately the metabolic products are eliminated mainly in the bile.

Methyprylon is a white powder that, like glutethimide, is soluble in alcohol. Unlike glutethimide, methyprylon is moderately soluble in water. It is a short intermediate-acting hypnotic agent that has effects similar to corresponding barbiturates. Because this drug offers no significant advantage over the barbiturates, it has not had widespread clinical use.

The absorption of methyprylon has not been extensively investigated, although oral absorption of this drug might be less erratic than that of glutethimide because of its less pronounced hydrophobicity.

Methyprylon is extensively metabolized and conjugated with glucuronic acid. The resulting glucuronide is excreted in the urine as well as in the bile. Like glutethimide, methyprylon stimulates the hepatic microsomal enzyme system and is therefore contraindicated in cases of intermittent porphyria.

FIG. 25-8. Structure of methyprylon.

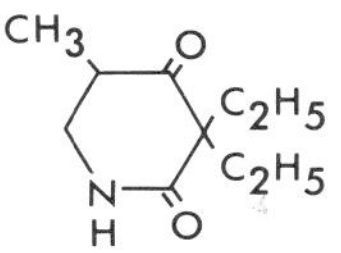

As with glutethimide and all of the above CNS depressants, methyprylon may produce habituation, tolerance, and physical dependence. Withdrawal symptoms resemble those described for barbiturates and other CNS depressants.

METHAQUALONE

Methaqualone, a 2,3-disubstituted quinazolinone, is an efficacious sedative/hypnotic agent. As such, it is characterized by a rapid onset of action and a duration of 4 to 8 hours.

Methaqualone is an interesting compound insofar as its pattern of use and abuse over the years typifies several similar drugs. As with glutethimide, when methaqualone was first introduced it was thought to be a "safe" sedative/hypnotic agent, reportedly being relatively free from addiction liability and abuse potential. Methaqualone was therefore freely prescribed for a few years until its inherent dangers became readily apparent owing to its widespread use and abuse. Methaqualone is, if anything, even more addictive than barbiturates and is characterized by a withdrawal syndrome that may include severe grand mal seizures (*see* Chap. 26).

Partly owing to the once indiscriminate dissemination of methaqualone, this drug has long been a popular drug of abuse with a reputation for producing a highly euphoric condition with minimum sedation and, under certain conditions, as an effective aphrodisiac. In fact, abuse of methaqualone is thought by some to have reached epidemic proportions. Given the highly addictive nature of this substance and its considerable inherent toxicity, this dangerous situation must be fully controlled.

Major Actions

Pharmacologically, methaqualone has a wider spectrum of action than the barbiturates and many of the above agents. In addition to its sedative/hypnotic and anticonvulsant actions, this drug has appreciable antitussive and antispasmodic activity. Like the barbiturates, methaqualone has no analgesic activity.

FIG. 25-9. Structure of methaqualone.

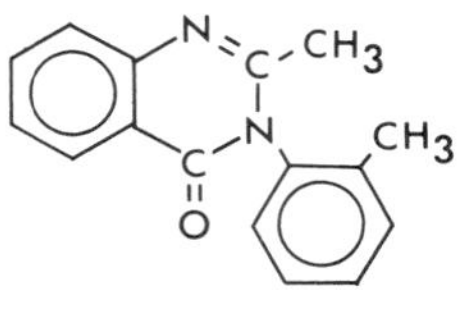

Absorption, Metabolism, and Excretion

Methaqualone is rapidly and completely absorbed after oral administration. Metabolism proceeds by hydroxylation by the P-450 microsomal enzymes, followed by conjugation and urinary elimination. Although methaqualone causes microsomal enzyme induction in experimental animals, this effect is less pronounced than that of the barbiturates, and methaqualone has been administered to patients with intermittent polyporphyria with no complications.

Adverse Effects

In addition to the abuse potential and addiction liability, other side-effects include hangover, dizziness, uticaria, and paresthesias. A methaqualone overdose can be characterized by muscle spasms and convulsions, symptoms not associated with barbiturate overdose. Obviously, methaqualone-induced convulsions cannot be managed with barbiturates; neuromuscular blocking agents such as succinylcholine are much better suited for this condition.

Hemodialysis is usually ineffective as a means of removing methaqualone from the bloodstream, and forced diuresis is seldom effective. Therefore treatment of methaqualone overdose is essentially supportive.

FLURAZEPAM

Flurazepam is a benzodiazepine derivative. Unlike other drugs of this class, flurazepam is generally used as a sedative/hypnotic agent rather than as an anxiolytic or anticonvulsant primarily because of pharmacokinetic factors: Flurazepam is rapidly inactivated in the body, and hangover effects are thus minimized due to its short duration of action. Flurazepam is by far the safest of the sedative/hypnotic agents in this section and is widely used, having largely replaced many of the above drugs in treating insomnia.

The overall pharmacologic profile of flurazepam and its putative mechanism of action are presented below.

ANTIANXIETY AGENTS

All commonly used anxiolytic drugs have sedative/hypnotic properties, and most sedative/hypnotic drugs have antianxiety effects. Certain novel anxiolytic compounds (which have yet to be introduced into clinical medicine) are reportedly devoid of sedative effects, indicating that sedation and anxiolysis are distinct pharmacologic effects.

Anxiety is an unpleasant emotion associated with feelings of fear and apprehension, often accompanied by physical symptoms such as sweating, dizziness, epigastric distress, constriction of the throat and chest, and difficulty in breathing. Anxiety neurosis is therefore not a purely neuropsychiatric disorder, and an understanding of anxiolytic pharmacotherapy is essential not only for psychiatrists, but also for general physicians.

BENZODIAZEPINES

At present, benzodiazepines are the most widely used anxiolytic drugs. Owing to the efficacy and safety inherent in these drugs, they have largely replaced classic anxiolytic drugs such as barbiturates and meprobamate. Members of this class of drugs include diazepam (Valium), chlordiazepoxide (Librium), and flurazepam (Dalmane), along with hundreds of chemically related compounds, most of which have never been widely used clinically.

Chemistry

Table 25-3 lists the most commonly used benzodiazepines, along with their structures and dosages. These drugs may be chemically subdivided into two groups: the 2-amino-4-oxides (*e.g.*, chlordiazepoxide) and the 1,3-dehydro-2-ketones (*e.g.*, diazepam). These compounds are all efficacious antianxiety agents; the only major pharmacologic differences relate to their potencies and durations of action. Potency is generally not an important clinical consideration because dosages can be manipulated to compensate for this variable. The most pharmacologically significant variable of benzodiazepine derivatives is their duration of action. As opposed to sedative/hypnotic pharmacotherapy, which is best suited by drugs having short to intermediate durations of action, longer-acting drugs are preferred in the treatment of anxiety because more stable blood concentrations can be maintained during chronic administration.

Absorption, Metabolism, and Excretion

All of the clinically used benzodiazepines are well absorbed after oral administration. Peak blood levels are attained after 2 to 4 hours. These drugs distribute well into most body tissues because of their high degree of lipophilicity. The plasma half-life values vary considerably between different benzodiazepines; for example, for diazepam the half-life is 20 to 40 hours, whereas that for lorazepam is 12 hours. This is an important clinical consideration in selecting a particular compound for a given therapeutic use: Shorter-acting compounds are preferred as hypnotics, whereas long-acting agents may be better suited for treating anxiety.

Most benzodiazepines undergo similar metabolic fates, depending on the available functional groups. Metabolism occurs primarily in the liver. Flurazepam, which has a diethylamine function at N_1, undergoes desthylation and deamination followed by conjugation with glucuronic acid. Oxazepam and lorazepam, which have a hydroxyl group at C3, can be directly conjugated and thus rapidly inactivated and excreted. Nitrazepam, with a nitro group at C7, is subjected to reduction of this group followed by acetylation of the resulting amine group. This process is accompanied by demethylation at N_1 and hydroxylation at C3. Metabolism of chloridazepoxide proceeds by demethylation and yields desmethylchlordiazepoxide, which, along with its oxidized derivative, is pharmacologically active and extends the duration of action of an ingested dose of the parent compound. Elimination of diazepam is biphasic, having one component with a half-life of a few hours and a second phase with a much longer half-life of 20 to 50 hours. Demethylation of diazepam also yields a pharmacologically active metabolite, and therefore its duration of action is extended. Diazepam is finally eliminated after being hydroxylated at C3, yielding a product with enhanced lipophilicity that may be excreted in the urine or be conjugated with glucuronic acid.

Major Actions

Benzodiazepines depress the excitability of neurons in the CNS, an effect they have common with many other hypnotics and anticonvulsants. In contrast to the antiolytic actions of barbiturates and other CNS depressants, however, the anxiolytic actions of certain benzodi-

---

LEO H. STERNBACH, 1908– . Austrian-born American pharmacologist. Discovered the first antianxiety agents derived from benzodiazepine in the mid-1950s. Has conducted further research on the benzodiazepines as well as on many other drugs.

LOWELL ORLANDO RANDALL, 1910– . American pharmacologist. Extensive research on the biochemistry and toxicology of many groups of drugs, including the initial work on the benzodiazepines in the 1960s.

TABLE 25-3. Benzodiazepine Derivatives

Drug	Trade Name	Structure	Anxiolytic Dosage/Frequency
Diazepam	Valium	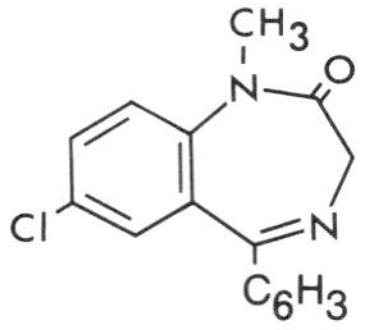	2–10 mg 2–4 times/day
Chlordiazepoxide	Librium	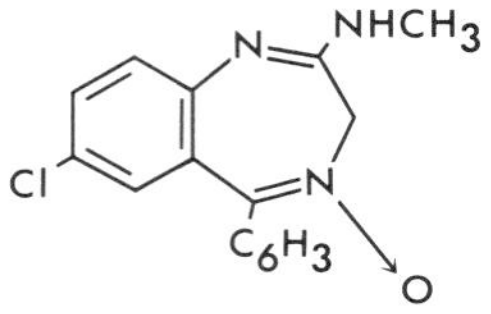	5–10 mg 3–4 times/day
Flurazepam	Dalmane	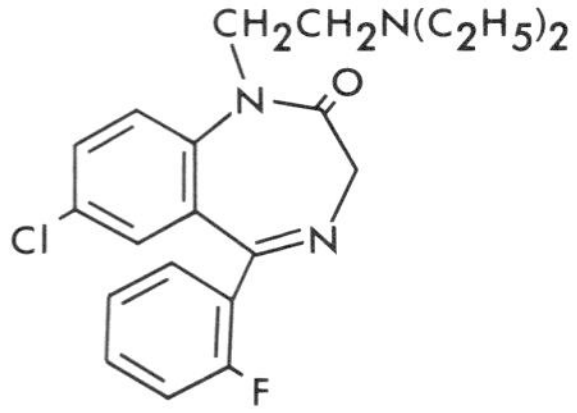	15–30 mg*
Nitrazepam	Mogadon	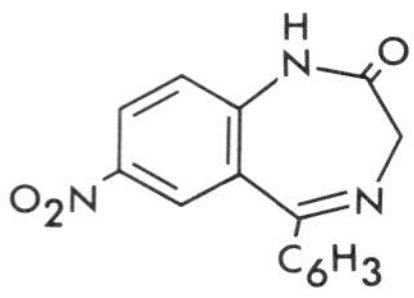	5–10 mg*
Lorazepam	Ativan	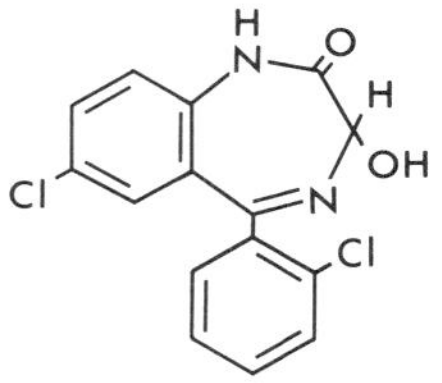	1 mg 3–4 times/day
Oxazepam	Serax	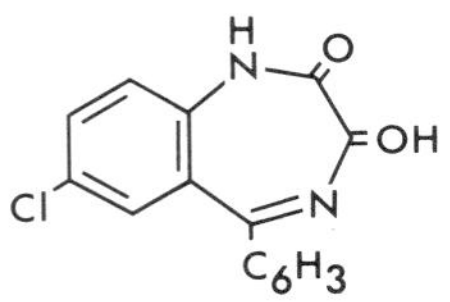	10–30 mg 3–4 times/day

* Hypnotic dosage.

azepines are exhibited at doses that do not have pronounced hypnotic or ataxic effects, although these side-effects are seen in a small percentage of patients. The benzodiazepines are reportedly superior to meprobamate and to the barbiturates in terms of anxiolytic efficacy. Like many other CNS depressants, the benzodiazepines are effective anticonvulsants and are currently the treatment of choice in managing certain types of seizures. The benzodiazepines also have muscle relaxant properties and exhibit antidepressants properties.

Mechanism of Action

Until recently, the molecular mechanism of action of the benzodiazepines was unknown. The classic theory of action, arrived at largely by analogy to other CNS depressants, assumed that benzodiazepines, being highly lipophilic compounds, reduced neuronal excitability simply by dissolving in nerve membranes and thereby rendering them less capable of propagating action potentials. This theory, however, failed to explain several characteristics of benzodiazepine action, which distinguish benzodiazepines from most other CNS depressants.

A quantum leap in the understanding of the mechanism of benzodiazepine action was the discovery, in 1977, of "benzodiazepine receptors" in mammalian brain tissue. Benzodiazepine binding was found to have several characteristics that have come to be thought of as criteria for the definition of pharmacologically or physiologically relevant receptors. The most compelling evidence that supports the existence of pharmacologically relevant benzodiazepine binding sites is the strong correlation between the affinities of several benzodiazepines for these binding sites and their clinical or behavioral potencies.

The discovery of high-affinity saturable binding of benzodiazepines to mammalian brain tissue not inhibited by any known neurotransmitter or neuromodulator has been widely construed as *a priori* evidence for some endogenous ligand for which these "benzodiazepine receptors" exist, the logic here being identical to that which led to the discovery of endogenous morphinelike substances, the "endorphins."

Implied here is that benzodiazepines may act by binding to receptors for such an endogenous substance. Theoretically, benzodiazepines may act either as agonists or antagonists at these receptors. Thus in the case of their anxiolytic effects, the endogenous molecule might function to produce anxiety, in which case benzodiazepines would act antagonistically to ameliorate anxiety; alternatively if the endogenous molecule itself served to reduce anxiety, benzodiazepines would mimic this effect and act as agonists.

Recent evidence supports the contention that the unique multiplicity of actions exhibited by the benzodiazepines might be explicable in terms of multiple, functionally distinct subpopulations of binding sites. The existing data indicate that at least two populations of benzodiazepine binding sites have equal affinities for flunitrazepam and other benzodiazepines but widely disparate affinities for other anxiolytics, such as the triazolopyridazines. The implication of this observation is that a particular subpopulation of benzodiazepine binding sites mediate the characteristic anxiolytic effects of these drugs and that classic benzodiazepines are unable to distinguish between this population of receptors and other populations and therefore exhibit other actions in addition to anxiolytic effects. Conversely certain triazolopyridazines bind selectively to that subpopulation of benzodiazepine receptors that mediate anxiolytic effects, and these drugs therefore have a selective anxiolytic action.

Adverse Effects

There is significant overlap among the toxicities, side-effects, and addiction potential of many CNS depressants. The benzodiazepines are, in other respects, quite different from other drugs of this class. They are considerably safer than the barbiturates. Massive overdoses of benzodiazepines have, in the absence of other drugs, never been reported to cause death and in some cases fail to produce even a loss of consciousness. Benzodiazepines, unlike barbiturates, do not markedly stimulate the hepatic microsomal enzyme system. However, caution should still be exercised with patients who suffer from intermittent porphyria.

The benzodiazepines have certain side-effects in common with the barbiturates. They have been reported to cause paradoxic excitation and, in some cases, to impair motor function. In addition, the benzodiazepines have respiratory depressant effects that must be considered in cases of marginal pulmonary function.

Although early claims indicated that diazepam was a panacea devoid of addiction liability, more recent evidence suggests that long-term use of large doses of benzodiazepines may be accompanied by tolerance and dependence. Overall, however, the benzodiazepines seem to have considerably less addiction liability than the barbiturates and other CNS depressants, although chronic administration of all sedative/hypnotic and anxiolytic agents, including the benzodiazepines, must be done cautiously.

NONBENZODIAZEPINE ANXIOLYTICS

Although the use of barbiturates and meprobamate has declined considerably since the introduction of the benzodiazepines, these drugs are still occasionally prescribed for the relief of anxiety. Meprobamate, as noted earlier, is a dicarbamate that has sedative/hypnotic anxiolytic and muscle relaxant actions. As an anxiolytic, it actually has no advantage over certain barbiturates while being equally dangerous in terms of its addiction liability and toxicity.

Hence, the still widespread use of this drug in the pharmacotherapy of anxiety is not entirely justifiable.

Absorption, Metabolism, and Excretion

Meprobamate is well absorbed after oral administration, achieving peak plasma concentrations within 3 hours. Meprobamate has an intermediate duration of action, with a plasma half-life of about 10 hours.

Metabolism of meprobamate proceeds by means of hydroxylation and conjugation followed by urinary excretion of the resulting glucuronide. Meprobamate causes induction of the hepatic microsomal enzymes and is therefore contraindicated with intermittent polyporphyria.

Adverse Effects

As noted above, meprobamate can produce tolerance and physical dependence. The associated withdrawal syndrome is of the CNS depressant type, being accompanied in extreme cases by convulsions and possibly even resulting in death.

Allergic reactions to meprobamate occur infrequently and may include erythematous cytopenia, urticaria, and nonthrombocytopenic purpura. In addition, meprobamate has reportedly produced aplastic anemia, although this particular sequela is quite rare.

Moderate doses of pentobarbital, amobarbital, and phenobarbital have been used to treat anxiety and are reported to be equal, if not superior, to meprobamate in anxiolytic efficacy. As described above, however, the barbiturates are associated with a fair number of adverse effects and are generally thought to be inferior to the benzodiazepines in the treatment of anxiety. The most important considerations are the disparity between the barbiturates and benzodiazepines with respect to their therapeutic indices and the addiction liability associated with use of barbiturates, which is considerably greater than that which seems to characterize the benzodiazepines. Further, the barbiturates produce a greater degree of sedation than do the benzodiazepines when given in anxiolytic doses.

CONCLUSION

The foregoing consideration emphasizes the general trend in pharmacology toward development of more *specific* drugs. With respect to anxiolytic pharmacotherapy, the ideal drug would be an efficacious antianxiety agent that has no sedative/hypnotic properties. Given the possibility, alluded to above, that these may be mechanistically distinct pharmacologic effects, the development of such a drug would appear to be feasible. Indeed, certain novel anxiolytics (*e.g.*, the triazolopyridazines) seem to conform to this ideal. The next few years will undoubtedly witness the introduction of these and similar drugs into clinical medicine.

FURTHER READING

1. Blackwell B: Psychotropic drugs in use today: The role of diazepam in medical practice. JAMA 225:1637, 1973
2. Kales A, Kales J: Sleep disorders. *N Engl J Med* 290:487, 1974
3. Katz RS: Sedatives and tranquilizers. *N Engl J Med* 286:757, 1972
4. Lasagna L: Drug therapy: Hypnotic drugs. *N Engl J Med* 287:1182,1972

CHAPTER 25 QUESTIONS

(*See* P. 7 for Full Instructions)

Select the One Best Answer

1. Chloral hydrate
   A. is reduced directly to an inactive alcohol.
   B. is useful as an anesthetic agent.
   C. is contraindicated in patients receiving disulfiram.
   D. is irritating to the gastrointestinal tract.
   E. in toxic doses produces muscle spasms.

2. Which of the following barbiturates is an orally effective antiepileptic agent at doses that produce little sedation?
   A. Secobarbital
   B. Pentobarbital
   C. Phenobarbital
   D. Thiopental
   E. Amobarbital

3. Phenobarbital
   A. produces a parkinsonian-like syndrome.
   B. is effective in the treatment of anxiety.
   C. demonstrates cross-dependence with morphine.
   D. has a greater safety factor than diazepam.

E. is useful for treating hyperkinetic syndrome.

4. Diazepam is used clinically for each of the following EXCEPT
   A. treatment of anxiety.
   B. premedication in surgery.
   C. production of muscle relaxation.
   D. suppression of status epilepticus.
   E. chronic treatment of schizophrenia.

A = 1,2,3; B = 1,3; C = 2,4; D = 4; E = All

5. Compared to phenobarbital, diazepam has
   1. a more selective effect on the limbic system.
   2. a greater skeletal muscle relaxant effect.
   3. a faster effect intravenously in status epilepticus.
   4. a greater potency for inducing liver microsomal enzymes.

6. Phenobarbital and thiopental are both
   1. effective within 5 minutes after intravenous administration.
   2. able to diminish the responsiveness of the respiratory center to carbon dioxide.
   3. metabolized completely to inactive metabolites by the liver.
   4. able to produce stage III anesthesia.

7. Chloral hydrate and pentobarbital are both
   1. addicting agents.
   2. effective hypnotic agents.
   3. excreted mainly as inactive products.
   4. metabolized to highly active metabolites.

8. Therapy for severe secobarbital intoxication detected early includes
   1. respiratory support.
   2. gastric lavage.
   3. cardiovascular support.
   4. pentylenetetrazol

9. Common over-the-counter preparations for sleep induction may contain
   1. antihistamines.
   2. sympathomimetic amines.
   3. antimuscarinic agents.
   4. xanthines.

26

LEO E. HOLLISTER

Drugs of Abuse

One person's social drug is another's drug of abuse. One person's treatment may be another's treat. When we speak of "drug of abuse," we make a judgment. On the other hand, "drug dependence" refers to a biologic phenomenon. The one term is socially defined, according to local custom; the other term is universal. Perhaps "drugs used for nonmedical purposes" or "drugs of social use" or "recreational drugs" would be better, but these terms are less familiar. In any case, the term "drug of abuse" creates a paradox by including marijuana and excluding alcohol and nicotine. In this chapter, I shall deal with opiates, sedatives, stimulants, hallucinogens, and marijuana—those drugs most widely "abused" at present.

HISTORICAL PERSPECTIVES

Even the most primitive people have developed some potion that can produce a changed outlook on the world. Alcohol use goes back as far as recorded history. The Greeks administered nepenthes, possibly a form of opiate, to troubled people. Cannabis use has been recorded by Herodotus. Other drugs have a more recent history. Coffee use in the Middle East was not very prevalent until the 15th century, although tea had been used in the Orient for a much longer time. Tobacco was a New World plant, as was coca, which had been used by the Indians of the Andes for about as long as their history has been recorded. Hallucinogenic substances have been discovered by almost every culture. Thus man seems to have a drive to find materials that alter one's senses, for mystical or healing purposes or for relief of tedium, hunger, and hard work.

Drugs have been used in the United States for as long as the country has existed. Tobacco use quickly caught on among the colonists and became a major agricultural crop, and it remains so today. Spirits were distilled easily and provided a cheap method of intoxication. An attempt to control the individual production of such beverages led to the Whiskey Rebellion. The first epidemic of opiate use followed the widespread medical use of opium during the Civil War. On the other hand, drugs such as hallucinogens and cannabis are relatively new to our culture. The present fad for their use can be traced to the 1950s and early 1960s through the writings of Aldous Huxley and the preachings of Timothy Leary.

Thus nonmedical use of drugs is a worldwide phenomenon, the patterns of use fluctuating with new laws or altered customs. Given such a history, it is little wonder that most sensible persons do not talk about the elimination of drug abuse but simply aim to reduce illicit drug use to some reasonable amount.

HIERARCHIES OF DRUG USE AND ABUSE

PERMISSIVE DRUGS

Each culture has its special drugs. In the United States, the three national drugs are caffeine, nicotine, and alcohol. Habituation to each is widespread, some citizens having the dubious distinction of taking all three drugs simultaneously! Yet few of us even think of these as drugs. Our attitude to these drugs is almost completely permissive. Caffeine is available to children in the form of cola-containing beverages and to adults as colas plus the ubiquitous coffee and tea. Because caffeine is a mild stimulant, its action is not likely to be discernible during the working day; rather, it may become more apparent in the form of a sleepless night following a dinner finished with too many cups of coffee.

Nicotine is available in a number of different forms of tobacco smoking, along with recently revived intranasal and buccal forms. Although a strong campaign is currently being waged to discourage the use of cigarettes, with a discouraging lack of success among young people, the objection is not primarily to the nicotine effect but to the inhalation of noxious matter that accompanies the combustion of tobacco. Although large acute doses (*e.g.*, 60 mg) of nicotine could kill a person, the constant doses taken by smokers, and the tolerance that develops, allow that much or more to be taken daily with relatively few physiological effects. Smoking is associated with an increased number of deaths from various diseases, but it is questionable whether the pharmacologic effects of nicotine in cigarettes contribute directly to this harmful effect. The addicting effect of nicotine has, however, been increasingly recognized as a major factor in continued cigarette smoking despite the well-known health hazards associated with it.

By far the most dangerous of our national drugs is ethyl alcohol (*see* Chap. 27), a drug addicting in every sense of the word. Apparently our society values the beneficial aspects of the use of alcoholic beverages more than it fears the evil consequences, for they are readily available to all adults in unlimited quantities. Alcohol is primarily a CNS depressant: It produces enough "disinhibition" to achieve the desired social facility, although this is attended by impairment of function. Much could be said for and against the use of alcoholic beverages, but the fact is that we accept their use and their presumed benefits as well as their dangers of abuse. No serious attempt has been made to prohibit use of alcoholic beverages since the universally disregarded Eighteenth Amendment to the United States Constitution was repealed in 1933.

PRESCRIPTIVE DRUGS

Prescriptive drugs are those used therapeutically and those readily available when prescribed by physicians. Drugs of this type constitute some of the most widely prescribed and used drugs in our country.

The *opiate analgesics* are among the most valuable drugs in medical practice; no physician would attempt to practice without them (*see* Chap. 32). A great variety of natural derivatives have been extracted from crude opium and many synthetic analogues manufactured. The natural opiates morphine and codeine have remained major drugs, codeine being nearly irreplaceable. The development of a growing class of opioids with mixed agonist–antagonist activity may eventually lead to compounds that will replace morphine for analgesia and will be virtually free from dependence liability.

Barbiturates, in use for almost 70 years, are enormously useful in clinical practice, having sedative, hypnotic, muscle relaxant, anticonvulsant, and anesthetic effects in different forms of varying doses (*see* Chap. 25). Except for their continued use as anticonvulsants (phenobarbital) or as intravenous (i.v.) induc-

---

ALDOUS LEONARD HUXLEY, 1894–1963. British novelist, essayist, and poet. Member of a distinguished family that includes his brothers Julian A. Huxley, the biologist, and Andrew F. Huxley, who won the Nobel prize in 1963. In the 1950s Huxley experimented with and described the effects of psychedelic drugs.

TIMOTHY LEARY, 1920– . American psychologist and author. Moved from psychology to psychedelic experience in the 1960s. Ran for governor of California in 1969–70.

tion agents or anesthetics (thiopental or methohexital sodium), barbiturates are rapidly being replaced by the *benzodiazepines*. Several drugs of this class are now marketed in the United States for most of the same indications as the barbiturates. The benzodiazepine diazepam remains the most widely prescribed drug in most developed countries, although its use is declining.

Amphetamines have been used as stimulants for more than 40 years and as appetite suppressants for nearly as long (*see* Chap. 17). These drugs have strong sympathomimetic effects and are more potent than caffeine. A number of amphetamine analogues have been produced as appetite suppressants: diethylproprion, phenmetrazine, and others. Some of these analogues have also been abused.

PROSCRIPTIVE DRUGS

Proscriptive drugs include those that have been placed under special controls because of a great amount of illicit or illegal use. The situation at present is rapidly changing owing to recent laws that expand the list of controlled drugs. Proscriptive drugs would include those with medical value, such as opiates, sedatives, and stimulants, used for nonmedical purposes and usually obtained from some illicit source. They would also include drugs such as marijuana and the hallucinogens, for which no medical uses have yet been established and whose sources of supply, under prevailing laws, are largely illicit.

CONCEPTS OF TOLERANCE AND DEPENDENCE

Tolerance to and *dependence* on drugs are closely linked. Without tolerance to a drug, physical dependence is most unlikely.

TOLERANCE

Several possible mechanisms of tolerance to a drug may be distinguished. *"Behavioral" tolerance* is best exemplified by chronic alcoholics who even with high plasma levels of ethanol may appear to be functioning normally. *"Metabolic" tolerance* may ensue with enzyme induction (*see* Chap. 4). Meprobamate is such an example where its rate of hydroxylation is doubled after 1 week of use. When such drugs are clinically used over long periods, patients either experience a loss of the initial effects or a need to increase the dose to maintain them. If the difference between the therapeutic dose of a drug and that which may result in physical dependence is small (with meprobamate, this may be as low as a factor of 2 or 3), "metabolic" tolerance may rapidly place the patient in danger of becoming physically dependent. *"Immune" tolerance* may develop from the formation of antibodies to the drug. Most drugs are low molecular weight substances not ordinarily antigenic, but when bound to protein they may act as haptens. Antibodies to many have now been demonstrated, although their role in development of tolerance is not entirely clear. *"Pharmacodynamic" tolerance* results when a reduced effect is observed due to the development of compensatory or other homeostatic mechanisms. Because pharmacodynamic tolerance is linked conceptually with physical dependence, it will be discussed further below.

DEPENDENCE

Two types of dependence are recognized, *psychological* and *physiological*, although the boundaries between the two are sometimes difficult to define. Psychological dependence is manifested by a strong craving for the drug, but not necessarily with the appearance of physical signs of withdrawal when the drug is stopped abruptly. Physical dependence is defined as the appearance of psychological and physical symptoms of withdrawal, as exemplified by the well-known withdrawal reactions that occur in heavy users of alcohol, opiates, sedatives, or stimulants. Psychological dependence is seen in all persons who develop physical dependence, although the converse is not true.

The social drugs caffeine and nicotine or "abused" drugs such as marijuana, hallucinogens, or amphetamines in small doses produce largely psychological dependence. The consequence of stopping these drugs is the loss of comfort they may provide. Physical symptoms, such as headache and listlessness, have been associated with caffeine withdrawal. Sudden withdrawal of nicotine may provoke anxiety. Physical dependence to opiates has long been recognized, manifested by the withdrawal syndrome: sneezing, sweating, runny nose, shivering, gooseflesh, muscle aching, abdominal cramps, and diarrhea. Proof that delirium tremens is solely due to physical dependence on ethanol has been firmly established only about 30 years ago. A short time later, similar physical dependence was shown to follow barbiturate use. Both syndromes were manifested by apprehension, sweating, tachycardia, tremors, mental confusion, hallucinations, and occasionally convulsions.

A scheme that explains how tolerance and later physical dependence develop is shown in Table 26-1. This scheme could be modified to include changes in drug receptor sensitivity or even possibly the displacement of endogenous ligand. In any case, homeostatic mechanisms in the body produce tolerance and then physical dependence and withdrawal signs. The latter generally are opposite to the usual pharmacologic actions of the drug.

SPECIFIC TYPES OF DRUGS OF ABUSE

HEROIN AND OTHER OPIATES

Although heroin is the most notorious of all abused opiates, other drugs that share many of its pharmacologic properties may also be subject to abuse (*see* Chap. 32). Hundreds of thousands of doses of morphine and codeine are administered daily for medical purposes with little consequent abuse. Synthetic drugs that resemble opiates, the opioids, are represented primarily by meperidine, methadone, dextropropoxyphene, and pentazocine.

Heroin is the preferred drug for street use. Although morphine seems to be in most respects its full equivalent, a mystique about heroin makes it preferable. Codeine is not a widely abused drug because large doses cause too many unpleasant side-effects, such as itching from release of histamine (*see* Chap. 51).

Most opioids were introduced as narcotics less prone to cause addiction. This belief was rapidly dissipated in the case of meperidine, although its abuse has been restricted largely to those with easy access to it, such as physicians, nurses, and other health personnel. Methadone, a potent narcotic quite useful as a substitute for morphine when patients are intolerant of morphine, is highly addicting. D-Propoxyphene most resembles methadone chemically. Despite an undeservedly wide clinical use, instances of abuse are rare, undoubtedly due to its extreme lack of potency. A long search for drugs with mixed agonist–antagonist actions and less potential for abuse is now paying off. Pentazocine was the first such drug of the benzomorphan type. Hallucinogenic side-effects limit its tendency to abuse, and withdrawal reactions have been relatively mild. At present, a whole series of drugs with mixed agonist–antagonist actions are being marketed (nalbuphine, buprenorphine, butorphanol) that appear to be virtually devoid of dependence liability.

TABLE 26-1. Scheme of Possible Sequence of Tolerance–Withdrawal–Dependence

Assume	[a] drug x to be a CNS depressant [b] a neurohumor c to be a CNS excitant
Initially	x blocks c, producing *sedation*
Block of	c derepresses enzyme e synthesis
Increased	e compensates for block of c
Increased	c restores equilibrium, *tolerance*
Increased	x must be taken to obtain desired effect of sedation; repeated through several cycles, yielding marked increases of e and c
Withdrawal	of x in presence of increased e and c produces marked *excitement,* unmasking *physical dependence*

History

There are references to an opiumlike drink in Greek mythology. Until relatively recently, opium was most widely used in the Orient and the Near East. For many years, China was the leading user of opium, although from all available reports, its use on the Chinese mainland has declined to the vanishing point under the present political regime. Not only has Indochina been one of the leading areas of opium production, but for many years Saigon was a leading opium port. Therefore the great exposure to opium of American troops in Vietnam should not have been unexpected. In addition, the economy of many other areas of the world depends heavily on cultivation of the opium poppy, so that attempts to reduce the supply of opium are usually frustrated.

The widespread use of opium for treating wounds during the American Civil War led to the first of several "epidemics" of opiate use. It was estimated that 4% of Americans used opiates during the post-Civil War period. Just before World War I, the estimate had dropped to 1 in 400 adults, but its rate of use was so alarming as to merit the passage of the Harrison Narcotic Act. From the end of World War II until 1964, the prevalence of heroin use was relatively constant, but a new epidemic followed the wake of increased nonmedical use of many drugs. At present, the number of heroin addicts in the United States is estimated to be around 400,000, as compared to an estimated 700,000 persons in 1972. Present trends, unfortunately, show an increase.

Chemistry

Morphine was first isolated from opium early in the 19th century; a little less than a century ago it was found that a diacetyl derivative (heroin) could be produced by exposing it to acetic anhydride. Heroin was actually a Bayer trade name, just like aspirin, but both are now definitely generic. After opium has been harvested in growing areas, it is converted to morphine at one of the nearest transshipment points. Conversion to heroin can occur at any number of changing locales as the morphine makes its way to markets in the United States and Western Europe. A yield of 1 kg of 90% to 98% pure heroin might be expected from conversion of 12 kg of high-grade opium. Scarcely does such pure material reach the consumer; usually it is first diluted considerably either with inert materials, such as lactose or talc, or with other drugs, such as quinine or barbiturates.

Pharmacologic Considerations

Since heroin is about three times more potent than morphine it is a more acceptable illicit drug. Heroin is also more water soluble, affording a more rapid onset of action by i.v. injection. Monoacetylmorphine and morphine are active metabolites, readily passing into the brain and possibly accounting for its increased potency. Heroin is excreted as conjugated or unconjugated morphine, which is the substance actually measured by urine tests. As with most drugs, duration of action depends somewhat on dose, with most street doses lasting for 3 to 5 hours. Thus the addicted person is never very far removed from withdrawal symptoms.

Tolerance to opiates is well known. Many symptoms of the opiate withdrawal syndrome resemble those of increased cholinergic activity. Although withdrawal may be quite uncomfortable, it is rarely life-threatening. The need for ever-increasing amounts of drug to maintain the expected euphoriant effects, as well as the discomfort of withdrawal, have the expected consequence of strongly reinforcing the addiction once it has started. The prevalent belief is that both immediate reward (in the form of relief of physical or psychic pain) and the act of self-administration are strong reinforcing factors in opiate addiction.

The role of the endorphins in opiate addiction is uncertain. One hypothesis is that endorphins might be deficient in some persons, leading them to take opiates as a form of "substitution" therapy. At present, no evidence for such an endorphin deficiency exists. Further, the demographic pattern of opiate addiction is not consistent with some predisposition that might be equally distributed in the population.

Toxicity

Death from inadvertent overdose (always a possibility when an i.v. dose of an unknown material is injected) is probably due to acute respiratory depression accompanied by pulmonary edema with a highly viscid proteinaceous fluid. Such deaths rank high in the 15- to 25-year-old age group in such cities as New York. This syndrome is treated by prompt administration of a morphine antagonist (naloxone), endotracheal intubation, intermittent positive pressure oxygen, and antibiotics for any complicating pneumonitis. Many other medical complications are associated with heroin use, principally owing to lack of aseptic techniques in its administration. These include hepatitis B infection (the majority of chronic users) and a multitude of infections, notably bacterial endocarditis.

Etiologic and Epidemiologic Considerations

The notion of drug "fiends" that persisted until fairly recently has been largely supplanted by the illness model of drug addiction. Use of drugs is construed as an attempt by certain persons to attain pharmacologic relief from anxieties and depressions. One wonders whether the drug addict might not best be considered an "exploitee," preyed on by those who exploit human folly. In any case, addiction to heroin and other drugs is a complex interplay between many factors: personal, environmental, and pharmacologic.

Since the end of World War II, two rather stable patterns of opiate addiction have existed in the United States. The larger group was confined to the ghettos of northern cities and affected primarily persons who, for whatever reason, had not been assimilated fully into society: blacks and Puerto Ricans in Harlem, blacks in Detroit or Chicago, or Chicanos in Los Angeles. A much smaller group was found in the rural South, with addition to opiate-containing cough syrups. Estimates of the total number of addicts in the country ranged between 75,000 and 200,000 until a few years ago.

Accurate estimates of the number of users of narcotics are difficult to determine. For every person addicted, perhaps two or three others use opiates only occasionally—the so-called chippers. Estimates of addicts are often based on the number of deaths due to overdose or to the number of persons applying for treatment programs, both rather indirect measures subject to many extraneous influences. At any given time, probably many fewer than one half of all addicts are in some treatment program.

Treatment

The detoxification of a patient on opiates follows the same principles as that for most other types of drug detoxification. First, a longer-acting drug, preferably one that can be administered orally, is substituted and the patient stabilized on a dose that prevents abstinence symptoms. Methadone admirably meets the requirements for such a drug. Second, the substituted drug is withdrawn gradually, more slowly as doses become low, the withdrawal phase taking from a few days to 3 weeks.

Clonidine (*see* Chaps. 17 and 36), a presynaptic central alpha-adrenergic receptor agonist used therapeutically as an antihypertensive agent, alleviates the opiate-withdrawal syndrome. Presumably the action of the drug decreases the release of norepinephrine and many of the disturbances of the autonomic nervous system associated with withdrawal. Whether this drug suppresses abstinence as well as methadone does has not yet been determined. Its major advantage is that, unlike methadone, it has no narcotic action and is not addicting.

Two contrasting styles of treatment have been used for opiate-dependent individuals. The most widely used approach is *methadone maintenance*. The main idea behind this treatment is that methadone, given once daily by mouth, is more active and longer lasting than most other opiates. The person's dependent need for drug is sustained without interfering with his activities. He does not feel sleepy (the "nod"), nor is he obliged to sustain his dependence with criminal activity. Drug treatment is never given alone but accompanied by sustained efforts at social and vocational rehabilitation. The cost of such treatment for each patient is usually not more than a few hundred dollars per year. Problems have arisen with diversion of methadone with "take home doses" and with difficulty in maintaining frequent clinic attendance once rehabilitation has been accomplished. Moralistic objections concern the desirability of maintaining drug dependence, yet methadone treatment is generally preferable to maintenance of heroin dependence. A methadonelike drug with a much longer duration of action, methadyl acetate (L-acetyl-α-methadol, LAAM) may obviate some of the difficulties mentioned above. Some problems with toxicity have delayed its release for general use.

Additional pharmacologic treatments under investigation include narcotic antagonists to render opiate use unrewarding. Naltrexone, unlike naloxone, is a narcotic antagonist that is highly active orally and longlasting. Depending on the size of the single dose, narcotic blockade can be affected from 24 to 72 hours. Although the drug seems ideal, its acceptance by patients has generally been poor. A long-acting depôt form of the drug would be highly desirable.

Psychosocial approaches include drug-free programs, which are variations of therapeutic communities, as pioneered for opiate users by Synanon. They assume that drug use is symptomatic of some emotional disturbance or inability to cope adequately with life. The most common technique uses peer group pressures, emphasizing confrontation. Other techniques include variations on group or individual psychotherapy, didactic approaches, alternative life-styles through work or communal living, and meditative techniques such as transcendental meditation, Zen, or hypnosis. Treatment may last for months or years with costs depending on the degree to which professional staff is used.

As each treatment approach has a self-selected clientele, it is difficult to compare results. More chronic users of opiates seem to prefer methadone maintenance, whereas those with shorter histories of drug use seem more amenable to the drug-free approach. Unfortunately proponents of each treatment have become markedly polarized.

BARBITURATES AND OTHER SEDATIVES

History

Barbiturates have been used medically for most of this century, being one of the most widely prescribed classes of drugs (*see* Chapter 25). The experimental demonstration of physical dependence to barbiturates in the early 1950s led to a decline in their use, especially after the development of new barbiturate surrogates (often only technically "nonbarbiturates") or new chemicals with sedative properties labeled "tranquilizers" or "antianxiety drugs." Thus newer drugs such as glutethimide (a barbiturate surrogate more dangerous than its analogue, phenobarbital), meprobamate, chlordiazepoxide and its congeners, and more recently methaqualone have to some extent replaced the barbiturates in clinical practice.

Pharmacology

Phenobarbital, amobarbital, pentobarbital, secobarbital, and thiopental are the barbiturates most often used medically (*see* Chap. 25). Meprobamate (*see* Chap. 25) is a relatively weak sedative, with a span of action similar to that of secobarbital. Methaqualone and glutethimide (*see* Chap. 25) are also weak drugs with relatively short durations of action. Chlordiazepoxide, diazepam, and other drugs of the benzodiazepine series are more potent and much longer acting.

Those who abuse sedatives do so to obtain a rapid but fairly brief state of intoxication, not too unlike that caused by alcohol. Seemingly, then, the drugs most likely to be abused would be those that are rapidly absorbed and have a short span of action. These requirements are well met by secobarbital, pentobarbital, or amobarbital, and by meprobamate, methaqualone, or glutethimide. Drugs with a longer half-life such as phenobarbital or the benzodiazepines do not lend themselves well to repeated bouts of intoxication. *Thus, the biological half-life of the drug seems to have an important bearing on its potential for abuse.* For various reasons, including easier availability and cheaper price, secobarbital sodium is the preferred street drug.

Most abuse of sedatives is by oral ingestion, and the effect from secobarbital occurs rather quickly: primarily a drunken state akin to alcohol intoxication, with relief of tension, euphoria, and later sleepiness. By titrating the dose, users can maintain a constantly intoxicated state during the day but "sleep it off" at night. Tolerance develops rapidly so that the dose must be constantly raised to attain the same effects. Tolerant persons can take with impunity normally lethal doses up to 1 to 2 g daily. When such dose levels are reached, severe withdrawal reactions that resemble delirium tremens may occur. Like delirium tremens, these withdrawal reactions are life threatening if not treated appropriately. The principles of treatment are the same as those with most other types of withdrawal from drugs: *substitution* of a pharmacologically equivalent drug (usually phenobarbital), *gradual withdrawal* of the substituted drug, and *supportive treatment*.

Toxicity

Chronic intoxication of animals with barbiturates has produced abnormal histologic changes in the brain, but such changes have not been established in humans. Withdrawal reactions or inadvertent overdosage are the major hazards of sedative abuse. Because these drugs are commonly used by alcoholics, the combination having synergistic respiratory depressant effects, unintentional suicides have occurred. Their concurrent use with heroin seems to be a major factor in "overdose" deaths attributed to heroin.

Epidemiology

Instances of iatrogenic abuse have been reported periodically for many years. The extent to which patients for whom sedatives are prescribed overuse or "abuse" these agents is uncertain. Because diazepam is the most widely prescribed drug of this type, it has been the subject of most speculation. Judging by the number of case reports in the medical literature of dependence on this drug compared with the degree of its use, one might conclude that such events are rare. Judging by the number of journalistic stories of diazepam abuse, one might judge that a veritable epidemic of such dependence is occurring. The best guess is that the problem occurs much more commonly than is reported in the medical literature and much less commonly than is reported in the press.

Recently so-called low-dose dependence on benzodiazepines after prolonged treatment has been a concern. The withdrawal syndromes as described are subtle and often resemble those symptoms for which the patient was originally treated. They also tend to be long lasting. Benzodiazepines act through well-identified and relatively specific receptors in the brain whose sensitivity might be changed by prolonged occupancy. Whether this mode of action makes these drugs different from other sedatives has not been decided. Much more study of this phenomenon is needed.

Most sedative abuse is by young people using supplies from the illicit market. Secobarbital and methaqualone remain favorites, although diazepam is used as it becomes available. Why some users may prefer drugs of this type, commonly called "downers," to stimulants (uppers) is unknown. Many use either, depending on availability, or may use one to counter the effects of the other. Sedatives may also be used in a pattern of multiple drug use involving other sedative drugs such as alcohol, marijuana, or heroin.

Treatment of Sedative Abuse

The same treatment model might be applied to sedatives as to alcohol abuse, considering their pharmacologic similarities. The social context of use, including sedatives in a pattern of polydrug use, is somewhat different, however, so whether similar treatment would be equally effective is uncertain.

AMPHETAMINES AND STIMULANTS

History

The stimulant effects derived from chewing coca leaves were discovered by folk pharmacologists in the Andes centuries ago. The active component cocaine, discovered in 1860, is a local anesthetic (*see* Chap. 20). Although cocaine has little chemical resemblance to the amphetamines and more modern stimulants, its pharmacologic actions are quite similar.

Chemical analogues of epinephrine and norepinephrine were known before the identity of either hormone was established. Medical use of amphetamine dates from 1935, and shortly thereafter most of the common indications were discovered (*see* Chap. 17). Racemic amphetamine was quickly replaced by dextroamphetamine and other homologues such as methamphetamine. Newer homologues include methylphenidate, phenmetrazine, diethylproprion, and pipradol.

Chemistry and Pharmacology

Most amphetamines or their surrogates have a phenethylamine structure (*see* Chap. 17). Yet this structure is not found in cocaine, which has remarkably similar pharmacologic actions (*see* Chap. 20). Both amphetamines and cocaine act as indirect central and peripheral sympathomimetics. The mode of action of amphetamines on dopamine and norepinephrine is complex. Amphetamine increases the release of catecholamines (dopamine and norepinephrine) presynaptically, blocks their reuptake, and weakly and reversibly blocks monoamine oxidase. Additionally the phenethylamine structure of amphetamines may act as a direct adrenergic agonist. The usual central effects are alertness, tremor, and increased deep tendon reflexes. The mechanism for appetite suppression, which is only temporary, is not clear.

Methamphetamine is the most widely abused preparation possibly because it is more easily made in the illicit market. It is usually sold as the raw chemical (slang term "crystal"). Most d-amphetamine reaching the illicit market is delivered from marginal pharmaceutical houses.

The familiar clinical effects of mild oral doses, such as an increased sense of well-being (euphoria) and perhaps a slight degree of nervousness, are quite different from those obtained from the massive doses (50—5000 mg/day) taken intravenously by confirmed users. Such doses would be fatal in intolerant subjects, who have died from as little as 120 mg intravenously. After i.v. injection, users report an immediate "rush" characterized by general sensations of tingling (said to be something like an orgasm). Great alertness and feelings of confidence and power follow. Users develop repetitive masticatory movements or writhing movements of the extremities. As effects subside over a few hours, a new dose may be taken. Such repetitive dosing (a "run") may last a week or more, during which time sleeping and eating are minimal. Exhaustion at the end of a run is followed by withdrawal ("coming down" or "crashing") characterized by marked depression and restlessness. Withdrawal often is so painful that the user seeks relief by taking downers, such as barbiturates or heroin. The latter drug is so effective that many heroin addicts are first initiated into its use as a treatment for a crash reaction from shooting amphetamines.

Epidemiology

The exact extent to which drugs of this class are abused is not really known. Two patterns of abuse exist: oral and i.v. Oral abuse often originates from initial use of the drug either self-administered to enhance performance or prescribed by physicians to assist weight reduction. The consequences of this pattern of abuse are seldom great. A larger number of users quite early administer the drug intravenously, the desired effect being the "rush." Although there are some pure "speed freaks," often this pattern of amphetamine use is associated with multiple drug abuse.

Tighter controls over manufacture and strong persuasion against its medical use have reduced prescription of amphetamines. The reduction in amphetamine abuse, however, has not been proportionate to the decreased medical use. More likely, reduced use stems from increased use of alternative stimulants.

The encouraging decline in amphetamine abuse has been paralleled by an ominous increase in cocaine abuse. Cocaine has attained a certain cachet among middle- and upper-class circles as well as among those who find it a ready substitute for street amphetamine. The drug has a low margin for safety, so that mucosal absorption through the nose ("sniffing") is preferred to oral or i.v. administration.

Cocaine mimics all the effects of amphetamines but creates them more quickly (unless amphetamines are taken intravenously) and more intensely. Its plasma half-life is comparatively short, which is consistent with a shorter span of clinical action than the amphetamines. Most effects of cocaine are no longer apparent after 2 to 4 hours. Contrary to the mythology of the drug-using world, cocaine is dangerous, and fatalities have occurred from its use.

Phenmetrazine, although promoted only as an anorexiant, enjoys wide popularity as a drug of abuse. Allegedly it increases sexual performance and is highly valued among the young for that alleged effect. Whether its effects are very much different from those of amphetamines is highly questionable.

Treatment

No specific pharmacologic or psychological treatment programs have been devised. Patients using amphetamines to treat a prevailing depression may be better treated with conventional antidepressant drugs. Some who have experienced psychotic reactions may have been destined to become schizophrenic, especially if the psychosis is long lived. Antipsychotic drugs would then be the treatment of choice. Psychological approaches to treatment would be similar to those described for addiction to opiates.

Toxicity

Amphetamine abusers frequently develop a paranoid psychosis during its use. Symptoms may appear rapidly after a rather small total dose, and when full blown the state resembles naturally occurring schizophrenia more closely than any other drug-induced condition. Persistence of abnormal brain function and sleep disturbances may last for months after termination of a run.

Amphetamine abuse may lead to an irreversible necrotizing arteritis that resembles periarteritis nodosa. It is often fatal, providing some credence to the popular slogan "speed kills." As amphetamines are often taken intravenously with unsterile apparatus, users of this drug are exposed to the same infectious complications as heroin users, as well as to the hazards of embolic phenomen from "excipients."

HALLUCINOGENS

History

Almost every society, however primitive, has found some bark, skin, leaf, vine, berry, or weed that contains "hallucinogenic" materials. Although the fortuitous discovery of the amazing properties of lysergic acid diethylamide (LSD) occurred in a chemical laboratory 4 decades ago, it was a case of art imitating nature. Similar compounds were known in morning-glory seeds, and drugs such as mescaline and psilocybin had long been used by North and Central American Indians in the form of cactus buttons or magical mushrooms. Deliriants, such as the materials in belladonna (*Datura stramonium*), were also known to ancient man.

Hallucinogens rarely produce hallucinations, and other terms such as "psychedelic" or "psychotomimetic" are equally inappropriate. Hallucinogens are taken for many reasons but especially to provide new ways of looking at the world or new insights into personal problems. The former action implies varying degrees of perceptual distortion, whereas the latter implies mood changes and increased introspection. Drug users seemingly will use any drug that alters thinking or mood, including deliriants such as the synthetic central anticholinergic drug Ditran or organic solvents taken by inhalation. The prototypic hallucinogenic drug is LSD because of the extent of its use, because it represents a family of drugs that are similar, and because it has been most carefully studied.

Chemical and Pharmacologic Considerations

Lysergic Acid Diethylamide and Related Drugs. LSD is based on the lysergic acid nucleus (*see* Fig. 51-2), within which one may discern resemblances to the phenethylamine structure of mescaline and the indolethylamine structure of psilocybin and to biogenic amines such as norepinephrine and dopamine, in the case of phenethylamines, and 5-hydroxytryptamine (serotonin), in the case of the indolethylamines. Whether these chemical resemblances account for the similar action of the three types of drugs or for the mechanism of action mediated by effects on brain biogenic amines is still not certain.

Hallucinogens of the LSD type, like marijuana, are of very low acute toxicity, and deaths from overdose are rare. Their mode of action is uncertain, despite much experimental study. At the neurophysiological level they induce a state of hyperarousal of the CNS. Neurochemically, LSD seems to work mainly through serotonergic systems, decreasing serotonergic activity. Early, it was believed that LSD might act postsynaptically as a false transmitter, weakening the action of serotonin by replacing the normal transmitter. More recently, LSD has been thought to act on a presynaptic serotonergic receptor, this stimulation impeding the release of serotonin.

The effects of LSD, mescaline, and psilocybin are so similar that most persons regard them as a specific group of hallucinogens. The ratio of dose between LSD and psilocybin or mescaline is about 1:250 and 1:4000, respectively. LSD may be one of the most potent pharmacologic materials known. It is equally effective when taken orally or by injection, and thus the former route is preferred.

The usual doses of LSD in humans (1–2 mg/kg) produce a series of somatic, perceptual, and psychic effects that overlap each other. Dizziness, weakness, tremors, nausea, and paresthesias are prominent somatic symptoms. Blurred vision, distortions of perspective, organized visual illusions (hemeralopia) or "hallucinations," and less discriminant hearing are common perceptual abnormalities, as is the hallmark of hallucinogenic activity, a *change in time sense*.

Some of the psychic effects are similar to those observed with large doses of marijuana, but they are usually much more intense. Physiologically, LSD produces signs of sympathetic overactivity and central stimulation, in contrast to marijuana, which has a marked sedative action. Drug effects develop usually within 30 minutes of ingestion, the duration varying with the dose. As with most drugs of this type, the phenomena experienced may vary considerably owing to the personality of the drug taker, the expectations of the drug taken, and the experimenters or the circumstances under which the drug is taken. Waxing and waning of effects are typical.

A series of amphetamine analogues with varying alphabetical chemical designations (DOM, also called "STP," MDA, MMDA) are also hallucinogenic. In most respects they fit into the LSD group of drugs, although they are more potent than mescaline, which they resemble chemically.

The Deliriant Hallucinogens. The deliriant hallucinogens, exemplified by scopolamine or a series of synthetic anticholinergic drugs with strong CNS activity, produce marked mental disorganization; usually the experience is terrifying and not fully remembered, and residual confusion may last for days. Stramonium-containing cigarettes, proprietary remedies that contain scopolamine or atropine, and the Datura plant itself have been used by those who prefer to use drugs of this type.

Phencyclidine. Phencyclidine (PCP, "angel dust") is one of the series of phenylcyclohexamines. Phencyclidine was introduced in 1957 as a "dissociative anesthetic," that is, one that causes no loss of consciousness but makes patients insensitive to pain owing to a separation of their bodily sensations from their minds. Soon after its use, emergent psychotomimetic effects were noted. By 1965 the drug (trade named "Sernyl") was abandoned for human use but continued to be marketed as a highly effective anesthetic (trade named "Sernylan") for veterinary use. Another homologue, ketamine, supplanted phencyclidine for human use and remains in use today (*see* Chap. 28).

In initial street use in 1967, PCP quickly gained a bad reputation. Subsequently it was usually mislabeled, being passed off as LSD, THC, or some other hallucinogen. Since the mid-1970s, however, phencyclidine has been accepted as a "drug of abuse" under its own label.

Phencyclidine reduces the reuptake of dopamine, supporting clinical observations that it provides the best model psychosis for schizophrenia. The drug is unique among hallucinogens in that animals given a choice of self-administering it by pressing a lever will continue to do so, just as they do with heroin, cocaine, or some barbiturates. The clinical effects are multiple and are dose dependent. Detachment, disorientation, mania, numbness, dysarthria, ataxia, nystagmus, and hypertension are clinical manifestations that help to distinguish it from the LSD-type hallucinogens.

Overdoses have been fatal, as contrasted with no direct fatalities from drugs of the LSD group. Phencyclidine, being a weak base, is secreted into the stomach (*see* Chap. 3) and can be removed by continual nasogastric suction. Acidification of the urine to *p*H 5.5 hastens PCP excretion. Antipsychotics given during the acute period of intoxication may aggravate the situation; diazepam is a better choice and may protect against seizures. Some users experience a prolonged schizophrenialike psychosis and may require sustained treatment with antipsychotic drugs.

Toxicity

A number of adverse psychological consequences of hallucinogenic drug use have been reported. Most common is a panic reaction associated with a "bad trip." Panic reactions are often best managed by simple sedation with a barbiturate or with benzodiazepine rather than with a phenothiazine; simple "talking down" often sufices, if one has the time. Acute psychotic or depressive reactions may be evoked, but these generally occur in patients strongly predisposed. Errors of judgment may lead to reckless acts that may threaten life; everyone on these drugs should be monitored by someone who is not.

Epidemiology

In the late 1950s, most hallucinogens were regarded as laboratory curiosities, but under the spell of Huxley, Leary, and the lay press their alleged benefits for opening minds created an explosive increase in their use. This epidemic has partially waned as the popularity of PCP has grown. LSD began to fall from favor when it was appreciated as being synthetic and not a "natural" like mescaline. Virtually all street "mescaline" is mislabeled LSD. PCP is a much more widely used hallucinogen than LSD. Indeed, in some areas, use of PCP approaches epidemic proportions. The trade-off is a poor one, for PCP is a bad drug, just as it was described when drug-abusers first tried it.

Treatment

Except for treating specific complications, no systematic program of treatment has been defined specifically for this class of drugs. The most successful way to have people stop using these drugs is to separate them from the drug culture, which is not feasible unless voluntarily accepted.

MARIJUANA

History

Marijuana is one of the oldest of all socially used drugs, its use being recorded several millennia ago. It may also be the most frequently used drug; current estimates vary between 200 to 300 million users throughout the world. During the past two decades, a remarkable increase in the social use of this drug has occurred in western society, so that today an estimated 40 million people in the United States, mostly youth, have used the drug, but only a small proportion regularly. This recent trend has stimulated renewed interest in its pharmacologic effects, especially as they may relate to socially undesirable consequences.

Chemical and Pharmacologic Considerations

Of the three principal cannabinoids in marijuana—cannabidiol, tetrahydrocannabinol (THC), and cannabinol—only THC has been proved definitely to be active. Two isomers of THC exist in marijuana: the delta-1 isomer accounts for about 99% of the total THC, whereas the delta-6 isomer often cannot be clearly identified in chemical analyses. A number of other THC isomers and analogues have been synthesized and have varying degrees of activity.

The availability of synthetic delta-1-THC, as well as chemical techniques for quantifying its content in marijuana, has made possible pharmacologic studies that provide some, but not complete, precision in dose. The bioavailability of smoked THC is about 20%, variable fractions being lost in side-stream smoke or exhaled from the respiratory dead space. Relatively little is lost by pyrolysis. The efficiency of delivery of a dose by smoking seldom exceeds 40% even with the most adroit smoker. Sharing cigarettes reduces the loss from side-stream smoke. Oral doses of THC are only one third as bioavailable as smoked material.

When it is smoked, THC is absorbed rapidly and effects appear within minutes. If the marijuana is of low potency, effects may be subtle and brief. Seldom do they last longer than 2 to 3 hours after a single cigarette, although users prolong effects by repeated smoking. Symptoms after oral administration appear within 15 minutes to 2 hours, but they last much longer than do those from smoking. Duration of symptoms corresponds poorly, however, to the plasma drug levels.

The mechanism of action of THC is still unknown. Investigations have been unsuccessful in linking its action to several neurotransmitters, and its high lipid solubility suggests that it might act on cell membranes rather than on any specific receptors.

Clinically, marijuana has a biphasic effect, with initial symptoms of "stimulation" and euphoria followed later by sleepiness and dreamlike states. These effects are highly dose dependent, ranging from a brief and mild high with minimal sleepiness to a prolonged intoxication with many features similar to psychotomimetic drugs.

The major physiological effects of marijuana are reddening of the conjunctivae, increased pulse rate, muscle weakness, and some uncoordination. Perceptual and psychic changes predominate and may include uncontrollable laughter, difficulty in concentration or thinking, depersonalization, dreamlike states, slowing of the time-sense, visual distortions or illusions, and less discriminant hearing. Almost all psychological tests show impairment if the dose is high enough; if the task is difficult enough, even small doses induce impairment.

Marijuana has a unique profile of pharmacologic actions: It does not fit into some existing category of drugs, such as hallucinogens, sedatives, stimulants, or anticholinergics. It most resembles the combined effects of hallucinogens and alcohol, which may explain its great popularity.

Toxicity

Lethal doses of THC in animals are almost astronomical in size. No fatalities have been proved from use of marijuana in humans. The drug certainly ranks as one of the safest intoxicants.

Tolerance develops with continued frequent use of the drug but with ordinary social use is not a recognizable phenomenon. A mild physical withdrawal syndrome has been described, but dependence is most often of the psychological type. The mechanism of tolerance has not been defined, but it does not appear to be metabolic.

The potential health hazards of marijuana are of continuing concern. A number of *in vitro* studies suggest impairment of cell-mediated immunity, but the clinical significance is unknown. Chromosomal damage, another *in vitro* effect, seems to be no worse than with many acceptable drugs. Effects on pregnancy and fetal development, as they are with most other drugs, are uncertain. One is often impressed by the development in young users of an "amotivational syndrome," in which the youngster "drops out." Still, it is difficult to say whether the decision to drop out is part of a conscious change in life-style that also includes marijuana use or whether the drug actually causes the changed attitude. Most authorities agree that the use of this drug by immature persons could be a psychological hazard. Brain damage has been described in animals, but the findings are controversial. Endocrinologic effects have been described, suggesting diminished sexual functioning in men. Bronchopulmonary disorders would probably occur among smokers of marijuana just as they do among those who smoke tobacco. Ability to operate machinery (*e.g.*, a motor car) is very likely to be impaired during acute intoxication with marijuana.

Marijuana has a long history of use as a therapeutic agent, and some of its uses are currently being reinvestigated. Most promising are its possible benefits as an antiemetic, particularly for vomiting induced by some anticancer drugs, and in treating glaucoma, bronchial asthma, and spasticity. Many other therapeutic uses are also being studied. Synthetic homologues of THC are being devised to separate the desired from the undesired properties, which ironically include the mental effects so sought by social users of the drug.

Epidemiology

The dramatic increase in marijuana use closely followed increased hallucinogenic use. As far as one can tell, the same general influences are obtained, supplemented by the symbolic value of marijuana as a sign of revolt by the young. Marijuana is preferred to the hallucinogens by many, who describe its effects as "mellow," presumably signifying a milder and more pleasant type of reaction.

The number of users continues to rise, but patterns of use vary as greatly as those for alcohol. Many people use marijuana only on social occasions. Others may avoid it during the workweek but indulge on weekends, although not in a typical "binge" pattern. Still others may use the drug daily but only at the end of the workday. The percentage of true "potheads," those who use the drug several times a day and who remain in a permanent state of intoxication, is unknown but is probably no more than that of users of alcohol who become alcoholics.

Marijuana probably will remain as a social drug, although acceptance by society is still incomplete. Efforts at reducing the criminal penalties for possession and use have had partial success, but attempts at full legalization seem to be entirely fruitless.

Treatment

Few users seek treatment, although many who have stopped using the drug have been pleasantly surprised at their increased clarity of thinking. Although marijuana has been alleged to be a substitute for alcohol, it is more commonly used along with alcohol; alcoholism complicating marijuana use is rare. Marijuana may also be used in a pattern of multiple drug use, in which case treatment may be needed for the more serious drugs being taken.

FURTHER READING

1. Lewin L: Phantastica. Narcotic and Stimulating Drugs. Their Use and Abuse, p 335. New York, E P Dutton, 1931
2. Pradhan SN, Dutta SN: Drug Abuse. Clinical and Basic Aspects, p 598. St. Louis, C V Mosby, 1977
3. Schuckit MA: Drug and Alcohol Abuse. A Clinical Guide to Diagnosis and Treatment, p 211. New York, Plenum, 1979

4. Nahas GG, Paton WDM: Marihuana: Biological Effects, p 777. London, Pergamon Press, 1979
5. Ray OA: Drugs, Society and Human Behavior, 2nd ed, p 457. St. Louis, C V Mosby, 1978

CHAPTER 26 QUESTIONS

(*See* P. 7 for Full Instructions)

Select the One Best Answer

1. Each of the following agents can produce tolerance *and* physical dependence EXCEPT
   A. methadone.
   B. naloxone.
   C. alcohol.
   D. meprobamate.
   E. chlordiazepoxide.

2. Which of the following drugs is a highly effective opioid analgesic with mixed agonist–antagonist properties but has virtually no abuse potential?
   A. *d*-Propoxyphene
   B. Buprenorphine
   C. Pentazocine
   D. Naltrexone
   E. Methadone

3. Each of the following lists a drug that, when taken in marked overdosage, would be correctly managed with the associated treatment EXCEPT
   A. alcohol—fructose.
   B. opiates—naloxone.
   C. amphetamine—haloperidol.
   D. barbiturates—supportive treatment.
   E. hallucinogens—diazepam.

4. Chronic intoxication with high doses of amphetamine frequently produces
   A. gum hyperplasia.
   B. toxic psychosis.
   C. constipation.
   D. activation of peptic ulcer.
   E. respiratory depression.

5. Each of the following pairs of drugs exhibit cross-dependence EXCEPT
   A. heroin and methadone.
   B. meperidine and chlordiazepoxide.
   C. diazepam and ethanol.
   D. paraldehyde and chloral hydrate.
   E. methaqualone and pentobarbital.

A = 1,2,3; B = 1,3; C = 2,4; D = 4; E = All

6. Convulsions from withdrawal of alcohol in addicted persons can be prevented by
   1. chloral hydrate.
   2. paraldehyde.
   3. barbiturates.
   4. morphine.

7. Which of the following pairs of drugs exhibit cross-dependence?
   1. Ethanol and chlordiazepoxide
   2. Morphine and methadone
   3. Meprobamate and pentobarbital
   4. Meperidine and haloperidol

8. Which of the following drugs produces both psychological dependence and physical dependence?
   1. LSD
   2. Alcohol
   3. Marijuana
   4. Barbiturates

9. Immediate signs of cocaine overdosage would include
   1. sedation.
   2. pupillary dilatation.
   3. hypotension.
   4. tachycardia.

10. In which of the following is a drug of abuse correctly associated with its characteristic medical complication?
    1. Phencyclidine—prolonged schizophrenic-like illness
    2. Heroin—bronchopulmonary disorders
    3. Amphetamine—necrotizing arteritis
    4. Marijuana—hepatitis B infection

HAROLD KALANT

27 Alcohols and Disulfiram

THE ALCOHOLS

ETHANOL

History and Uses

Ethanol (grain alcohol) has been known in almost all parts of the world since prehistoric times. Formed naturally by yeast fermentation of starch or sugar in fruits, grains, potatoes, or sugar cane, alcohol in many countries is permitted for human consumption only in natural form. Ethanol for industrial use is produced mainly by organic synthesis from ethylene.

Although brandy and whiskey were considered "stimulants," alcohol is really a hypnotic and anesthetic drug used very little in modern medicine except as a solvent for some drugs given in liquid form (tinctures). Most alcohol consumption by humans is for nonmedical purposes: with meals, in social gatherings, for relaxation, or as "problem drinking."

Within the last few years, several epidemiologic studies have suggested that moderate daily alcohol consumption may protect against myocardial infarction. This is, however, not yet certain.

Chemistry

The aliphatic alcohols form a homologous series beginning with methanol (wood alcohol):

CH_3OH
METHANOL

$CH_3{-}CH_2OH$
ETHANOL

$CH_3{-}CH_2{-}CH_2OH$
N-PROPANOL

$CH_3{-}CH(OH){-}CH_3$
ISOPROPANOL

The first three are completely soluble in water, in all proportions, but as the carbon chain length increases water solubility decreases, and octanol (eight carbons) is almost insoluble. These higher alcohols, along with methanol, are used mainly in industry.

Alcoholic Beverages. Only ethanol is used for human consumption, although trace amounts of methanol, higher alcohols, aldehydes, and esters are present as the "congeners" that give different alcoholic beverages their distinctive tastes and aromas. Fermentation stops when the alcohol concentration becomes high enough to inhibit the yeast; beers contain only 3% to 6% alcohol by weight and table wines about 10% to 15%.

Distillation can increase the alcohol concentration greatly, and in most countries the law sets limits on the content that may be sold. In the United States, proof spirit is 50% alcohol by volume; in Britain and Canada it is about 57%. An American whiskey is usually 90% proof (10 under proof) and therefore contains 45% alcohol by volume, or about 36 g of ethanol/dl. Canadian whiskey is usually about 40% ethanol by volume, or 32 g/dl. One 12 oz bottle of beer, $1\frac{1}{2}$ oz of whiskey or gin and 5 oz of table wine all contain roughly about the same amount of ethanol.

Absorption, Distribution, and Elimination

Alcohol is absorbed by simple diffusion across any mucosal surface. This occurs in the stomach but is faster across the thinner mucosa of the small intestine, so that anything that delays gastric emptying (*e.g.*, food, exercise, and anticholinergic drugs) will retard absorption of ethanol. Reduction of visceral blood flow, excessive dilution of the ingested alcohol, or any variable that reduces the ethanol concentration gradient across the mucosa will also slow its absorption. Fastest absorption occurs with an intragastric concentration of 20% to 30%; less than this reduces the diffusion rate, whereas higher concentrations may delay gastric emptying by causing irritation and pylorospasm.

Ethanol diffuses rapidly from the blood across all capillary walls and cell membranes and equilibrates with the *total* body water, including the CSF and urine. Ethanol dilution methods can therefore be used for measuring body water. The vapor pressure of ethanol in the alveolar air is in equilibrium with that in the plasma; this is the basis of the Breathalyzer test. The amount of ethanol eliminated in breath, sweat, and urine is, however, usually less than 5% of the ingested dose. The rest is metabolized chiefly in the liver.

Metabolism

The first step in alcohol metabolism takes place mostly in the liver and consists of NAD-dependent oxidation, first to acetaldehyde and then to acetate: Alcohol dehydrogenase (ADH) is located in the soluble cytoplasm, whereas acetaldehyde dehydrogenase (AcDH) is located in the mitochondria. Ethanol oxidation sharply reduces the activity of the tricarboxylic acid cycle (Krebs cycle) so that much of the acetate diffuses back into the cytoplasm. The NADH can be reoxidized to NAD either by the mitochondrial respiratory chain or by cytoplasmic redox reactions such as conversion of pyruvate to lactate. Ethanol oxidation therefore results in output of small amounts of acetaldehyde and large amounts of acetate and lactate from the liver into the peripheral circulation. Conversely, infusion of pyruvate or fructose can speed up alcohol oxidation by reoxidizing NADH to NAD.

Ethanol can be oxidized *in vitro* by a peroxidative reaction with the cytochrome P-450 system in liver microsomes (MEOS). This reaction appears to be negligible in alcohol oxidation *in vivo*, except possibly at very high blood alcohol concentrations and in chronic heavy drinkers whose livers have increased amounts of smooth endoplasmic reticulum. Minute amounts of ethanol are conjugated with sulfate or glucuronate or esterified with fatty acids.

Blood Alcohol Curve. Liver alcohol dehydrogenase shows quasi-zero-order (saturation) kinetics at blood alcohol levels (BAL) above 25 mg/dl. There are differences between individuals and in the same person at different times, but on average a 70-kg man can oxidize about 10 g of ethanol per hour. Therefore, after a single dose, the BAL usually rises to a peak level in 30 to 90 minutes, depending on the dose, falls steadily at an average rate of 15 to 20 mg/dl/hr until it reaches 20 to 25 mg/dl, then falls off exponentially. However, the higher the peak value of the curve, the greater the slope of its pseudolinear falling portion (Fig. 27-1).

Interaction with Other Drugs

The ADH reaction can function readily in the reverse direction as an aldehyde reductase. Therefore chloral hydrate (trichloracetaldehyde) competes with both ethanol and acetaldehyde for their respective dehydrogenases, and chloral and alcohol therefore potentiate each other. Large doses of thyroxine, chlorpro-

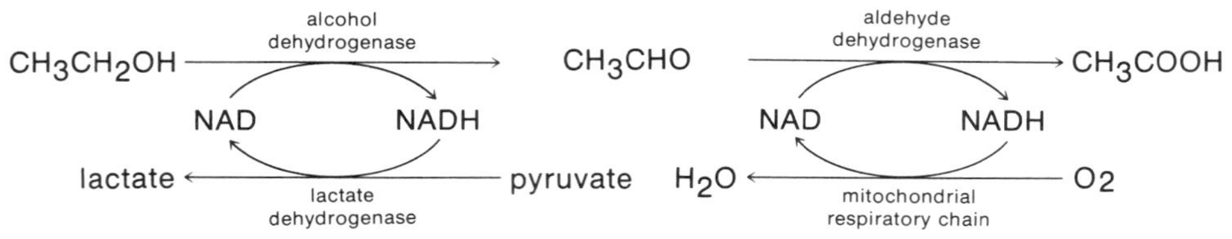

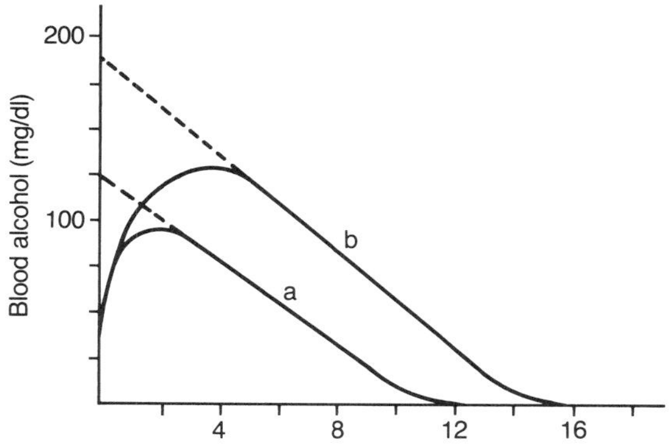

FIG. 27-1. Hypothetical blood alcohol curves that would be found after ingestion of ethanol in a dose of 1.0 (*a*) or 1.5 (*b*) g/kg on an empty stomach. The broken lines indicate extrapolation of the zero-order portion of each curve back to zero time, to give the theoretic initial concentration (vertical intercept) from which the volume of distribution can be calculated.

mazine, and various other drugs may impair the oxidation of ethanol by inhibiting alcohol dehydrogenase.

Acutely, ethanol can interfere with the binding of many drugs (*e.g.*, pentobarbital, warfarin, meprobamate) to cytochrome P-450, and this may be partly responsible for slowing their biotransformation. Chronic heavy drinking increases, however, the amount of cytochrome P-450 in the liver and may therefore increase the rate of metabolism of these drugs and shorten their half-lives (*see* Chap. 8).

ACTIONS

Three types of pharmacologic effects of ethanol can be distinguished: those caused by a direct action of ethanol on cell membranes; disturbances resulting from ethanol metabolism; and stress reactions secondary to severe intoxication.

Direct Effects on Cell Membranes

Like hypnotic, sedative, and general anesthetic agents, ethanol dissolves in the lipids of the cell membrane, making the lipids more mobile ("fluidization") but at the same time making the membrane more dense and mechanically stable. This interferes with three processes that require the membrane to undergo rapid reversible changes in structure:

1. *Rapid changes in Na^+ and K^+ flux*, the basis of the action potential, are impaired. Nerve impulse conduction and muscle contraction (smooth, skeletal, and cardiac) are therefore depressed at fairly high alcohol concentrations. The smaller the nerve fiber diameter, the greater is the effect at a given alcohol concentration.
2. *The inward movement of membrane-bound Ca^{++}* in association with the action potential is also reduced by ethanol. Therefore Ca^{++}-dependent processes, such as neurotransmitter release at the axon terminal, and muscle contraction (smooth, skeletal, and cardiac), are decreased.
3. *Active transport of Na^+, K^+, and amino acids* is decreased by inhibition of the membrane ATPase, especially when the enzyme has been sensitized by catecholamines. This inhibitory action of alcohol also reduces Na^+-linked processes such as reuptake of norepinephrine into sympathetic nerve endings (*see* Chap. 17).

In the CNS, these changes lead to decreased neuronal activity, reflected in lower turnover of acetylcholine, lower ATP utilization and lower oxygen consumption. Effects are more marked in polysynaptic than in monosynaptic pathways. Thus spinal reflexes, primary afferent sensory input, and basic motor pathways are affected only at very high alcohol levels, while modulatory systems such as the reticular activating system, limbic system, extrapyramidal motor pathways, and hypothalamus are sensitive to much lower levels.

Typically, small doses of alcohol (1–2 drinks) cause relaxation and mild sedation, along with centrally mediated autonomic changes: cutaneous vasodilatation, tachycardia, and increased gastric acid secretion and motility. The sedation is usually accompanied by reduced conscious control over emotional expression, so that the person may become talkative, jovial, aggressive, or morose, according to his underlying mood. Small doses do not hinder higher intellectual processes if there is no time limit and may even improve them by reducing nervous tension. However, complex reactions involving rapid decisions are impaired even by small doses. Other early changes include positional nystagmus and positive Romberg sign when the eyes are closed.

With higher doses, when the blood alcohol level is 100 mg/dl or higher, secretion of vaso-

---

MORITZ HEINRICH ROMBERG, 1795–1873. Berlin pathologist and neurologist. Known for Romberg's disease: facial hemiatrophy (1846), Romberg's sign for tabes dorsalis (1846), and Romberg's masticatory spasm (1840). Has been described as the founder of scientific neurotherapy in Germany.

pressin is inhibited, causing diuresis of variable intensity. Oxytocin secretion is also inhibited; ethanol infusion has been used clinically to stop premature labor, although it is no longer recommended for this purpose because of possible harmful effects on the fetus. Motor incoordination becomes marked, with slurred speech, motor ataxia, and loss of balance. Analgesia occurs, and the intoxicated person may burn himself with a cigarette without noticing. Tendon reflexes are sometimes increased initially by loss of descending inhibitory control at the spinal synapses, but at high blood alcohol levels the reflexes disappear. Mental processes are progressively slowed; attention span is reduced. Finally, sleep progresses to coma at levels of 250 mg/dl or higher.

Disturbances Owing to Alcohol Metabolism

NADH, formed during ethanol oxidation, modifies other NAD-linked enzyme reactions in the liver cytoplasm and mitochondria. For example, oxidation of fatty acids is inhibited, and phosphoglyceraldehyde is reduced to glycerolphosphate that is esterified with fatty acids to form triglycerides, giving rise to hyperlipemia and fatty liver. Also, condensation of the unoxidized fatty acyl-CoA molecules gives rise to increased ketone body formation.

Conversion of pyruvate to lactate interferes with gluconeogenesis, and the fasting subject may exhibit hypoglycemia. The excess lactate passes into the blood, contributing to metabolic acidosis. It also inhibits renal tubular clearance of urate and thus can precipitate attacks of gout.

Secondary Effects Owing to Stress

Loss of emotional control during intoxication may cause excitement, anger, fighting, and other stressful behavior. With deeper intoxication, including coma, respiratory depression and fall in effective blood volume (owing to peripheral vasodilatation), hypoxia may result. In both cases, stress-induced catecholamine release may cause hepatic glycogenolysis, mobilization of free fatty acids from adipose tissue, and reduced visceral blood flow. The latter may help explain why large doses of alcohol reduce drug metabolism in the liver.

Acute Toxicity

Death from acute ethanol poisoning is usually due to respiratory depression at a blood alcohol level of 500 mg/dl or higher. If respiration is maintained artificially, death can result from direct inhibition of myocardial contractility at a BAL of about 1 g/dl.

These effects can occur at considerably lower levels in people who are also using other depressant drugs. Barbiturates and other sedatives, major and minor tranquilizers, antihistamines, cannabis, and tricyclic antidepressants may be additive or synergistic with ethanol, mainly because of interaction in the nervous system (*see* Chap. 8).

Treatment of Acute Toxicity. Because even the most severe acute toxic effects of ethanol are reversible, treatment essentially comprises maintaining respiration, blood pressure, and body temperature until the ethanol has been removed by metabolism or by hemodialysis. Stimulants have very little place in therapy.

Chronic Toxicity

Although light use of alcohol *may* have some protective effect against myocardial infarction, regular heavy use significantly increases the risk of illness and death from a number of causes, including alcoholic hepatitis and cirrhosis, peripheral nerve degeneration, alcoholic cardiomyopathy, cancer of the pharynx, hypertension, stroke, and trauma. These effects may in part be due to impaired absorption of water-soluble vitamins and amino acids from the intestine, to stress associated with repeated intoxication, or to the effects of alcohol metabolism. For example, increased alcohol dehydrogenase activity generates more NADH, which requires more oxygen for its reoxidation in the mitochondria. At the same time, intoxication impairs gas exchange in the lungs and reduces oxygen transport in the blood. These factors combine to reduce pO_2 at the hepatic venous end of the liver sinusoid to a point that may result in hypoxic damage to the liver cells next to the terminal hepatic vein. Extensive or repeated damage of this type may provoke alcoholic cirrhosis, first described by Laennec.

Recently it has been recognized that women who drink alcohol during pregnancy are at risk of giving birth to infants with the *fetal alcohol syndrome*. This syndrome is characterized by a combination of congenital anomalies, of which the most important are low birth weight and continuing retardation of development during infancy and childhood, defects in the upper lip and palate, an increased frequency of congenital defects in the heart, and mental retardation. The minimum amount of alcohol required to produce these effects and the pathogenetic mechanisms are not yet known.

RENÉ THÉOPHILE HYACINTHE LAENNEC, 1781–1826. French physician. Remembered for Laennec's cirrhosis of the liver associated with chronic alcoholism, Laennec's sign in bronchial asthma and his invention of the stethoscope, described in 1819.

OTHER ALCOHOLS

Methanol

Methanol (wood alcohol, CH_3OH) has very similar pharmacologic actions to ethanol but is only about half as potent. Its special toxicity arises from its oxidation by alcohol dehydrogenase to yield formaldehyde, which in turn is oxidized to formic acid. These metabolites are toxic to the retina and optic nerve and may cause permanent blindness. The formate also gives rise to metabolic acidosis, which is sometimes fatal.

Treatment requires rapid correction of the acidosis by i.v. $NaHCO_3$ solution and elimination of the remaining unoxidized methanol by hemodialysis. An alternative method is to give small doses of ethanol, which competitively inhibits oxidation of the methanol. The latter is then gradually lost in the urine.

Higher Alcohols

Small amounts of propanols, butanols, pentanols, and their corresponding aldehydes and esters are found in alcoholic beverages, making up the so-called "congeners" or "fusel oil." Some evidence suggests that they may enhance ethanol toxicity. When the higher alcohols are drunk in place of ethanol, either alone or mixed with gasoline, benzene, and other organic solvents, the treatment is basically the same as for ethanol or methanol poisoning.

ALCOHOLISM

Although alcoholism is now widely considered a disease, it is perhaps best viewed as a form of *conditioned behavior*. If alcohol is used repeatedly and in large amounts to obtain relief from problems that the person does not know how to solve in other ways, drinking becomes a firmly established and automatic behavioral response to all sorts of difficulties. Unfortunately, alcohol seldom solves the original problems and usually gives rise to new ones.

As a form of acquired behavior, alcoholism should not be expected to have a single cause. Recent evidence suggests that there may be a hereditary predisposing factor. Parental and prevailing social attitudes toward drinking and drunkenness, personal emotional conflicts, availability and relative cost of alcohol, and the drinking practices of one's friends have a great deal to do with the amount of alcohol used by society as a whole and by an individual within it. In the United States and Canada, about 85% of all adults drink alcohol; about 6% of these drink enough to be considered alcoholics.

COMPLICATIONS

The consequences of alcoholism include high rates of automobile and other accidents, loss of work productivity and earnings, family and social conflict, and high incidence of certain diseases. There are three main pharmacologic problems.

1. Oxidation of ethanol yields 7 kcal/g. Because it is possible to derive well over half the daily caloric requirement from alcohol, the rest of the alcoholic's diet tends to be reduced. Deficiency of protein and vitamins is common and may lead to peripheral neuritis, Wernicke's disease, Korsakoff's psychosis, and pellagra.
2. The direct effects of alcohol on cell membrane functions in the liver, gastrointestinal tract, and other organs are probably related to the production of liver cirrhosis, folate deficiency anemia, alcoholic cardiomyopathy, and other diseases.
3. Chronic exposure of the brain to high concentrations of alcohol gives rise to adaptive changes that result in tolerance and physical dependence.

TOLERANCE AND DEPENDENCE

The depressant effects of ethanol provoke an adaptive response, characterized by hyperexcitability of the affected neurons. Thus the nervous system functions relatively normally in the continued presence of the drug, and the subject is said to be *tolerant*. The dose-response (D-R) curve is shifted to the right, that is, larger doses are needed to produce the same degree of effect. *Metabolic tolerance*, or faster elimination of the ethanol, may contribute to this shift of the D-R curve, but *functional tolerance* of the nervous system is the most important component.

Tolerance can develop "acutely," that is, within the duration of action of a single dose of ethanol. This fact was recognized more than 60 years ago by Mellanby, who observed that the drinker was more intoxicated at a given blood alcohol level (BAL) during the rising part of the

---

Sergei Sergeivich Korsakoff, 1853–1900. Russian psychiatrist. Best known for his description of Korsakoff's psychosis in 1877—the psychosis and polyneuritis found in chronic alcoholism—he also established the concept of paranoia. One of the founders of Russian psychiatry, he did much to encourage less harsh restraints in the treatment of mental patients and developed a mental disease classification scheme.

blood alcohol curve than at the same BAL during the falling part. However, this acute tolerance is of short duration. In chronic heavy drinkers, the tolerance is of greater degree and lasts much longer.

When the ethanol is withdrawn, the changes in the nervous system are left unbalanced, and the hyperexcitability is revealed. This constitutes an alcohol withdrawal reaction, relieved by taking more alcohol; the person is therefore said to be physically dependent on alcohol (*see* Chap. 26).

Withdrawal Reactions. The withdrawal reaction can range from mild to very severe. After a single episode of intoxication, signs of mild hyperexcitability are found for a few hours, coinciding with the "hangover." After prolonged intoxication for days or weeks, withdrawal symptoms usually include sleeplessness, tremor, increased reflexes, sweating, and loss of appetite. In more severe reactions there may be hallucinations and convulsions. The most severe type (*delirium tremens*) includes, in addition, fever, delirium, intense hyperactivity, and tachycardia, which may end in cardiovascular collapse and death. Treatment usually includes sedation, fluid replacement, and avoidance of environment disturbance. Phenytoin (*see* Chap. 29) is not always effective against convulsions in these patients, and phenothiazines (*see* Chap. 24) may worsen the clinical situation. Diazepam is perhaps the most widely favored drug because it has both sedative and anticonvulsant effects (*see* Chap. 25). Chlormethiazole has the same advantages and is widely used in Europe and various other parts of the world, although not yet in the United States. Propranolol (*see* Chap. 18) and lithium (*see* Chap. 22) are being investigated at present for possible therapeutic value against tremor and other milder withdrawal symptoms.

DISULFIRAM

CHEMISTRY AND METABOLISM

Disulfiram, or tetraethylthiuram disulfide, consist of two molecules of diethyl-dithiocarbamate (DDC), probably the pharmacologically active material, joined through a disulfide bond. It is split in the body to give DDC, which in turn is broken down to yield the carbon disulfide that appears in the breath.

ACTIONS AND USE

Disulfiram is a vulcanizing agent. Rubber workers who used it found that they became violently ill if they drank alcohol. This reaction was caused by inhibition of acetaldehyde dehydrogenase. Thus oxidation of ethanol led to an accumulation of acetaldehyde in the blood, causing intense flushing, tachycardia, nausea, vomiting, and circulatory collapse. If an alcoholic treated with disulfiram knows that such consequences are likely to follow drinking, he is more resolute in his resolve to avoid alcohol. Disulfiram is absorbed from the gastrointestinal tract, begins to act in 2 to 4 hours, and reaches maximum effect in 12 to 24 hours. Some patients, after starting on disulfiram therapy, lose their will to take it; to prevent this, clinical trials of an allegedly long-acting parenteral form of disulfiram have been conducted, but the results are unclear.

TOXICITY

Disulfiram inhibits other enzymes and may interfere with the metabolism of other drugs by the liver. It inhibits dopamine β-hydroxylase (*see* Chap. 13), thus interfering with catecholamine synthesis. This may account for such symptoms as weakness, dizziness, and cardiac arrhythmias seen in some patients. Skin allergies and toxic psychoses occasionally occur. Many patients complain of headache, sexual impotence, and tiredness, but it is unclear whether these are due to the disulfiram or to the strain of learning to live without alcohol.

RELATED DRUGS

A number of other drugs cause disulfiram-like reactions to alcohol. Citrated calcium carbimide has a similar, more rapid, and shorter action. It is also less severe, probably because dopamine β-hydroxylase is not affected. Animal charcoal and tolbutamide (*see* Chap. 46) may also provoke similar reactions to alcohol, and physicians should warn patients given these drugs.

FURTHER READING

1. Israel Y, Mardones J (eds): Biological Basis of Alcoholism. New York, Wiley-Interscience, 1971

2. Kalant H, Kalant OJ: Drugs, Society and Personal Choice. Toronto, General Publishing, 1971
3. Kalant H, LeBlanc AE, Gibbins RJ: Tolerance to, and dependence on, some nonopiate psychotropic drugs. Pharmacol Rev 23:135–191, 1971
4. Kissin B, Begleiter H (eds): The Biology of Alcoholism: Volume 1 (Biochemistry); Volume 2 (Physiology and Behavior); Volume 3 (Clinical Pathology). New York, Plenum Press, 1971, 1972, 1974
5. Majchrowicz E, Noble EP (eds): Biochemistry and Pharmacology of Ethanol. New York, Plenum Press, 1979
6. Rosett HL: The effects of alcholol on the fetus and offspring. In Kalant OJ (ed): Alcohol and Drug Problems in Women. New York, Plenum Press, 1980
7. Seeman P: The membrane actions of anesthetics and tranquilizers. Pharmacol Rev 24:583–655, 1972
8. Wallgren H, Barry H III: Actions of Alcohol. Amsterdam, Elsevier, 1970

CHAPTER 27 QUESTIONS

(*See* P. 7 for Full Instructions)

Select the One Best Answer

1. Each of the following represents a demonstrated clinical use of ethyl alcohol EXCEPT
   - *A.* ready source of i.v. calories.
   - *B.* production of nerve damage in trigeminal neuralgia.
   - *C.* diagnostic aid in gastric secretion.
   - *D.* antifoaming agent in pulmonary edema.
   - *E.* coronary dilator for treating angina pectoris.

2. The treatment of choice for alcoholic withdrawal and the prevention of delirium tremens is
   - *A.* chlorpromazine.
   - *B.* phenytoin.
   - *C.* diazepam.
   - *D.* meprobamate.
   - *E.* methadone.

3. Each of the following is true in methanol intoxication EXCEPT
   - *A.* blindness is a common sequela.
   - *B.* marked acidosis occurs.
   - *C.* prompt administration of ethyl alcohol is beneficial.
   - *D.* the pathologic changes are due to metabolic products of methanol.
   - *E.* respiration is generally stimulated.

4. The most important and fundamental characteristic of alcoholism is
   - *A.* the development of metabolic tolerance, that is, increased rate of ethanol oxidation in the liver.
   - *B.* disturbance of nutrition owing to the high caloric contribution of the ingested alcohol.
   - *C.* the potentially life-threatening withdrawal reactions, including delirium tremens.
   - *D.* the use of alcohol as a conditioned response to problems or situational stimuli that the drinker can no longer deal with in other ways.
   - *E.* its role as a prelude to the use of benzodiazepines, opiates, and other drugs.

5. Ethanol
   1. stimulates gastric acid secretion.
   2. has an antianxiety effect.
   3. yields about 7.0 kilocalories per gram when metabolized.
   4. is a safe, practical, general anesthetic agent.

A = 1,2,3; B = 1,3; C = 2,4; D = 4; E = All

6. Ethyl alcohol
   1. is used to treat poisoning with methyl alcohol.
   2. produces hypnotic effects that are potentiated by the concomitant administration of chlorpromazine (Thorazine).
   3. can predispose to lactic acidosis if consumed while taking phenformin (DBI).
   4. stimulates ADH release.

7. Disulfiram (Antabuse) inhibits
   1. dopamine β-hydroxylase.
   2. alcohol dehydrogenase.
   3. aldehyde dehydrogenase.
   4. pseudocholinesterase (plasma).

8. Methyl alcohol is
   1. a depressant of the central nervous system.
   2. a solvent used in oral liquid drug preparations.
   3. usually toxic because of its metabolic products.
   4. seldom lethal when taken orally.

9. Convulsions from withdrawal of alcohol in addicted persons can be suppressed by
   1. paraldehyde.
   2. chloral hydrate.
   3. diazepam.
   4. morphine.

JORDAN D. MILLER
RONALD L. KATZ

28 General Anesthetic Agents

The earliest use of drugs for the suppression of pain during surgery cannot be easily identified. Alcohol and opiates were known in antiquity, and some even suggest that the removal of Adam's rib while he was asleep was an early example of general anesthesia. Before the use of anesthetics, operations were torturous, and the length and success of the surgery were related more to the patient's constitution than to other factors. Speed during surgery was essential. Mortality rates of 50% or greater were common. Predictable and relatively safe relief from the pain of surgery awaited the use of ether, chloroform, and nitrous oxide in the mid-19th century. Although the use of these and a host of other agents spread rapidly, the science of anesthesia progressed slowly. Only in the last 50 years have major changes occurred. The use of sodium pentothal as an induction agent in the 1930s and the introduction of muscle relaxants in the 1940s date the modern era of anesthesia. The medical specialty of anesthesiology developed after World War II, partly out of the need that arose during the war. Although the modern era began in the 1930s, the regular use of open-drop ether continued into the 1960s.

Many of the major advances in surgery have had to await the development of anesthetic techniques. A simple example is the development of the endotracheal tube that made feasible positive pressure ventilation and therefore intrathoracic surgery.

Horace Wells, 1815–1848. Dentist in Hartford, Connecticut. In 1844 was the first to use nitrous oxide inhalation anesthesia in dentistry. Wells believed that nitrous oxide was superior to ether.

Crawford Williamson Long, 1815–1878. Physician in Danielville, Georgia. In 1842 used ether anesthesia during the surgical removal of a cystic tumor on the neck. This was the first use of a general anesthetic, but Long did not publish his procedure until 1849.

William Thomas Green Morton, 1819–1868. Boston physician. In 1846 used ether anesthesia in the removal of a vascular tumor of the neck at Massachusetts General Hospital. Played a major role in promoting the use of ether on which he held a patent for 14 years.

GENERAL ANESTHESIA: A DEFINITION

General anesthesia can be divided into five components: amnesia, loss of consciousness, analgesia, loss of reflexes (both sensory and autonomic), and muscle relaxation. Although all drugs used as anesthetics are aimed at producing at least one of these effects, the agent termed the "general anesthetic" is the one that produces amnesia, analgesia, and loss of consciousness. A complete anesthetic agent is one that can produce all of the effects by itself. The extent to which a general anesthetic possesses each of the above characteristics varies among agents. Modern anesthesia combines a variety of drugs in an attempt to use the best properties of each and to minimize the unnecessary or harmful side-effects. Thus ether, which will produce all of the above effects, is generally not used alone. Modern anesthesia would combine ether, nitrous oxide, muscle relaxants, and drugs to suppress some of the autonomic reflexes, all in an attempt to produce the smoothest and least detrimental depression of the patient.

At present, there are two classes of general anesthetics: those administered by inhalation and those given by injection. The largest class by far is the inhalational general anesthetic class.

MECHANISM OF ACTION

The specific site of action in the CNS on which anesthetics work is uncertain. Some general anesthetics inhibit the reticular activating system before blocking other areas. The reticular activating system is that portion of the CNS that receives nonspecific sensory input and is responsible for initiating and maintaining alert wakefulness. Unconsciousness may be related to the suppression of this system. It is known that synaptic transmission is slowed by general anesthesia and, since the reticular activating system has a great number of synapses, would be most susceptible to blockade.

The cellular site of action of anesthetics is unknown. Pauling and Miller proposed that all inhalational anesthetics act as a nidus for "water crystals" or "clathrates"; the crystal formation interferes with neural transmission. This theory remains to be proved because clathrates have never been demonstrated to exist under conditions likely to be found in the body.

The more soluble an agent is in a lipid, the lower the concentration necessary for it to produce general anesthesia. Although this variable may be related to the need of an anesthetic agent to cross lipid membranes, it does not indicate the cellular site of action of the anesthetic. Recent evidence has supported the hypothesis that anesthetics act by expanding lipid layers (*i.e.*, cell membrane) in which they dissolve. Pressure can counteract this effect. Lipid solubility does not predict or guarantee which agents will be anesthetic.

SIGNS AND STAGES OF ANESTHESIA

The depth of ether anesthesia was divided by Guedel into sequential stages and planes of anesthesia. Although not used in its entirety by modern anesthesiologists, this classification of the sequence of events is useful. Analgesia and amnesia (stage 1) precede the loss of consciousness, followed by delirium or stage 2. During this period vomiting and violent combative behavior may occur. To avoid this excitement stage, short-acting barbiturates, such as sodium pentothal, are given intravenously before most anesthetics (*see* Chap. 25). (The use of sodium pentothal has gained wide acceptance for this purpose.) Barbiturates, although technically general anesthetics, have too narrow a therapeutic ratio to be used as the sole agent.

Stage 3, surgical anesthesia, formerly was subdivided into four planes that are no longer relevant. For example, muscle relaxation or apnea was formerly used to define different planes. Today these effects are produced by specific drugs, thus making the plane concept outdated. Another reason for abandoning the plane concept is that the effects of general anesthetics depend on the sensory input as well as on the concentration of the agent being used. Thus respiratory and cardiovascular depression are much greater with low sensory input when the patient is anesthetized but surgery has not begun. After surgical stimulation, both variables tend to be less depressed, and the patient appears to be in a lighter plane. Therefore a patient's level reflects a balance between anesthetic depression and surgical stimulation.

The stages described above for general anesthesia can apply to any depressant of the CNS. Hypoxia, or decreased cerebral blood flow, can produce each of the stages but with more permanent damage. During a cardiac arrest, the adequacy of external cardiac massage can be evaluated by that stage of "general anesthesia" the patient appears to have achieved. The return of reflexes, corneal and respiratory particularly, are signs of improving cerebral perfusion.

The awakening from general anesthesia is the reverse of the induction process. Patients first regain reflexes, may go through a short excitement stage, and come to analgesia and full wakefulness. The shorter the recovery time, the safer it is for the patient.

The minimum goals of anesthesia are amnesia, analgesia, and ideal operating conditions for the surgeon, which frequently requires muscle relaxants that may make evaluation of somatic reflexes difficult. However, autonomic reflexes, such as blood pressure and heart rate, are a good guide to the depth of anesthesia. Increases in blood pressure and heart rate with surgical stimulation indicate inadequate depth of anesthesia, and thus the concentration of the anesthetic is increased. If, on the other hand, the blood pressure falls, the anesthetic concentration is decreased.

Recently the therapeutic concentration or ED_{50} for inhalational anesthetics has been assessed. Minimum alveolar concentration (MAC) is the alveolar tension at which 50% of the patients move when a surgical stimulus is applied. The conditions under which this is measured require that patients receive no premedication, no barbiturate for induction, and no supplementation at any time. All of these factors would tend to decrease the concentration of anesthetic necessary for adequate surgical anesthesia. Thus under clinical circumstances, MAC may be an overestimate. The concept of an ED_{50} or MAC is useful in comparing pharmacologic effects of different anesthetic agents.

It has been found that MAC is additive; thus if 0.5 MAC halothane (0.38%) of 0.5 MAC nitrous oxide (50%) are used, the patient appears to be at 1 MAC. MAC is also age dependent: the younger the patient, the higher the concentration of anesthetic necessary. Finally the patient's temperature is important: Hyperthermic patients require more anesthetic; those who are hypothermic require less. MAC values for general anesthetics are found in Table 28-1. MAC is only a guideline, however, and represents the concentration at which 50% of the patients will be too lightly anesthetized for surgery. Further, MAC is the alveolar concentration, not the delivered concentration. As can be seen in Figure 28-1, the alveolar concentration may be much lower than the concentration delivered from the anesthesia machine, particularly for agents with high solubility or those delivered for a short period. The concentration listed applies to an atmospheric pressure equal to 760 mm Hg. Whereas MAC is commonly reported in concentration, actually the anesthetic tension or partial pressure is important. Therefore, when atmospheric pressure differs significantly from 760 mm Hg, as may occur in a hyperbaric chamber or at altitude, the partial pressure expressed in millimeters of mercury is the correct value. Thus, at 2 atm, nitrous oxide MAC is 760 mm Hg, or 50%. At 1 atm it is still 760 mm Hg, but it requires 100% nitrous oxide, an unobtainable goal. Conversely, at a higher altitude where atmospheric pressure is 600 mm Hg, halothane MAC is still 6 mm Hg but 1% rather than 0.76% at sea level.

TABLE 28-1. Physical Contents and Formula of Anesthetic Agents

Agent	Blood/ Gas	MAC		Fat/ Blood	P Vapor 20° C mm Hg	Formula
		%	*mm Hg*			
Chloroform	9.1	0.37	2.7	26	160	$CHCl_3$
Cyclopropane	0.46	10	76	13	—	C_3H_6
Diethyl ether	12	2	15	5	443	$(C_2H_5)_2O$
Enflurane	1.9	1.68	13	36	174	$CHF_2—O—CF_2CHFCl$
Ethylene	0.14	80	610	9	—	C_2H_4
Fluroxene	1.4	3.4	26	—	286	$CF_3CH_2—O—CH{=}CH_2$
Halothane	2.3	0.76	6	60	243	$CF_3CHBrCl$
Isoflurane	1.4	1.3	10	45	260	$CHF_2—O—CHClCF_3$
Methoxyflurane	12	0.16	1.2	49	24	$CH_3—OCF_2CHCl_2$
Nitrous oxide	0.43	100	760	3	—	N_2O
Trichloroethylene	9	0.22	1.7	—	—	$CHCl{=}CCl_2$

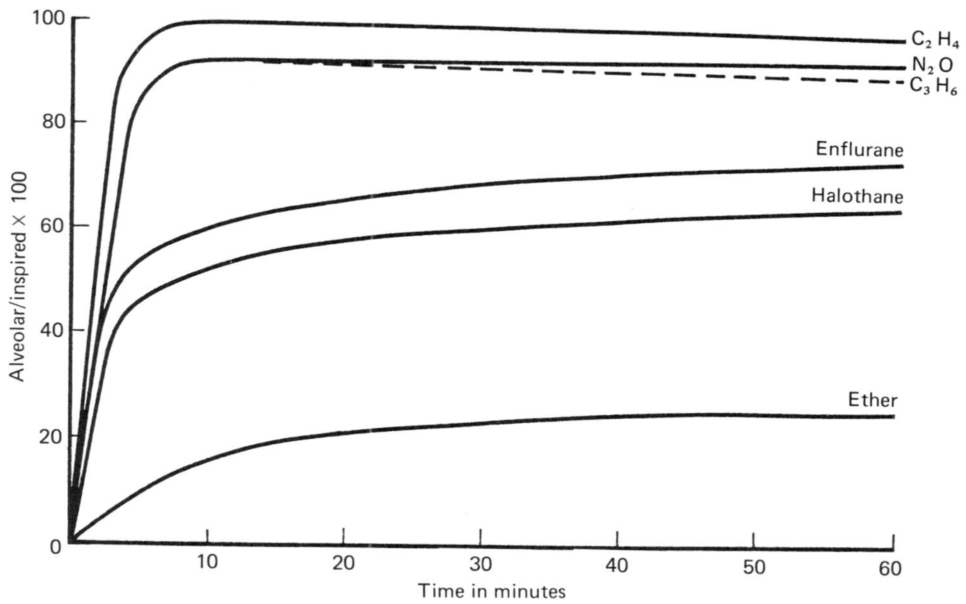

FIG. 28-1. Alveolar concentration of anesthetics as a fraction of the inspired tension during the first 60 minutes of anesthesia.

UPTAKE

The depth of anesthesia depends on the tension or partial pressure (expressed in millimeters of mercury) that reaches the brain. This in turn depends on the arterial tension at equilibrium with the alveolar tension: The higher the tension in the alveoli, the more rapid the induction. The tension in the alveoli depends on the administered tension and solubility of the anesthetic. The more soluble the anesthetic is in blood, the more agent is removed from the alveoli and the lower the alveolar tension; the less soluble the agent is in blood, the more rapidly the alveolar tension approaches that of the inspired gas. As a result, the less soluble the agent, the more rapidly the brain (which again is in equilibrium with the blood) will reach the anesthetic tension. With anesthetics, it is important to realize that the dose does not matter. Thus ether, which is very soluble, will have many more molecules in the blood before reaching an anesthetic level (or tension) than a less soluble agent, even though both agents have the same MAC.

A second factor that determines uptake is ventilation. The greater the ventilation of the alveoli, the more anesthetic is delivered to the alveoli and the more rapid the induction. This factor is most important early in the induction of anesthesia, when uptake by the blood is most rapid. It is also more important for soluble agents than for insoluble ones.

A third important factor is blood flow. The higher the flow through the lungs, the more agent is removed from the alveoli, and thus the tension is low.

The initial inspired tension is a fourth factor that influences uptake. If the tension is higher than that needed for maintenance anesthesia, the brain will reach anesthetic levels more rapidly. This is called *overpressure*, and although used for most agents, it is of greatest importance with those that are soluble. Thus ether, which requires a brain tension of about 14 mm Hg, may initially be administered at an inspired tension of 140 mm Hg to allow for its great solubility and uptake into the blood. Nitrous oxide needs almost no overpressure because its solubility is so low. Halothane may initially be administered at two to three times the maintenance concentration to speed its onset of action.

Awakening from anesthesia is the reverse process. The less soluble an agent, the more completely it is removed from the blood in one passage through the lungs, and thus the more rapid the awakening.

Anesthetics are metabolized, in some cases as much as 35% of the administered dose. This process is slow, however, and of no clinical significance as far as induction or awakening. The metabolic products, however, may be toxic (discussed below under Methoxyflurane and Halothane). That inhalation anesthetic agents are metabolized is a relatively recent concept;

for years the classic concept was that these agents were eliminated unchanged.

The solubility of most anesthetics in tissues is equal to that in blood, except for fat. Fat acts as a storehouse for anesthetics and may account for a delay in awakening of patients from agents with high solubility.

ANESTHESIA MACHINE

Flowmeter

The anesthesia machine diagramed in Figure 28-2 is composed of several gas sources that can be either tanks of compressed gas, such as oxygen or nitrous oxide, or, in modern operating rooms, wall sources of these two gases. The pressure is reduced from these sources, and the final pressure supplied to the flowmeters is about 6 lb/sq in. The most common flowmeter is controlled by a needle valve. An indicator or float sitting in a carefully calibrated tube indicates the rate of flow of the gas. Each tube is calibrated for a specific gas. The gases are then collected and leave the machine at a common site. Volatile anesthetics, those that are liquid at room temperature, can be accurately vaporized by one of several means, the simplest being the copper kettle. Oxygen from a flowmeter is bubbled through the liquid in the kettle. The vapor reaches equilibrium and is collected in the common outflow from the machine. The concentration of vapor that leaves the kettle depends on the vapor pressure of the liquid (Equation 1):

$$\text{cc vapor} = \frac{P_{vap} \times \text{cc } O_2}{P_{atm} - P_{vap}}, \qquad 1$$

where P_{vap} = vapor pressure of liquid (mm Hg) and P_{atm} = atmospheric pressure (mm Hg).

Since the evaporation of the vapor requires energy in the form of heat, the liquid tends to cool. To prevent great changes in the temperature of the liquid, the copper kettle is attached to the metal of the anesthesia machine, which acts as a large heat sink and stabilizes the temperature of the liquid. The advantage of a copper kettle is that it can be used with any volatile anesthetic and does not require frequent calibration. It is, however, temperature dependent, and if the temperature changes rapidly it can deliver concentrations of an anesthetic very different from the one expected (*e.g.*, if enflurane is used at a temperature of 18°C, vapor pressure = 198, but at 28°C, it is 357). Once the vaporizer output is calculated for the oxygen flow, the final anesthetic concentration is that figure divided by the diluent gases coming from the oxygen and nitrous oxide flowmeters. Thus 100 ml of oxygen into the copper kettle filled with enflurane yields 26 ml of enflurane vapor at 18°C. If the oxygen flow is 1 liter/min and nitrous oxide flow is 1.5 liters/min, the final enflurane concentration is 1%.

Temperature and Flow Compensated Vaporizer

A simple system that does not require these calculations is the temperature and flow compensated vaporizer. Several of these are available (Fig. 28-3). In this system, the total gas flow from the machine is passed through the input, then divided into two streams, one passing through the anesthetic liquid and the other bypassing the chamber that holds the liquid. As the temperature increases and, thus the vapor pressure of the liquid increases, a bimetallic strip acts as a valve and decreases flow through the volatile anesthetic. As a result a steady output concentration is maintained. These systems suffer from several disadvantages: They

FIG. 28-2. Diagramatic representation of the flowmeters and copper kettle of an anesthetic machine.

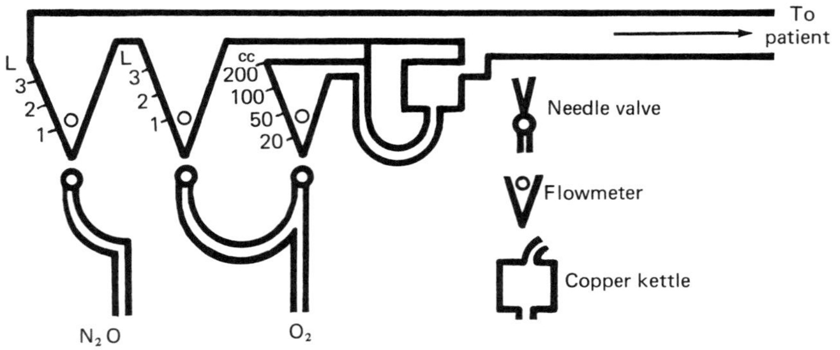

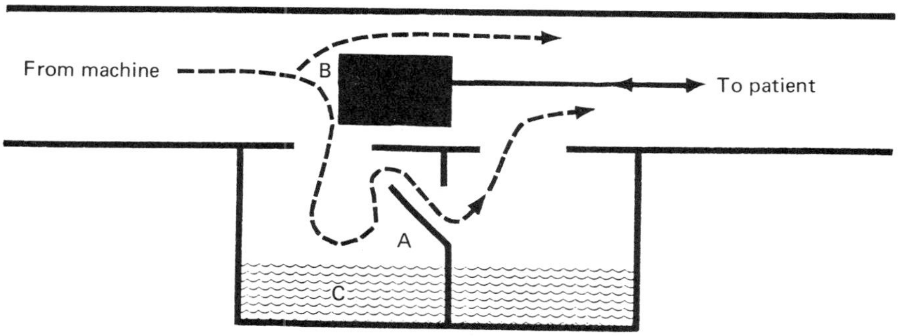

FIG. 28-3. Path of anesthetic gases in a temperature-compensated vaporizer. (*A*) Bimetalic strip. (*B*) Slide to occlude path of gases through vaporizer. (*C*) Anesthetic liquid.

can be used only with one specific anesthetic vapor. In addition, they must be calibrated very frequently, and any mechanical defect might lead to a massive overdose. If the bimetallic strip is stuck in the open position, for instance, the patient might receive an unacceptably high concentration. These systems are, however, growing in popularity because of the ease with which they can be used. There are other types of vaporizers, but the two kinds listed above are the most frequently used.

ANESTHESIA CIRCUITS

Closed Systems

A variety of anesthetic circuits are available. The most commonly used circuit is diagramed in Figure 28-4. Gas leaving the anesthesia machine enters a circle with two one-way valves. An inflatable bag allows the patient to breathe spontaneously or to be ventilated by the anesthesiologist who squeezes the bag. A simple pop-off valve allows excess gas to leave the circuit. A cannister containing soda lime absorbs the carbon dioxide present in any rebreathed gas. If the gas flow into the circuit just equals the uptake of oxygen and the anesthetic agent, the system is called "closed." The exact concentration the patient is breathing is not known, since the uptake of each gas occurs independently. Cyclopropane is almost always administered by a closed system because the anesthetic is extremely explosive as well as expensive. The danger of explosion is significantly decreased because little of the cyclopropane enters the room.

Semiclosed or Partial Rebreathing System

A semiclosed or partial rebreathing system is one in which more gas enters the circle than is taken up by the patient. Generally 2 to 6 liters/min is used. The patient does rebreathe some previously exhaled gas, but the inspired concentration approaches that which the machine delivers. Absorption of CO_2 is important to prevent increased CO_2 in the inspired gas. The advantage of the closed and semiclosed systems is that dry gas that comes from the machine gains moisture both from the CO_2 absorber and from water vapor in the tubing. Thus secretions in the tracheobronchial tree do not get as thick and tenacious and are less likely to cause obstruction. This is particularly important in infants and children, especially when an endotracheal tube bypasses the normal humidifiers of the upper airways.

Nonrebreathing System

The nonrebreathing system does not use a circle or CO_2 absorber but depends on an extremely high fresh gas flow to keep the patient from accumulating CO_2. There are many such systems, but probably the simplest one is an Ayre's T piece. In its most basic form the fresh gas must enter at two to three times the patient's minute ventilation to prevent rebreathing of exhaled gas or inhalation of room air. This tends to dry the patient's respiratory tract, is extremely wasteful of anesthetics, and is a pollutant of the operating room environment. The advantages of this system are that it is simple and allows rapid changes in inhaled concentration, and therefore a more rapid change in anesthetic depth. To avoid the high flows necessary for this system, various nonrebreathing valves have been designed to allow one to use flows that match the ventilation of the patient and still prevent rebreathing. However, the flows are still larger than those needed in the semiclosed circle. This and other difficulties tend to make nonrebreathing valves less commonly used than the circle absorption system.

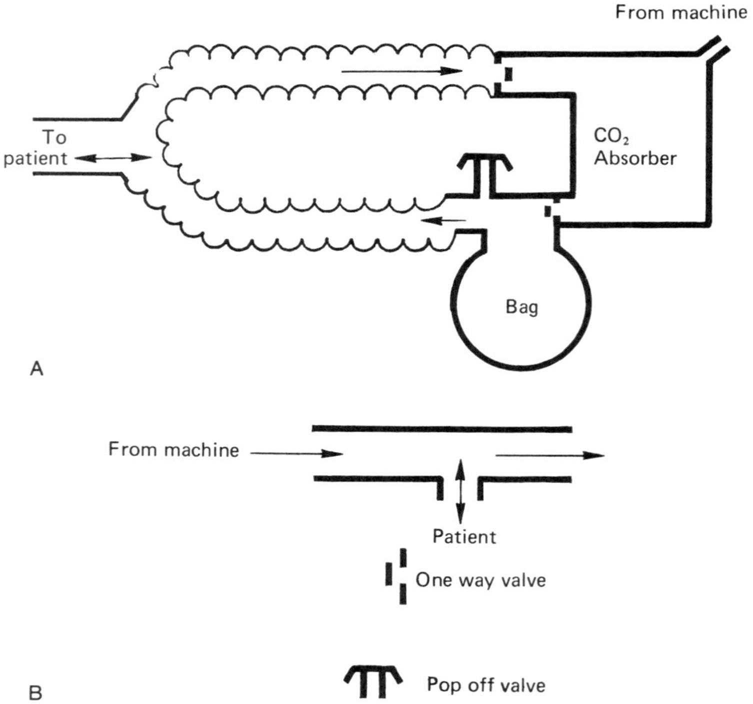

FIG. 28-4. (*A*) Diagramatic representation of a circle system. (*B*) Diagram of an Ayre's T-piece.

At present, anesthesiologists are attempting to prevent the buildup of anesthetic vapors in the operating room. Recently several papers have discussed the increased incidence of spontaneous abortion in pregnant women who work in operating rooms. In addition, a decreased attention span and other signs of depressed mental function have been observed in the operating team after prolonged inhalation of anesthetics. Most systems for removing anesthetic agents from the operating room pass the excess vapors into a suction that carries them away.

FLAMMABLE AGENTS

It is common to classify anesthetic agents in terms of flammability. In general, the use of flammable agents has decreased markedly as new, more satisfactory nonflammable agents have become available. The flammable agents require special care in handling, not only during transport and storage but also during administration in the operating room. In the operating room all possibility of sparks either from electrical equipment or static electrical discharges must be eliminated. All switches must be at least 5 feet above the floor or of special construction. All electrical outlets must have special design to prevent a spark during connection of equipment. Electric cautery may not be used. This requirement has handicapped many surgeons. All personnel and equipment must be interconnected through conductive flooring so that no static electric charges can build up. All high-voltage equipment must be 5 feet above the floor or in specially constructed cases. Many hospitals are unwilling to spend the extra money for these precautions as well as for the increased insurance costs. Many anesthesiologists are unwilling to accept the extra risk to their patients and themselves, and, in the absence of well-documented advantage, have given up the flammable agents.

The following classification of anesthetic agents starts with those most commonly used and progresses to those least commonly used.

NONFLAMMABLE AGENTS

Nitrous Oxide—MAC 100%; Blood/Gas Ratio 0.43

One of the oldest agents available, nitrous oxide is the only inorganic substance currently used for anesthesia. Nitrous oxide is one of the least soluble anesthetics, and thus its onset of action is extremely rapid; awakening is similarly fast. A primary limitation is the concentration that can be administered and still allow an adequate concentration of oxygen (MAC of 100%). Therefore, nitrous oxide is not used alone except when the patient is very ill and MAC may be 70% to 80%. It is, however, an ideal supplemental anesthetic. In the "balance technique," barbiturates with or without narcotics or neuromuscular blocking agents (muscle relaxants) are used to supplement nitrous oxide. Balanced anesthesia can produce adequate anesthesia for all forms of surgery. The nitrous oxide primarily provides amnesia and analgesia, whereas the barbiturate and narcotic add depression of reflexes as well as analgesia and sleep. The neuromuscular blockers add muscle relaxation.

Nitrous oxide is also used with other more potent inhalation agents, allowing a lower concentration of the latter to be used. This may offer several advantages over the use of the more potent agent alone. If nitrous oxide is used to supplement a slower inhalational agent, both onset of surgical anesthesia and awakening are more rapid. In addition, nitrous oxide is less depressant to both the cardiovascular system and respiratory system than most of the inhalational agents currently available. As a result, nitrous oxide combined with other inhalational agents produces less cardiovascular and respiratory depression than does an equal depth of anesthesia produced by a single inhalational agent.

Because nitrous oxide is used in such high concentrations (50–70%) and its solubility in blood is greater than that of nitrogen, it will replace nitrogen in any air pockets in the body. This generally is of no consequence, but in bowel obstructions the volume of gas in the bowel may increase twofold in only 2 hours of administration of nitrous oxide, making it difficult to replace the bowel in the abdomen. Similarly, after injection of air into the ventricles of the brain during a pneumoencephalogram, nitrous oxide inhalation may dangerously raise the cerebrospinal fluid pressure and cause decreased blood flow to the brain or even herniation of the brain stem.

Halothane (Fluothane)—MAC 0.76%; Blood/Gas Ratio 2.3

Since its introduction in 1956, halothane has become one of the most widely used anesthetics and is a potent agent that produces total anesthesia on its own. However, muscle relaxation is poor at normally used concentrations. When muscle relaxation is needed, neuromuscular blockers must be used. While depressant to the cardiovascular system and capable of lowering the blood pressure, there is a fall in peripheral resistance before a decrease in cardiac output. The addition of nitrous oxide (and hence a lowering of the concentration of halothane required for anesthesia) makes for less depression of the blood pressure at equal depths of anesthesia. (This is partially through increased systemic vascular resistance.) Awakening is rapid and usually uneventful. Laryngeal reflexes are obtunded early, and laryngospasm (reflex closure of vocal cords) is rarely a problem.

Respiration under halothane becomes rapid and shallow, but the Pco_2 may be only minimally elevated, especially if light anesthesia is maintained. The addition of nitrous oxide to supplement halothane will also help to maintain a normal Pco_2. Controlled ventilation is frequently needed, however, to maintain a normal Pco_2 and certainly is needed for deeper anesthesia or if muscle relaxants are used. Narcotics decrease the rate and increase the depth of respiration under halothane, but the overall alveolar ventilation is decreased and Pco_2 increased. Halothane exerts potent relaxant effects on smooth muscle. The bronchospasm of asthma is diminished by deep halothane anesthesia, and if bronchospasm occurs under anesthesia or is an expected problem halothane is an excellent choice. It will also relax the smooth muscle of the pregnant uterus, having the undesirable side-effect of excessive blood loss during parturition.

A potential problem with halothane is that it sensitizes the myocardium to the arrhythmogenic properties of catecholamines (*see* Chap. 17). Thus there may be cardiac arrhythmias secondary to exogenous catecholamines (injected by surgeon or anesthesiologist) or by endogenously released catecholamines owing to increased carbon dioxide tension or drugs. This limits the amount of catecholamines or local anesthetics with catecholamines that can be used during operations.

The occurrence of nodal rhythm under halothane is very common and usually presents no undesirable effects to the patient. The patient reverts spontaneously to normal sinus rhythm with the end of anesthesia, if not before.

A rare, often fatal, complication of halothane anesthesia is "halothane hepatitis." It has not been reported in children. "Hepatitis." is preceded by fever, usually 3 to 10 days postoperatively, and there are two theories as to its etiology. One theory is that an as-yet-unidentified metabolite binds to a cell protein, sensitizing the cell to autoimmune destruction. This theory has led to the common practice of avoiding repeated exposure to halothane. However, the incidence of hepatitis is so low that if no previous evidence of halothane hepatitis exists, there is no contraindication of its use. A second view is that the anaerobic metabolism of halothane in a patient with previous enzyme induction is responsible. There is now an animal model for this latter theory, and thus it is gaining in popularity.

Enflurane (Ethrane)—MAC 1.68%; Blood/Gas Ratio 1.9

Introduced clinically in 1972, enflurane is similar in effect to halothane but is less potent and soluble. However, it produces better muscle relaxation than does halothane, even at light levels of anesthesia. Enflurane has a somewhat irritating odor and may cause coughing and bronchospasm during light levels of anesthesia. Not infrequently a muscle relaxant is needed for intraabdominal operations, although in smaller doses than with halothane. Again nitrous oxide is almost always used to allow a lower concentration of enflurane and thus diminish cardiovascular and respiratory depression, which is similar in extent to that seen with halothane. Sensitization to catecholamines is significantly lower than that seen after halothane administration, and it has become the agent of choice for managing patients with phenochromocytoma. In addition, increased P_{CO_2} does not produce cardiac arrhythmias as it does with halothane. Hepatitis has not been reported with this agent, but only further experience will establish this difference. Metabolism of enflurane is low, but inorganic fluoride is produced and blood levels rise postoperatively. Although the rise is much smaller and of shorter duration than that seen after methoxyflurane, it may be sufficient to damage further an already compromised kidney. Seizures (both physical and on electroencephalogram) have been seen during the use of this agent. The deeper the anesthetic and the lower the P_{CO_2}, the more frequent is their occurrence. At commonly used concentrations and with close to normal P_{CO_2}, however, this is not a problem. The mechanism of the seizure activity is unknown. Awakening is usually rapid and uneventful, although nausea appears to be somewhat more common than after halothane administration.

Isoflurane (Forane)—MAC 1.3 Blood/Gas Ratio 1.4

This agent, the least soluble of the volatile anesthetics, has not yet been used enough to determine its proper place, but it may have some advantages over other volatile anesthetics. A potential benefit is its slow rate of metabolism. Inorganic fluoride is released, but at a slower rate than that seen after enflurane, and not much quicker than that seen after halothane; thus the risk of hepatitis or renal damage should be minimal. Although its somewhat irritating odor may delay induction, making it no faster than halothane, its low solubility speeds awakening. It potentiates the neuromuscular blocking agents about as well as enflurane but does not sensitize the heart to catecholamines, and rhythm disturbances are uncommon. It does not cause seizures and thus is preferable to enflurane. Cardiac output is better maintained with isoflurane than with either halothane or enflurane, although stroke volume is decreased. (This is compensated for by an increased heart rate.) Blood flow to skin and muscle increases markedly, and maintenance of flow to important organs such as the brain may be no better than that seen with other agents. Barring problems not yet apparent, this agent may find widespread use.

Methoxyflurane (Penthrane)—MAC 0.16%; Blood/Gas Ratio 12

Methoxyflurane is the most potent agent currently available, but, because of its high blood solubility, overpressure is needed during induction. The use of nitrous oxide and frequently doses of barbiturates early in the anesthetic help to produce a rapid onset of surgical anesthesia. Awakening, however, cannot be similarly facilitated and is therefore quite slow. Methoxyflurane is a complete anesthetic that produces good muscle relaxation at usual levels of anesthesia. In addition, it sensitizes the myocardium minimally to the effects of catecholamines. Its analgesic effect is quite marked, and even before loss of consciousness methoxyflurane produces profound analgesia. Patients awaken relatively free of pain. It has been used in labor to decrease pain over prolonged periods by periodic breathing of its vapor. The main reason for its lack of favor is that it is metabolized (over many days) to inorganic fluoride. Metabolism is prolonged because the drug is avidly stored in fat. If the fluoride level is high enough, methoxyflurane causes a high-output renal failure that may progress to total renal failure. Although usually reversible, total renal failure is too high a price to pay for methoxyflurane's limited advantages. Obese patients under deep anesthesia and undergoing long procedures are most susceptible to renal failure because they receive a large total dose and take a long time to excrete the agent.

Fluroxene (Flumar)—MAC 3.4%; Blood/Gas Ratio 1.5

Fluroxene was introduced shortly before halothane and has been eclipsed by it. The compound is flammable at concentrations greater than 4%. If used with nitrous oxide, which decreases the amount of fluroxene necessary, it may be possible to use fluroxene below the explosive range. Most anesthesiologists believe that this risk is unacceptable, however, and therefore this agent is treated as flammable. Fluroxene does offer certain advantages: It does not sensitize the myocardium to catecholamines or to increased Pco_2; blood pressure is better maintained than with the other halogenated agents; and respiratory depression seems to be less marked. If fluroxene hepatitis exists in humans, it is much rarer than with halothane. Finally, awakening is rapid, but nausea is quite common. Fluroxene is no longer available in the United States.

Trichloroethylene (Trilene or Trimar)—MAC 0.22%; Blood/Gas Ratio 9

Trichloroethylene is rarely used in this country except as an inhalational analgesic during labor. It is metabolized to trichloracetic acid but not in sufficient quantity to be toxic. If used in a circle system with soda lime to absorb exhaled carbon dioxide, this agent decomposes to phosgene and carbon monoxide, both extremely toxic agents; decomposition is facilitated by increased temperature. Cranial nerve palsies occasionally develop and are probably due to decomposition products. Trichloroethylene must be used in a nonrebreathing system that does not require carbon dioxide absorption with soda lime. At excessively deep levels of anesthesia, cardiac arrhythmias may occur. At the levels required for light anesthesia, however, arrhythmias are rare.

Chloroform—MAC 0.37%; Blood/Gas Ratio 9.1

Its hepatotoxicity, plus the availability of better agents, has virtually eliminated its use from anesthesia.

FLAMMABLE AGENTS

Diethyl Ether—MAC 2.0%; Blood/Gas Ratio 12

Diethyl ether is rarely used alone because of its extremely slow induction time and recovery. It stimulates respiratory secretions, necessitating the use of belladonna drugs preanesthesia. The cardiovascular system is less depressed than with the halogenated agents, and in this respect diethyl ether is similar to fluroxene. The release of endogenous catecholamines is responsible for this. Respiration is initially stimulated but is depressed at deeper anesthetic levels. Since muscle relaxation is good, this drug can be used without muscle relaxants. To allow faster recovery, however, diethyl ether is generally used along with nitrous oxide. Only small amounts of neuromuscular blockers are needed to produce adequate muscle relaxation for intraabdominal surgery. Nausea and vomiting occur over a prolonged period, even with light levels of ether. As a result, diethyl ether has poor public acceptance. Properly managed, however, it is at least as safe as any other agent, and some anesthesiologists believe it still has some qualities that make it superior to other agents currently available.

Cyclopropane—MAC 10%; Blood/Gas Ratio 0.47

Cyclopropane has gone out of favor because of its explosive nature. It supports the blood pressure, however, and may even cause moderate hypertension, even at deep levels of anesthesia. The pulse rate generally falls as a baroreceptor response to the hypertension, and if atropine is given to increase heart rate, multifocal ventricular premature contractions occur frequently. Cyclopropane is the most potent anesthetic sensitizer of the myocardium to catecholamines. In the presence of an increased Pco_2, cardiac arrhythmias occur frequently. Spontaneous respiration with this agent will result in an increased Pco_2; thus controlled ventilation is often necessary except at the lightest levels of anesthesia. Cyclopropane increases skin blood flow, but this does not usually result in increased blood loss during surgery. Operations may be somewhat slowed, however, due to the need for greater hemostasis during skin incision. Because of its high cost and its extreme flammability, cyclopropane is administered in a closed-circle system.

Ethylene—MAC 80%; Blood/Gas Ratio 0.14

Ethylene is similar to nitrous oxide, but its flammability far outweighs any small benefits obtained by the slightly lower solubility and greater potency. It is rarely used today.

Divinyl Ether

Divinyl ether is primarily used for rapid induction before ether anesthesia. If used for longer than 30 minutes it leads to hepatic necrosis. It is rarely used.

INTRAVENOUS AGENTS

Ketamine (Ketalar or Ketaject)

The only true general anesthetic administered by means other than inhalation, ketamine produces profound somatic anesthesia but no muscle relaxation, and most reflexes are maintained. Patients exhibit protective reflexes, maintain their own airway and normal respiration, and display corneal reflexes. The patient seems awake but disconnected from the environment. The term *dissociative anesthesia* is used to describe this state. The agent produces variable hypertension and tachycardia that may cause problems. Ketamine seems particularly useful during diagnostic procedures because it allows a well-maintained airway. When a patient is hypotensive and hypovolemic, this agent maintains the blood pressure while other measures are being instituted to correct the primary problem. Difficulties inherent in its use, however, include the production of hallucinations that may be remembered by the patient as extremely unpleasant, inadequate anesthesia for deep pain such as intraabdominal surgery, and a long sleep time that cannot be hastened relative to the length of the surgical anesthesia. The dose is 2 to 4 mg/kg, intravenously, or 5 to 10 mg/kg intramuscularly. Additional doses are given when the patient shows signs of responding to pain.

NARCOTIC-OXYGEN

In some situations, primarily in open-heart surgery, large doses of narcotics (morphine 1–3 mg/kg or fentanyl 50–150 μg/kg) may be used as an anesthetic agent. Although amnesia is not guaranteed, patients do not experience discomfort during surgery and will not be uncomfortable if properly prepared preoperatively. Frequently muscle relaxant drugs are used to prevent the muscle rigidity seen with these high doses of narcotics, as well as to give optimal operating conditions. Cardiovascular depression is minimal, although venous dilatation can occur and may require large infusions of fluid to maintain venous return. Hormonal responses to surgical stimulation are at least as well suppressed with this regimen as with other general anesthetic techniques. The use of supplemental agents to produce amnesia such as nitrous oxide, diazepam, or lorazepam is associated with cardiovascular depression similar to that produced by other techniques. Ventilation is required both intraoperatively and postoperatively for 12 to 48 hours until the narcotic is either metabolized or excreted. Shorter-acting narcotics are currently being investigated and may make this form of anesthesia more popular.

For detailed descriptions of agents used to supplement anesthesia, *see* the chapters on barbiturates (Chap. 25), neuromuscular blocking agents (Chap. 19), narcotics (Chap. 32), and tranquilizers (Chap. 24).

PREANESTHETIC MEDICATION

The goal of the anesthesiologist is to bring the patient to the operating room in a state of carefree wakefulness. To reach this goal, many agents have been given for preoperative medication. Combinations of barbiturates, narcotics, and minor tranquilizers, even antihistaminics with sedative properties, have been used. Since there is no one best agent, the most commonly used agents are barbiturates, such as secobarbital, tranquilizers, such as diazepam, droperidol, hydroxyzine, and agents of mixed properties, such as promethazine.

Belladonna alkaloids (atropine or scopolamine; *see* Chap. 16) are used less frequently now that salivary secretions are less of a problem with new agents as compared to ether or cyclopropane. When used, the dose in adults is 0.4 to 0.6 mg of scopolamine and 0.6 to 0.8 mg of atropine.

Narcotics are frequently used for preanesthetic medication and may be useful in the early postoperative period to prevent pain on awakening from the anesthetic.

FURTHER READING

1. Dripps, RD, Eckenhoff JE, Vandam LD: Introduction to Anesthesia: The Principle of Safe Practice. Philadelphia, W B Saunders, 1972
2. Miller RD: Anesthesia. New York, Churchill Livingstone, 1981
3. Schwartz H, Ngai SH, Papper EM: Manual of Anesthesiology for Residents and Medical Students. Springfield, Illinois, Charles C Thomas, 1962
4. Wylie WD, Churchill-Davidson HC: A Practice of Anesthesia. Chicago, Year Book Medical Publishers, 1971

CHAPTER 28 QUESTIONS

(See P. 7 for Full Instructions)

Select the One Best Answer

1. If each of the following general anesthetic agents is inhaled at its concentration that eventually will produce stable stage III, plane 3 anesthesia, which agent will show the most rapid approach of the alveolar concentration to the inhaled concentration?
   A. Halothane
   B. Ethyl ether
   C. Chloroform
   D. Vinyl ether
   E. Cyclopropane

2. Neuromuscular blocking agents are least likely to be required when the anesthetic agent is
   A. nitrous oxide.
   B. halothane.
   C. cyclopropane.
   D. ether.
   E. thiopental.

3. In terms of the inspired gas concentration, the most potent of the inhalation anesthetic agents is
   A. halothane.
   B. diethyl ether.
   C. cyclopropane.
   D. methoxyflurane.
   E. chloroform.

4. Each of the following is true for ketamine EXCEPT
   A. it has some sympathomimetic activity.
   B. it produces minimum cardiovascular depression.
   C. its onset of action is rapid.
   D. it generally causes respiratory depression.
   E. it produces analgesia without unconsciousness.

5. Which of the following physiological factors would be most limiting to the rate of induction of anesthesia with an agent having a blood/gas partition coefficient of 15?
   A. Blood flow through the lungs
   B. Cardiac output
   C. Blood flow through the brain
   D. Respiratory rate
   E. Alveolar ventilation

A = 1,2,3; B = 1,3; C = 2,4; D = 4; E = All

6. Nitrous oxide (N_2O)
   1. possesses high blood solubility.
   2. may produce hypoxia during induction and recovery.
   3. produces good muscle relaxation.
   4. possesses marked analgesic activity.

7. Postanesthetic vomiting is a frequent occurrence after anesthesia with
   1. halothane.
   2. cyclopropane.
   3. thiopental.
   4. diethyl ether.

8. At a concentration of 1 MAC halothane may cause
   1. depression of myocardial contractility.
   2. bradycardia by a direct action on the sinoatrial node.
   3. bradycardia by indirect parasympathomimetic action.
   4. peripheral vasodilation.

9. The heart is sensitized to epinephrine-induced arrhythmias by
   1. trichloroethylene.
   2. chloroform.
   3. methoxyflurane.
   4. ether.

10. There is a hazard of producing liver injury when the anesthetic agent is
    1. vinyl ether (Vinethene).
    2. chloroform ($CHCl_3$).
    3. halothane ($CF_3CHBrCl$).
    4. cyclopropane (C_3H_6).

29

MARK A. GOLDBERG

Antiepileptic Drugs

The term epilepsy, used synonymously with convulsive disorder or seizure disorder, is applied generally to a syndrome characterized by brief, recurrent, paroxysmal episodes of disturbed central nervous system function, usually with alteration in the state of consciousness. Epilepsy is not a disease but a complex syndrome of disturbed central nervous system function that can occur as a symptom of a wide variety of pathologic processes that affect the brain. A tumor or laceration of the brain, a defect in a single enzyme, or a metabolic disturbance elsewhere in the body all can manifest themselves by seizures. Therefore, all patients who have seizures require a careful neurologic evaluation to seek out possible correctable causes.

Epilepsy is a common disorder with a prevalence rate of approximately 1%. If untreated, it may be socially, psychologically, and physically devastating to the patient. Fortunately, about 80% of all patients can be adequately controlled by drug therapy.

CLASSIFICATION OF SEIZURES

A number of classifications of epileptic seizures have been proposed, and the World Health Organization (WHO) classification is the most widely accepted and will be used in this textbook. Older terms continue to be used, however, and will be given in parentheses. Classification is of great importance in drug therapy because drugs that are effective in certain types of seizures may be ineffective against others.

GENERALIZED SEIZURES WITHOUT FOCAL ONSET

Tonic–Clonic (Grand Mal)

The most common seizure type encountered clinically, the tonic–clonic (grand mal) seizure represents a common response of the central nervous system to many genetic or pathologic processes. Characteristically, the patient has no warning or recollection of preceding events. Initially there is generalized tonic activity with flexion of the upper extremities and forced extension of the lower extremities. Urinary incontinence may occur. The tonic phase is followed by a clonic phase in which there is generalized tremulousness followed by rhythmic contraction of the arms and legs. This phase gradually subsides and the patient recovers consciousness. The entire event usually lasts several minutes. During the seizure the patient may become cyanotic and have apneic periods interspersed with normal respiratory patterns; blood pressure rises, heart rate increases, and the pupils become widely dilated. These responses result from discharge of the sympathetic nervous system and return to normal soon after the seizure.

Absence (Petit Mal)

Occurring characteristically in young children after the age of 6, absence (petit mal) seizures frequently terminate spontaneously after adolescence. The seizures are very brief, lasting only seconds, and are characterized by brief staring during which the patient is unaware of his or her surroundings. There may be some movement of the eyelids but there is no gross motor activity. The patient usually recovers quickly and continues his or her previous activity. These attacks represent brief periods of unconsciousness during which time a child is unable to learn or interact socially, and can therefore result in apparent personality changes and learning difficulties. There are no known structural abnormalities of the central nervous system associated with typical absence seizures.

PARTIAL SEIZURES (FOCAL SEIZURES)

Partial Motor Seizures

Seizures that begin as and may be entirely limited to movement of one side of the body or even one extremity or that begin on one side and then gradually spread to the other side, becoming generalized, are known as partial motor seizures. This type of seizure represents more limited cortical abnormalities or indicates the presence of inhibitory mechanisms that may limit its spread. Consciousness may not be lost if the seizure does not spread. Partial sensory seizures may also occur, although they are rare. All of these have the potential of becoming generalized, but the term *partial seizure* is maintained if a focal origin is discernible.

Complex Partial Seizures (Psychomotor or Temporal Lobe Seizures). These are partial seizures with extremely varied and complex symptoms. The mesial anterior temporal lobe is the most common site of origin. Usually there is a preceding aura, which may be an olfactory hallucination. During the attack the patient may continue to stand or carry out some semipurposeful activity but is out of contact with his or her environment and does not understand if spoken to. The patient may perform relatively complex activities during the attack or simply stare vacantly into space. Symptoms of temporal lobe epilepsy are extremely varied and complex and are frequently misinterpreted as abnormal behavior rather than an epileptic event.

A number of other seizure types are recognized, especially in young children. These types, which are frequently unresponsive to the usual anticonvulsants, are relatively rare and beyond the scope of the present discussion.

EDUCATION OF THE PATIENT AND THE FAMILY

It is extremely important that the patient understand the nature of the illness at a level appropriate to his or her educational background. The family too should learn to accept the illness without excessive limitation of activities or unnecessary attention. Unfortunately, many persons associate epilepsy with insanity or mental retardation, and only through education will the patient and family be able to accept the social problems that may arise because of the seizure disorder. Patient cooperation and understanding are of critical importance in the management of epilepsy because a physician will rarely witness even a single seizure and must depend on reports of the patient and family for a description of the seizure and for keeping records of seizure frequency.

PRINCIPLES OF DRUG THERAPY

The underlying principle of anticonvulsant therapy is to select the appropriate agent for the type of seizure the patient is having and then to gradually increase the dose of medication until seizure control is achieved or toxicity prevents further increases in dose. The dose increments should be small with sufficient time between dosage adjustments to evaluate fully the effectiveness of the preceding change. Measurements of serum concentrations of anticonvulsants serve as a useful guide to predicting therapeutic effect and toxicity, but ultimately clinical criteria are the most useful (Table 29-1). If seizure control is not obtained and toxicity is approached, a second anticonvulsant drug would be added without withdrawing the first agent. Occasionally additional anticonvulsants may be needed to

TABLE 29-1. Antiepileptic Drugs

Generic Name	Trade Name	Serum Concentration*	Half-Life†
		µg/ml	*hr*
Phenytoin	Dilantin	10–20	24 ± 6
Phenobarbital	‡	15–30	96 ± 24
Primidone	Mysoline	8–12	6 ± 3
Ethosuimide	Zarontin	40–120	48 ± 12
Carbamazepine	Tegretol	6–12	20 ± 5
Clonazepam	Clonopin	. . . .	24 +
Valproic acid	Depakene	>40	8 ± 2

* Serum concentration usually associated with therapeutic effectiveness and minimal toxicity.

† Approximate half-life in adults. There may be considerable individual variation, and values may be influenced by other drugs. Values tend to be age dependent and are considerably lower in children.

‡ Many manufacturers supply phenobarbital as the generic drug.

achieve good control. Careful monitoring of serum concentrations is especially important in the early stages of therapy to ensure that the patient is complying with the physician's instructions and to identify any patients with unusual patterns of drug metabolism. Failure to take medications properly (noncompliance) is perhaps the most common single cause of drug failure in patients with epilepsy and may be due to lack of understanding or complex psychosocial factors. Unusual metabolic patterns may be genetically determined or may result from the addition to the patient's therapy of other drugs that can affect the metabolism of anticonvulsants (drug interactions).

Hematopoietic depression and hepatic and renal damage are the most serious toxic effects associated with the use of anticonvulsants. Therefore, appropriate blood tests and urinalysis should be done at regular intervals, especially when a new drug is added to the patient's therapy.

Using combinations of anticonvulsants at the outset is not recommended because adverse effects that occur after initiation of two new drugs cannot be ascribed accurately to either and may necessitate discontinuing both.

EXPERIMENTAL EPILEPSY

EXPERIMENTAL MODELS

Ideally, understanding the molecular mechanisms involved in the genesis of epilepsy would permit the design of specific drugs to prevent seizures. Unfortunately, in spite of substantial progress in recent years, this is not yet possible. The most rewarding studies of epileptogenesis and anticonvulsant action have depended on the development of a number of experimental models of epilepsy that can be investigated by electrophysiologic and pharmacologic techniques.

Electrically induced seizures can be produced by either a single supramaximal shock or repeated exposure to small subthreshold doses of electric current given over a number of weeks. The latter method, known as kindling, has been of particular value because it induces a chronic condition in which seizures will occur spontaneously, much as in human epilepsy. A chronic seizure disorder may also be produced by creating a lesion in the cerebral cortex by direct trauma such as a stab wound or application of Dry Ice. More subtle lesions can be produced by application of heavy metals such as aluminum or cobalt to the cortex. Seizures can be produced by drugs administered systemically or directly to the surface of the brain. An example of the latter is penicillin, which has been used extensively to study the cellular changes that accompany seizures. Another drug, pentylenetetrazole, produces seizures that can be prevented by drugs used to prevent absence seizures in humans.

MEMBRANES AND SYNAPSES

The fundamental mechanism underlying neuronal function is the controlled passage of cations, primarily sodium, potassium, and calcium, through cell membranes. There is considerable evidence, derived from studies of experimental models, of defects in the membrane regulation of ion fluxes in some forms of seizures. Inhibition of Na^+-K^+ ATPase, the enzyme believed to function as the Na^+-K^+ "pump," will result in seizures by allowing an increase of intracellular sodium and a decrease in potassium within the cell. Defective control of the channels through which cations cross cell membranes can also result in unstable, readily depolarized neurons and is implicated in some types of experimental epilepsy.

In addition to abnormalities in ionic conductance, there is evidence that impaired synaptic transmission can result in depolarization of long chains of neurons resulting in epileptic discharges. A number of convulsant poisons (*e.g.*, picrotoxin) are known to antagonize the inhibitory neurotransmitter gamma-aminobutyric acid (GABA) and are thought to induce seizures by preventing normal inhibitory brain mechanisms. Other convulsants act by depleting brain GABA through inhibition of its synthesis. Drugs that are GABA agonists or increase GABA concentration are anticonvulsants. Relatively little is known about the role of other neurotransmitters in epilepsy. Although the aforementioned mechanisms have been found in some types of experimental epilepsy, no specific abnormality in membrane ion conductance or neurotransmission had been shown in human epilepsy.

SPECIFIC ANTICONVULSANT AGENTS

The first effective anticonvulsant agents to be used in clinical medicine were salts of hydrobromic acid introduced in the mid-19th century. Although bromides are effective to a limited degree, they cause serious toxic problems, and there is no indication for their use today. Most currently used antiepileptic agents are organic substances with relatively similar molecular structures (Fig. 29-1).

PHENYTOIN

Introduced into clinical medicine by Merritt and Putnam in 1938, this compound has proved remarkably effective in the treatment of several types of epilepsy and is often considered the drug of choice for tonic–clonic seizures. Although a number of potentially toxic side effects have been described, phenytoin is a relatively safe agent that meets many of the criteria of the ideal anticonvulsant.

HIRAM HOUSTON MERRITT, 1902–1979. American physician. Has worked on the relationship of blood, cerebrospinal fluid, nervous system infections, and anticonvulsants. Between 1937 and 1939 he and T. J. Putnam discovered the anticonvulsant activity of phenytoin and established its effectiveness in humans.

TRACY JACKSON PUTNAM, 1894– . American neurologist. Published papers on the treatment of hydrocephalus, multiple sclerosis, and other neurological disorders.

CHARLES LOCOCK, 1799–1875. London obstetrician. Known for his report, in 1857, on the effectiveness of potassium bromide for treatment of epilepsy. Also noteworthy for having attended at the birth of all Queen Victoria's children.

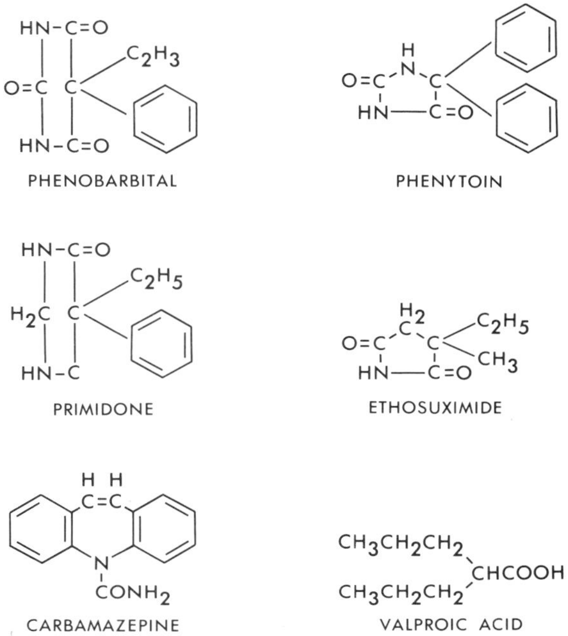

FIG. 29-1. Structural formulae of anticonvulsants.

Action

Phenytoin is highly effective in the treatment of generalized tonic–clonic, partial motor, and partial complex epilepsy but has no value in typical absence attacks. Its major effect is to reduce the extension of the seizure from the epileptogenic focus to normal surrounding neurons, preventing their activation and therefore the spread of the seizure. Phenytoin inhibits post-tetanic potentiation and prevents development of chains of rapidly firing neurons. The drug has little suppressant effect on the epileptogenic focus itself and produces little change in normal neurons. In usual therapeutic concentrations it does not impair consciousness or produce significant mental change.

A number of theories on the molecular basis of phenytoin's action have been proposed. In general, the drug appears to stabilize excitable cell membranes including those of peripheral nerve, skeletal and cardiac muscle, and central neurons. Under certain experimental conditions phenytoin stimulates the enzyme Na^+-K^+ ATPase, resulting in more active extrusion of sodium from the cell. The importance of this effect on the anticonvulsant action of phenytoin is a matter of controversy, however. The drug also reduces sodium conductance in cell membranes with a consequent decrease in intracellular sodium ion. This action tends to lower the excitability of neurons and prevent depolarization. Phenytoin inhibits the phosphorylation of specific synaptic proteins; this inhibition is accompanied by a decrease in norepinephrine release, which could result in polysynaptic neuronal firing. No specific receptor for phenytoin has been identified, but the drug has been found to bind strongly to membrane protein and phospholipids, which may account for the membrane stabilization that occurs. Many studies have been conducted on the mechanisms of action of phenytoin and many effects have been detected; which is responsible for its anticonvulsant action has not yet been determined.

Clinical Pharmacology

In recent years the development of a number of analytical techniques has permitted the routine measurement of serum concentrations of most anticonvulsants, and a much better understanding of the requirements for clinical control of seizures has emerged. When a patient begins the usual oral dosage of 300 to 400 mg daily (5 mg/kg of body weight in children), adequate serum levels may not be achieved for 5 to 7 days and effective seizure control cannot be expected before that. A serum concentration of 10 to 20 μg/ml correlates best with anticonvulsant activity and minimal toxicity and is usually considered the therapeutic range. With serum concentrations between 20 and 30 μg/ml, some toxicity may be apparent. Above 30 μg/ml toxicity is present in most patients and may become severe enough to limit the patient's functioning and necessitate lowering the dose. Once adequate levels of phenytoin are achieved, they tend to remain fairly stable as long as the patient maintains the same daily intake. If rapid seizure control is required, loading doses of up to 1000 mg in divided doses may be used the first day and 500 mg on the second day, and then usual maintenance levels of 300 to 400 mg/day instituted. Drug levels in the therapeutic range may be reached in 1 to 2 days. As the half-life in the serum is 16 to 24 hours, the medication may be taken only once a day after therapeutic levels are achieved. Although serum concentrations may fluctuate slightly, in most patients they will remain within the therapeutic range. Phenytoin administered intramuscularly is slowly and irregularly absorbed, and reliable blood levels may not be achieved.

Metabolism

Phenytoin is metabolized by hepatic microsomal enzymes, and the parahydroxyphenyl compound is the principal metabolite in humans. This inactive metabolite is very soluble and is excreted rapidly by the kidney. The enzymes responsible for this metabolic transformation are saturable at levels not much greater than those used clinically. Consequently, a small increase in dose may result in enzyme saturation and a disproportionate elevation in serum concentration with an increased frequency of toxicity. The dose must be regulated carefully in patients whose serum concentrations are in the upper range. Other drugs that stimulate hepatic microsomal enzymes may increase the detoxification of phenytoin resulting in lower serum levels and poor antiepileptic control. In addition, phenytoin may stimulate the rate of metabolism of other drugs. These drug interactions can be extremely complex and vary greatly among individual patients. It is therefore important to determine the serum concentrations of phenytoin in patients receiving other medications. Approximately 90% of phenytoin in the serum is bound to plasma proteins, principally albumin. Patients with liver disease or other conditions causing hypoalbuminemia may require smaller doses of the drug. Several drugs (*e.g.*, nonsteroidal anti-inflammatory agents and valproic acid) may displace phenytoin from albumin binding sites, resulting in unpredictable changes in serum levels.

Adverse Effects

The toxic effects of phenytoin are of three types: allergic, dose-related toxicity, and chronic toxicity.

Allergic Reactions. A few patients have severe allergic reactions to phenytoin. Characteristically, symptoms begin 2 to 3 weeks after the institution of therapy. Pruritus, fever, and skin rash are the most common complaints, and eosinophilia usually is seen. In some persons a severe allergic reaction may occur, with exfoliation of the skin, hepatic toxicity, and bone marrow depression with pancytopenia. Because of the severity of some allergic reactions to phenytoin, the drug must be withdrawn immediately after symptoms appear. Owing to the long half-life, symptoms may continue to progress for a short time after withdrawal of the agent, which is usually the only therapy needed. Patients may require antihistamines for symptomatic relief, and occasionally glucocorticosteroids are necessary in cases of severe allergic toxicity.

Dose-Related Toxicity. More commonly experienced are acute dose-related toxic symptoms. These include nystagmus with blurring of vision or diplopia, ataxia, and dysarthria, and with blood levels of 40 μg/ml or greater, stupor or coma may occur. Occasionally, seizure frequency increases when toxic levels of phenytoin are attained. Acute ataxic symptoms usually can be reversed by lowering the serum level to the range of 10 to 20 μg/ml.

Chronic Toxicity. As more and more patients have taken this agent over 20 years, a number of chronic toxic effects have been described. A very common one, especially in children, is gingival hyperplasia, which in some instances may cause painful bleeding gums. In most patients good oral hygiene will prevent this condition from becoming a serious side effect, but occasionally surgical intervention is necessary. Hirsutism occurs frequently, especially in young girls, and, although not a serious effect, is aesthetically disturbing. More serious chronic toxic side effects include folic acid deficiency due to interference with absorption of folic acid from the small intestine. Hypocalcemia and osteomalacia occur, probably because of interference with absorption of calcium from the intestine and to increased metabolism of vitamin D by the liver. A syndrome resembling systemic lupus erythematosus has been described in patients taking anticonvulsants. Although these toxic effects are potentially serious, they are rarely encountered clinically.

Finally, the incidence of birth defects, especially cleft palate, is statistically higher among the children of women who took phenytoin during their pregnancies. Pregnant patients should not receive this drug if their seizures can be controlled with other drugs.

Several other hydantoin derivatives are effective in controlling seizures, but they are associated with a number of adverse reactions and their use is no longer recommended.

CARBAMAZEPINE

An inostilbene that is chemically related to the tricyclic antidepressant compounds (*see* Chap. 22), carbamazepine has been in use as an anticonvulsant for approximately 15 years. Despite its clinical acceptance, much less is known about its pharmacologic action than that of phenytoin.

Action

Carbamazepine is effective in generalized tonic–clonic, partial motor, and partial complex epilepsy and has been found to be useful in trigeminal neuralgia. Although the compound is comparable in efficacy to phenytoin, its high cost and potential serious toxicity limit its use. Relatively few laboratory studies have been conducted on its mechanism of action, but the results of those that have been done suggest that carbamazepine is quite similar to phenytoin. It depresses polysynaptic discharges and inhibits post-tetanic potentiation. The drug inhibits seizure discharges induced by electroshock, penicillin, and aluminum compounds but not those produced by pentylenetetrazole. At higher concentrations it decreases sodium conductance in neural membranes. Carbamazepine also inhibits the reuptake of norepinephrine by presynaptic endings but to a much lesser degree than the tricyclic antidepressants. No interaction with GABA has been reported.

Clinical Pharmacology

Effective seizure control can be correlated with serum concentrations of 6 to 12 μg/ml. At higher concentrations, toxicity frequently occurs. The dose required to achieve these serum concentrations varies considerably among individuals; in practice a starting dose of 400 mg is used, and the dose is increased by 200 mg increments until seizure control is achieved. Carbamazepine has a serum half-life of approximately 24 hours under steady-state conditions, which are reached within about 5 days of treatment. The drug frequently can be administered on a once-a-day basis; however, because of marked individual variation in half-life, it usually is administered twice a day without significant fluctuation in serum concentration.

Metabolism

Carbamazepine undergoes biotransformation to a number of metabolites, the most important of which is the 10,11-epoxide that has some anticonvulsant activity. As with other compounds metabolized by hepatic enzyme systems, carbamazepine metabolism can be influenced by other drugs, including other anticonvulsants. The most important interaction is with phenytoin, which consistently lowers carbamazepine levels. The effect of carbamazepine on phenytoin concentration appears to be more variable. Because of the individual variation in rates of metabolism and the lack of data for many potentially interacting agents, the serum concentration of carbamazepine should be determined whenever another drug is added to a patient's treatment. Approximately 75% of serum carbamazepine is bound to serum protein, but no clinically important interactions resulting from protein binding have been reported.

Adverse Effects

Dose-Related Toxicity. Many patients experience blurred vision, a feeling of disequilibrium, and sedation with serum levels higher than 10 μg/ml. These symptoms can usually be reversed by lowering the dose.

Idiosyncratic Effects. Several cases of aplastic anemia have been reported in patients receiving carbamazepine. This tends to occur early in the course of therapy and may be irreversible. Careful monitoring of blood count, platelet count, and serum iron on a weekly basis for the first 3 months of therapy has been recommended, with periodic blood counts thereafter. Occasional renal and hepatic toxicity also occur, and appropriate biochemical investigations are indicated. The syndrome of inappropriate antidiuretic hormone release has been reported in some patients taking carbamazepine. If symptomatic hyponatremia occurs, carbamazepine therapy should be discontinued.

BARBITURATES

Many commonly used barbiturates (*see* Chap. 25) possess some anticonvulsant activity but generally produce excessive sedation at therapeutic dosage levels to be useful clinically. Phenobarbital is the principal exception and has emerged as one of the safest and most widely used anticonvulsant agents.

Action

Phenobarbital is effective in treating tonic–clonic, partial motor, and partial complex seizures but ineffective in typical absence seizures. Phenobarbital is particularly useful in controlling febrile convulsions in children and convulsions associated with withdrawal from sedative agents such as barbiturates and alcohol. In contrast to other barbiturates, phenobarbital has a selective depressant action on the motor cortex and can suppress seizure activity at an epileptogenic focus at a concentration that does not produce generalized sedation. In contrast to phenytoin, phenobarbital increases the threshold of normal cells and can prevent seizures induced by both pentylenetetrazol and electroshock. It may increase presynaptic inhibition and therefore decrease repetitive firing of neurons in the epileptogenic focus. Phenobarbital has no effect on cells outside the central nervous system or on sodium and calcium transport at therapeutic concentrations.

Clinical Pharmacology

Absorption of phenobarbital on oral ingestion is slow, and steady-state blood levels are reached in approximately 2 to 3 weeks after onset of therapy. Its half-life in adults is 48 to 96 hours and is somewhat shorter in children. Clinical anticonvulsant activity is best correlated with serum levels of 15 to 30 μg/ml, but many patients can tolerate higher serum levels. Toxic manifestations occur regularly above levels of 40 μg/ml. Once adequate serum concentrations are reached, they tend to remain fairly constant as long as oral intake is maintained. The usual oral starting dose in adults is 100 mg/day, and 100 to 150 mg/day is usually adequate to achieve therapeutic serum levels. In children approximately 4 mg/kg will achieve therapeutic serum levels. As a consequence of phenobarbital's long half-life, this amount can be taken as a single daily dose. Intramuscular phenobarbital is absorbed into the blood more rapidly than is phenytoin and can be used when oral intake is limited. Intravenous phenobarbital can be used safely if administered slowly.

Metabolism

Phenobarbital is a potent stimulator of hepatic microsomal enzymes and can affect the metabolism of other drugs, such as anticoagulants. It does not appreciably alter blood levels of phenytoin when both drugs are given. Phenobarbital is metabolized in humans to the inactive parahydroxyphenyl derivative, which may then be conjugated with glucuronic acid and excreted by the kidney. Approximately 25% of phenobarbital is excreted unchanged in the urine. About 50% of phenobarbital is bound to plasma proteins, principally albumin, but displacement from binding is of little clinical significance except in neonates, where it may interfere with bilirubin binding.

Adverse Effects

Phenobarbital is an extremely safe agent, although many patients develop mild sedation initially, tolerance usually develops to this side-effect but not to the anticonvulsant activity. At higher blood levels of phenobarbital (greater than 40 μg/ml) sedation, ataxia and blurring of vision may occur but can be reversed easily by lowering the dosage of phenobarbital. Toxic serum levels of phenobarbital may result in a

---

ALFRED HAUPTMANN, 1881– German neurologist. In 1912 reported on several years of experience in the use of phenobarbital—"Luminal"—in treatment of epilepsy. At the same time, others were describing its use as a sedative and hypnotic.

paradoxical increase in seizures, especially in children.

Allergic reactions to phenobarbital may occur, usually manifested by pruritus and urticarial skin eruptions. The severe dermatologic, hematologic, and hepatic complications encountered with phenytoin rarely occur with phenobarbital. Chronic toxicity is relatively rare although some of the syndromes encountered with hydantoin derivatives may occasionally be found with this drug.

Mephobarbital differs from phenobarbital by the addition of one methyl group, and it is partially metabolized to phenobarbital. It is unknown whether the intact molecule has anticonvulsive activity of its own, but its actions and toxicity are quite similar to those of the parent compound. Mephobarbital is much more expensive than phenobarbital.

Primidone

Although not an authentic barbiturate, primidone is structurally very similar. It is effective in partial complex epilepsy, tonic–clonic seizures, and partial motor seizures. Recent evidence has indicated that it is metabolized to phenobarbital and phenylethylmalonamide, both of which have anticonvulsant activity. Patients on usual doses of primidone may achieve serum levels of phenobarbital similar to those encountered when that drug is used alone, and there is little indication for the use of primidone and phenobarbital in the same patient. The presence of primidone and its active metabolites makes clinical correlation between serum level and clinical control difficult, but measurements of phenobarbital levels provide an estimate of patient compliance.

The initial use of the agent is associated with sedation, and it is best to start with low doses, gradually increasing the dose. In children the dose requirements are quite variable, but 5 to 10 mg/kg daily is recommended. Toxicity of this agent is similar to that of phenobarbital.

Other barbiturate derivatives commercially available do not have the specific anticonvulsant properties of the agents discussed above and produce their anticonvulsant effect only at hypnotic dosage levels. They therefore have no place in the treatment of epilepsy.

SUCCINIMIDES

Several substituted succinimides have been introduced in recent years for treating absence attacks (petit mal epilepsy). Ethosuximide is an excellent drug for absence seizures, controlling 80% to 90% of symptoms. It is ineffective in tonic–clonic and partial motor epilepsy.

Actions

Electrophysiological studies have suggested that absence seizures result from the synchronization of both excitatory and inhibitory neurons within the brain stem and mesial reticular activating system. These agents may act by increasing postsynaptic inhibition and preventing the propagation of seizure activity by way of thalamocortical projections. The succinimides have little effect on electrically induced seizures in experimental animals but are potent antagonists to the seizures produced by pentylenetetrazol. No good evidence relates its actions to ionic fluxes or specific neurotransmitters.

Clinical Pharmacology

Ethosuximide is rapidly absorbed from the gastrointestinal tract. Peak serum levels are achieved in 1 to 2 hours and fall off very slowly thereafter. Its half-life is approximately 30 hours in children and 55 hours in adults. This drug is converted by hepatic microsomal enzymes into several metabolites that result from the oxidation of side-chains of the parent molecule. Maximum clinical control is achieved with doses of approximately 10 to 20 mg/kg, and clinical control is correlated with serum levels of 40 to 120 μg/ml. Clinical control in petit mal seizures may be related to the severity of the disorder, and, unlike in other types of seizures, monitoring of the electroencephalogram has proved to be useful in evaluating seizure control. Because of its relatively long half-life, ethosuximide can be given in two divided doses daily to children and in a single dose to adults. Treatment usually begins with a single capsule (250 mg) a day and is increased gradually.

Adverse Effects

Ethosuximide is a relatively safe drug, although transient leukopenia occurs occasionally. Although usually of a minor nature, more severe pancytopenia has been reported. Dose-related symptoms of toxicity include gastrointestinal upset, sedation, headache, and occasional allergic manifestations. Complete blood counts should be obtained periodically, especially early in the course of treatment.

Methsuximide and Phensuximide are both effective in suppressing absence seizures but are less efficacious than ethosuximide. Because of the higher incidence of serious side-effects with these two agents, they are less commonly used and are reserved for refractory cases.

BENZODIAZEPINES

A number of compounds of the chemical class benzodiazepine have been introduced as antianxiety agents and hypnotics (*see* Chap. 20). Many of these compounds possess some anticonvulsant activity at appropriate serum concentrations. Only two, diazepam and clonazepam, have been used extensively as anticonvulsants. The use of diazepam is limited to i.v. use in status epilepticus and is discussed below.

Clonazepam

Effective in absence seizures and minor motor attacks that occur primarily in children, clonazepam is also useful in myoclonus, a type of involuntary muscular contraction that may be accompanied by loss of consciousness. As with other benzodiazepines, it is thought to act at specific receptor sites within the CNS, but there is little evidence to differentiate specific anticonvulsive effects from its general sedative properties.

Clonazepam is rapidly absorbed from the gastrointestinal tract with a half-life of approximately 24 hours. It undergoes biotransformation to a number of metabolites, several of which have anticonvulsive activity and relatively long half-lives. A serum concentration of greater than 25 ng/ml has been associated with anticonvulsant effect, but relatively little data exist on this subject primarily because of the difficulty in measuring serum concentrations of this class of drugs.

There is relatively little toxicity other than dose-related sedation and ataxia with this agent. In contrast to most other antiepileptic drugs, however, a relatively high degree of tolerance to the anticonvulsant effect has been noted in some patients receiving this agent over a long period. Therefore, increasing doses are frequently necessary to maintain therapeutic effectiveness.

VALPROIC ACID

Recently introduced, valproic acid differs both chemically and in action from most of the other anticonvulsant agents. Chemically it is a branch-chain fatty acid that does not contain a nitrogen group in contrast to the other agents (Fig. 29-1).

Action

Valproic acid has a broader spectrum of action than the other anticonvulsants in that it is effective against the two major categories of generalized seizures—tonic–clonic and absence. It is also useful in treating minor motor seizures and myoclonus but is relatively ineffective in treating partial seizures. Many of the studies of its mechanisms of action relate to its ability, in high concentrations, to inhibit the enzymes responsible for the degradation of GABA, resulting in increased brain levels of this inhibitory neurotransmitter. GABA does not increase significantly in brain at clinically used concentrations, leading to some question as to whether this effect is clinically significant. It has no action on any tissues outside the central nervous system.

Clinical Pharmacology

Valproic acid is rapidly absorbed after oral administration, reaching peak serum levels in 2 hours; serum levels then decline rapidly, and the average half-life in adults is approximately 8 hours. As a consequence of this short half-life, three to four doses a day are needed. It is customary to start at approximately 10 mg/kg and to increase the dose as needed to a maximum of 60 mg/kg. Because of valproic acid's rapid half-life, correlation between serum level and therapeutic effectiveness is of limited value, although a level of 40 μg/ml suggests patient compliance.

Metabolism

Valproic acid is oxidized to several shorter chain fatty acids not known to have anticonvulsant activity. Valproic acid may inhibit the rate of metabolism of phenobarbital, resulting in higher serum concentrations of phenobarbital with consequent increase in toxicity. Valproic acid is highly bound to serum protein and competes with phenytoin for binding sites. As a consequence of displaced binding, serum phenytoin levels are frequently reduced in patients taking valproic acid, but free phenytoin levels remain unchanged. These complex interactions make monitoring serum levels in patients taking valproic acid difficult.

Adverse Effects

Dose-Related Toxicity. Nausea and gastrointestinal irritation are common side-effects that can be minimized by increasing the dose slowly or by giving the drug with food. Reducing the dose frequently relieves these side-effects. Sedation and ataxia rarely occur with this drug.

Reportedly valproic acid interferes with platelet function, but the clinical consequence of this action is uncertain.

Idiosyncratic Reaction. A number of reports have indicated that valproic acid is associated with acute hepatic necrosis, usually resulting in death. This effect seems to occur more frequently in children who have been under treatment for several months. Often this toxic effect is manifested quite abruptly, and the course is a fulminant one. As a minimum, frequent measurement of liver function has been recommended during the first several months of therapy with valproic acid. Because of the danger of this toxic effect, many clinicians prefer to reserve valproic acid for patients whose seizures are refractory to other forms of therapy. The exact incidence of hepatic necrosis and possible predisposing factors are unknown.

A number of other agents are used as secondary agents in treating refractory epilepsy or specific unusual types of seizures. Their use should be reserved for the special conditions for which they have reportedly been helpful. They are of little value in most forms of epilepsy.

TREATMENT OF STATUS EPILEPTICUS

Status epilepticus (acute repetitive seizures) is a medical emergency that results from continuous or repetitive generalized tonic–clonic seizures. Serious brain damage occurs with untreated status epilepticus, and the degree of potential danger is related to the duration of the seizures. Several methods of treating this condition have been used, all of which have advantages and disadvantages. The essential principle of therapy is that the patient should be given large doses of the appropriate anticonvulsant by the i.v. route. The use of i.m. or p.o. drugs in small doses is usually ineffective and serves only to complicate therapy.

Three anticonvulsants are used extensively.

1. Intravenous *diazepam* in doses of approximately 10 mg administered slowly will usually stop the seizures. However, the duration of action of this agent after i.v. administration is short, and recurrence of seizures within 30 minutes to 1 hour is common. Its usefulness is therefore limited to emergency care until more definitive therapy can be undertaken.
2. Large doses of *phenobarbital* given by slow i.v. infusion are usually effective in controlling status epilepticus. In practice an adult can receive 250 mg of phenobarbital over 2 to 3 minutes, a dose that can be repeated in 30 minutes if control is not achieved. Higher doses are rarely needed. This procedure is usually safe, but respiratory depression may occur, and physicians should be prepared to treat this complication. The principal disadvantage of this therapy is that it produces deep sleep in most patients that may persist for 24 hours.
3. Intravenous *phenytoin* can be effective in controlling grand mal seizures in some patients. Large doses of the agent are, however, needed to achieve therapeutic blood levels, and the potential for cardiac toxicity and hypotension exists from the rapid i.v. injection of this drug. When used, a loading dose of 1000 mg is given very slowly at the rate of 50 mg/minute, preferably with ECG and blood pressure monitoring. If hypotension or changes in cardiac rhythm occur, the administration of drug should be immediately discontinued. This therapy has the advantage of producing relatively little sedation, but its effectiveness in stopping seizures is variable.

These therapies are directed toward stopping the acute repetitive phase of seizures, but maintenance therapy is usually needed and should be instituted shortly after the acute phase has subsided. Patients refractory to the above treatment have a dire prognosis; if seizures persist over several hours despite vigorous i.v. therapy, such patients should be placed under general anesthesia. Maintenance of general anesthesia for more than 60 to 120 minutes is rarely needed, and longer-acting anticonvulsants should be administered in addition. The halogenated general anesthetics are potentially harmful to the patient with status epilepticus because they may produce EEG abnormalities and seizures.

FURTHER READING

1. Eadie MJ, Tyler JH: Anticonvulsant Therapy. London, Churchill-Livingstone, 1980
2. Glaser G, Penry K, Woodbury D (eds): Antiepileptic Drugs: Mechanisms of Action. New York, Raven Press, 1980
3. Pinder RM, Brogden RN, Speight TM, Auery GS: Sodium valproate: A review of its pharmacological properties and therapeutic efficacy. Drugs 13:81–123, 1977
4. Woodbury DM, Penry JK, Pippenger CE: Antiepileptic Drugs, 2nd ed. New York, Raven Press, 1982

CHAPTER 29 QUESTIONS

(See P. 7 for Full Instructions)

Select the One Best Answer

1. Each of the following agents is used therapeutically to suppress epileptic seizures EXCEPT
   A. diazepam.
   B. reserpine.
   C. diphenylhydantoin.
   D. phenobarbital.
   E. ethosuximide.

2. An agent characterized by its clinical usefulness in treating trigeminal neuralgia and grand mal epilepsy is
   A. ethyl alcohol.
   B. diphenylhydantoin.
   C. phenobarbital.
   D. lidocaine.
   E. primidone.

3. A child who suffers brief periods of absence and who presents an EEG pattern of 3/sec spike and wave forms should benefit from the administration of
   A. phenytoin.
   B. ethosuximide.
   C. primidone.
   D. metharbital.
   E. corticotropin.

4. Select the correct pairing of a drug with its therapeutic indication.
   A. Phenobarbital—petit mal epilepsy
   B. Diazepam—status epilepticus
   C. Ethosuximide—focal motor epilepsy
   D. Phenytoin—narcolepsy
   E. Trimethadione—grand mal epilepsy

A = 1,2,3; B = 1,3; C = 2,4; D = 4; E = All

5. Both phenytoin and phenobarbital generally suppress
   1. petit mal seizures.
   2. jacksonian seizures.
   3. psychomotor seizures.
   4. grand mal seizures.

6. Phenytoin
   1. can produce cardiovascular collapse when administered intravenously.
   2. may prevent the spread of seizure discharge by suppressing posttetanic potentiation.
   3. can produce megaloblastic anemia.
   4. induces enzymes that metabolize corticosteroids.

7. Drugs effective in the control of grand mal and focal motor epilepsies include
   1. phenobarbital.
   2. primidone.
   3. phenytoin.
   4. trimethadione.

8. Hypersensitivity reactions reported with phenytoin include
   1. a clinical syndrome resembling mononucleosis.
   2. lupus erythematosus.
   3. hepatic necrosis.
   4. erythema multiforme.

9. Both phenytoin and phenobarbital
   1. are useful in the treatment of tonic–clonic (grand mal) seizures.
   2. depress normal *and* epileptogenic neurons.
   3. induce hepatic microsomal enzymes.
   4. act as membrane stabilizers.

10. Both valproic acid and ethosuximide
    1. are associated with hepatic necrosis.
    2. have produced leukopenia or pancytopenia.
    3. are useful in tonic–clonic seizures.
    4. are useful in absence (petit mal) attacks.

11. Agents useful in partial complex seizures include
    1. phenobarbital.
    2. carbamazepine.
    3. phenytoin.
    4. primidone.

CHARLES H. MARKHAM

30

Antiparkinson Drugs

In the last 15 years, significant advances have been made in the treatment of Parkinson's disease, resulting from the use of levodopa (L-dopa), now usually combined with a peripherally acting dopa decarboxylase inhibitor, and synthetic dopamine agonists. Amantadine hydrochloride (Symmetrel) and anticholinergic agents combined with levodopa have also helped. To understand how these drugs work, it is necessary to look at the disease itself and at anatomical and biochemical processes in the basal ganglia.

The etiology of Parkinson's disease is unknown in most patients. The disease may follow, however rarely, viral encephalitis as it did with the great influenza pandemics during World War I. Infrequently, it may result from multiple small vascular lesions. A recent study of identical twins, one of whom had Parkinson's disease, appears to rule out heredity as a cause for the typical disease. The attrition of nerve cells in the aging process, including those in the substantia nigra, may partly explain its prevalence in middle-aged and elderly persons.

The main symptoms of Parkinson's disease are a 3 to 6/sec tremor of a limb when that part of the body is at rest; rigidity, a relatively unremitting low-grade muscular contraction that the patient feels as stiffness or awkwardness, and the physician detects as an increased tone as the involved limb is moved; and akinesia, a hesitancy in initiating a movement, changing its speed or direction and carrying it to completion. Other symptoms include flexed posture and a soft voice with reduced volume and disturbed rhythm. Slowly progressive dementia also afflicts about one third of patients.

Excluding dementia (due to a gradual loss of cortical neurons), these symptoms have one lesion in common—loss of the large pigmented cells in the substantia nigra. Other changes in

---

The drug therapy of Parkinson's disease is presented in more detail than most other topics because it is an example of the successful rational application of the findings of basic medical research to a human disease process in the CNS.

Sir James Parkinson, 1755–1824. First described paralysis agitans in 1817 in his "Essay on the Shaking Palsy." Was a suburban London physician who reported on six cases, three of these his own patients and three persons he had observed on the street. Paralysis agitans was first called "Parkinson's disease" by Jean Martin Charcot in 1862.

the substantia nigra and elsewhere in the basal ganglia depend on the particular etiology of the parkinsonism.

SOME ANATOMY AND BIOCHEMISTRY

The large pigmented nigral neurons contain melanin, manufacture dopamine, and have unmyelinated axons 0.1 to 0.2 microns in diameter, which project to two nearby nuclei, the caudate and putamen. These structures, together termed the striatum, have the highest concentration of dopamine in the CNS (*see* Chap. 21). Striatal dopamine is contained in irregular varicose presynaptic terminals.

In the early 1960s, Hornykiewicz and his colleagues in Vienna first showed the dopamine content in the striatum and nigra to be very low in Parkinson's disease. Levodopa decarboxylase (*see* Chap. 17), the dopamine synthesizing enzyme, and homovanillic acid, the main dopamine metabolite, are also diminished in the striatum in Parkinson's disease. These findings led to a trial of replacement therapy with large oral doses of levodopa, the precursor of dopamine that crosses the blood–brain barrier.

The main steps in dopamine neurotransmission are as follows. Dopamine is decarboxylated from levodopa within the nigrostriatal neuron and is held in storage vesicles in the synaptic terminal. Free dopamine within the nigrostriatal neuron is apparently degraded by the mitochondrial enzyme monoamine oxidase (MAO). The nigrostriatal neuron releases dopamine, a probable inhibitory transmitter, into the presynaptic cleft. Multiple branching of the dopaminergic axons suggests one nigral cell acts on many striatal neurons, probably the medium-sized spiny neurons (*see* below). After presumably causing a hyperpolarization of the receptor cell, the dopamine is released from the receptor site to be taken up into the presynaptic terminal or inactivated (0-methylated) by catechol-O-methyl transferase (COMT). With the very slow conduction velocity related to the very small axonal diameter of the nigrostriatal dopamine, it seems likely that natural stimulation of substantia nigra neurons exerts a delayed and possibly prolonged release of dopamine in the striatum, suggesting that dopamine serves a tonic, sustaining influence rather than exerting an abrupt, phasic effect on motor control.

The striatum contains other neurotransmitters either altered in Parkinson's disease or during its treatment: acetylcholine (ACh), gamma amino butyric acid (GABA), and serotonin (5HT). ACh concentration in the striatum is significant, as is the activity of acetylcholinesterase (AChE) and choline acetylase (*see* Chaps. 13–16). It now seems likely that all, or almost all, the ACh is formed and released within the striatum by one group of interneurons. Choline acetylase activity is reduced abut 50% in Huntington's chorea, a disease with major loss of striatal neurons. Although ACh, or its forming or inactivating enzymes, has not been conclusively shown to be abnormal in Parkinson's disease, anticholinergic drugs clearly benefit parkinsonian symptoms (*see* Chap. 16). This suggests that decreased striatal dopamine in this disease may allow striatal ACh interneurons to be relatively overactive and anticholinergic agents to correct this imbalance in part.

GABA, an inhibitory neurotransmitter, and its forming enzyme glutamic acid decarboxylase (GAD) are also important in striatal function. In untreated Parkinson's disease, GAD activity is reduced in the striatum to less than 50% of the control mean, whereas in Parkinson's disease chemically treated with levodopa it is normal. In Huntington's chorea, GABA is low in the striatum, globus pallidus, and substantia nigra, and GAD activity is reduced to 10% to 20% of control in the striatum. This suggests that GABA may be formed and released by a class of neurons in the striatum and that parkinsonian nigrostriatal dopamine deficiency may lead to elevated GAD activity.

Striatal 5HT is mildly decreased in Parkinson's disease. Serotonin is concentrated in nerve cell terminals and is converted there from its precursor by 5-hydroxytryptophan decarboxylase, which is apparently the same enzyme as dopa decarboxylase. The cell bodies of the serotonin-containing neurons lie in the midbrain and pontine raphé nuclei not far from the dopaminergic neurons in the midbrain. Why serotonin is decreased in the striatum in Parkinson's disease is unknown, but it may be from death of some of these cells. Administration of 5-hydroxytryptophan, the precursor of serotonin, does not significantly change human parkinsonian symptoms.

Two peptides, substance P and encephalin,

OLEH HORNYKIEWICZ, 1926– . Polish-born pharmacologist and neurochemist working in Vienna who first demonstrated low levels of dopamine in the caudate nucleus and striatum in Parkinson's disease. With his clinical colleagues, observed a clear but transient benefit from dopa given intravenously to patients with Parkinson's disease.

are found in cell bodies in the striatum, and at least one, substance P, is released in the substantia nigra where it exerts an excitatory influence on dopaminergic neurons. It is unknown whether these peptides are altered in Parkinson's disease.

It is now possible to study the cellular makeup of the striatum. In most cases of Parkinson's disease, cells die in the substantia nigra, but many symptoms are attributable to failure of dopamine delivery to specific sites in the striatum. The striatum has several morphologic cell types (Fig. 30-1). Medium-sized spiny neurons constitute about 96% of the striatal neurons; they have many spines on their branched dendrites.

Recent investigations with horseradish peroxidase and other substances transported intraaxonally in a retrograde fashion from nerve terminal to cell body indicate that at least 40% to 50% of the medium-sized spiny neuron axons terminate in the substantia nigra and have axon collaterals ending in the globus pallidus and the striatum itself. These are GABAergic neurons that inhibit neurons in the substantia nigra and globus pallidus. The terminations and the neurotransmitters of the remaining medium-sized spiny neurons are unknown.

ACh is formed and released within the striatum by one class of interneuron. The morphologic type has not yet been determined, but the cells are few in number despite the fact that ACh, AChE, and choline acetylase are present in high concentration.

Electron microscopic and Golgi studies combined with lesions of the thalamus and cortex have shown that both of these sites have afferents to the striatum that terminate predominantly on dendritic spines of medium-sized spiny cells. Another study using electron microscopy combined with autoradiography has shown dopaminergic terminals ending on dendritic spines of medium-sized spiny neurons. And other studies using electrophysiological techniques have shown transsynaptic influence on single striatal output cells from the cortex, thalamus, and the nigral area.

At the risk of oversimplification, one might conclude the following.

FIG. 30-1. Diagrammatic view of a frontal section through basal ganglia with emphasis on pathways to and from the striatum. Neural somas that contain presumed inhibitory neurotransmitters are dark; open ones contain excitatory transmitters.

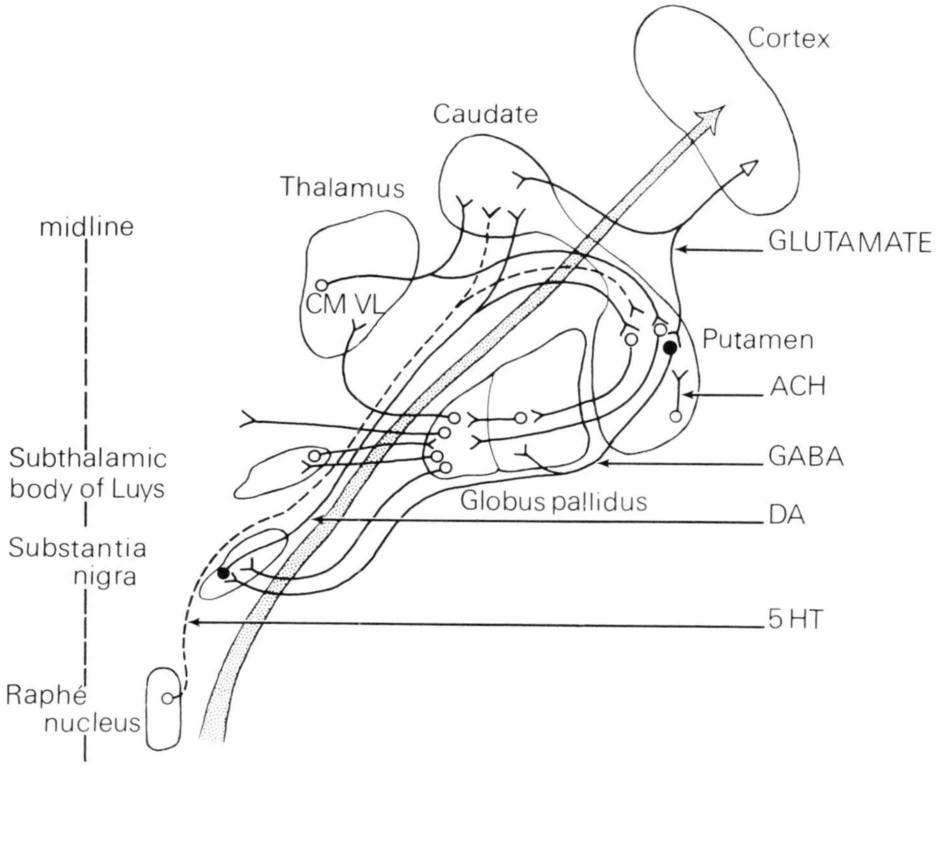

1. There are at least four inputs to the striatum: from the cortex, thalamus, the raphé nucleus of the midbrain, and the substantia nigra. Dopamine is the neurotransmitter for the nigrostriatal path, serotonin for the ascending fibers from the midbrain raphé nuclei, and glutamate for the corticostriatal projection.
2. The cortical and thalamic inputs terminate largely on dendrites of the medium spiny cells, often on the same cells. The dopaminergic cells in the nigra send axons to the striatum that branch repeatedly before terminating on cells with dendritic spines. These cells may be the same as those receiving thalamic and cortical terminations.
3. The medium-sized spiny neurons constitute about 96% of the striatal cells. At least one half of these are output cells that terminate in the substantia nigra and globus pallidus and contain and release the inhibitory transmitter GABA. GABAergic terminals contact dendrites of DA cells in the substantia nigra.
4. Some striatal interneurons produce and release ACh.

RESPONSE TO INJURY OF THE SUBSTANTIA NIGRA

When a lesion is made in the substantia nigra in an experimental animal, some cells die, axons going to the striatum and elsewhere are severed, and striatal dopamine content decreases.

Several changes occur that may also develop in Parkinson's disease.

1. Vigorous sprouting of the remaining or possibly damaged dopaminergic cells takes place near the injury. Nearby areas, including such aberrant sites as capillaries and scar tissue, receive many terminals filled with dopamine.
2. With loss of some striatal endings following death of their distant cell bodies in the nigra, some postsynaptic terminals become vacated, and neighboring intact nigrostriatal presynaptic endings may sprout to cover them. Depending on the pattern of loss of presynaptic terminations, postsynaptic sites may have either too few or too many new presynaptic terminations. Depending on the pattern of new growth in the nigrostriatal path, therapeutic elevation of brain dopamine could either do little good, help certain symptoms, or produce signs of local overdosage (choreoathetosis; *see* below).
3. Adrenergic and serotoninergic neurons in the CNS have also been shown to sprout vigorously in response to injury and to have grown into postsynaptic sites previously covered by presynaptic endings with entirely different transmitters. If similar aberrant reinnervation takes place in Parkinson's disease, striatal receptors, formerly dopaminergic, might be reinnervated by ACh or serotoninergic endings. Some of the variations in clinical symptoms or in therapeutic response to different drugs may be due to such variations in regrowth (*see* below).
4. Some terminals may make the "wrong" neurotransmitter. Regenerating dopaminergic terminals, for example, seem to make norepinephrine. Further, serotoninergic terminals, regenerating or not, appear to be able to convert dopa to dopamine.
5. When the dopaminergic nigrostriatal pathways are partially degenerated in the rat, there is hyperactivity of the remaining dopaminergic neurons. This compensating mechanism may also be a factor in human parkinsonism. Overt symptoms arise in experimental animals when dopamine cells are reduced to about 25% of their normal number.
6. Denervated dopamine receptors may become hypersensitive to dopamine.

DRUGS

Several drugs are known to improve the symptoms of human Parkinson's disease: levodopa; dopamine agonists such as bromocriptine and apomorphine; anticholinergic medications; and amantadine hydrochloride (Symmetrel). Other drugs such as diphenhydramine HCl (Benadryl) are occasionally helpful. Still others can produce a state that resembles naturally occurring Parkinson's disease, including the phenothiazines and haloperidol (*see* Chap. 24) (possibly by blocking the postsynaptic dopamine receptor site) and reserpine (by interfering with dopamine storage in the presynaptic terminal).

DOPA

The rationale for using levodopa has been presented above. Following oral intake, some is destroyed in the stomach. Decreasing gastric acidity, increasing gastric and upper intestinal motility, and even gastrectomy favor absorption. Passage through the small intestinal wall is enhanced by dopa decarboxylase inhibitors, suggesting that this enzyme is in the intestinal mucosa. About 20% of orally administered levodopa reaches the peripheral circulation intact. In the first passage through the liver, more dopa is degradated, mainly by catechol-O-methyltransferase (COMT). In the peripheral circulation, dopa is free in the plasma or bound to plasma proteins and is found in red blood cells. Following a single i.v. injection, levodopa is maintained at reasonably stable blood levels for several hours.

Only about 1% to 2% of orally administered levodopa enters the CNS because further loss to dopa decarboxylase occurs in crossing the brain capillary endothelium (blood–brain barrier). Dopa is converted to dopamine within the cell bodies and synaptic terminals of the nigrostriatal cells. When large doses of levodopa are given, however, or when some of the nigral cells have died, some dopamine may be formed in serotoninergic terminals or elsewhere.

In 1967 Cotzias administered levodopa in large amounts (many grams a day) to patients with parkinsonism and effected a remarkable reduction in symptoms. His results were confirmed by other neurologists, but side-effects of nausea and vomiting, a dyskinesia best characterized as choreoathetosis, and, infrequently, postural hypotension or organic confusion have limited the usefulness of the drug. Fortunately, none of the side-effects has proved lethal or persistent.

In the early 1970s, dopa was first administered with dopa decarboxylase inhibitors that acted almost entirely at sites outside the brain. These loci include the gut, liver, and the brain capillary endothelium. Such combined therapy allowed the dose of dopa to be decreased by 75% to 80%. The incidence of nausea and vomiting and postural hypotension was much reduced. Combined therapy with Sinemet (carbidopa and levodopa) and Madopa (benserazide and levodopa) has almost supplanted use of levodopa alone.

Sinemet is used worldwide and Madopa is available in most of the world except the United States. The unavailability of Madopa in the United States is unfortunate because an appreciable number of patients with Parkinson's disease respond better on this therapy than on Sinemet (Fig. 30-2).

George Constantin Cotzias, 1918–1977. Greek-born American physician. Studies of the effects of manganese poisoning led to work on Parkinson's disease and the first long-term, effective treatment with levodopa.

Sinemet therapy is usually started at one fixed combination tablet of the 25/100 or 10/100 size (10 mg carbidopa and 100 mg levodopa) taken two or three times a day with food. Every 1 to 2 weeks the dosage is increased until a daily dosage of 1000 mg of dopa is reached, or to the point that side-effects (*see* below) become troublesome. Sinemet may be further increased to as high as 2000 mg. Sinemet tablets of 25/250 size are usually used for higher doses. To achieve the optimum balance between therapeutic benefits and side-effects, the dosage should be adjusted every 3 to 4 months. Both the physician and the patient must be knowledgeable about the nuances of drug action and cooperate actively with each other.

Parkinsonian symptoms usually improve after 3 to 4 weeks on levodopa therapy alone and a shorter time on Sinemet. Improvement may continue for as long as 1 year. Of the major parkinsonian symptoms, akinesia and rigidity are most helped, and tremor somewhat less frequently. At 1 year about 10% of compliant patients are symptom-free, 80% are markedly improved, and 10% are worse or have little improvement. After 10 years of treatment, most patients show progression of the underlying Parkinson's disease. However, some are still nearly symptom-free, and more than half are better than before levodopa had been started. This is the first time any medical treatment has interrupted the progressive worsening of Parkinson's disease. Up to 1967, people with primary Parkinson's disease had about three times greater likelihood of dying at a given age than did the average person. Present mortality figures indicate that patients with primary parkinsonism who take levodopa daily on an optimum schedule have about the same life expectancy as their nonparkinsonian contemporaries.

Adverse Effects

The side-effects of levodopa are troublesome. The concomitant administration of peripheral dopa decarboxylase inhibitors with levodopa usually reduces nausea, vomiting, and postural hypotension probably because these drugs allow a 75% to 80% reduction in levodopa dosage. Postural hypotension is rarely a persistent problem, however, and if not controlled by concomitant use of dopa decarboxylase inhibitors, fludrocortisone acetate can be used.

Choreoathetosis (involuntary pulling of the head to one side, or facial grimacing or restless movements of a limb) may develop after the patient has been on levodopa for 3 to 12 months.

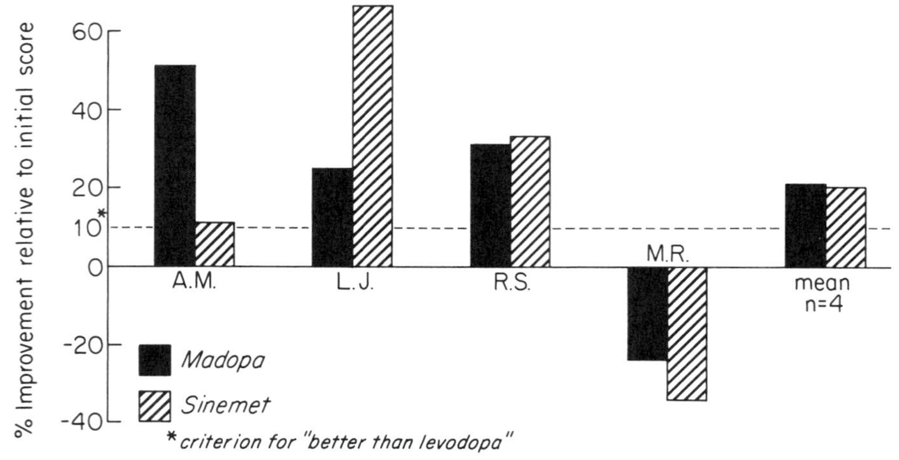

FIG. 30-2. Four patients showing four different types of responses to madopa and Sinemet. Improvement greater than 10% (*dotted line*) must be shown before the judgment "better than levodopa" is made. Relative to levodopa baseline, patient A.M. shows greater improvement in disability on madopa therapy; L.J. has greater improvement on Sinemet; R.S. shows equal improvement on either madopa or Sinemet; and M.R. is worse on either. Mean for this group of 4 patients is 21% improved on madopa and 20% improved on Sinemet, illustrating that equal means can conceal varying responses. The four classes of responses shown here are approximately equally represented in the total group of 20 patients studied. (Diamond SG, Markham CH, and Treciokas LJ: A double-blind comparison of levodopa, madopa and Sinemet in Parkinson disease. Ann Neurol 3:267–272, 1978)

Because it is often difficult for patients to distinguish between levodopa-induced dyskinesia and parkinsonian tremor, the physician should see the patient and decide. Choreoathetosis usually occurs at a dosage just above that needed to control the parkinsonian symptoms, and thus is dealt with by reducing the daily intake. Rarely, however, choreoathetosis develops at the same dosage needed to treat the parkinsonian symptoms and then constitutes a real therapeutic challenge. Choreoathetosis does not benefit from peripherally acting dopa decarboxylase inhibitors. The disorder is probably due to too much dopamine activity on some striatal receptors. It occurs always, or almost always, when there is partial loss of either nigrostriatal terminations (as in Parkinson's disease) or of some striatal cells (as in Huntington's chorea).

Behavioral alterations from levodopa are relatively infrequent except in those patients who have preexisting organic dementia. Patients may become more confused, or euphoric, or may become less inhibited, including in their sexual behavior. Levodopa has reportedly improved depression or made it worse but probably does neither.

An "on–off" effect may occur in parkinsonian patients who have been on levodopa therapy for several years. The "off" response, a repeated, abrupt, and unanticipated worsening of parkinsonian symptoms, occurs over a few minutes and may benefit from levodopa taken at more frequent intervals or by use of bromocriptine (Parlodel) or pergolide (*see* below). The "off" response is thought to be due to a great reduction in dopamine-containing nigrostriatal neurons or to a dopamine receptor abnormality. Patients who show an "off" response may show an "on" response—a remission of parkinsonian symptoms within a few minutes, usually after taking a dose of dopa.

Treatment

When should levodopa therapy be initiated? Opinions differ on this issue: Those in favor of delaying therapy until symptoms are significantly disabling do so because they observe a worsening in their patients' conditions after several years of levodopa treatment. The duration of therapy, however, is concomitant and confounded with the duration of this progressive disease. A recent study separating the effects of duration of disease and years of levodopa therapy (Markham and Diamond, 1981) found that it is not decreased levodopa efficacy over time but rather the progression of the disease itself that accounts for the increasing disability in Parkinson patients (Fig. 30-3). Thus, delaying therapy simply fails to improve

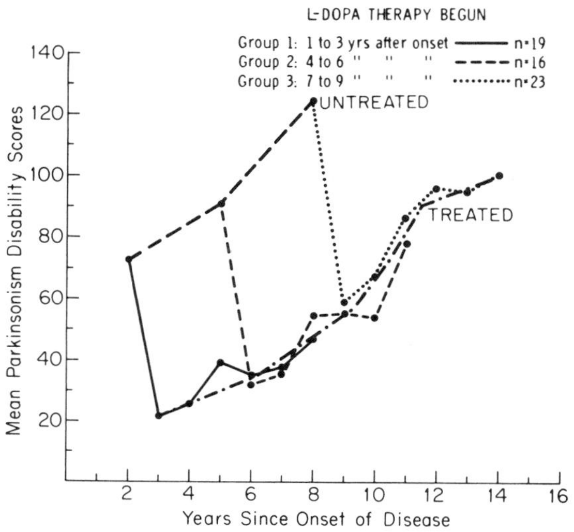

FIG. 30-3. Line connecting prelevodopa scores of the three groups is a projection of disease progression when untreated with levodopa. Line through treated points shows progression of disease with levodopa treatment. Difference between treated and untreated state is highly significant ($p < 0.0005$, paired *t*-tests). There is no difference between treated groups at the same duration of disease. Withholding levodopa does not improve the later state and fails to alleviate symptoms in early years. (Markham CH, Diamond SG: Evidence to support early levodopa therapy in Parkinson disease. Neurology (NY) 31:125–131, 1981)

disability in the early years of the disease without conferring any benefit to the patient's later years. Consequently levodopa should be initiated as soon as a patient is willing to start a medicine that needs frequent dosage adjustments and that must be taken many times a day for years.

DOPAMINE AGONISTS

Bromocriptine (Parlodel), pergolide mesylate, lisuride, and apomorphine have strong dopaminergic activity. Bromocriptine has proved very useful in a limited number of patients, particularly those suffering from the "off–on" effect or who must take dopa very frequently. Bromocriptine must be used with dopa. Pergolide and lisuride are still investigational drugs but offer much promise. Apomorphine is not clinically useful because it must be given parenterally.

ANTICHOLINERGIC AGENTS

Belladonna alkaloids and certain synthetic preparations such as trihexyphenidyl (Artane), benztropine (Cogentin), procyclidine (Kemadrin), and ethopropazine (Parsidol) have long been known to improve parkinsonian tremor and rigidity (*see* Chap. 16). Usually this improvement is mild to moderate, but in a patient with severe Parkinson's disease, withdrawal may lead to a significant increase in invalidism and even death from pneumonia.

As noted above, the striatum has very high concentrations of ACh. Because striatal ACh does not diminish after lesions of the cortex, thalamus, and midbrain, the major inputs to the striatum, its source is probably one class of striatal interneurons. This view is supported by immunologic demonstration of choline acetylase in certain striatal neurons.

In Parkinson's disease there appears to be a relative or absolute increase in striatal ACh and an absolute decrease in striatal dopamine. Either elevating the dopamine concentration or interfering with ACh use helps parkinsonian symptoms. More than half the patients do better on a combination of the two approaches.

Adverse Effects

The main adverse effects of the anticholinergic agents are organic confusion, including hallucinations, delirium, and urinary retention. Hallucinations and delirium are more common in patients with some degree of preexisting organic dementia and are especially likely to occur in persons recovering from operations or intercurrent illnesses. Urinary hesitancy or retention almost exclusively occurs in middle-aged or elderly men with narrowed bladder necks due to prostatic hypertrophy. Urinary retention and organic confusion can usually be dealt with by reducing the daily dosage of the anticholinergic agent or changing to another preparation. Benztropine and ethopropazine are more likely to produce these side-effects and procyclidine, somewhat less so.

AMANTADINE HYDROCHLORIDE (SYMMETREL)

Amantadine hydrochloride was originally introduced as an antiviral agent (*see* Chap. 70). Its antiparkinsonian properties were serendipitously discovered when one patient with influenza and Parkinson's disease noticed an improvement of tremor and rigidity while taking amantadine. Since this observation, amantadine has been shown to benefit symptoms (especially tremor) in many patients with parkinsonism; about one fourth of patients find this a useful adjunct to levodopa therapy.

Mode of Action and Dosage

The mode of action of amantadine is uncertain. Clinical observations of adverse effects such as decreased salivation and urinary hesitancy suggest it has a mild anticholinergic action. Experimental evidence shows, however, that it releases dopamine from synaptic storage sites and increases GABA levels in the striatum and substantia nigra. Side-effects of livido reticularis and grand mal convulsions (the latter occurring only at 2 to 3 times the recommended dosage limit of 300 mg/day) also indicate that amantadine has an action other than anticholinergic.

Adverse effects are further discussed in Chapter 70.

PROPRANOLOL (INDERAL)

Beta-adrenergic blocking agents such as propranolol may suppress parkinsonian resting tremor as well as postural tremor. If parkinsonian tremor is particularly severe and does not respond to the drugs discussed above, propranolol therapy should be considered.

SURGERY

Specific operations may occasionally help certain parkinsonian symptoms, particularly when combined with subsequent drug therapy. Stereotaxic thalamotomy, in which surgical lesions are made in the ventrolateral thalamus, has largely been replaced by levodopa therapy because thalamotomy and other operations do not help akinesia, ultimately the most disabling parkinsonian symptom. A few patients, however, have persistent or progressive tremor that may best be treated by a unilateral operation opposite to the side of the most severe tremor, and then by levodopa therapy thereafter.

FURTHER READING

1. Diamond SG, Markham CH, Treciokas LJ: A double-blind comparison of levodopa, Madopa and Sinemet in Parkinson disease. Ann Neurol 3:267–272, 1978
2. Diamond SG, Markham CH, Treciokas LJ: Long term experience with L-dopa: Efficacy, progression and mortality. In Birkmayer W, Hornykiewicz O (eds): Advances in Parkinsonism, Fifth International Symposium on Parkinson's Disease, Vienna, 1975, pp. 444–455. Basel, Editiones Roche, 1976
3. Isselbacher KJ et al: Harrison's Principles of Internal Medicine, 9th ed, pp 1997–1999. New York, McGraw-Hill, 1979
4. McDowell FH, Markham CH (eds): Recent Advances in Parkinson's Disease, Contemporary Neurology Series, p 245. Philadelphia, F A Davis, 1971
5. Markham CH, Diamond SG: Evidence to support early levodopa therapy in Parkinson disease. Neurology 31:125–131, 1981
6. Walton JN: Brain's Diseases of the Nervous System, 8th ed, pp 587–600. Oxford, Oxford University Press, 1977

CHAPTER 30 QUESTIONS

(See P. 7 for Full Instructions)

Select the One Best Answer

1. Which of the following agents, administered orally, will ameliorate the symptoms of Parkinson's disease?
   A. Chlorpromazine
   B. Dopamine
   C. Haloperidol
   D. Amantadine
   E. Reserpine
2. Symptoms of parkinsonism can be relieved by oral administration of each of the following EXCEPT
   A. benztropine.
   B. levodopa.
   C. diphenhydramine.
   D. trihexyphenidyl.
   E. pyridoxine (vitamin B_6).
3. A drug that may improve the therapeutic response to levodopa in Parkinson's disease when given concurrently is
   A. guanethidine.
   B. thiothixene.
   C. carbidopa (α-methyldopa hydrazine).
   D. pyridoxine.
   E. trifluoperazine.
4. Pharmacologic agents that may either produce or exacerbate the extrapyramidal signs of Parkinson's disease include each of the following EXCEPT
   A. physostigmine (eserine).
   B. reserpine.
   C. chlorpromazine.
   D. trihexyphenidyl.
   E. haloperidol.

A = 1,2,3; B = 1,3; C = 2,4; D = 4; E = All

5. Parkinsonism is a frequent side-effect of
   1. haloperidol.
   2. lithium carbonate.

   3. trifluoperazine.
   4. imipramine.

6. Which of the following agents is effective in the treatment of postencephalitic parkinsonism?
   1. Trihexyphenidyl
   2. Methantheline
   3. Benztropin
   4. Atropine methylnitrate

7. Levodopa therapy may
   1. reverse CNS toxicity of manganese.
   2. exacerbate peptic ulcers.
   3. cause paranoid dreams.
   4. cause excessive salivation.

8. The large doses of levodopa used in the treatment of Parkinson's disease may
   1. be reduced when α-methyldopa hydrazine is added to the therapy.
   2. produce nausea and vomiting for which phenothiazine compounds are recommended as treatment.
   3. produce increased cardiac ischemia, which is alleviated by treatment with propranolol.
   4. produce miosis, which is a beneficial effect in persons also afflicted with narrow-angle glaucoma.

31

HAROLD E. PAULUS

Drugs for Rheumatic Diseases

The drugs used to moderate the pain, swelling, heat, and general discomfort of acute and chronic inflammatory conditions are called the *analgesic, antipyretic, antiinflammatory* agents. These compounds differ from the narcotic analgesics (*see* Chap. 32) in that they are not addicting and have little effect on the central recognition of pain; instead they appear to act peripherally, suppressing inflammatory processes that trigger pain receptors of peripheral nerves. They are particularly useful for treating musculoskeletal discomfort and headaches but are ineffective for severe pain or pain of cardiac or visceral origin. Most nonsteroidal antiinflammatory drugs also tend to restore an elevated body temperature toward normal, hence their designation as antipyretics. They are most frequently prescribed for patients with chronic inflammatory arthritis—for example, rheumatoid arthritis, ankylosing spondylitis, osteoarthritis, and gout—and primarily in this context are the *salicylates, acetaminophen, phenylbutazone, indomethacin,* and *colchicine* discussed. Except for acetaminophen, each has significant gastrointestinal toxicity that may be considered a general characteristic of these drugs. Although they have no analgesic or antiinflammatory activity, the drugs used to decrease plasma uric acid concentrations in patients with gout—*probenecid, sulfinpyrazone,* and *allopurinol*—are also discussed. Gold compounds and penicillamine are included as examples of rheumatoid-arthritis-modifying drugs. Corticosteroids are discussed in Chapter 47.

TARGETS OF DRUG THERAPY IN CHRONIC INFLAMMATION

Inflammation is the normal protective response to tissue injury, restoring the host to its former healthy state. Normally, the tissue-damaging stimulus initiates a series of biochemical, immunologic, and cellular events that proceed through apparently well-regulated steps, culminating in tissue repair and restoration of function. When healing is completed, the inflammatory response ceases until needed again. The sequence of events in inflammation is as follows (Table 31-1): The prime cause of the inflammation either directly or through mediators (such as antigen–anti-

TABLE 31-1. Targets for Therapy of Chronic Inflammatory States

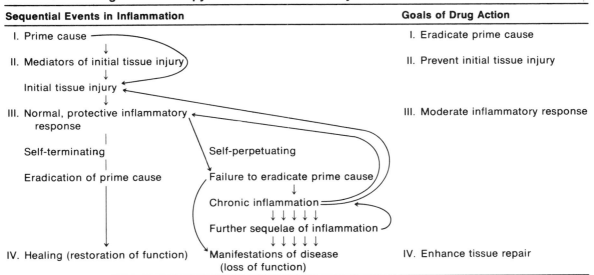

Sequential Events in Inflammation		Goals of Drug Action
I. Prime cause		I. Eradicate prime cause
↓		
II. Mediators of initial tissue injury		II. Prevent initial tissue injury
↓		
Initial tissue injury		
↓		
III. Normal, protective inflammatory response		III. Moderate inflammatory response
Self-terminating	Self-perpetuating	
Eradication of prime cause	Failure to eradicate prime cause	
	↓	
	Chronic inflammation	
	↓ ↓ ↓ ↓ ↓	
	Further sequelae of inflammation	
↓	↓ ↓ ↓ ↓ ↓	
IV. Healing (restoration of function)	Manifestations of disease (loss of function)	IV. Enhance tissue repair

body–complement complexes) produces the initial injury to the tissue. The injured tissue then releases mediators that initiate the complex cellular and biochemical events of normal inflammation. Usually these events result in the elimination of the prime cause, followed by healing and restoration of function. If the prime cause cannot be eradicated, however, the various mediators of inflammation enhance tissue injury and magnify the damage produced by the prime cause. The consequence is chronic inflammation, which results in the manifestations of disease and ultimately in loss of function. This formulation of chronic inflammatory disease suggests that treatment may be directed at four targets (Table 31-1).

1. *Eradication of the prime cause* could be expected to result in healing or scar formation. This may occur even if the disease has been present for many years, as is seen when tuberculosis or syphilis is adequately treated with an effective antibiotic. When dealing with diseases of unknown etiology, a "disease" may merely be a common clinical expression of injury produced by any of a number of prime causes; for example, the disease "pneumonia" may be caused by *Diplococcus pneumoniae*, *Staphylococcus aureus*, or one of a number of other microorganisms. If treatment is aimed at the prime cause, it must be specific. None of the drugs currently available for the management of inflammatory arthritis even remotely approaches the goal of eradicating the prime cause, but if such a drug were found it might be effective only in a few patients with a particular diagnosis.
2. The second possible target for drug therapy is *prevention of initial tissue injury*. A drug of this type might be unable to eliminate the prime cause but in some way would completely prevent it from producing tissue injury and thus would circumvent the events of the normal inflammatory response. Such a drug could not be expected to "cure" the disease and indeed might allow wider dissemination of the prime cause because it masks the prime cause from the effects of the normal inflammatory response. As a corollary to this, however, it would not interfere with established inflammatory responses, nor would it suppress the body's response to ordinary environmental challenges. Tetanus antitoxin is an example of a therapeutic agent acting on this target; it prevents tetanus without destroying the causative bacterium or interfering with the normal immune or inflammatory mechanisms. For the inflammatory arthritides, the investigational cytotoxic immunosuppressive drugs (*see* Chap. 70) may fall in this category. They appear to interfere with the normal immunologic response (which in this case is misguided and results in tissue damage) against the prime cause, preventing the initiation of the inflammatory sequence by these immunologic mediators. Cyclophosphamide may prevent the progression of destructive joint erosions in pa-

tients undergoing effective treatment with it. As might be expected, however, if there is no effect on the prime cause, the disease recurs when the immunosuppressive therapy is discontinued. The gold salts and D-penicillamine may also fall in this category.

3. If it is impossible to eradicate the cause of the disease or to prevent tissue injury and the resultant inflammatory response, attempts may be made to *moderate the inflammatory response* to suppress at least some of the manifestations of established inflammation. Aspirin, indomethacin, phenylbutazone, corticosteroids, and all of the nonsteroidal antiinflammatory agents are included in this category. They may be expected to relieve, in varying degrees, some of the symptoms and signs of inflammation, regardless of its cause. A major advantage of these drugs is that they do not interfere with the normal immunologic response, although a truly effective antiinflammatory drug, such as high doses of corticosteroid (*see* Chap. 47), substantially disarms the recipient in his daily battle to protect himself against his environment. Despite treatment with these agents, tissue injury continues, the disease progresses, and disability continues to become more severe. The available drugs cover a wide spectrum of effectiveness, varying from almost complete suppression of inflammation by large doses of prednisone to minor symptomatic improvement by small doses of salicylates. Each available drug may have serious side-effects that prevent its use in a substantial number of patients. A number of new drugs (Table 31-2) of this type have been introduced during the past decade, and others are being developed. They give the clinician more flexibility in patients who do not tolerate, or who fail to respond to, the more traditional agents.
4. Treatment of chronic inflammation may be directed at the reparative and healing process that occurs as the terminal event in normal inflammation; drug therapy might be used to *enhance tissue repair*. Drugs of this type might be particularly useful in degenerative processes. Unfortunately, so little is known about the regulation of these reparative processes that this problem has not even begun to be approached by pharmaceutical chemists and experimental pharmacologists. No drug that acts in this area is available at present, and none is under active investigation.

TABLE 31-2. Some Antiinflammatory Drugs

			Side-Effects	
Drug	**Dose Range**	**Half-Life**	***Dyspepsia and Peptic Ulcer***	***Others***
Heterocarboxylic acids	*mg/day*	*hr*		
Aspirin (Acetylsalicylic acid)	1000–6000	4–15	++++	Tinnitus
Magnesium choline salicylate	1500–4000	4–15	+	Tinnitus
Salicylsalicylate	1500–5000	4–15	+	Tinnitus
Phenylacetic acids				
Ibuprofen	1200–3200	2	++	—
Fenoprofen	1200–3200	1	++	—
Ketoprofen	100–400	2	++	—
Naphthaleneacetic acids				
Naproxen	250–750	13	+	—
Indoleacetic acids				
Indomethacin	50–200	3–11	++++	Headache
Sulindac	300–400	16	++	—
Pyrrolealkanoic acids				
Tolmetin	800–1600	1	++	—
Pyrazolon derivatives				
Phenylbutazone	200–800	40–80	+	Blood dyscrasias
Oxyphenbutazone	200–800	40–80	+	Blood dyscrasias
Oxicam				
Piroxicam	20	30–86	+	
Colchicine				
	1 or 2 intravenously Oral—*see* text	24–36	+	Diarrhea, nausea, vomiting

The rapidly acting nonsteroidal antiinflammatory compounds have no effect on the causes of inflammation, but their importance as symptomatic therapy is attested to by the huge quantities of these drugs used. They moderate the activity of inflammation within the first few days of administration and are effective only while blood levels are sustained. Unless the underlying inflammatory condition has already subsided spontaneously, their withdrawal is soon followed by a recurrence of signs and symptoms. They appear to act late in the events of the inflammatory cascade and have little or no discernible effect on immune defenses. Because inflammation appears to be a multifaceted defense system with many mechanisms for arriving at the same end-state, it is likely that these drugs interfere with all of the mediators in the more distal aspects of the inflammatory process rather than specifically affecting only one or two mediators. Evidence for this is supplied each time a new mediator is discovered. Thus the clinically useful antiinflammatory drugs have been found to uncouple oxidative phosphorylation, inhibit the release of hyaluronidase and β-glucuronidase from isolated rat liver lysosomes, inhibit phosphatase and cathepsins, and inhibit the induction of inflammation by kinins. They also inhibit cyclooxygenase, thus interfering with the transformation of arachadonic acid (via) endoperoxides) to prostaglandins, prostacyclin, and thromboxanes. Arachadonic acid metabolites, prostaglandins, and thromboxanes help to mediate inflammation, among a myriad of other activities (*see* Chap. 53). Each of these effects has been considered to be their mode of action, but as additional mediators of inflammation are described, the clinically useful antiinflammatory agents may also be active against them.

ANTIINFLAMMATORY ANALGESICS

SALICYLATES

Willow and poplar barks that contain salicin have long been used to treat sepsis, pain, gout, and fever. Salicylic acid was first synthesized in 1860 and aspirin (acetylsalicylic acid) in 1899. Today, aspirin is one of the least expensive and most widely used drugs in the world. About 30 tons of aspirin are consumed daily in the United States. Even though salicylates have such an ancient heritage and are so casually used, they continue to be the prototype of the nonsteroidal, antiinflammatory, antirheumatic drug and are still the yardstick that newer agents are assessed against. The fairly frequent occurrence of fatal salicylate intoxication in children emphasizes that salicylates are potent drugs that deserve the same careful administration as other potentially dangerous pharmacologic agents.

Chemistry

The parent compound, salicylic acid, and its methyl ester, methyl salicylate (oil of wintergreen), are local irritants and are used only as keratolytic agents (*see* Chap. 69) or as counterirritants for topical application to the skin. Sodium salicylate and aspirin are useful analgesic antipyretic antiinflammatory agents, and aspirin is the prototype compound for this group.

Pharmacology

Aspirin has a broad spectrum of pharmacologic activities. In therapeutic concentrations (0.5–2.0 mM) salicylates uncouple mitochondria oxidative phosphorylation, and at much higher concentrations they may inhibit cellular oxidative enzymes, prevent the activation of kinin-forming enzymes, and antagonize peripheral effects of kinins (*see* Chap. 55). In sensitized animals, they inhibit the release of histamine and modify the effects of intradermal histamine injections; in addition, the response to 5-hydroxytryptamine is inhibited, both in experimental animals and in humans. In experimental animals, high doses of salicylates may suppress antibody production, interfere with antigen–antibody aggregation, and stabilize capillary permeability in the presence of immunologic insults. Blood coagulation may be slowed by increasing the prothrombin time, and aspirin decreases platelet adhesiveness. Since salicylate is an organic acid tolerated in rather high plasma concentrations, it competes with other organic acids in the renal tubules (*see* Chap. 3).

Aspirin also is an effective antagonist of the enzyme prostaglandin synthetase, which is responsible for the production of prostaglandin E_1 (*see* Chap. 53). Because prostaglanding E_1 inhibits gastric acid secretion, the inhibition of

FIG. 31-1. Salicylates.

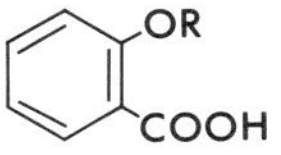

'SALICYLATES'
R=H. SALICYCLIC ACID
R=$COCH_3$, ASPIRIN

prostaglandin synthesis by antiinflammatory drugs may be the common factor responsible for their gastric toxicity. Salicylates decrease blood glucose concentrations in diabetic patients, but high levels may elevate blood glucose levels in normal subjects. Very high doses stimulate the release of corticoids from the adrenal cortex. Aspirin is thought to acetylate a lysyl residue of human serum albumin irreversibly.

Salicylates bind rather tightly to albumin and also to erythrocytes. They may displace other drugs from albumin binding sites and are known to increase protein-free levels of coumarin, thus enhancing its anticoagulant effects (*see* Chap. 8). Salicylates may also interfere with the binding of thyroxin by thyroxin-binding prealbumin, thus decreasing plasma protein-bound iodine levels without decreasing normal concentrations of free circulating thyroxin.

Analgesia. Salicylates are particularly effective for relieving pain due to headache, myalgia, and arthralgia but relatively ineffective for visceral or cardiac pain. Their major effect probably is related to peripheral antiinflammatory activity or to an effect on pain receptors; a subcortical CNS site of analgesic action has been suggested but not demonstrated conclusively. Important, and in contrast with the narcotic analgesics, analgesic doses of aspirin do not disturb mentation, nor are they addicting. For pain of musculoskeletal origin, however, they are much more effective than narcotics; indeed, patients with chronic inflammatory arthritis rarely become addicted to narcotic drugs.

Antipyresis. Salicylates lower the body temperature in febrile patients but have no effect on normal body temperature, an effect due to normalization of temperature-sensitive neurons in the hypothalamus, whose function appears to be depressed by pyrogens in the febrile patient. Sweating generally is associated with reduction of fever in salicylate-treated patients. Paradoxically, salicylate poisoning may cause fever when increased oxygen consumption is caused by uncoupling of oxidative phosphorylation.

Antirheumatic and Antiinflammatory Actions. Salicylates are the most widely used therapeutic agents in rheumatoid arthritis and rheumatic fever. They markedly reduce painful joint swelling and fever but do not affect the ultimate course of either disease. The degree of suppression of inflammation increases with the plasma concentration of salicylate even beyond the point of toxicity. Thus patients with severe inflammatory arthritis often tolerate tinnitus and other mild manifestations of toxicity to obtain the increased antiinflammatory effects associated with plasma levels of about 30 to 35 mg/dl. The usual optimal subtoxic level is in a range of 20 to 30 mg/dl. The mechanism of their antiinflammatory action is probably related to some of the factors discussed above. The antiinflammatory activity of salicylates has been demonstrated in induced inflammation in experimental animals and documented in patients with rheumatoid arthritis.

Uricosuric Action. Salicylates affect renal tubular reabsorption and secretion of uric acid (*see* Chap. 3). In low doses (1–2 g/day) tubular secretion of uric acid is inhibited, and serum uric acid concentrations are increased. In doses that cause serum salicylate concentrations of greater than 20 mg/dl, salicylates also inhibit tubular reabsorption of uric acid. The net effect of this inhibition is an enhanced excretion of uric acid; hence, serum uric acid concentrations decrease. However, because more effective and less toxic uricosuric drugs are available, salicylates are no longer used for this purpose.

Decreased Platelet Adhesiveness. Aspirin inhibits platelet aggregation by acetylating platelet cyclooxygenase irreversibly. (Nonacetylated salicylates inhibit platelet aggregation only minimally.) As little as 300 mg of aspirin may produce an antiaggregation effect that is still detectable 4 to 6 days after ingestion. The prophylactic use of this anticoagulant effect is being explored in patients predisposed toward myocardial infarction and cerebrovascular accidents.

Absorption and Metabolism

Aspirin is readily absorbed from the stomach and the small intestine. It is rapidly and completely hydrolyzed to salicylate by a plasma esterase, and within 90 minutes acetylsalicylic acid concentrations in the plasma are insignificant because all of the aspirin has been converted to salicylate. Plasma salicylate levels are not a simple function of the dose ingested because several of the major pathways of drug metabolism (conversion to salicylurate and formation of a glucuronide) become saturated at higher doses. Therefore the time required to excrete half of a large dose of salicylate is longer than that needed to excrete half of a small dose.

In addition, above a certain point, there is a nonlinear rise in the blood concentration of salicylate with small increments in the dose. Further, the renal excretion of unmetabolized salicylate increases when the urine is alkaline and decreases when the urine is acid (*see* Chap. 3), approaching zero when its pH is five or less. Because of genetically determined variations in the metabolism of salicylate, serum concentrations attained by different people taking the same weight-adjusted dose of aspirin may vary up to fivefold. Salicylate induces its own metabolism (*see* Chap. 8); after 3 weeks of administration, serum salicylate levels are substantially lower than at the end of the first week. Because the serum salicylate concentration associated with optimal antiinflammatory effect is rather critical, therapeutic doses of salicylate must be determined individually for each patient, using serum salicylate concentrations as a guide.

Adverse Effects

Gastric intolerance, in the form of epigastric discomfort, nausea, anorexia, or heartburn, is common in patients who take fairly large doses of aspirin chronically. Increased occult fecal blood loss during salicylate administration is well documented; it can be minimized by administering aspirin in a solution of sufficient buffer capacity to neutralize gastric acidity completely. The important role of acid in the gastric irritation produced by aspirin has been confirmed by studies in achlorhydric subjects who had fewer mucosal erosions and less occult blood loss than did normal subjects given the same aspirin dose. These studies suggest that the toxic effects are predominantly local and are supported by animal studies that were unable to relate gastric toxicity to plasma salicylate concentrations. Ethanol ingestion may increase the occult blood loss induced by aspirin.

Tinnitus and decreased auditory acuity are reliable early signs of salicylate toxicity in adults. In persons with normal hearing, persistent tinnitus is present only when serum salicylate concentrations are greater than 20 mg/dl and this has been used as a guide for individualization of aspirin dosage. Unfortunately, many older patients have preexisting hearing loss and cannot perceive tinnitus, while children may fail to appreciate it. In these two age groups, serum salicylate concentration should be used to individualize drug dosage. Both the tinnitus and deafness associated with high salicylate concentrations are readily reversible when the drug is withdrawn.

Reversible hepatocellular toxicity has been observed in a small number of children and in a few patients with systemic lupus erythematosus who had therapeutic plasma salicylate concentrations. These abnormalities of liver function apparently are rather unusual and disappear when the drug is withdrawn. Because salicylates avidly bind to plasma proteins, they may enhance the effect of other drugs displaced from their protein binding sites by salicylate (*see* Chap. 8); examples include coumarin anticoagulants, phenytoin, the oral hypoglycemic agents, and phenylbutazone. Nephrotoxicity has been observed with chronic ingestion of combinations of salicylate and phenacetin, but there is no convincing evidence that prolonged use of aspirin alone has any irreversible effect on the kidney. Serious allergic reactions to aspirin may be manifested as asthma, hypotension, and hives. The syndrome of rhinitis and nasal polyposis has also been attributed to aspirin hypersensitivity.

Salicylate Poisoning. Because of their ubiquity, salicylates frequently cause serious intoxication in children (*see* Chap. 72). Hyperventilation, severe acidosis, irritability, psychosis, fever, coma, and cardiovascular collapse may occur with salicylate poisoning and may be complicated by gastrointestinal hemorrhage owing to local gastric irritation and the hypoprothrombinemic and antiplatelet activities of aspirin. Gastric lavage, alkalinization, diuresis, and intensive supportive measures are necessary to treat salicylate poisoning. Because of the peculiarities of salicylate metabolism, elevated plasma levels may fall very slowly.

The characteristic disturbance of acid–base balance by salicylate toxicity may be explained as follows. Therapeutic concentrations of salicylate increase oxygen consumption and CO_2 production by uncoupling oxidative phosphorylation. Increased ventilation compensates for the increased CO_2 production. With slightly higher salicylate concentrations (greater than 35 mg/dl), the respiratory center is stimulated, causing hyperventilation and respiratory alkalosis; if these salicylate concentrations persist, renal excretion of bicarbonate, sodium, and potassium returns the blood *p*H toward normal, resulting in compensated respiratory alkalosis but also decreasing the reserve buffering capacity of the system. With further increase in salicylate concentrations above 50 mg/dl, the medullary respiratory center is depressed. Hypoventilation, combined with increased CO_2 production, causes respiratory acidosis with increased plasma P_{CO_2} and decreased *p*H, but this cannot be adequately buffered because of the earlier compensatory excretion of cations (to correct the respiratory alkalosis). Acidosis is enhanced by the substantial concentrations of organic acids of salicylate and acetylsalicylate and the accumulation of lactic, pyruvic, and acetoacetic acids due to salicylate-induced disturbance of carbohydrate metabolism. Coma, cardiovascular collapse, impaired tissue oxygenation, and impaired renal function all add to the acidosis and contribute to a fatal outcome in severe salicylate poisoning.

Preparations and Dosage

Aspirin is the most commonly used salicylate. Buffered preparations may dissociate more readily in the stomach but do not contain sufficient buffer to neutralize the gastric contents. Enteric-coated aspirin tablets are often better tolerated, but in some persons may be incompletely absorbed. The usual dosage form is the 300-mg tablet. Combinations with propoxyphene, codeine, or phenacetin (acetophenetidin) are often used for treating headaches and pain syndromes. Salicylamide has little or no antipyretic, analgesic, or antiinflammatory effect but shares the potential for gastrointestinal irritation with other members of the salicylate family. Salicyl salicylate, choline magnesium salicylate, sodium salicylate, and magnesium salicylate may be used to administer nonacetylated salicylates.

For the relief of mild pain, aspirin and other forms of salicylate are effective in doses of 0.3 to 0.9 g every 3 to 4 hours. Fever usually can be relieved with similar doses. For intensive antiinflammatory therapy, plasma concentrations of 20 to 30 mg/dl should be maintained as discussed above.

PARA-AMINOPHENOL DERIVATIVES

PHENACETIN AND ACETAMINOPHEN

The parent compound for this group of drugs is acetanilid, but it is no longer used because of excessive toxicity. Phenacetin and acetamino-

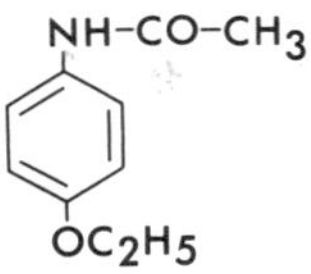

PHENACETIN

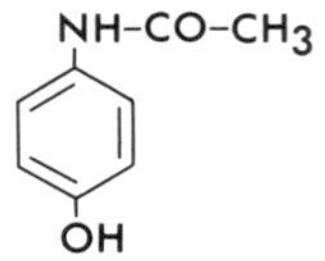

ACETAMINOPHEN

phen are useful for their antipyretic and analgesic effects but have no antirheumatic or antiinflammatory activity. Their major advantage is their lack of gastrointestinal side-effects. Phenacetin was widely used in combination with aspirin and caffeine as a mild analgesic, but its use has been largely abandoned owing to occasional occurrence of chronic interstitial nephritis and papillary necrosis in association with chronic use of high doses of the combination product. Acetaminophen, used as a substitute for salicylates in patients who have peptic ulcer disease or who for other reasons are unable to tolerate aspirin, is bound to plasma protein to a much smaller extent than are the salicylates. A minor metabolite may cause the formation of methemoglobin; this is seen more frequently with phenacetin than with acetaminophen and rarely causes clinical problems. Excessive doses of acetaminophen may be associated with severe hepatic toxicity.

PYRAZOLON DERIVATIVES

Antipyrine and aminopyrine are phenylpyrazolon derivatives first used during the 19th century. Although they are effective analgesic antipyretic antiinflammatory drugs, antipyrine and aminopyrine are no longer used clinically, because they occasionally cause fatal agranulocytosis. Antipyrine is frequently used in drug metabolism studies (*see* Chap. 4).

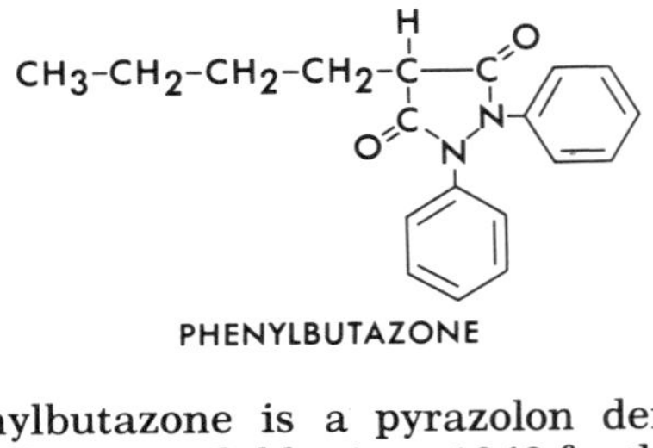

PHENYLBUTAZONE

Phenylbutazone is a pyrazolon derivative that has been available since 1949 for the treatment of inflammatory musculoskeletal conditions. Although it has analgesic and antipyretic effects, its major virtue is its potent antiinflammatory activity. Because of its occasional serious toxicity, phenylbutazone is generally used as a secondary drug in patients unresponsive to or unable to tolerate aspirin or other nonsteroidal antiinflammatory drugs. It is particularly effective in patients with ankylosing spondylitis, psoriatic arthritis. Reiter's syndrome and bursitis, tendonitis, and tenosynovitis. Phenylbutazone is also somewhat effective in the treatment of thrombophlebitis, pericarditis, and pleurisy and is especially effective in treating acute gout.

PHARMACOLOGY

The analgesic and antipyretic effects of phenylbutazone are less marked than those of salicylates, and it is not used for these purposes. It is nearly as potent as the corticosteroids in its antiinflammatory effects in experimental models of inflammation. The mechanism of its antiinflammatory action is probably similar to that of the salicylates: It is rapidly and completely absorbed from the gastrointestinal tract, with peak plasma levels being obtained in about 2 hours. Phenylbutazone is slowly metabolized in the liver to oxyphenbutazone and a metabolite with moderate uricosuric properties. Its biologic half-life in humans is about 72 hours owing to marked reabsorption of the un-ionized molecule in the distal renal tubules. Both phenylbutazone and its metabolites are highly bound to plasma proteins. With maximum therapeutic doses of 400 to 600 mg daily, the albumin binding sites for phenylbutazone become saturated. A further increase in dosage considerably increases the unbound drug fraction in plasma and increases the frequency of untoward side-effects. Displacement interactions may occur (*see* Chap. 8), and chronic administration of phenylbutazone induces hepatic microsomal enzymes (*see* Chap. 8), increasing its rate of metabolism. Sodium retention occurs frequently and occasionally causes clinically apparent edema, but this can be minimized by use of a low salt diet. This drug should be avoided in patients with borderline cardiac function.

ADVERSE EFFECTS

Gastrointestinal side-effects of nausea, epigastric discomfort, or vomiting are fairly frequent, and peptic ulcers may occur or may perforate or bleed during phenylbutazone therapy. Renal or hepatic dysfunction occurs rarely. Bone marrow failure (less than 1 in 50,000 patients treated) may develop abruptly and has resulted in a number of deaths from aplastic anemia or agranulocytosis. Because of its fairly common less serious side-effects and its rare association with lethal bone marrow failure, phenylbutazone is generally used only for relatively short courses of therapy, and blood counts should be followed closely.

PREPARATIONS AND DOSAGE

Phenylbutazone is available in 100-mg tablets. For treatment of acute gout or acute bursitis, the usual dose is 100 mg every 4 to 6 hours. For ankylosing spondylitis, 100 or 200 mg daily often suffices.

Oxyphenbutazone is also available in 100-mg tablets. It has the same properties as phenylbutazone, and its dosage is similar.

INDOLEACETIC ACIDS

INDOMETHACIN

A systematic study of indoleacetic acid compounds resulted in the development of indomethacin as an antiinflammatory drug, and it has been available for prescription since 1965.

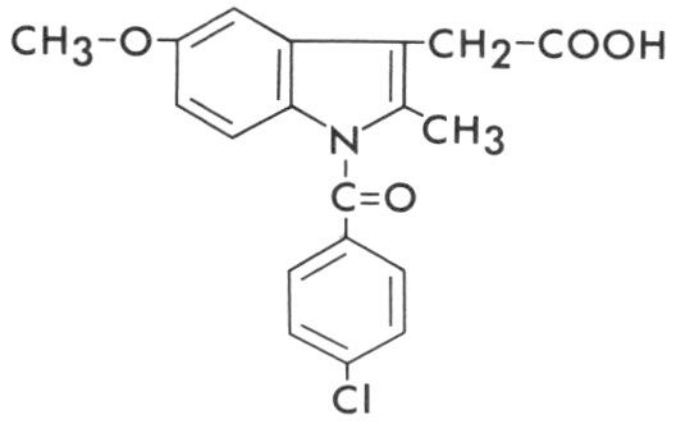

INDOMETHACIN

Its therapeutic spectrum is similar to that of phenylbutazone, to which it is preferred because it has not caused fatal bone marrow suppression.

Pharmacology

Indomethacin was originally synthesized as a potential antiserotonin drug. It is an effective antipyretic agent and may be useful in the treatment of fever due to lymphoma or other malignancies. It has little or no intrinsic analgesic activity and relieves pain only in inflammatory conditions. Indomethacin is an exceptionally potent antiinflammatory agent and, in animals, inhibits carrageenin-induced edema and exudate formation, adjuvant-induced polyarthritis, and urate-induced synovitis. Its exact site of action is not known, but, in common with other acidic antiinflammatory drugs, it uncouples oxidative phosphorylation in isolated liver mitochondria. Indomethacin is one of the most effective inhibitors of prostaglandin synthetase clinically available (*see* Chap. 53).

Absorption, Excretion, and Metabolism

In humans, indomethacin is rapidly absorbed. Peak blood levels are reached in 30 to 60 minutes in fasting subjects, but a prior meal slows absorption and flattens the peak. It is initially distributed or eliminated rapidly, and serum concentrations decrease by 50% within $1^1/_2$ to $2^1/_2$ hours. After this rapid initial decrease, serum half-life is about 8 to 10 hours, perhaps because of substantial enterohepatic recirculation. Indomethacin serum concentrations are higher on the second day of administration but thereafter do not continue to increase with continued administration of the same dose. This agent is 90% to 95% bound to plasma proteins. Indomethacin is primarily excreted by the kidney as several inactive conjugation products. Probenecid substantially decreases the rate of urinary excretion and results in higher serum indomethacin concentrations.

Adverse Effects

Side-effects occur in nearly half of the patients taking indomethacin, and about 20% are unable to continue its use. Indomethacin shares the problem of gastric toxicity with aspirin and phenylbutazone but causes less gastrointestinal blood loss than aspirin when evaluated by ^{51}Cr-labeled red blood cell studies. Unique among the antiinflammatory drugs in its CNS effects, indomethacin produces a feeling of "muzziness" in some patients, whereas severe drug-related headaches prevent other patients from continuing its use. Serious hypersensitivity to the drug, neutropenia, and hepatotoxicity are very rare.

Therapeutic Uses

Indomethacin is moderately effective in treating rheumatoid arthritis, but salicylates are usually preferable. It is as effective as phenylbutazone for treating ankylosing spondylitis, the rheumatoid variants, acute gout, and the bursitis and tendonitis syndromes. It is also useful for treating patients with osteoarthritis of the hip.

Preparations and Dosage

Indomethacin capsules contain 25 mg or 50 mg. For acute inflammation of gout or bursitis, up to 200 mg daily in divided doses may be used for a few days. For chronic inflammation of ankylosing spondylitis or rheumatoid arthritis, 25 mg every 6 to 24 hours is used. Side-effects are less frequent if the drug is given with meals and the dose is increased gradually. A sustained release preparation is available in 75-mg capsules given every 12 to 24 hours.

OTHER NONSTEROIDAL ANTIINFLAMMATORY DRUGS

Many new antiinflammatory drugs have been developed during the past decade. Some of those currently marketed in the United States and elsewhere are listed in Table 31-2. Others include meclofenamate, diflunisol, flufenamic acid, alclofenac, and flurbiprofen. These newer agents tend to cause gastric toxicity less frequently than do aspirin and indomethacin, and some patients may respond better to one drug than to others. The clinical activity of effective doses of these drugs is similar to that of aspirin and indomethacin, although they vary somewhat in the ratio of analgesic to antiinflammatory activity. Drugs with longer half-lives may be given one or three times daily, thus improving patient compliance with dosing recommendations.

COLCHICINE

Symptomatic antiinflammatory therapy of gout was practiced long before hyperuricemia and urate crystal deposits were first described by Garrod in 1848. Extracts of the autumn crocus were recommended for articular pain in the 6th century A.D., and the alkyloid colchicine was isolated in 1820 by Pelletier and Coventou.

ROBERT KOCH, 1843–1910. German bacteriologist. A pioneer in his field, Koch developed many standard microbiologic techniques. Was the first to obtain a pure culture of *Bacillus anthracis*. Discovered the causative agents of Asiatic cholera (1883) and the way in which bubonic plague and sleeping sickness were transmitted. Also worked on rinderpest, malaria, and tuberculosis. In 1890 discovered that gold compounds suppressed *Mycobacterium tuberculosis in vitro*. Received the Nobel Prize in 1905.

WILLIAM HYDE WOLLASTON, 1766–1828. English physician, chemist, and physicist. Discovered urates in tophi around 1797 but is probably best remembered for his investigation into electricity, the physics of light, crystallography, and minerology. He discovered palladium and rhodium and invented the camera lucida.

ALFRED BARING GARROD, 1819–1907. English physician. Worked especially on gout. Established that uric acid was a normal blood constituent and in 1848 published a method for detecting elevated levels in gouty patients. In 1890 was appointed physician-extraordinary to Queen Victoria.

HIPPOCRATES, c. 460—c. 377 B.C. Greek physician. Founder of the Cos school of medicine, his ideas are known through some 60 works, many probably by his followers. Usually described as the father of Western medicine, Hippocrates emphasized that disease was a natural phenomenon and medicine should be based on observation, not superstition. His works contain descriptions of many recognizable diseases, including gout.

GALEN, c. 129–c. 200. Hellenistic physician. Physician to Emperor Marcus Aurelius, Galen was a great diagnostician, prolific writer, and great systematizer. He added much personal observation and experiment to the Greek medical corpus and until the 16th century remained the master of Western medicine. Among his observations is a description of tophi.

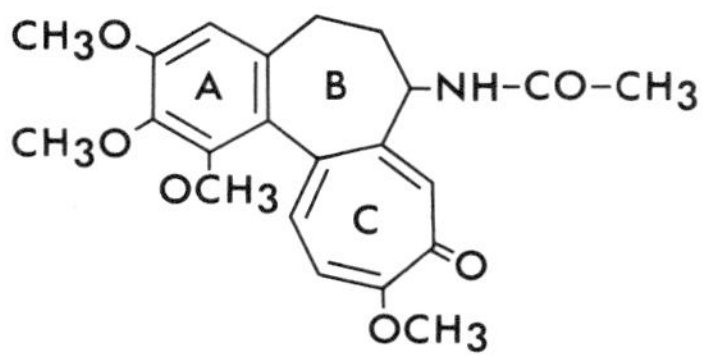
COLCHICINE

Colchicine is used primarily in gouty arthritis and occasionally in pseudogout (calcium pyrophosphate crystal-induced arthritis) and familial Mediterranean fever prophylaxis, but it is of little use in other conditions. The drug has several possible antiinflammatory effects on polymorphonuclear leukocytes: disaggregation of subunit proteins of microtubules; suppression of glucose oxidation; reduced phagocytosis, chemotaxis, kinin generation, and metabolic activity. *In vivo* the net effect is decreased local lactic-acid production and lysosomal enzyme liberation, thereby interrupting part of the inflammatory process of gout.

Colchicine is not an analgesic and has no effect on metabolism, excretion, or solubility of urate, but it abolishes the pain of acute gout entirely by its antiinflammatory action. This agent may be given intravenously in a dose of 1 mg or 2 mg in 15 ml of 5% glucose in water, with a maximum of 5 mg in any 24-hour period, or it may be given orally in a dose of 0.6 mg/hr until symptomatic relief is obtained or gastrointestinal toxicity occurs (maximum dose, 6 to 10 mg in 24 hours).

Dramatic improvement in the exquisite pain, swelling, and inflammation of acute gout usually occurs within 6 to 12 hours after the initiation of intensive therapy; complete recovery of joint function occurs within 24 to 48 hours. Colchicine, 0.6 mg every 8 to 24 hours, is frequently given prophylactically, even though the underlying hyperuricemia is not altered by this drug.

The primary symptoms of colchicine overdosage are abdominal pain, nausea, vomiting, and diarrhea that may become bloody owing to a hemorrhagic gastroenteritis. With severe toxicity, paralysis develops and death is usually due to respiratory arrest. Significant amounts of colchicine are excreted in the bile and reabsorbed in the intestine, perhaps partly explaining the prominence of intestinal symptoms with overdosage.

Preparations and Dosage

Colchicine is available as 0.5 or 0.6 mg oral tablets or a sterile solution (0.5 mg/ml). Dosage is described above.

DISEASE-MODIFYING ANTIRHEUMATIC DRUGS

Disease-modifying antirheumatic drugs are a diverse group of compounds that share a common pattern of clinical response when used to treat rheumatoid arthritis. Thus their administration does not result in any immediately recognizable clinical benefit, but after weeks or months of continuous administration subtle clinical benefit may appear, and with continued administration complete suppression of some or all disease manifestations may occur. Suppression of laboratory evidence of disease sometimes also occurs, but if the drug is withdrawn, disease manifestations gradually recur. All of the available disease-modifying agents were developed for other purposes. Because their use is frequently associated with serious, and sometimes fatal, toxicity, they are reserved for patients with severe, progressive, or life-threatening disease. Gold compounds and D-penicillamine are discussed below. Other disease-modifying antirheumatic agents include hydroxychloroquine and chloroquine (*see* Chap. 67), azathioprine, cyclophosphamide, chlorambucil, methotrexate, and levamisole (*see* Chap. 71).

GOLD COMPOUNDS

Sulfhydryl-containing organic gold compounds were first used to treat arthritis in the 1920s, but their value in rheumatoid arthritis was not established until a large double-blind trial by the Empire Rheumatism Council in 1960. Gold therapy is indicated in patients with adult and juvenile rheumatoid arthritis or psoriatic arthritis, whose disease is progressive and has been poorly controlled by nonsteroidal anti-inflammatory drugs and conservative management.

Pharmacology

Aurothiomalate (Myochrysine) and aurothioglucose (Solganol) are the most commonly used preparations (Fig. 31-2). Both are water soluble, 50% gold by weight, and are given intramuscularly in a dose of 50 mg weekly. The oil-based suspension of aurothioglucose is less rapidly absorbed than is the aqueous solution of aurothiomalate. An orally absorbed gold preparation, auranofin, is undergoing clinical trials but is not yet available for general use; it is lipid soluble, 30% gold by weight, and appears to be effective in a dose of 6 mg daily.

The mechanism of action of gold compounds in rheumatoid arthritis is not known. Gold com-

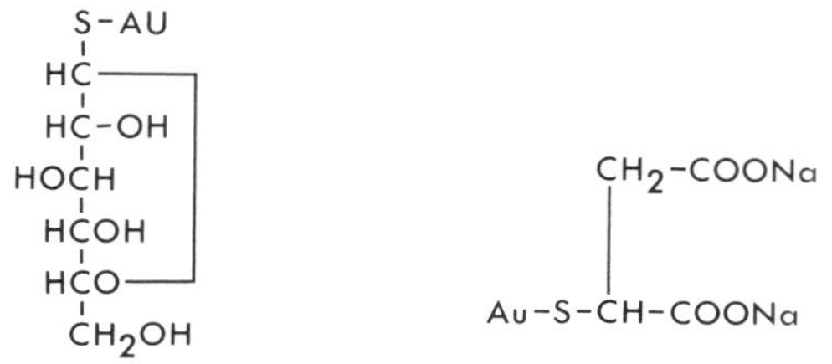

FIG. 31-2. Gold salts. (Left) Aurothioglucose. (Right) Aurothiomalate.

pounds inhibit lysosomal enzymes either directly or by membrane stabilization, and human lymphocyte responses to mitogens and antigens are inhibited in culture conditions. Additionally, monocyte participation in cell-mediated *in vitro* responses is impaired by gold. In patients receiving gold therapy, however, there is no evidence of generalized suppression of cellular or humoral immune responses or of inflammatory responses. Nevertheless gold reduces the progression of joint erosions and often produces major improvement and occasionally remission in patients with rheumatoid arthritis.

Distribution and Excretion

Studies with radiolabeled gold compounds demonstrate prolonged total body retention of gold with both the i.m. and p.o. preparations; 30% of the injected isotope is retained 4 months after a dose of aurothiomalate. Gold concentrations are easily measured in plasma, where it is predominantly bound to albumin, but there is no generally accepted relation between plasma gold concentrations and clinical benefit or toxicity. Gold is excreted both in the urine and in the stool, predominantly in urine for the injectable preparations and predominantly in stool for auranofin.

Adverse Effects

Toxicity that requires discontinuation of gold therapy occurs in 30% to 50% of patients. In responsive patients without toxicity, gold is continued indefinitely, although the frequency of injections gradually may be decreased to every second, third, or fourth week. Important side-effects include pruritic rashes (15–25%), proteinuria due to an immune complex-mediated membranous glomerulonephritis (10–20%), stomatitis (5–10%), and hematologic abnormalities (1–2%). Although rare, thrombocytopenia, aplastic anemia, or pancytopenia due to gold may be fatal. To monitor for early signs of toxicity, complete blood cell counts and urine protein determinations are done before each gold injection.

Preparations and Dosage

Aurothiomalate and aurothioglucose are available in single- and multiple-dose vials containing 50 mg/ml for i.m. administration. Initial dosage is 5 or 10 mg, increased at weekly intervals to 25 mg and then to 50 mg. Weekly administration of 50 mg is continued until major clinical benefit is seen, when the frequency of administration may be gradually decreased to maintenance injections every 3 or 4 weeks.

D-PENICILLAMINE

Penicillamine, a metabolite of penicillin, is a structural analogue of crysteine. D- and L-isomers are formed, but only the D-isomer is used clinically. Because D-penicillamine chelates heavy metals, its first use was to reduce tissue levels of copper in Wilson's disease. It is also used to treat lead and mercury poisoning and cysteinuria. This drug was first used to treat rheumatoid arthritis in the early 1960s, but widespread acceptance and use did not occur until after its efficacy was documented by a large, double-blind, placebo-controlled trial in 1973.

Pharmacology

D-Penicillamine is orally absorbed with peak blood levels developing in about 1 hour. It is

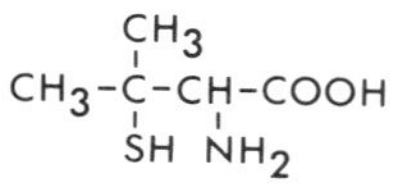

PENICILLAMINE

metabolized to a disulfide and excreted in both urine and feces; 60% is excreted within 24 hours, and very little can be detected in blood 48 hours after a dose. Its mechanism of action in rheumatoid arthritis is unknown. In addition to its ability to chelate heavy metals, D-penicillamine may, under certain conditions, inhibit collagen fibril cross-linking, dissociate macroglobulins, and block replicating viral RNA.

Despite major structural, metabolic, and pharmacologic differences, the time-course of efficacy and the spectrum of toxicity of D-penicillamine are very similar to that of the gold compounds. The starting dose of 250 mg daily is increased by 250 mg/day at 2- to 3-month intervals until clinical improvement is detected or a total daily dosage of 750 to 1000 mg is reached. The onset of clinical response is delayed and gradual, but complete remissions may occur in some patients. The dose may be reduced slightly for maintenance therapy, but the drug is continued indefinitely unless there is toxicity or a loss of efficacy. In controlled comparisons, D-penicillamine and gold are equally effective. Relapse occurs within 6 months after its withdrawal.

Adverse Effects

Toxicity that requires cessation of therapy occurs in 30% to 60% of patients and is more frequent with higher doses. Dermatitis (12–25% of patients); anorexia, nausea, vomiting, diarrhea (12–20%); dose-dependent thrombocytopenia (5–10%); neutropenia or aplastic anemia (rare); and proteinuria due to reversible immune complex-mediated glomerulonephritis (10–20%) are seen. Autoimmune syndromes develop rarely during D-penicillamine therapy of both Wilson's disease and rheumatoid arthritis but improve after the drug is withdrawn; examples include myasthenia gravis, polymyositis, Goodpasture's syndrome, and systemic lupus erythematosus. To minimize morbidity, patients should be seen every 1 to 2 weeks while taking D-penicillamine. A complete blood cell count, urinanalysis, and quantitative platelet count should be done at each visit to monitor for early signs of toxicity.

Preparations

D-Penicillamine is available as 125-mg and 250-mg tablets and capsules. Dosage is described above.

URATE LOWERING DRUGS

The hyperuricemia responsible for gout may be pharmacologically controlled by increasing uric acid excretion or by decreasing uric acid production.

URICOSURIC DRUGS

Urate is filtered by the renal glomeruli, reabsorbed in the proximal tubule, and then secreted by the distal tubule. Substances that decrease distal tubular urate secretion produce hyperuricemia; examples are organic anions such as lactate or salicylate in low doses and most diuretics. Substances that decrease proximal tubular reabsorption increase renal uric acid clearance and lower serum uric acid levels. Salicylates in high doses, phenylbutazone, sulfinpyrazone, and probenecid are among the drugs that have been found to inhibit the renal tubular transport of urate. Small doses of these agents decrease urate clearance, presumably by inhibiting its secretion, but larger doses also block reabsorption and thus have a net uricosuric effect. Probenecid and sulfinpyrazone are the two most frequently used uricosuric agents (Fig. 31-3).

Probenecid is available as 0.5-g oral tablets. Dosage is regulated by following the serum uric acid concentration and may vary from 0.5 to 2.5 g daily in divided doses. The drug is readily absorbed, and peak plasma levels are achieved in 2 to 4 hours, whereas the half-life varies from 6 to 12 hours. It is generally well tolerated, but it must be given for many years because it has no effect on the underlying cause of the patient's hyperuricemia. Gastrointestinal discomfort and hypersensitivity are the most common side effects, but are rarely serious. Uricosuric drugs should be avoided in patients who have renal calculi since the increased clearance of urate tends to exacerbate stone formation. Probenecid also effectively blocks renal tubular secretion of penicillin (*see* Chap. 59). Similarly, by interfering with tubular excretion, probenecid also increases serum levels of penicillin derivatives cephalosporins (except cephalordine), paraaminosalicylic acid, dapsone, salicylate, pantothenic acid, acetazolamide, furosemide, thiazides, indomethacin, naproxen, and sulfinpyrazone. It also inhibits biliary excretion of indomethacin, methotrexate, and rifampin, further enhancing their blood levels. The ability of probenecid to interfere with renal and biliary transport of organic acids appears to extend to the central nervous system, where it blocks the transport of various substances including norepinephrine, homovanillic acid, and dopamine. Probenecid also inhibits the hepatic metabolism of azathioprine to 6-mercaptopurine by glutathione-5-transferase and the glucuronidation of naproxen by the liver, thus increasing plasma concentrations of these drugs.

Sulfinpyrazone is a modification of the urico-

FIG. 31-3. Uricosuric drugs: probenecid and sulfinpyrazone.

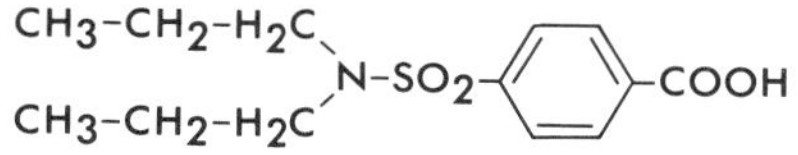

PROBENECID

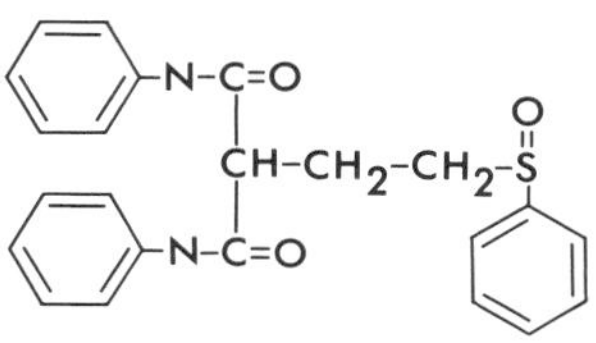

SULFINPYRAZONE

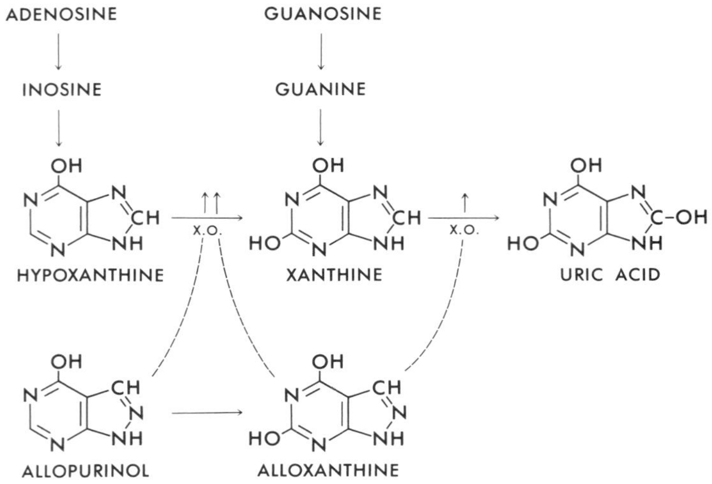

FIG. 31-4. Purine metabolism by xanthine oxidase and its inhibition by allopurinol.

suric metabolite of phenylbutazone. Its action is similar to that of probenecid, and it has no antiinflammatory or analgesic properties. The drug is available in 100-mg tablets; one tablet is usually given every 6 to 24 hours depending on the serum uric acid concentration. Gastrointestinal irritation is somewhat less frequent, and bone marrow suppression has not been reported with sulfinpyrazone despite its ancestry.

INHIBITORS OF URATE SYNTHESIS

The immediate metabolic precursor of uric acid is xanthine, formed from hypoxanthine by the enzyme xanthine oxidase and oxidized to uric acid by the same enzyme (Fig. 31-4). Allopurinol is a structural isomer of hypoxanthine. It competitively inhibits these metabolic reactions and thus reduces the production of uric acid. Inhibition of xanthine oxidase increases the concentrations of xanthine and hypoxanthine in the urine, but these two oxypurines are somewhat more soluble than uric acid, and there have been only a few reports of xanthine crystal deposits in patients treated with allopurinol (100–500 mg daily in divided doses). Allopurinol is particularly useful in patients with impaired renal urate clearance owing to renal failure or chronic diuretic ingestion and is indicated in patients with renal calculi. The drug is generally well tolerated and only rarely causes hypersensitivity skin rashes or mild gastrointestinal toxicity.

Neither the uricosuric agents nor allopurinol has any antiinflammatory or analgesic effects, and neither is useful for treating the inflammation of gouty arthritis. Thus in gout the therapy for inflammation is separated completely from the therapy for the underlying cause of the inflammation. Effective treatment of gout necessitates the use of an antiinflammatory agent and a uric acid lowering agent. Unless both are used, the patient with gout cannot be treated optimally.

FURTHER READING

1. Bunch TM, O'Duffy JD: Clinical pharmacology. Series on pharmacology in clinical practice, 6. Disease-modifying drugs for progressive rheumatoid arthritis. Mayo Clin Proc 55:161–179, 1980
2. Klinenberg JR: Current concepts of hyperuricemia and gout. Calif Med 110:231–243, 1969
3. Paulus HE, Furst DE: Aspirin and nonsteroidal antiinflammatory drugs. In McCarty DJ (ed): Arthritis and Allied Conditions, 9th ed, pp 331–354. Philadelphia, Lea & Febiger, 1979

CHAPTER 31 QUESTIONS

(*See* P. 7 for Full Instructions)

Select the One Best Answer

1. Each of the following is a valid therapeutic indication for the use of salicylates EXCEPT
   A. fever.
   B. headache.
   C. rheumatoid arthritis.
   D. pain of peptic ulcer.
   E. athlete's foot.

2. Salicylate intoxication is characterized by all of the following EXCEPT
   A. fever.
   B. mental confusion.

C. hyperventilation.
D. increased metabolic rate.
E. swollen joints.

3. The most effective agent for the treatment of an acute attack of gout is
   A. aspirin.
   B. probenecid.
   C. acetaminophen.
   D. colchicine.
   E. phenytoin.

4. Allopurinol will produce each of the following EXCEPT
   A. a reduction of tophi in chronic gout.
   B. increased excretion of xanthine.
   C. enhanced uric acid excretion.
   D. decreased plasma concentration of uric acid.
   E. enhancement of 6-mercaptopurine effect.

A = 1,2,3; B = 1,3; C = 2,4; D = 4; E = All

5. Aspirin
   1. may be effective as an antipyretic agent by inhibition of prostaglandin synthetase in the CNS.
   2. may be effective as an analgetic agent by both a central and a peripheral action.
   3. in therapeutic doses may cause gastrointestinal bleeding.
   4. in toxic doses produces respiratory stimulation followed by respiratory depression.

6. Both aspirin and acetaminophen
   1. produce gastric irritation and bleeding.
   2. relieve mild to moderate integumental pain.
   3. suppress joint inflammation that accompanies rheumatic fever.
   4. promote heat loss by a central mechanism.

7. Urinary excretion of uric acid is usually increased
   1. during sodium salicylate therapy for rheumatoid arthritis.
   2. during aspirin therapy for the fever of a "cold."
   3. during probenecid therapy for tophaceous gout.
   4. during hydrochlorothiazide therapy for hypertension.

8. Both phenylbutazone and probenecid
   1. may produce urate stones when administered to a gouty patient.
   2. are effective for treatment of an acute attack of gout.
   3. can reduce tophi.
   4. prolong the half-life of penicillin.

9. Both penicillamine and gold compounds can cause
   1. bone marrow suppression.
   2. gastric irritation.
   3. proteinuria.
   4. rash.

10. Both penicillamine and gold compounds
   1. act by inhibiting prostaglandin synthesis.
   2. cause increased uric acid excretion.
   3. are antipyretic.
   4. have a delayed onset of benefit in rheumatoid arthritis.

32

DON H. CATLIN

Opioids: Agonists, Antagonists, and Mixed Antagonist–Agonists

Great pain is a powerful and dominating sensory experience that seriously interrupts the integrity of the body and mind and compels one to seek relief. The experience preempts all other events and signifies that something is internally wrong. Sometimes the cause is obvious and other times obscure. In either case, the physician must intervene. The drugs described herein are analgesics that relieve great pain. They have other important effects, too, but their principal use is to relieve the suffering, anguish, and anxiety that accompanies great pain. Minor aches and pains are treated with the nonopioid analgesics (*see* Chap. 31).

The opioids are divided into the agonists, the antagonists, and the mixed antagonist–agonists. Morphine, the prototype narcotic agonist, produces analgesia, respiratory depression, inhibition of gastrointestinal motility, and effects on the central nervous, gastrointestinal, hormonal, and cardiovascular systems. Narcotic agonists can also produce tolerance, physical dependence, and psychological dependence (*see* Chap. 26).

Antagonists are essentially devoid of pharmacologic effects in normal persons. If administered just before a dose of an agonist, however, antagonists completely block its effects, and if administered just after an agonist they reverse its effects. If antagonists are administered to someone physically dependent on opioids, they produce, within minutes, a highly specific withdrawal syndrome.

The antagonist–agonists share properties of both the agonists and antagonists (Table 32-1). The predominating effects are determined by the previous opioid exposure of the person. In naive subjects, antagonist–agonists act like agonists; hence they can be used to relieve great pain. In the patient who is dependent on an agonist, they often, but not always, produce a withdrawal syndrome.

SOURCE

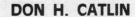

The word *opium* is derived from the Greek word for "juice" and refers to the dried juice of the poppy plant (*Papaver somniferum*). Opium contains a great many chemically distinct alkaloids. *Morphine,* named after the Greek god of dreams Morpheus, and *codeine* are the most important. Morphine is obtained commercially from opium because it is laborious and expen-

TABLE 32-1. Comparative Features of Opioid Agonists and Antagonist–Agonists

Nonproprietary Name	Trade Name	Dose*	Duration of Action	Most Common Route of Administration†	Schedule‡
		mg	*hr*		
Morphine		10	4	P	II
Heroin		5	3	P	I
Codeine		120	4	O	II
Hydromorphone	Dilaudid	1.5	4	O	II
Oxymorphone	Numorphan	1.5	4	P	II
Levorphanol	Levo-dromoran	2	4	P	II
	Meperidine and chemically related agents (phenylpiperidines)				
Meperidine	Demerol	100	3	P	II
Alphaprodine	Nisentil	30	1.5	P	II
Anileridine	Leritine	30	3	P	II
Fentanyl	Sublimaze	0.2	0.4	P	II
	Methadone and Propoxyphene				
Methadone	Dolophine	7.5	5	O	II
Propoxyphene	Darvon	§	4	O	IV
	Opioid antagonist–agonists				
Pentazocine	Talwin	40	3	O	IV
Butorphanol	Stadol	2	4	P	NC
Nalbuphine	Nubain	10	4	P	NC
Buprenorphine	Temgesic	0.4	5	P	NC

* Doses and durations are approximations (±25%) and refer to the subcutaneous route of administration. The doses listed produce about the same degree of analgesia at the peak of action as does the standard, 10-mg morphine sulfate.

† NC = not classified; O = oral; P = parenteral.

‡ Controlled Substances Act: *See* Chapter 12.

§ Not available in parenteral dosage form.

sive to synthesize *de novo*. Heroin (diacetylmorphine) does not occur naturally but is readily synthesized from morphine. A great many other semisynthetic opioids are prepared from morphine and other opium alkaloids. Synthetic opioids, like meperidine and methadone, are synthesized from simple precursors.

TERMINOLOGY

For many years, the term *opiate* was used to designate morphine, codeine, and other morphinelike substances derived from opium alkaloids. More recently with the development of totally synthetic morphinelike drugs, the word opiate was replaced by *opioid*. Herein, the term opioid will be used generically to designate an exogenous substance that is chemically similar to morphine, specifically binds to receptors, and produces a spectrum of activity similar to, but not necessarily identical to, that of morphine. Although the term narcotic is commonly used to denote a strong analgesic, the term is inaccurate and should be abandoned. A *narcotic* is defined as a drug that produces profound sleep and relieves pain, yet conventional doses of opioids do not produce profound sleep. Also the term narcotic is increasingly used by the legal profession to denote any substance that produces drug dependence.

CHEMISTRY AND STRUCTURE–ACTIVITY RELATIONSHIPS

The opioids (Fig. 32-1) are structurally similar. Morpine is a pentacyclic compound that contains an N-methylpiperidine ring (ring e, Fig. 32-1) and a benzene ring (ring a, Fig. 32-1) with a phenolic hydroxyl group at C3. The pKa of the nitrogen in morphine is 9.8. Thus morphine (and most other opioids) are more than 90% protonated and carry a positive charge at physiologic *p*H. Most opioids are highly lipid soluble and widely distributed. There are five asymmetric carbon atoms in morphine. Natu-

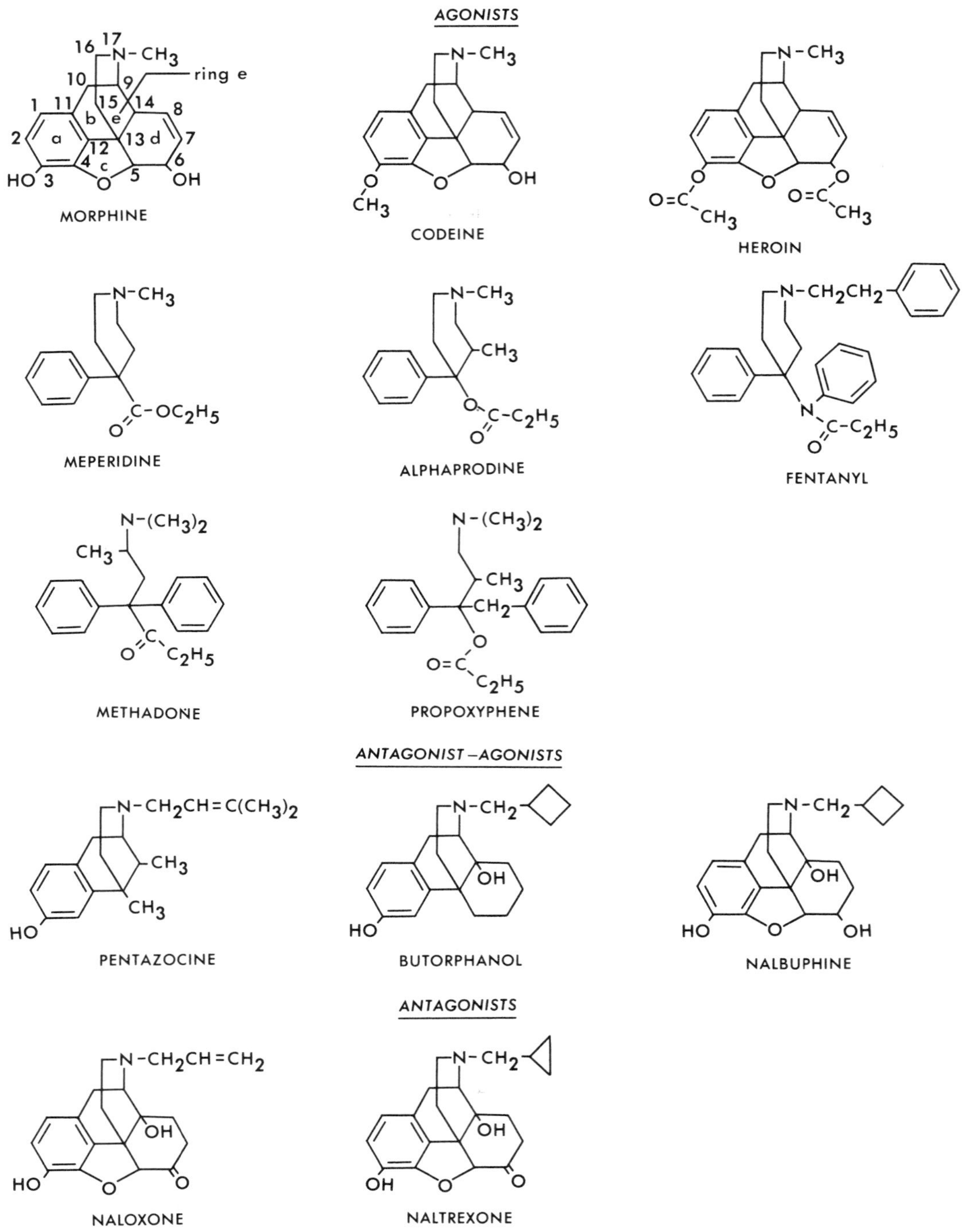

FIG. 32-1. Structures of selected opioids.

ral morphine is levorotary; the dextrorotary enantiomer is not pharmacologically active. The pharmacologic activity of most opioids is due to the levorotary anantiomer.

The structural requirements for an opioid have been studied by modifying various portions of the molecule and side-chain. Small changes in the structure may result in profound alterations in pharmacologic activity. Modification at the 3 and 6 position of morphine results in codeine, heroin, and many other opioids. The phenylpiperidine series, which includes meperidine, demonstrates that rings b, c, and d are not required for opioid activity. Methadone may appear to be an exception because it lacks a piperidine ring; however, three-dimensional models reveal that stearic factors hold the nitrogen and oxygen adjacent to each other, thus closely approximating a six-membered piperidine ring. The most interesting structural modification is the substitution of an alkyl group for the N-methyl group; this change converts morphine, an agonist, to naloxone, an antagonist.

ACTIONS OF AGONISTS: MORPHINE

The actions of all opioid agonists and the agonistic actions of the antagonist–agonists are similar. The actions of morphine, the prototypic agent for this group, are described in detail. Distinguishing characteristics of other agents are discussed under Clinical Pharmacology below.

CENTRAL NERVOUS SYSTEM

The most important effects of morphine are mediated in the central nervous system. Morphine is the most efficacious analgesic known: It relieves great pain regardless of the source and is the standard by which all other powerful analgesics are compared.

The analgesia is closely related to sedation and euphoria. If left unstimulated, patients appear to be calm and sleepy but may be readily aroused. Euphoria usually does not accompany the first few doses of morphine but after several doses or days of continuous use is often present. The first few doses of morphine often produce nausea and sometimes vomiting. These effects tend to be positional. Vomiting is less common in the supine position, whereas movement and walking are likely to elicit both nausea and vomiting. Normal volunteers who do not have pain but are given morphine to study its effects usually dislike morphine because it inhibits their ability to think clearly and to concentrate.

A most intriguing aspect of morphine is the qualitative character of the analgesia it produces. Patients will often say "the pain is still present, but it doesn't hurt anymore." They mean that the awareness of the pain is still present, it has not been obliterated, but there is no physical discomfort or disagreeable sensation. One interpretation of these reports is that morphine affects the perception of pain, not the original sensation of the pain at its source. Evidently, it is the *perceived consequences* or *meaning of pain* to the individual—not simply the physical discomfort—that is the important element in morphine-induced analgesia. This contrasts markedly with the nonopioid analgesics that act peripherally (*see* Chap. 31).

RESPIRATORY SYSTEM

At doses that produce analgesia, morphine depresses the rate and depth of respirations by acting on the respiratory center. A decreased respiratory rate is more readily detected than a decreased tidal volume. Both result in an increased Pco_2 and a decreased Po_2. Respiratory depression is the principal limiting adverse effect.

CARDIOVASCULAR SYSTEM

The cardiovascular effects of morphine are influenced by the patient's clinical condition. In those with pain and a normal cardiovascular system, morphine produces a small decrease in systolic blood pressure and heart rate, but cardiac index and myocardial contractility are not altered. Morphine does not have a pronounced effect on the myocardium. The net effect on the peripheral vascular system is vasodilation resulting from venous and arterial dilation. Peripheral vascular resistance is lowered and cutaneous blood flow increased. These peripheral effects are probably due to a decreased sympathetic tone that results from a diminished central sympathetic outflow.

The cardiovascular effects of morphine are more variable and complex in patients with acute myocardial infarction and pain. Hemodynamic studies in these patients usually show no change in cardiac index and pulmonary wedge pressure, but pulmonary vascular resistance and mean pulmonary artery pressure are often increased. About one third of patients with acute myocardial infarcts who receive morphine experience a modest decrease in blood pressure. A marked but transient decrease in blood pressure occurs in a few patients; there is no simple way to predict which patients will have this response.

GASTROINTESTINAL SYSTEM

The first recorded use of opium was for the treatment of dysentery, but other agents have largely supplanted its use for treating diarrhea. The opioids increase the tone of gastrointestinal smooth muscle and cause intermittent spasm of the musculature. They increase tone in the pylorus, anal sphincter, and ileocecal valve. The results of all these actions are delayed gastric emptying and passage-time, increased fluid absorption, and constipation. These effects are mediated partly by a local direct action on the myenteric plexus and by the CNS.

Morphine also constricts the sphincter of Oddi, increasing pressure in the bile ducts. The effect of opioids on sphincters is partially reversed by atropine and more completely by naloxone. The effect on the bile ducts is a relative contraindication to the use of opioids in patients with biliary tract obstructions.

OTHER SYSTEMS

Opioids suppress the cough reflex. Morphine constricts the pupil probably at the Edinger–Westphal nucleus. Pupillary constriction is one of the most easily recognized and reliable signs of an opioid effect. Morphine increases the tone of the bladder detrussor muscle and also the urethral sphincter. The former may result in an urge to urinate; however, the usual effect on the urinary tract is a tendency to retain urine. Morphine has a variety of endocrine effects, the most constant being to increase plasma concentrations of growth hormone, prolactin, and vasopression. Morphine also releases histamine (*see* Chap. 51).

ADVERSE EFFECTS

Adverse effects of the agonists and mixed antagonist–agonists are largely extensions of their basic actions. Nausea, vomiting, respiratory depression, and increased pressure in the biliary tract are always considered to be adverse effects. Sedation and euphoria, however, may be adverse or desirable, depending on the clinical circumstances. Similarly, the constipating action of opioids is unwanted except when being used to treat diarrhea. Allergic phenomena have been attributed to the opioids but are not common. Anaphylactoid reactions have been reported rarely. Various disease-states increase the sensitivity of a person to the effects of opioids. Some are predictable, such as the increased sensitivity of patients with emphysema and chronic obstructive pulmonary disease to opioid-induced respiratory depression. Patients with hepatic disease are more sensitive because of reduced drug clearance. Patients with an altered level of consciousness, resulting either from other drugs or CNS injury, are more sensitive to the CNS depressant effects of opioids. Opioids aggravate gastrointestinal symptoms in some types of inflammatory bowel disease.

TOLERANCE, PHYSICAL DEPENDENCE, AND PSYCHOLOGICAL DEPENDENCE

A characteristic of all opioid agonists and antagonist–agonists is the development of *tolerance* and *physical and psychological dependence* (*see* Chap. 9). Tolerance develops to most of the effects of opioids: One consequence is a reduced area under the time-action curve. The effect can usually be restored by increasing the dose. Tolerance to the euphoric effects of agents such as heroin explains why drug abusers require successively higher doses to obtain the desired effects. Opioid tolerance is primarily due to adaptive changes at the cellular level with a possible contribution from altered pharmacokinetics.

Physical and psychological dependence describes states where a drug is needed for normal physiologic and psychological function. The dependent state is revealed by withdrawing the drug (or giving an antagonist to an addict under the influence of an opioid) and observing the characteristics signs and symptoms of withdrawal, including back, flank, and leg pain, chills, nausea, vomiting, dilatation of the pupils, and increased respiratory rate and blood pressure. Drug-seeking behavior is a prominent part of the syndrome in persons prone to drug abuse. In an addict, the morphine abstinence syndrome typically begins 6 to 12 hours after the last dose. The intensity peaks at about 36 hours and is largely over by 72 hours. Other opioid agonists and antagonist–agonists have a different spectrum of symptoms and time-course. A remarkable feature of the dependent state is that the entire abstinence syndrome may be precipitated within minutes of administering an antagonist. Precipitated withdrawal is similar to natural withdrawal except the time-course is compressed into 1 to 2 hours.

There is a high degree of cross-tolerance and cross-physical dependence among the opioids. This is one basis for treating heroin addiction with methadone. Because cross-tolerance is rarely complete, there is some rationale for trying a different agent when a person develops a high degree of tolerance to the analgesic effect of another agent. Essentially no cross-tolerance or dependence exists between the opioids and the barbiturates, alcohol, amphetamines, or cocaine.

The processes underlying tolerance and physical dependence begin with the first dose of an opioid; however, the rate at which they develop is highly variable. Dose and frequency of administration are important variables, but other individual factors are also important. Some persons, for example, may experience a mild withdrawal syndrome after only 2 to 3 days of morphine, whereas others will have little withdrawal after 2 weeks of therapy. A remarkably high degree of tolerance may occur. Thus tolerant persons experience few effects after a dose that is more than 10 times greater than a conventional dose in a nontolerant person.

OPIOID ANTAGONISTS

Naloxone, the prototype, is the only currently available antagonist with virtually no agonistic actions. Its effects depend entirely on the recent exposure of the person to opioid agonists or antagonist–agonists. In the normal person naloxone has very few, if any, unequivocal effects. Even a very high dose (25 mg parenterally) produces only drowsiness. In contrast, if a person is experiencing the acute effects of a recently administered opioid, a small dose (0.4 mg) of naloxone reverses these effects. Rarely the reversal will be accompanied by a transient increase in blood pressure to higher than normal levels. If naloxone is administered before an agonist, it will block the effects of the agonist. This is a useful investigational technique and a potential approach to the treatment of heroin addiction.

EFFECTS IN PHYSICALLY DEPENDENT PATIENTS

If a patient has received a sufficient number of closely spaced doses of an opioid agonist to be physically dependent, a small dose of naloxone will precipitate a moderate or severe withdrawal syndrome. The syndrome begins within 2 to 3 minutes, peaks at 15 to 30 minutes, and is over in 1 to 2 hours. The intensity and duration of the precipitated abstinence syndrome depend on the dose of naloxone and the degree of physical dependence.

ANTAGONIST–AGONISTS

One of the most elusive goals of opioid research for many years has been to develop a compound that possesses the strong analgesic properties of morphine yet is devoid of the dependence-producing and addiction liability properties. This goal has not yet been achieved, but the antagonist–agonists represent considerable progress in this direction. This group of drugs, sometimes referred to as mixed antagonist–agonists, combine the properties of both agonists and antagonists. Their effects depend on the patient's history. In patients who have not recently received opioids, they have the typical effects of other agonists; however, if the patient has received a sufficient dose of an agonist to be physically dependent, the mixed compounds usually precipitate a mild withdrawal syndrome.

The first compound in this series, nalorphine, is of historical interest only because it causes psychotomimetic effects at analgesic doses. The first clinically useful drug in this class was *pentazocine*, an agonist with mild antagonist properties. In 1980, two more compounds, *nalbuphine* and *butorphanol*, were approved for the relief of moderate to severe pain. The agonistic properties of pentazocine are similar to morphine. Its principal effects are analgesia, respiratory depression, sedation, and delayed gastric emptying. Pentazocine produces less euphoria and pupillary constriction than does morphine. Evidence suggests that the dose-response curve of respiratory depression flattens (a ceiling) at high doses. Naloxone reverses the respiratory depression, but relatively high doses may be needed. In contrast to morphine, pentazocine usually increases blood pressure and heart rate. These effects, plus increased pulmonary artery pressure and cardiac work, are observed in patients with recent myocardial infarctions, thus pentazocine is relatively contraindicated in this circumstance. Pentazocine is a weak antagonist and will precipitate a mild withdrawal syndrome in patients dependent on morphine or other agonists. Patients switched from morphine to pentazocine should be done so cautiously.

Pentazocine may be administered orally or parenterally. The s.c. route is not recommended because pentazocine is irritating to tissues. Equianalgesic i.m. doses of morphine and pentazocine are 10 and 40 to 50 mg, respectively. The oral:i.m. potency ratio is estimated to be 2:1 to 3:1.

The adverse effects of pentazocine are similar to those of morphine with one important exception: Pentazocine produces psychotomimetic symptoms. These are variously described as racing, hyperactive, and bizarre thoughts; vivid dreams; feelings of doom, depersonalization, and anxiety; and overt visual hallucinations. These symptoms may occur at recommended doses and are quite common at higher doses; thus the therapeutic index of pentazocine is low. The abuse potential of pentazocine is less than that of morphine. Some cases of physical dependence have been reported in patients receiving parenteral pentazocine. The physical signs of pentazocine withdrawal are quite mild even after heavy parenteral abuse. However, drug-seeking behavior is common after withdrawing from parenteral or oral pentazocine. Psychological dependence may be a serious problem with some patients.

The early experience with butorphanol and nalbuphine indicates that they are quite similar to pentazocine. Currently they are available only for parenteral administration.

MECHANISM OF ACTION

OPIOID RECEPTORS

The competitive reversal of opioid agonistic effects by naloxone and the remarkable degree of structural and conformational similarity between the agonists and antagonists stimulated a search for receptors. Abundant evidence now suggests that the initial event in the steps that result ultimately in an observable opioid effect is an interaction of drug with opioid receptors. These receptors have not been isolated in a chemically pure form, but their composition includes proteins and lipids. Both opioid agonists and antagonists presumably bind to the same receptor; the antagonists compete with the agonist for the site but do not initiate changes that result in a pharmacologic response.

Cell membrane opioid receptors specifically bind all types of opioids. The active isomers bind to receptors, the inactive isomers and nonopioids do not show specific, high-affinity binding. Distribution studies show that opioid receptors are located in many areas of the nervous system and in several peripheral tissues. High densities are found in areas of the brain known to mediate physiological responses affected by the opioids.

Multiple Opioid Receptors

A growing body of knowledge supports the hypothesis that there are multiple opioid receptor subtypes. Opioid agonists and antagonist–agonists can be divided into three groups based on the spectrum of their pharmacologic effects in animals. *In vitro* studies also suggest that there are three opioid receptor subtypes: One classification system designates the morphine subtype (μ), the ketocyclazocine subtype (k), and the N-allylnorphenazocine (σ) subtype. Morphine is considered to be an agonist at the μ receptor only and naloxone an antagonist at all three receptors. The mixed agents are more complex. Pentazocine may be an antagonist at the μ receptor and an agonist at the k and σ receptors. Most other opioids available for clinical use have not been characterized in terms of receptor subtypes.

The multiple opioid receptor hypothesis may explain some confusing aspects of opioid pharmacology. The observation that some opioids (*e.g.*, pentazocine) produce hallucinations whereas others (*e.g.*, morphine) do not is explained if each receptor subtype mediates different effects. Similar reasoning explains why there is more than one type of opioid withdrawal syndrome. Further, an opioid could be an antagonist at one receptor and an agonist at another. The hypothesis also explains why some opioids do not suppress the morphine abstinence syndrome. Other explanations, however, can account for these observations. All the opioids, for example, might act at one receptor but produce different subsequent steps that result in different response spectra.

ENDORPHINS

The term *endorphin* is a contraction of the words *endogenous* and *morphine* and refers to endogenous peptides that have morphinelike effects. Herein, endorphin will be used generically to refer to either the natural endogenous morphinelike peptides or to closely related synthetic analogues.

The search for endorphins was stimulated by the discovery of receptors in human brain with opioid specificity and the observation that electrical stimulation of selected brain nuclei produced analgesia that could be partially reversed by naloxone. These findings suggested that endogenous morphinelike substances might exist. The first endorphins to be isolated and characterized were the pentapeptides: H-Tyr-Gly-Gly-Phe-Met-OH and H-Try-Gly-Gly-Phe-Leu-OH. These endorphins are referred to as methionine enkephalin and leucine enkephalin, or simply as enkephalins. The term *enkephalin*, which means "in the head," is incorrect now because the pentapeptides are found in many peripheral tissues; nevertheless the term is commonly applied and will continue to be used until an alternative is accepted. In various test systems, the activity of the enkephalins is similar to that of morphine, and the effects are reversed by naloxone.

PRO-ACTH/β-LPH (PRO-OPIOCORTIN)

Chronologically the elucidation of the structure of methionine enkephalin led to the observation that the identical sequence of amino acids also occurs at residues 61–65 of the 91 residue anterior pituitary hormone β-lipotropin (β-LPH). β-LPH itself is initially synthesized as one segment of a prohormone called pro-ACTH/β-LPH or pro-opiocortin (Fig. 32-2). The prohormone is a large glycoprotein divided into three segments: ACTH, β-LPH, and a 16,000 dalton third fragment called 16K fragment. Like other prohormones, pro-opiocortin has several pairs of basic amino acids. Cleavage at these sites releases ACTH, β-LPH, and other peptides. The principle endorphins located within pro-opiocortin are β-endorphin (β-LPH_{61-91}) and methionine enkephalin (β-LPH_{61-65}). ACTH and β-LPH are precursors for several biologically active peptides, but they are not endorphins.

β-ENDORPHIN (β-EP)

β-EP, the C-terminal 31 amino acids of β-LPH, is one of the most important endorphins. It is obtained by cleavage from β-LPH and is relatively resistant to further degradation. β-EP is about 50 times more potent than morphine in receptor binding assays and bioassays and possesses the full spectrum of morphinelike activity when tested under appropriate circumstances.

CHARACTERISTICS OF THE ENDORPHIN SYSTEM

The newly discovered system is complex and not well understood. Some of the most widely accepted observations are outlined below. Pro-opiocortin is synthesized *de novo* in the hypothalamus, pituitary, and placenta. ACTH and β-LPH (or β-EP alone) are also found in several brain nuclei; however, they are probably transported to these sites rather than synthesized there. In the anterior pituitary, ACTH and β-LPH (or β-EP alone) are found in the same secretory granules, and β-EP and ACTH appear to be released simultaneously and in equimolar quantities from the pituitary. Plasma levels of ACTH and β-EP increase after stressful stimuli and metyrapone (*see* Chap. 47) and decrease after administration of glucocorticoids. Diseases characterized by high plasma level of ACTH also have high levels of β-EP.

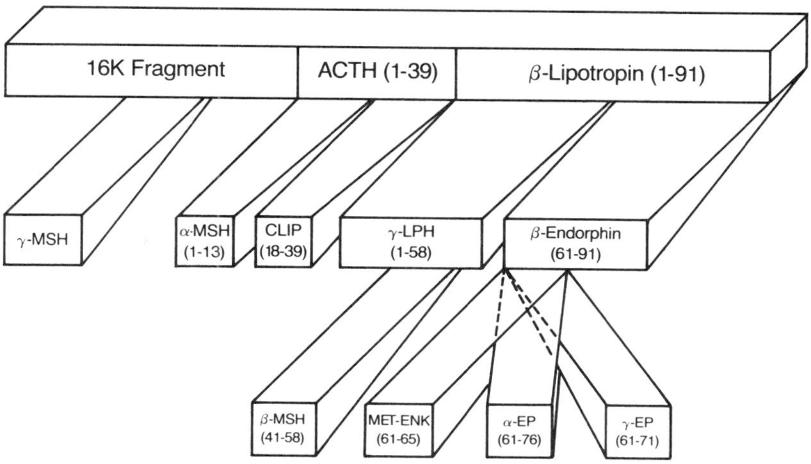

FIG. 32-2. Schematic representation of pro-opiocortin. The 16,000 dalton (*16K*) fragment contains within it γ-melanocyte stimulating hormone (*γMSH*). ACTH contains α-MSH and corticotropinlike intermediate lobe peptide (*CLIP*). β-LPH contains γ-lipoprotein (*γ-LPH*), β-MSH, β-EP, methionine enkephalin (*MET ENK*), α-endorphin (*α-EP*), and γ-endorphin (*γ-EP*). (Partially adapted from Nakanishi et al: Nature (Lond) 278:423, 1979)

RELATION BETWEEN β-EP AND THE ENKEPHALINS

A particularly interesting yet puzzling aspect of the endorphin system is the relation between the enkephalins and β-EP. Even though methionine enkephalin is contained within β-EP, β-EP is not the biologic precursor of methionine enkephalin. The enkephalins are derived by proteolysis from separate precursors. The enkephalins and β-EP are not found in the same cells. The enkephalins are distributed more widely than β-EP: They occur in many brain areas but not in the anterior pituitary. They are found in relatively high concentration in the spinal cord, sympathetic ganglia, pancreas, and gastrointestinal tract. Large amounts and multiple forms are found in the adrenal gland, in glandular cells, and in chromaffin granules. In the nervous system, enkephalins are located in nerve terminals and cell bodies.

Studies on delineation of receptor subtypes indicate that β-EP binds to the μ receptor and the δ (delta) receptor. (The relation between the δ receptor and the previously discussed k and σ receptors is unclear.) Both enkephalins bind to the δ receptor but not to the μ receptor. Conversely, morphine shows high affinity at the μ receptor but not at the δ receptor. This and other evidence suggest that an opioid receptor may have two close, but nonoverlapping, binding sites, one that accommodates morphine and the other the enkephalins. In this model β-EP binds simultaneously to both sides.

FUNCTIONS OF THE ENDORPHIN SYSTEM

The endorphin system comprises two major components: one represented by β-EP and the other by the enkephalins. Too little information about the system does not allow a functional classification of the components. β-EP has many of the characteristics of a neurohormone: anatomically, chemically, and functionally it is related to ACTH. Like ACTH, is has a multiplicity of actions but no obvious target-organ like the adrenal gland. When β-EP or the enkephalins are centrally administered (as opposed to being released), the effects of the β-EP last hours whereas the effects of the enkephalins last only minutes. The enkephalins fulfill most of the characteristics of a neurotransmitter: They are found at synapses and released by depolarizing stimuli. A specific synaptic inactivating enzyme has not, however, been identified as yet. Other aspects of the system indicate that both components can function as neuromodulators.

The endorphin system is so widespread and complex that it is unlikely to subserve any single function. Unsurprisingly it has been implicated in a variety of pathophysiologic states such as pain, obesity, psychiatric disease, and endocrinopathies. It may also play a role in regulating blood pressure, temperature, and respiration.

Many aspects of clinical pain are so mystifying that it is tempting to invoke the endorphin system to explain many complex phenomena. Acupuncture and placebo analgesia could be mediated by endorphins. Although there are some animal data implicate endorphins in these phenomena, and in pain in general, the direct evidence is still meager.

METABOLISM AND PHARMACOKINETICS

The metabolism and pharmacokinetics of morphine are reasonably representative of the opioids. The principal metabolite of morphine is morphine-3-glucuronide. Four other minor metabolites have been identified. No metabolite is pharmacologically active. The kidney is the main organ of excretion. The ratio of metabolites to morphine in urine is about 9:1. The pattern of hepatic metabolism, glucuronide formation, and renal excretion is similar for most of the opioid agonists and for naloxone.

The $T\frac{1}{2}_{\alpha}$ and $T\frac{1}{2}_{\beta}$ (*see* Chap. 5) of most of the agonists and antagonists that have been studied are 1 to 5 minutes and 1.5 to 3 hours, respectively. The V_d ranges from 3 to 5 liters/kg, and drug clearance is about 15 ml/min/kg. Most agonists and antagonists are less active by the oral than the parenteral route mainly due to high first-pass metabolism. The oral bioavailability of most opioids is low.

The relation between plasma concentration of opioids and various effects is complex. Plasma levels are not routinely monitored in clinical practice. No known pharmacokinetic interactions result in altered kinetics of the opioids, but a few potential interactions have been studied. In contrast, by delaying gastric emptying, opioids probably alter the absorption of many drugs (*see* Chap. 8). The $T\frac{1}{2}_{\beta}$ of meperidine is two times longer in patients with hepatic disease than in normal subjects. Thus altered pharmacokinetics is one explanation for the increased sensitivity of patients with hepatic disease to meperidine. The kinetics of other opioids are also likely altered by hepatic disease.

CLINICAL PHARMACOLOGY, USES, AND EFFICACY

TREATMENT OF PAIN

The selection of a potent analgesic depends on the clinical pharmacology of the drug, the characteristics of the pain, and the clinical state of the patient. Acute great pain requires a parenteral agent, whereas chronic pain is usually treated with an oral agent. A long duration of action is desirable for chronic pain, whereas a short-acting agent may be satisfactory for some types of intermittent pain.

A single dose or a short (2–3 day) course of morphine will not result in clinically significant physical dependence. After 1 to 2 weeks a withdrawal syndrome will occur, but the symptoms are readily tolerated by many patients and often they will not associate the symptoms with opioid withdrawal. In marked contrast, the physician must be constantly vigilant for the few patients who will complain about the symptoms and ask for more opioids. Patients with a history of drug abuse or an obvious propensity to abuse drugs should not receive morphine and other highly addicting agonists unless absolutely necessary.

The drug of choice for most types of severe pain is morphine, the most efficacious parenteral analgesic. In patients without recent exposure to opioids, the average analgesic dose is 7.5 mg. Elderly patients and patients with hepatic disease, CNS disease, or other debilitating conditions should receive a smaller initial dose. The dose may be increased rapidly if the initial dose is insufficient. The choice of a route of administration depends on the urgency of the clinical situation. The onset of analgesia occurs about 30 minutes after s.c. administration and 15 minutes after i.m. administration. Morphine may be given slowly intravenously if a more rapid onset of action is needed, but the patient must be constantly observed for cardiorespiratory complications.

The duration of analgesia is one of the most important factors that determine the choice of an analgesic. The duration of analgesia after alphaprodine administration is only 1.5 hours, for example; thus it is used for brief procedures and labor pain but is not satisfactory for most types of clinical pain. The mean duration of analgesia for morphine and meperidine is 4 and 3 hours, respectively. This difference is clinically significant to the patient and more convenient for nursing staff. Because of the many factors that contribute to individual variability of drug response, it is impossible to predict the duration of analgesia for a person; therefore an approximate duration should be estimated for each patient by assessing the quality of the analgesia at various times during the dosing interval.

Since the ratio of ED_{50}s for analgesia and respiratory depression is about the same in the opioid series, there is little advantage to using one agent over another with respect to the problem of providing analgesia without respiratory depression.

Mild pain is treated first with nonopioids (*see* Chap. 31). The next more potent agent is usually an opioid such as codeine, meperidine, or dihydromorphine, or a combination of an opioid and a nonopioid. There are many combinations from which to choose: The combinations of aspirin or acetaminophen with codeine are common. The rationale for combining an opioid and a nonopioid is that they have different mechanisms of action and may therefore be additive.

The most efficacious opioid for oral administration is methadone. It provides excellent analgesia, and its duration of action (5–6 hours) is longer than that of all other available agents. Methadone has an important disadvantage in that it produces a greater degree of physical dependence than do other agents commonly prescribed by the oral route. Methadone is primarily used for patients with cancer pain.

TREATMENT OF OTHER CONDITIONS

The ability of the opioids to suppress the cough reflex and to diminish the propulsive activity of the gut makes them effective agents for the treatment of cough and diarrhea. Morphine is frequently used in combination with other measures to treat pulmonary edema. This acute life-threatening condition is principally due to cardiac decompensation; hence the treatment is complex and uses various combinations of drugs and procedures. Why morphine is effective in pulmonary edema is unclear but probably relates to vasodilatation, respiratory depression, sedation or some combination of these effects. Another specialized use of morphine and a few other opioids is in anesthesiology. Very high doses (1–2 mg/kg) of morphine provide excellent analgesia with minimal or no cardiac depression; hence some anesthesiologists use morphine as the principal or only analgesic for certain times of cardiovascular surgery.

TREATMENT OF HEROIN AND RELATED DEPENDENCIES

Specialized drug abuse treatment clinics use methadone as a substitute for heroin and other abused opioids because methadone will suppress the heroin abstinence syndrome. Heroin and morphine will only suppress the signs and symptoms of heroin withdrawal for 6 to 10 hours, whereas methadone will suppress the syndrome for at least 24 hours and often 48 hours. The other advantage of methadone is that it can be given orally, thus eliminating the problems associated with maintaining drug abusers on parenteral agents.

Methadone maintenance refers to a plan whereby a person who is dependent on heroin is stabilized on a high dose of methadone, usually between 40 and 60 mg/day, for an indefinite period. During this time the person does not need to engage in drug-seeking behavior and thus is more responsive to various nonpharmacologic treatment modalities. Methadone detoxification refers to a declining schedule of doses that usually begin at about 40 mg and taper to 0 over a period ranging from 3 to 4 days up to several months (*see* Chap. 9).

DISTINGUISHING CHARACTERISTICS OF SELECTED AGONISTS

Heroin, readily synthesized from morphine by acetylation, is classified in schedule I (*see* Chap. 12) because of its high potential for abuse. There is no accepted medical use for heroin in the United States. Heroin has an earlier onset of analgesia than does morphine and a shorter duration of action but is not more efficacious as an analgesic. It is highly euphorigenic and therefore is preferred by drug addicts. Heroin is deacetylated to monoacetylmorphine and morphine. Its greater lipid solubility than morphine probably accounts for its greater euphorigenic effect.

Codeine is widely prescribed for mild pain and for cough. As an analgesic it is considerably less potent than morphine, since parenteral doses of 120 mg are needed to approximate the analgesia produced by 10 mg of morphine. Such high parenteral doses of codeine are toxic and rarely prescribed. An important advantage of codeine is its relatively high oral to parenteral potency ratio. Oral doses of 15 to 30 mg produce analgesia that lasts about 4 hours. Codeine is metabolized by the liver to morphine and morphine conjugates and is excreted by the kidney. It has a low addiction liability.

Meperidine is a widely prescribed potent analgesic usually administered intramuscularly but also efficacious by the oral route. Intramuscular doses of 100 mg are equivalent to 10 mg of morphine. Evidence suggests that meperidine produces less constriction of the sphincter of Oddi than does morphine. Meperidine, usually causes more nausea, vomiting, and hypotension but less constipation. The toxicity of meperidine includes CNS excitation characterized by tremulousness, twitches, and occasionally seizures. Tolerance does not develop to the excitant effects. The first-pass metabolism of meperidine is about 50%, and the T½ is about 3 hours. Normeperidine, a principal metabolite, accumulates in renal failure and may be responsible for CNS excitation. MAO inhibitors sometimes potentiate the CNS depression produced by meperidine.

Alphaprodine is principally used in obstetrics and minor surgical procedures because of its short duration of action. There are no special advantages to *anileridine*, and it is not widely used.

Methadone is one of the most important opioid agonists because of its efficacy as an oral analgesic and because of its usefulness in treating addiction to other opioids. Although not as euphorigenic as heroin or morphine, methadone does produce a high degree of physical dependence and should not be prescribed for minor ailments. A major problem and distinguishing characteristic of methadone is its prolonged withdrawal syndrome. In contrast to morphine, withdrawal from methadone lasts for many days to weeks. The methadone withdrawal syndrome is less intense than is the morphine syndrome, but its protracted nature leads to a high degree of recidivism. Consequently methadone should not be chronically prescribed as an analgesic except in patients with a limited life expectancy or unusual and complicated pain syndromes. The oral analgesic dose of methadone is 5 to 10 mg. Methadone is also effective parenterally but is rarely used by this route. Methadone is well absorbed from the gastrointestinal tract and undergoes extensive biotransformation to demethylated and cyclic metabolites excreted in urine and bile. The plasma T½ is 15 to 20 hours. Rifampin induces the metabolism of methadone (*see*

Chap. 8), an interaction that can lead to a loss of efficacy of methadone.

Propoxyphene, a complex, controversial agent, is often maligned because many controlled studies have failed to demonstrate a significant difference between a placebo and a low dose (32 mg) of propoxyphene. At a higher dose (64 mg), propoxyphene provides analgesia equivalent to, but not superior to, other agents such as aspirin and acetaminophen. Higher doses (120 mg) produce good analgesia but a greater degree of toxicity. Despite the controversy about its efficacy, propoxyphene is one of the most widely prescribed agents.

Respiratory depression and euphoria are usually not prominent if the dose of propoxyphene is less than the maximum recommended daily dose of 480 mg. There is a mild abstinence syndrome following abrupt withdrawal of propoxyphene after prolonged administration of 300 to 600 mg/day. Toxic doses cause respiratory and CNS depression occasionally complicated by delusions, hallucinations, and seizures. The combination of propoxyphene plus hypnotics, tranquilizers, or ethanol may produce a serious overdose. Deaths have occurred when excessive quantities of propoxyphene were taken alone or in combination with these other agents. Most of the deaths are the result of deliberate self-overdose or abuse. Propoxyphene is available as the hydrochloride or napsyalate salt and in combination with acetaminophen, aspirin, and codeine. The combinations are prescribed more frequently than is propoxyphene alone.

Fentanyl is a highly potent analgesic that has achieved widespread use in surgical analgesia. Its rapid onset and short duration of action (15–30 minutes) make it useful for surgical procedures. It is usually administered in combination with a major tranquilizer to produce a type of anesthesia known as neuroleptanalgesia (*see* Chap. 28).

ANTAGONISTS

The principal therapeutic use of *naloxone* is to reverse the adverse effects of an excessive dose of an agonist. Naloxone is sometimes given to patients in coma of undetermined etiology to discover if opioids are the cause of the coma. It is also widely used to investigate the endorphin system. *Naltrexone* is an investigational long-acting antagonist that has the advantage of activity after oral administration. Its potential usefulness in treating heroin addiction is under investigation.

CHAPTER 32 QUESTIONS

(*See* P. 7 for Full Instructions)

Select the One Best Answer

1. Morphine
   - A. decreases serum amylase.
   - B. enhances the response to diuretics.
   - C. decreases CSF pressure.
   - D. relieves the pain of biliary colic.
   - E. is less effective than codeine in depressing the cough reflex.
2. Tolerance develops to each of the following effects of narcotic analgesics EXCEPT
   - A. euphoria.
   - B. constipation.
   - C. respiratory depression.
   - D. analgesia.
   - E. sedation.
3. Methadone
   - A. has antagonistic effects similar to naloxone.
   - B. is diacetyl-morphine.
   - C. penetrates the blood–brain barrier better than morphine.
   - D. orally is a weak analgesic agent.
   - E. produces negligible gastrointestinal effects.
4. Naloxone
   - A. is a general respiratory stimulant.
   - B. has a longer duration of action than does morphine.
   - C. has both agonist and antagonist properties.
   - D. will precipitate barbiturate withdrawal.
   - E. has been used to treat compulsive narcotic abusers.
5. In a patient predisposed to asthma, morphine-induced bronchospasm could be alleviated by
   - A. atropine.
   - B. aminophylline.
   - C. propranolol.
   - D. methadone.
   - E. phenylephrine.

A = 1,2,3; B = 1,3; C = 2,4; D = 4; E = All

6. Codeine
   1. may produce excitement and convulsions in children.
   2. produces greater depression of the cough reflex than morphine.
   3. is partially metabolized to morphine.

4. is as efficacious as morphine for the relief of severe visceral pain.

7. Which of the following agents produces significant analgesia and also suppresses the cough reflex?
   1. Codeine
   2. Meperidine
   3. Methadone
   4. Dextromethorphan

8. Morphine
   1. depresses respiratory and vasomotor centers.
   2. produces a vasodepressor effect by releasing histamine.
   3. delays gastric emptying time and slows propulsion of food along intestinal tract.
   4. stimulates the chemoreceptor trigger zone of the medulla oblongata.

9. Nalorphine will
   1. depress respiration.
   2. antagonize heroin-induced respiratory depression.
   3. antagonize meperidine induced respiratory depression.
   4. antagonize phenobarbital-induced respiratory depression.

10. As a preanesthetic agent, meperidine may cause
   1. respiratory depression.
   2. increased biliary duct pressure.
   3. tachycardia.
   4. nausea.

BERTRAM G. KATZUNG

33 Cardiac Glycosides

The term "cardiac glycosides" describes a group of compounds of similar chemical structure that increase the contractility of heart muscle, an effect most useful in the failing heart. In addition, these agents have effects on the electrical properties of the myocardium that are of both therapeutic and toxic importance. Since the best known members of the group are derived from plants of the genus *Digitalis*, the terms *digitalis*, *digitalis glycosides*, and *cardiac glycosides* are used interchangeably for all members of the class. Because of the low therapeutic index of the glycosides and the varying pathophysiology of cardiac failure, there is much interest in alternative therapeutic measures. Such alternatives may include vasodilators (hydralazine, nitrates; *see* Chap. 35), alpha-adrenergic blocking agents (prazosin; *see* Chap. 18), and beta-adrenergic stimulants (dobutamine, prenalterol; *see* Chap. 17), and new inotropic agents (*e.g.*, amrinone, discussed later in this chapter).

SOURCE

Plant. Digitalis leaf, digoxin, digitoxin, and deslanoside are derived from the purple and the white foxglove (*Digitalis purpurea* and *D. lanata*); ouabain and strophanthin from various species of *Strophanthus*. The sea onion or squill, the lily of the valley, the oleander, and *Helleborus* species are botanic sources of other glycosides.

Animal. Certain butterflies and some toads contain glycosides.

HISTORY

Although digitalis glycosides have been used for various purposes for more than 3000 years, an English physician and botanist, William Withering, was the first to describe the main indications and actions of an extract of digitalis leaf. His monograph *An Account of the Foxglove and Some of Its Medical Uses, with Practical Remarks on Dropsy and Other Diseases*

WILLIAM WITHERING, 1741–1799. English physician, botanist, and mineralogist. Learned from folk medicine that foxglove, containing digitalis, could be used to treat dropsy. First to link dropsy and heart disease. A genus of Solanaceae, *Witheringia*, is named for him.

(1785) contains a surprisingly accurate account of the main effects of digitalis extracts on patients with heart failure.

CHEMISTRY

A cardiac glycoside molecule consists of an *aglycone* or *genin,* which possesses the same pharmacologic activity as the whole molecule combined chemically with one or more sugars (Fig. 33-1). An aglycone has a steroid nucleus with an α, β, unsaturated 5- or 6-member lactone ring attached at the C-17 position. The basic pharmacologic properties of all aglycones are similar. The attached sugars are important in determining the absolute potency, solubility, absorbability, rate of onset, duration of action, and plasma and tissue protein-binding properties of the glycosides.

PATHOPHYSIOLOGY OF HEART FAILURE

The actions of digitalis are best described in the context of the disease in which it is used. Heart failure is defined simply as cardiac output inadequate for the needs of the body. The type of failure that responds best to digitalis therapy is the chronic, low-output form caused by conditions such as atherosclerosis or hypertension. Although the biochemical lesion has not been defined, the major physiologic manifestation of failure is well shown by the *ventricular function curve* (Fig. 33-2). The reduction in mechanical performance can be detected in almost any inotropic measure: *peak contractile tension* or shortening, *rate of tension development* or of shortening, *stroke volume,* and *cardiac output.* This primary defect results directly in symptoms such as easy fatigability and shortness of breath and evokes the compensatory responses of sympathetic discharge (tachycardia, increased arterial and venous tone), renal salt and water retention (edema of peripheral tissues and lungs), and hypertrophy of the cardiac musculature.

INOTROPIC EFFECTS OF DIGITALIS

The primary therapeutic effect of digitalis in heart failure is to increase cardiac contractility at all fiber lengths (Fig. 33-2). This is a direct effect on the myocardial cell (*see* below) and in favorable situations occurs without any increased vascular tone. In fact, improved cardiac output allows reduced compensatory sympathetic tone and decreased preload and afterload. Because of the decreases in afterload and fiber length, the increase in output (external work) is not accompanied by an equivalent increase in oxygen consumption, and an improvement in efficiency (external work per unit of oxygen consumption) results. Similarly, improvement of renal blood flow allows the excretion of retained edema fluid. Normal myocardium also manifests a positive inotropic response to these drugs. However, in this case, compensatory reflexes prevent supernormal cardiac output, and no increased efficiency is seen.

ELECTRICAL EFFECTS OF DIGITALIS

As indicated in Table 33-1, digitalis has various effects on the electrical properties of cardiac

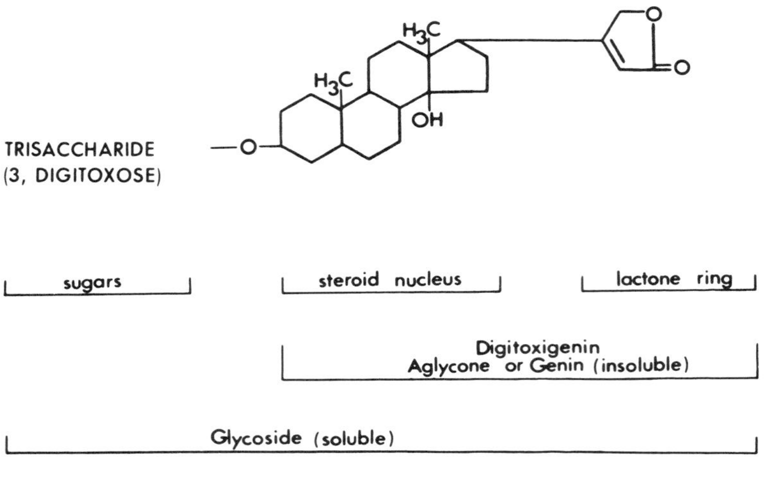

FIG. 33-1. A typical cardiac glycoside (digitoxin).

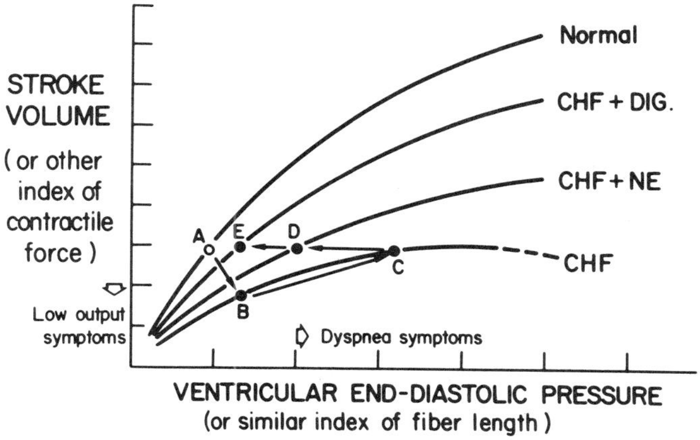

FIG. 33-2. Schematic ventricular function curves. Point "A" on the "normal" curve shows the operating point for the nonfailing myocardium. The congestive heart failure (*CHF*) curve reflects the decreased contractile performance at all fiber lengths; point "B" shows the increase in end-diastolic pressure resulting from decreased ejection fraction in the decompensated heart. When compensatory mechanisms become involved, salt and water are retained, moving the operating point to "C," and sympathetic tone to the heart is increased, shifting contractile performance upward to the CHF + NE (norepinephrine) function curve. This allows a shift of the operating point to a shorter fiber length and end-diastolic pressure (point "D"). The increased vascular tone associated with sympathetic discharge, however, usually prevents a return to normal end-diastolic pressure. Use of digitalis (*CHF + DIG* curve) provides an additional increase in contractile force, further shifting the curve towards normal. Because sympathetic reflexes may then be reduced or abolished, vascular tone decreases, end-diastolic pressure decreases (point "E"), and cardiac size decreases.

muscle. At low-to-moderate doses, these effects are chiefly parasympathetic actions on the heart and can be partially blocked by atropine.

In the sinoatrial (SA) node, automaticity is slowed by both direct (membrane) and indirect (parasympathomimetic) actions. In the atrial musculature a decrease in action potential duration and in effective refractory period are the major actions. At the atrioventricular (A-V) node, slowed conduction and increased refractory period are prominent. Below the level of the A-V node, relatively little digitalis effect is observed at subtoxic concentrations except for a small increase and then decrease of action potential duration.

CARDIAC TOXICITY OF DIGITALIS

Mechanical toxicity of digitalis is not usually a major clinical problem because electrical toxicity precedes it. Experimentally, however, digitalis has slowed relaxation and may lead to contracture at high doses. Electrical toxicity may simulate every known cardiac arrhythmia but takes two major forms: decreased or *blocked A-V conduction* and increased abnormal or *ectopic automatic activity*. The latter effect can occur anywhere in the heart but is especially dangerous when it occurs in the Purkinje system or ventricular fibers. In this situation, the degree of toxicity may vary from occasional extrasystoles (premature ventricular depolarizations) through bigeminal rhythm to rapid unifocal or multifocal ventricular tachycardia and fibrillation. This automatic activity probably arises from a type of oscillatory depolarizing afterpotential (*see* Fig. 33-4), which results from intracellular calcium overload (*see* Mechanism of Action, below).

MECHANISM OF CARDIAC ACTION

Figure 33-3 provides a schematic diagram of the functional unit of cardiac cells, the sarcomere. The normal sequence of events in contraction of the sarcomere involves

1. excitation—an action potential that occurs in the sarcolemma;
2. coupling of excitation to the internal contractile process (excitation contraction (EC) coupling)—involves the influx of calcium ions through gated channels in the membrane. This calcium apparently triggers the release of additional calcium from the sarcoplasmic reticulum, which initiates

TABLE 33-1. Summary of Effects of Cardiac Glycosides on the Heart

Effect	Atria	A-V Node and Bundle	Ventricles
Direct digitalis effects	**Contractile force increased***	**Refractory period lengthened**	**Contractile force increased**
	Refractory period lengthened	**Conduction velocity decreased**	Refractory period shortened
	Conduction velocity decreased		Marked increase in automaticity
	Automaticity slightly increased		
Indirect digitalis effects (increased vagal tone)	Refractory period shortened	**Refractory period lengthened**	No effect
	Conduction velocity increased	**Conduction velocity decreased**	
Electrocardiographic changes	P changes	PR interval increased	QT shortened; T and ST depressed
Adverse irregularities	Extrasystoles	A-V depression or block	Fibrillation
	Tachycardia		Extrasystoles
			Tachycardia

* Therapeutically important actions are set in **bold face type.**

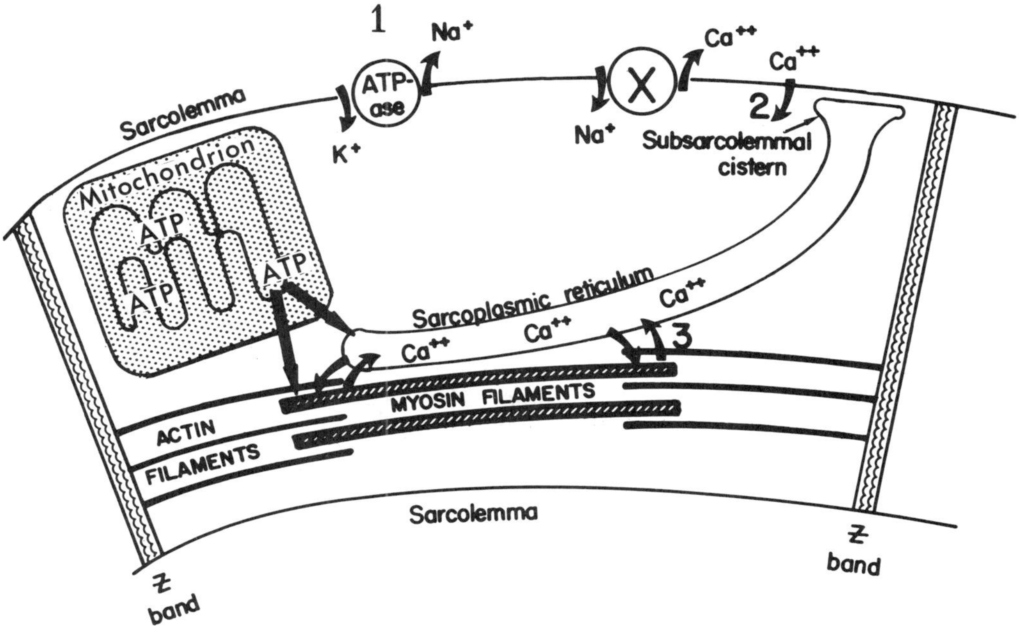

FIG. 33-3. Functional components of the cardiac sarcomere. Digitalis is known to inhibit Na^+/K^+-ATPase (process 1). It may also act directly on sarcolemmal calcium channels (process 2), allowing more calcium to flow into the cells with each depolarization and thereby triggering greater release of internal calcium. Digitalis has also been reported to increase release of calcium from internal stores (process 3) for the *same* stimulus. The net result is an increase of free calcium during the contractile phase of the cardiac cycle with increased tension development and shortening of the actinmyosin filaments.

3. sliding of the tension-generating actin-myosin filaments;
4. the whole process is supported by ATP, generated primarily in the mitochondria for driving the Na^+/K^+-ATPase pump, the sarcoplasmic reticulum calcium sequestration machinery, and the tension-generating process itself in the actin-myosin filaments.

ATP production is not significantly changed in treated or untreated congestive heart failure, nor is any change in the contractile machinery detectable; therefore the positive inotropic action of digitalis must be mediated through an increase in calcium in the region of the contractile proteins. The mechanism for this increase in free calcium is not completely clear. Digitalis has a well-documented *inhibitory action on Na^+/K^+ATPase*. (However, a few scientists believe that the positive inotropic action of the drug may occur at concentrations too low to inhibit the enzyme—concentrations that may actually stimulate it.) Inhibition of Na^+/K^+-ATPase does not directly increase intracellular calcium, however, as evidenced by the fact that some other ATPase inhibitors, such as oligomycin, have no positive inotropic action. Decreased activity of the "sodium pump" does lead to increased intracellular sodium, which can result in decreased expulsion of calcium ions by the Na–Ca exchange carrier, designated "X" in Figure 33-3. This secondary increase in intracellular calcium might be the immediate cause of digitalis' effect. Two other possible sites of action have been proposed for digitalis: The *transmembrane calcium influx* that occurs during action potentials has been reported to increase, and *increased calcium release from the sarcoplasmic reticulum* has also been described. Although digitalis undoubtedly does inhibit Na^+/K^+-ATPase, these two possible sites of action have not been disproved. Since the three mechanisms are not mutually exclusive, it may be that each plays a role.

The pretoxic ECG effects of the cardiac glycosides (*see* Table 33-1) result from a combination of the parasympathomimetic action, referred to above, and the increased intracellular calcium caused by direct action of the agents. Parasympathomimetic effects account for most of the supraventricular changes, including sinoatrial slowing and A-V block (prolonged P-R interval). On the other hand, the shortening of the QT or ST segment, and associated T-wave changes, are manifestations of shortening of the action potential of ventricular cells, an effect that results from increased potassium permeability. This permeability change is another result of increased intracellular calcium concentration and may be observed before arrhythmias occur.

The major toxic arrhythmogenic effects of digitalis have been convincingly shown to involve excessively high intracellular calcium levels that may undergo oscillatory variations, resulting in both membrane (electrical) and actin-myosin (contractile) oscillations. If the membrane oscillations reach threshold, they trigger action potentials (Fig. 33-4) and increase the cardiac rate. Since increased rate facilitates calcium influx and more overload, this process quickly becomes regenerative, which partially explains the very low therapeutic index of the digitalis agents. These effects may involve increased sympathetic outflow from the CNS but also occur in denervated and catecholamine-depleted tissue.

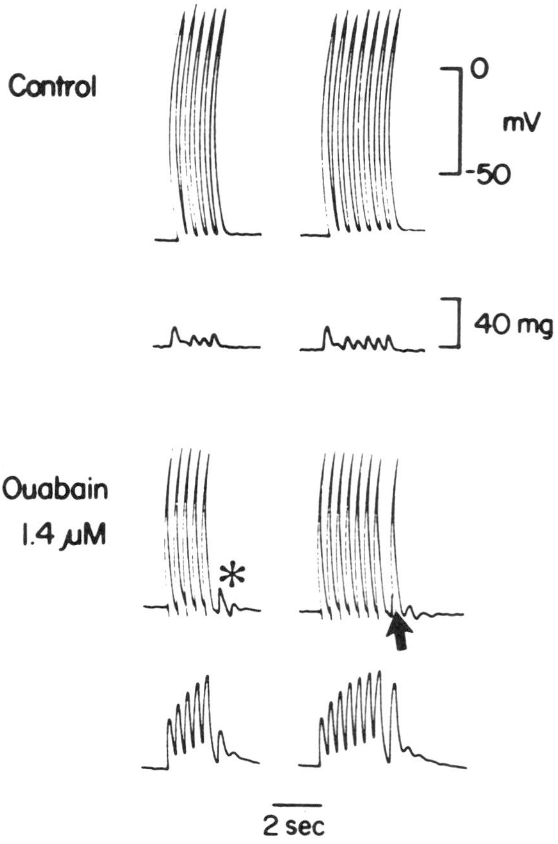

FIG. 33-4. Effects of a cardiac glycoside on transmembrane electrical activity and on contractility. The recording was made at slow speed on a chart recorder to display slow events. The upper panel shows the action potentials (upper trace) and contractions (lower trace) that result from trains of stimuli applied to an isolated strip of guinea pig ventricular myocardium. The lower panel shows the same variables after exposure to a toxic dose of ouabain. Contractile tension increases markedly. In addition, electrical oscillations are seen after the action potential trains. In the first train (five stimuli), they do not reach threshold (asterisk), but after the second train (seven stimuli), the first oscillatory afterpotential elicits a full action potential (*arrow*). (Record provided by Dr. H. Karagueuzian.)

OTHER ACTIONS OF DIGITALIS

Because digitalis blocks membrane-bound Na^+/K^+-ATPase in all tissues, it may be able to reduce ATPase-dependent secretion in several types, such as renal tubules, choroid plexus, and ciliary body. Unfortunately the effect is not sufficient in any of these structures to be clinically useful.

CLINICAL PHARMACOLOGY

HEART FAILURE

Digitalis has been used in every form of congestive heart failure, but, as noted above, its effectiveness is not uniform. In particular, it is not very useful when failure is of the high-output type, as in thyrotoxicosis, beriberi, or arteriovenous shunt. It is also ineffective when failure is associated with an acute inflammatory carditis. Failure associated with very high preload (pulmonary wedge) or afterload (arterial) pressures respond better to the use of vasodilators or diuretics than to digitalis. Finally, some evidence suggests that significant tolerance develops to the therapeutic actions of digitalis, so that chronic use is attended by a decreasing therapeutic safety margin. Nevertheless these agents are still the mainstay of therapy for "uncomplicated" failure associated with chronic rheumatic valvular disease and atherosclerotic coronary insufficiency and for failure secondary to hypertension if it persists after correction of the arterial pressure.

ATRIAL ARRHYTHMIAS

Atrial fibrillation is an arrhythmia that results from chaotic reentry of impulses traveling through the atrial musculature (see Chap. 34). Under these conditions, the A-V node is bombarded by many hundreds of impulses per minute. Most impulses are extinguished in the upper part of the node because of its relative refractoriness, caused by prior incompletely conducted impulses. The ventricular rate is therefore a function of the number of impulses that succeed in traveling through the A-V node and may be as high as 150 to 250/minute, especially during periods of high sympathetic tone. Digitalis very effectively limits ventricular rate in this arrhythmia because its electrical effects on the A-V node—both parasympathomimetic and direct—tend to increase the refractory period and reduce conduction velocity. Because this action is usually accompanied by at least some positive inotropic effect, the net result is therapeutically useful.

ATRIAL FLUTTER

Digitalis is used to treat atrial flutter. The partial A-V block usually present in this condition can be increased and then maintained by the use of digitalis. Sometimes the heart spontaneously reverts to normal sinus rhythm or to well-controlled atrial fibrillation. If neither occurs, quinidine therapy (*see* Chap. 34) or direct-current electrical cardioversion may be tried.

PAROXYSMAL TACHYCARDIA

Rapid digitalization is one of many procedures that may be effective in paroxysmal atrial or supraventricular tachycardia. Its effectiveness is probably the result of its vagal-stimulating effects on the atrial muscle and the A-V node. It is essential to establish that the condition is not the result of digitalis overdose.

ELECTROCARDIOGRAPHIC CHANGES

Therapeutic doses of digitalis (one third to one half the lethal dose) cause characteristic electrocardiographic changes, listed below in the order of most common occurrence. The ECG is sometimes useful in determining if a patient has received recent glycoside therapy.

T-wave changes occur in which the T wave becomes small, isoelectric, or inverted. At the same time the ST segment frequently becomes depressed and often falls below the isoelectric line. Unfortunately these changes have no predictable relation to the adequacy of the therapeutic dose or the imminence of toxicity.

Lengthened PR interval is associated with slower or delayed A-V condition.

Shortened QT interval is the result of the shortening of the plateau phase of the transmembrane action potential.

P-wave changes are presumably caused by the complex action of the glycosides on the atria.

With higher doses of digitalis, the above changes are exaggerated, and electrocardiographic patterns are appropriate to the drug-induced arrhythmias.

PREPARATIONS, ADMINISTRATION, AND DOSAGE

Only the most popular glycosides or glycosides whose properties are of special interest are discussed. Since the therapeutic ratio of all glycosides is the same, selection must be based on criteria such as rate of onset, duration, absorbability, and bioavailability.

PREPARATIONS

Digoxin, U.S.P., the main glycoside from the white foxglove, *D. lanata*, is by far the most commonly prescribed agent for oral use. It is also available in parenteral form and has a fairly rapid onset of action when given intravenously (Table 33-2). It is also favored when rapid digitalization is required. Digoxin is a pure crystalline compound, and the bioavailability of the oral form is now monitored to ensure therapeutic equivalence.

Digitoxin, U.S.P., is the main cardiac glycoside from the purple foxglove, *D. purpurea*. It is the most completely absorbed and the longest acting of the commonly available agents (Table 33-2). It is also available for i.v. use, but its slow rate of onset of action nullifies any rationale for its use by this route. The crude preparation *D. purpurea* (digitalis leaf) is also available and has pharmacokinetic and pharmacodynamic properties identical to those of digitoxin. Because it is a mixture, digitalis leaf must be commercially standardized by bioassay to a consistent content of active glycoside (Table 33-3). It is difficult to rationalize the use of this traditional preparation now that pure agents have been fully standardized and proved by decades of clinical use.

Ouabain and *deslanoside* are two additional pure digitalis glycosides available for parenteral use (Table 33-2). Ouabain is slightly faster in its onset of action than is digoxin, whereas

TABLE 33-2. Characteristics of Common Cardiac Glycosides

Drug	Gastrointestinal Absorption	Route of Administration	Latency	Time to Maximum Effect	Half-Life	Digitalizing Dose	Maintenance Dose
	%			*hr*			
Ouabain	—	i.v.	5–10 min	½–2	21 hr	0.25–0.50 mg	—
Deslanoside	—	i.v.	10–30 min	1–2	36 hr	1.2–1.6 mg	—
Digoxin	—	i.v.	10–30 min	1½–5	36 hr	0.75–1.25 mg	—
Digoxin	50–75	p.o.	1½–4 hr	6–8	36 hr	2.0–3.0 mg	0.25–0.5 mg
Digitoxin	—	i.v.	½–2 hr	8	4–6 days	1.0–1.5 mg	—
Digitoxin	90–100	p.o.	2–6 hr	4–12	4–6 days	1.0–1.5 mg	0.1–0.2 mg
Digitalis leaf	40	p.o.	2–6 hr	12–24	4–6 days	1.0–2.0 g	0.12 g

deslanoside, a precursor of digoxin, has digoxin's properties. Ouabain represents the most water soluble of the clinically available digitalis glycosides. It is inactive by the oral route.

ADMINISTRATION AND DOSAGE

Except in an emergency, when speed rather than maximum safety is the prime consideration, or when poor absorption is expected, cardiac glycosides should be given orally. When minutes are vital, a crystalline glycoside may be given by i.v. injection. Absorption from subcutaneous and i.m. sites is irregular.

Because the therapeutic ratio of the cardiac glycosides is small, optimal dosage is particularly desirable. A detailed knowledge of pharmacokinetic factors that influence dosage is important to ensure this. For this reason, thorough familiarity with one pure glycoside, preferably digoxin, is advisable. This agent is incompletely but reliably absorbed from the gastrointestinal tract, significantly bound to plasma proteins, and excreted in the urine. Its half-life, which averages 35 to 40 hours (Table 33-2), is altered in renal disease. Algorithms based on creatinine clearance are available for predicting the dosage required in patients with impaired renal function.

Glycosides are sometimes administered orally in two stages. For *initial digitalization* (of a patient who has not recently received the drug), the glycoside is administered at a rate designed to cause its accumulation within the body. This dosage scheme is continued until the desired therapeutic aim is attained or toxic effects emerge. Since the dose that causes a given therapeutic effect varies among people, the procedure of initial digitalization is equivalent to an individual biologic assay. Once the desired effect is obtained, *maintenance dosage* is initiated. This dose also varies and is selected to maintain optimal therapeutic effect.

TABLE 33-3. Approximate Equivalents of Glycoside Preparations from *D. purpurea*

Powdered digitalis, *U.S.P.* (leaf of *D. purpurea*), 0.1 g ≡ 1.0 *U.S.P.* unit
Digitalis tincture, *N.F.*, 1.0 ml ≡ 0.1 g digitalis leaf
Digitoxin injection, *U.S.P.*, 0.1 mg ≡ 0.1 g digitalis leaf

ADVERSE EFFECTS OF TOXICITY

The therapeutic index of cardiac glycosides is between two and three, one of the lowest indices of all commonly used therapeutic agents. Consequently adverse effects are not rare. Even in hospitalized patients, up to 30% of those treated with cardiac glycoside reportedly experience some potentially serious toxicity.

GASTROINTESTINAL EFFECTS

Anorexia, nausea, and vomiting are frequently the first signs of intoxication. Although crude digitalis leaf can cause gastric and intestinal irritation, most of these effects are the result of direct drug action on the brain stem vomiting center. In addition, abdominal discomfort, pain, diarrhea, and cramps may be experienced.

NEUROLOGIC EFFECTS

Diverse adverse effects have been described, including headache, malaise, drowsiness, and neuralgic pain; mental symptoms include delirium, convulsions, and confusion. Visual effects are fairly common: blurred vision and white, yellow, green, or red colored perception have been reported.

CARDIAC EFFECTS

Cardiac arrhythmias are by far the most dangerous of digitalis toxic effects. As noted above, digitalis overdose can simulate every known cardiac arrhythmia. Some of the more common forms are described below.

Extrasystoles

Atrial, junctional, and ventricular extrasystoles occur. Multifocal premature ventricular depolarizations are a particularly serious form because they may presage ventricular fibrillation. A special form of coupled ventricular extrasystoles in which each normal sinus beat is followed by a ventricular ectopic depolarization is called bigeminy (twinning of normal and extrasystolic beats) and suggests digitalis intoxication when prior drug intake of a patient is unknown.

Atrioventricular Block

Partial or complete heart block (electrical dissociation of atria and ventricles) occurs, presumably owing to an extension of the therapeutically useful effects of digitalis on the A-V bundle. Propagation in the A-V bundle ceases. Atrial tachycardia with heart block is a classic rhythm of digitalis intoxication.

Tachycardia

Tachycardia, both atrial and ventricular, occurs and is usually considered an indication to discontinue treatment. Ventricular tachycardia is more dangerous because it may precede ventricular fibrillation, an arrhythmia that is the usual cause of death after an overdose of digitalis.

A digitalis dose adequate to control fibrillation or flutter may be toxic to the myocardium controlled by sinus rhythm. To prevent the emergence of adverse effects, digitalis therapy is stopped a few days before elective electrical conversion.

TREATMENT OF INTOXICATION

Because the therapeutic index of the glycosides is low and their duration of action long, and because treatment involves a clinical compromise between an effective therapeutic dose and one that causes adverse effects, intoxication is fairly common. Mortality among those with demonstrable adverse effects has been reported to be as high as 20%. Discontinuation of treatment must be considered as soon as the first adverse effects appear. For many, this is the only "treatment" required, and once these adverse effects disappear the glycoside may be resumed at a lower dose. Careful clinical observation during the period of initial digitalization is crucial.

A reduction in serum potassium sensitizes the myocardium to digitalis. If hypopotassemia occurs, for example, as a result of coincidently pursued diuretic or steroid therapy, toxic effects may become manifest following standard digitalis dosage. Under these circumstances the carefully controlled oral or, if necessary, parenteral administration of potassium may be effective in reducing intoxication within 1 hour. Parenteral injections must be made with extreme caution because too rapid injection can cause asystole or fibrillation. The administration of potassium is contraindicated when disturbances of conduction are detected. Elevated calcium levels predispose to digitalis toxicity, probably by contributing to intracellular calcium overload. Attempts to reduce toxicity by chelation, as with disodium versenate, have not been successful, partly because of the direct toxicity of the chelating agent.

Any antiarrhythmic drug can be used for drug therapy of digitalis intoxication, but lidocaine, phenytoin, and propanolol are the most popular (*see* Chap. 34). They are used in digitalis arrhythmias as in any other type.

DC countershock (cardioversion) frequently makes arrhythmias *worse* in the digitalized heart. This treatment therefore should be reserved only for ventricular fibrillation (which cannot be treated by any other method).

ALTERNATIVES TO DIGITALIS THERAPY

As noted above, the poor therapeutic index of the cardiac glycosides has encouraged the search for substitute therapies. Some of these involve dilation of blood vessels (hydralazine, nitrates, prazosin), an action that decreases cardiac preload, afterload, or both. The reduced oxygen requirement that results from this maneuver may allow a dramatic degree of compensation by the cardiac contractile mechanism. Dopamine and beta-adrenergic stimulants may improve cardiac performance by a combination of cardiac stimulation with vasodilation.

Amrinone is a new investigational inotropic agent that has no effect on digitalis or adrenergic receptors but a significant positive inotropic effect on the heart in patients with congestive heart failure. Its mechanism of action is unknown, as is its clinical safety.

FURTHER READING

1. Braunwald E, Ross J Jr, Sonnenblick EH: Mechanisms of Contraction of the Normal and Failing Heart. Boston, Little, Brown & Co., 1968
2. Marks BH, Weissler AM (eds): Basic and Clinical Pharmacology of Digitalis. Springfield, Illinois, Charles C Thomas, 1972
3. Mason DT: Afterload reduction and cardiac performance: Physiologic basis of systemic vasodilators as a new approach in treatment of congestive heart failure. Am J Med 65:106–125, 1978
4. Smith TW: Digitalis glycosides. N Engl J Med 288:719–722, 942–946, 1973

CHAPTER 33 QUESTIONS

(See P. 7 for Full Instructions)

Select the One Best Answer

1. The primary action of digitalis in the therapy of congestive failure is
   - A. diuresis.
   - B. A-V nodal blockade.
   - C. vagal blockade.
   - D. increased cardiac contractile force.
   - E. decreased central venous pressure.

2. Digitalis glycosides may be effective in the treatment of each of the following EXCEPT
   - A. atrial fibrillation.
   - B. atrial flutter.
   - C. congestive heart failure.
   - D. edema in the nephrotic syndrome.
   - E. paroxysmal atrial tachycardia.

3. Which of the following indicates the correct order of rank for duration of action after oral administration (from longest to shortest duration)?
   - A. Digoxin > digitoxin > ouabain
   - B. Digitoxin > digoxin > ouabain
   - C. Digitoxin > ouabain > digoxin.
   - D. Ouabain > digitoxin > digoxin.
   - E. Ouabain > digoxin > digitoxin.

4. The potential for cardiac toxicity of digitalis is increased by each of the following EXCEPT
   - A. triamterene.
   - B. ethacrynic acid.
   - C. chlorothiazide.
   - D. meralluride (a mercurial diuretic).
   - E. cortisol in high dose.

5. Digitalis pretreatment is recommended before attempting conversion of atrial fibrillation to normal sinus rhythm in order to
   - A. reduce the toxic effects of DC electroshock "cardioversion."
   - B. depress ectopic pacemakers.
   - C. suppress the gastrointestinal side-effects of quinidine.
   - D. protect against excessively high ventricular rate when quinidine is given.
   - E. produce a vasoconstrictor effect to maintain blood pressure.

A = 1,2,3; B = 1,3; C = 2,4; D = 4; E = All

6. Actions of digitalis on cardiac electrical activity may include
   1. slowed A-V conduction.
   2. slowed SA nodal rate.
   3. increased ectopic automaticity.
   4. increased atrial flutter rate.

7. Which of the following actions of digoxin are correctly matched with an appropriate therapeutic indication for that action?
   1. Increased vagal tone—paroxysmal atrial tachycardia
   2. Increased maximum velocity of shortening of ventricular muscle—congestive heart failure
   3. Prolonged refractory period of the A-V node—atrial flutter
   4. Increased ventricular automaticity—complete heart block

8. Agents that will increase cardiac output in the presence of cardiac failure induced by propanolol are
   1. dopamine.
   2. digoxin.
   3. isoproterenol.
   4. glucagon.

9. Effects of digitoxin resulting from an action on the central nervous system include
   1. vomiting.
   2. bradycardia.
   3. anorexia.
   4. diuresis.

10. The treatment of digitalis toxicity may justifiably include the administration of
    1. propanolol.
    2. calcium gluconate.
    3. potassium chloride.
    4. chlorothiazide.

BERTRAM G. KATZUNG

34

Antiarrhythmic Drugs

Antiarrhythmic drugs are used to control or to cure cardiac arrhythmias. *Arrhythmias* are defined as disorders of rate, rhythm, origin, or conduction of impulses within the heart. They are common manifestations of functional and anatomic cardiac disease. Various studies have estimated their incidence at 10% to 25% during digitalization of hospitalized patients, 20% to 50% in general anesthetic procedures, and 80% to 90% in patients with acute myocardial infarction. In fact, ventricular arrhythmias are the major cause of death following myocardial infarction.

PATHOPHYSIOLOGY OF ARRHYTHMIAS

The factors that precipitate arrhythmias may include ischemia with resulting hypoxia and *p*H and electrolyte abnormalities, excessive fiber stretch, excessive discharge of, or sensitivity to, autonomic regulator substances, and exposure to foreign chemicals such as digitalis and other potentially toxic substances. However, all arrhythmias result from one or a combination of the following fundamental conditions.

1. Abnormal impulse formation: automaticity defects.
2. Abnormal propagation of impulses: conduction defects.

The quantitative description of these defects requires an understanding of the electrical activity of cells in different parts of the heart and the way this electrical activity is propagated (Fig. 34-1).

DETERMINANTS OF AUTOMATICITY

The frequency of discharge of a spontaneously discharging cardiac cell is determined by the slope of phase 4 of the transmembrane electrical potential as well as by several other factors, as suggested in Figure 34-2. Normally the phase 4 slope of cells outside the normal pacemaker, the sinoatrial (SA) node, is less than that of SA cells. Under conditions conducive to arrhythmias, Purkinje or other cells may develop a steeper phase 4 slope and take over

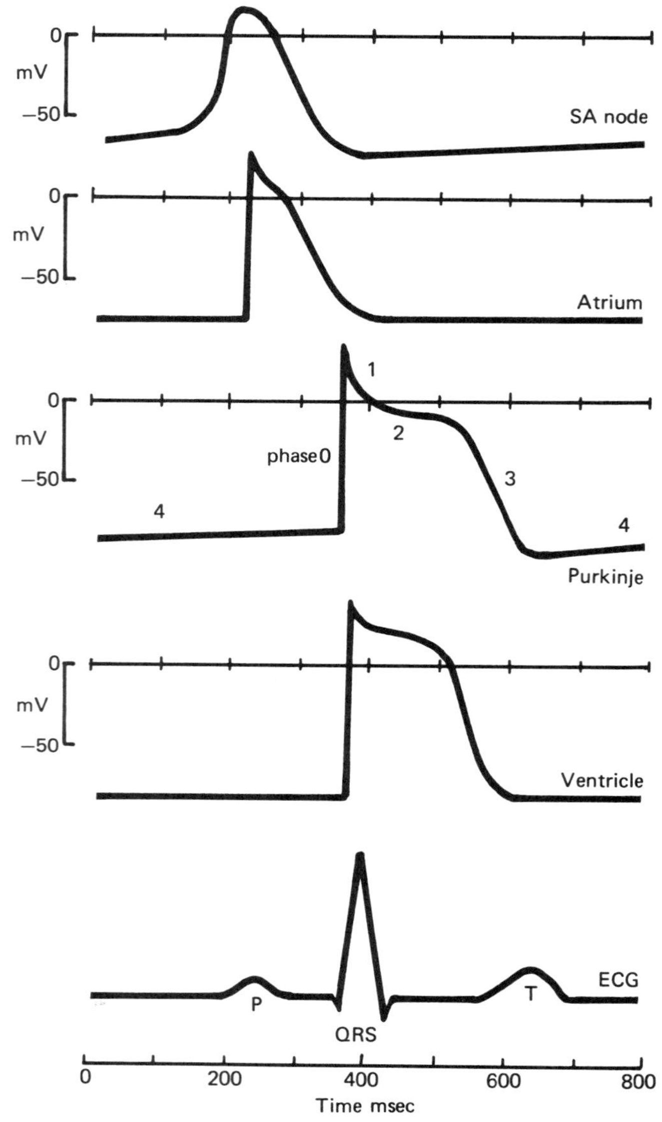

FIG. 34-1. Schematic drawing of typical transmembrane potential recordings from several areas of the heart and their relation in time to the electrocardiogram (*ECG*). The sinoatrial (*SA*) node recording is characterized by slow action-potential upstroke, low overshoot at the peak of the depolarization, and relatively rapid depolarization between action potentials (diastolic depolarization). The atrial action potentials differ primarily in their faster upstroke and flat (nonpacemaker) diastolic potential. The Purkinje fiber recording shows the conventional numbering for identifying the various phases of cardiac action potentials. Note that this fiber demonstrates a slow but definite pacemaker depolarization during phase 4, that is, it is a latent pacemaker. The ventricular pattern differs from that of a Purkinje fiber in having a stable diastolic potential and a somewhat shorter action potential duration. The ECG record illustrates the correlation of the P wave with atrial activity, the P–R interval with the A–V conduction delay, the QRS complex with ventricular depolarization, and the Q–T interval with the ventricular action potential duration.

pacemaker function—that is, they become ectopic pacemakers. Increased catecholamine concentration, depolarization, hypoxia, and hypokalemia are potential causes of increased phase-4 automaticity. In addition, agents that increase intracellular calcium, such as digitalis and catecholamines, may evoke oscillatory afterpotentials (Chapter 33). These afterpotentials are an important cause of extrasystoles. Common arrhythmias resulting from ectopic automaticity include ventricular escape rhythms, premature ventricular beats, and probably some ventricular tachycardias.

DETERMINANTS OF CONDUCTION

The excitability of electrically excitable cells is inversely proportional to the stimulus current required to change the membrane potential from its resting level to the threshold potential at which an all-or-none spike occurs. The effective refractory period is that time which must elapse after the start of one action potential before a second propagated action potential can be elicited. Once an action potential has been elicited, the ability of a cardiac cell to propagate the impulse can be estimated from the

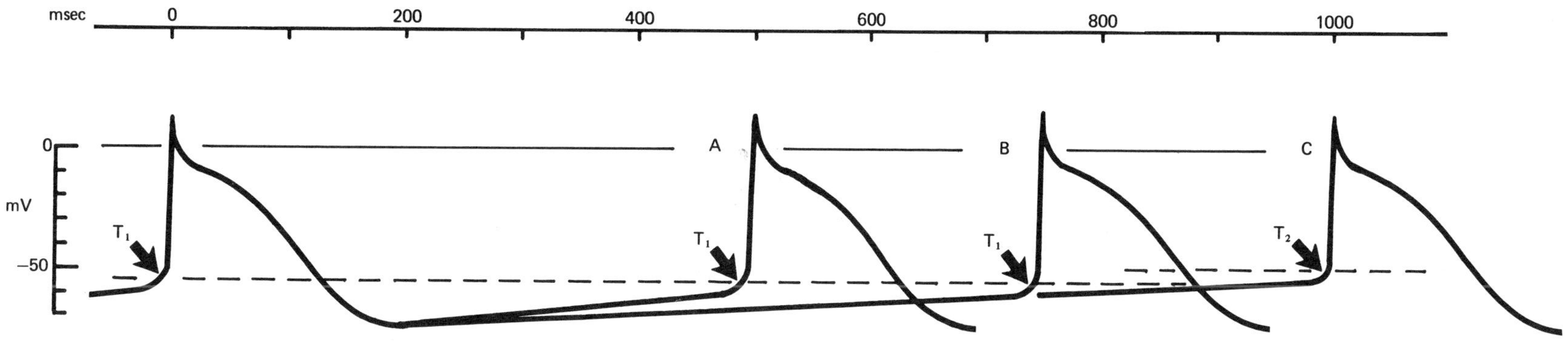

FIG. 34-2. Schematic representation of pacemaker activity in a Purkinje fiber. Trace A indicates the pretreatment condition in which diastolic depolarization causes threshold (T_1) to be reached every 500 msec, corresponding to a rate of 120 beats/min. Under the influence of a drug that slows diastolic depolarization (Trace B), the threshold is reached every 750 msec, corresponding to a rate of 80 beats/min. Trace C shows the effect of a drug such as quinidine that changes the threshold to a more positive potential (T_2) in addition to slowing diastolic depolarization. The combination of these two effects results in further slowing of the ectopic rate to 1 beat/sec or 60 min. Other variables also influence pacemaker rate, but phase 4 slope (diastolic depolarization) and threshold potential are the most important ones in determining antiarrhythmic drug effect on pacemakers.

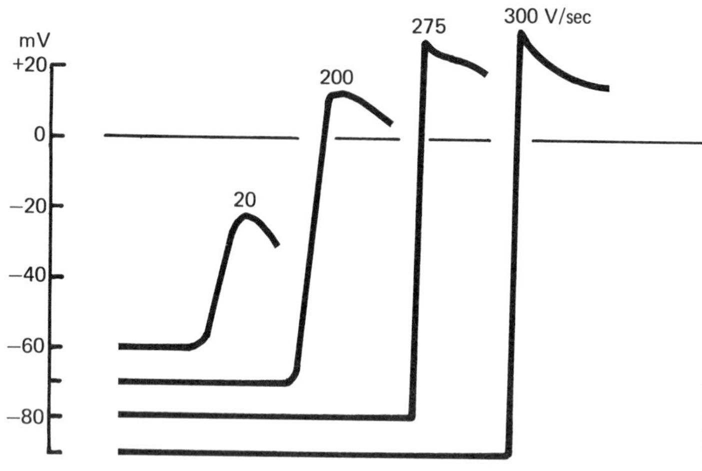

FIG. 34-3. Dependence of action potential upstroke velocity (numbers at each action potential peak, volts per second) and amplitude on the previous level of resting potential for a typical myocardial cell. Note that at resting potentials more negative than −80 mV, upstroke velocity stabilizes at a maximum level. At resting potentials less negative than −80 mV, upstroke velocity falls precipitously, declining to zero at −45 to −50 mV.

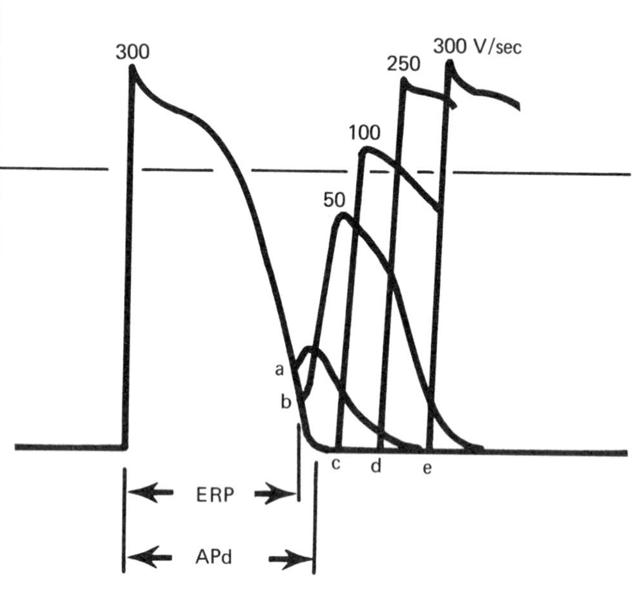

FIG. 34-4. Dependence of action potential upstroke velocity and amplitude on recovery time following the preceding action potential. Stimuli that arrive before completion of the effective refractory period (*ERP*) produce only a small, nonpropagated response (trace a). A stimulus arriving immediately after completion of the ERP results in a very small, slowly conducted response (trace b). Both of these early responses may occur before complete repolarization and are therefore depressed by the low "resting" potential at the time they are elicited according to the mechanism shown in Fig. 34-3. Even after full repolarization, however, an early extrasystole, *e.g.*, trace c, will be associated with slow upstroke and low amplitude, showing that these variables depend on recovery time as well as one membrane potential. In normal tissue, recovery requires only 10 to 20 msec. In depressed tissue, however, recovery may need 100 msec or more.

slope of phase 0—the maximum rate of depolarization—and the amplitude of the action potential. Both of these variables are measures of the sodium ion current that flows into the cell. As shown in Figures 34-3 and 34-4, these quantities are controlled by two major variables: The level of resting membrane potential, and the time allowed for recovery of the sodium mechanism following previous activity. Depressed "fast" conduction (Table 34-1) results from moderate depression of these variables.

Recent studies of severely depressed myocardium (such as that found in the region of a recent myocardial infarct) suggest that conduction may persist at resting potentials too positive to allow any sodium-dependent ionic currents. This conduction involves the slow response action potential, is very slow indeed (Table 34-1), and depends on an inward current of calcium ions.

Depression of conduction can lead to significant cardiac malfunction. Simple slowing or block results in such recognized arrhythmias as A-V blockade and bundle-branch block. More complex arrhythmias such as paroxysmal atrial tachycardia, A-V nodal tachycardias, and many ventricular tachycardias seem to result from the phenomenon of reentry (Fig. 34-5). In reentry, the arrhythmia depends on an intermediate degree of conduction depression; either normalization or further depression abolish the unidirectional block on which reentry depends. Further, the effective refractory period of the tissue in the circuit must be shorter than the conduction time.

EFFECTS OF IONS

The level of extracellular potassium ion (K_o) is important in modulating automaticity and conduction. Ectopic automaticity is suppressed by adequate or elevated K_o because the ion tends to reduce the slope of phase 4 (diastolic depolarization), especially in Purkinje fibers. Conduction velocity may be depressed by elevated K_o since increased K_o tends to reduce the resting membrane potential (Fig. 34-3) and to prolong the recovery time for the sodium conductance mechanism (Fig. 34-4). Normal cardiac rhythm implies minimal automaticity (outside the normal SA nodal pacemaker) but optimal conduction velocity. Thus increasing K_o might reduce ectopic automaticity but impair conduction.

MODES OF THERAPY OF THE ARRHYTHMIAS

Major modes of therapy include electrical pacemakers and DC electroshock ("cardioversion"), autonomic manipulation through drugs that stimulate or suppress normal autonomic regulatory mechanisms in the heart (*see* Chaps. 13–20), and direct pharmacologic manipulation of cardiac cell membrane properties. The major antiarrhythmic agents act via the last mechanism, including quinidine, procainamide, disopyramide, lidocaine, phenytoin, propranolol, amiodarone, and verapamil. Bretylium, an agent used only for the acute treatment of postmyocardial infarction arrhythmias, probably acts by reducing the release of catecholamines in the myocardium.

MODES OF ANTIARRHYTHMIC DRUG ACTION

Most antiarrhythmic agents reduce ectopic automaticity (Table 34-2) probably by reducing influx of the depolarizing cations sodium and calcium. Thus one obvious mechanism for their beneficial effects is the suppression of abnormal pacemakers. Arrhythmias caused by reentry mechanisms can be abolished in several ways (Fig. 34-5). Purely depressant effects on either "depressed fast" conduction or "slow" conduction (Table 34-1) may halt propagation and convert unidirectional block to bidirectional block. Prolongation of the effective refractory period could also precipitate bidirectional conduction block. Finally, improvement of conduction might convert a unidirectional

TABLE 34-1. Types of Cardiac Action Potentials

Types of Potential	Resting Potential	Conduction Velocity	Major Ion	Blocked By
	mV	*m/sec*		
Normal fast	−100 to −75	0.2 to 3	Sodium	Quinidine or lidocaine
Depressed fast	−76 to −60	0.05 to 0.2	Sodium	Lidocaine or quinidine
Slow	−65 to −40	0.01 to 0.05	Calcium	Verapamil

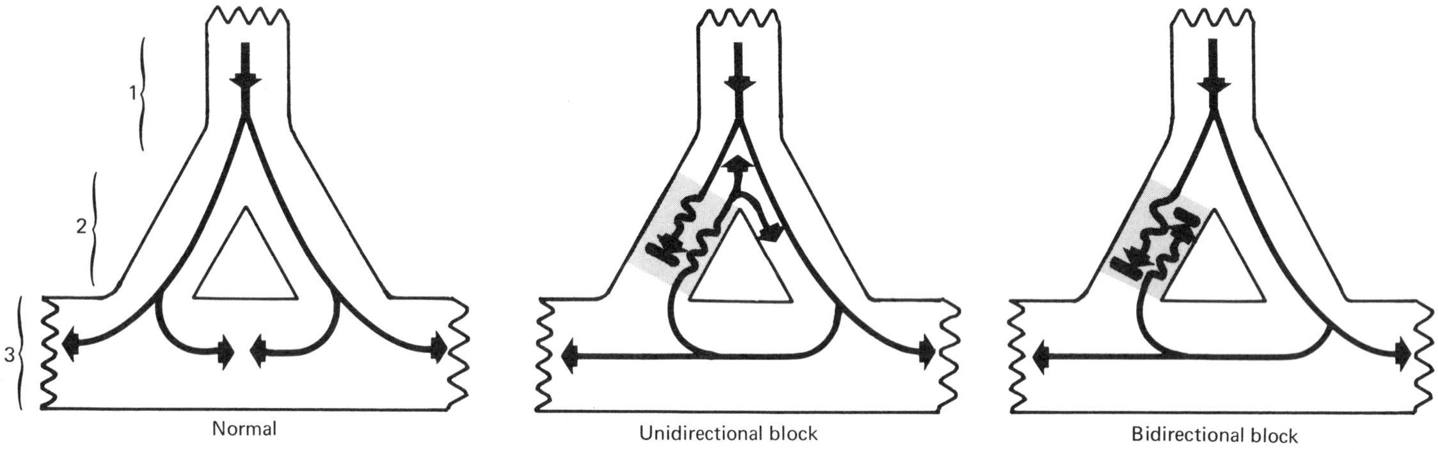

FIG. 34-5. Conduction patterns in a main Purkinje fiber (*1*), terminal Purkinje branches (*2*), and ventricular wall (*3*). (*Left*) Diagram shows how a normally conducted impulse would spread in the myocardium. (*Center*) Disease or drug toxicity may cause unidirectional conduction block. In this case the descending impulse in the left-hand branch enters a partially blocked or refractory (area (*shaded*) and is extinguished. The impulse from the right-hand branch, arriving somewhat later, can traverse the region and therefore reenters both the main fiber and the right branch, resulting in reexcitation and an arrhythmia. (*Right*) More severe depression of the Purkinje branch may result in bidirectional conduction block. Now the depressed area (*shaded*) will not conduct in either direction, thus reentry is prevented.

TABLE 34-2. Major Cardiac Effects of Antiarrhythmic Drugs

Drug	Action	ECG Changes
Quinidine, procainamide, disopyramide	Atria: decreased automaticity	Increased P-P
	A-V node: increased refractory period (direct)	
	Decreased conduction velocity (direct)	Increased P-R
	Increased conduction velocity (antivagal)	Decreased P-R
	His–Purkinje system: decreased automaticity	Decreased ectopic rate
	Ventricles: increased action potential duration	Increased QT
	Decreased conduction velocity	Increased QRS
Lidocaine, phenytoin	Atria: decreased automaticity (high doses or high serum K)	
	A-V node: no effect, facilitation, or depression of conduction	No effect, decreased or increased P-R
	His–Purkinje system: decreased automaticity	Decreased ectopic rate
	Decreased conduction velocity in depressed fast cells	
Propranolol	Atria: decreased SA automaticity	Increased P-P
	A-V node: decreased conduction velocity	Increased P-R
	His–Purkinje system: decreased automaticity	Decreased ectopic rate
Amiodarone	Atria, His–Purkinje system, and ventricles:	
	Increased action potential duration and refractory period	Increased QT
Verapamil	Atria: decreased SA automaticity (may be marked)	Increased P-P
	A-V node: decreased conduction velocity (may be marked)	Increased P-R
	His–Purkinje system, ventricular muscle: depressant effects minimal in normally polarized cells, marked in severely depressed (slow response) cells	

block to bidirectional conduction. All these effects would abolish reentry.

Conduction velocity is depressed in a *use-dependent* fashion by most antiarrhythmic agents; that is, membrane activity (as in a rapid tachycardia) facilitates more depressant drug effect. Further, most agents have a greater depressant effect in depolarized tissue than in normal myocardium.

Most antiarrhythmic agents increase the duration of the effective refractory period relative to the action potential duration (ERP/APd ratio). The result of this action is to prevent action potentials from occurring very close to a preceding one. Such "closely coupled" extrasystoles are more likely to be conducted abnormally and are therefore more likely to set up reentry circuits. Thus an increased ERP/APd ratio would reduce the incidence of reentry arrhythmias.

Because these effects tend to be more marked in partially depolarized tissue, the antiarrhythmic drugs may be considered *selective depressants*, that is, they abolish activity in damaged cells while leaving activity in normal cells relatively unaffected. Assuming that the total mass of damaged tissue is not too large, complete suppression of both automaticity and conduction in a localized area could result in abolition of both ectopic pacemaker and reentry arrhythmias.

QUINIDINE

Quinidine, the optical isomer of quinine (*see* Chap. 67), is obtained from the bark of the cinchona tree indigenous to South America and Indonesia. The use of cinchona extracts in cardiac disease resulted from the observation that the treatment of malaria with cinchona occasionally brings relief of coexisting cardiac arrhythmias.

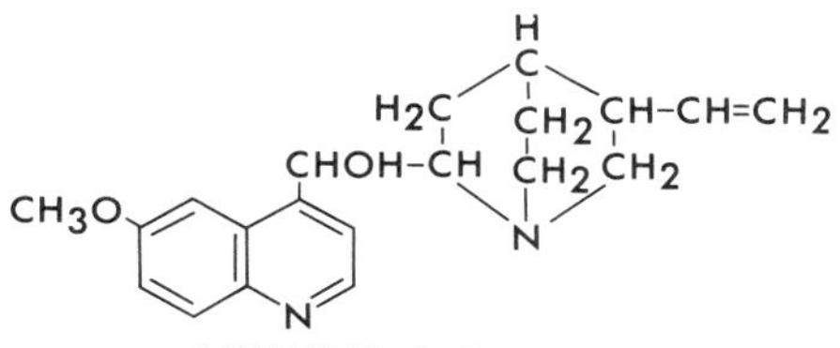

l-QUININE, D-QUINIDINE

Karl Frederik Wenckebach, 1862–1940. Viennese physician. In 1914 reported treatment of cardiac arrhythmia with quinine—on the patient's suggestion. Also remembered for his mechanical theory of cardiac pain in coronary occlusion (1928).

ACTIONS

Cardiac Effects

The major cardiac effects of quinidine (Table 34-2) on automaticity and conduction are depressant; the depression of automaticity is more marked in ectopic pacemakers (*e.g.*, Purkinje fiber) than in the SA node. Quinidine depresses excitability and increases the ERP/APd ratio. These actions are direct ones, exerted on the cardiac cell membrane.

Quinidine also has indirect effects on the heart that result from anticholinergic and antiadrenergic actions. Of these two autonomic effects, the anticholinergic one is more commonly seen. The only significant manifestation of this anticholinergic action is the occasional appearance of cardiac vagal blockade with increased A-V conduction velocity and sinus tachycardia.

In the presence of atrial fibrillation, A-V conduction time cannot be directly measured, but an antivagal effect on this variable is easily detected from an increased ventricular rate. These effects are readily prevented by prior administration of digitalis (*see* Chap. 33). When given in higher doses, quinidine can depress cardiac contractility.

Extracardiac Effects

Quinidine has no therapeutically useful extracardiac effects. It mimics its isomer, quinine, in having antimalarial, antipyretic, and oxytocic properties as well as modest stabilizing effects on the end-plate of skeletal muscle. In each of these effects, however, it is weaker than quinine.

MECHANISM OF ACTION

Quinidine reduces phase-4 depolarization slope in pacemaker cells probably through reduction of diastolic sodium influx. The result is reduction or abolition of ectopic pacemaker function. The drug also appears to reduce the transfer of sodium across the cell membrane during phase 0 of the action potential. This action occurs at all resting membrane potentials, and only extremely long recovery times can alleviate the depression. As a result, conduction velocity is decreased and refractory period prolonged. The effects on sodium influx are coincident with a decreased efflux of potassium. The reduction in potassium efflux may be responsible for the increased action potential duration and prolonged QT interval commonly observed after quinidine administration.

ABSORPTION, METABOLISM, AND EXCRETION

Quinidine, well absorbed from the gastrointestinal tract, is strongly bound (80%) to plasma proteins and is finally excreted in the urine, largely in the form of hydroxylated metabolites. The half-life of the parent compound in the plasma is 4 to 7 hours and is more likely to be prolonged in patients with congestive heart failure than in those with renal disease.

PREPARATIONS AND DOSAGE

Quinidine is almost always administered orally. The sulfate (U.S.P.) salt generally is used, although gluconate and polygalacturonate salts are available. Doses of 0.2 to 0.6 g may be given 4 to 6 times/day depending on the therapeutic goal or the appearance of serious toxicity. The therapeutic plasma concentration is 3 to 5 μg/ml. Quinidine gluconate injection, U.S.P., is soluble quinidine for i.v. use. Its administration is rarely justified because it is accompanied by a high incidence of untoward effects.

ADVERSE EFFECTS AND TOXICITY

Cardiac

At high plasma concentrations, quinidine may be a powerful cardiac depressant. It may cause depression of contractility, resulting in significant reduction of cardiac output, pacemaker arrest, and conduction block. Through nonhomogeneous impairment of condition, it may even precipitate cardiac arrhythmias, including ventricular fibrillation. These adverse effects are much more likely to occur at high serum potassium levels (greater than 5 mEq/liter) than at low ones.

Extracardiac

The most common side-effects of quinidine are gastrointestinal (nausea, vomiting, diarrhea). Along with quinine (and aspirin), quinidine may cause cinchonism (headache, dizziness, tinnitus). This drug is associated with occasional hypersensitivity reactions that may take the form of skin rash, angioneurotic edema, or thrombocytopenic purpura.

PROCAINAMIDE

Early in the development of local anesthetics it was found that procaine, an ester, had significant antiarrhythmic effects. Because procaine is so rapidly metabolized, the amide derivative, procainamide, was developed for cardiovascular applications.

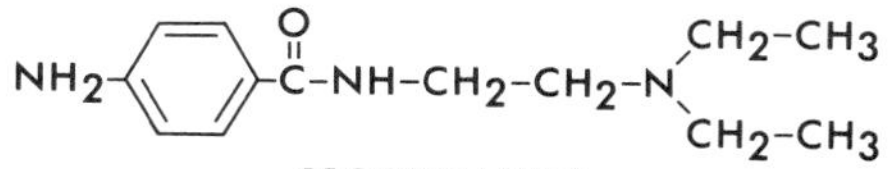

PROCAINAMIDE

ACTIONS

In almost every respect, procainamide can be considered equivalent to quinidine (Table 34-2): It reduces ectopic pacemaker rate, slows conduction velocity, and may increase the ERP/APd ratio. Like quinidine, it is sometimes associated with accelerated A-V conduction or sinus tachycardia. These effects can be prevented by digitalis administration.

ABSORPTION, METABOLISM, AND EXCRETION

Procainamide is well absorbed after oral administration and is excreted primarily by the kidneys. About 50% of the administered dose is metabolized. It has a half-life of 3 to 6 hours. The primary metabolic product, *n*-acetylprocainamide (NAPA), also has considerable antiarrhythmic action.

PREPARATIONS AND DOSAGE

Procainamide hydrochloride, U.S.P. (Pronestyl), is usually given orally in doses of 0.25 to 0.5 g, 3 to 4 times/day. A parenteral preparation is available, administered intramuscularly or intravenously. The therapeutic plasma level is 5 to 10 μg/ml.

ADVERSE EFFECTS AND TOXICITY

The adverse cardiac effects of procainamide, like its therapeutic effects, resemble those of quinidine but do not include cinchonism. Extracardiac effects include gastrointestinal upsets, hypotension (especially if given parenterally), and dizziness. Occasionally, a lupus erythematosuslike syndrome and agranulocytosis have been reported. The acetylated metabolite (NAPA) is said to have a slower onset of lupuslike complications.

DISOPYRAMIDE

Disopyramide is another quinidinelike antiarrhythmic. Its therapeutic cardiac effects can be considered equivalent to those of quinidine (Table 34-2).

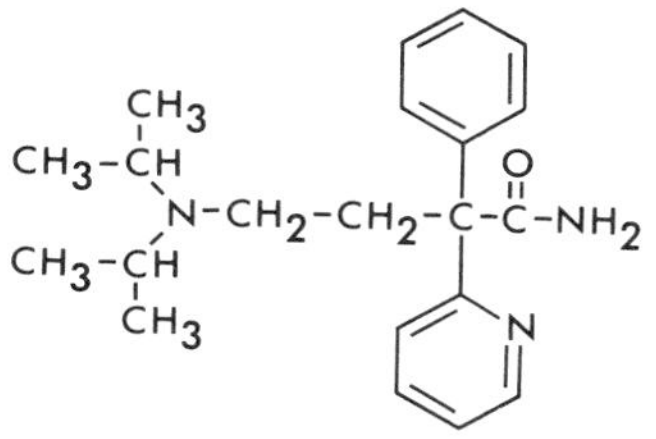

DISOPYRAMIDE

ABSORPTION, METABOLISM, AND EXCRETION

Disopyramide is readily absorbed after oral administration. It is partially protein bound in the plasma, metabolized, and excreted in the urine. Its half-life is 6 to 8 hours, considerably longer in patients with renal disease.

PREPARATION AND DOSAGE

Disopyramide phosphate, U.S.P. (Norpace), is currently available only for oral use; a parenteral preparation is available outside the United States. Usual dosage is 400 to 800 mg/day in divided doses. The therapeutic plasma level is about 3 μg/ml.

ADVERSE EFFECTS AND TOXICITY

As noted above, the cardiac effects of disopyramide resemble those of quinidine. In patients with preexisting myocardial insufficiency, disopyramide may precipitate severe cardiac failure. Disopyramide has more marked anticholinergic effects than either quinidine or procainamide and should be used with caution, if at all, in patients with glaucoma or urinary retention.

LIDOCAINE

Lidocaine has been an important local anesthetic for many years (*see* Chap. 20). It is also one of the most popular antiarrhythmic drugs for the acute treatment of ventricular arrhythmias and for arrhythmias caused by digitalis.

ACTIONS

In ordinary clinical use, the cardiac actions of lidocaine are more marked on the ventricles than on the atria. In general, the SA and A-V nodes are relatively resistant to depression by lidocaine, although occasional reports of severe bradycardia or A-V blockade have appeared. Under some circumstances, facilitation of A-V conduction has been reported. Experimentally one can readily demonstrate depression of conduction in Purkinje fibers and ventricular myocardium (Table 34-2). Like the previously described agents, lidocaine effectively reduces pacemaker activity in the ventricles.

MECHANISMS OF ACTION

The mechanism of the depressant action of lidocaine is similar, but not identical to, that of quinidine. The cell membrane is stabilized by inhibition of sodium influx. However, the inhibition of phase 0 sodium conductance is much greater at high rates (short recovery times) and is much more marked at low (less negative) membrane potentials than at high ones. The ERP/APd ratio is increased. Therefore lidocaine has minimal effects on conduction velocity of normal beats at slow heart rates. Early extrasystoles, on the other hand, especially in partially depolarized tissue, are very slowly conducted or abolished by the drug (Table 34-1, depressed fast potentials). Thus lidocaine is a highly selective depressant.

PREPARATION AND DOSAGE

Lidocaine hydrochloride, U.S.P. (Xylocaine), lignocaine, B.P., is inactive by the oral route (*see* Chap. 20) and is always given parenterally. The drug has a short half-life (cardiac effects last 15 to 30 minutes, elimination half-life is about 2 hours) and is therefore given either intermittently or by continuous infusion. When given intermittently, an initial i.v. dose of 1 to 2 mg/kg every 5 to 10 minutes usually yields effective plasma levels (1 to 5 μg/ml). Smaller supplements may be given every 30 minutes. Continuous infusions of 20 to 60 μg/kg/min may be used to achieve the same result.

ADVERSE EFFECTS

When limited to total doses of less than 300 mg and plasma levels of 5 μg/ml, serious toxicity from lidocaine is rare. Although electrical and contractile cardiac depression may occur (especially in the presence of high serum potassium concentration), most of the reported toxicity is restricted to the CNS (*see* Chap. 20).

PHENYTOIN

Phenytoin, an antiepileptic agent (*see* Chap. 29) has clear antiarrhythmic effects and is occasionally prescribed for its cardiac effect. It is not, however, considered the drug of choice for any arrhythmia.

ACTIONS

The major cardiac effects of phenytoin resemble those of lidocaine (Table 34-2). At low concentrations, the drug appears to be less depressant on atrial function (including SA and A-V nodes) than quinidine, and at plasma potassium concentrations less than 4 mEq/liter it appears to depress contractility less than the prototype agent. It is more effective in arrhythmias caused by digitalis than in other types of arrhythmias.

PREPARATIONS AND DOSAGE

Phenytoin sodium, U.S.P. (Dilantin), can be given orally or parenterally. The antiarrhythmic plasma concentration is 5 to 15 μg/ml. When used parenterally, doses of 100 mg are given intravenously every 5 minutes until the arrhythmia is abolished or until 10 doses have been given unless toxicity occurs first.

ADVERSE EFFECTS

The most common acute adverse effects of phenytoin are due to its action on the CNS (*see* Chap. 29). However, cases of cardiovascular collapse and cardiac arrest have been reported after i.v. use of this drug as an antiarrhythmic agent.

PROPRANOLOL

Propranolol is an important beta-adrenergic receptor blocking agent (*see* Chap. 18). It is listed here because one of its approved applications is in the therapy of arrhythmias. Probably a direct membrane stabilizing action augments the beta-adrenergic receptor blocking effect in causing a net antiarrhythmic effect. As indicated in Table 34-2, most of propranolol's direct effects are similar to those of quinidine and procainamide. It lacks the anticholinergic (indirect) effect of these two agents.

AMIODARONE

Amiodarone is not yet approved for use in the United States but is under intensive investigation in a number of clinical centers. Because it may be used when all other drugs fail, amiodarone is included here.

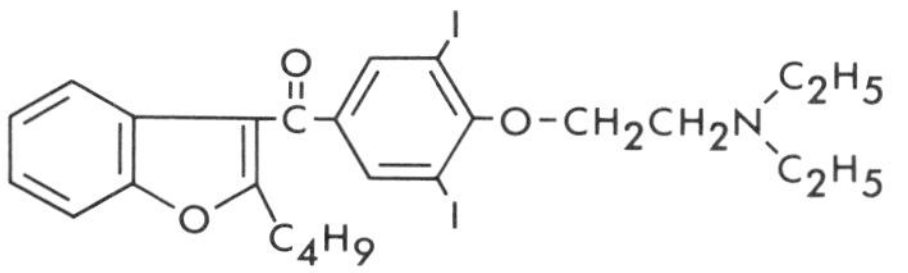

AMIODARONE

ACTIONS

Amiodarone has only modest depressant effects on normal pacemaker rate. It appears to depress action potential upstroke velocity, and conduction velocity. It also significantly prolongs action potential duration, perhaps through a change in potassium permeability. This action would be expected to prolong the effective refractory period.

PREPARATIONS AND DOSAGE

Amiodarone is an investigational agent that has been given by the i.v. and oral routes. Dosage for the oral route is 200 to 800 mg/day. The therapeutic plasma concentration range is not yet known. The elimination half-life is thought to be several weeks.

ADVERSE EFFECTS

Amiodarone induces many toxic effects. Because of its extremely long half-life, it is highly cumulative in the body, and caution in its use is essential. Most commonly reported effects are thyroid disorders (both hypothyroidism and hyperthyroidism), microcrystalline deposits in the eye, and pigmentation of the skin.

VERAPAMIL

Verapamil is a representative of a large group of drugs that interfere with transmembrane calcium current. Although only recently approved for use in the United States, it has been extensively used in Europe for more than a decade.

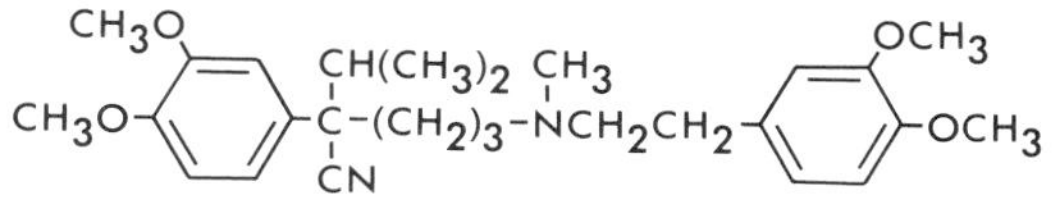

VERAPAMIL

ACTIONS

The major effect of verapamil is to *reduce transmembrane calcium flux* into cardiac and smooth muscle cells. Since contraction in both tissues depends on calcium influx, cardiac contractility is reduced and blood vessels are dilated. The cardiac action is highly use dependent (increased by an increased rate) and selective for depolarized tissue. Therefore the "slow response" (Table 34-1) is easily suppressed with verapamil.

PREPARATIONS AND DOSAGE

Verapamil is approved for use against supraventricular tachycardias in the United States. Parenteral and oral use have been extensively studied in Europe. Dosage is 0.05 to 0.1 mg/kg intravenously or 160 to 240 mg/day orally, in divided doses. The elimination half-life is 3 to 7 hours.

ADVERSE EFFECTS

The major toxicity of verapamil is a direct extension of its therapeutic effect: depression of cardiac function and hypotension. Sinoatrial arrest and A-V blockade have been reported. (Both nodes depend highly on calcium influx for normal electrical function.)

CLINICAL CONSIDERATIONS

EFFECTS OF ANTIARRHYTHMIC DRUGS ON THE ELECTROCARDIOGRAM

Since the electrocardiogram (ECG) provides a convenient measure of some electrical properties of the heart, it is an important tool for diagnosing arrhythmias and monitoring the effects of therapy. Some of the ECG effects of the antiarrhythmic drugs are summarized in Table 34-2.

The ECG manifestations of the cardiac effects of quinidine include increased P-P or R-R interval (slowing of rate); increased QT (prolonged action potential duration)—a very sensitive variable; increased QRS duration (slowing of intraventricular conduction); and, if direct effects predominate, a prolongation of the P-R interval (slowing of A-V conduction). If the indirect (antivagal) effect dominates, a decreased P-R interval may be observed. The effects of procainamide and disopyramide on the ECG are very similar to those of quinidine. With all three drugs, prolongation of the QRS interval by more than 30% is associated with an increased incidence of drug-induced arrhythmias and is avoided by stopping or decreasing the dosage.

The ECG effects of propranolol and verapamil differ from those of quinidine and procainamide because A-V conduction is uniformly depressed by the former agents and the ventricular action potential is not prolonged. Therefore propranolol and verapamil consistently prolong the P-R interval but have little effect on the QT interval.

The effects of lidocaine and phenytoin on the ECG are different from all of the above. Neither drug has notable effects on the ECG of normal sinus rhythm when given in low doses. In ventricular tachycardia, however, a reduced ectopic rate or conversion to normal sinus rhythm may be expected. In some cases of depressed A-V or intraventricular conduction, these agents may improve conduction and thereby normalize the ECG.

CLINICAL USE OF THE ANTIARRHYTHMIC DRUGS

As noted previously, use of antiarrhythmic drugs represents only one of several modes of treating arrhythmias. In selecting a specific antiarrhythmic drug, the following guidelines are representative. Quinidine remains the broad-spectrum antiarrhythmic of choice for most chronic atrial arrhythmias and many ventricular arrhythmias. Supraventricular tachycardias that involve abnormal conduction pathways are especially responsive to verapamil.

Procainamide and disopyramide are useful for chronic therapy in those patients who do not respond well or cannot tolerate quinidine. They are also recommended for the treatment of lidocaine-resistant arrhythmias following myocardial infarction.

Lidocaine is the most popular agent for the management of acute ventricular arrhythmias, especially those due to myocardial infarction. Because it must be given parenterally, it is used almost exclusively in hospitalized patients.

Propranolol is used only occasionally because of the hazard of excessive cardiac depression. However, it is extremely effective in controlling ventricular rate in the presence of very high atrial rates owing to its ability to depress A-V conduction.

Phenytoin, although available for decades, is still a poorly understood antiarrhythmic drug. Therefore, it is reserved for those arrhythmias that are refractory to all other therapies. For the same reason, its use as an antiarrhythmic is usually restricted to hospitalized patients. Amiodarone, which has been notably successful in some clinical studies but disappointing in others, is also reserved at present for arrhythmias refractory to all other treatment.

INTERACTIONS OF ANTIARRHYTHMIC DRUGS WITH OTHERS

The actions of quinidine, procainamide, and disopyramide can be significantly enhanced by a number of tranquilizer, antidepressant, and antihistamine drugs. In fact, these drug groups are occasionally used for their antiarrhythmic effects.

Quinidine (but apparently not procainamide or disopyramide) reduces the volume of distribution of digoxin and may increase the blood level of the cardiac glycoside twofold or more. Serious digitalis toxicity may result, although the quinidine would be expected to counter its cardiac effects to some extent. Quinidine has little or no effect on the blood levels of other cardiac glycosides.

Quinidine may also increase the effects of oral anticoagulants such as warfarin (*see* Chap. 42); therefore prothrombin levels should be monitored carefully in patients who receive both drugs.

Propranolol, because of its beta-adrenergic receptor blocking effects, predictably interacts with beta-adrenergic stimulants (*see* Chaps. 17,18).

Phenytoin, when used chronically, accelerates the metabolism of some drugs by the liver. Conversely, isoniazid has been reported to interfere with the hepatic metabolism of phenytoin. Large doses of phenytoin have reportedly displaced coumarin-type anticoagulants from plasma protein binding sites.

Finally, most of the antiarrhythmic drugs, including lidocaine, have two interactions in common: Their depressant actions on both electrical and mechanical functions of the heart are increased when serum potassium is high (greater than 5 mEq/liter); and all of these agents can augment or prolong the skeletal muscle paralysis produced by neuromuscular blocking drugs such as *d*-tubocurarine and succinylcholine (*see* Chap. 19).

FURTHER READING

1. Warnowicz MA, Denes P: Chronic ventricular arrhythmias: Comparative drug effectiveness and toxicity. Prog Cardiovasc Dis 23:225–236, 1980
2. Wit AL, Rosen MR: Cellular electrophysiology of cardiac arrhythmias, Parts 1 and 2. Concepts Cardiovasc Dis 50:1–6, 7–12, 1981
3. Zipes DP, Troup PJ: New antiarrhythmic agents: Amiodarone, aprindine, disopyramide, ethmozin, mexiletine, tocainide, verapamil. Am J Cardiol 41:1005–1024, 1978

CHAPTER 34 QUESTIONS

(*See* P. 7 for Full Instructions)

Select the One Best Answer

1. Clinical usefulness in treating both digitalis-induced ventricular arrhythmias and grand mal epilepsy best characterizes
   A. lidocaine.
   B. phenobarbital.
   C. sodium bromide.
   D. phenytoin.
   E. propranolol.

2. Sinus tachycardia can be treated with all of the following EXCEPT
   A. phenylephrine.
   B. digoxin.
   C. methacholine.
   D. propranolol.
   E. atropine.

3. The most probable mechanism of an arrhythmia induced by a toxic dose of quinidine is
   A. inhibition of Na/K-ATPase.
   B. increased automaticity of latent pacemakers.
   C. cholinergic effects on the SA node.
   D. reduced conduction velocity resulting in unidirectional block.
   E. decreased effective refractory period causing unidirectional block.

4. An agent useful in the treatment of both supraventricular arrhythmias and propranolol-induced cardiac failure is
   A. glucagon.
   B. digoxin.
   C. quinidine.
   D. lidocaine.
   E. procainamide.

5. Drugs commonly used for the treatment of cardiac arrhythmias also may have any of the following effects EXCEPT
   A. Cholinergic blocking effects.
   B. Adrenergic blocking effects.
   C. Ganglionic blocking effects.
   D. Local anesthetic effects.
   E. Anticonvulsant effects.

A = 1,2,3; B = 1,3; C = 2,4; D = 4; E = All

6. The effects of quinidine on heart muscle include
   1. decreased contractility.
   2. slowed atrial conduction.
   3. widened QRS.
   4. decreased ventricular refractory period.

7. Quinidine intoxication may result in
   1. tinnitus.
   2. thrombocytopenic purpura.
   3. diarrhea, nausea, and vomiting.
   4. ventricular arrhythmias.

8. Procainamide
   1. can cause a lupus erythematosus-like syndrome.
   2. may cause asystole in patients with partial or complete heart block.
   3. toxicity includes premature ventricular contractions.
   4. decreases membrane responsiveness.

9. Drugs that can abolish reentry arrhythmias include
   1. quinidine.
   2. phenytoin.
   3. lidocaine.
   4. verapamil.

10. Which of the following antiarrhythmic substances must be given parenterally?
   1. Quinidine
   2. Phenytoin
   3. Potassium
   4. Lidocaine

35

JOHN A. BEVAN

Antianginal and Vasodilator Drugs

In some diseases of the blood vessels, the blood flow to, and, in consequence, the oxygen supply and nutrition of, certain organs or regions of the body becomes inadequate. Metabolites accumulate. If the diminution in blood supply is other than temporary or is not adequately treated, cellular viability is threatened and serious symptoms and signs occur. The most important clinical entity included in this group is ischemic heart disease associated with a compromised blood flow to the myocardium. Angina pectoris is the most commanding symptom. Peripheral vascular disease associated with vascular insufficiency most importantly of the brain and skeletal muscles of the lower limbs is the other condition where vasodilator therapy may be advantageous.

In the absence of any therapy specific to the disease process, diminution in blood flow may be ameliorated pharmacologically in two ways: blood flow to the deprived tissues may be increased; or the metabolic requirements of the cells supplied by the diseased vascular bed may be reduced. Drugs that act by both mechanisms are described herein. The most important group of vasodilators, the *nitrites*, are often very effective in treating angina because they reduce the oxygen demands of the heart by a vasodilator action on the peripheral circulation. The β-adrenergic receptor blocking agent *propranolol* is helpful in angina because it reduces myocardial oxygen requirements by reducing the sympathetic drive to the myocardium; at the same time, it increases coronary blood flow to diseased or ischemic parts of the myocardium. A group of drugs usually described as vasodilators act either by reducing sympathetic drive to the blood vessel or by directly relaxing vascular smooth muscle through various molecular mechanisms.

NITRITES AND NITRATES

A group of inorganic and organic nitrites and organic (but not inorganic) nitrates shares the ability to relax all smooth muscle, particularly that found in the blood vessel wall but including that in the bronchi and in the gastrointestinal tract, including the biliary system. The actions of nitrites and nitrates are the same. These drugs differ in their rate of onset, duration of action, potency, and mode of administration.

ACTIONS

Nitrites relax smooth muscle by direct action. The word "direct" is used because the effect does not depend on muscle innervation and is not mediated by means of known types (adrenergic, cholinergic, and histaminergic) of pharmacologic receptors. These drugs may act by increasing cellular levels of cyclic GMP via the formation of an intermediate nitric oxide (NO), which has marked relaxant properties. The nitrites act as physiological antagonists to all drugs and nervous influences that increase smooth muscle tone. Fortunately, not all smooth muscle is equally sensitive to nitrites and nitrates. Doses can be given that reduce the tone of the circulation without noticeably affecting other systems and, within the circulation, certain regional vascular beds without significantly affecting others.

Within the cardiovascular system, muscle tone in the resistance and capacitance vessels is reduced. The consequence of this on the circulation as a whole varies widely and depends not only on the dose, preparation, and rate of administration of the drug but on the patient's compensatory capacity (*see* below) and developed tolerance to the drug. Venous dilation results in decreased venous return, with subsequent reduced filling of the heart. Both right and left end-diastolic pressures are reduced. This effect, combined with a usually modest reduction in systemic and pulmonary arteriolar resistance, leads to a fall in systemic arterial pressure and a reduced ventricular afterload. This is followed by activation of compensatory arterial baroreceptor and other reflexes. When, for example, amyl nitrite is given to the young adult, the heart rate increases modestly, and both systolic and diastolic arterial pressures fall. The fall in diastolic pressure reflects the change in total peripheral resistance that occurs mainly in the coronary, cerebral (including meningeal and retinal), and skin vessels. The fall in systolic pressure is the result of an increased venous capacity and the consequent decreased venous return and cardiac filling. Tachycardia is a compensatory mechanism. The effect of these drugs on the circulation is more pronounced in the vertical than in the horizontal position. Thus the final response to the drug is the net result of many interacting primary and compensatory factors.

"Monday morning disease"—Those exposed to nitroglycerin at work, e.g., in munitions factories during World War II, develop tolerance to its physiological effects, but symptoms can reappear after a weekend at home.

Myocardial oxygen consumption is related to cardiac work. The indirect effects of the nitrite on the myocardium resulting from peripheral vasodilation—decreased heart size resulting from decreased ventricular and diastolic pressure, and thus resistance to ventricular ejection, and decreased systolic pressure and myocardial afterload—would tend to decrease myocardial oxygen consumption. The reflex sympathetically mediated compensatory changes would increase the work of the heart and heart oxygen needs. These would mitigate against, but never completely negate, the immediate effects of the nitrite on heart function.

Although nitrites do dilate coronary blood vessels and this action may, in the healthy young adult, contribute to an increased coronary blood flow, in the diseased heart, when myocardial ischemia itself acts as a potent dilator mechanism through the local production of metabolic products, this effect is probably unimportant. Direct nitrite action is, however, probably the primary mechanism in the treatment of vasospasm (*see* below), a disease of middle-sized arteries. Such vessels are not influenced by the accumulation of local metabolites.

PREPARATIONS AND DOSAGE

Many preparations are available (Fig. 35-1). Some representative ones are described below in order of decreasing rate of onset and increasing duration of action. Nitrites are explosive and for safety are made up into large bulky tablets with a large amount of excipient.

Amyl nitrite, N.F., is inflammable and volatile. It is prepared in glass pearls that are crushed and the contents inhaled. It acts within 5 to 15 seconds and lasts for 5 to 10 minutes. The dose is 0.1 to 0.3 ml by inhalation. Some consider these effects too brief to be valuable therapeutically.

Glyceryl trinitrate, *U.S.P.* (nitroglycerin, trinitrin TNG), and isosorbide nitrate are administered as sublingual tablets because they are well absorbed through the buccal mucosa. Since there is no significant difference between these drugs administered sublingually, nitroglycerin, because of its economy, is the drug of choice for treating an acute anginal attack and its prophylaxis. Latency of action is less than 3 min; effects last up to 30 minutes. The doses of nitroglycerin and isosorbide are 0.2 to 0.6 mg and 5 mg sublingually, respectively. For maximum rapidity of action, the tablet may be crushed between the teeth and flushed around

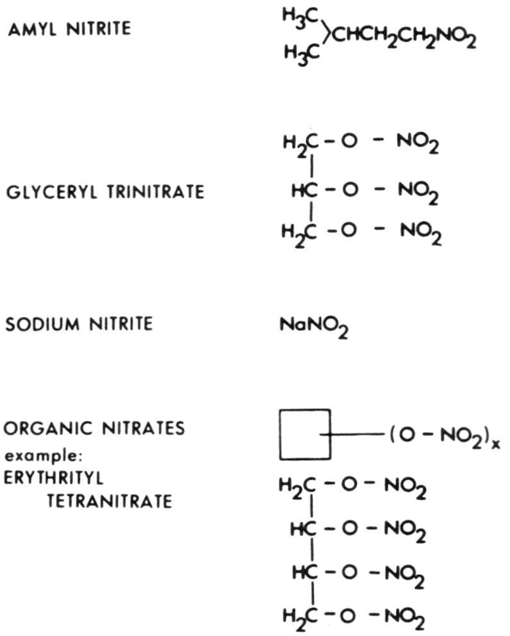

FIG. 35-1. Some representative nitrites.

the buccal cavity with the tongue. These drugs are considerably less effective when swallowed because, after absorption, they must pass through the liver where they are metabolized during one passage by glutathione organic nitrate reductases to inactive products before reaching their site of action. Fresh tablets must be used because the drugs are inactivated easily and even deteriorate after fairly optimal storage for prolonged periods. Tablets should be temporarily kept in the refrigerator and carried around in a stoppered dark container.

There are many oral sustained-release formulations and some for topical application. Although not initially accepted, nitrites administered topically in large amounts have been shown to cause *significant hemodynamic change* and to be valuable therapeutically. Dosage, however, must be carefully adjusted.

Sodium nitrite, U.S.P, is taken orally. It is effective within 5 to 20 minutes, and its action is maintained for 1 to 2 hours. Because of its toxicity (*see* below), it is rarely used except intravenously in the treatment of cyanide poisoning.

Organic nitrates—such as, erythrityl tetranitrate, mannitol hexanitrate, and pentaerythritol tetranitrate—are complex organic molecules that contain 4 to 6 nitrate groups. Their effects are slow in onset but persist for 3 to 6 hours. There is little reason for selecting one over another, and there are a variety of preparations for use. Only when administered in high dose have circulatory changes and therapeutic efficacy over a long period been demonstrated. Unfortunately such doses often result in some side-effects or tolerance to their pharmacologic actions.

CLINICAL USES

Angina Pectoris

The pain of angina pectoris is one of ischemia resulting from a relative hypoxia of the myocardium. It often occurs during physical or mental stress and, in some cases, during rest. Vasospasm of the coronary arteries appears to be a feature of the latter form—variant (Prinzmetal) angina—as well as a component of the more classic disease-state. In both diseases atherosclerosis may play an important role.

The flow of blood through the coronary arteries that run on or near the surface of the heart is little affected by pressure changes within the heart itself. In contrast, blood flow through the vessels that ramify within the heart muscle, especially those subjacent to the endocardium, is greatly influenced by pressure in the ventricle and within the myocardial wall. Most flow occurs during diastole and is related to the difference between diastolic aortic and intramyocardial pressures. This flow is jeopardized in angina pectoris and must be increased relative to the needs of the heart muscle.

In most studies of patients with angina, nitrites have been found to cause little change in net total coronary flow. Evidence suggests, however, that because of redistribution effects, regional flow through ischemic areas is improved. Although the mechanism is not clear, the nitrites, by increasing flow through large epicardial channels, even if they are diseased, may preferentially increase flow through subendocardial vessels that are dilated by local ischemia when the load on the heart is reduced.

An atheromatous lesion in a large coronary artery is equivalent to a fixed or constant narrowing of the blood vessel. This constriction tends to dominate the resistance pattern of the vessel so that flow is not primarily controlled by changes in arteriolar diameter. Consequently adaptation of the vascular bed to extremes of changes in aortic pressure (perfusion pressure) is poor. Pathologic constriction of a larger coronary vessel results over the long term in collateral vessel growth and changes in the overall pattern of blood flow; an area of myocardium that receives its blood supply through a comparatively normal artery may be linked to a poorly vascularized area. One consequence is that the heart is not uniformly vascularized and some parts, for example, those at rest that receive only a marginal supply, might during stress "steal" blood from a normally vascularized section and vice-versa. The consequences of such changes can be diminished by decreasing at the same time the global and regional myocardial oxygen requirements of the heart muscle, particularly when compensatory changes are not brisk.

Nitrites are used to abort or shorten an impending anginal attack and to prevent or reduce the incidence of attacks. Amyl nitrite or glyceryl trinitrite dramatically relieves anginal pain and, when taken during the prodromal symptoms or immediately before conditions known to precipitate angina (*e.g.*, exercise), may abort an attack. Some patients prefer isosorbide.

Prolonged administration leads to tolerance, although tolerance to adverse effects usually develops before that to therapeutically useful actions. Despite this, in clinical practice tolerance is rarely a therapeutic problem. Sudden withdrawal of nitrites has resulted in death probably due to coronary vasospasm. The original sensitivity returns rapidly when the drug is withheld. Cross-tolerance between preparations is not absolute.

Administration of long-acting nitrites is of value in the long-term prophylaxis of anginal attacks. The apparently well-established opinion that nitrites are contraindicated in the acute treatment of myocardial infarction has recently been challenged. The effectiveness of nitrites is obviously dose dependent. If their peripheral vascular actions lower aortic pressure too much, many of their advantageous actions are offset by a reduction in coronary perfusion pressure and hence flow. The optimum compromise must be achieved. In practice this depends on the dose used and the timing of its administration. These are usually decided by the patient by a process of trial and error. However, since adequacy of treatment is largely in the hands of the patient, he must be well instructed in the objectives of therapy.

Thomas Lauder Brunton, 1844–1916. London physician. In 1867 administered amyl nitrite, known as a vasodepressor, to relieve anginal pain. Also worked with digitalis. One of the founders of modern pharmacology.

Heart Failure

The performance of the left ventricle is closely related to the resistance encountered by ventricular outflow during systole. Thus an inappropriately high resistance to ejection might actually, particularly in the failing heart, lead to increased ventricular volume and then to reduced stroke volume. Nitrites reduce ejection impedance and ventricular preload, resulting in decreased left ventricular filling pressure and consequently ventricular filling. Patients with congestive heart failure associated with high left ventricular filling pressure and resistance to ventricular outflow would benefit from such an action. Nitrites have been used effectively on these variables over a period of many months. The use of nitrites for this condition reflects the growing acceptance of dilator therapy in heart failure.

Other Uses

Nitrites have been used to relieve *biliary spasm* and that of the *urinary tract*.

ADVERSE EFFECTS

Fainting

Particularly in the hypertensive patient and during warm weather, the response to nitrites may be exaggerated or prolonged. The patient may faint or exhibit prolonged hypotension, effects that are an exaggeration of the drugs' therapeutic action in a poorly adapting circulation. With practice, however, most patients learn to adjust dosage remarkably well to their individual needs and circumstances.

Headache

Nitrites may cause a painful throbbing headache associated with the dilation of cerebral or meningeal vessels and an increased cerebrospinal pressure. Tolerance to this frequently develops before that to other therapeutically advantageous cardiovascular effects.

Methemoglobinemia

Nitrites oxidize the ferrous iron of hemoglobin to the ferric form that does not carry oxygen. A functional anemia results. Although this is usually a disadvantageous effect of nitrites, this formation is used to treat cyanide poisoning.

Cyanide poisoning occurs under various circumstances: industrial—metallurgy, chemical synthesis; and domestic—insecticides, silver polish, and as result of the ingestion of fruit, particularly apricot kernels and preparations such as *laetrile* that are derived from these. Deaths allegedly due to cyanide poisoning have been reported in all these circumstances. Cyanide reacts with cellular cytochrome oxidase to inhibit respiration. In the presence of methemoglobin, and because cyanide has greater affinity for methemoglobin, the cytoplasm oxidase–cyanide complex dissociates and forms cyanomethemoglobin, restoring cellular respiration. Thiosulfate is then given to detoxify the hemoglobin through the formation of thiocyanate ion. This treatment supposedly protects against several lethal doses of cyanide.

The principle of treatment is to form methemoglobin as rapidly as possible in the body. In the adult, sodium nitrite (0.3–0.5 g) is administered intravenously over several minutes in 10 to 15 ml of saline, followed by sodium thiosulphate (10–15 g) given slowly intravenously and very diluted (up to 50 ml) over 10 to 15 minutes. This schedule can be repeated at half dosage if subsequently indicated by the emergence of symptoms.

PROPRANOLOL

β-Adrenergic receptor blocking agents, in particular propranolol, are now established agents in the therapy of angina pectoris. Only those features of the action of this drug related to the treatment of angina are described herein. (For other actions, *see* Chaps. 18, 34, 36.)

ACTIONS

Blockade of tonic sympathetic activity to the heart by β-adrenoceptor blockade results in negative inotropic and chronotropic effects, reducing oxygen requirements. The augmentation of myocardial activity during stress or exercise is thus minimized by such treatment. The effects of blockade of the β-adrenergic receptors on the coronary vasculature are complex and vary with the size of the vessels. Propranolol may exacerbate variant angina by increasing the spastic state of the coronary arteries responsible for this condition. Propranolol is believed by some to alter distribution of coronary blood flow, resulting in improved flow to ischemic areas.

Propranolol blocks the reflex compensatory stimulation of the heart—tachycardia and increased contractility that results from nitrite-induced and its own self-induced hypotension—thus reducing the effective dose of nitrite required and prolonging the therapeutically advantageous effect. There is some therapeutic advantage, especially if side-effects associated with β-adrenergic receptor blockade are obtrusive, in using a β_1 adrenoceptor antagonist (*see* Chap. 18).

DOSAGE AND ADMINISTRATION

Propranolol is usually indicated in patients with angina pectoris due to coronary artery disease who take nitrites daily. It reduces the number of times the patient will need to take the nitrite and lowers the effective dose. The dosage of propranolol varies widely and must be determined in each patient. Significant tolerance does not seem to develop. The drug is usually contraindicated in the treatment of failing myocardium because propranolol reduces compensatory supportive sympathetic drive, and thus exacerbates the underlying condition. It also depresses atrioventricular conduction, which limits its use in any condition complicated by some degree of A-V block. Because of functional rebound effects, the drug should not be withdrawn abruptly. Other general considerations are discussed in Chapter 34.

OTHER DRUGS USED IN ANGINA PECTORIS

Many agents reputedly are effective coronary vasodilators and thus are used to treat angina pectoris. Many of these drugs, including ethyl alcohol, nicotinic acid, nicotinyl tartrate, theophylline derivatives, androgens, and vitamin E, are considered by most cardiologists to be totally ineffective.

Dipyridamole (Persantin) causes coronary artery and arteriolar dilation by antagonizing the uptake of adenosine released from the hypoxic myocardium. Adenosine is a potent vasodilator and a physiological regulator of coronary blood flow. Despite the lack of convincing proof of therapeutic advantage of this drug as a prophylactic, it is prescribed by many physicians. Dipyridamole interferes with platelet function by potentiating prostacycline action (*see* Chap. 53).

VASODILATOR DRUGS

Drugs used to treat vascular insufficiency to organs other than the heart cause vasodilation by various mechanisms. It seems unlikely that pharmacologic action can improve the consequences of a mechanical obstruction by merely acting on existing blood vessels, yet some believe that improvement in some patients does occur. This brings into question the pathology proposed for these diseases.

α-ADRENERGIC RECEPTOR BLOCKING AGENTS

Because α-adrenoceptors are predominant in the cutaneous circulation, the effect of tonic sympathetic neurogenic activity on this part of the circulation should be effectively inhibited by α-adrenergic receptor blocking agents (*see* Chap. 18). These drugs exhibit some additional direct vasodilator properties whose basis is unknown. Although these agents are of considerable scientific interest, their clinical usefulness in vascular insufficiency is essentially restricted to the treatment of that in the limbs, particularly the skin, and is seriously limited by the adverse effects they cause. *Tolazoline* (Priscoline), *phentolamine* (Regitine), and *azapetine* (Ilidar) have all been used.

β-ADRENOCEPTOR AGONISTS

β-Adrenoceptors are preponderant in the vascular bed of skeletal muscle. Although the flow through this bed is regulated mostly by the metabolic products of muscular exercise, β-receptor agonists are used to treat reduced blood flow. *Isoxsuprine hydrochloride* and *nylidrin hydrochloride*, the best known in this class, are similar in action to isoproterenol but are orally active, act longer, and have direct smooth muscle relaxant properties. Some claim that their long-term administration may hinder the progress of disease.

PAPAVERINE

Papaverine is an opium alkaloid that relaxes vascular muscle irrespective of the cause of the contraction and possibly even when in spasm. Papaverine is believed to inhibit phosphodiesterase activity and adenosine uptake into the muscle cells. Local adenosine release may be related to the active dilation of the blood vessel wall. Papaverine is used to manage the spasm of collateral vessels after embolization in the limbs and the pulmonary circulation, and primary spasm in pulmonary and cerebral vessels.

Papaverine hydrochloride, U.S.P., is dispensed as tablets and sustained-release capsules and for systemic injection. The recommended dose is 100 to 300 mg three or four times daily.

VASODILATOR DRUGS AND HEART FAILURE

Reduced ventricular afterload is important in treating moderate to severe heart failure (*see* Nitrites above). Nitroprusside (*see* Chap. 36), nitrites, hydralazine, and prazosin (*see* Chap. 18)—and possibly the converting enzyme inhibitor captopril (*see* Chap. 55) that inhibits the coincidentally raised plasma renin levels in these conditions—have all been claimed to be efficacious. The role of such therapy, particularly their possible combination with positive inotropic drugs (*see* Chap. 33), awaits careful assessment.

FURTHER READING

1. Aronow WS: Use of nitrates and antianginal agents. In Needleman P (ed): Organic Nitrates: Handbuch der Experimentellen Pharmakologie Vol 40, pp 163–174. Berlin, Springer–Verlag, 1975
2. Coffman JD: Vasodilator drugs in peripheral vascular disease. Am J Hosp Pharm 32:1276–1281, 1975
3. Hillis LD, Braunwald E: Coronary artery spasm. N Engl J Med 13:695–702, 1978
4. Murad F, Arnold WP, Mittal CK et al: Properties and regulation of guanylate cyclase and some proposed functions for cyclic GMP. Adv Cyclic Nucleotide Res 11:175–204, 1979

CHAPTER 35 QUESTIONS

(See P. 7 for Full Instructions)

Select the One Best Answer

1. An attack of angina pectoris is most rapidly relieved by
   A. pentaerythritol tetranitrate.
   B. aminophylline (theophylline ethylenediamine).
   C. amyl nitrite.
   D. procaine amide.
   E. guanethidine.

2. All of the following agents have been implicated in the production of methemoglobinemia EXCEPT
   A. pentaerythritol tetranitrate.
   B. primaquine.

C. sulfanilamide.
D. amyl nitrite.
E. phenacetin.

3. The therapeutic effectiveness of nitrites in the treatment of angina pectoris is primarily the result of
A. decreased coronary sinus pressure associated with coronary vein dilation.
B. an absolute increase in myocardial blood flow.
C. an augmentation of metabolite-induced vasodilation.
D. decreased cardiac work associated with decreased cardiac preload and afterload.
E. decreased coronary resistance.

A = 1,2,3; B = 1,3; C = 2,4; D = 4; E = All

4. Angina pectoris may be effectively treated with
1. caffeine.
2. propranolol.
3. ethyl alcohol.
4. nitroglycerin.

5. A therapeutic sublingual dose of glyceryl trinitrate (nitroglycerin)
1. frequently produces a headache.
2. generally produces marked methemoglobinemia.
3. usually dilates capacitance vessels.
4. generally decreases coronary flow in patients with angina pectoris.

6. Propranolol is often used in conjunction with nitrites in the treatment of angina because it
1. reduces the effect of released endogenous catecholamine on the coronary circulation.
2. antagonizes some of the reflex circulatory consequences of nitrite administration.
3. uncouples the interrelationship between myocardial metabolic activity and vascular dilation.
4. prevents the consequences of surges of sympathetic activity on the myocardial workload.

7. Which of the following drug actions on the indicated tissues would *not* be expected to cause vasodilation?
1. Papaverine on pulmonary muscular arteries
2. Beta-adrenoceptor antagonists on skeletal muscle arterioles
3. Hydralazine on renal vascular bed
4. Cocaine on oral mucosal membrane arterioles

MATTHEW E. CONOLLY

36

Antihypertensive Drugs

Treatment, especially in younger patients, must begin with a thorough evaluation to eliminate any surgically remediable lesion. However, most patients presenting with elevated blood pressure prove to have essential hypertension; lifelong treatment with an ever expanding array of blood pressure lowering agents awaits them. Such drugs have done much to lower cardiovascular mortality and morbidity since reduction of blood pressure became a reality 30 years ago.

It is common to hear of the "stepped approach" to hypertension therapy in which, starting with diuretics, successive ranks of antihypertensive drugs are used. Although this approach has pragmatic value, especially if hypertension clinics are manned by paramedical personnel, in reality hypertension is far too complex and the drugs far too subtle in their effects for such an approach to be intellectually satisfying or clinically ideal. The aim of the clinician treating hypertension should be to understand each drug, the way in which it works, and the likely side-effects, so that combinations of drugs can be chosen judiciously and tailored to each person to provide as much pressure control with as few side-effects as possible (Table 36-1).

DRUGS AVAILABLE FOR TREATING HYPERTENSION

DIURETICS

More commonly in North America than in Europe, diuretics form the starting point and foundation of antihypertensive therapy. Their effect is to reduce blood volume by promoting loss of salt and water through the kidneys. Secondarily, they may change the ionic composition of the vasculature, altering the reactivity of arteriolar smooth muscle. Experience has shown that, although effective in many cases, such treatment is not wholly benign, and serious complications may arise from diuretic therapy. In Chapter 40, the mechanism of action of the diuretics and their side-effects are described systematically.

Clinical Use of Diuretics in Hypertension

In most patients, a cheap and simple thiazide will suffice. Except for furosemide, the dose-response curve for these drugs is flat, and no extra hypotensive effect will be obtained by increasing the dose to levels higher than those generally recommended. With furosemide, however, in order to achieve a diuretic effect in

TABLE 36-1. Drug Interactions That Reduce Antihypertensive Efficacy

Hypotensive Agent	Interfering Drug	Mechanism
1. Adrenergic neuron blocking drugs	Tricyclic antidepressants Amphetamine	Inhibition of neuronal uptake
2. Methyldopa	Amphetamine	Uncertain
3. Clonidine	Amphetamine	Uncertain
2. Diuretics (especially furosemide)	Nonsteroidal antiinflammatory agents	?Inhibition of a prostaglandin-dependent mechanism in kidney.
3. Propranolol	Nonsteroidal antiinflammatory agents	?Inhibition of a prostaglandin-dependent mechanism
4. Furosemide	Probenecid	Blockade of tubular secretion of furosemide into tubular lumen

the face of compromised renal function, doses of up to 1000 mg may be needed. With the advent of metolazone, it has become possible to combine a powerful thiazide-type diuretic with a powerful loop diuretic to produce an additive, if not a synergistic, effect. This also is useful in patients with compromised renal function.

Used alone, the hypotensive effect of diuretics is modest. They are, however, an invaluable and often necessary concomitant of therapy with other agents, particularly if the effectiveness of the other agent becomes diminished over time because of salt and water retention.

ADRENERGIC NEURON BLOCKING DRUGS

Of the many that have been synthesized, only one adrenergic neuron blocking drug, *guanethidine,* has been available for many years in the United States. However, *bethanidine,* which has much more convenient pharmacokinetic characteristics, has just been released in this country. A third agent, *bretylium,* now regarded as obsolete in treating hypertension, is making a comeback, this time as an antiarrhythmic agent.

This class of drugs reduces blood pressure by preventing the release of norepinephrine from postganglionic sympathetic nerves (*see* Chaps. 13, 18). This is accomplished by preventing the influx of calcium ions into the nerve terminal, which is the usual sequel to the arrival of a nerve impulse and an essential element in excitation–secretion coupling. Guanethidine, unlike some members of this group, also causes depletion of neuronal norepinephrine stores. The mechanism by which this occurs is unknown. Although this may be unimportant with respect to establishing neuronal blockade, it may be important as one explanation for the fact that patients on guanethidine therapy much less commonly develop tolerance to its effects than patients on bethanidine therapy, for example.

To block adrenergic transmission, these drugs have to gain access to the interior of sympathetic nerve terminals. They enter this compartment by "riding" the neuronal uptake$_1$ mechanism that normally serves to restore released norepinephrine to the nerve terminal from which it originated. Therein lies the basis for the only important drug interaction that involves this class of agent, for the tricyclic antidepressant agents specifically block uptake$_1$ (*see* Chap. 13, 22). In consequence, coadministration of such antidepressants to patients taking adrenergic neuron blocking drugs will lead to abolition of pressure control. If the two classes of drugs must be given together, pressure control can be restored by increasing the dose of the antihypertensive agent, since the antagonism by the antidepressant is competitive in nature and the adrenergic neuron blocking drugs do not cross the blood barrier to any appreciable degree. Toxicity is rare because they are so exclusively concentrated in the intraneuronal pool. However, the nature of their action in obliterating the body's sympathetic responses gives rise to numerous adverse effects.

Adverse Effects

Postural Hypotension. When neither the peripheral resistance nor the volume of the capacitance vessels can be regulated properly, abrupt changes in blood pressure may occur on standing and after exercise. Typically, patients present with symptoms of orthostatic faintness or syncope, but occasionally the complaint may not be of giddiness but of extreme weakness. It is important for the physician routinely to measure blood pressure in the patient lying down (when pressure control may be poor), standing, and after exercise when he is on adrenergic neuron blocking drug therapy.

Fluid Retention. Reduction of sympathetic drive reduces cardiac output and may of itself precipitate cardiac failure. Renal blood flow also falls. In addition, however, another important mechanism operates. Normally the level of sympathetically mediated venoconstriction is considerable: This functional "sphincter" is an important regulator of hydrostatic pressure in the capillary bed, and when it is paralyzed blood volume may expand uncontrollably. Clinically this manifests itself as a loss of pressure control despite maintenance of a previously effective dose of the drug in question. It is important to recognize such an event for what it is, since the correct therapeutic response is to add a diuretic, not to increase the dose of the sympatholytic agent.

Diarrhea. Diarrhea is encountered with guanethidine much more than with any of the other drugs in this group; thus its mechanism presumably is not just withdrawal of sympathetic inhibition from the gut. The explosive and watery nature of this very disabling side-effect has led to the suggestion that a serotonergic mechanism may be involved.

Sexual Function. Paralysis of the sympathetically innervated internal sphincter of the bladder allows retrograde ejaculation. The emotional anguish associated with this can lead to psychogenic impotence. Strictly, such impotence should not be attributed to the drug becuse the genesis of an erection is a parasympathetic function, but this knowledge is small consolation to the patient.

Clinical Use

Owing to the disabling nature of the adverse effects, these powerful antihypertensive drugs have come to be regarded as agents of last resort. Guanethidine is particularly awkward to manipulate because the half-life of the drug in the neuronal pool is about 5 days. This means that on a fixed dose the full effect will not be seen for almost 3 weeks and that it would take the same time for the consequences of overdose to dissipate fully. However, with the other drugs now available (bethanidine has a half-life of 12 hours), this should not be necessary. Given the kinetics mentioned above, guanethidine obviously can be given once a day, and this simplification of dosage may be an important factor when compliance is uncertain. Guanethidine may be used alone but more commonly is given with a diuretic. If other drugs are needed, guanethidine should be combined with a beta-blocking drug or a vasodilator rather than with a centrally acting sympatholytic such as clonidine or methyldopa, because the modulation of sympathetic tone by a centrally acting sympatholytic agent would probably be obliterated by the peripheral presynaptic effect of adrenergic neuron blockade.

VASODILATORS

Although in the form of hydralazine vasodilator therapy has been available for 25 years, only since its use as part of a triple regimen and only since newer, more potent agents have become available has such treatment developed fully.

Rapid vasodilation lowers blood pressure but, in so doing, causes a reflex increase in heart rate and cardiac output. This is subjectively uncomfortable, and, for the patient with ischemic heart disease, potentially dangerous. Additionally vasodilation, by changing intrarenal hemodynamics and possibly by increasing the flow of blood into the peripheral capillary bed, causes salt and water retention with increased extracellular fluid volume. This is especially true of those agents that dilate the arterial circulation but have little effect on the veins, such as hydralazine and diazoxide. As a result of these hemodynamic changes, the hypotensive effect of vasodilators alone is short lived, and to maximize the benefit of vasodilator therapy these agents must be combined with beta-adrenoceptor blockers and a diuretic as described above. For those paients unable to tolerate beta blockers, clonidine (*see* below) has been substituted with some success.

HYDRALAZINE

Hydralazine exerts a direct relaxant effect on vascular smooth muscle. Initial enthusiasm has been tempered by the problems mentioned above and by its toxicity. Given in high enough doses, hydralazine causes lupus erythematosuslike clinical features (or at least unmasks the lupus diathesis) in susceptible patients. Hydralazine is metabolized by acetylation, and those patients particularly at risk are the slow acetylators (*see* Chaps. 4, 6). However, it has become conventional practice, since acetylator status is not usually determined, never to give more than 200 mg/day, at which level the lupus problem does not usually arise.

In patients with normal renal function, the half-life is no more than 4 hours, and consequently the drug must be given three to four times per day. In renal failure, the dose should be reduced because about half is normally excreted unchanged. A parenteral form is available and may be used intravenously or intramuscularly in the emergency control of severe hypertension, although it has been superceded largely by sodium nitroprusside (*see* below) in this context.

DIAZOXIDE

Formerly available as an oral medication, diazoxide has been found to be unsuitable for long-term therapy because, more so than the other thiazides to which it is structurally related (even though it exerts no diuretic effect), it has a marked diabetogenic effect. Additionally it, like other vasodilators, causes pronounced fluid retention. It has survived, however, as an injectable drug to be used in the emergency reduction of high blood pressure. When given rapidly intravenously, a significant bolus of unbound diazoxide remains in a small segment of the circulating blood volume. Only this fraction of the administered drug, of course, is free to act on the vascular smooth muscle. When given this way, pressure reduction is rapid and lasts for up to 12 hours. The drug solution is highly alkaline, and thus it is imperative that extravasation of the injectate into the tissues should not occur.

PRAZOSIN

Unlike the other agents in this section that act directly on vascular tissues, prazosin causes vasodilation by blocking the postsynaptic α_1 adrenoceptor (*see* Chap. 18). It is active when given by mouth, with a half-life of less than 5 hours, so that it is given in divided doses throughout the day. There is a pronounced and poorly understood "first dose effect" with prazosin whereby the initial dose causes an exaggerated hypotensive effect. To avoid syncopal attacks on this account, the patient should be advised to take the first dose just before going to bed. Apart from this phenomenon, no serious side-effects appear to be associated with prazosin, and to date no significant toxicity has emerged. The usual daily dose extends up to about 20 mg.

MINOXIDIL

Available in the United States since 1980, Minoxidil is the most potent oral vasodilator known and represents a major advance in drug treatment of severe hypertension. It has proved to be a viable alternative to nephrectomy in hypertensive patients with end-state renal disease. For a long time, there was concern that myocardial lesions seen in dogs treated with minoxidil might occur in humans, but in conventional doses, at least (which range up to 40 mg/day in divided doses), this does not seem to be a problem. Indeed the only concern associated with minoxidil (except those common to all vasodilators described above) is hypertrichosis, which obviously limits its usefulness in women. Increased hair growth on the face, arms, and legs can be marked. It usually regresses over 2 to 6 months once the drug is withdrawn.

SODIUM NITROPRUSSIDE

The most powerful of the vasodilators, sodium nitroprusside must be given by i.v. infusion. Its onset and offset of action are both extremely rapid, so that the infusion rate can be regulated on a minute-by-minute basis to provide "finger-tip" control of the blood pressure. The infusion rates used range from 15 to 500 μg/min. Because sodium nitroprusside is light sensitive, it should be used as a freshly prepared solution, shielded from direct light. Care must be observed with prolonged use because nitroprusside gives rise to cyanide; although this is metabolized to thiocyanate, both are toxic, and levels of both should be monitored. Thiocyanate is excreted in the urine and thus is especially prone to accumulate in patients with renal failure. Cyanide toxicity can be treated with cobalt-based chelating agents, such as hydroxycobalamin.

NITROGLYCERIN

Within the last 2 years, i.v. nitroglycerin has become commercially available in the United States. It claims to be more beneficial on compromised coronary hemodynamics than nitroprusside, but this remains controversial. Nitroglycerin acts almost as rapidly as does nitroprusside and also has a very short half-life (1–4 minutes). It is rapidly metabolized and of course will not give rise to cyanide or thiocyanate. Its merits vis à vis nitroprusside have not yet been established.

CENTRALLY ACTING HYPOTENSIVE AGENTS

Drugs that lower blood pressure through an action on the central nervous system include the now little used *reserpine, methyldopa, clonidine,* and *guanabenz.* Each by a different mechanism reduces the intensity of centrally generated sympathetic drive. Reserpine causes a central and a peripheral depletion of neuronal norepinephrine, thereby reducing sympathetic tone. The relative importance for reserpine of the central versus the peripheral action has never been firmly established. Methyldopa, clonidine, and guanabenz in contrast, reduce transmission solely by stimulating inhibitory α_2 receptors within the vasomotor center. The effect of this is to inhibit norepinephrine release from the adrenergic neurons, which leads to a marked reduction of efferent sympathetic traffic from the central nervous system. Peripherally this is manifested in low circulating catecholamines and in "reset" sympathetic responses. To achieve this result, methyldopa has to enter the sympathetic nerves and be metabolized to, and stored as, the false neurotransmitter methylnorepinephrine. Animal experiments using agents that inhibit central dopa decarboxylase have indicated clearly that if the production of methylnorepinephrine is blocked, methyldopa ceases to have a hypotensive effect. Clonidine and guanabenz, in contrast, are direct agonists of the α_2 adrenoceptors, and the hypotensive effect is (in normal therapeutic concentrations; *see* below) directly related to plasma concentrations, and presumably cerebrospinal fluid concentrations.

Given the common areas of action, it is not surprising that these drugs share many pharmacologic properties. For instance, unlike that seen with adrenergic neuron blocking drugs, pressure reduction is relatively independent of body position, so that orthostatic symptoms are very uncommon. Because all drugs reduce sympathetic tone, they all may lead to cardiac failure in a patient whose cardiac function is so compromised that he depends on increased adrenergic drive to ward off decompensation (*see* Chap. 18). However, the risk of this seems to be less than with beta-adrenoceptor blocking agents. Mental depression may occur with all these drugs and was particularly prominent with reserpine in the early days of its use, when daily doses of many milligrams were used. Sedation is common to all these agents, and, manufacturers' claims notwithstanding, may be persistent. Dry mouth, also a centrally mediated adverse effect, occurs with all three. Extrapyramidal side-effects may occur with reserpine and methyldopa but not with clonidine or guanabenz.

RESERPINE

Reserpine should be regarded as a moderately potent and useful hypotensive agent. It is little used today, however, having been replaced by newer agents that cause fewer side-effects than were seen when reserpine was used in the excessive doses of the 1950s and early 1960s. In daily doses of up to 10 mg, nasal congestion was more than a trivial inconvenience and depression of suicidal proportion was all too common. For this reason, the use of reserpine declined, and now it is rarely prescribed except as a component of various diuretic–vasodilator combinations in which the daily dose rarely exceeds 0.3 mg. Even in this form, reserpine came under a cloud when a report from the Boston Collaborative Study suggested a link between reserpine and breast cancer, an allegation subsequently withdrawn for lack of corroborative evidence.

Reserpine had another useful role in the treatment of hypertension: the emergency reduction of severe hypertension. An i.m. injection of up to 10 mg would produce a smooth and sustained fall in blood pressure. Newer and more fashionable agents have, however, appeared in that field also, and the production of parenteral reserpine was discontinued on economic grounds.

METHYLDOPA

Methyldopa remains one of the most potent and widely used hypotensive agent in the world. Its blood-pressure-lowering effect was discovered accidentally during a systematic study of aromatic amino L-acid decarboxylase inhibitors in humans. Absorption is rapid, incomplete, and variable both within and between subjects. Since its hypotensive effect depends on an active metabolite, it is not surprising that there is no relation between plasma level and effect.

The metabolite methylnorepinephrine appears in the urine in amounts similar to its natural counterpart, and its continuing excretion for several days after a single dose of methyldopa is consistent with the view that it is responsible for the hypotensive action that persists long after methyldopa itself has been eliminated. A parenteral form of methyldopa, an ester, is available but is not very effective because hydrolysis of the ester is so incomplete. The normal oral dose ranges up to 2.5 to 3.0 g/day in divided doses.

The hemodynamic profile of methyldopa is characterized by attenuation, not obliteration, of normal cardiovascular reflex responses. The pressure overshoot seen in the Valsalva response still occurs but is reduced. Peripheral resistance is reduced in the lying position and does not increase as expected on standing, but because it remains fairly constant there is little or no postural fall in pressure. Orthostatic symptoms are extremely rare. Although cardiac output falls, because renal vascular resistance falls, renal blood flow and renal function remain unchanged.

Adverse Effects

In only a very small proportion of patients are adverse effects serious, but because methyldopa is so widely used the problem cannot be disregarded. The most serious form of toxicity is liver damage. Most commonly, an illness clinically and biochemically indistinguishable from acute viral hepatitis occurs, but obstructive jaundice, chronic active hepatitis, and massive (sometimes fatal) hepatic necrosis have all been reported. They may appear after several years of uneventful therapy. Usually the condition remits once methyldopa is withdrawn. An impression exists that once hepatotoxicity has occurred, a second exposure to methyldopa may cause much more severe liver damage, so this should be avoided.

Of great scientific interest, but of less clinical importance, is the development of a positive direct Coombs' test (rarely progressing to frank hemolytic anemia) in up to 25% of patients receiving more than 2 g of methyldopa per day. It takes about 120 days (the life of a red cell) from the start of therapy for the positive Coombs' test to develop, and about as long after the cessation of methyldopa therapy for it to disappear. If not recognized for what it is, a positive Coombs' test may cause confusion during grouping and cross-matching procedures. A positive antinuclear factor may develop in some patients, but only three methyldopa-related cases of recognizable lupus erythematosus have been reported.

CLONIDINE

Accidentally discovered to be hypotensive when its vasoconstrictor (nasal decongestant) properties were being explored, clonidine is a remarkably potent drug whose daily dose is usually measured in micrograms. The drug is well absorbed and extensively metabolized before excretion. The time-course of its hypotensive effect seems to follow fairly closely the plasma concentration until high levels are reached (equivalent to a daily dose of about 5 mg). At these concentrations, as the drug level rises beyond a certain point, the blood pressure also begins to increase. The late pressor effect may be due to the emergence of a significant peripheral α_1-receptor-mediated vasoconstriction, whereas at lower (hypotensive) concentrations, the central α_2 (hypotensive) effect predominates.

Hemodynamically, clonidine closely resembles methyldopa. Cardiovascular reflexes are attenuated, not blocked. The hemodynamic adaptation to exercise is qualitatively normal but is "reset" to a lower baseline. Renal blood flow is preserved because the fall in renovascular resistance matches the fall in cardiac output.

Clinically clonidine has proved to be as effective as methyldopa. As noted above, it causes very similar side-effects. Interestingly, some patients intolerant of methyldopa may fare better on clonidine therapy, and *vice versa*.

Adverse Effects

No serious toxic effect has been linked to clonidine. Severe rebound hypertension is, however, one problem much more commonly encountered after clonidine is abruptly withdrawn than after methyldopa. This condition is characterized by clinical and biochemical features of a severe hyperadrenergic state. It may take 2 to 3 days to resolve spontaneously but will respond immediately to the reintroduction of clonidine, preferably parenterally. The cause is unknown but may represent the consequence of normal neurotransmission resumption in an area of the brain that has developed "denervation hypersensitivity" during clonidine-induced inhibition of neurotransmission in the vasomotor center. All patients on clonidine therapy must be warned of this risk. Patients thought to be unreliable tablet-takers should be given another drug.

GUANABENZ

Guanabenz was introduced in the United States in 1982. It appears to be very similar to clonidine in terms of efficacy and side-effects. It has a longer half-life and may be given in doses up to 30 mg twice a day. Its longer half-life may make guanabenz less likely to cause rebound hypertension if it is suddenly withdrawn.

BETA-ADRENOCEPTOR BLOCKING DRUGS

A chance observation made during the early evaluation of a now obsolete beta-adrenoceptor blocking agent (pronethalol) in ischemic heart disease led to one of the most important advances in the treatment of hypertension. Although the means by which beta-adrenoceptor blockade lowers blood pressure remains uncertain, all such drugs will lower blood pressure in many hypertensive patients, regardless of their ancillary pharmacologic properties. Numerous theories have been advanced to explain how beta blockade could lower blood pressure. The link is not obvious, because if propranolol, for example, is given acutely, the manifestations of beta blockade, such as bradycardia and reduced cardiac output, appear immediately but the blood pressure does not fall. Some other changes in the homeostatic mechanisms are obviously required. Peripheral resistance, which rises acutely, falls with prolonged dosing, but the mechanism underlying this is unknown.

One of the earliest theories advanced was that a downward resetting of the baroceptors occurred. No data have emerged to support this contention.

Beta blockade reduces renin release from the juxtaglomerular apparatus. About 10 years ago, interest was aroused by the suggestion that, among nonrenovascular hypertensive patients, those characterized by high plasma renin activity might represent the subset for whom beta blockade was uniquely the treatment of choice. However, later studies have shown that patients with low plasma renin activity will respond equally well, albeit requiring larger doses.

The difference in responsiveness between patients with high renin and low renin persists throughout the dose range studied. In both groups of patients the relation between dose and response throughout the range studied is log linear. This is an important observation since many authors have suggested that a very modest dose of propranolol, such as 420 mg/day, should be accepted as an arbitrary upper dose level. The form of the dose-response curves, however, makes it clear that the maximum hypotensive effect has not been reached even at 960 mg/day.

The possibility that beta blocking drugs may work by some central mechanism has certain attractions, and for propranolol, at least, some animal data support the idea. However, not every beta blocking drug crosses the blood–brain barrier so readily. Thus the validity of the suggestion is somewhat doubtful.

Finally it has been proposed that blockade of presynaptic β-receptors may reduce norepinephrine release from the postganglionic sympathetic nerves. However, data on plasma norepinephrine levels in patients taking beta blocking drugs have been very inconsistent. At present, therefore, how beta blocking drugs lower blood pressure is unknown; nevertheless an attractive feature of their hypotensive effect is that pressure control is uniformly good, regardless of posture, and there is no further fall after exercise. This fact, associated with the usually low incidence of adverse effects and relative lack of disturbance of sexual function in men, makes beta-adrenoceptor blocking drugs especially useful in young patients. Side-effects do, of course, occur but are usually an obvious consequence of the known effects of beta blockade and can thus be avoided by judicious patient selection.

Adverse Effects

Cardiac Failure. Cardiac failure will arise in patients who depend on sympathetic stimulation to maintain adequate contractility. Should beta blocking agents be needed regardless of the patient's cardiac status, failure often can be controlled by the concomitant administration of digitalis and diuretics (*see* Chaps. 33, 40).

Heart Block. Both atrial and atrioventricular conduction are far more susceptible to sympathetic modulation than is conduction in the ventricles. Thus first-degree A-V block may increase to second degree and progress to total A-V block under the influence of this class of drugs. Progression from first- to third-degree block is unlikely to happen without warning so that, if indicated on other grounds, beta-adrenoceptor blocking agents could be used in first- but not second-degree heart block with a fair degree of safety.

Intermittent Claudication. Whether because of reduced cardiac output or loss of the beta-adrenergic component of vasodilatation (probably the former), claudication commonly becomes worse.

Bronchial Asthma. Beta-adrenoceptor-mediated function is important in maintaining relaxation of bronchial smooth muscle and, in those patients in whom it is a factor, in suppression of release of mediators of bronchoconstriction from mast cells. Clearly beta blockade only makes asthma worse. An attempt has been made to avoid this problem by developing cardioselective (β_1) blockers, but unfortunately this selectivity is a *relative* one and is only really pronounced at low doses (*see* Chap. 18). It is not safe to assume that cardioselective agents will not dangerously compromise a patient's respiratory function.

Hypoglycemia. The effect of coadministration of beta-adrenoceptor blocking drugs with insulin or oral antidiabetic therapy, on hypoglycemia is commonly misunderstood. Beta blockade does not worsen hypoglycemia but may prolong the recovery time because mobilization of glycogen is a beta-adrenoceptor mediated process. Another misconception is that the symptoms of hypoglycemia are masked. A more correct perspective is to regard them as altered. True, the tachycardia and tremor are suppressed, but sweating is a *cholinergically* mediated sympathetic function and this becomes the dominant and most easily recognizable warning sign.

Exacerbation of Renal Failure. Still controversial is whether, in susceptible persons, reduced cardiac output may cause a sufficient fall in renal blood flow to produce or exacerbate renal failure. Beta-adrenoceptor blocking agents should be carefully introduced into the treatment of patients where this may be possible.

Intrinsic Sympathomimetic Activity. Generally intrinsic sympathomimetic activity (ISA) is of no significance. Certainly it has no proven value in protecting against cardiac failure or bronchial asthma. *Pindolol*, the beta blocker with the greatest intrinsic sympathomimetic activity, will, above a dose of about 40 mg/day, cause a reversal of any hypotensive effect achieved by lower doses as the ISA becomes more apparent.

Central Nervous System Effects. Hallucinations, vivid dreams, and altered sleep patterns may be associated with lipid-soluble drugs in this class.

Miscellaneous Toxic Effects. The most important toxic effect thus far is the mucocutaneous reaction to *practolol*. In its most severe form, this reaction has involved zerophthalmia, leading sometimes to corneal perforation and blindness, a serous otitis media sometimes causing deafness, a sclerosing peritonitis occasionally causing intestinal obstruction, and a lupus-like skin rash. The mechanism for this rare but disastrous toxicity remains unknown. The reaction has not occurred with any other beta blocker, and practolol is no longer used in humans. Psoriasis may be markedly worsened by all beta blockers.

Pronethalol, the first beta blocker used clinically, was withdrawn because of tumor development in mice. Subsequent study, however, failed to confirm any tumor-producing potential in pronethalol. One other beta blocker, tolamolol, has also been withdrawn from clinical use because of animal tumor development.

INDIVIDUAL BETA-ADRENOCEPTOR BLOCKING DRUGS

Propranolol. A nonselective agent without intrinsic sympathomimetic activity (ISA), propranolol is the yardstick by which other beta blockers are measured. It is subject to extensive and very variable first-pass metabolism so that in moderate-sized doses (80 mg 6 hourly), plasma levels may vary up to twenty-fold between patients. Doses used have ranged up to 4.0 g/day, but a more common maximum (arbitrary) is about 1.0 g/day. All of the side-effects listed above may occur with propranolol. Its biochemical half-life is about 3 hours, but the *biological* half-life is about 6 to 8 hours, so that twice-a-day administration is often appropriate.

Oxprenolol. Almost identical to propranolol, oxprenolol possesses a small and unimportant degree of ISA.

Acebutolol. *In vitro* acebutolol behaves as a cardioselective agent, but in clinical circumstances this is not so apparent, possibly because of an active nonselective metabolite. The drug is about 40% metabolized.

Pindolol. Pindolol exhibits marked ISA, which is the outstanding feature of this partially metabolized nonselective beta blocker.

Nadolol. Nadolol is characterized by a long half-life, readily allowing once-a-day treatment for hypertension. Nadolol is not metabolized but is excreted unchanged in the urine. Dosage adjustment is therefore necessary in renal failure.

Metoprolol. Through 1981, metoprolol represented the only β_1-selective agent available in the United States. It is extensively metabolized with a chemical half-life of around 4 hours.

Atenolol. A cardioselective agent with a longer half-life (around 9 hours), atenolol is excreted largely unchanged, and thus dosage adjustment in renal failure is appropriate. Once-a-day treatment for hypertension is adequate. This is now one of the most widely used beta-blocking drugs worldwide.

Clinical Use

There is no way to predict which hypertensive patients will respond well to these agents. Selection of an individual beta blocker is largely a matter of personal preference, remembering that at high doses the ISA of pindolol becomes obtrusive and that the cardioselectivity of the β_1 specific agents is lost. No good data indicate that patients who do not tolerate one will fare better on another. Use of an agent with a long enough half-life to allow once-a-day therapy will improve compliance in some patients.

Although beta-adrenoceptor blockade may be used as the sole form of therapy, if the dose required is large this becomes expensive and adverse effects become more likely. Commonly, therefore, drugs of this class are used as one component of a multiple drug regimen in which they are combined with a vasodilator and a diuretic. This is a particularly felicitous combination in that beta blockers prevent the reflex tachycardia that makes vasodilator therapy unpleasant for many patients, and diuretics prevent the fluid retention that vasodilators and beta blockers may cause. Such a regimen is often extremely effective and allows the use of low doses of each of the three components. Its use has been increased recently by the advent of new, potent vasodilators.

Abrupt withdrawal of beta blockers should be avoided because some data suggest that during prolonged blockade the number of beta receptors may increase (as though the end-organs were denervated). This may cause what amounts to a hyperadrenergic state, potentially hazardous to patients with ischemic heart disease.

ANTAGONISTS OF THE RENIN–ANGIOTENSIN SYSTEM

Although the renin–angiotensin system has long been known to be important in many hypertensive patients and in many experimental models of hypertension, only within the last 10 years have experimental drugs become available for blocking this system, and only within the last 6 months have effective agents been available to the practicing clinician. The actions, clinical uses, and adverse effects of saralasin and captopril, both used to lower blood pressure, are discussed in Chapter 55.

CHOICE OF ANTIHYPERTENSIVE AGENTS

The development of antihypertensive agents has been one of the major advances of the past 25 years, for hypertension, untreated, certainly qualifies as one of the "captains of the men of death."

The clinician treating a hypertensive patient in whom no surgically correctable lesion exists must accept the fact that he will have to steer his patient through life-long therapy. His choice of drugs must be tempered by his evaluation of the patient's reliability (long-term compliance may be as low as 50% and some drugs are dangerous when abruptly withdrawn) and the existence of other diseases (such as asthma and arterial insufficiency). He must pay heed to the ability of the patient to metabolize or excrete the drugs he chooses.

Traditionally in the United States, treatment begins with a diuretic, but this may not always be good. Young patients respond less well, and a few may develop paradoxical hypertension because of a brisk renin response. Sexual function in men may be impaired. Metabolic disturbances such as hypokalemia, hyperglycemia, and hyperuricemia are well known, but hyponatremia, especially in elderly persons, may occur. Less well recognized are subtle changes in lipid metabolism that, over 30 or 40 years, may have an adverse effect on the development of atheroma. Clearly, therefore, it is not unreasonable, especially in younger patients, to consider starting with one of the more potent agents. Many fare extremely well on a beta-blocking agent. Fewer tolerate the centrally acting drugs as well because of sedation, dry mouth, and depression, although this is not universally so. If single drug therapy does not work or requires doses large enough to cause unacceptable side-effects, then combination therapy based on the considerations set out above should be used. Usually only when the full potential of these has been exploited without success are adrenergic neuron blocking drugs used, especially in elderly persons. It is still too early to say how captopril should be used. At present, considerations of toxicity cause us to use it only when all reasonable alternatives have failed or when evidence of renin–angiotension involvement is clear. However, particularly when second-generation drugs of this type with less toxicity are developed, this view may change.

FURTHER READING

1. Apostolides AY, Cutter G, Kraus J: Impact of hypertension information on high blood pressure control between 1973 and 1978. Hypertension 2:708–713, 1980
2. Franklin SS, Conolly ME, Tuck ML: Hypertension. In Gonick MC (ed): *Current Nephrology*, pp 225–294. Boston, Houghton–Mifflin, 1979

CHAPTER 36 QUESTIONS

(See P. 7 for Full Instructions)

Select the One Best Answer

1. Which of the following compounds will lower the blood pressure during an attack of hypertension caused by pheochromocytoma?
   A. Methyldopa
   B. Reserpine
   C. Phentolamine
   D. Levodopa
   E. Tripelennamine

2. Which of the following drugs is paired with an incorrect side-effect?
   A. Prazosin—postural hypotension with the first dose
   B. Clonidine—rebound hypertensive crisis following abrupt withdrawal of the drug
   C. Guanethidine—postural hypotension
   D. Chlorothiazide—hypouricemia
   E. Reserpine—depression

3. An agent useful in treating both hypertensive crisis and hypoglycemia caused by an insulinoma is
   A. glucagon.
   B. epinephrine.
   C. hydrochlorothiazide.
   D. sodium nitroprusside.
   E. diazoxide.

4. In the event of hypertensive crisis, a rapid lowering of blood pressure could be achieved by parenteral administration of each of the following EXCEPT
   A. trimethaphan.
   B. diazoxide.
   C. sodium nitroprusside.
   D. guanethidine.
   E. prazosin.

A = 1,2,3; B = 1,3; C = 2,4; D = 4; E = All

5. Drugs effective as chronic therapy in lowering the blood pressure in essential hypertension may act by
   1. blocking catecholamine release from the sympathetic nerve endings.
   2. blocking peripheral alpha-adrenergic receptors.
   3. stimulating alpha-adrenergic receptors in the brain.
   4. stimulating peripheral beta-adrenergic receptors.

6. In the treatment of hypertension,
   1. hydralazine lowers blood pressure without causing reflex tachycardia.
   2. phenoxybenzamine is useful in patients with pheochromocytoma.
   3. diazoxide is suitable for chronic use.
   4. chlorothiazide may supplement the antihypertensive effect of other agents.

7. Guanethidine
   1. may produce severe postexercise hypotension.
   2. is more likely to cause orthostatic hypotension than is methyldopa.
   3. can cause diarrhea.
   4. causes extrapyramidal effects.

8. Methyldopa
   1. inhibits dopa-decarboxylase.

2. causes norepinephrine depletion in sympathetic nerves.
3. is metabolized to active pressor metabolites.
4. is an effective antihypertensive agent that produces postural hypotension infrequently.

9. Clonidine may cause
   1. a marked fall in blood pressure.
   2. troublesome dry mouth.
   3. rebound hypertension when given in high doses.
   4. rebound hypertension when abruptly withdrawn.

10. Diuretics such as hydrochlorothiazide
    1. are totally benign.
    2. in a few patients may cause a paradoxical rise in blood pressure.
    3. may cause hyponatremia, potassium retention and hypoglycemia.
    4. may cause hyponatremia, hypokalemia, hyperuricemia, hyperglycemia, and an elevated triglyceride level.

37 Drugs Used to Treat Hyperlipidemia

MARY J. MALLOY
JOHN P. KANE

Hyperlipidemia may be defined as a pathologic elevation of content of one or more of the macromolecular complexes of lipid and protein (lipoproteins) of plasma. This is reflected by an elevated plasma cholesterol and/or plasma triglyceride level.

The rationale for treating hyperlipoproteinemia is based on the observation that high levels of certain lipoproteins in serum contribute to the formation and progression of atheromata and on the association of severe hypertriglyceridemia with the risk of acute pancreatitis.

Hyperlipidemia has been repeatedly identified as one of the most important epidemiologic risk factors for accelerated development of atherosclerosis, most notably coronary artery disease. The lipoproteins that contain the B-100 apolipoprotein are the species implicated in atherogenesis, including low-density (LDL), intermediate-density (IDL), and very low-density (VLDL) lipoproteins. The lipid found in the atherosclerotic plaque is delivered to the site by these lipoproteins. Interaction of the B-100 apoprotein with a mucopolysaccaride in the artery wall may contribute to accumulation of lipoprotein lipids. High density lipoproteins (HDL) apparently enhance removal of cholesterol from the artery wall, and low levels of these lipoproteins are correlated with increased risk of atherosclerosis. There are apparently multiple subspecies of HDL, which differ in their ability to participate in this centripetal transport of cholesterol. Definitive analysis of the effect of normalization of lipoprotein levels on the rate of atherogenesis must await primary intervention studies of long duration. However, the results of several more brief dietary and drug intervention studies suggest that a significant reduction of morbidity or mortality from coronary vascular disease may be realized by such therapy. For example, the size of tendon xanthomata in patients with familial hypercholesterolemia decreases when the level of serum cholesterol is normalized, and hence deposits of lipid in arterial walls may respond similarly.

Since hyperlipidemia in humans occurs in a number of phenotypic forms that display highly individual responses to therapy, understanding of the fundamentals of the biochemistry of lipoproteins is essential to definitive diagnosis and the selection of a rational therapeutic regimen.

TABLE 37-1. Human Plasma Lipoproteins*

Electrophoretic Mobility	Ultracentrifugal Designation	Principal Lipids in Quantitative Order	Approximate Diameter
			nm
α_1	High-density lipoprotein (HDL)	Cholesterol Phospholipid	8–10
β	Low-density lipoprotein (LDL)	Cholesterol Phospholipid	21
Pre-β	Very low-density lipoprotein (VLDL)	Triglyceride Cholesterol Phospholipid	30–100
No mobility in most systems	Chylomicrons (normally absent from plasma after an overnight fast)	Triglyceride Phospholipid Cholesterol	>100

* Lipoproteins were first recognized as macromolecular complexes in 1929 by Michel Macheboeuf of the Pasteur Institute. The principal species were first delineated ultracentrifugally by John Gofman of the Donner Laboratory of the University of California, Berkeley, in the early 1950s.

LIPOPROTEIN METABOLISM

Except for free fatty acids (FFA) and lysolecithins bound to albumin, the plasma lipids are carried in lipoprotein complexes, pseudomicellar in structure, having a hydrophobic lipid-filled core region surrounded by a monolayer of amphiphilic lipids and apoproteins. Some biochemical characteristics of the principal classes of human plasma lipoproteins are presented in Table 37-1. Chylomicrons, which form in the intestinal epithelial cells, carry triglyceride of dietary origin. VLDL originate in liver and transport triglyceride of endogenous origin. Each of these lipoproteins contains apoproteins of very large molecular weight (B apoproteins) that behave like intrinsic proteins of membranes. The B proteins associated with VLDL and chylomicrons are different: intestinal B protein, B-48, is found in chylomicrons and their remnants; VLDL contains B-100, as does its daughter particle, LDL, which is formed from VLDL remnants by the liver. LDL also contains B-74 and B-26, complementary apoproteins apparently derived from B-100. In addition to the B apoproteins, a number of small proteins also are associated with the lipoproteins, many of which are known to have important roles in their metabolism.

Chylomicrons, the largest species of lipoprotein, emerge into the lymph spaces adjacent to the intestinal cells and at once begin to exchange surface components with HDL, a process that continues as they move through the lymphatic ducts to the thoracic duct and into the blood stream. A similar process of exchange with HDL occurs with the newly secreted VLDL from liver. A common pathway of hydrolysis by the lipoprotein lipase (LPL) system delivers fatty acids derived from these lipoproteins to tissues. LPL is known to exist in at least two forms with different molecular weights and substrate affinities. One of the small apolipoproteins, apo C-II, and heparin are cofactors for LPL. Insulin induces increased activity of this enzyme.

As hydrolysis progresses, core triglycerides are depleted and particle diameter decreases, resulting in "remnant" lipoproteins. Chylomicron remnants are removed by liver where they are disassembled completely. Uptake of remnants apparently depends on their recognition by specific receptors on the hepatocytes. Apolipoproteins E-3 and E-4 and apo B are important in this process. VLDL remnants are further catabolized in liver, and the end-products, LDL, are released into plasma. The clinical phenomenon of the "beta shift" (increased LDL as hypertriglyceridemia resolves) and the increased levels of LDL associated with increased VLDL secretion are thus explained by the formation of LDL from VLDL.

High-affinity receptors on cell membranes mediate the catabolism of LDL by adsorptive endocytosis. Apo B is degraded to amino acids and the cholesteryl esters of the LDL core hydrolyzed to free cholesterol, which is used to form cell membranes. The cholesterol entering the cell in this way supresses cholesterol biosynthesis and leads to down regulation of the

Michel Macheboeuf—isolated first lipoprotein (HDL) at the Pasteur Institute, 1929.

John Gofman—made striking advances in the field by introduction of analytical ultracentrifugation in the 1950s.

LDL receptors. At least two other pathways exist for the catabolism of LDL: a low-affinity uptake by many cell types, probably by bulk fluid endocytosis; and uptake of chemically altered LDL by macrophages.

HDL arise from the catabolism of chylomicrons and, in nascent bilayer disc form, from the liver. In addition to their important role in centripetal transport of cholesterol, HDL serve as carriers for the C apolipoproteins, are involved in the degradation of bacterial endotoxins, and exert an inhibitory effect against certain species of trypanosomes. Catabolic pathways for these lipoproteins appear to exist in liver and some peripheral tissues.

CLINICAL DISORDERS OF HYPERLIPOPROTEINEMIA

The most clinically applicable classification of disorders of plasma lipoprotein metabolism is based on the classes of lipoproteins abnormally elevated. Each phenotypic pattern can arise as a primary genetic abnormality or as the result of some other pathologic process (secondary hyperlipidemia). Before considering therapy, this distinction must be made, since treatment of the underlying disorder, if possible, is indicated in secondary hyperlipidemia.

GENETIC DISORDERS ASSOCIATED WITH HYPERTRIGLYCERIDEMIA (HYPERLIPEMIA)

Deficiency of lipoprotein lipase or its cofactor (apolipoprotein C-II) is a rare recessive trait that can cause severe hypertriglyceridemia (chylomicrons predominate) with resultant hepatosplenomegaly, pancreatitis, and eruptive xanthomata. Estrogens intensify the lipemia. Treatment is entirely dietary, with total fat intake reduced to 10% of calories or less. Medium-chain triglycerides may be added for palatability because they bypass transport in chylomicrons. Fat-soluble vitamins and 5 g of polyunsaturated fat per day should be included in the regimen.

Endogenous (hyperprebetalipoproteinemia) and mixed lipemia (prebetalipoproteins and chylomicrons both elevated) probably result from a number of genetically determined disorders, at least some of which involve impedance in mechanisms of removal of circulating triglyceride. The lipemia is aggravated by any factor that increases the secretion of VLDL from liver, such as insulin resistance with obesity, alcohol, and estrogens. Clinical findings may include eruptive xanthomata and pancreatitis. Treatment is dietary, with fat restriction, weight reduction, and avoidance of alcohol. Although serum triglyceride levels usually approach normal on this regimen, drug treatment may occasionally be needed. Clofibrate or gemfibrozil may lower the triglyceride levels in plasma when moderate elevations of VLDL are present, but they may be less effective if the lipemia is mixed. Nicotinic acid tends to be effective even in the face of severe mixed lipemia.

Multiple lipoprotein-type (combined) hyperlipidemia is a common heredofamilial disorder in which affected persons may have increased levels of VLDL, LDL, or both. The pattern may also change with time in an individual patient's serum. The elevations are usually moderate, and factors known to increase hypertriglyceridemia do so in these patients as well. Because risk of coronary disease is increased, both dietary and drug intervention are indicated. Weight reduction and restriction of saturated fat and cholesterol are of some value, but most patients need drug therapy. Those with lipemia respond to nicotinic acid or clofibrate, and those with elevated LDL to bile acid binding resins. Persons with elevations of both LDL and VLDL levels may require combined drug regimens.

Familial dysbetalipoproteinemia is a condition in which remnant particles accumulate in plasma. The E-3 and E-4 isoforms of apolipoprotein E are absent. Heterozygotes may show intensification of hyperlipemia from other causes. Homozygotes frequently have tuberous or tuberoeruptive xanthomata or planar xanthomata of the palmar creases. They are often obese, have impaired glucose tolerance, and have increased risk for atherosclerotic coronary and peripheral vascular disease. Management includes weight reduction, reduced cholesterol intake, and minimal use of alcohol. The few patients in whom weight reduction does not produce satisfactory response may be given clofibrate in doses as low as 0.5 to 1.0 g/day or nicotinic acid, 1 to 2 g/day.

SECONDARY HYPERTRIGLYCERIDEMIA

Secondary causes of hypertriglyceridemia include diabetes mellitus, uremia, corticosteroid excess, exogenous estrogens, alcohol ingestion, nephrosis, glycogen storage disease, hypopituitarism and acromegaly, hypothyroidism, and immunoglobulin–lipoprotein complex disorders. Management of hypertriglyceridemia depends on adequate treatment of the underlying disorder. Because coronary artery disease is particularly prevalent in patients with chronic nephrotic syndrome, treatment of the hyperlipidemia *per se* would seem to be indicated. Diet is of little value. Bile acid binding resins and nicotinic acid appear to be the drugs of choice. (Clofibrate may cause myopathy in these patients, even in small doses.)

GENETIC DISORDERS ASSOCIATED WITH HYPERCHOLESTEROLEMIA

Familial hypercholesterolemia is a mendelian dominant trait that occurs in about 1 in 500 people in the heterozygous form. Levels of LDL are high at birth and tend to increase during childhood. Tendinous xanthomata often appear in early adulthood, and coronary atherosclerosis occurs prematurely. The underlying defect is a deficiency of LDL receptor sites on cell membranes, homozygotes having none and heterozygotes about half the normal number. Some patients have combined heterozygosity with one gene for absent receptor activity and an allele for defective binding. These persons are severely affected and have aggressive coronary artery disease. The homozygous state is even more catastrophic, with death from coronary atherosclerosis often occurring in childhood. Portocaval shunt or repeated plasmapheresis along with a combined drug regimen is only partially effective in treating the homozygote. However, in the compliant heterozygote, the combination of a bile acid binding resin and nicotinic acid with a diet low in cholesterol and saturated fat completely normalizes levels of LDL.

Less well-defined types of hypercholesterolemia also occur in kindreds, some of which show marked response to low saturated fat, low cholesterol diets. Drug therapy may be needed, however.

SECONDARY HYPERCHOLESTEROLEMIA

Secondary hypercholesterolemia is associated with hypothyroidism, nephrosis, immunoglobulin disorders, porphyria, anorexia nervosa, and cholestasis. Cholesterol levels generally fall during treatment of the underlying disorder. In those patients with cholestasis who develop neuropathy, bile acid binding resins may be of use, but plasmapheresis is the most effective treatment. Clofibrate actually causes increased levels of cholesterol in these patients. In nephrosis, the treatment of choice appears to be a bile acid binding resin in combination with nicotinic acid.

HYPOLIPIDEMIA

Although deficiency of HDL is an important risk factor for coronary artery disease, it has not yet been established whether measures that increase levels of total HDL will inhibit the atherogeneic process. Because only certain subspecies of HDL may be involved in the centripetal transport of cholesterol, factors that increase total levels of HDL may not necessarily be beneficial. The reported HDL lowering effect of probucol would appear to severely limit its usefulness. Further, propranolol also lowers HDL levels, but this must be weighed against the need for its cardiovascular effects in an individual patient.

TREATMENT

OVERVIEW

Institution of an appropriate diet is the first measure in treating any form of hyperlipidemia. A "universal" diet should be prescribed that includes achieving and maintaining ideal body weight; reducing total fat by restricting saturated fat to less than 10% of total calories; reducing cholesterol intake to less than 250 mg/day; making up caloric difference with carbohydrate; and avoiding alcohol if hypertriglyceridemia is present. Moderate supplementation of fat-soluble vitamins should be prescribed. In those patients with familial hypercholesterolemia, other resistant forms of hyperbetalipoproteinemia, or severe lipemia, drug therapy will be needed in addition to the dietary intervention. The diet should be continued to achieve the full potential of the drugs.

BILE ACID BINDING RESINS

Mechanism of Action

These cationic resins are not absorbed, and they bind bile acids electrostatically in the lumen of the intestine. Ninety-eight percent of the bile acid normally secreted in the bile is reabsorbed in the enterohepatic circulation during each pass. When the resins are given, bile acid excretion is increased up to tenfold. This is associated with increased cholesterol synthesis by the liver, but, increased uptake of LDL by high-affinity receptor-mediated endocytosis is reflected in an increased fractional catabolic rate of LDL.

Preparations and Dosage

Granules of cholestyramine, U.S.P., and colestipol come in packets of 4 and 5 g, respectively or in bulk. The usual starting dose is 16 to 20 g/day in three doses with meals. The therapeutic effect usually increases with the dose. Although most patients are managed with 24 to 25 g daily, some can tolerate up to 32 g under close supervision. Patients should be encouraged to mix the granules in fruit juice or other fluid or with semifluid foods to increase their palatability.

Indications

The resins are of use only in patients who have elevated LDL levels. If concomitant VLDL elevation is present, the resins may cause even higher levels of serum triglyceride. If levels of LDL are only moderately increased, the starting dose of resin may be effective. Maximum doses are necessary to treat more severe cases. The levels of LDL fall only about 20% in patients with heterozygous familial hypercholesterolemia who receive the maximum dose, whereas smaller doses may produce much larger decrements in patients with less severe types of hypercholesterolemia. The resins may also be used in combination with nicotinic acid for patients with familial hypercholesterolemia or combined hyperlipidemia. The resins are also useful in treating digitalis toxicity and in managing cholestasis (*see* Chap. 38).

Toxicity

Few systemic side-effects occur because the resins are not absorbed. Constipation and a bloating sensation are easily reversed by bran or other sources of fiber. In patients with cholestasis or bowel disease, malabsorption of fat or fat-soluble vitamins and hypoprothrombinemia may occur. Special attention should be given to vitamin-K intake in subjects who receive coumarin or indandione-type anticoagulants.

The resins bind certain drugs, including digitalis glycosides, warfarin, thyroxin, and ascorbic acid. Absorption of iron and perhaps other drugs may be impaired. The possibility of binding of drugs must be considered, regardless of electrostatic charge, since certain neutral and even cationic species may be bound. This problem is averted if other drugs are given 1 hour before the resin. Occasionally patients may develop dry, flaking skin, which is easily managed by applying lanolin. There may be a small risk of increased cholelithiasis, especially in obese patients, because of the altered composition of bile micelles produced by the resins.

NICOTINIC ACID (NIACIN)

Mechanism of Action

The ability of nicotinic acid, but not its amide, to reduce levels of LDL, VLDL, and chylomicrons appears to be due to inhibition of secretion of VLDL by liver. VLDL turnover is decreased, and amino acid incorporation into its protein moiety is inhibited. The efficiency of VLDL triglyceride removal by the LPL pathway is also increased. In addition to these effects on VLDL, nicotinic acid affects cholesterol metabolism by mobilizing sterol from tissue pools, increasing sterol excretion and decreasing biosynthesis. The drug does not alter LDL turnover but rather appears to reduce LDL levels by decreasing the secretion of its precursor, VLDL, from liver. It also causes a decreased fractional catabolic rate of HDL, particularly HDL_2, hence significantly increasing levels of HDL in plasma.

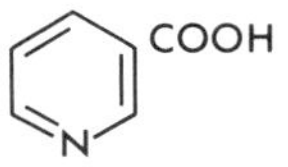

NICOTINIC ACID

Nicotinic acid is absorbed readily from the intestine. A number of metabolites are formed in the body, including nicotinamide, methyl nicotinamide, N-methyl-2-pyridone-5-carboxamide, N-methyl-2-pyridone-3-carboxamide, and nicotinuric acid, which are excreted along with unmodified nicotinic acid in urine.

Preparations and Dosage

Niacin, N.F., is available in tablets of 0.1, 0.5, and 1.0 g. Treatment is usually initiated with 0.1 g daily, divided into three doses, given with meals. The daily dose may then be increased by 1.0 g each month up to a maximum of 7.5 g. Whereas gastric irritation occurs infrequently at a daily dose of 3 g, nausea may limit the dose at some point below the maximum dosage. Nonsystemic antacids should be given when gastric irritation occurs.

Indications

Nicotinic acid is used to treat endogenous and mixed hypertriglyceridemia, usually in a dose of 1.5 to 3.5 g/day. When used in combination with a bile acid sequestrant in the treatment of heterozygous familial hypercholesterolemia, nicotinic acid, 6 to 7.5 g daily, normalizes LDL levels. In other forms of hyperbetalipoproteinemia, lower doses (1 to 3 g/day) are generally adequate.

Toxicity

Nicotinic acid causes a harmless cutaneous vasodilatation, a flushing sensation that can be minimized if the initial dose is 100 mg every 8 hours and is increased slowly. Tachyphylaxis occurs within a few days with each increment of dose. Because it is prostaglandin mediated, the flushing can be reduced by 300 mg of aspirin about 30 minutes before each dose of nicotinic acid. Nicotinic acid may potentiate the action of antihypertensive drugs.

Biochemical evidence of hepatic parenchymal dysfunction in the form of elevated serum glutamic-oxalacetic and glutamic-pyruvic transaminase and, less commonly, alkaline phosphatase levels may occur. These changes are reversible upon withdrawal of the drug. Abnormal retention of sulfobromophthalein (bromsulfalein) may also be observed. Bilirubin levels are usually normal, and no consistent abnormality of hepatic histology is present. The frequency of abnormalities of hepatic function appears to be greater in patients who receive aluminum nicotinate. Abnormalities of liver function tend to be mild.

Mild hyperuricemia may occur in about one fifth of patients but is usually not symptomatic unless there is preexisting gout. A reversible (except in some patients with latent diabetes) hyperglycemia may occur in some persons. Gastric irritation, responsive to nonsystemic antacids, is somewhat more common. Patients with history of peptic ulcer should be observed carefully for recrudescence. An occasional patient may develop acanthosis nigricans, but this condition clears upon withdrawal of the drug. Skin rash, pruritus, and icthyosis occur uncommonly. Rarely, macular degeneration has been described, not clearly related to the drug. Occasionally, patients develop cardiac arrhythmias.

CLOFIBRATE (ETHYL CHLORPHENOXYISOBUTYRATE)

Mechanism of Action

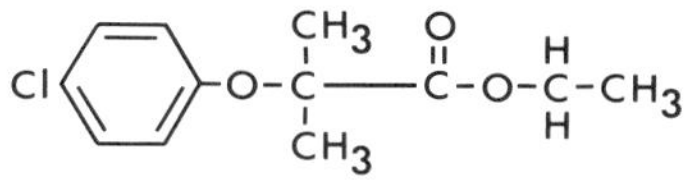

CLOFIBRATE

Clofibrate is the ethyl ester of parachlorophenoxyisobutyric acid. The ester bond is hydrolyzed in plasma and body tissues to yield the free anion bound to proteins, principally albumin. It has a half-life of 12 hours and is largely excreted in urine, principally as glucuronide. The clofibrate anion tends to displace free fatty acids from albumin and may affect the binding of other drugs to albumin (*see* Chap. 8). Clofibrate apparently acts chiefly by increasing LPL activity and may also increase hepatic fatty acid oxidation. Inhibition of hepatic cholesterol biosynthesis is probably secondary to other alterations in lipoprotein metabolism.

Preparations and Dosage

Clofibrate is available in capsules of 0.5 g. The usual dose is 1 g every 12 hours.

Indications

Clofibrate is used to treat moderate endogenous hypertriglyceridemia, mildly increased levels of LDL, and, most important, familial dysbetalipoproteinemia. Patients with familial dysbetalipoproteinemia may respond well to doses of 0.5 g to 1 g daily. Clofibrate is less effective if chylomicronemia is present and has little or no effect in familial hypercholesterolemia. Current practice suggests that drug treatment is not indicated in any patient with endogenous hyperlipemia whose serum triglyceride level is less than 500 mg/dl.

In a significant number of subjects, a fall in VLDL levels will be accompanied by an increase of LDL, a catabolic product of VLDL. This "β shift" phenomenon occurs when the triglyceride level declines in response to the drug but plasma cholesterol levels remain at approximately the pretreatment value. Patients with β shift should either be treated with nicotinic acid or a bile acid binding resin should be added to the therapeutic regimen to decrease LDL levels.

Toxicity

Moderate elevations of serum glutamic aminotransferase activity, hepatomegaly, leukopenia, skin eruptions, nausea, diarrhea, decreased libido, impotence, and muscle pain associated with elevated muscle creatine phosphokinase activity have been described in patients receiving clofibrate. Myopathy, occasionally involving myocardium, is most likely to occur in patients whose serum albumin levels are low. Activities of coumarin, indandione anticoagulants, and sulfonylureas may be potentiated through displacement (*see* Chap. 8). The dosage of anticoagulants should be reduced by one third to one half when initiating therapy with clofibrate until the appropriate individual dose is determined. Reactivity of platelets may be decreased. Lithogenicity of bile, especially in obese patients, is increased. Cardiac arrhythmias occur infrequently. The drug may have modest carcinogenic potential for gastrointestinal tissues and may increase the risk of thromboembolic disease. Therapy with clofibrate is contraindicated in uremia unless blood levels of the drug can be monitored. Increases in blood urea nitrogen and serum potassium may occur.

GEMFIBROZIL

Mechanism of Action

Gemfibrozil, a congener of clofibrate, is absorbed quantitatively from the intestine. It is bound tightly to plasma protein and has a half-life of 90 minutes in circulation. Gemfibrozil is excreted in bile and may be reabsorbed from the intestine. About 70% is excreted by the kidney. It decreases levels of VLDL in plasma due to improved efficiency of intravascular lypolysis. Gemfibrozil also decreases the pool of precursor free fatty acids available to the liver for synthesis of VLDL triglycerides by inhibiting lipolysis in adipose tissue. HDL levels are increased moderately.

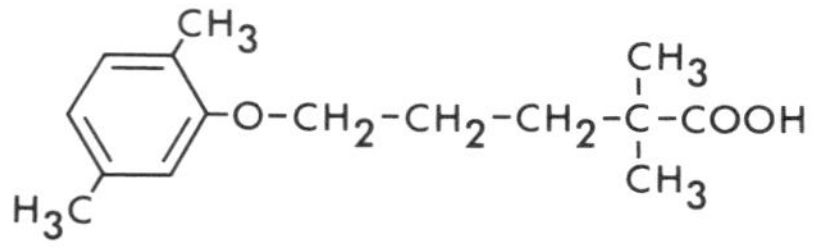

GEMFIBROZIL

Preparation and Dosage

Gemfibrozil is available in capsules of 300 mg. The usual dose is 600 mg every 12 hours.

Indications

Gemfibrozil is used to treat hypertriglyceridemia under the same circumstances as clofibrate.

Toxicity

Skin eruptions and gastrointestinal and muscular symptoms similar to those associated with clofibrate have been observed. Some patients have elevated levels of transaminase or alkaline phosphatase activity in blood. Blood dyscrasias have also been described. Gemfibrozil potentiates the action of coumarin or indandione anticoagulants.

BETA SITOSTEROL

A plant sterol, beta sitosterol is poorly absorbed and impedes the absorption of cholesterol. Thus it affects LDL levels only to the extent that dietary cholesterol contributes to LDL cholesterol in an individual patient. This effect is variable, but serum cholesterol is usually not reduced by more than 20%.

Side-effects are rare. Beta sitosterol is used to produce modest lowering of cholesterol in patients with mild hypercholesterolemia, given in doses of 3 to 6 g/day. Its use is contraindicated in betasitosterolemia, a condition that mimics familial hypercholesterolemia.

NEOMYCIN

Neomycin inhibits intestinal cholesterol absorption and produces decreased pools of exchangeable cholesterol in the body and a moderate reduction of serum cholesterol levels in many patients with hypercholesterolemia. Dosage is usually 0.5 to 2.0 g/day. Diarrhea and abdominal cramps are encountered in some patients. Bacterial or fungal suprainfection may occur. Malabsorption of fat could occur in patients with preexisting gastroenteric disease, and absorption of digitalis glycosides is impaired. Less than 1% of the administered dose is absorbed from normal intestine, but a greater fraction may be absorbed through diseased bowel, leading to specific toxicity (*see* Chap. 61). Neomycin should not be given to patients with impaired renal function.

D-THYROXINE

D-Thyroxine, an isomer of L-thyroxine, is thought to act by increasing the conversion of cholesterol to bile acids. It appears to retain some hypercalorigenic activity, which may cause increased cardiac work and induce angina. D-Thyroxine has only limited effect in the treatment of hyperlipidemia. For this reason and because it may cause fatal cardiac arrhythmias, D-thyroxine is no longer indicated.

COMBINED DRUG THERAPY

Combined drug treatment has been useful when a single drug fails to normalize LDL levels in familial hypercholesterolemia; when VLDL levels increase significantly during treatment of hypercholesterolemia with bile acid sequestrants; and when levels of LDL and VLDL are elevated. Clofibrate, in combination with the resins, is sometimes effective in lowering levels of VLDL but has little, if any, complementary effect on LDL levels. Nicotinic acid, when used alone, is much more effective than clofibrate in lowering levels of triglycerides and also decreases LDL levels. When used with the resins, nicotinic acid has a marked complementary effect in decreasing levels of LDL. This combination completely normalizes levels of LDL in heterozygous familial hypercholesterolemia and usually normalizes levels of VLDL in patients who have increased levels of this lipoprotein while taking the resins.

The complementary action on LDL most likely reflects decreased production of VLDL, the LDL precursor, induced by nicotinic acid and the effect of the resin on increased LDL catabolism. The toxicity or side-effects of this regimen are only those observed when the drugs are given singley. Long-term adherence to the regimen has shown that the effect on lipoprotein levels is sustained and that no new side-effects or toxicity develops. An added benefit may be that nicotinic acid causes significant increases in levels of HDL.

Nicotinic acid and the resin can be given together because niacin, although it is an anion, does not bind to the resin. Simultaneous administration of these drugs is of additional benefit in those patients who complain of gastric irritation when taking nicotinic acid because the resins have significant acid-neutralizing properties.

When this combination is used to treat patients who have increased levels of LDL and VLDL, 1.5 to 3.0 g/day of nicotinic acid is usually effective. However, to normalize levels of LDL in familial hypercholesterolemia, a median daily dose of 6.5 g of nicotinic acid is needed in combination with 24 or 30 g/day of cholestyramine or colestipol, respectively.

Other drugs that may have some complementary effect with the resins in treating hypercholesterolemia are neomycin and beta sitosterol. The reductions in LDL levels produced by these combinations are, however, relatively smaller than with the resin-nicotinic acid regimen.

FURTHER READING

1. Coronary Drug Project Research Group: Clofibrate and niacin in coronary heart disease. J Am Med Assoc 231:360, 1975
2. Einarsson K, Hellstrom K, Leija B: Bile acid kinetics and steroid balance during nicotinic acid therapy in patients with hyperlipoproteinemia types II and IV. J Lab Clin Med 90:613, 1977
3. Fredrickson DS, Goldstein JL, Brown MS: The familial hyperlipidemias. *In* Stanbury JB, Wyngaarden JB, Fredrickson DS (eds): The Metabolic Basis of Inherited Disease, 4th ed, pp 604–655. New York, McGraw–Hill, 1978
4. Havel RJ, Goldstein JL, Brown MS: Lipoproteins and lipid transport. *In* Bondy PK, Rosenberg LE (eds): Metabolic Control and Disease, pp 393–467. Philadelphia, WB Saunders, 1980
5. Havel RJ, Kane JP: Drugs and lipid metabolism. Annu Rev Pharmacol 13:287, 1973
6. Kane JP, Malloy MJ: Treatment of hypercholesterolemia. Med Clin N Amer 66:537, 1982
7. Kane JP, Malloy MJ, Tun P et al: Normalization of levels of low density lipoproteins in serum of patients with heterozygous familial hypercholesterolemia with a combined drug regimen. N Engl J Med 304:251, 1981
8. Levy RI, Fredrickson DS, Shulman R et al: Dietary and drug treatment of primary hyperlipoproteinemia. Ann Intern Med 77:267, 1972
9. Lewis B: The Hyperlipidaemias: Clinical and Laboratory Practice. Oxford, Blackwell Scientific, 1976
10. Miettinen TA: Effects of neomycin alone and in combination with cholestyramine on serum cholesterol and fecal steroids in hypercholesterolemic subjects. J Clin Invest 64:1485, 1979

CHAPTER 37 QUESTIONS

(*See* P. 7 for Full Instructions)

Select the One Best Answer

1. Each of the following statements is true EXCEPT
   A. clofibrate is effective in the treatment of certain types of hyperlipidemia.
   B. cholestyramine is effective in reducing the pruritus that accompanies biliary obstruction.
   C. dextrothyroxine decreases the biosynthesis of cholesterol.
   D. nicotinic acid commonly produces generalized flushing.

E. heparin forms an inactive complex with protamine.

2. The agent that reduces the plasma lipoprotein concentration by decreasing production is
   A. cholestyramine.
   B. nicotinic acid.
   C. *d*-thyroxine.
   D. heparin.
   E. ethyl alcohol.

3. Certain forms of hypertriglyceridemia may respond favorably to therapy with
   A. estrogen.
   B. ethyl alcohol.
   C. clofibrate.
   D. cholestyramine.
   E. glucocorticoids.

4. When a patient's serum cholesterol level is more than 400 mg/dl and the triglyceride level is less than 150 mg/dl, it can be assumed, in the absence of cholestasis, that the patient's blood contains an elevated level of
   A. chylomicrons.
   B. very low density lipoproteins.
   C. intermediate density lipoproteins.
   D. low density lipoproteins.
   E. high density lipoproteins.

5. For a patient with severe endogenous or mixed lipemia, medical recommendations might include each of the following EXCEPT
   A. abstinence from alcohol.
   B. avoidance of estrogens.
   C. consumption of at least 60 ml of alcohol per day.
   D. restriction of total caloric intake.
   E. treatment with nicotinic acid.

A = 1,2,3; B = 1,3; C = 2,4; D = 4; E = All

6. Cholestyramine
   1. is most effective in patients with high serum triglyceride.
   2. inhibits cholesterol synthesis at the level of mevalonate formation.
   3. inhibits lipoprotein synthesis by blocking amino-acid incorporation into protein.
   4. is effective in reducing plasma cholesterol in essential hypercholesterolemia.

7. Sodium dextrothyroxine
   1. does not have a calorigenic action.
   2. may precipitate angina pectoris.
   3. is not associated with arrhythmias.
   4. promotes the catabolism of cholesterol.

8. Drugs that primarily affect levels of low density lipoproteins include
   1. bile acid binding resins.
   2. neomycin.
   3. sitosterol.
   4. clofibrate.

9. For almost all kinds of hyperlipoproteinemia, dietary modifications should include
   1. restriction of cholesterol.
   2. restriction of total calories to achieve ideal body weight.
   3. restriction of saturated fats.
   4. increased protein from animal sources.

Drugs That Affect the Gastrointestinal System

38

JEREMY H. THOMPSON

Drugs that affect the gastrointestinal tract act mainly on its muscular and glandular tissues directly, or indirectly by way of the endocrine or autonomic nervous system. These drugs are best discussed by grouping them according to their major therapeutic indications.

DRUGS THAT AFFECT APPETITE

STIMULANTS

Many drugs, mostly alkaloidal in nature and with no other property than a *bitter taste,* are occasionally used to *stimulate the appetite.* Their small success is due entirely to reflex vagal stimulation. *Alcoholic drinks, appetizers,* and highly-spiced *hors d'oeuvres* are more valuable. *Vitamin preparations* and *iron* are worthless except in the rare case of true deficiency, and *thyroid hormones* and *insulin* may be valuable in anorexia nervosa.

SUPPRESSANTS (ANOREXIANTS)

There are many causes of obesity, and before anorexiants are used care must be taken to exclude all specifically treatable causes, such as endocrine disorders. The anorexiant or anoretic drugs (those that lead to loss of appetite) should be used only as adjuncts in the management of overweight due to excessive calorie consumption. Thus they should be used as part of a long-term patient "contract" along with motivational and psychological support and most important, reduction of calorie intake. Anorexiants elevate the patient's mood and make him more tolerant of the dietary restrictions. They also suppress the feelings of hunger by an unknown action. Among the proposed mechanisms of action are stimulation of the satiety center in the medial hypothalamus; blockade of impulses reaching the "eating center" in the lateral hypothalamus; and elevation of plasma free fatty acid levels, which in turn depress the "eating center." The amphetamine group of drugs, once widely used, is now obsolete, having been replaced by other sympathomimetic agents, among which *diethylpropion hydrochloride, phenmetrazine hydrochloride,* and *fenfluramine* are most popular. Although these drugs are used frequently, they are ineffective over long periods and are of no value without conscientious food restriction. All anorexiants possess some adverse effects, and no drug therapy can produce greater weight loss than proper dieting.

DRUGS THAT AFFECT THE STOMACH

CARMINATIVES

Carminatives are predominantly mild mucosal irritants that relieve discomfort of the stomach due to gaseous distention by relaxing the cardiac sphincter. Aniseed, camphor, cinnamon, dill, ginger, glycyrrhiza (liquorice), peppermint, sassafrass, and spearmint are used, particularly in chewing gums, but are of doubtful value. Peppermint oil (often used in antacids) is a weak antispasmodic agent. Methylpolysiloxane (simethicone), often formulated with antacids, is reputedly a mild carminative.

EMETICS

Many drugs, if taken by mouth in too large a quantity or too concentrated a solution, excite reflex nausea and vomiting. The induction of emesis may be a therapeutic necessity, for example, in the treatment of poisoning (*see* Chap. 72). *Locally acting and centrally acting* emetics are available. Hypertonic salt solutions (usually sodium chloride), copper and zinc sulfate solutions, and mustard solutions act locally because of their osmotic pressure or their irritant properties. The uncontrolled use of hypertonic solutions of sodium chloride may lead to fatal hypernatremia. Derivatives of the opium alkaloids (particularly apomorphine) and syrup of ipecac stimulate vomiting by an action on the brainstem (*see* Chap. 72).

ANTIEMETICS

Antiemetics are used to control nausea and vomiting. Vomiting may be dangerous; if uncontrolled, it can lead to exhaustion of the patient, with dehydration, *p*H and electrolyte abnormalities, aspiration of vomitus into the tracheobronchial tree, and esophagogastric bleeding or rupture. *Nausea and vomiting are only symptoms and should not be treated without the underlying cause being determined.* Phenothiazine compounds depress the medullary chemoreceptor trigger zone; common examples are chlorpromazine hydrochloride, prochlorperazine maleate, and promazine hydrochloride (*see* Chap. 23). H_1-Blockers (*see* Chap. 51) in common use are buclizine hydrochloride, diphenhydramine hydrochloride, and meclizine hydrochloride. They act centrally on the eighth nerve and its connections presumably by their anticholinergic properties. Some nonphenothiazine, nonantihistaminic antiemetics are available that act on the medullary chemoreceptor trigger zone. *Trimethobenzamide hydrochloride* (Tigan) and *Diphenidol hydrochloride* (Vontrol) are popular.

Experimentally, metoclopramide and marijuana (Δ-9-THC) offer some promise.

Adverse Effects

Adverse effects of the phenothiazine and nonphenothiazine compounds are discussed elsewhere (*see* Chap. 23). *Trimethobenzamide* may produce drowsiness, headache, diarrhea, muscle cramps, dizziness, and alterations of mood. Rarely, hypotension, blurred vision, bone marrow depression, jaundice, convulsions, and extrapyramidal symptoms may appear. It may be a weak teratogen. Trimethobenzamide suppositories contain benzocaine, which may produce hypersensitivity reactions. *Diphenidol* may produce nausea, indigestion, headache, nervousness, drowsiness, and, rarely, hypotension. Anticholinergiclike symptoms (xerostomia, blurred vision, urinary retention, increased intraocular tension, visual and auditory hallucinations, and confusional states), urticaria, and various other skin rashes in sensitive patients may also develop.

DIAGNOSTIC AGENTS

Histamine and betazole hydrochloride (Histalog) are discussed in Chapter 51 and azuresin in Chapter 77.

DIGESTANTS

The digestants are a group of replacement drugs that supply a deficiency of a normal component of gastrointestinal secretion. Once popular, their exact place in therapy is now questionable.

Hydrochloric acid may be supplied in two forms. Diluted hydrochloric acid N.F. (Acidulin) is a 10% solution that should be administered by glass drinking tube or straw to avoid contact with the teeth. *Betaine hydrochloride* (Normacid) is a formulation of 400 mg of betaine hydrochloride that contains the equivalent of 1.0 ml of dilute HCl, 32.4 mg of pepsin, and 110 mg of methylcellulose. The formulation is said to release HCl slowly within the stomach, paralleling the release of acid that occurs during digestion. *Pepsin* is commonly supplied as a powder prepared from the oxyntic gland area of the fresh stomach of the hog (Pepsin N.F.) *Dehydrocholic acid* N.F. (Decholin) and *sodium dehydrocholate* N.F. (Decholin sodium) increase the volume of bile secreted (choleresis). Their administration may aid the absorption of fat and fat-soluble vitamins in those conditions associated with partial biliary obstruction. Both agents are contraindicated in complete biliary obstruction and may aggravate the pruritus associated with poor bile formation. Sodium dehydrocholic acid is also used to determine the arm-to-tongue circulation time in certain conditions where the velocity of blood flow may be altered.

Pancreatic extracts may benefit patients with cystic fibrosis, adult pancreatic insufficiency, and selected postgastrectomy syndromes. They should be given with an appropriate low-fat, high-protein diet. Efficacy is highly variable between different preparations and their cost. *Pancreatin* N.F., a cream-colored, amorphous powder obtained from the fresh pancreas of the hog or ox, contains amylase, lipase, and trypsin. *Pancrelipase* (Cotazym) is a concentrate of ox pancreatic enzymes standardized by lipase content. Some proprietary pancreatic extracts are enriched with bile salts, cellulases, collagenase, or elastase. In the very rare patient who lacks both bile and pancreatic enzyme secretion, each component should logically be supplied separately. Since release from enteric-coated tablets is capricious, pancreatic extracts should be given with food, milk, or alkali in an attempt to buffer the gastric contents, thereby reducing inactivation of the enzyme. Cimetidine (*see* Chap. 51) is far more beneficial, however. Dosage of enzymes is variable, and treatment should be directed at restoring weight and a feeling of well-being and converting the volume, consistency, and odor of stools to normal. Children may develop buccal irritation, ulceration, or perianal soreness, and, on rare occasions, allergy to the animal-derived protein may occur. Gout may develop rarely, presumably because of the high purine content of the drugs. *Choline dihydrogen citrate* (Monichol) may be effective as a lipotropic agent in patients with hepatic cirrhosis.

CHENODEOXYCHOLIC ACID (CHENIC ACID)

Chenic acid is naturally occurring, primary dihydroxy bile acid under clinical investigation to promote solubilization of cholesterol in bile and the dissolution of cholesterol-containing gall stones. About 10 million Americans have significant cholesterol gall-stone disease. Chenic acid is most effective in patients with mild symptoms but of no value in treating pure pigment, or high calcium-containing, stones. Chenic acid may also be valuable in reducing serum triglyceride levels in patients with hypertriglyceridemia (*see* Chap. 37). Formation of cholesterol gall stones occurs when the bile becomes supersaturated with cholesterol; several mechanisms are possible, including excessive bile salt loss (ileal disease), decreased bile salt synthesis, and excessive formation/secretion of cholesterol.

Several effects of chenic acid have been described, but its precise mechanism of action in reducing net hepatic secretion of cholesterol, thereby promoting dissolution of stones within the biliary system, is not known. For example, chenic acid reduces primary bile salt synthesis in the liver, impairs cholesterol absorption from the intestine, and impairs HMG-Co reductase (the rate limiting enzyme for cholesterol synthesis) and cholesterol 7α-hydroxylase activity in the liver. Chenic acid does not increase total exchangeable body cholesterol or phospholipid secretion but does increase bile salt pool size twofold. With doses up to about 1 *g/day*, chenic acid is almost completely absorbed in the small bowel, whereas higher doses saturate the ileal absorption mechanism and produce diarrhea; a large crystal size reduces absorption. First-pass clearance of chenic acid is about 60% with doses of 400 mg.

Chenic acid is secreted into bile. In animals, particularly primates, it is degraded by colonic bacteria into lithocholic acid, which after reabsorption is hepatotoxic (bile duct proliferation, periportal infiltration). Hepatotoxicity from lithocholic acid is probably never seen in humans because chenic acid epimerizes in the bowel lumen to ursodeoxycholic acid, which is not a preferred precursor for lithocholic acid, and because humans possess an avid pathway (sulfation) of lithocholic acid detoxification not present in animals.

Side-effects are minimal. Diarrhea may develop with doses greater than 1 g/day. Transient elevations of serum SGOT and alkaline phosphatase have been reported, but their significance is not known. Partially solubilized gall stones may migrate, producing obstruction. Chenic acid is expensive.

The usual dose is 14 to 16 mg/kg/day, but in obese patients 18 to 20 mg/kg/day may be needed. Preferably, the drug should be given at bedtime, since its action is prolonged by enterohepatic circulation with overnight fasting.

Therapy will probably be needed for 6 to 24 months; 20% to 40% of patients will reform stones if effective therapy is discontinued. Unanswered questions are the need, safety, and efficacy of chenic acid therapy after stones have dissolved and its use in women of child-bearing age or in those taking oral contraceptive steroids.

The potential long-term effect of chenodeoxycholic acid on cholesterol and triglyceride metabolism, on the development of atherosclerosis, or on liver function is not known. Patients have been given the drug for up to 4 years. Chenic acid probably should be reserved for use in older patients, particularly those who are a poor operative risk, and those with small cholesterol stones, a functioning gall bladder, and patent bile ducts.

DRUGS FOR PEPTIC ULCER DISEASE

A "peptic ulcer" is a sharply circumscribed loss of mucosa and muscularis mucosa in those segments of the digestive tract exposed to gastric juice that contains hydrochloric acid and pepsin. "Stress" ulcers, occurring acutely in patients after severe head injury, burns, or trauma or with severe renal, hepatic, or respiratory disease must also be considered, even though the lesion does not typically penetrate the muscularis mucosae. The cause of these different ulcers is unknown, but it is generally believed that gastric acid and the proteolytic enzyme pepsin are required for the maintenance and persistence of an ulcer; Schwartz's dictum—"no acid, no ulcer"—is still valid for the most part.

Peptic ulcers develop when there is an imbalance between acid/pepsin secretion and mucosal "resistance." Thus increased acid/pepsin secretion, reduced mucosal resistance as championed by Grossman, or the two conditions acting simultaneously may lead to ulcer formation. With gastric ulcer disease, impaired mucosal resistance with bile reflux and acid back diffusion may be etiologically more important than other factors; in duodenal ulcer disease, however, an increased number of parietal cells and vagal overactivity resulting in augmented acid production are probably more important. Interestingly the incidence of peptic ulcer disease is falling, but the reason is not apparent.

Morton Irvin Grossman, 1919–1981. American gastroenterologist. Worked especially on the physiology of nutrition and gastrointestinal hormones.

Numerous drugs and therapeutic maneuvers (Table 38-1) have been used to manage peptic ulcer disease, the aims being to relieve pain, to promote healing, to prevent recurrences, and to reduce complications (bleeding, perforation, chronicity). Drugs are only a part of therapy that should include emotional support, rest, and the withdrawal (when possible) of certain drugs (Table 38-2). A full understanding of the application of treatment will be facilitated by an understanding of normal gastric secretion.

MECHANISMS AND CONTROL OF GASTRIC SECRETION

Gastric juice is a highly complex fluid, but for the purpose of this chapter only hydrochloric acid, pepsin(ogen), and mucosubstances will be discussed.

Hydrochloric Acid

Acid is secreted by the parietal cells. The total number of parietal cells (parietal cell "mass") varies widely, but generally normal adults possess about 1 billion cells and can secrete about 22 mEq of acid/hr. The corresponding values for subjects with duodenal and gastric ulcers are 1.8 billion cells and 42 mEq of acid and 0.8 billion cells and 18 mEq of acid, respectively. Even though there is great variation around these means, patients with chronic duodenal ulcer disease tend to secrete more acid than do normal subjects both at rest and after test stimuli.

The quantity of gastric acid secreted at any moment depends on the interplay of many stimulatory and inhibitory factors. Classically, gastric acid secretion has been divided into two periods, *interprandial* (interdigestive, basal, spontaneous) and *postprandial* (digestive, stimulated) secretion. Postprandial secretion is further separated into *cephalic*, *gastric*, and *intestinal* phases; this is an artificial division that indicates only the region in which a given stimulus acts.

In humans, *interprandial* secretion contains varying amounts of hydrochloric acid. The *cephalic* phase of postprandial secretion is mediated by the vagus nerves. Vagal impulses generated by the thought, sight, smell, taste, or swallowing of food produce acid release by direct cholinergic stimulation of parietal cells, and indirectly by the release of pyloric gland area gastrin. Additionally, vagal (cholinergic) impulses "sensitize" the parietal cells to gastrin and other stimulants. Gastric secretion in the *gastric phase* of postprandial secretion has

TABLE 38-1. Drugs and Maneuvers Used to Treat Peptic Ulcer Disease

Drug/Maneuver		Comment
Hyposecretory Drugs		
Hydrochloric acid:	H_2-receptor antagonists	Cimetidine has recently achieved great popularity, even surplanting antacids. However, questions still remain as to its precise role in therapy. *See* Chapter 51.
	Anticholinergic agents*	Because gastric secretion and gastric emptying are under vagal cholinergic (muscarinic) control, anticholinergic drugs have been proposed as adjuncts to antacids in the treatment of duodenal ulcer. Oral doses of anticholinergic drugs giving minimal and tolerable systemic side-effects fail to produce significant diminution of acid secretion or prolongation of gastric emptying. On the other hand, large doses of many anticholinergic drugs reduce gastric acid output and gastric emptying but only in the face of varying degrees of systemic parasympathetic blockade. Anticholinergic drugs do not alter the incidence of duodenal ulcer complications or recurrence. Once popular, their clinical use is limited. They may be valuable in controlling nocturnal hypersecretion of acid, since systemic side-effects of parasympathetic blockade may be tolerable because they occur during sleep. They should be used combined with antacids only if antacids have failed to control symptoms and if no contraindications (glaucoma, prostatic hypertrophy, pyloric stenosis) to their use are present (*see* Chapter 16). They should be given 15 to 30 minutes before antacids or food.
	Sedatives/tranquilizers*	The popular concept that "stress" and emotional and physical factors stimulate the vagal motor nuclei prompted the widespread use of these agents in duodenal ulcer. These agents have little, if any, effect on acid secretion and should be reserved for those patients with concomitant anxiety, restlessness, or insomnia.
Pepsin(ogen):	Anticholinergic agents*	*See* previous comment.
Neutralizing Drugs		
Hydrochloric acid:	Antacids	By far the most commonly used drugs. *See* text.
Pepsin(ogen):	Antipepsins*	Some limited use in gastric ulcer. *See* text.
Drugs that Augment Mucosal "Resistance"		
Licorice-derived:	Carbenoxolone	Effective in ulcer disease but has significant side-effects. *See* text.
	Deglycyrrhizinated licorice*	Has no effect on mucous production but possesses weak antispasmodic and antacid activity, presumably because of the added ingredients. *See* text.
	Gefarnate†	Possibly of some benefit in gastric ulcer. *See* text.
Bismuth salts:	Tri-potassium dicitratobismuthate (TBD)	Possesses several actions; augments mucosal "resistance," chelates pepsins, stimulates mucous production, and has antacid properties. *See* text.
Alginates:		Hydrophilic compounds derived from polyuronic acids in seaweeds. They precipitate in an acid medium, forming a sticky gel that adheres to the mucosa. They are frequently added to antacids.
Sex hormones:	Stilbestrol‡	Increases the production of gastric mucosubstances and enhances the rate of epithelial cell renewal. It accelerates the healing of duodenal (but not gastric) ulcers in men and reduces the relapse rate. Synthetic estrogen therapy is not generally suitable because unpleasant feminizing effects develop.
Miscellaneous Drugs and Maneuvers		
	Hormones†	Somatostatin, secretin, glucagon, cholecystokinin/pancreozymin, and calcitonin possess potent antiulcer or antisecretory properties and may become therapeutically important in humans.
	Metoclopramide†	May reduce gastric reflux by "coordinating" antral emptying.

(*continued*)

TABLE 38-1. *(Continued)*

Drug/Maneuver	Comment
Miscellaneous Drugs and Maneuvers	
Prostaglandins†	Endogenous and exogenous prostaglandins, particularly of the E series (*see* Chap. 53), protect the gastric mucosa of animals against various ulcerogens (aspirin and other nonsteroidal anti-inflammatory agents, boiling water, absolute ethanol, acids, alkalis, and bile salts) and possibly promote healing. *15,15-methyl prostaglandin* E_2 and *16,16-dimethyl prostaglandin* E_2 are orally active agents being evaluated in ulcer disease. They depress gastric acid secretion, gastrin release, gastric mucosal blood flow, and gastric emptying. Additionally they increase mucous and bicarbonate secretion and reduce acid back-diffusion. Clinically they produce diarrhea.
Urogastrone†	A 52-amino acid polypeptide similar to epidermal growth factor and isolated from human urine. It depresses acid output in animals after parenteral administration.
Sulglycotide†	Isolated from porcine duodenal mucosa; reduces peptic activity. Little clinical promise.
Sulpiride†	Depresses gastrin release. Of doubtful therapeutic potential.
Carbonic anhydrase inhibitors, zinc salts, cholestyramine, deep x-ray therapy, and gastric freezing‡	Generally obsolete because of limited potency and significant side-effects.
General Measures	
Hospitalization	
Bed rest	
Avoidance of specific drugs (*see* Table 38-2)	
Diets or dietary restrictions*	

* Of some limited value.
† Experimental/investigational therapy.
‡ Obsolete.

the same components and is activated by both vagal impulses and vagovagal reflexes. The *intestinal phase* of postprandial secretion is relatively unimportant; it is mediated by intestinal gastrin and other less well-defined humoral agents.

Cyclic adenosine 3′,5-monophosphate (cyclic AMP) is the final link in gastrin-induced secretion. Histamine (and related agents) induces copious gastric acid secretion, and accumulating evidence suggests that this autacoid may play a role in normal gastric secretion. Almost certainly acetylcholine, histamine, and gastrin all have direct input onto the parietal cell.

When the parietal cells are stimulated to secrete, they produce isotonic hydrochloric acid (165 mN) in which the concentration of hydrogen ions is a million times that in the plasma. The mechanism whereby this intense concentration occurs is unknown, but the overall change can be represented as follows.

$$H_2O + CO_2 \xrightarrow{\text{Carbonic Anhydrase}} (H)^+ + (HCO_3)^- \qquad 1$$

The $(H)^+$ accompanied by $(Cl)^-$ is transported into the gastric lumen, and the $(HCO)^-$ passes to the extracellular fluid where it is balanced by sodium. In the small bowel the $(H)^+$ reacts under normal circumstances with biliary, intestinal, and pancreatic bicarbonate, as indicated below, and is absorbed.

$$(H)^+ + (HCO_3)^- \rightarrow H_2O + CO_2 \qquad 2$$

Since equation 2 is the exact opposite of equation 1, there is no overall net alteration in extracellular *p*H as a result of gastric acid secretion and its subsequent intestinal absorption. However, if gastric juice is lost from the body, for example, by vomiting, gastric suction, or severe diarrhea, metabolic alkalosis may result.

TABLE 38-2. Some Drugs Contraindicated in Patients with Peptic Ulcer Disease

Drug	Comment
ACTH	*See* Corticosteroids
Alcohol (ethanol)	Produces gastritis but probably does not stimulate gastric acid secretion. May increase acid back-diffusion
Anticoagulants	Facilitate ulcer bleeding
Aspirin and other salicylates	Increase acid back-diffusion, produce mucosal irritation, leading to erosions and bleeding. Ulcerogenic after parenteral administration. Interfere with blood coagulation
Caffeinated beverages (tea, coffee, cola)	*See* xanthines
Corticosteroids	Diminished tissue resistance; exhibit antiinflammatory action; produce "defective" mucus.
Ethacrynic acid	May produce gastric ulceration
Nonsteroidal antiinflammatory drugs (*e.g.*, phenylbutazone)	Use may result in gastroduodenal ulceration. May increase acid back-diffusion. Ulcerogenic on parenteral administration
Para-aminosalicyclic acid (PAS)	Mucosal irritation, erosions, and bleeding
Phenacetin	*See* PAS
Probenecid	*See* PAS
Reserpine	Gastroduodenal ulceration
Tobacco smoking	Reduces rate of ulcer healing. Reduces pancreatic bicarbonate output and increases duodenogastric reflux. Increases mortality from ulcer disease
Xanthine alkaloids	Gastric acid secretory stimulants through interaction with cyclic AMP

Pepsin(ogen)

The proteolytic enzyme pepsin is produced from pepsinogen. There are two separate immunochemical pepsinogen groups: Group I pepsinogens limited to the zymogen (chief) cells and mucous neck cells of the oxyntic gland area; and group II pepsinogens also present in these cells and additionally located in mucous neck cells of the pyloric gland area and in Brunner's glands.

Johann Conrad von Brunner, 1653–1727. Swiss anatomist at the University of Heidelberg. Discovered Brunner's glands in the duodenum in 1672 and in 1683 observed the effects of experimental removal of the pancreas and spleen.

Pepsinogens comprise pepsin and peptide moieties; the terminal moiety is an inhibitor of proteolytic activity. The pepsin-inhibitor complex dissociates about *p*H 5.4, but not until the *p*H falls to about 4.0 is the inhibitor gradually inactivated autocatalytically by digestion, with progressive development of full peptic activity. Pepsin (molecular weight about 35,000) is maximally active about *p*H 2.0. During the basal state, pepsin stores remain intact, and the small continuous secretion is probably an "overflow" from continued synthesis. The most powerful stimuli to pepsin secretion are vagal (cholinergic) stimulation and histamine and gastrin administration.

About 50% of patients with duodenal ulcer disease have an elevated plasma pepsinogen-I concentration. Hyperpepsinogen-Iemia is inherited as an autosomal dominant trait. At least two other traits have been discovered in duodenal ulcer disease: rapid gastric emptying and antral G-cell hyperfunction.

Mucosubstances

Gastric mucin is the viscous secretion of the stomach that serves to protect the mucosa. No conclusive evidence, however, suggests that this is so. Gastric mucus is a heterogenous secretion derived from the surface epithelium columnar cells and the mucous neck cells of the cardiac, oxyntic, and pyloric gland areas. Secretion of alkaline mucus is spontaneous and is increased by mechanical irritation of the mucosa and by both sympathetic and parasympathetic nervous system stimulation. No simple test quantitates differences in mucosal "resistance."

ANTACIDS

Antacids probably still remain the cornerstone of therapy. Some physicians have replaced antacids with cimetidine, but both are equally active, and the side-effects and cost of the H_2-receptor antagonist do limit its popularity.

Mechanism of action

Antacids diminish the quantity of free hydrochloric acid in the stomach. The rationale for using antacids includes that ulcers do not occur when acid is not present; peptic activity decreases with increasing *p*H; operations that reduce acid output may cure ulceration; and antacids prevent experimental ulceration in animals. Antacids diminish the free acid concentration by three main mechanisms.

1. *Direct neutralization of preformed acid.* This phenomenon has been amply seen both *in vivo* and *in vitro* and is the most important mechanism of action of antacids. Common antacids contain a weak basic moiety, which is sufficient to elevate the gastric *p*H above 4 (*see* below) but not strong enough to damage the mucosal surface. Examples of antacids that act thus are sodium bicarbonate and magnesium oxide.
2. *Buffering of preformed acid.* Examples of antacids that act by this mechanism are magnesium trisilicate and sodium citrate. Antacids vary widely with respect to buffering capacity, and the volume of antacid required to yield optimal buffering varies from patient to patient. Generally, persons who hypersecrete require more antacid than do those who hyposecrete.
3. *Absorption of hydrogen ions and adsorption and inactivation of pepsin.* Both have been demonstrated with aluminum antacids and with some anion exchange resins; aluminum antacids may also bind bile acids.

In addition to these three primary mechanisms of action, some new antacid formulations contain *alginates* (Table 38-1), *simethicone* (a mixture of liquid dimethylpolysiloxanes that acts as a defoaming agent, lowering surface tension and allowing gas bubbles to coalesce), *local anesthetics* (possibly reducing gastrin release or ulcer pain), and *peppermint oil* (a weak antispasmodic). *Thus antacids act locally within the stomach and are effective only as long as they remain there. Antacids have no inhibitory effect on the parietal cells, and consequently their effects are only temporary.*

Principles of Therapy

Antacids are used to raise the gastric *p*H to about 4.0 or greater, so that peptic activity is reduced and the *p*H of the intra-lumenal contents is less irritating to the mucosa and ulcer crater. Complete neutralization of gastric acid by antacids is not desirable because more rapid gastric emptying will result, and possibly more rebound acid secretion due to excessive release of gastric gastrin. The efficiency of an antacid depends on the amount of acid secreted per unit of time, the neutralizing capacity of the antacid, and the rapidity of gastric emptying. Antacids given in the fasting state will neutralize the gastric contents for about 30 to 60 minutes, and after meals for about 2 to 3 hours. Consequently one of the most important factors in treating acute peptic ulcer disease is adequate hourly antacid therapy, which may be difficult to achieve, and a compromise of 40 and 80 mEq of liquid antacid 1 and 3 hours after meals, and at bedtime, for patients with gastric and duodenal ulcers, respectively, may result in greater patient compliance. For maintenance therapy, antacids should be given about 1 hour after meals rather than before meals because this regimen yields more prolonged acid neutralization. In practice, unfortunately, many patients limit their antacid ingestion to times of pain.

Classification

Antacids are conveniently classified into *systemic* and *nonsystemic* groups, depending on their degree of absorption.

The cationic fraction of systemic antacids does not form insoluble basic compounds in the bowel lumen but is absorbed and may produce alkalosis and an expanded extracellular fluid volume. Such alkalosis is enhanced by chloride loss (vomiting, gastric suction, or diarrhea) and by sodium absorption. Nausea, vomiting, diarrhea, abdominal pain, irritability, occipital headaches, insomnia, myalgia, and tetany may develop. Acute alkalosis may produce paralytic ileus and electrocardiographic abnormalities. *Sodium bicarbonate* is the only systemic antacid used; it has limited application because of its side-effects.

Nonsystemic antacids are either not absorbed or are poorly absorbed, and are therefore therapeutically preferable. Typical examples are basic compounds of *magnesium* and *aluminum; calcium* salts (*e.g.*, calcium carbonate) are still available, but they should not be used because they stimulate gastrin release. Other less efficient "antacids" are *milk, anion exchange resins*, and *gastric mucin*.

The sodium content of most nonsystemic antacids is 3 to 10 mg/dl. Thus 2 to 3 g of sodium will be ingested daily during conventional therapy (unless low sodium-containing preparations are used), a situation that may compromise cardiovascular, hepatic, and renal function in patients with disease of these systems. Contamination of antacids by pathogenic yeasts, molds, and bacteria has been described as a source of potential infection, and several cases of brucellosis have been reported in patients drinking infected milk in whom antacids had reduced the antimicrobial properties of gastric juice.

A plethora of antacids are available, many

formulated with sedatives, tranquilizers, and other antacids or drugs with questionable pharmacologic properties. Table 38-3 lists the properties and adverse effects of some common antacids.

Uses

At least $100 million and £20 million are spent annually on antacids in the United States and United Kingdom, respectively. Most sales are

TABLE 38-3. Properties, Dosage, and Adverse Effects of Some Common Antacids

Antacid	Properties	Dose	Adverse Effects and Comment
Sodium bicarbonate USP (baking soda)	Rapid onset and short duration of action because of high solubility. 1.0 g neutralizes about 12 mEq of acid. Cheap, but taste, color, and cost have been added in proprietary preparations.	300 mg–2 g hourly	Sodium bicarbonate is almost totally absorbed, thus presenting the body with excess sodium and alkali (systemic alkalosis). This may be detrimental to those with diminished renal reserve or sodium retention. Sodium bicarbonate has a very short duration of action owing to rapid gastric emptying. Additionally, rebound acid secretion may be seen. Gastric distention from CO_2 production may rarely produce perforation. *Sodium bicarbonate is not recommended for use as an antacid.*
Precipitated calcium carbonate USP (precipitated chalk)	More prolonged duration of action to sodium bicarbonate. Cheap. 1.0 g neutralizes about 2 to 3 mEq of acid. Converted into calcium chloride, carbonate, and phosphate, which react in the small bowel with dietary fatty acids to form insoluble soaps that produce constipation. About 10% of the calcium is absorbed.	1.0–2.0 g hourly	An inexpensive potent antacid now probably obsolete because of its stimulatory properties in gastric secretion. Certainly oral calcium produces increased acid secretion in the fasting or fed state, after single or repeated dosage, both in patients with ulcer disease and in normal subjects; stimulation of gastrin release is probably responsible. Calcium carbonate tends to produce nausea and constipation, and it has a chalky taste. Chronic therapy, particularly in conjunction with sodium bicarbonate, may result in the milk–alkali (Burnett's) syndrome due to hypercalcemia. If recognized early in subjects with normal renal function, the syndrome may resolve on discontinuing therapy. However, if unrecognized, it may progress to renal failure and metastatic calcification. Symptoms of the milk–alkali syndrome include nausea, anorexia, malaise, vomiting, weakness, lethargy, myalgia, polydipsia, and polyuria. Parathormone secretion may be depressed.
Magnesium hydroxide USP (milk of magnesia)	Insoluble, 8% aqueous suspension with *p*H of about 10.6. Magnesium chloride, formed on hydrochloric acid neutralization, is highly soluble and in the small bowel acts as an osmotic laxative. 1.0 ml neutralizes about 3 mEq of acid.	5.0–15.0 ml hourly	All preparations may produce laxation. With each preparation, about 5% to 10% of the magnesium is absorbed. This is of little import in patients with satisfactory renal function. However, hypermagnesemia with hypotension and respiratory arrest may develop if renal function is impaired. Some recently introduced concentrated magnesium antacids must be taken in lower doses to minimize diarrhea and sodium and magnesium overloading.
Magnesium oxide USP	Converted into magnesium hydroxide in the stomach and thus acts slowly. 1.0 g neutralizes about 30 mEq of acid.	250 mg hourly	*See* magnesium hydroxide.

Charles Hoyt Burnett, 1913–1967. American physician. Milk–alkali syndrome had already been described in 1923, but Burnett was the first to show, in 1949, how it could be reversed by decreasing the intake of milk and alkaline salts.

(continued)

TABLE 38-3. (*Continued*)

Antacid	Properties	Dose	Adverse Effects and Comment
Magnesium trisilicate USP	Contains 20% magnesium trisilicate and 40% silicon dioxide. 1.0 g neutralizes about 15 mEq of acid. Slow acting. Gelatinous silicon dioxide, liberated with formation of magnesium chloride in the stomach, may protectively coat the ulcer crater and adsorb acid and pepsin.	1 g hourly	*See* magnesium hydroxide. May chelate drugs intralumenally. About 7% of the silica may be absorbed and produce renal calculi.
Aluminum hydroxide gel USP	A varying mixture of aluminum oxide, hydroxide, and carbonate. Thus 1.0 g neutralizes between 0.5 and 2 mEq of acid, and different proprietary preparations may elicit different responses. Aluminum hydroxide neutralizes and absorbs hydrochloric acid, precipitates and inactivates pepsin, increases gastric mucous production, and is a mild astringent and a demulcent. Proteins, peptides, amino acids, and some dietary organic acids reduce its neutralizing capacity. The aluminum chloride formed on hydrochloric acid neutralization does not depress the gastric *p*H below 3.5. In the small bowel it reconverts to the hydroxide, subsequently forming insoluble complexes with dietary phosphates.	400 mg of the dried material or 15 ml of the gel, hourly	Tends to produce nausea and anorexia. Constipation is common and is due to the production of insoluble aluminum phosphate concretions and to a direct smooth muscle relaxant effect of the aluminum ion. Loss of dietary phosphate may result in hypophosphatemia, hypophosphaturia, and hypopyrophosphaturia, with general fatigue and muscle weakness, particularly in the shoulder girdle area, and in osteomalacia with hypercalcemia. The gastrointestinal absorption of tetracycline antibiotics, isonicotinic acid hydrazide, and chlorpromazine is depressed; a chelate is formed with tetracyclines. Chronic treatment may result in iron-deficiency anemia. In renal failure, the administration of aluminum hydroxide may produce plasma aluminum levels of 53 mg/liter. Aluminum-induced phosphate binding can be a useful therapeutic adjunct in patients on chronic renal dialysis. However, aluminum may be toxic under these circumstances.
Aluminum phosphate gel NF	Aqueous suspension of 4% to 5% aluminum phosphate. Similar to aluminum hydroxide except that it does not bind phosphates.	10–30 ml hourly	Nausea, anorexia, and constipation.

(*continued*)

TABLE 38-3. (*Continued*)

Antacid	Properties	Dose	Adverse Effects and Comment
Dihydroxyaluminum aminoacetate NF	Insoluble but rapid acting. 1.0 g buffers about 4 to 8 mEq of acid.	0.5–2.0 g hourly	Nausea, anorexia, and constipation.
Aluminum carbonate	A varying mixture of 4.9% to 5.3% aluminum oxide and 2.4% carbon dioxide. Similar to aluminum hydroxide but binds phosphate more readily. 1.0 ml neutralizes between 1.2 and 1.5 mEq of acid.	600 mg hourly	Nausea, anorexia, and constipation. May be a more efficient binder of phosphate than aluminum hydroxide.
Milk	A poor antacid but relatively available and palatable.		Tends to produce acid rebound. When taken with calcium carbonate, milk may produce the milk–alkali syndrome (*see* calcium carbonate).
Anion exchange resins	Poor antacids but effective acid adsorbers. Rarely used.		Bulky, costly, and possess an offensive odor and a gritty taste.
Gastric mucin	An alcoholic precipitate of hog stomach. An inefficient acid neutralizer that is rarely used.		Costly and has an offensive odor and taste.

over-the-counter preparations. The exact benefits of antacid therapy in relief of pain and promotion of healing are still somewhat controversial since, in double-blind controlled trials, placebos have also been shown effective. Some of the poor responses to antacids may reflect poor compliance (cost, side-effects, patient acceptancy, palatability). Antacids are effective only if taken chronically, and the rapid relief of ulcer pain (usually occurring within days of starting therapy) is not an indication for reduction in dosage. Relief of ulcer pain and healing do not go hand in hand. Antacids are most efficacious in acute ulceration; nonsystemic antacids are preferred over systemic antacids, and aqueous drugs are preferred over tablets or powders. Tablets must be fully chewed but are usually not as effective acid neutralizers as are liquids. Patients vary in the proportion of constipating antacid required to offset the effects of laxative preparations. Thus fixed dosage ratios should not be used. When antacids are prescribed, dosage should be determined by the milliequivalents of neutralizing capacity rather than by an arbitrary volume or number of tablets.

Because of its disadvantages and the availability of more effective drugs, the routine use of *sodium bicarbonate* should be limited. Oral sodium bicarbonate is, however, used in neutralizing gastric contents before endoscopy, in temporarily combating systemic acidosis, to produce urinary alkalinization in the treatment of gout or urinary infections, or to prevent crystalluria (*see* Chap. 64).

Magnesium trisilicate, hydroxide, and *oxide* are effective but slow-acting hydrochloric acid neutralizers. Magnesium trisilicate is usually considered superior to the other two owing to the added action of the silicon dioxide. However, magnesium hydroxide and oxide react with gastric acid more rapidly than does the trisilicate.

Aluminum preparations are slow acting and, because of their constipating property, should be combined with a magnesium preparation. Aluminum phosphate gel should be used if phosphate loss is to be avoided. Aluminum hydroxide, or preferably aluminum carbonate, may be used to treat phosphate nephrolithiasis or to control the blood phosphate level in renal insufficiency.

Apart from their use in peptic ulcer disease, antacids are valuable in Mendelson's syndrome, reflux esophagitis, the dyspepsia and heartburn of pregnancy, and some cases of nonspecific diarrhea or constipation. In pancreatitis, antacids may be of value after initial treatment with nasogastric suction has been completed. By neutralizing gastric acid, antacids indirectly reduce pancreatic secretion by reducing duodenal secretin release.

Dosage

There is little consensus as to how often and in what dosage antacids should be given, or for how long they should be administered. Clinical studies have been complicated by difficulty in quantitating the degree of ulcer healing even when using endoscopy, and often by poor patient compliance. Further, evaluation of therapies is difficult because of the high relapse rate in ulcer disease. For example, relapse rates of 65% to 80% within 1 year have been reported. Moreover, endoscopy has shown that about 20% of ulcers recur asymptomatically.

In acute gastric ulcer disease, antacids should probably be prescribed in doses of 40 mEq/hr during the waking hours until the ulcer has healed. If healing has not taken place within 3 months of adequate medical therapy, surgery is probably indicated.

In acute duodenal ulcer, antacids should probably be prescribed in doses of about 80 to 160 mEq/hr. After symptoms have ameliorated, a similar dose can be given 1 and 3 hours after meals and at bedtime for an additional 4 to 8 weeks during the time of epithelialization.

In hypersecreting patients who fail to respond, cimetidine or hospitalization and antimuscarinic agents (*see* below) are probably indicated.

ANTIPEPSINS

Antipepsins are drugs that inhibit peptic activity independent of changes in gastric *p*H. Some *aluminum*, *magnesium*, and *bismuth* antacids may absorb or inactivate pepsin, and *amylopectin sulfate* (Depepsen), the sodium salt of sulfated potato amylopectin, inhibits peptic activity by complexing with tissue proteins, reducing their digestability. Amylopectin sulfate may also complex pepsin directly. The usual dose of depepsen is 500 mg every 4 hours. It may be of some value in gastric ulcer, but results in patients with duodenal ulcer are not encouraging.

Curtis Lester Mendelson, 1913– . American physician. Specialist in obstetrics and gynecology. In 1946 described Mendelson's syndrome, a pneumonitis produced by aspiration of the stomach contents during obstetric anesthesia.

LIQUORICE COMPOUNDS

Two separate drugs have been prepared from liquorice: *carbenoxolone sodium* and *deglycyrrhizinated liquorice*.

CARBENOXOLONE SODIUM

Carbenoxolone sodium is the water soluble, disodium salt of the hemisuccinate of β-glycyrrhetinic acid, synthesized from a glycoside extracted from liquorice root.

Mode of Action

Carbenoxolone sodium acts on the mucosa, and, because absorption occurs primarily in the stomach, poor results were initially obtained in the treatment of duodenal ulcer disease. *In vivo*, carbenoxolone sodium lengthens the life span of the gastric mucosal epithelial cells, effectively prolonging the synthesis and secretion of mucosubstances. It also increases the volume of mucus produced and increases its "effectiveness." Carbenoxolone sodium depresses pepsin secretion, reduces acid back-diffusion, and possibly augments secretin release. *In vitro*, carbenoxolone sodium inhibits human pepsins 1, 3, and 5 and inhibits the activation of total pepsinogens in mucosal extracts.

Carbenoxolone sodium has antiinflammatory activity due to stimulation of adrenal 11-hydroxycorticosteriod production. It also leads to sodium chloride and water retention and hypokalemia owing to an intrinsic aldosterone-like activity, and possibly through displacement of endogenous aldosterone from plasma.

Absorption, Metabolism, and Excretion

Despite the stomach's large size, carbenoxolone sodium is absorbed rapidly from it when the *p*H is 2 or less. The initial plasma maximum at about 1 hour is followed by a second maximum at about 4 hours due to enterohepatic circulation. At therapeutic plasma levels (10–100 μg/ml), the drug is more than 99.9%

bound to plasma proteins, with 83% being associated with the albumin fraction and 17% with the globulin fraction, explaining its low V_d. Binding to serum albumin occurs at two different classes of binding sites with apparent association constants of 10^7 and 3×10^6, respectively. It is metabolized to inactive glucuronide and sulfuric acid conjugates, which are excreted in the bile. Less than 2% of the drug and its metabolites are excreted in the urine.

Adverse Effects

Carbenoxolone sodium possesses several important side-effects, particularly of a mineralocorticoid nature and probably should not be used in patients over 65 years of age. Both salt and water retention producing edema, hypertension, and hypokalemia develop in up to 50% of patients. Some control of these effects can be achieved with thiazide diuretics and potassium supplements; aldosterone antagonists should not be used because they also antagonize the effect of carbenoxolone sodium on ulcer healing. Significant hypokalemia may develop rapidly, particularly with excessive dosage and poor patient supervision. Hypokalemia leads to anorexia, weakness, and fatigue and rarely to congestive heart failure, renal tubular necrosis, and rarely quadriparesis.

Patients on carbenoxolone sodium therapy must be monitored (BP, serum K) every 1 to 2 weeks. Elevation of serum transaminases and alkaline phosphatase activity, a decrease in plasma C-reactive protein, and myopathies and myoglobinuria occur rarely.

Salt and water retention, edema, hypertension, and hypokalemia with muscle weakness also occur after excessive consumption of liquorice.

Clinical Use

Carbenoxolone sodium seems to be effective in accelerating the healing of gastric and duodenal ulcers. For gastric ulcers, its effect appears to be similar to that obtained by hospitalization and bed rest, but the two treatments are not additive.

Preparations and Dosage

Carbenoxolone sodium is available in the United Kingdom, and in the United States as *biogastrone* for gastric ulcer disease, *biogastrone electuary* for peptic esophagitis, and *duogastrone*, a position release form for duodenal ulcer disease. Duogastrone is formulated in a special gelatin capsule that supposedly releases the active ingredient in the pyloric antrum for discharge into the duodenum. The usual dose for gastric ulcer is 100 mg every 8 hours for 1 week followed by 50 mg every 8 hours until the ulcer heals. In duodenal ulcer the dose is 50 mg every 6 hours 20 minutes before food. Potassium supplements are needed to offset hypokalemia, particularly when thiazide diuretics are also used; antacids can be given in addition if response is slow.

DEGLYCYRRHIZINATED LIQUORICE

Glycyrrhizinic acid is the basic moiety of carbenoxolone sodium responsible for both therapeutic and adverse effects. The efficacy of deglycyrrhizinated (about 1–3% glycyrrhizinic acid) liquorice alone (Ulcedal-R) or with bismuth subnitrate 100 mg, aluminum hydroxide gel 100 mg, light magnesium carbonate 200 mg, sodium bicarbonate 100 mg, and powdered frangula bark (Caved-S) is controversial. The drug possesses weak antispasmodic activity and minimally depresses hydrochloric acid secretion but has no effect on mucus production. It is substantially free of side-effects, but its activity is low.

GEFARNATE

Gefarnate (geranyl farnesylacetate) is a synthetic terpene that contains a number of isoprene units, the basic fragments from which pentacyclic ring structures such as steroids can be synthesized and with which the triterpenoid carbenoxolone bears some structural resemblances. It was originally extracted from the white-headed cabbage. Gefarnate (200–400 mg every 8 hours) may possess the beneficial effects of carbenoxolone on gastric ulcer disease but without the side-effects of the liquorice preparation; clinical trials in Europe have been contradictory. It has no benefit in duodenal ulcer disease.

BISMUTH SALTS

Tri-potassium di-citrato bismuthate (TDB) is an ammoniacal suspension of a complex colloidal solution that contains chelated bismuth. Its precise mode of action is not known, but it inhibits experimental ulcer formation in animals and has beneficial effects in both human gastric and duodenal ulcer disease.

TBD reacts at *p*H 2.5 to 3.5 with mucoproteins in the ulcer bed to generate a mucinlike protective layer of bismuth oxide. Additionally

TDB is a weak antacid, inhibits pepsin by chelation, stimulates mucus production, and delays gastric emptying.

Bismuth is not absorbed, and its side-effects are minimal; the oral mucosa and dentures may be stained black, and stools will become black, possibly to be confused with melena. Some patients complain of dry mouth or the drug's ammoniacal odor.

The usual dosage is 5 ml diluted with 15 ml of water every 6 hours to be drunk 30 to 60 minutes before antacids or meals and 2 hours after the last meal of the day, for 4 weeks. In resistant cases the dose can be increased to 10 ml diluted similarly every 4 hours. Nothing else should be taken by mouth for 30 minutes after administration.

MEDICAL TREATMENT OF PEPTIC ULCER DISEASE

The aims of medical therapy are similar regardless of anatomic location: *relief of pain, promotion of healing, prevention of recurrence* and *prevention or control of complications.* Ulcer healing depends on chronic drug-mediated control of gastric secretions, plus other therapeutic approaches such as hospitalization, bed rest, cessation of smoking, and possibly dietary restrictions, psychotherapy, sedation, and tranquilization. Treatment regimens should be multifaceted and individually tailored. Patients should be given some insight into their disease, particularly its tendency to recur.

The traditional Sippy diet is obsolete, and there is little evidence that "bland" diets are more advantageous than "regular" diets. Foods are poor antacids, but they increase the duration of action of antacids; the eating of regular meals is more important than their content. Three meals a day are less stimulating to gastric secretion than small frequent feedings. Milk should be used for nutrition rather than as an antacid because it stimulates gastric acid secretion owing to its protein and calcium content. If possible, caffeine-containing beverages (coffee, tea, colas, *e.g.*) should be omitted (Table 38-2). Although tobacco smoking impedes the healing of peptic ulcers and increases the incidence of complications, any benefit achieved through cessation of smoking during treatment of an acute attack may not offset the associated anxiety and tension generated by such a change.

BERTRAM WELTON SIPPY, 1866–1924. Chicago physician. In 1915 published his diet for gastric and duodenal ulcer.

Gastric Ulcer

Ideally, all gastric ulcer patients should be hospitalized initially to ensure maximal medical therapy and to confirm the benignancy of the lesion. In addition, hospitalization, bed rest, cessation of tobacco smoking, and ulcerogenic drugs are exceedingly important adjuncts to full antacid therapy. *Cimetidine, carbenoxolone sodium,* and *bismuth* are considered by some gastroenterologists to be of greater benefit than antacids. The role of deglycyrrhizinated liquorice, depepsen, and other agents is less clear.

Duodenal Ulcer

Cimetidine has revolutionized the treatment of duodenal ulcer disease to where many consider it the drug of choice even though antacids are equally effective. In practice, cost, patient preference, and side-effects usually dictate the choice. Once cimetidine is withdrawn, symptoms rapidly recur, and the patient reverts to pretherapy condition; some ulcers may redevelop asymptomatically during treatment. Certain questions still remain, particularly with respect to the long-term use of cimetidine and its role with or without other drugs such as antacids and anticholinergics. It is unknown which drug, if any, yields the most rapid healing rate, reduces the incidence of complications, and diminishes the likelihood of relapse.

Stress Ulcer

Therapy is still controversial, but antacids are probably preferred over cimetidine by most authorities since they apparently reduce the incidence of bleeding.

Drug Interactions with Antacids

The absorption and excretion of many drugs could theoretically be influenced by antacids (Table 38-4). Since most antacids are sold "over-the-counter," often taken for no specific symptoms or for prescribed drug-induced symptoms, and often considered (erroneously) inert, their possible participation in drug interaction therapy failures should be remembered. It is considered prudent that drugs be given 30 to 60 minutes before antacids in an attempt to minimize interference with therapy.

DRUGS ACTING ON THE INTESTINES: CATHARTICS

Cathartics (Greek—*katharsis,* purification) are used to promote passage of feces. They are divided classically into *intestinal smooth mus-*

TABLE 38-4. Some Important Drug Interactions with Antacids

Mechanism	Primary Drug	Antacid	Comment
Reduced tablet disintegration dissolution	Digitalis glycosides	Most common agents	Reduced bioavailability of digitalis
	Tetracycline antibiotics	Sodium bicarbonate	Reduced bioavailability of tetracycline
Reduced drug ionization	Naproxen	Several antacids	Reduced bioavailability of naproxen
Intralumenal chelate formation	Tetracycline antibiotics	Calcium, magnesium, and aluminum antacids	Reduced bioavailability of tetracycline
	Iron, chlorpromazine, dietary phosphate	Aluminum hydroxide	Reduced absorption of primary agent
Reduced drug stability	Tetracyline antibiotics	Aluminum hydroxide	Antacid inactivates the antibiotic
Increased drug stability	Acid-labile penicillins	Antacids	More penicillin available for absorption
Delayed gastric emptying	INAH	Aluminum hydroxide	Reduced bioavailability of INAH
Increased rate of gastric emptying	Levodopa	Magnesium hydroxide	Increased bioavailability of levodopa since less destroyed in stomach
	Salicylates	Most antacids	Increased bioavailability of primary drug since passed to site of maximal absorption more rapidly
Urinary alkalinization	Quinidine, amphetamine	Most antacids	Increased tubular reabsorption of primary drug
	Salicylates	Most antacids	Decreased tubular reabsorption of primary drug

cle stimulants, fecal mass softeners, and *lubricants;* parasympathomimetic agents (*see* Chap. 16) are not included. Recent evidence suggests, however, that, excluding the lubricant cathartics, all agents act primarily to *increase the intraluminal content* of fluid and therefore indirectly to increase peristalsis. Thus the classic separation of cathartics as referred to above, although useful conceptually, bears little relation to their mode of action. The terms *aperient, laxative, purgative,* and *drastic* are sometimes used to describe the magnitude of cathartic action. A small dose of some cathartics produces an aperient or laxative effect (a few formed feces without griping), whereas a larger dose produces purgation (loose, watery feces, usually accompanied by griping abdominal pain). The *drastic cathartics* (croton oil, jalap, colocynth, and podophyllum) all produce severe mucosal irritation and gastroenteritis, and are obsolete.

Constipation (delayed passage of fecal matter through the intestine) is a functional disturbance of the gastrointestinal tract, different from dyschesia (difficulty in defecation). Humans are commonly obsessed with the possible evils associated with retained feces, and bowel-conscious subjects fear that harm will come if they do not defecate daily. Thus cathartics are widely abused by the laity—so widely abused, in fact, that many people, particularly the elderly, have become habituated to their daily dose of "salts." In the United States, more than $300 million is spent annually (in 1979) on greater than 700 different proprietary preparations. Physicians more commonly treat symptoms of cathartic overdose (abuse) than symptoms requiring cathartics.

Physiological Principles

Three important "colonic" functions are discussed briefly with respect to the effects of cathartics; *smooth muscle activity, water and electrolyte absorption and secretion,* and *bacterial action.*

Approximately 9 liters of fluid and undigested or partially digested food (roughage) reaches the cecum of an adult each day. In the ascending and transverse colons the intestinal contents are slowly mixed and concentrated by the absorption of electrolytes and water. Absorption is highly efficient, since normally only about 100 ml of fluid of the 9 liters delivered is passed daily with stool. In this absorption process, sodium enters the mucosal cell passively; it is then pumped (Na^+/K^+ ATPase-dependent) through the basolateral membrane against an electrochemical gradient into the extracellular fluid, generating an osmotic gradient that draws in water (Fig. 38-1).

Generally, circular muscle contraction delays intestinal transit by increasing resistance to flow, whereas circular muscle relaxation shortens intestinal transit. For example, opioids (*see* Chap. 32) produce constipation by inducing circular smooth muscle spasm, and the "smooth muscle stimulant" cathartics castor oil and phenolphthaline produce, paradoxically, circular smooth muscle relaxation.

Several times a day, and usually as a response to meals, the contents of the transverse colon are transported into the descending colon and proximal rectum by strong colonic contractions (gastrocolic reflex). Here the semisolid food residue (feces) arouses the defecation reflex, which is a local reflex that involves sacral segments of the spinal cord. If the defecation reflex is inhibited (by higher centers), the stimulus subsides. Although defecation can occur independently of any higher center control, in normal persons the act is assisted and usually accompanied by skeletal muscle participation. The diaphragm descends to its position of full inspiration while concomitantly the glottis closes, and contraction of the intercostal muscles increases both the intrathorasic and intraabdominal pressures. These skeletal muscle contractions produce, in sequence, an abrupt rise in arterial pressure, almost total cessation of right heart venous return with a rise in pe-

FIG. 38-1. Schematic representation of catharic actions

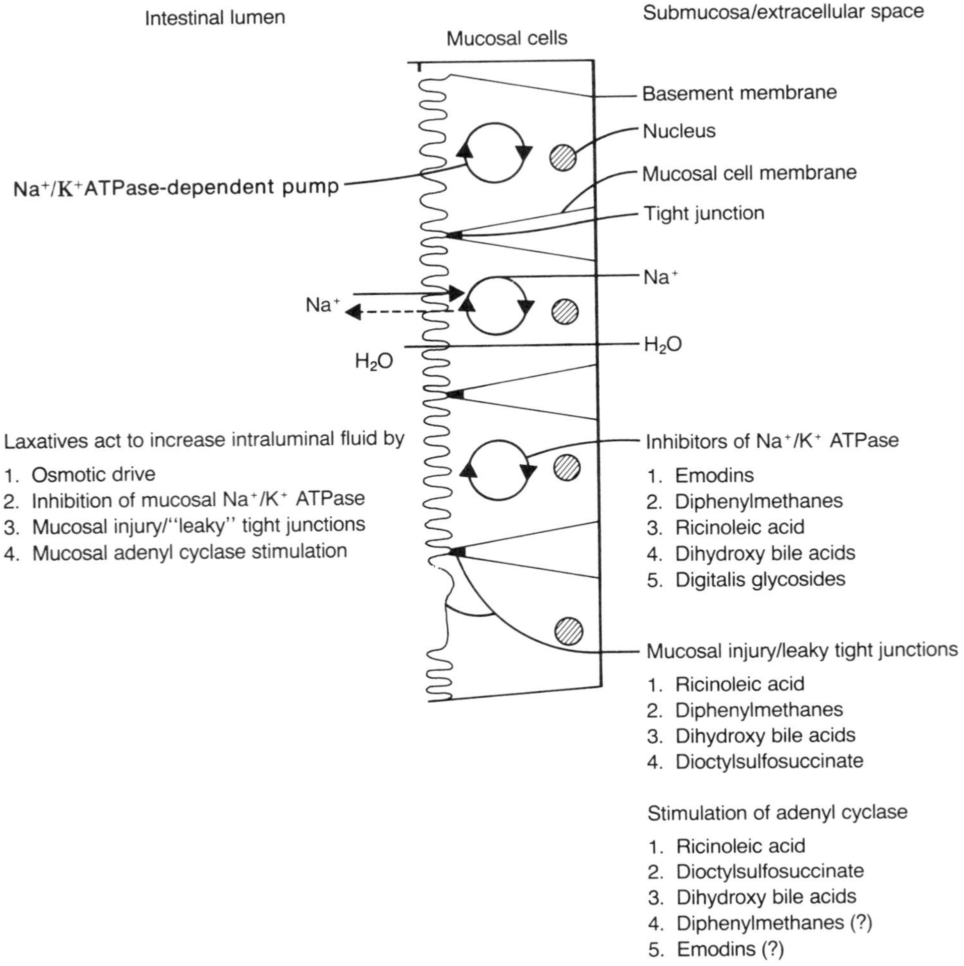

ripheral venous pressure, and a fall in arterial pressure. During intense skeletal muscle contraction, the intraabdominal pressure may rise to 200 mm Hg or more.

Bacterial action in the colon is responsible for activation of cathartics secreted in the bile as glucuronides (bisacodyl) or present as naturally inactive compounds (anthraquinones).

Mode of Action

All cathartics (except some specific lubricants and some suppositories that produce rectal distention through release of CO_2 or peroxide) probably produce their effect by leading to an accumulation of fluid intraluminally (an hydrophoric effect). This may be accomplished (Fig. 38-1) by an osmotic drive; by the depression of mucosal Na^+/K^+ ATPase with diminished absorption of Na^+; by loss of mucosal Na^+ intraluminally through either "leaky" tight junctions or disruption of mucosal cells; or possibly by a cholera-toxin-like action, activation of mucosal adenyl cyclase, with resulting mucosal "secretion" of water and electrolytes. Fluid and electrolyte changes develop in both the large and small bowel with laxative use. Fecal fluid content of 200 to 300 ml usually results in some obvious softening of stool; fecal fluid values of greater than 300 ml usually result in diarrhea.

Some laxatives may have additional modes of action. Osmotic agents, for example, may also lead to smooth muscle stimulation through release of cholecystokinin (CCK), and autacoids such as prostaglandins and vasoactive intestinal polypeptide (VIP) [*see* Chap. 55]), and magnesium ions may have some unique stimulant properties. Bulk laxatives and a high-residue diet reduce intestinal transit time by retaining fluid intraluminally and are thus the most "physiologic" ("natural") stimulators of peristalsis and the best "regulators" of patients with constipation.

An adequate intake of roughage and fluid, a nonsedentary existence, and obeying the call to stool are the best prophylactic measures against constipation. Cheap sources of roughage are cereals, whole grain breads, leafy vegetables, whole fruits, and raw carrots.

Adverse Effects of Cathartics

Some important effects common to many cathartics are discussed below. Adverse effects specific to individual cathartics are discussed with each drug.

Nonspecific Symptoms

Bloating, anorexia, headaches, vague, diffuse, crampy hypogastric pain or discomfort, flatulence and various other symptoms may develop that may either confuse diagnostic attempts or lead to use of other drugs, particularly additional over-the-counter preparations.

Habituation. Although the occasional taking of a cathartic is relatively safe, continued use can lead to a habit not easily broken. After a reasonably complete cathartic action, the large bowel from the ascending colon distally may be completely empty of food residue, and several days may pass before a further normal bowel movement can occur. If the patient and physician do not realize the normality of this delay, further cathartic exposure is common, leading, after several weeks, to drug dependence and habituation. With habituation, the normal reflex mechanisms that initiate defecation are lost, necessitating continual reliance on cathartics. With chronic cathartic abuse a condition of "cathartic colon" may result where the large bowel is atrophic, ulcerated, atonic, and dilated with loss of haustrations.

Withdrawal. Patients dependent on cathartics exhibit withdrawal symptoms when their stimulant is withheld. Anorexia, bloating, irritability, dizziness, weakness, myalgias, occipital headaches, depression, general malaise, and insomnia are typically produced in various combinations. It is not certain whether these symptoms develop primarily from bowel irritation or from stress. In most cases, however, symptoms are relieved by a simple tapwater enema.

Electrolyte Disturbances

Chronic cathartic exposure may lead to colonic mucosal injury (proctocolitis) and water and electrolyte disturbances. Dehydration may be severe, and electrolyte (sodium, potassium, magnesium, chloride, bicarbonate) loss can produce significant symptoms or interfere with concomitant drug therapy. Hypokalemia develops in up to 50% of subjects taking cathartics in excess, with weakness, skeletal muscle disorders, or renal tubular necrosis resulting; digitalis intoxication commonly appears (*see* Chap. 33). Hyponatremia may be severe enough to generate hyperreninemia and aldosterone secretion (*see* Chap. 40).

ANTHRAQUINONE (ANTHRACENE, EMODIN) CATHARTICS

Actions

Anthraquinone cathartics obtained from numerous plants (cascara, senna, rhubarb, and aloe) or synthetically (danthron) contain vari-

(*Text continues on p. 400*)

TABLE 38-5. Some Major Cathartics

Drugs	Sources and Properties	Adverse Effects	Preparations and Single Dose
Anthraquinone Cathartics			
Cascara sagrada ("sacred bark")	Bark of *Rhamnus purshiana.* Contains 1%–2% emodin.	Purgation with large doses. Excreted in human milk. Melanosis coli seen with chronic use	Aromatic *Cascara sagrada* fluid extract USP (plus magnesium oxide) 1 to 2 ml orally. *Cascara sagrada* fluid extract NF 1 to 2 ml orally. Cascara tablets NF 300 mg orally.
Senna	Dried leaves of plants *Cassia acutifolia* (Alexandria senna) and *C. angustifolia* (*Trinnevelly senna*).	As for *Cascara*	Senna syrup NF 8 ml orally. Senna fluid extract NF 2 ml orally. Various costly proprietary preparations (*e.g.,* syrup of figs, castoria, sennokot).
Aloe	Juice of the plant *Aloe perryi.* Most irritating of all emodins.	As for *Cascara*	Various costly proprietary preparations (*e.g.,* Carter's Little Pills, Hinkels Pills).
Rhubarb (Rheum)	Dried rhizome and roots of *Rheum officinale.* Not obtained from garden rhubarb.	As for *Cascara*	Rhubarb fluid extract, 0.6 to 1.2 ml orally
Danthron	Synthetic drug (1,8-dihydroxy-anthraquinone) related chemically to senna, but only $^1/_{10}$ as potent.	Purgation with large doses	Danthron (Dorbane) 150 to 300 mg orally
Diphenylmethane Cathartics			
Phenolphthalein	Synthetic cathartic. Partially refined (yellow) phenolphthalein produces greater laxation than refined (white) phenolphthalein because it is more water repellent. Acts in small and large bowel by depressing Na^+/K^+ATPase and by opening "tight" junctions. About 20% absorbed, conjugated, and renal excreted, where it colors alkaline urine pinkish red. Laxation produced in 6 to 12 hours.	*See* text	Phenolphthalein NF (white phenolphthalein) tablets, 60 to 180 mg orally. Various costly proprietary preparations for children are formulated in candy or chewing gum
Bisacodyl	Synthetic agent resembling phenolphthalein. Absorbed in upper intestine, glucuronated in liver, and excreted in bile, active ingredient hydrolyzed in colon from the conjugate by bacteria. Depresses Na^+/K^+ATPase. Action by suppositories can be blocked by anesthesia of the mucosa. Formed feces produced 1 hour or 8 to 12 hours after suppository or oral administration, respectively.	Purgation with large doses. Suppositories may produce a burning sensation in the rectum.	Bisacodyl (Dulcolax) 5 mg enteric-coated tablets and 10 mg suppositories. Ten to 15 mg orally and 10 mg by suppository.

(*continued*)

TABLE 38-5. *(Continued)*

Drugs	Sources and Properties	Adverse Effects	Preparations and Single Dose
Oxphenisatin	Synthetic agent resembling phenolphthalein.	Oxyphenisatin acetate has been withdrawn from the market due to its propensity in causing hepatic necrosis and fibrosis. No notable adverse effects have been reported using oxyphenisatin dihydrochloride.	Oxyphenisatin dihydrochloride (Lavema) 10 to 20 mg as an enema.
Oils and Softeners			
Castor oil (Oleum ricini)	A fixed oil, a triglyceride of unsaturated ricinoleic acid and glycerol obtained from the castor bean *Ricinus communis.* It should not be confused with the poisonous toxalbumin ricin obtained from the castor bean. Hydrolyzed by pancreatic and intestinal lipases to glycerol and ricinoleic acid (a C_{18} aliphatic monohydroxy fatty acid) that forms alkaline ricinoleates, which are readily absorbed and act on the small bowel within 2 to 4 hours. Castor oil is also used on the skin as an emolient. Its laxative effect may be due to direct mucosal toxicity or via stimulation of adenyl cyclase.	Retards gastric emptying. May produce pelvic congestion; therefore contraindicated during menstruation and pregnancy.	Castor oil USP, 15 to 60 ml orally. Aromatic castor oil NF, 15 to 60 ml orally.
Dioctyl sulfosuccinate	An anionic surface-active emulsifying and wetting agent that lowers surface tension, allowing water to penetrate the fecal mass. May act in addition by depressing Na^+/K^+ATPase and by increasing mucosal adenyl cyclase activity. It is not digested or absorbed. May increase the absorption of concomitantly administered agents. Full effects not seen for 1 to 3 days.	Gastrointestinal irritation.	Dioctyl sodium sulfocuccinate NF, 25 to 120 mg four times daily. Dioctyl calcium sulfosuccinate NF, 25 to 100 mg four times daily.
Poloxalkol	A nonionic surface-active agent composed of a propylene oxide polymer plus ethylene oxide. Similar to dioctyl sulfosuccinate.		Dose 200 mg to 1 g

ous oxymethylquinones present partly in the free form but principally as inactive polar glycosides (Table 38-5). The glycosides are slowly hydrolyzed in the small bowel and more rapidly in the colon, at least in part by bacterial enzymes (β-glucuronidases), with the liberation of their principal active substances, emodin (trioxymethylanthraquinone) and chrysophanic acid (dioxymethylanthraquinone). Several other active anthraquinones are usually present in each drug, and consequently a wide variation in potency occurs depending on the anthraquinone content and on their ease of liberation from the inactive glycoside precursor. For example, two isomeric glycosides, sensosides A and B, have been isolated from senna preparations, the use of which ensures a reasonably standardized preparation. However, purified anthraquinone compounds of other stimulant cathartics are not as potent as the crude preparations generally used because they may contain other active ingredients or because they are less soluble in the intestinal lumen.

The emodins reach the large bowel initially by passage through the lumen. After the active principle has been hydrolyzed (*see* above), it produces laxation and is partially absorbed. The absorbed portion is cleared through the bile and after secretion may act on the small and large bowel a second time. Danthron acts in the small bowel since it does not require bacterial degradation to become activated. The principal action of the emodins is probably to inhibit Na^+/K^+ ATPase (Fig. 38-1), thus reducing net sodium (and water) absorption. In very high doses they may stimulate Auerbach's plexus directly. Chrysophanic acid has little or no cathartic action. It is pigment that, when excreted, colors alkaline urine red and acid urine yellow.

The anthraquinones tend to produce griping, with laxation 5 to 8 hours after administration.

PHENOLPHTHALEIN

Adverse Effects

Phenolphthalein (Table 38-5) is relatively nontoxic, but occasionally hypersensitivity reactions occur. With severe hypersensitivity, diarrhea, cardiovascular and respiratory distress, and syncope may be seen in association with skin rashes. With mild hypersensitivity, skin rashes only are seen, and these usually take the form of erythema nodosum and a polychromatic, deep pink to purple, macular rash, which may be pruritic and burning. The macular rash may progress to ulceration but usually heals rapidly, leaving a residual dusky pigmentation. In some cases pigmentation may persist for years. On reexposure to phenolphthalein, the areas of pigmentation or the nonpigmented sites of previous rashes tend to become involved. A malabsorption syndrome, with atrophic villi demonstrable on intestinal biopsy, is a rare adverse effect of long-term ingestion.

LEOPOLD AUERBACH, 1828–1897. German physician and anatomist. Reported his observations on the Auerbach ganglion cells and plexus of sympathetic nerves within the muscle layers of the intestinal wall in 1862 and 1863. May have introduced the prefix "karyo" in 1874.

SALINE (OSMOTIC) CATHARTICS

Actions

Saline (osmotic) cathartics comprise small molecular, water-soluble compounds that are slowly or incompletely absorbed from the intestinal lumen. Consequently water is retained in the lumen through osmotic pressure, and peristalsis is stimulated indirectly by the semifluid fecal bulk. Additionally some saline cathartics, such as magnesium sulfate, may act by releasing cholecystokinin/pancreozymin and other intestinal hormones that stimulate pancreatic and small intestinal secretions and reduce absorption of sodium chloride. The efficiency of osmotic cathartics depends on their rate and degree of absorption and their osmotic pressure. Osmotic pressure depends on the molecular weight of the drug and the number of ions into which it dissociates in solution. Saline cathartics stimulate the small bowel and usually act within 3 to 6 hours. The differences among osmotic cathartics depend on rapidity of action, taste, and cost. Some popular preparations are indicated in Table 38-6.

The osmotic effect is not greater if both, rather than one, of the ions are nonabsorbable because if the cation is nonabsorbable, an equivalent amount of anion is retained in the bowel lumen to maintain balance, and *vice versa*. Catharsis results irrespective of the tonicity of the administered agent. If the cathartic is given in a hypotonic or hypertonic solution, excessive intestinal water absorption or loss, respectively, results, the draught becoming isotonic with plasma in the stomach and duodenum. Hypertonic saline cathartics may cause nausea and vomiting from pyloric sphincter spasm. Up to 20% of the magnesium

TABLE 38-6. Some Popular Osmotic Cathartics

Drug	Properties	Dose
Magnesium sulfate USP (epsom salt)	Bitter tasting	15 g
Milk of magnesia USP	A 7% to 8% aqueous suspension of magnesium hydroxide. Slow acting since it has to be converted into soluble salts.	15 ml
Sodium sulfate NF (Glauber's salt)	Cheap but impalatable.	15 g
Sodium phosphate NF	Dibasic sodium phosphate. Pleasant tasting.	4–10 mg
Potassium sodium tartrate NF (Rochelle salt)	Pleasant tasting	10 g
Potassium bitartrate NF (Cream of tartar)	Pleasant tasting	2 g
Lactulose	Sweet taste, nausea, abdominal cramps, diarrhea	15–30 ml

cation from magnesium cathartics can be absorbed. Symptoms of hypermagnesemia may thus develop in subjects with compromised renal function.

LACTULOSE

Lactulose (Chronulac) is a synthetic disaccharide available on prescription for treating constipation. Each 15 ml contains 10 g of lactulose and small quantities of other sugars such as galactose and lactose. Lactulose is not hydrolyzed by intestinal enzymes but is degraded by colonic enzymes to galactose and fructose, and then further degraded to lactic, acetic, and formic acids and CO_2; the low molecular-weight acids generate an osmotic drive, and the low *p*H may facilitate colonic propulsion. The cathartic response to lactulose in normal persons is similar to the laxation produced in a patient with lactase deficiency after drinking a glass of milk.

Lactulose commonly produces flatulence, crampy abdominal pains, and diarrhea. The drug is more expensive than other osmotic agents and should be used with caution in diabetics because it contains some digestible sugars. Patients may find the drug nauseously sweet. The usual dose of lactulose is 15 to 30 ml daily.

BULK CATHARTICS AND LUBRICANTS

Bulk cathartics (Table 38-7) are natural and semisynthetic polysaccharides and celluloses that primarily stimulate peristalsis indirectly by their water content and their content of unabsorbable, undigestible fiber. They also absorb water, swell, and assume an emollient gel-like consistency that lubricates the fecal mass, facilitates its passage, and may carry bile acids to the colon where they could alter fluid absorption.

Liquid petrolatum is probably obsolete. It has numerous unpleasant side-effects.

OTHER CATHARTIC PROCEDURES

Enemas and glycerine suppositories have been used to treat constipation.

Enemas

Rectal distention by enemas (sodium phosphate or biphosphate, tap water, soapy water, saline, olive oil, or cotton seed oil) is effective in softening feces and producing laxation. Rapid rectal distention is dangerous and in elderly persons may precipitate cardiac failure. A tap-water enema should not be larger than 500 to 1000 ml. An enema, when properly administered, comes closer to imitating a normal bowel movement than any of the cathartic drugs, since it usually empties only the descending colon and rectum.

Phosphate enemas may lead to significant calcium loss and a lowering of serum calcium levels.

USE OF CATHARTICS

Cathartics should never be given to patients suffering from undiagnosed abdominal pains or intestinal obstruction. Many young children with abdominal pain become sulky, irritable, and fractious and, because they fear a cathartic, will keep silent. How often are fretful children given a "good dose of salts?"

Cathartics are used frequently for conditions other than constipation. A partial list is presented in Table 38-8. With functional constipation—the most common disease that requires active cathartic administration—the lowest effective dose should be used, and drugs should be withdrawn as soon as dietary and other habits are initiated. Practically, many over-the-counter preparations are formulated with multiple ingredients.

TABLE 38-7. Some Popular Bulk Cathartics and Lubricants

Drug	Source and Properties	Adverse Effects	Preparations and Dosage
Bran fiber	A biproduct of wheat milling containing 15% to 25% indigestible cellulose	Should be taken with sufficient water to avoid acute esophagointestinal obstruction.	Bran cereal, cookies, and muffins are regularly used at breakfast but usually in homeopathic doses.
Celluloses	Grayish–white fibrous hydrophilic powders that swell in water, producing an opalescent, viscous solution.	*See* bran fiber.	Methylcellulose USP and sodium carboxymethyl-cellulose USP, 2 to 4 g daily.
Plantago seed	Cleaned, dried, ripe seed of *Plantago psyllium*. Contains natural mucilage. Highly effective in psychological constipation and functional bowel syndromes.	*See* bran fiber. Some preparations contain a carbohydrate as a dispersing agent and sodium, possibly posing problems for some diabetics or patients on low salt diets, respectively.	Plantago seed NF, 1 to 5 g three times daily.
Agar (Agar agar)	Dried hydrophilic colloid from *Gelidium cartilagineum* containing hemicelluloses that partially hydrolyse to D-galactose and 3,6-anhydro-L-galactose. At 25°C absorbs five times its weight of water.	*See* bran fiber.	Agar USP, 4 g, three times daily
Mineral oil (Liquid petrolatum)	Complex mixture of indigestible petroleum hydrocarbons mainly of the methane series. Acts primarily as a lubricant and also as an emulsifying agent augmenting fecal bulk.	Sequesters fat-soluble vitamins, reducing their absorption, and delays gastric emptying. Dosage is difficult to control, resulting in anal leakage, fissure in ano, pruritus ani, and reduced healing of anorectal wounds (*e.g.,* following hemorrhoidectomy). When inadvertently inhaled into the lungs (particularly in the elderly), produces lipoid pneumonia. Is minimally absorbed, producing a foreign body giant cell reaction in lymph nodes and liver, among other organs.	Mineral oil USP, 10 to 50 ml orally. Mineral oil emulsion. NF, 10 to 50 ml orally.

DRUGS ACTING ON THE INTESTINES: CHELATING AGENTS

Cholestyramine is an insoluble anion resin that has a strong affinity for complexing with cholates (bile salts). Thus it is of some value in reducing the intense pruritus that often accompanies biliary cirrhosis and all types of chronic cholestatic jaundice.

Actions

After oral administration, the resin exchanges chloride for cholates in the intestinal lumen and forms insoluble bile salt complexes subsequently lost in the feces. With the enterohepatic bile salt circulation broken, bile salts are synthesized from cholesterol, and, in most patients exposed to cholestyramine, a 20% to 80% reduction in serum cholesterol levels develops within a few weeks. This cholesterol reduction is usually, however, not maintained.

Adverse Effects

Gastrointestinal upsets are common, especially during early therapy, and patients may balk at the drug's offensive odor. High doses may produce steatorrhea, and theoretically hyperchloremic acidosis is possible from excessive chloride absorption. Cholestyramine prevents fat-soluble vitamin absorption and may chelate

TABLE 38-8. Some Applications of Cathartic Drugs

Preparation of bowel for radiography or surgery
Preparation of bowel for endoscopy
Diagnosis and treatment of intestinal parasites
Adjunct agents in toxicology, particularly drug and some cases of food poisoning
Postoperatively, after abdominal and hernia operations
Induction of labor and postpartum
Prevention of excessive straining at stool (with associated rise in arterial blood pressure) in patients with hypertension, cerebral or coronary arteriosclerosis, and pulmonary embolism, for example
During convalescence from myocardial infarction, pulmonary embolism, cerebral hemorrhage, among other diseases
Treatment of hepatic precoma and coma
Cerebral edema (hypertonic magnesium sulfate)
Functional constipation

other drugs (phenylbutazone, barbiturates, thyroxine, digitalis glycosides, anticoagulants, clindamycin, thiazide diuretics) given orally. It may increase the absorption of calcium and, with chronic therapy, yield significant folic-acid deficiency.

Preparations and Dosage

Cholestyramine resin, U.S.P., (Questran) is given in a dose of 4 g every 8 hours.

Uses

Cholestyramine is valuable in treating cholate pruritus that occurs in primary biliary cirrhosis and all types of chronic cholestatic jaundice. Its value in controlling hypercholesterolemic states is not yet clear. It is very effective in controlling diarrhea after ileal resections of less than 100 cm. It may be of some value in treating hyperlipoproteinemias, porphyria cutania tarda, and erythropoietic protoporphyria. Occasionally cholestyramine is effective in controlling the diarrhea of Crohn's disease.

DRUGS ACTING ON THE INTESTINES: ANTIDIARRHEA AGENTS

Diarrhea is a symptom associated with too rapid a passage of fecal material and the frequent passage of semisolid or liquid feces. In all cases of severe or prolonged diarrhea, no matter what the cause, the rapid and complete correction of water and electrolyte loss is of the utmost importance. Antidiarrheal agents are primarily used to manage self-limiting diarrheal disorders. Their value in chronic disorders is less apparent.

BURRILL BERNARD CROHN, 1884– . New York gastroenterologist. Described the use of aluminum hydroxide as an antacid in the treatment of peptic ulcer in 1929, and in 1932 delineated regional ileitis.

SEDATIVES

The opiates (*see* Chap. 32) have been used for many years in the symptomatic control of diarrhea. *Paregoric* (camphorated tincture of opium), 4 ml as required; *laudanum* (tincture of opium), 0.3 to 0.6 ml as required; and *codeine sulphate,* 16 to 32 mg as required, are popular. Addiction and tolerance (*see* Chap. 32) often develop rapidly with the opiates. These drugs act by causing circular smooth muscle spasm, contraction of the anal sphincter, and central depression of the defecation reflex. Their use should be avoided in ulcerative colitis and acute inflammatory bowel disorders because they may lead to toxic megacolon. In patients with hepatic disease, hepatic coma may be precipitated.

Diphenoxylate hydrochloride (Lomotil) is a synthetic opiumlike drug combined with atropine (0.0025 mg) to minimize abuse. The usual dose is 5 mg three times daily, and it is the most useful agent on the market. It has low addictive potential but, otherwise, all the potential side-effects of opiates (*see* Chap. 32). Withdrawal symptoms may occur.

Loperamide hydrochloride (Imodium) is similar to diphenoxylate. It may act on intestinal nerve endings or ganglia. Reported side-effects for this new agent have been few: Anorexia, vomiting, skin rashes, crampy abdominal pains, and dry mouth have been reported.

ANTISPASMODICS

The use of antispasmodic agents to treat diarrhea is discussed in Chapter 16.

HYDROPHILICS

The hydrophilics may incorporate water, forming a gelatinous mass. *Psyllium hydrophilic mucilloid* with dextrose (Metamucil), *psyllium seed* with dextrose (Serutan), and *polycarbophil* plus thihexinol, an anticholinergic (Sorboquel), are of value. Other drugs have been used, largely on an empiric basis.

DEMULCENTS

Some *bismuth, calcium,* and *magnesium* salts may exhibit mild demulcent activity (relieves irritation). Bismuth subcarbonate, U.S.P., 2 g orally as required; calcium carbonate, U.S.P., 2 g orally as required; and magnesium oxide, U.S.P., 1 g orally as required, are popular.

ADSORBENTS

A variety of adsorbents have been used, but their value is questionable. They supposedly adsorb irritants, reduce mucus secretion, and bind water. *Activated charcoal,* U.S.P., 1 to 6 g orally as required; and *kaolin,* N.F. (aluminum silicate), 30 g every 3 hours, are popular. *Kaopectate* (a mixture of 20% kaolin, pectin, and hydrated aluminum silicate) is both a demulcent and an adsorbent. The usual dose is 15 to 30 ml as required. Many of these preparations contain neomycin (*see* Chap. 60) in addition, and their value is doubtful. Liberal quantities of pectin are found in apples.

FURTHER READING

1. Binder HJ: Pharmacology of laxatives. Annu Rev Pharmacol 17:355–367, 1977
2. Brogden RN, Pinder RM, Sawyer PR et al: Tripotassium di-citrato bismuthate: A report of its pharmacologic properties and therapeutic efficacy in peptic ulcer. Drugs 12:401–411, 1976
3. Ewe K: The physiological basis of laxative action. Pharmacology (Suppl 1) 20:2–20, 1980
4. Fordtran JS, Morawski SG, Richardson CT: In vivo and in vitro evaluation of liquid antacids. N Engl J Med 288:923–928, 1973
5. Grossman MI: Physiologic abnormalities in duodenal ulcer: A brief review. Brain Res Bull (Suppl 1) 5:37–38, 1980
6. Hurwitz A: Antacid therapy and drug kinetics. Clin Pharmacokinet 2:269–280, 1970
7. Thompson JH: Gastrointestinal disorders—Peptic ulcer disease. In Rubin AA (ed): Search for New Drugs, pp 116–199. New York, Marcel Dekker, 1972
8. Van Berge-Henegouwen GP, Hofmann AF, Gaginella TS: Pharmacology of chenodeoxycholic acid. I. Pharmaceutic properties. Gastroenterology 73: 291–299, 1977
9. Van Berge-Henegouwen GP, Hofmann AF: Pharmacology of chenodeoxycholic acid. II. Absorption and metabolism. Gastroenterology 73:300–309, 1977

CHAPTER 38 QUESTIONS

(*See* P. 7 for Full Instructions)

Select the One Best Answer

1. The most effective antiemetic agent for treatment of drug-induced nausea and vomiting due to stimulation of the chemoreceptor trigger zone is
   A. atropine.
   B. diphenhydramine.
   C. chlorpromazine.
   D. pentobarbital.
   E. apomorphine.

2. Which of the following antacids would be most likely to produce acute depression of mentation in a patient with poor renal function?
   A. Sodium bicarbonate ($NaHCO_3$)
   B. Magnesium trisilicate ($Mg_2Si_3O_8$)
   C. Calcium carbonate ($CaCO_3$)
   D. Aluminum hydroxide ($Al(OH)_3$)
   E. Glycine ($H_2NCH_2CO_2H$)

3. Gastric ulceration may be exacerbated by each of the following EXCEPT
   A. phenylbutazone.
   B. propantheline.
   C. corticosteroids.
   D. ethyl alcohol.
   E. 5-fluorouracil.

4. Agents used in the treatment of acid peptic disease include each of the following EXCEPT
   A. propantheline.
   B. magnesium trisilicate.
   C. phenobarbital.
   D. indomethacin.
   E. cimetidine.

5. Adynamic ileus can be an undesirable consequence of therapy with
   A. reserpine.
   B. mecamylamine.
   C. magnesium sulfate (epsom salt).
   D. phentolamine.
   E. neostigmine.

A = 1,2,3; B = 1,3; C = 2,4; D = 4; E = All

6. Agents used for assessing the completeness of gastric vagotomy include
   1. caffeine.
   2. insulin.
   3. betazole.
   4. 2-deoxyglucose.

7. Sodium bicarbonate is therapeutically desirable in

1. neutralizing gastric acid before endoscopy.
2. combating systemic acidosis.
3. minimizing the development of crystalluria with sulfonamide therapy.
4. the long-term treatment of duodenal ulcer disease.

8. Which of the following orally administered agents should be avoided by a person with a duodenal ulcer?
   1. Aspirin
   2. Indomethacin
   3. Phenylbutazone
   4. Phenobarbital

9. Undesirable side-effects resulting from the chronic use of mineral oil include
   1. CNS depression.
   2. granuloma formation in the bowel.
   3. impaired renal function.
   4. decreased absorption of vitamins A and D.

10. Cathartic drugs that must be metabolized to act include
    1. lactulose.
    2. castor oil.
    3. cascara sagrada.
    4. methylcellulose.

RALPH E. PURDY

39 Drugs That Affect Uterine Contractility

PHYSIOLOGY

Uterine muscle is organized into branching bundles of electrically coupled cells that exhibit continuous myogenic activity. The membrane potential of myometrial cells fluctuates rhythmically, giving rise to a burst of action potentials at the crest of each slow wave oscillation. Thus the rhythmic electrical activity is converted into phasic contractile responses that involve the entire uterus.

Estrogen enhances spontaneous uterine activity as well as the response to pharmacologic stimulation. Thus the degree of phasic contraction fluctuates during the menstrual cycle. During the first two trimesters of pregnancy, the uterus is quiescent and less sensitive to oxytocic agents, partly because of low levels of plasma estrogen. During the final 5 to 6 weeks of pregnancy, however, estrogen production increases progressively, with the most rapid increase occurring during the final 20 days of gestation. This increase in estrogen production, which increases uterine contractility and sensitivity, contributes to parturition. In some species, progesterone reduces myometrial contractility and sensitivity and is responsible for pre-term uterine quiescence. A similar role for this hormone in human pregnancy has not been established.

OXYTOCIN

PHYSIOLOGICAL CONSIDERATIONS

Oxytocin and vasopressin are two octapeptide hormones released from the posterior pituitary (*see* Chap. 43). Kamm and coworkers first separated and characterized these hormones in 1928. In the early 1950s, Vincent duVigneaud determined the structure of and synthesized oxytocin. The major physiological role of oxytocin is to stimulate contraction of the uterus and the myoepithelial cells of the mammary glands. During labor, many factors work together to cause a progressive increase in the strength and duration of uterine contraction, and consequently a progressive dilation of the cervix. Cervical dilation sends sensory im-

Oliver Kamm, 1888– . American chemist. In 1928 reported the separation of vasopressor and oxytocic factors of the pituitary posterior lobe.

pulses to the hypothalamus, causing the release of pituitary oxytocin. Oxytocin further enhances uterine contraction and cervical dilation as one component of a complex positive feedback process.

Oxytocin also causes milk ejection or "let down" in lactating mammary glands. Milk is continuously produced in the mammary alveoli, which are surrounded by myoepithelial cells. Suckling stimulates oxytocin release, which contracts the myoepithelial cells, expressing the milk from the alveoli into larger mammary ducts and sinuses where it becomes available to the infant.

METABOLISM AND EXCRETION

Oxytocin is metabolized in liver and kidney by proteolytic enzymes (oxytocinases). It is also destroyed in the gastrointestinal tract and is therefore not effective by the oral route. The onset of action of oxytocin is very rapid, and its duration of action lasts a few minutes. During pregnancy and lactation, oxytocinase activity is found in plasma, uterus, placenta, and lactating mammary gland, and the duration of action of oxytoxin is even shorter.

MECHANISM OF ACTION

The initial event in the uterine and myoepithelial response to oxytocin is the occupation of specific oxytocin receptors located on the cell membranes. The resulting contractile response occurs because of increased free intracellular calcium. However, the events between receptor occupation and elevation of calcium are unknown. Oxytocin may work in conjunction with endogenous prostaglandins to produce its effect.

The responsiveness of the nonpregnant uterus and pregnant uterus in the first two trimesters to oxytocin is low. Responsiveness increases progressively, however, during the last trimester, an increase owing to nonspecific changes in the uterus caused by estrogen and to an estrogen-induced increase in the number of oxytocin receptors.

PHARMACOLOGIC USES AND ADVERSE EFFECTS

Oxytocin is used to induce labor at term by increasing both the frequency and the force of uterine contractions. In view of the enhanced sensitivity of the uterus at term, caution in selecting patients for oxytocin use is advisable. Unusually strong contractions can occur that could rupture the uterus or cervix or harm the fetus. Sustained contracture would cause fetal asphyxiation.

Oxytocin may be administered after the third stage of labor to increase phasic contraction. This hastens the delivery of the placenta and diminishes uterine bleeding.

Oxytocin is used to facilitate breast feeding but is not very successful. It helps only those cases where the milk ejection reflex to suckling is insufficient.

Large amounts of oxytocin may cause hypotension, particularly in deeply anesthetized patients. The antidiuretic hormonelike activity of oxytocin is weak. During prolonged infusion, however, water intoxication, convulsions, and coma can occur.

PREPARATIONS AND DOSAGES

Each milliliter of oxytocin injection, Pitocin (Parke–Davis), and Syntocinon (Sandoz) possesses an oxytocin activity equal to 10 USP Posterior Pituitary Units. For induction of labor, 10 units of oxytocin are infused intravenously in 1 liter of 5% dextrose at a rate of 5 mU/min for 5 minutes, gradually increasing the rate to 20 mU/min during the next 15 minutes, if necessary. In the control of postpartum bleeding, 3 to 10 units are given, and this may be repeated intramuscularly in 30 minutes. In an emergency a slow i.v. injection of 0.6 to 1.8 units (diluted with 3 to 5 ml of isotonic saline or 5% dextrose) may be used.

Oxytocin nasal spray, 40 U/ml, may be used to facilitate breast feeding; a single application of the spray is taken 2 to 3 minutes before breast feeding. Oxytocin citrate buccal tablets (Parke–Davis), 200 units, may also be used to facilitate breast feeding.

ERGOT ALKALOIDS

ACTIONS AND PROPERTIES

The natural ergot alkaloids are obtained from the fungus *Claviceps purpurea* that infects rye grain. Over many centuries, epidemics characterized by dry gangrene, convulsive episodes, and severe uterine contractions have occurred in populations that consume the infected rye. The first report of ergot's medical use to quicken childbirth was that by John Stearns in 1807.

The most important actions of the ergot alkaloids include stimulation of vascular and uterine smooth muscle. Two alkaloids, *ergonovine* and *methylergonovine*, are powerful uterine stimulants but possess only weak vasoconstrictor activity. Thus they are used as oxytocic agents. Both drugs are effective either orally or parenterally, and the onset of action after oral, i.m., and i.v. administration is 10 minutes, 7 to 8 minutes, and less than 1 minute, respectively. The duration of action lasts several hours. These drugs are administered after delivery of the placenta to control uterine bleeding. When the degree of uterine contraction is suboptimal, sufficient drug is administered to cause a sustained nonphasic contraction. These drugs may also be used to facilitate uterine involution that occurs over the first 4 to 5 weeks after parturition.

The adverse effects of ergonovine and methylergonovine include nausea, vomiting, blurred vision, and headaches. Because of their weak vasoconstrictor activity, these drugs can also cause hypertensive crises, particularly in patients with hypertension or preeclampsia. These drugs are contraindicated before birth of the fetus.

PREPARATION AND DOSAGE

Both ergonovine maleate (Ergotrate Maleate; Lilly) and methylergonovine maleate (Methergine; Sandoz) are available in solution, 0.2 mg/ml in 1-ml containers, and tablets, 0.2 mg. To control uterine bleeding, 0.2 mg is injected intramuscularly. This is repeated every 2 to 4 hours as needed; in emergencies 0.2 mg can be given intravenously. The oral dose is 0.2 to 0.4 mg every 6 to 12 hours for 2 days postpartum, but longer if needed.

PROSTAGLANDINS

Prostaglandins (PGs) are ubiquitous substances and participate in numerous physiological processes (*see* Chap. 53), including human parturition. The uterus is particularly sensitive to PGs, and, in contrast to oxytocin and the ergot alkaloids, these substances can induce labor any time during pregnancy. The concentrations particularly of PGE and PGF in maternal blood and amniotic fluid increase at the time of parturition; and inhibition of PG synthesis, for example, with indomethacin decreases PG concentrations, followed by a reduction in uterine contractility. Inhibition of PG synthesis has been successfully used experimentally to prevent premature labor.

Prostaglandins are currently used as abortifacients between the 12th week and the end of the second trimester. They increase the strength and rate of uterine phasic contractions, and abortion is usually completed between 11 and 20 hours.

Prostaglandins enter the maternal blood regardless of their route of administration, and adverse effects occur frequently. Nausea, vomiting, diarrhea, and transient hyperpyrexia occur in 40% to 60% of patients. Antiemetic and antidiarrheal therapy should be used prophylactically.

PREPARATIONS AND DOSAGES

Dinoprostone (PGE_2; Prostin E_2 [Upjohn]) is available as a uterine suppository of 20 mg. It should be inserted high in the vagina and repeated every 3 to 4 hours until delivery of the fetus.

Dinoprost tromethamine (PGF_2 alpha tromethamine; Prostin F_2 alpha injectable [Upjohn]), 5 mg/ml, may be given by transabdominal intraamniotic instillation. After an appropriate volume of amniotic fluid is withdrawn, 10 to 40 mg of dinoprost tromethamine can be injected.

Also available is carboprost tromethamine (15 methyl PGF_2 alpha; Prostin/M15 [Upjohn]), 0.25 mg in 1-ml containers. The addition of a methyl group at C-15 (*see* Chap. 53) increases the duration of action; 0.25 mg is given intramuscularly and repeated every $1^1/_2$ to $3^1/_2$ hours depending on the uterine response. A total of 12 mg should not be exceeded.

UTERINE RELAXANTS

Infant mortality is greater after premature delivery. Thus in selected patients, prolongation of pregnancy may be an important clinical goal. Unfortunately, prevention of premature labor and delivery usually requires pharmacologic intervention, and the following have been used.

ALCOHOL

Alcohol is infused intravenously over 2 hours in doses that provide blood levels of 0.09% to

---

JOHN STEARNS, 1770–1848. American physician. In 1808 introduced the use of ergot into obstetrics.

0.16%. Additional maintenance doses are administered intravenously or orally to maintain these levels for at least 6 hours. The therapy is repeated when needed. Pregnancy can be prolonged from one to several days by this means.

The mechanism by which alcohol inhibits labor has not been clearly established, but there appear to be two components: Alcohol inhibits the release of oxytocin and may also directly suppress uterine contractility. The most obvious adverse effect of alcohol therapy is inebriation which, at the high blood levels required, occurs in nearly all patients. Nausea and vomiting are also common. Alcohol crosses the placental barrier readily, and alcohol intoxication of the fetus can occur, causing central nervous system depression, hiccups, excessive heat loss, hypoglycemia, and acidosis in the newborn infant.

BETA ADRENERGIC AGONISTS

Stimulation of uterine β_2-adrenergic receptors inhibits uterine contraction by initiating adenylate cyclase activity, (*see* Chap. 17, 50) and ultimately lowers the concentration of free intracellular calcium.

Agents that preferentially activate β_2 receptors, such as salbutamol and terbuline, produce less tachycardia and hypotension than do β_1 agonists (*see* Chap. 17) and are therefore preferable.

Although the use of beta agonists to prolong pregnancy is still largely experimental, this approach appears promising. The beta agonist isoxsuprine, for example, has been used successfully to prolong pregnancy up to 12 weeks. Complete inhibition of uterine contractions is obtained by i.v. infusion, which is followed over 1 to 2 days with an i.m. injection and finally oral administration of maintenance doses.

FURTHER READING

1. Anderson NC: Physiologic basis of myometrial function. Semin Perinatol 2:211, 1978
2. Caritis SN, Edelstone DI, Mueller–Heubach E: Pharmacologic inhibition of preterm labor. Am J Obstet Gynecol 133:557, 1979
3. Challis JRG: Endocrinology of late pregnancy and parturition. In: Greep RO (ed): Reproductive Physiology, III: International Review of Physiology, Volume 22, p. 277. Baltimore, University Park Press, 1980
4. MacDonald PC, Porter JC, Schwarz BE, Johnston JM: Initiation of parturition in the human female. Semin Perinatol 2:273, 1978
5. Tepperman HM, Beydoun SN, Abdul–Karim RW: Drugs affecting myometrial contractility in pregnancy. Clin Obstet Gynecol 20:423, 1977

CHAPTER 39 QUESTIONS

(See P. 7 for Full Instructions)

Select the One Best Answer

1. The most serious of the side-effects of ergotamine would be
   - *A.* nausea and vomiting.
   - *B.* LSD-like CNS effects.
   - *C.* dry gangrene of fingers and toes.
   - *D.* hypertension.
   - *E.* stimulation of the heart.
2. A potent stimulant of uterine contractility active after oral administration is
   - *A.* oxytocin.
   - *B.* prostaglandin $F_{2\alpha}$.
   - *C.* bradykinin.
   - *D.* angiotensin.
   - *E.* ergonovine.
3. An agent that has direct vasoconstrictor activity, oxytocic activity, and therapeutic value against migraine headaches is
   - *A.* angiotensin.
   - *B.* oxytocin.
   - *C.* ergotamine.
   - *D.* vasopressin.
   - *E.* propanolol.
4. Ergonovine produces all of the following effects EXCEPT
   - *A.* peripheral vasoconstriction.
   - *B.* elimination of the pain of migraine headache.
   - *C.* increased blood flow in uterine vasculature.
   - *D.* uterine contraction after oral administration.
   - *E.* blockade of serotonin (5-HT) receptors.

A = 1,2,3; B = 1,3; C = 2,4; D = 4; E = All

5. Ergotamine tartrate
   1. is effective for treating migraine.
   2. effects on blood vessels may be antagonized by propanolol.
   3. is a powerful uterine muscle stimulant.
   4. does not penetrate the blood–brain barrier.
6. Preterm labor may be delayed by the administration of
   1. indomethacin.
   2. terbutaline.
   3. ethanol.
   4. dinoprostone (PGE_2).

40

DAN A. HENRY
JACK W. COBURN

Diuretics

Diuretics are agents that increase the urinary excretion of sodium chloride and water. Generally these drugs are useful when sodium chloride and water have been retained, usually with edema formation, but they also can be valuable in certain nonedematous conditions. To understand the mechanisms of action of various diuretics and the adverse effects that may arise with their use, it is important to review the physiology of the renal excretion of salt and water.

RENAL PHYSIOLOGY

SODIUM

In an adult male the normal glomerular filtration rate (GFR) is about 125 ml/min or 180 liters/day. Large quantities of sodium chloride and other solutes are contained in the glomerular filtrate. Under normal conditions about 99% of the sodium (Na^+) and water is reabsorbed, resulting in a urine output of about 0.5 to 1 ml/min. Sodium is reabsorbed by the proximal tubule (65–70%), the ascending loop of Henle (20–25%), and the distal tubule and collecting duct (5–10%). Factors that affect Na^+ reabsorption by the proximal tubule are shown schematically in Figure 40-1. Within the lumen, the Na^+ (Fig. 40-1) concentration is 140 mM compared to 20 mM in the cell. Since an intracellular voltage of −70 mV is generated by the active extrusion of Na^+ at the peritubular membrane, Na^+ will enter the cell passively down an electrochemical gradient. To preserve electrical neutrality, 80% of the Na^+ is reabsorbed with chloride (Cl^-), whereas 20% of Na^+ is coupled with active secretion of H^+, resulting in the reabsorption of $NaHCO_3$. At the peritubular membrane, Na^+ is actively transported from the cell against both electrical and concentration gradients, probably by means of an Na^+-K^+ activated ATP-ase. In contrast, the cells of the ascending limb of the loop of Henle act to reabsorb Cl^- actively, whereas Na^+ follows passively. The specific fraction of filtered Na^+ that is excreted depends on various factors, including effective circulating intravascular volume, aldosterone levels, and the hemodynamics of the peritubular capillaries.

Robert Franklin Pitts, 1908–1977. American physiologist. Did extensive research on the physiology of the kidney and of diuretic therapy, the control of electrolyte and acid–base balance.

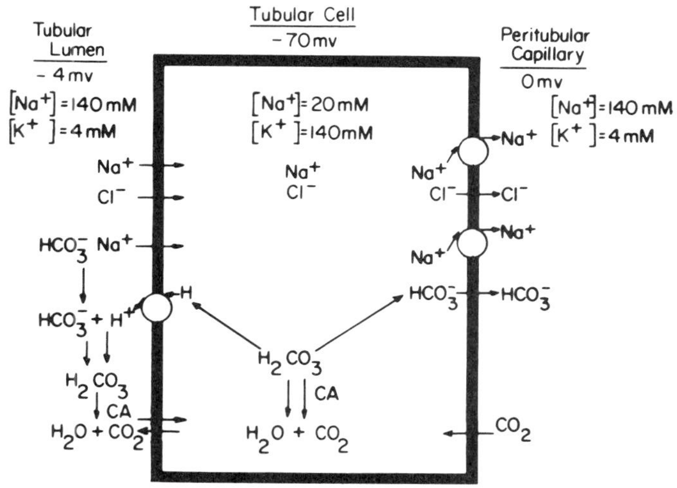

FIG. 40-1. Schematic illustration of the reabsorption of NaCl and $NaHCO_3$ by the proximal renal tubular cell. Sodium entry into the cell is linked either to passive chloride movement or to active extrusion of H^+ from the cell. The latter results in the reabsorption of HCO_3 through the action of carbonic anhydrase (*CA*) along the brush border. On the contraluminal surface, Na^+ is actively transported from the cell against electrochemical gradients, with either Cl^- or HCO_3^- accompanying the Na^+. The approximate concentrations of Na^+ and K^+ in the different compartments are indicated as $[Na^+]$ and $[K^+]$; the approximate electrical potentials are noted above.

POTASSIUM

The kidney plays the major role in the maintenance of potassium (K^+) balance. Total K^+ excretion varies with changes in its dietary intake. The K^+ filtered at the glomerulus is almost entirely reabsorbed in the proximal tubule and the loop of Henle. The distal tubule is the primary site for regulating K^+ secretion, which accounts for most, if not all, of the K^+ in the final urine. In the distal tubule (Fig. 40-2) there is a transepithelial potential gradient of −40 mV with the tubular lumen negative. Since the cellular K^+ concentration is about 140 mM and is 4 mM within the lumen, there is a tendency for passive movement of K^+ out of the cell, down both electrical and chemical gradients. This passive movement of K^+ is opposed by the capacity of the cell to transport K^+ actively into the cell at the luminal membrane. This active transport is particularly evident during K^+ depletion. Potassium excretion can be augmented by an increased rate of flow within the distal tubule; increased sodium delivery to the distal tubule; any factor, such as nonreabsorbable anions (*e.g.*, carbenicillin or sulfate), that causes the transepithelial potential difference to increase with the lumen more negative; increased aldosterone secretion; and alkalosis.

ACID–BASE BALANCE

The kidney contributes to acid–base balance by regulating the concentration of the principal plasma buffer, HCO_3^-. It does this by reabsorbing the filtered HCO_3^- and by excreting the 50 to 100 mEq of H^+ generated each day. About 85% of filtered HCO_3^- is reabsorbed in the proximal tubule and 10% to 15% in the distal tubule and collecting duct. As shown in Figure 40-1, intracellular CO_2 combines with H_2O under the influence of carbonic anhydrase to form H_2CO_3. The H_2CO_3 then dissociates into H^+ and HCO_3^-. The H^+ is secreted into the lumen in exchange for Na^+, which is absorbed; the HCO_3^- within the cell then diffuses into the peritubular capillary with Na^+. The H^+ secreted into the

FIG. 40-2. Schematic representation of K^+ secretion by the distal tubular cell. Potassium may be secreted from the cell into the lumen down its electrochemical gradients by simple diffusion; with potassium depletion, K^+ is actively reabsorbed by the cell. At the contraluminal surface, the maintenance of a high intracellular K^+ concentration is linked to an active Na^+ pump, with the extrusion of Na^+ from the cell.

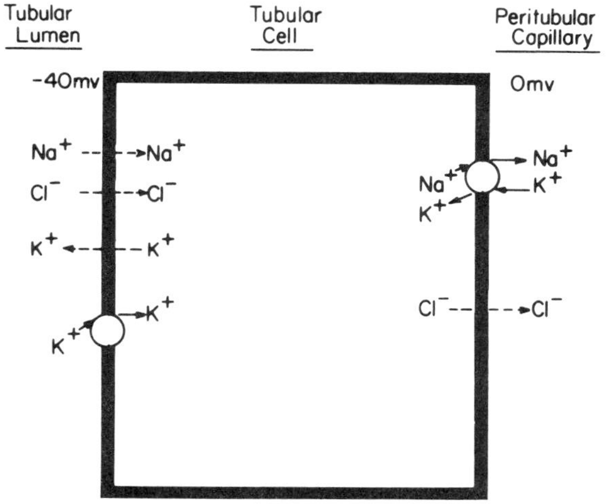

lumen combines with filtered HCO_3^- to form H_2CO_3, which forms H_2O and CO_2 under the influence of the carbonic anhydrase present in the brush border membrane; the CO_2 readily diffuses into the cell. The net result is the reabsorption of the filtered $NaHCO_3$.

In metabolic alkalosis, a frequent complication of diuretic use, plasma HCO_3^- is elevated and blood *p*H is increased. The factors that lead to an increase in the reabsorption of HCO_3^- and maintain this elevated HCO_3^- and the alkalosis include extracellular volume depletion; mineralocorticoid excess; K^+ depletion; and increased Pco_2.

URINARY CONCENTRATION AND DILUTION

The countercurrent mechanism, discussed in detail in standard physiology textbooks, enables the kidney to form a concentrated urine—one that is hypertonic in relation to plasma—or to generate hypotonic urine. The formation of a hypertonic urine (Fig. 40-3) depends on achieving an increment in the osmolality within the interstitium of the medulla by the countercurrent mechanism. In the presence of ADH, which acts on the collecting tubule to increase the permeability to water, urine becomes concentrated to a maximum of 1200 mOsm/kg. The kidney's capacity to dilute urine (Fig. 40-3) depends on an adequate delivery of Na^+ and Cl^- to the distal diluting segments (the ascending limb of Henle's loop and early distal tubule); the active reabsorption of Na^+ and Cl^- in these sites that are impermeable to water; and suppression of ADH secretion so that water cannot be reabsorbed by the collecting duct. The active transport of Na^+ and Cl^- in the ascending limb of Henle's loop is the driving force for generating dilute tubular fluid. The minimum urinary osmolality the kidney can achieve is 25 to 50 mOsm/kg.

PLASMA OSMOLALITY

The osmolality of the plasma (P_{Osm}) is equal to the sum of all individual solutes present in the plasma. The normal P_{Osm} is 275 to 290 mOsm/kg; since most plasma solutes are salts of Na^+, the osmolality can be estimated conveniently as twice the plasma Na^+ concentration. The plasma osmolality is maintained within narrow limits by variation of water excretion of equal water intake less insensible water loss; thus, in a steady state, water output (urine + insensible losses) equals intake. When there is excess water ingestion, the secretion of ADH is inhibited, and the kidney responds by diluting the urine and excreting "free water." This excretion of free water is referred to as "free water clearance" (C_{H_2O}), or the theoretical amount of solute-free water excreted per unit time. Conceptually the urine flow (V) can be viewed as having two components: an amount equal to osmolal clearance (C_{Osm}), which represents the volume of urine necessary to excrete all the solutes in a urine with an osmolality equal to that of plasma; and a component that is solute-free water or free water clearance (C_{H_2O}). If the urine osmolality is 140 mOsm/kg, the plasma osmolality is 280 mOsm/kg, and the urine volume is 2 liters/day, then the C_{H_2O} is 1 liter/day.

$$V = C_{Osm} + C_{H_2O} = \frac{U_{Osm} \times V}{P_{Osm}} + C_{H_2O}$$

$$2 \text{ liters} = \frac{140 \text{ mOsm/kg} \times 2 \text{ liters}}{280 \text{ mOsm/kg}} + C_{H_2O}$$

$$C_{H_2O} = 1 \text{ liter}$$

If the free water intake minus insensible losses of H_2O (about 600 ml/day) exceeds the free water clearance, the plasma osmolality and serum Na^+ concentration will fall.

URIC ACID

Uric acid is formed from the metabolism of purine nucleotides. Since the pK_a of uric acid is 5.7, it circulates primarily as sodium urate, which is highly soluble. The urate is handled entirely by the proximal tubule, where it can be reabsorbed, secreted, and even reabsorbed again. Its net absorption parallels the reabsorption of Na^+. There is increased reabsorption of both Na^+ and urate in many conditions with depletion of extracellular fluid volume or in edematous states with sodium retention.

OSMOTIC DIURETICS

An *osmotic diuretic* is a solute that increases urine flow by its being nonreabsorbable; it obligates the excretion of water by its osmotic effect. To act as an osmotic diuretic, a substance must have the following properties: be freely

---

Homer William Smith, 1895–1962. American physiologist. Described the diodrast clearance test in 1938. Worked on the evolution of the kidney and vertebrate comparative physiology.

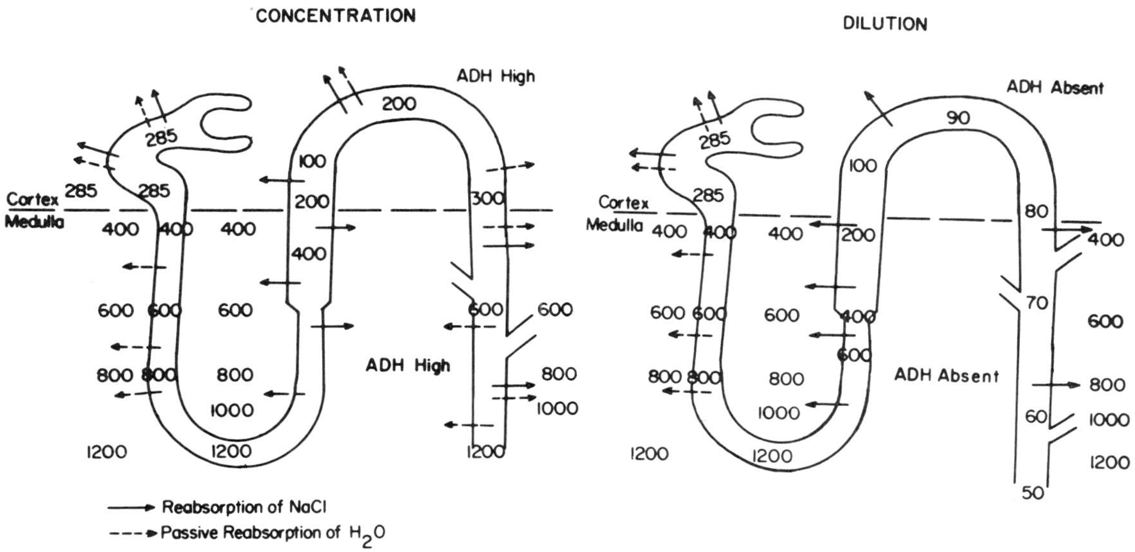

FIG. 40-3. The countercurrent mechanism for the production of either concentrated or diluted urine by the kidney. (*Left*) The mechanism for generating concentrated urine in the presence of high levels of antidiuretic hormone (*ADH*). A hypertonic medullary interstitium is generated by the active transport of Na^+ and Cl^- into the interstitium in the thick limb of Henle's loop, which is impermeable to water. In the distal tubule and collecting duct, ADH renders the tubular lumen permeable to water and urea; therefore, water and urea pass down their concentration gradients into the interstitium. The result is the generation of urine with an osmolality that is increased relative to the interstitium. (*Right*) The schema for maximal urinary dilution when ADH secretion is inhibited. Under these circumstances, Cl^- and Na^+ are transported from the ascending limb of Henle's loop and distal tubule, which are impermeable to water, creating diluted tubular fluid. Without ADH, the distal tubule and collecting duct remain impermeable to H_2O, resulting in the excretion of a large volume of hypotonic urine.

filterable at the glomerulus; be pharmacologically inert with a primary effect to raise the osmolality of the tubular fluid; and undergo limited reabsorption by the renal tubules (*i.e.*, be a nonreabsorbable solute). A common clinical example of an osmotic diuresis is that which occurs in uncontrolled diabetes mellitus. Glucose is present in concentrations in the filtrate so high that the filtered load of glucose exceeds the reabsorptive capacity of the tubule (TmG); the unreabsorbed glucose acts as a nonreabsorbable solute or osmotic diuretic.

MANNITOL

Mannitol is the prototype of an exogenous osmotic diuretic.

Chemistry and Mechanism of Action

After its i.v. injection, mannitol, a six-carbon sugar with molecular weight of 182, is distributed in the extracellular space, thereby raising the osmolality of the extracellular fluid. Because of this effect, water moves from the intracellular to extracellular space to equalize the osmolality. Within the kidney, mannitol may cause dilation of the afferent arteriole, resulting in an increased renal blood flow. Mannitol is freely filterable through the glomerular capillary membrane and is not reabsorbed. It inhibits the passive reabsorption of water in the proximal tubule and the loop of Henle and thereby causes an osmotic diuresis. Mannitol can result in the excretion of as much as 28% of filtered water, whereas the fractional Na^+ excretion is substantially less. By increasing solute excretion, mannitol inhibits both the maximal diluting and concentrating capacities of the kidney (Fig. 40-4).

Clinical Uses and Indications

Mannitol is often used to prevent the onset of acute renal failure. Conditions commonly predisposing to acute renal failure include a severe crush injury with the release of myoglobin, the presence of free hemoglobin in plasma after either mismatched transfusion or intravascular hemolysis, and acute hyperuricemia. In these conditions, mannitol may act by its

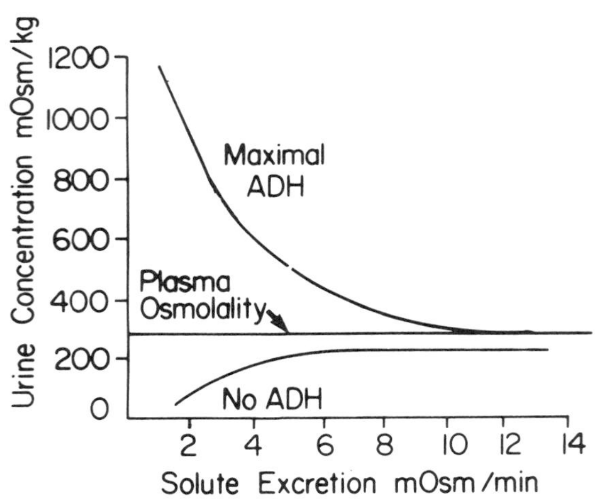

FIG. 40-4. The osmolality or concentration of urine, either with maximal urinary concentration (maximal ADH) or maximal urinary dilution (no ADH), as the solute excretion is increased. When an osmotic agent such as mannitol is given, the solute excretion rate increases, lowering the maximal concentrating ability and raising the minimum diluting capability of the kidney.

ability to inhibit water reabsorption; thus it dilutes the toxic agent within the tubular fluid and maintains urine flow. It may also prevent a decreased renal blood flow observed with those conditions. Many physicians also give an injection of mannitol (12.5 to 25 g) to any patient with acute oliguric renal failure who does not respond to the correction of hypotension and to the replacement of body fluid deficits.

Mannitol can also be used to treat cerebral edema. It increases the osmolality of the plasma and thereby withdraws intracellular water from the brain and cerebrospinal fluid.

Adverse Effects

As a result of its ability to expand extracellular fluid volume, mannitol should be used with great caution in patients with cardiac decompensation.

THIAZIDES AND THIAZIDELIKE DRUGS

Chemistry

Chlorothiazide is the prototype of a large number of compounds of the benzothiadiazide class that have a similar mode of action and effectiveness when each is given in optimal dosage. The classification, usual dosages, and site of action of the thiazides and other commonly used diuretics are given in Table 40-1. The benzothiadiazides are derivatives of sulfonamides and have the general formula illustrated in Fig. 40-5; they are often referred to collectively as "thiazide diuretics."

Absorption, Metabolism, and Excretion

The thiazides are rapidly absorbed from the intestinal tract and exert their action after 1 to 2 hours. They are primarily excreted by the kidney. The duration of action for chlorothiazide is 6 to 8 hours and for hydrochlorothiazide, 12 to 18 hours. Chlorthalidone, metolazone, and polythiazide have a longer duration of action. With the exception of metolazone, these diuretics are not effective if the glomerular filtration rate is below 20 to 30 ml/min.

Mechanism of Action and Physiological Effects

Thiazide diuretics inhibit sodium reabsorption in the cortical segment of the ascending limb of Henle's loop and the early distal tubule (Fig. 40-6). They also inhibit carbonic anhydrase but not by an amount believed to be of physiological significance. Metolazone may also inhibit the reabsorption of Na^+ in the proximal tubule to a small degree; this action is not due to the inhibition of carbonic anhydrase. In maximal doses, the thiazide diuretics can cause the excretion of 3% to 5% of filtered Na^+ and water. Because they do not affect the reabsorption of Na^+ in the medullary ascending limb of Henle's loop, the maximal concentrating ability is not impaired; however, thiazide diuretics do reduce the diluting capacity because they inhibit Na^+ reabsorption in the cortical diluting segment.

These diuretics can cause a marked kaliuresis as a result of the increased flow to the distal nephron and as a result of increased aldosterone levels that enhance the secretion of K^+. Increased aldosterone secretion may arise secondary to the volume depletion produced by diuretic use, but in certain edema-forming states, such as congestive heart failure, liver disease with ascites, and the nephrotic syndrome, aldosterone levels are often increased before diuretic therapy. These diuretics can reduce the renal excretion of uric acid, possibly as a result of extracellular volume depletion, which leads to increased proximal tubular reabsorption of urate. They may also have a direct effect to reduce uric acid secretion; urinary calcium excretion is also decreased primarily owing to extracellular volume depletion that results in enhanced reabsorption of both sodium and calcium more proximally in the tu-

TABLE 40-1. Classification, Usual Dosages, and Actions of Commonly Used Diuretic Agents

Category of Diuretic	Specific Diuretic Agent	Usual Dosage*	Action: Onset	Action: Duration	Mechanism and Principal Site of Action
Thiazide-type diuretics	Chlorothiazide	500–1000 mg/day	1 hr	6–8 hr	Inhibition of Na^+ reabsorption at cortical ascending limb of loop of Henle and early distal tubule
	Hydrochlorothiazide	50–100 mg/day	2 hr	12–18 hr	
	Polythiazide	1–4 mg/day	2 hr	24 hr	
	Trichlormethiazide	4–8 mg/day	2 hr	24 hr	
	Chlorthalidone	50–100 mg/day	2 hr	24 hr	
	Metolazone	2.5–20 mg/day	2 hr	24 hr	
Loop diuretics	Furosemide	40–160 mg/day	30 min	6–8 hr	Inhibition of active Cl^- reabsorption at ascending limb of loop of Henle
		10–80 mg i.v.	5 min	2–3 hr	
	Ethacrynic acid	50–150 mg/day	30 min	6–8 hr	
		20–100 mg i.v.	15 min	2–3 hr	
Potassium-sparing diuretics	Spironolactone	100–200 mg/day	12–72 hr	2–3 days	Competitive inhibitor of aldosterone at distal tubule
	Triamterene	100–300 mg/day	2 hr	12–16 hr	Inhibition of Na^+ reabsorption and K^+ and H^+ secretion at distal tubule
	Amiloride	5–10 mg/day	2 hr	24 hr	
Carbonic anhydrase inhibitors	Acetazolamide	250–1000 mg/day	1 hr	6–8 hr	Carbonic anhydrase inhibitor at proximal tubule

* Oral unless indicated otherwise.

bule. The thiazides may enhance bone reabsorption directly or indirectly by increasing the sensitivity to parathyroid hormone, although these latter effects are probably weak.

The thiazides may stimulate hydrogen ion secretion and bicarbonate generation and thereby initiate and maintain a state of metabolic alkalosis. The following factors are responsible for this metabolic alkalosis.

1. The contraction of extracellular volume due to diuretics may result in a constant pool of HCO_3^- in a reduced volume of extracellular fluid. This arises from the excretion of fluid rich in Cl^- but free of HCO_3^-; thus there is "contraction alkalosis."
2. The increased delivery of Na^+ to the distal tubule in the presence of increased aldosterone levels.
3. The direct enhancement of H^+ secretion.
4. The development of K^+ depletion, which enhances proximal HCO_3^- reabsorption.

Hyperglycemia is occasionally seen during thiazide therapy, particularly in persons with latent or mild diabetes mellitus. The hyperglycemia may be related to hypokalemia, which decreases the release of insulin, but other factors may also contribute.

Adverse Effects

Hypokalemia. Hypokalemia is particularly serious in two groups of patients: those receiving digitalis in whom hypokalemia may increase the susceptibility to digitalis-induced arrhythmias; and those with severe liver disease in whom hypokalemia may precipitate hepatic encephalopathy and even coma. The degree of K^+ depletion is variable but often quite small. Thus K^+ supplements are needed prophylactically in patients receiving digitalis (Table 40-2), in those with known arrhythmias, and in those with severe liver disease. Potassium supplements are also needed if symptoms of K^+ depletion develop or if the serum K^+ falls below 3.5 mEq/liter. The usual dose of K^+ as KCl is 20 to 80 mEq/day.

Volume Depletion. As a result of increased salt and water excretion, thiazide therapy may lead to depleted intravascular volume, even when edema or ascites is present. Symptoms include weakness, malaise, and orthostatic dizziness. The glomerular filtration rate may fall with a subsequent rise in serum urea nitrogen and creatinine levels (prerenal azotemia). Treatment is usually to discontinue the diuretic tem-

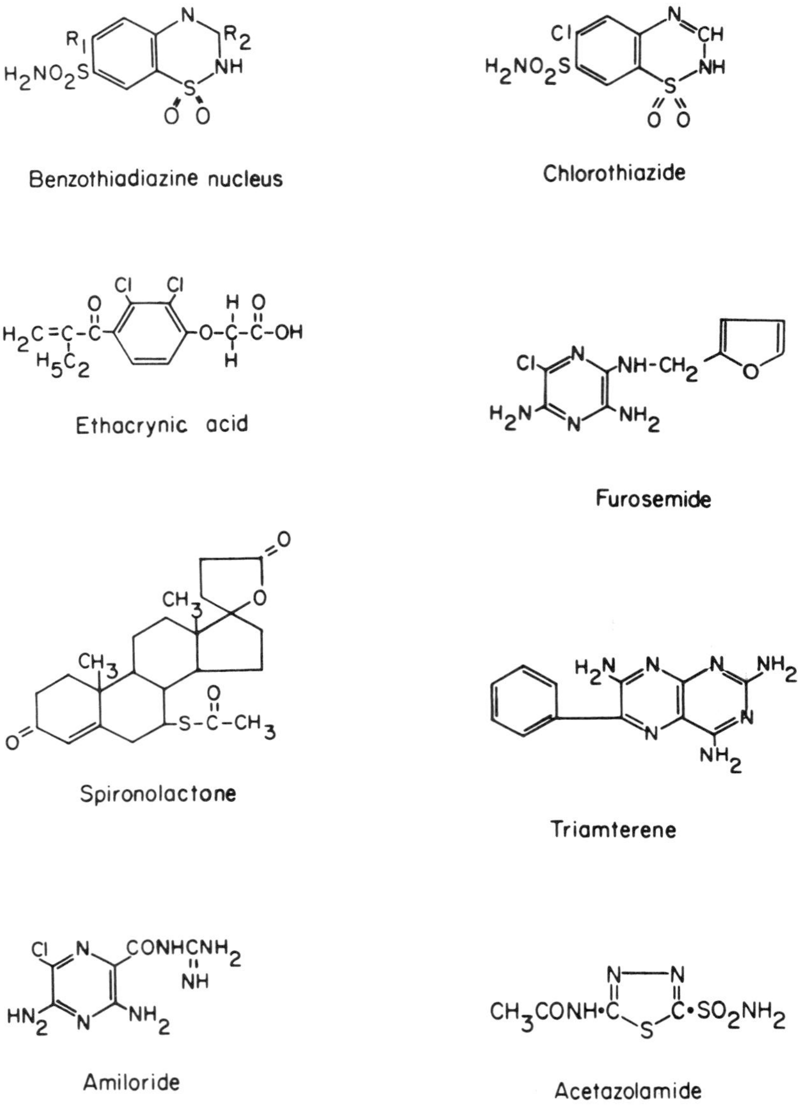

FIG. 40-5. A structural formula for the major diuretics discussed in the text. The other thiazide diuretics have the basic benzothiadiazine structure but with different radicals substituted for R1 and R2.

porarily and occasionally to replace deficits of extracellular fluid volume.

Hyperuricemia. Hyperuricemia may occur but usually does not require treatment unless associated with gout.

Hyperglycemia. A diabetic patient may require more insulin.

Hyponatremia. Hyponatremia will develop if water ingestion exceeds the ability of the kidney to excrete free water (C_{H_2O}). Thiazides cause inhibition of free water excretion by several mechanisms.

1. By impairing the renal diluting ability by direct interference with Na^+ transport along the diluting segment.
2. By causing volume depletion, which leads to increased proximal reabsorption of Na^+ and a consequent decrease in solute delivery to the distal tubule. The presence of increased ADH levels caused by volume depletion may lead to a further decrease in excretion of free water.
3. By causing hypokalemia. Such K^+ depletion may facilitate the intracellular movement of Na^+, leading to extracellular volume depletion, which can enhance ADH secretion.

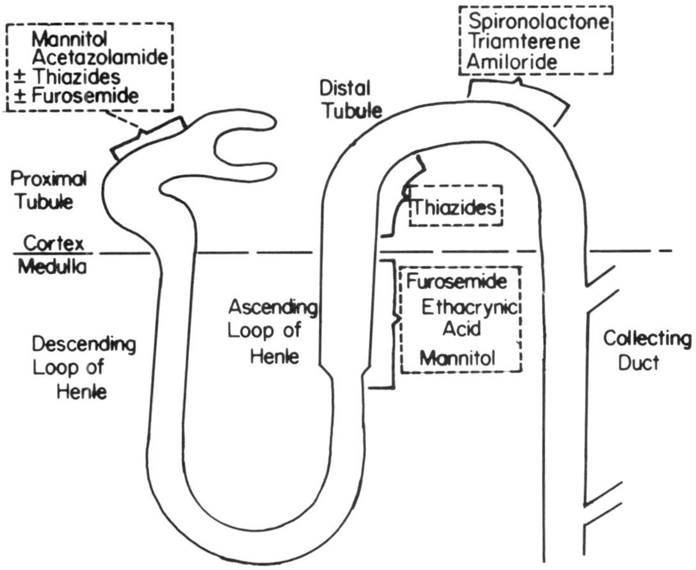

FIG. 40-6. Schematic illustration of the probable sites of action of various diuretics discussed in the text.

Diuretic-induced hyponatremia is generally treated by restricting water intake, since the administration of salt may be hazardous, particularly in patients with edema.

Hypercalcemia. When a patient receiving thiazide diuretics develops hypercalcemia, he should be evaluated for the presence of primary hyperparathyroidism.

Metabolic Alkalosis. Metabolic alkalosis is usually not treated. However, in patients with concomitant respiratory failure and in whom the metabolic alkalosis may cause further respiratory depression by raising the P_{CO_2}, therapy should include K^+ and even extracellular volume repletion. When metabolic alkalosis develops in a patient with severe edema, repletion of extracellular volume may be hazardous; instead, acetazolamide or even exogenous HCl should be given.

Other Side-Effects. Other side-effects include a rise in serum lipid levels, pancreatitis, allergic interstitial nephritis, and various skin rashes.

LOOP DIURETICS

Furosemide and ethacrynic acid act on the cells of the thick ascending limb of Henle; they are the most potent diuretics available. Even though they differ chemically (Fig. 40-5), their actions are similar and will be considered together.

Ethacrynic acid is an unsaturated ketone de-

TABLE 40-2. Adverse Interactions of Drugs with Commonly Used Diuretics

Drug	Diuretic	Adverse Effect or Mechanism
Digitalis	All diuretics except spironolactone, triamterine, and amiloride	Increased sensitivity to digitalis toxicity associated with hypokalemia
Lithium	Thiazides and loop diuretics	Increased lithium toxicity due to reduced lithium excretion
Aminoglycoside antibiotics	Ethacrynic acid and furosemide	Increased risk of ototoxicity
	Furosemide	Possible increased risk of nephrotoxicity
Potassium salts	Spironolactone, triamterene, and amiloride	Hyperkalemia
Corticosteroids	All diuretics except spironolactone, triamterene, and amiloride	Additive K^+ loss

* GFR = glomerular filtration rate.

rivative of aryloxyacetic acid, and furosemide is a derivative of sulfanilamide.

Absorption, Metabolism, and Excretion

Furosemide is readily absorbed from the intestinal tract. When it is given orally, a diuretic response occurs within 30 minutes and persists for 6 to 8 hours. When given intravenously, it acts within 5 minutes and lasts for 2 to 3 hours. Furosemide is about 95% bound to plasma proteins. It is lost from the body through urine and feces. Urinary elimination is by proximal tubular secretion.

When given intravenously to normal subjects, about 10% to 15% of a dose is excreted in the feces. This percentage can reach 60%, however, when the agent is given to a patient with renal failure. Since the natriuresis is more closely related to the concentration of furosemide in the tubular lumen than to its plasma concentration, higher doses are needed in patients with renal failure when tubular secretion of furosemide is decreased. This decrease in secretion is likely due to the accumulation of uremic metabolites that inhibit its secretion and to a decreased mass of functioning tubular cells.

Ethacrynic acid is readily absorbed from the gastrointestinal tract. It is strongly bound to plasma proteins. After its i.v. injection, about one third is excreted by the liver and two thirds by the kidney.

Mechanism of Action and Physiological Effects

Ethacrynic acid and furosemide act by inhibiting the active transport of Cl^- at the ascending limb of Henle. Normally, 25% to 30% of filtered NaCl is reabsorbed in this segment. In high dosage, these agents can block this reabsorption and result in the excretion of as much as 30% of filtered Na^+. Furosemide may also have a small effect on proximal tubular function by inhibiting carbonic anhydrase. By causing renal vasodilation, the loop diuretics may also increase renal blood flow.

Since the reabsorption of NaCl in the thick ascending limb is essential for both the concentration and the dilution of urine, these agents, when given in high doses, may cause the excretion of isotonic or only minimally hypotonic urine. Potassium excretion is increased as a result of increased flow to the distal tubule and increased aldosterone secretion, which is stimulated by depletion of extracellular fluid volume. As with the thiazides, these agents can increase magnesium excretion, but, in contrast, they increase the renal excretion of calcium by inhibiting calcium resorption by the ascending loop of Henle. When given intravenously, furosemide increases venous capacitance, a feature that makes it useful in treating pulmonary edema even without a natriuretic effect.

Adverse Effects

As a result of the very considerable effectiveness of ethacrynic acid and furosemide, severe depletion of extracellular fluid volume and electrolyte disturbances are common adverse effects. Similar to the thiazides, these agents can cause hyponatremia, hypokalemia, hyperuricemia, hypomagnesemia, metabolic alkalosis, and carbohydrate intolerance; the last occurs less commonly than during treatment with a thiazide-type diuretic.

Gastrointestinal disturbances are the most common side-effect, with reports of nausea, vomiting, and diarrhea. A serious and rare complication of ethacrynic acid is the development of vertigo, deafness, and tinnitus, seen most frequently in patients with severe impairment of renal function and who have received very large doses.

Furosemide may also cause ototoxicity, with symptoms similar to those produced by ethacrynic acid. It can increase the ototoxic potential of aminoglycosides; both reversible and irreversible hearing impairment and tinnitus have been reported after its parenteral use. Usually these problems occur when furosemide is infused rapidly in patients with severely impaired renal function and in whom other drugs known to be ototoxic have been given. Other side-effects of furosemide include allergic reactions, particularly in patients with known sensitivity to sulfonamide, allergic interstitial nephritis, hepatic dysfunction, and blood dyscrasias.

POTASSIUM-SPARING DIURETICS

Spironolactone, triamterene, and amiloride may inhibit urinary K^+ excretion. They are used predominantly in combination with other diuretics to decrease K^+ loss.

SPIRONOLACTONE

The structure of spironolactone is shown in Figure 40-5. It is readily absorbed from the intestinal tract and is rapidly and extensively metabolized. The primary metabolite is canrenone. Spironolactone and its metabolites are excreted chiefly in the urine but also in the bile. It has a relatively slow onset of action and often requires a 12- to 72-hour lapse before a diuresis occurs.

Spironolactone is a competitive inhibitor of aldosterone at the distal tubule. Aldosterone normally stimulates Na^+ reabsorption and the secretion of K^+ and H^+, and spironolactone inhibits these effects. Spironolactone is not a very potent diuretic when given alone because it acts primarily on the distal tubule, where only 5% of filtered Na^+ is normally reabsorbed. Besides preventing K^+ loss, spironolactone can be used in patients with primary aldosteronism (Conn's syndrome) because it blocks the effect of excess aldosterone.

The major adverse effect of spironolactone is the development of hyperkalemia, which usually occurs when a patient is also given supplemental potassium or when spironolactone is given to a patient with impaired renal function. Most physicians do not give supplemental potassium to a patient receiving spironolactone. Other adverse effects include the development of hyponatremia, especially when spironolactone is given with other diuretics, gynecomastia, impotence in males, and menstrual irregularities. The development of gynecomastia is a major factor limiting its long-term use in the medical management of primary aldosteronism.

TRIAMTERENE

Triamterene is a pteridine compound with a structure that resembles folic acid and the antimalarial diaminopyrimidines. It can be administered only by the oral route and is rapidly absorbed. Triamterene has a latency before its effect of 2 hours and duration of action of 12 to 16 hours. This drug acts directly on distal tubular transport, independent of aldosterone. It decreases the distal tubular secretion of K^+ by reducing the potential difference between the tubular cell and the lumen. As with spironolactone, only minimal natriuresis is produced, and triamterene is never used as the sole diuretic. The major adverse effect is the development of hyperkalemia. As with spironolactone, K^+ supplements should not be given to patients on triamterene therapy, and triamterene should not be used in patients with renal insufficiency.

AMILORIDE

Amiloride has been recently released in the United States and is widely used in Europe. After its oral administration, 15% to 20% of amiloride is absorbed. It is almost completely excreted in the urine. It can also be given parenterally. Its main action is to inhibit the distal tubular secretion of K^+ and H^+. This agent inhibits K^+ secretion by decreasing the transepithelial potential difference, but it may also directly affect K^+ secretion independent of Na^+ transport. Its major side-effect is the development of hyperkalemia.

OTHER DIURETICS

ACETAZOLAMIDE

Acetazolamide is a sulfanilamide with the structure shown in Figure 40-5. It is readily absorbed from the intestinal tract and excreted by the kidney. After a latency of 1 hour, it acts for 6 to 8 hours. Acetazolamide is a noncompetitive inhibitor of the enzyme carbonic anhydrase, which is important in the proximal tubular reabsorption of HCO_3^-. This inhibition of $NaHCO_3$ reabsorption causes increased HCO_3^- excretion, with a consequent fall in plasma HCO_3^-, and the loss of HCO_3^- buffer leads to hyperchloremic metabolic acidosis. Acetazolamide enhances the distal tubular secretion of K^+ by increasing the distal delivery of Na^+ and the nonreabsorbable anion HCO_3^-. The presence of nonreabsorbable HCO_3^- increases the negative potential difference across the lumen, which enhances the movement of both K^+ and H^+ from the tubular cells into the lumen.

Acetazolamide is rarely used as a diuretic because it is relatively ineffective and causes metabolic acidosis, a predictable complication of its continued use. Carbonic anhydrase is also present in the eye, and its inhibition reduces the rate of formation of aqueous humor, leading to a fall in intraocular pressure. This action makes acetazolamide useful in the management of glaucoma. As a result of its ability to cause a HCO_3^- diuresis, acetazolamide is also useful in treating metabolic alkalosis or when there is a need to alkalinize the urine (with cystinuria or acute hyperuricemia). Acetazolamide is also used occasionally in epilepsy.

The major adverse effect of acetazolamide is the development of hyperchloremic metabolic acidosis. Other side-effects include paresthesias, drowsiness, confusion, and hypokalemia.

ORGANOMERCURIALS

Organomercurials are included only for historical reasons, since they are rarely used today. They must be given parenterally and have numerous side-effects. (For more complete information, *see* earlier editions of this textbook.)

TICRYNAFEN

Ticrynafen is similar to the thiazides but, unlike these agents, is uricosuric. Due to the development of hepatic toxicity, this agent has been withdrawn from approved clinical use.

DIURETICS IN NONEDEMATOUS CONDITIONS

Diuretics are most commonly used in edema-forming states, such as congestive heart failure, liver disease with ascites, and nephrotic syndrome. By increasing salt and water removal, they are usually effective in treating edema. Diuretics are also useful in certain nonedematous conditions.

HYPERTENSION

Diuretics are usually the initial drug of choice in the treatment of hypertension. The mechanism of their antihypertensive effect is unclear; they act partly by volume depletion and partly by decreasing peripheral vascular resistance. Unless glomerular filtration rate decreases below 30 ml/min, thiazides may be more effective as antihypertensive agents than is furosemide. Spironolactone, amiloride, and triamterene are generally used only to prevent diuretic-induced potassium loss and hypokalemia (*see* Chap. 36). In patients with primary aldosteronism, spironolactone may be an effective antihypertensive agent, but its long-term use is limited by the toxicity noted above.

IDIOPATHIC HYPERCALCIURIA

Thirty percent to 50% of patients with recurrent calcium-containing kidney stones have idiopathic hypercalciuria. Thiazides can decrease the rate of kidney stone formation in these patients because they reduce urinary calcium excretion. They are also useful in patients with recurrent stones who have normal rates of urinary calcium excretion; urinary calcium decreases in these patients as well. The hypocalciuric action of the thiazides depends largely on extracellular volume depletion. If the patient consumes large quantities of salt (greater than 7–10 g/day), the hypocalciuric effect may not occur. Thus the use of thiazides in the management of hypercalciuria should include the prescription of a diet modestly restricted in sodium content.

HYPERCALCEMIA

In contrast to thiazides, the loop diuretics cause a marked increase in urinary calcium excretion by inhibiting calcium reabsorption in the ascending loop of Henle. In patients with severe hypercalcemia, treatment with i.v. saline and furosemide may be a useful emergency measure. Since furosemide will increase potassium and magnesium excretion, their concentrations must be monitored during such treatment. Because large doses of furosemide and saline are required, such treatment should be limited to patients with severe and symptomatic hypercalcemia. Treatment is usually carried out in an intensive care unit with a Foley catheter in place for the accurate collection and measurement of urinary electrolyte losses, which are needed to determine that the appropriate i.v. fluids are given as replacement.

NEPHROGENIC DIABETES INSIPIDUS

In nephrogenic diabetes insipidus, the nephron is unresponsive to the action of ADH. Consequently these patients excrete large volumes of very dilute urine. Thiazides are useful in reducing the urine volume to a modest extent; they are believed to act by causing extracellular volume depletion, which leads to the increased proximal reabsorption of Na^+ and water. A consequent decrease in the distal delivery of filtrate occurs, leading to reduced urine volume.

PROXIMAL RENAL TUBULAR ACIDOSIS (TYPE II RTA)

In proximal renal tubular acidosis, the proximal tubular reabsorption of HCO_3^- is defective, with a resultant increase in distal delivery of $NaHCO_3$, leading to losses of HCO_3^- in the urine and the consequent development of metabolic acidosis. Thiazides, by causing extracellular volume depletion and enhancing the proximal reabsorption of HCO_3^-, can reduce the urinary loss of HCO_3^-. Another explanation for the effectiveness of thiazides may be their hypocalciuric effect, which may lead to a slightly increased serum ionized calcium level;

this may reduce the secretion of parathyroid hormone (PTH). Since PTH can decrease the proximal reabsorption of HCO_3^-, a reduction in PTH secretion could enhance the proximal reabsorption of HCO_3^-.

SYNDROME OF INAPPROPRIATE ADH SECRETION (SIADH)

In SIADH, continued secretion of ADH is inappropriate for the degree of hypoosmolality that exists. This syndrome can arise from various disorders, many of which affect the central nervous system or the lungs. Since ADH inhibits the kidney's ability to excrete free water (C_{H_2O}), dilutional hyponatremia is an integral part of the syndrome. Normally a fall in serum osmolality inhibits the secretion of ADH. However, the "inappropriate" secretion of ADH persists.

Furosemide has been shown to be effective in the emergency treatment of severe, symptomatic hyponatremia that sometimes develops. Since furosemide abolishes the usual hypertonicity of the medullary interstitium, the kidney cannot generate a concentrated urine, even with the continued presence of ADH. As a result, there is decreased urine osmolality even approaching that of plasma. Because furosemide causes a significant loss of Na^+, this ion must be replaced quantitatively as i.v. hypertonic sodium chloride. This type of treatment is needed only for the treatment of acute and symptomatic hyponatremia; when the syndrome develops gradually and is without symptoms, water restriction is the only therapy needed.

URIC ACID NEPHROPATHY

Uric acid nephropathy can be a serious complication of myeloproliferative and lymphoproliferative diseases. It usually occurs when chemotherapy causes massive breakdown of tumor cells with the liberation of uric acid. The increased uric acid concentrations may result in uric acid deposits within the tubular lumen. Since sodium urate, with a pK_a of 5.7, is more soluble in an alkaline urine, measures to alkalinize the urine and decrease the concentration of urate in the tubular lumen are useful in preventing and managing intraluminal urate deposits. To alkalinize the urine, sodium bicarbonate may be given intravenously and acetazolamide added. Mannitol and i.v. fluids may also be given to dilute the tubular concentration of urate and enhance the flow within the tubule.

FURTHER READING

1. Kaloyanides GJ: Pathogenesis and treatment of edema with special reference to use of diuretics. In Maxwell MH, Kleeman CR (eds): Clinical Disorders of Fluid and Electrolyte Metabolism, 3rd ed. pp. 647–701. New York, McGraw-Hill, 1980
2. Martinez-Maldonado M, Eknoyan G, Suki WN: Diuretics in nonedematous states: Physiological basis for the clinical use. Arch Intern Med 131:797, 1973
3. Seely JF, Dirks JH: Site of action of diuretic drugs. Kidney Int 11:1, 1977

CHAPTER 40 QUESTIONS

(See P. 7 for Full Instructions)

Select the One Best Answer

1. The potential for cardiac toxicity of digitalis is increased by each of the following EXCEPT
   A. triamterene.
   B. ethacrynic acid.
   C. chlorothiazide.
   D. meralluride, a mercurial diuretic.
   E. cortisol.

2. Thiazide diuretics
   A. augment sodium excretion without significant loss of potassium.
   B. commonly produce orthostatic hypotension.
   C. are effective in nephrogenic diabetes insipidus.
   D. promote uric acid excretion.
   E. alleviate the symptoms of diabetes mellitus.

3. A female patient with a history of glaucoma and premenstrual epilepsy would be a candidate for treatment with
   A. chlorothiazide.
   B. triamterene.
   C. ethacrynic acid.
   D. acetazolamide.
   E. mannitol.

4. Each of the following associates a drug with one of its characteristics EXCEPT
   A. spironolactone—gynecomastia is a potential complication.
   B. triamterene—inhibits chloride reabsorption at the ascending limb of Henle.
   C. furosemide—can produce the excretion of as much as 30% of the filtered sodium.
   D. chlorothiazide—decreases sodium

chloride reabsorption in the distal convoluted tubule.
E. acetazolamide—metabolic acidosis is a frequent complication.

A = 1,2,3; B = 1,3; C = 2,4; D = 4; E = All

5. Acetazolamide
   1. competitively antagonizes carbonic anhydrase.
   2. produces metabolic acidosis.
   3. reduces intraocular pressure.
   4. is effective in the treatment of peptic ulcer.

6. Chronic use of furosemide may
   1. cause metabolic alkalosis.
   2. stimulate aldosterone output.
   3. cause hyperuricemia.
   4. cause hypovolemia.

7. Mannitol
   1. reduces cerebral edema.
   2. is an effective source of energy in the diabetic.
   3. is a poor natriuretic agent.
   4. is ineffective in metabolic alkalosis.

8. Which of the following agents may make the renal countercurrent multiplier system inoperative?
   1. Ethacrynic acid
   2. Hydrochlorothiazide
   3. Furosemide
   4. Acetazolamide

9. Thiazides cause a marked kaliuresis by
   1. increasing the sodium and water delivered to the distal tubule.
   2. decreasing the proximal tubule resorption of potassium.
   3. the increase in aldosterone secretion arising from thiazide-induced volume depletion.
   4. acidosis.

10. Both furosemide and hydrochlorothiazide
   1. may produce hypercalcemia as an adverse effect.
   2. decrease the minimum urinary diluting ability.
   3. decrease the maximum urinary concentrating ability.
   4. may cause hyponatremia as an adverse effect.

11. Potential complications of thiazide therapy include
   1. hyperglycemia.
   2. hyperuricemia.
   3. metabolic alkalosis.
   4. ototoxicity.

12. Metolazone differs from other thiazide and thiazide-like diuretics in that only metolazone
   1. can cause hypokalemia.
   2. is often effective when glomerular filtration rate is less than 25 ml/min.
   3. can cause metabolic alkalosis.
   4. can produce some inhibition of proximal reabsorption of sodium independent of carbonic anhydrase inhibition by the diuretic.

PETER LOMAX

41

Drugs Used in Anemia

The synthesis of hemoglobin and the formation of red blood cells are normally adjusted to allow for physiological losses and to maintain the body content at a steady level. If the loss of blood is excessive or the replacement mechanisms become defective, anemia develops.

Many dietary factors important for normal hematopoiesis, including iron, copper, cobalt, vitamin B_{12}, and folic acid, are commonly involved in the cause and treatment of anemia. It is important to consider carefully the type of erythropoietic substance required and why the deficiency has arisen before starting treatment. The precipitate use of an incorrect hematinic may obscure the correct diagnosis and render subsequent treatment difficult.

A list of agents commonly used in the treatment of anemia is presented in Table 41-1.

IRON

Iron is an essential component of the hemoglobin molecule. In most instances, anemia is the result of iron deficiency arising from chronic blood loss or inadequate dietary supplies. Typically, a microcytic, hypochromic anemia results. The mean corpuscular volume falls below the normal 80 μm^3, and the hemoglobin concentration may be reduced to 5–10 g/dl from the normal level of about 15 g/dl.

ABSORPTION AND METABOLISM

Many foodstuffs contain iron, and it can be adsorbed at all levels of the gastrointestinal tract, although the greatest amount enters through the duodenum. From 5% to 10% of dietary iron is absorbed in normal persons and about 20% in iron-deficient subjects. Most food iron is in the form of organic complexes, which are mainly broken down by gastric acid secretion, and ionized iron in the reduced ferrous state is liberated. Ferrous iron is oxidized to ferric iron and then bound by a protein acceptor (*apoferritin*) in the mucosal cell to form *ferritin*. Iron is carried in the body on a specific iron-binding protein, *transferrin*. The bound iron is carried to its functional sites, and free iron is liberated.

There do not appear to be any significant mechanisms for clearing the body of excess iron. The total content is regulated by control of the rate of absorption. How this is brought

TABLE 41-1. Preparations Commonly Used in Treating Anemia

Drug	Trade Name	Preparation	Dose
Oral iron preparations			
Ferroglycine sulfate complex	Ferronord	250-mg tablet	250 mg q 8 hr
Ferrous fumarate		200-mg tablet	600 mg daily
Ferrous gluconate		300-mg tablet or capsule; elixir containing 36 mg iron 5 ml	300 mg daily
Ferrous sulfate		300-mg tablet Syrup containing 40 mg/ml	300 mg q 8 hr 1 tsp q 8 hr (syrup)
Parenteral iron preparations			
Iron dextran injection	Imferon	Solution containing 50 mg iron/ml	2–5 ml, i.m. daily
Iron dextrin, dextriferron	Astrafer	Solution containing 20 mg iron/ml	20-mg initial dose increased to 100 mg over several days for slow i.v. injection
Vitamin B_{12} and folic acid			
Cyanocobalamin injection	Many designations	Solutions of 10, 30, 100, or 1000 μg/ml	30–250 μg, i.m. (for dosage schedule, *see* text)
Folic acid		5 mg tablet; solution of 15 mg/ml	0.1–30 mg, orally or parenterally, daily (*see* text)

about is not understood. The rate of absorption may depend on the availability of apoferritin or transferrin; this is the *mucosal block theory.* Alternatively the active transport of iron across the mucosa may depend on the level of tissue enzymes that regulate absorption. The transport and distribution of iron are summarized in Figure 41-1.

The normal iron stores in the adult are in the range of 0.5 to 1.5 g. These are mainly in the form of ferritin in the reticuloendothelial cells of the liver, spleen, and bone marrow. The iron stores are rapidly depleted in iron-deficiency anemia.

PREPARATIONS, USES, AND ADVERSE EFFECTS

Iron preparations are available for oral or parenteral administration.

The most common, least expensive oral drug is *ferrous sulfate.* The frequency of adverse effects from ferrous sulfate has led to the marketing of many iron-containing compounds for oral use. These compounds differ in their degree of absorption, and because even with the most effective preparations only about 10% to 15% is absorbed, an excess of the drug is usually administered. Oral therapy must be continued for about 6 months in patients with severe anemia. Because iron preparations are incompatible with many other drugs, they should be given alone.

All iron preparations are equally toxic when equivalent amounts of iron are administered. Acute toxic reactions are rare in adults, but serious acute poisoning in infants and children is fairly common. The treatment of acute iron poisoning is discussed in Chapter 72.

With usual doses, gastric distress, colic, and diarrhea are frequently related to the total dose administered and to psychological factors rather than to the particular iron salt used. Starting therapy with small doses (*e.g.*, 200 mg of dry ferrous sulfate every 8 hours) and gradually increasing the daily intake until the limit of tolerance is reached often allows adequate dosage without these adverse effects.

Parenteral therapy is rarely needed and should be used only when there are clear indications or there has been no response to oral administration. *Saccharated iron oxide* and *iron-dextran complex* are two of the iron preparations for i.v. or i.m. injection.

Local adverse effects near the injection site may include pain, discoloration, local inflammation, thrombophlebitis, and lymphadenopathy. Systemic intoxication occurs in a small number of patients, giving rise to headache, muscle and joint pain, syncope, nausea, vomiting, and dyspnea.

VITAMIN B_{12}

Vitamin B_{12}, or cyanocobalamin, is a cobalt-containing compound with a molecular weight of 1355 whose crystalline structure was determined by Hodgkin. One group of several cobal-

Thomas Hodgkin, 1798–1866. English physician. Best known for his description, in 1832, of the lymphoma that bears his name.

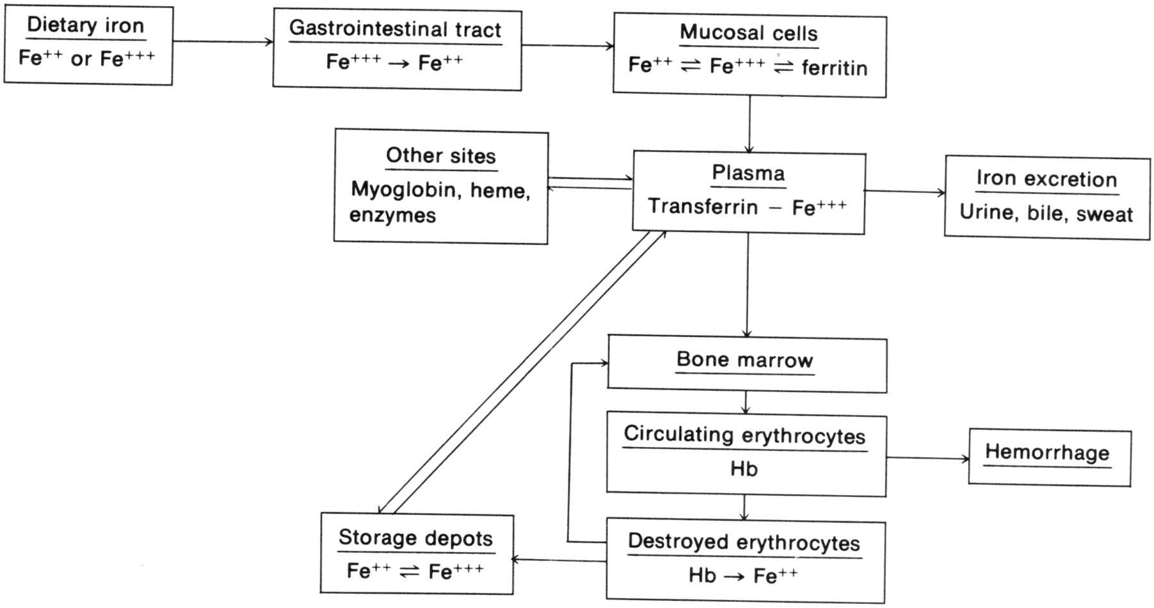

FIG. 41-1. Metabolism of dietary iron.

amins (*see* Chap. 73) all exhibit vitamin B_{12} activity. The vitamin is prepared commercially from liver (Minot and Murphy initially demonstrated the value of liver extracts in treating pernicious anemia) or from the growth of suitable microorganisms and is assayed spectrophotometrically.

ABSORPTION AND METABOLISM

Absorption of dietary vitamin B_{12} from the ileum requires the presence of a specific substance, the *intrinsic factor of Castle,* which is secreted by the gastric mucosa. Intrinsic factor appears to be a glycoprotein and is able to bind to vitamin B_{12} and in some way facilitate its absorption. In the blood the vitamin is bound to an α_1-glycoprotein and is widely distributed throughout the body tissues.

Daily requirements of vitamin B_{12} have been estimated at up to 5 μg, but there are considerable stores in the normal liver. The metabolic functions of the cobalamins have been studied in many biologic systems, particularly in bacteria. They act as coenzymes in a number of biochemical pathways. The systems significantly impaired by vitamin B_{12} deficiency in humans are DNA synthesis, proprionate catabolism, and the synthesis of methionine methyl groups.

Vitamin B_{12} deficiency arises from inadequate dietary intake or defective intestinal absorption. The most common deficient state is that due to absence of intrinsic factor in the gastric mucosa—Addisonian pernicious anemia. Less common malabsorption syndromes occur after gastrectomy from overgrowth of abnormal intestinal bacteria associated with conditions that produce intestinal stasis, parasitic infestations, and disorders of the bowel wall.

The major clinical manifestations of vitamin-B_{12} deficiency are megaloblastic macrocytic (pernicious) anemia, in which the peripheral blood contains large abnormal erythrocytes with a basophilic cytoplasm (DNA synthesis is impaired, so the replication and cell division are blocked and normoblasts fail to form); gastrointestinal symptoms from mucosal atrophy (glossitis, dyspepsia); and degenerative changes of the dorsal and lateral

---

George Richards Minot, 1885–1950. Boston physician. Won Nobel prize in 1934, with W. P. Murphy and G. H. Whipple, for work in the 1920s on liver therapy for pernicious anemia. Also discovered the relation between alcoholic polyneuritis and vitamin B deficiency.

William Parry Murphy, 1892– . Boston physician. Studied diabetes as well as blood disorders, and shared the 1934 Nobel prize with G. R. Minot and G. H. Whipple for their work on pernicious anemia.

William Bosworth Castle, 1897– . Boston physician. Known for Castle's principle of 1928, that pernicious anemia resulted from the stomach's inability to secrete an antipernicious anemia factor. Demonstrated efficacy of crude liver extracts in advanced sprue and iron therapy for hookworm-induced anemia.

columns of the spinal cord and of the peripheral nerves (subacute combined degeneration/combined system disease).

PREPARATIONS AND USES

Administration of vitamin B_{12} restores the blood picture to normal and arrests the development of neurologic damage. Usually the drug must be given by i.m. or s.c. injection. The object of treatment is repletion of body stores and the maintenance of an intake equal to the daily losses. Intensive treatment for the first 6 weeks leads to rapid clinical improvement. A dosage schedule of up to 250 μg daily for 10 to 15 days followed by 250 μg weekly for several months is frequently used. Thereafter, monthly injections of 100 μg are continued for the rest of the patient's life.

Oral administration of high doses of vitamin B_{12}, or of vitamin B_{12} plus animal intrinsic factor, has generally proved unreliable.

No toxic effects of vitamin B_{12} are known, and there are no known contraindications to its use.

FOLIC ACID

Folic acid is used generally to cover a group of pteroylglutamic acids. The pure compound is *pteroylmonoglutamic acid,* and in common use this is the compound referred to as folic acid (*see* Chap. 73).

ABSORPTION AND METABOLISM

Folates are present in most foodstuffs and are synthesized by many bacteria. Folic acid is readily absorbed from the gut, primarily in the proximal small intestine. The daily human requirement is about 50 μg.

In mammals folic acid is the precursor of coenzymes involved in single carbon transfer reactions and is therefore essential to all metabolic systems in which such transfer occurs. Folic acid and vitamin B_{12} are closely interrelated metabolically.

Deficiency arises in humans from malnutrition and from various malabsorption syndromes such as sprue. Malignant disease, hemolytic anemia, and pregnancy increase folic acid requirements so that a relative deficiency arises in these conditions. Certain metabolic inhibitors interfere with folic acid, and the megaloblastic anemia during administration of some anticonvulsant drugs may arise in this way (Chap. 29).

Folic acid deficiency leads to megaloblastic anemia indistinguishable from that due to vitamin-B_{12} deficiency. The gastrointestinal disorders, particularly glossitis and diarrhea, are prominent features of the syndrome. Unlike vitamin-B_{12} deficiency, however, neurologic damage does not occur.

THERAPEUTIC USES

Oral administration of folic acid will correct the hematologic defect in uncomplicated cases. The dose used depends on the severity of the anemia. The drug is administered by i.m. or deep s.c. injection if there is a malabsorption condition. The dose may need to be increased in patients taking chloramphenicol (*see* Chap. 61); in alcoholics; and in patients with uremia, tumors, rheumatoid arthritis, or hepatitis.

Initial therapy requires 1 mg daily, reduced to 0.1 mg for maintenance. Despite clinical evidence that this dose level is fully adequate, doses in the range of 10 to 30 mg/day continue to be recommended. Folic acid is nontoxic in humans.

The only therapeutic indication for folic acid is established deficiency. Particular care must be taken in establishing the correct diagnosis before starting therapy, especially in the patient with pernicious anemia, since folic acid will partially correct the hematopoietic defect and exacerbate spinal cord disease.

FURTHER READING

Bothwell TH, Charlton RW, Cook JD et al: From Metabolism in Man. Oxford, Blackwell Scientific, 1979

Smith EL: Vitamin B_{12}. New York, Wiley, 1965

Wintrobe MM, Lee GR, Boggs DR et al: Clinical Hematology. Philadelphia, Lea & Febiger, 1974

CHAPTER 41 QUESTIONS

(*See* P. 7 for Full Instructions)

Select the One Best Answer

1. Each of the following is characteristic of iron EXCEPT
   - A. the duodenum absorbs almost all of the ingested iron.
   - B. it is absorbed mainly in its reduced form.

C. its absorption is increased by acid.
D. an excess of systemic iron is eliminated from the body very slowly.
E. it occasionally causes constipation.

2. Folic acid
   A. should be included in any therapeutic regimen for managing anemia.
   B. must be given along with vitamin B_{12} in treating pernicious anemia.
   C. can induce a remission of the anemia of pernicious anemia, allowing the neurologic disease to progress.
   D. can induce a remission in the anemia of pyridoxine deficiency.
   E. is a specific for the anemia associated with *Diphyllobothrium latum*.

3. Vitamin B_{12}
   A. is synthesized in the liver.
   B. can cure pernicious anemia.
   C. is quite toxic in a dose of 1000 μg.
   D. deficiency results in cardiac failure.
   E. absorption occurs mainly in the duodenum.

4. Which of the following tends to cause black, tarry stools?
   A. Magnesium sulfate (Epsom salts)
   B. Magnesium hydroxide (milk of magnesia)
   C. Calcium carbonate
   D. Ferrous sulfate
   E. Castor oil

A = 1,2,3; B = 1,3; C = 2,4; D = 4; E = All

5. Vitamin B_{12}
   1. is the treatment of choice for pernicious anemia.
   2. is the usual treatment for megaloblastic anemia of pregnancy.
   3. may be effective orally in large doses for treatment of pernicious anemia.
   4. may be replaced by folic acid for treatment of pernicious anemia.

6. Microcytic hypochromic anemia usually responds to treatment with
   1. cyanocobalamin.
   2. folic acid.
   3. deferoxamine.
   4. ferrous sulfate.

7. Which of the following correctly matches a drug with the type of anemia it produces and the mechanism of the anemia?
   1. Acetysalicylic acid—iron deficiency anemia—chronic hemorrhage
   2. Chloramphenicol—aplastic anemia—bone marrow suppression
   3. Phenytoin—megaloblastic anemia—folic acid deficiency
   4. Primaquine—hemolytic anemia—glucose-6-phosphate dehydrogenase deficiency

8. Ferrous sulfate
   1. is an appropriate treatment for megaloblastic anemia.
   2. is only partially (10–25%) absorbed orally.
   3. seldom produces adverse side-effects.
   4. can be chelated by deferoxamine.

42

PETER LOMAX

Anticoagulants

The use of drugs that prolong the coagulation time of blood has become widespread in recent years. These agents have been used in many pathologic states, including venous thromboembolic conditions, coronary artery disease, cerebral artery disease, polycythemia, pulmonary hypertension, and various embolic phenomena, as well as in cardiac and vascular surgery, particularly when extracorporeal circulation is used.

In all instances of use other than surgical, there is debate about the indications for, and value of, anticoagulant therapy. Against the claimed efficacy of therapy in patients with coronary thrombosis, for instance, must be weighed the attendant mortality and morbidity resulting from the drugs themselves. On this point there is still a lack of reliable statistical information.

Table 42-1 presents a summary of the common anticoagulant agents.

NORMAL COAGULATION MECHANISMS

The arrest of hemorrhage after vascular trauma results from coagulation of the blood and such vascular factors as capillary retraction, arteriolar constriction, and the formation of platelet plugs at the puncture sites.

Normal coagulation depends on the formation of fibrin as the basis of the clot. This is the end-point of a series of reactions involving all the different components of the clotting system.

Blood coagulation is initiated by activation of either of two mechanisms: an intrinsic or blood mechanism, activated by surface contact of whole blood; and an extrinsic system involving tissue factors. These two systems eventually interact to form a common prothrombin-converting principle. The sequence of events involves a cascade of enzyme reactions of

TABLE 42-1. Common Anticoagulants

Drug	Trade Name	Time for Maximum Effect *hr*	Time for Recovery *hr*	Preparation	Dose* *mg*
Heparin sodium				For injection, solution of 1,000, 5,000, 10,000, 20,000, 40,000 *U.S.P.* IU/ml. Repository form in a gelatin complex containing 20,000 and 40,000 IU/ml	
Coumarin derivatives					
Bishydroxycoumarin	Dicumarol	36–48	84–108	25, 50, and 100 mg tablets and capsules	300
Ethylbiscoumacetate	Tromexan	18–30	36–60	150 and 300 mg tablets	900
Warfarin	Coumadin, Panwarfin, Prothromadin	36–48	84–108	2, 5, 7.5, 10, and 25 mg tablets. Also as powder for preparation of parenteral solutions	50
Indanedione derivatives					
Diphenadione	Dipaxin	48–60	96–168	1 and 5 mg tablets	20
Phenindione	Hedulin, Danilone, Dindevan	36–48	72–96	20, 50, and 100 mg tablets	200

* *See* text for detailed discussion of dosage.

which Figure 42-1 is a useful working model. The clotting factors are listed in Table 42-2.

Clinically useful anticoagulants act by inhibiting the action, or interfering with the formation, of one or more of these clotting factors.

HEPARIN

CHEMISTRY

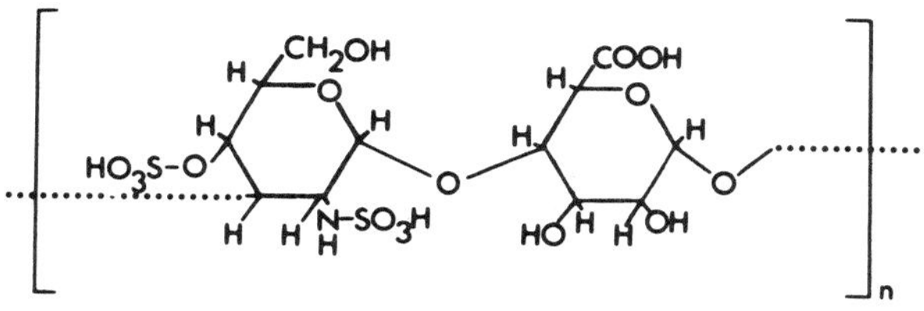

HEPARIN

Heparin is a mucopolysaccharide with a molecular weight between 10,000 and 12,000 daltons. The molecule comprises an alternating sequence of glucosamine and glucuronic acid. The hexose moieties are highly sulfated and carry a dense anionic charge.

The mast cells of the body contain heparin, which accounts for their characteristic metachromatic staining. Lung tissues are rich in heparin, and the drug is prepared commercially from the lungs or intestinal mucosa of cattle. The purified extract is assayed with sheep plasma and must contain at least 120 *U.S.P.* international units of anticoagulant activity per milligram.

TABLE 42-2. Clotting Factors: International Numbers and Synonyms

Clotting Factor	Factor and Synonym
I	Fibrinogen
II	Prothrombin
III	Thromboplastin (tissue)
IV	Calcium
V	Labile factor
	Proaccelerin
	Plasma Ac-globulin
VII	Stable factor
	Proconvertin
	Serum prothrombin conversion accelerator
	Co-thromboplastin
VIII	Antihemophilic globulin (AHG)
	Thromboplastinogen
IX	Plasma thromboplastin component (PTC)
	Christmas factor
X	Stuart–Prower factor
XI	Plasma thromboplastin antecedent (PTA)
XII	Hageman factor
XIII	Fibrin stabilizing factor
	Laki–Lorand factor

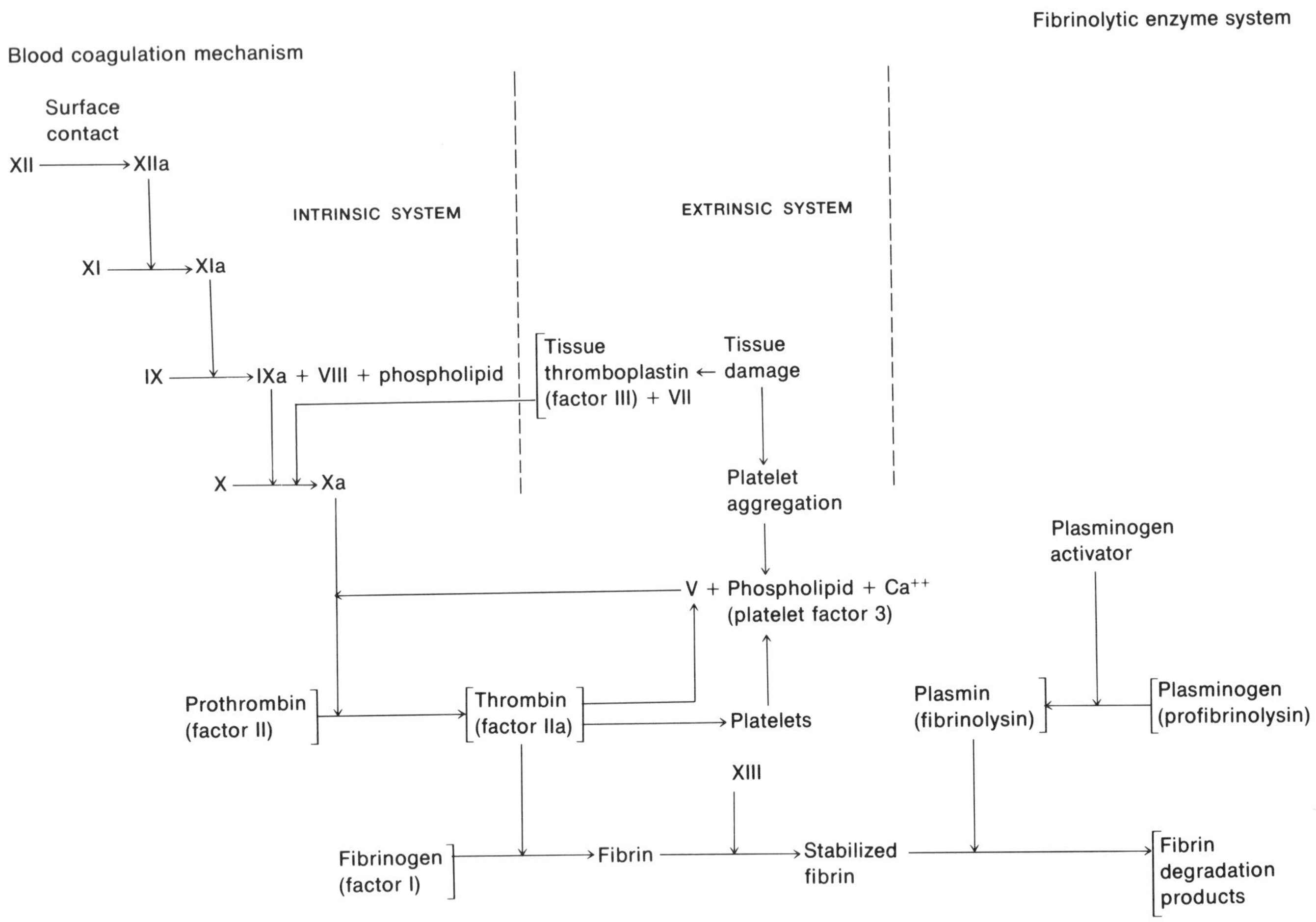

FIG. 42-1. Reactions involved in normal coagulation of the blood. Activated forms of the coagulation factors are indicated by the suffix "a."

MECHANISM OF ACTION

Heparin inhibits blood clotting both *in vivo* and *in vitro*. Whole blood clotting time, thrombin time, prothrombin time, and thromboplastin generation are suppressed. The activation of prothrombin is prevented, probably by interaction of heparin with clotting factors IX, X, and XI, and the catalytic action of thrombin on fibrinogen is blocked. These reactions require a naturally occurring plasma cofactor (an α_2-globulin, referred to as antithrombin III). Heparin also decreases the adhesiveness of platelets and inhibits thrombin-induced platelet aggregation.

The anticoagulant activity of heparin accounts for its effectiveness *in vitro*, but recent studies suggest that this is a minor part of its clinical and biologic actions. Anticoagulant activity is a property of only a few of the chains of commercial heparins. Heparin is a biochemical representative of a distinct class of compounds known as linear anionic polyelectrolytes. The polysaccharide chain, with multiple acidic groups giving them a highly negative charge, forms stable complexes and thus alters the activity of biologic proteins. The negative charge on cell surfaces is thus increased. This increase in the negative charge of the vessel wall (or on an intravascular prosthesis, graft, or transplant) largely may account for the clinical effectiveness of heparin in preventing thrombosis.

THERAPEUTIC USES

Heparin is destroyed in the gastrointestinal tract, and attempts at sublingual administration have not been effective. The drug must be given parenterally, and several techniques are available.

1. *Continuous i.v. infusion.* The anticoagulant effect is achieved immediately after i.v. injection. With the continuous drip method, an initial dose of 5,000 IU is given, and 20,000 to 30,000 IU is added to 1 liter of 5% glucose or 0.9% sodium chloride solution and given slowly over the next 24 hours (20–25 drops/min). This method has the advantage of maintaining steady blood levels of the anticoagulant, but it requires fairly constant attention, and in some cases the large fluid volume may be contraindicated by the patient's condition.
2. *Intermittent i.v. infusion.* A single i.v. injection of 5,000 IU is effective for about 3 hours. Decreased coagulability can be maintained using this dose every 3 hours or larger doses less frequently.
3. *Intramuscular injection.* Absorption is slower after i.m. injection, and the drug is not effective for 30 minutes, so that an initial i.v. dose is needed (5,000–10,000 IU) for immediate anticoagulation. A dose of 20,000 to 40,000 IU of heparin in 1 ml injected intramuscularly lasts 8 to 10 hours or longer. A respository form of the drug is available for i.m. injection. Large painful hematomas may occur with both types of preparation.
4. *Deep s.c. injection.* From 20,000 to 40,000 IU of heparin injected deeply subcutaneously can prolong coagulation up to 16 hours. An i.v. priming dose is needed initially for immediate anticoagulation. Hematoma formation and painful tissue induration are frequent occurrences.
5. *Low-dose therapy.* Much smaller doses of heparin (*e.g.*, 5,000 IU every 8 to 12 hours subcutaneously) than those needed to reduce blood coagulability to a therapeutic level are used to prevent venous thrombosis. Prophylaxis may be due to heparin complexing with antithrombin, which inhibits factor Xa. To avoid the high cost and inconvenience of treating patients unnecessarily, predictive indices have been developed for identifying patients at high risk of deep venous thrombosis. Jet-injected s.c. administration of low doses is less painful and simpler and faster to administer; intrapulmonary administration by aerosal may prove effective based on initial trials.

Larger than usual doses of heparin may be needed in febrile patients and in those to whom digitalis (*see* Chap. 33), antihistamines (*see* Chap. 51), or tetracyclines (*see* Chap. 61) are being given.

ADVERSE EFFECTS

The usual preparations of heparin are relatively nontoxic, and adverse effects are rare. The common danger is of spontaneous hemorrhage, particularly from a previously unsuspected lesion such as a peptic ulcer.

Other uncommon toxic reactions include hypersensitivity and anaphylactoid reactions, thrombocytopenia, fever, and alopecia development 3 to 4 months later. Alopecia is usually only transient.

Acute adrenal hemorrhage has been found

at autopsy in some patients who have died during heparin therapy, particularly when the drug has been administered for several days. Abdominal pain, nausea, and vomiting are signs of this syndrome. In addition to having their excessive coagulation defects monitored and corrected, such patients should be treated with cortisone.

HEPARIN ANTAGONISTS

In the event of minor bleeding during heparin therapy, withdrawal or reduction of dosage is sufficient. When major hemorrhage occurs, specific antagonists such as protamine sulfate are used (Table 42-3), which react with heparin to form stable inactive compounds.

Protamine sulfate is a low molecular weight protein rich in arginine and carrying a strong basic charge that reacts with the acidic heparin molecule. One milligram is equivalent to 1 mg of heparin and is given by slow i.v. injection as a 1% solution. The dose needed is based on the original dose of heparin. (The rate of metabolism of heparin is such that 50% of a given dose is removed in 30 minutes. Overdosage with protamine sulfate should be avoided because it possesses anticoagulant activity.

OTHER ACTIONS

Heparin decreases the plasma turbidity normally seen following a fat-containing meal. Absorbed fat is carried in the plasma bound to protein and forms particles of varying size, mainly consisting of protein-triglyceride complexes (the chylomicrons). Heparin releases a lipase from the capillary wall that breaks down the chylomicrons, and the free fatty acids liberated dissolve in the plasma (*see* Chap. 37). Heparin probably forms a component of this lipoprotein lipase and may act to bind the lipase to the substrate. Figure 42-2 illustrates these reactions. This lipemia-clearing action of heparin occurs with much lower doses than must be used for effective anticoagulant therapy. The clinical significance of this effect is uncertain at present.

Many other effects of heparin have been described, including antiinflammatory and antiallergic actions. These properties have been investigated for the treatment of bronchopulmonary disease but are not generally used clinically.

COUMARIN ANTICOAGULANTS

CHEMISTRY

The coumarin anticoagulants were discovered in 1941 when it was shown that *bishydroxycoumarin* was the compound present in spoiled

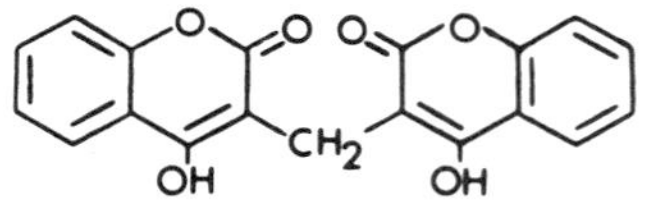

BISHYDROXYCOUMARIN

sweet clover, which led to the development of hemorrhagic disease in cattle. This compound was later synthesized. Since that time, many drugs have been investigated for anticoagulant activity, and the useful compounds fall into two groups: the *coumarin derivatives* and the *indanedione derivatives* (Fig. 42-3). The most widely used oral anticoagulant in the United States is *warfarin*. The commercial form is a

TABLE 42-3. Anticoagulant Antagonists

Drug	Trade Name	Preparation	Dose
Menadiol sodium diphosphate	Synkayvite, Kappadione	5 mg tablet; parenteral solution of 1–75 mg/ml	5–10 mg p.o.; 10–50 mg i.v. (5 mg/min)
Menadione	Vitamin K_3	1–10 mg tablets and capsules; oily solution 1 or 2 mg/ml for i.m. injection	1–2 mg/i.m.; 2–10 mg p.o.
Menadione sodium bisulfite	Hykinone	5 mg tablet; parenteral solution of 5–10 mg/ml	5–10 mg i.v.; 5–10 mg p.o.
Phytonadione	Vitamin K_1, Mephyton, Konakion, Mono-Kay	5 mg tablet; emulsion containing 10 or 50 mg/ml for parenteral injection in glucose solution	25–50 mg i.v. (slowly); 5 mg p.o.
Protamine sulfate		1% sterile solution for injection	1 mg for each 1 mg of heparin i.v. (slowly)

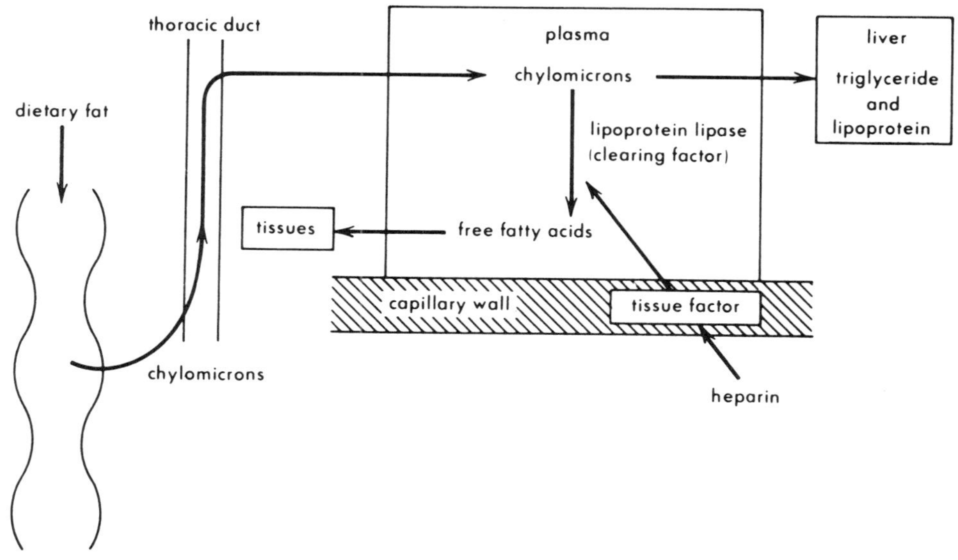

FIG. 42-2. Action of heparin in releasing lipase from the capillary wall.

racemic mixture of which the dextrorotatory (R-[+]-) enantiomorph is the more potent. Some of the drug interactions of the mixture are more prominent with the S-[−]-enantiomorph (*see* Chap. 8).

MECHANISM OF ACTION

The basic mechanism of action of all these compounds is the same, but the drugs differ widely in their rate of onset, duration of action, and recovery period. Their therapeutic action depends on their ability to suppress the formation of certain clotting factors. Prothrombin and factors VII, IX, and X are synthesized by the liver, and their production requires the presence of vitamin K as a coenzyme. Since the coumarins and indanediones structurally resemble vitamin K, they may act as antimetabolites or interfere with uptake of vitamin K by hepatic cells.

Delayed onset of the anticoagulant effect of these drugs occurs, since the normal plasma levels of clotting factors must decline before the synthesis deficiency becomes manifest. Because the coumarins have no direct effect on the clotting mechanisms, they are not effective *in vitro*.

FIG. 42-3. Hydroxycoumarin and indanedione anticoagulants.

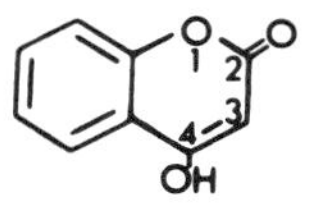

4-HYDROXYCOUMARIN

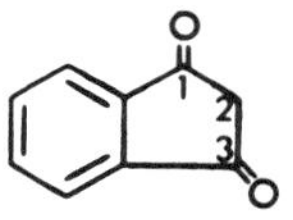

INDANE-1,3-DIONE

THERAPEUTIC USES

All coumarins and indanediones are effective by mouth. There is a wide variation in individual response to their action, however. Factors that influence the dose needed to attain an adequate depression of coagulation include absorption from the gastrointestinal tract, storage in the liver, rate of metabolism (which may vary tenfold or more from one patient to another), genetically determined resistance to the drug (*see* Chap. 6), and simultaneous therapy (*see* Chap. 8). Broad-spectrum antibiotics (which alter the intestinal flora and influence the production of vitamin K) and salicylates reduce the required dosage. Patients with decreased liver function show increased susceptibility to these anticoagulants.

These many factors render the question of dosage meaningless in terms of "milligrams per day." An average initial dose should be given and blood coagulability determined some hours later. Subsequent doses of the drug are based on the results of daily determinations of blood coagulation time. Once a steady daily dose has been established, less frequent blood tests are needed.

Long-term therapy is frequently used in patients in whom the dose of the anticoagulant has been stabilized initially in hospital. Such therapy is contraindicated in patients of low intelligence; in those who are unreliable about returning for blood checks; in chronic alcoholics; in pregnant women; in patients undergoing intensive salicylate therapy; and in patients with peptic ulcers, hepatic disease, renal failure, or a hemostatic defect.

Owing to the delayed onset of effect of the oral anticoagulants, heparin is administered along with the initial dose, and then, as the effect of the oral agent develops, the heparin is gradually terminated.

ADVERSE EFFECTS

Side-effects, other than hemorrhage, are rare in humans. Skin reactions, pyrexia, diarrhea, blood dyscrasias, hepatitis, and nephropathy have been reported, and fatalities have occurred.

Hemorrhage during therapy with the oral anticoagulants should be treated by withdrawal of the drug, which is all that is needed in minor cases. Severe hemorrhage may require the administration of vitamin K using an i.v. preparation such as *phytonadione sodium diphosphate*. The vitamin competes with the anticoagulant and restores formation of the plasma cofactors. The effect of vitamin K persists, however, for up to 2 weeks, and it may be difficult to reinstate coumarin or indanedione therapy.

In more serious hemorrhage, the transfusion of whole fresh blood may be indicated.

CONTROL OF ANTICOAGULANT THERAPY

The response of patients to anticoagulants is variable, and the effectiveness of these drugs may even vary at different stages of the condition under treatment. Further, absorption of oral anticoagulants is slow and erratic. These considerations pose a problem with respect to dosage. Anticoagulant thearpy is controlled, therefore, by routinely estimating the ability of the blood to coagulate, and the dose of the agents is adjusted so as to maintain the response within certain limits that have proved optimal in clinical trials. The physician's aim is to obtain an effective therapeutic result without spontaneous hemorrhage.

The patient undergoing anticoagulant therapy is continually on the brink of a hemorrhagic state, and frequent observation is imperative.

HEPARIN

Partial thromboplastin time (PTT), which is more sensitive and more reproducible, has largely replaced the whole blood clotting time (Lee–White method). The PTT should be maintained at twice the pretreatment level of 30 to 35 seconds. With intermittent administration of heparin, the test is made 1 hour before a scheduled dose. Monitoring of PTT is not required when low-dose therapy is used.

ORAL ANTICOAGULANTS

The original one-stage prothrombin time (Quick method) using a standardized tissue thromboplastin and a reference blood sample is the most reliable test. A standard curve is generated that relates coagulation time, in seconds, to percentage of normal prothrombin activity (Fig. 42-4); this partially compensates for differences in results from different laboratories. The patient should be instructed, however, to use the same laboratory to minimize variations. At the onset of treatment, the test should be done daily and the subsequent dose adjusted from the results. The coagulation time should be determined at least monthly in stabilized patients on long-term therapy. The coagulability is held at 20% to 25% of normal for optimum prevention of thrombosis, although prevention of spontaneous bleeding is usually the major determinant of dose.

Roger Irving Lee, 1881–1965. Boston physician. Developed a method for the study of blood coagulation time (1913) and studied the relation between calcium ions and coagulation time (1915).

Armand James Quick, 1894–1978. American hematologist. As well as for his methods for prothrombin clotting time (1935) and thromboplastin preparation (1938), Quick is known for his liver function test based on hippuric acid synthesis (1933) and his work on detoxication mechanisms.

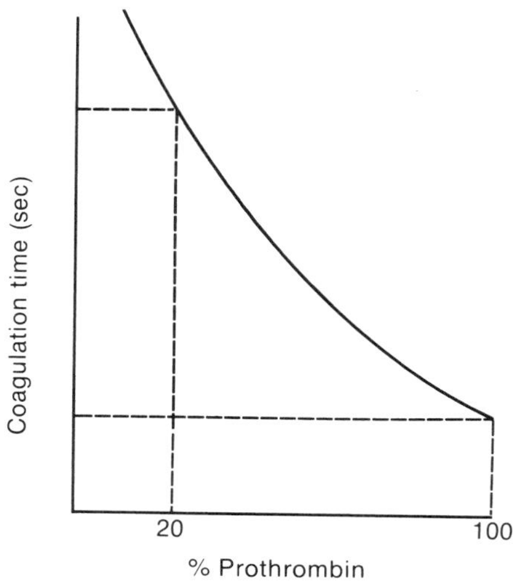

FIG. 42-4. Relation between prothrombin content and coagulation time obtained from serial dilutions of normal plasma. The percentage of prothrombin of test sample is read from the curve. For effective therapy the prothrombin level is held at approximately 20%.

ASPIRIN

Aspirin inhibits the cyclooxygenases ("prostaglandin synthetases") that form endoperoxides from arachidonic acid, and thus block the formation of thromboxane A_2 (TXA_2) and prostaglandin I_2 (PGI_2) (*see* Chap. 53). TXA_2 is a powerful activator of platelet aggregation, whereas PGI_2 is an antiaggregant present in the endothelium of the vessels. PGI_2 may be absent when the vessel wall is damaged by an atheromatous plaque. Empirical studies originally found that chronic administration of aspirin was valuable in the prophylaxis of myocardial infarction. A 3-year clinical trial in 1975 by the National Heart, Lung, and Blood Institute failed, however, to produce any evidence to substantiate this hypothesis. However, that study has been criticized on several counts, including dose of aspirin, time of administration, and patient selection. Further study of this question is needed.

FURTHER READING

1. Coon WW: Some recent developments in the pharmacology of heparin. J Clin Pharmacol 19:337, 1979
2. Coon WW, Willis PN: Some aspects of the pharmacology of oral anticoagulants. Clin Pharmacol Ther 11:312, 1970
3. Douglass AS: Anticoagulant Therapy. Oxford, University Press, 1962
4. Ingram GI: Anticoagulant therapy. Pharmacol Rev 13:279, 1961
5. Jaques LB: Heparin: An old drug with a new paradigm. Science 206:528, 1979
6. Suttie JW: Vitamin K Metabolism and Vitamin K-Dependent Proteins. Baltimore, University Park Press, 1980

CHAPTER 42 QUESTIONS

(*See* P. 7 for Full Instructions)

Select the One Best Answer

1. Dicumarol
   A. must be administered parenterally.
   B. is antagonized by protamine sulfate.
   C. has thrombolytic activity.
   D. is potentiated by barbiturates.
   E. reduces prothrombin formation.

2. Heparin is
   A. effective in the treatment of type I hyperlipoproteinemia (hyperchylomicronemia).
   B. the strongest naturally occurring base.
   C. commonly given for long periods without serious side-effects.
   D. inactivated both *in vivo* and *in vitro* by protamine sulfate.
   E. an inhibitor of histamine release.

3. The anticoagulant activity of dicumarol can be potentiated by each of the following EXCEPT
   A. clofibrate.
   B. aspirin.
   C. tetracycline.
   D. phenobarbital.
   E. tolbutamide.

4. Each of the following statements about heparin is correct EXCEPT
   A. hematoma formation can occur at the injection site.
   B. it can be used to detect a deficiency of tissue lipoprotein lipase activity.
   C. it is an effective anticoagulant *in vivo* and *in vitro*.
   D. it is commonly given orally.
   E. it can be antagonized by protamine.

A = 1,2,3; B = 1,3; C = 2,4; D = 4; E = All

5. Heparin
   1. is a naturally occurring substance found in tissues rich in mast cells.

2. has a plasma clearing effect *in vivo* and *in vitro*.
3. is a relatively short-acting inhibitor of prothrombin.
4. is fairly well absorbed orally.

6. Heparin
   1. binds strongly to protamine.
   2. is administered orally for a prolonged anticoagulant effect.
   3. rapidly inhibits blood coagulation when administered intravenously.
   4. is a neutral polypeptide.

7. Both heparin and dicumarol
   1. are effective *in vitro*.
   2. are antagonized by protamine.
   3. prevent the synthesis of prothrombin.
   4. prolong the one-stage prothrombin time (Quick).

8. The anticoagulant effect of dicumarol is *increased* by combined therapy with
   1. phenylbutazone.
   2. glutethimide.
   3. warfarin.
   4. menadione.

JEROME M. HERSHMAN

43 Hormones of the Hypothalamus and Pituitary Gland

HYPOTHALAMIC–PITUITARY PHYSIOLOGY

Hypothalamic neurons regulate production of pituitary hormones by secreting pituitary hormone stimulatory and inhibitory factors, which flow through the hypothalamic hypophyseal portal veins (Table 43-1). Five hypothalamic factors have been purified and are now regarded as hormones: *thyrotropin-releasing hormone* (TRH), gonadotropin-releasing hormone (LH-RH), somatostatin, corticotropin-releasing hormone (CRH), and growth hormone-releasing hormone (GH-RH).

When a pituitary hormone (Table 43-1) acts on its target gland to promote secretion, the hormone negatively feeds back on the pituitary and hypothalamus. For pituitary hormones that act on specific target glands, there appears to be only a releasing factor, for example, the relationship between TRH, thyroid-stimulating hormone (TSH), and thyroid hormone. On the other hand, pituitary hormones that do not act on a specific target gland, such as growth hormone, seem to be controlled by both hypothalamic-releasing and inhibiting hormones.

HYPOTHALAMIC–PITUITARY ANATOMY

The anatomical relation between the hypothalamus and the pituitary gland is seen in Figure 43-1. The hypothalamus joins with the pituitary stalk at the median eminence. The stalk connects the hypothalamus to the pituitary gland. The pituitary gland is divided into the anterior lobe, or adenohypophysis, and the posterior lobe, or neurohypophysis. Certain species such as the rat and dog also have an intermediate lobe.

The neurohypophysis receives neural elements from the hypothalamic paraventricular and supraoptic nuclei. The adenohypophysis receives communication solely by a network of capillaries (the portal system), originating in the median eminence of the tuber cinereum. These vessels form vascular trunks on the pituitary stalk and then split into smaller sinusoids, terminating in the adenohypophysis and

---

GEOFFREY WINGFIELD HARRIS, 1913– . British anatomist and physiologist. Many publications in endocrinology/neuroendocrinology.

TABLE 43-1. Anterior Pituitary Hormones and Hypothalamic Factors That Regulate Their Release

	Hypothalamic	
Anterior Pituitary Hormone	***Releasing Factor (RF)***	***Inhibiting Factor (IF)***
Growth hormone (GH)	GH-RH*	Somatostatin*
Prolactin	PRF (?TRH)	PIF (? Dopamine)
Thyrotropin (TSH)	TRH*	(? Somatostatin, ? dopamine)
Follicle-stimulating hormone (FSH)	LH-RH*	—
Luteinizing hormone (LH)	LH-RH*	—
Corticotropin (ACTH)	CRH*	—
Melanocyte-stimulating hormone (MSH)	MSH-RF	MSH-IF
β-Lipotropin	? CRF	—
β-Endorphin	? CRF	—

* Structure is known.

forming a transport system from hypothalamus to anterior pituitary, as described by G. W. Harris.

HYPOTHALAMIC HORMONES

THYROTROPIN-RELEASING HORMONE

Thyrotropin-releasing hormone is a tripeptide (Fig. 43-2) widely distributed in the brain and other tissues (pancreas, gastrointestinal tract, and reproductive organs). In the brain the highest concentrations are in the anterior and medial basal hypothalamus and the median eminence, regions known to be involved in control of TSH secretion. Its function in extrahypothalamic locations is unknown.

On injection into mammals TRH causes release of both TSH and prolactin through binding to specific receptors on the plasma membrane of the thyrotroph and the lactotroph in the anterior pituitary. The releasing effect of TRH on the thyrotroph is inhibited by thyroid hormones. Excessive circulating thyroid hormones, which occur in hyperthyroidism, block the stimulatory effect of TRH on TSH secretion.

In normal adults, as little as 10 μg of TRH intravenously produces a detectable increase in serum TSH, and 500 μg causes a maximum response (Figure 43-3). When given orally, about 50 times as much TRH is needed to produce the same effect as an i.v. dose. TRH is rapidly degraded in the blood, with a T½ of 5 to 10 minutes.

Many analogues of TRH have been synthesized. Addition of a methyl group in the 3-position on the histidine ring produces a derivative (3-methyl-TRH) that has three to eight times the biologic effect of TRH. Other substitutions or changes in the amino acid composition cause a loss of TRH activity.

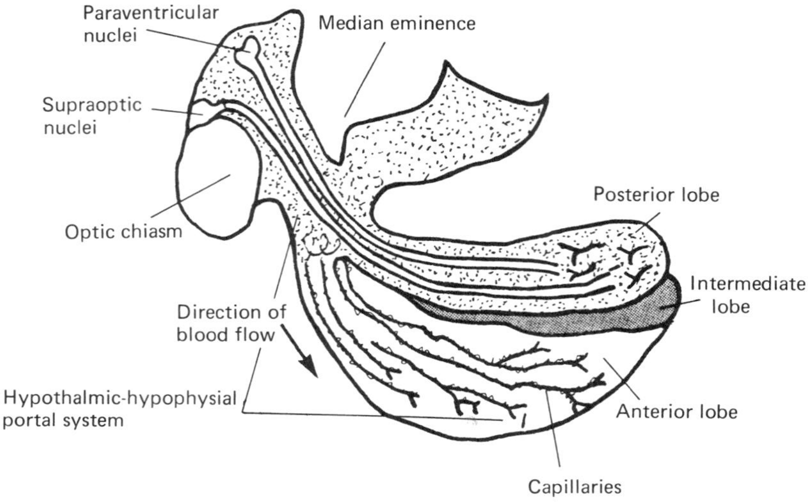

FIG. 43-1. Anatomical relation between the hypothalamus and the pituitary gland.

pGLU-HIS-PRO-NH_2
1 2 3

TRH

pGLU-HIS-TRP-SER-TYR-GLY-LEU-ARG-PRO-GLY-NH_2
1 2 3 4 5 6 7 8 9 10

LH-RH

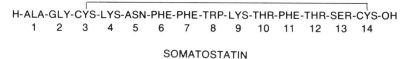

H-ALA-GLY-CYS-LYS-ASN-PHE-PHE-TRP-LYS-THR-PHE-THR-SER-CYS-OH
1 2 3 4 5 6 7 8 9 10 11 12 13 14

SOMATOSTATIN

FIG. 43-2. Amino-acid sequences of thyrotropin-releasing hormone (*TRH*), luteinizing hormone-releasing hormone (*LH-RH*), and somatostatin.

Clinical Applications of Synthetic TRH

Testing with synthetic TRH (protirelin) is useful in the diagnosis of mild or borderline thyroid disease. Thus failure of serum TSH to rise after giving TRH indicates hyperthyroidism. Additionally, in patients with exophthalmos without hyperthyroidism (euthyroid Graves' disease), failure of serum TSH to rise after TRH suggests the diagnosis, whereas an exaggerated response indicates impaired thyroid function and suggests the exophthalmos is related to Graves' disease. The TRH test is useful to monitor the effectiveness of TSH suppression in patients with nontoxic goiter or thyroid cancer who are being treated with thyroid hormone.

The TRH test is also used to evaluate TSH and prolactin reserve in patients with pituitary lesions and to help differentiate between pituitary and hypothalamic causes of hypothyroidism. A pituitary lesion is associated with reduced TSH secretion, whereas with hypothalamic lesions in the presence of an intact pituitary the peak response will be normal, although often delayed by 30 minutes.

FIG. 43-3. Serum TSH response to 500 μg TRH given i.v. to three normal subjects. The failure of response (flat curve) occurs in hyperthyroidism or in pituitary TSH deficiency.

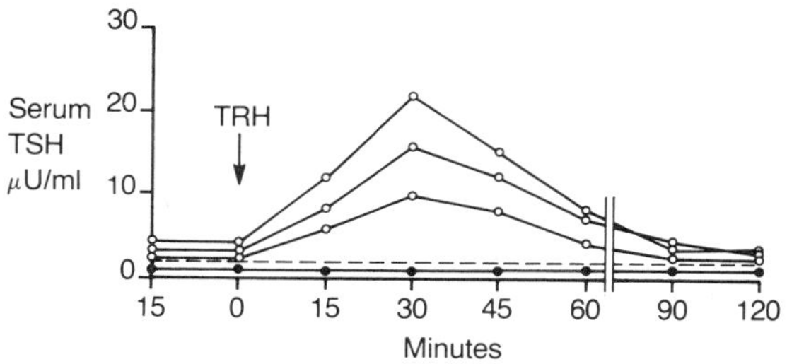

LUTEINIZING HORMONE-RELEASING HORMONE(LH-RH)

Luteinizing hormone-releasing hormone is a decapeptide (Fig. 43-2). Intravenous administration releases both luteinizing hormone (LH) and follicle-stimulating hormone (FSH), but the increment in LH is much greater than that of FSH. LH-RH has also been called LRF, LH-FSH-RH, and gonadotropin releasing hormone, GnRH, but LH-RH is the most commonly used abbreviation. LH-RH has a T½ of less than 5 minutes.

Intravenous LH-RH (25–100 μg) produces a prompt rise in serum LH that peaks in 20 to 40 minutes and a small rise in FSH; peak gonadotropin responses are proportional to the baseline serum levels of LH and FSH.

LH-RH is used to evaluate pituitary gonadotropin reserve in patients with pituitary and hypothalamic diseases when lesions of both regions have blunted responses. In patients with hypothalamic lesions, repeated injections of LH-RH will restore the pituitary sensitivity and increase the response. Injections of LH-RH cause ovulation in women and may be used to induce pregnancy in those with hypothalamic disorders. In men, repeated injections of LH-RH may stimulate spermatogenesis.

Modification of the molecule has resulted in more potent analogues. Replacement of glycine in position 6 by D-alanine or D-leucine and substitution of ethylamide for the terminal glycine amide result in analogues with 20 to 100 times the potency of the native decapeptide. These analogues reduce gonadotropin secretion by down-regulation of the LH-RH receptor. The resulting decreased testosterone secretion has induced remission in patients with metastatic prostate cancer. Analogues that inhibit the binding of LH-RH to its receptor are being tested for their effect as contraceptives in both men and women.

SOMATOSTATIN

Somatostatin (Fig. 43-2) is a tetradecapeptide isolated originally from the hypothalamus and shown to inhibit the release of growth hormone, TSH, insulin, glucagon, and renin. It is also present throughout the brain and spinal cord, in peripheral nerves, pancreatic islet D cells, and the gut (*see* Chap. 54). Somatostatin inhibits pancreatic and gastric exocrine secretion, splanchnic blood flow, and nutrient flux across the bowel. Because of its diffuse inhibitory activity, its potential beneficial effects are outweighed by its side-effects, and to date it has no established therapeutic use. Analogues with more selective effects are being tested.

CORTICOTROPIN-RELEASING HORMONE (CRH) AND GROWTH HORMONE-RELEASING HORMONE (GH-RH)

Corticotropin-releasing hormone is a 41-amino-acid peptide. It stimulates the release of both corticotropin and beta-endorphin from pituitary cells. In addition, it has sympathomimetic effects and behavioral effects to increase motor activity. CRH appears to be a hypothalamic mediator of stress responses. Its T½ is about 1 hour. Because it has only recently been discovered, its pharmacologic role has not been defined.

Growth hormone-releasing hormone is a 44-amino-acid peptide originally isolated from a human pancreatic tumor that caused acromegaly. The synthetic peptide appears to be identical with hypothalamic GH-RH. It has potential use for treating dwarfism caused by hypothalamic lesions.

OTHER HYPOTHALAMIC PEPTIDES

Other hypothalamic peptides may regulate pituitary hormone secretion. These peptides are also found in other organs, especially the gut (*see* Chap. 54) and include neurotensin, cholecystokinin, substance P, enkephalin, bombesin, vasoactive intestinal polypeptide, and angiotensin. The role of these peptides as neurotransmitters or neuromodulators is still unclear.

POSTERIOR PITUITARY HORMONES

VASOPRESSIN

Vasopressin (antidiuretic hormone, ADH) is a nonapeptide (Fig. 43-4) made in the supraoptic, paraventricular, and suprachiasmatic nuclei of the hypothalamus. It is transported along axons to the posterior pituitary where it is stored. Vasopressin is released in response to dehydration, hypertonicity of plasma, hemorrhage, and parturition. Vasopressin stimulates adenyl cyclase (*see* Chap. 50) in the distal convoluted tubules and renal collecting ducts to increase their permeability to water. This results in reabsorption of water and excretion of a concentrated urine. In addition, vasopressin causes contraction of splanchnic blood vessels and, in large doses, ACTH release. It affects memory and learning in experimental animals.

Arginine vasopressin is the natural ADH of humans, and lysine vasopressin (LVP), the ADH of pigs (Fig. 43-4). Desmopressin (DDAVP) is a potent, long-lasting antidiuretic relatively free of side-effects; elimination of the free amino group of position 1 (desamino) increases ADH activity, whereas substitution of D-arginine for L-arginine in position 8 markedly lowers pressor properties.

Vasopressin is used predominantly for therapy of diabetes insipidus. The diagnosis can be made by dehydrating the patient, measuring

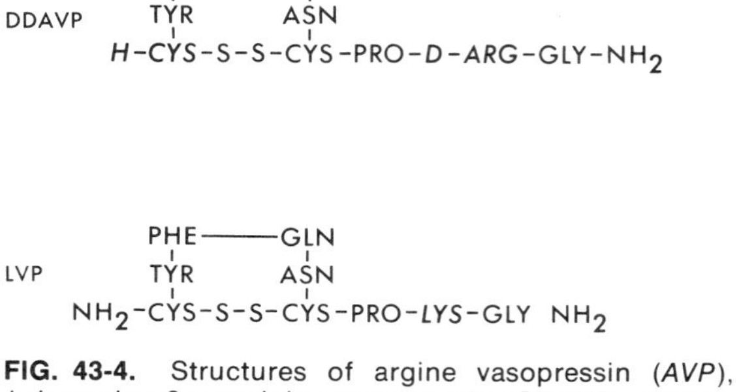

FIG. 43-4. Structures of argine vasopressin (*AVP*), 1-desamino-8-D-arginine vasopressin (*DDAVP*), and lysine vasopressin (*LVP*).

urinary osmolality, and then testing the response to exogenous vasopressin.

Intranasal *DDAVP* (10–20 μg) is the main therapy of diabetes insipidus. One dose lasts for about 12 hours. Intranasal *lysine vasopressin* is less potent and has a shorter duration of action than does DDAVP. *Aqueous vasopressin*, a partially purified neurohypophyseal extract, can be given by injection and can be suspended in oil to prolong its T½.

Oxytocin is the other hypothalamic nonapeptide stored in the posterior pituitary gland (*see* Chap. 39).

ANTERIOR PITUITARY HORMONES

THYROID-STIMULATING HORMONE

Thyroid-stimulating hormone is a glycoprotein (molecular weight of about 28,000 daltons) composed of two subunits: The alpha subunit is identical to that of FSH, LH, and chorionic gonadotropin (HCG); the beta subunit is specific for TSH. Human TSH has a potency of about 10 U/mg. Its secretion rate is about 80 mU/day and its plasma T½, about 50 minutes.

TSH is available as a partially purified hormone isolated from cattle pituitary glands. Its use as a diagnostic test to stimulate the thyroid gland of hypothyroid patients who lack TSH has been supplanted by the direct measurement of serum TSH levels. Serum TSH is low in hypothyroidism due to pituitary or hypothalamic lesions and elevated in hypothyroidism due to thyroid disease.

Bovine TSH is given intramuscularly to increase the thyroidal uptake of radioiodine in patients with thyroid cancer. Repeated administration of bovine TSH causes the formation of antibodies that neutralize its biologic effect.

TSH is also used to demonstrate the presence of normal thyroid tissue in patients with hyperfunctioning thyroid nodules that suppress the normal tissue; TSH increases the uptake of radioiodine in the suppressed normal tissue, which then shows up on a thyroid scan.

FOLLICLE-STIMULATING HORMONE

Follicle-stimulating hormone is a glycoprotein (molecular weight 28,000 daltons) made in the same pituitary cells that produce LH. Pure preparations contain 14,000 international units (IU)/mg. Its secretion rate varies with the menstrual cycle and increases severalfold after the menopause. Its T½ in plasma is about 4 hours. A significant fraction of FSH, perhaps 1/40 of the daily secretion, is excreted in the urine, so that human urine of postmenopausal women has been used as a source for its commercial preparation. The clinical preparation, *menotropin*, is an equal mixture of FSH and LH and is used for treating infertility in women who lack gonadotropin. Several injections will cause maturation of an ovarian follicle. Therapy is difficult and must be monitored by following serum estrogen levels. In men with infertility due to gonadotropin deficiency, therapy is even more difficult and somewhat impractical because daily injections must be given for about 2 months to induce spermatogenesis. Menotropin is very expensive.

LUTEINIZING HORMONE AND HUMAN CHORIONIC GONADOTROPIN (hCG)

Luteinizing hormone and hCG are very similar structurally and pharmacologically. The alpha subunits are identical. The beta subunits are similar, but hCG has a longer C-terminal tail. hCG has a much longer T½ (12 hours) than does LH (20 minutes). During pregnancy, large amounts of hCG are secreted by the placenta, and a large fraction of this is excreted in the urine. Thus the urine of pregnant women is an excellent source for commercial preparation of hCG.

Preparations of hCG have several uses. In the therapy of infertile women with hypogonadotropic hypogonadism, injections of hCG are given to cause ovulation after the follicles have been ripened with injections of FSH (menotropin) as described above. This therapy causes ovulation in about two thirds of the women. Unfortunately, multiple ovulation resulting in multiple pregnancies occurs in about 15% of cases.

hCG (1000–4000 units) will increase testicular secretion of testosterone. This therapy has been used for induction of puberty when puberty is delayed or absent because of pituitary or hypothalamic disease; however, because of the necessity for injections several times each week, therapy is impractical compared with injections of testosterone, which last for 2 to 4 weeks. hCG injections have also been used to facilitate descent of the testes in children.

GROWTH HORMONE

Growth hormone (GH, somatotropin) is a single-chain polypeptide (molecular weight,

21,5000 daltons) secreted by the somatotropes. Its plasma T½ is about 20 minutes, and the normal daily secretion rate is about 500 μg. The chronic effects of growth hormone include increased linear growth by stimulation of epiphyseal cartilage growth; increased synthesis of protein, DNA, and RNA; increased lipolysis; decreased glucose use by fat and muscle and increased hepatic gluconeogenesis; increased collagen synthesis; retention of calcium, sodium, and potassium; and lactogenesis. The growth-promoting effects of GH are mediated by *somatomedin*. Somatomedin refers to a family of growth factors, with molecular weights of 5,000 to 10,000 daltons, produced in the liver under the influence of GH.

GH is species specific, so that only human GH is active in humans. Human GH is prepared from human pituitaries collected at autopsies and preserved frozen or in acetone. It constitutes only 5% to 10% of pituitary wet weight, however. Recently human GH has been synthesized in bacteria by recombinant DNA techniques, which should solve the problem of its limited therapeutic availability.

The principal use of human GH is to promote growth in pituitary dwarfs, a condition recognized by stunted growth of young children. Specific testing shows failure of serum GH to increase after provocative tests. Therapy consists of injection of human GH intramuscularly three to seven times each week in a dose of 1 to 2 units. Purified human GH has a potency of 1 to 2 units/mg. With this therapy, growth rate accelerates about fourfold and reaches 4 to 7 cm/year. Therapy must be started before puberty and is effective as long as the epiphyses are open. Therapy is stopped when satisfactory height is achieved (about 60 inches, or 152 cm), when the epiphyses close, or when there is no further growth response, possibly due to the formation of antibodies. In children who lack other hormones, appropriate substitution therapy is also given. Adults who lack GH suffer no discernible adverse metabolic effects and thus are not treated with it.

PROLACTIN

Prolactin is a polypeptide hormone (molecular weight 21,000 daltons) secreted by the normal pituitary at levels of about 0.5 mg/day. Prolactin promotes milk formation, but its function in nonlactating women and in men is unclear. It has no therapeutic role. Prolactin has antireproductive effects by inhibiting the secretion of gonadotropins. Phenothiazines release prolactin through their antidopaminergic action.

ACTH, ENDORPHIN, LIPOTROPIN

Corticotropin (ACTH), β-lipotropin, and β-endorphin have various amino acid sequences in common (Fig. 43-5). ACTH, which includes the sequence of alpha-melanocyte-stimulating hormone (α-MSH), is discussed in Chapter 47. The function of β-lipotropin is unclear, but it includes the sequence of β-MSH. β-Endorphin is secreted in response to stress along with ACTH and β-lipotropin. The physiological effects of α- and β-MSH in humans are unknown, and the relative role of these substances as melanocyte-stimulators is unclear.

β-Endorphin binds very strongly to the opiate receptor and may well be a natural analgesic peptide (*see* Chap. 32). Synthetic β-endorphin has been tested for its analgesic effect and for psychiatric disorders with disappointing results. Thus far it has no therapeutic use.

HORMONE THERAPY FOR HYPOPITUITARISM

For patients with hypopituitarism, all of the hormonal deficiencies can be replaced with *glucocorticoids* for ACTH deficiency, L-*thyroxine* for TSH deficiency, and *testosterone* and *estrogen* for men and women, respectively, deficient in gonadotropins. Although restoration of fertility cannot always be achieved, therapy with gonadotropins is often successful, as described above.

FIG. 43-5. Structures of ACTH, β-lipotropin, β-endorphin, and related peptides and their parent molecule.

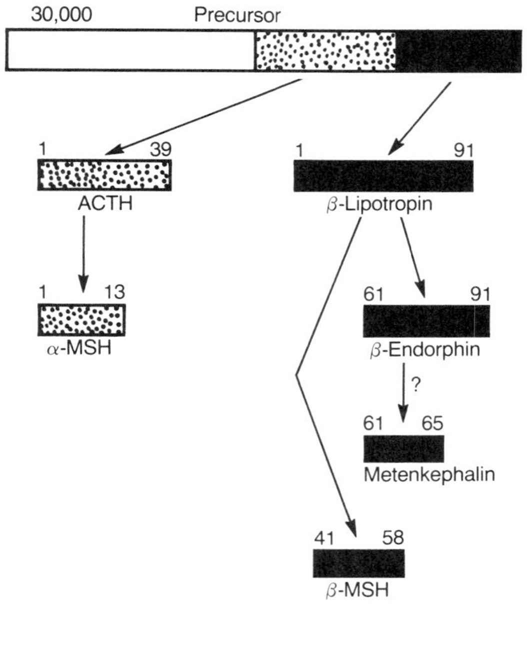

FURTHER READING

1. Carlson HE: Pituitary disease. In Hershman JM (ed): Endocrine Pathophysiology: A Patient Oriented Approach, 2nd ed. Philadelphia, Lea & Febiger, 1982
2. Eipper BA, Mains RE: Structure and biosynthesis of pro-ACTH/endorphin and related peptides. Endocr Rev 1:1, 1980
3. Guillemin R: Peptides in the brain: The new endocrinology of the neuron. Science 202:390, 1978
4. Hershman JM: Clinical application of thyrotropin-releasing hormone. N Engl J Med 299:886, 1974
5. Martin JB, Reichlin S, Brown GM (eds): Clinical Neuroendocrinology. Philadelphia, FA Davis, 1977
6. Ontjes DA, Walton J, Ney RL: Anterior pituitary gland. In Bondy PK, Rosenberg LE (eds): Metabolic Control and Disease, 8th ed, p 1165. Philadelphia, WB Saunders, 1980
7. Schally AV: Aspects of hypothalamic regulation of the pituitary gland. Science 202:18, 1978
8. Tolis G, Labrie F, Martin JB et al (eds): Clinical Neuroendocrinology: A Pathophysiological Approach. New York, Raven Press, 1979
9. Yen SSC, Jaffee RB (eds): Reproductive Endocrinology. Philadelphia, WB Saunders, 1978

CHAPTER 43 QUESTIONS

(See P. 7 for Full Instructions)

Select the One Best Answer

1. Vasopressin (ADH)
   A. increases sodium and water excretion.
   B. produces coronary vasodilation.
   C. stimulates ACTH secretion.
   D. is effective in nephrogenic diabetes insipidus.
   E. is produced by the posterior pituitary.

A = 1,2,3; B = 1,3; C = 2,4; D = 4; E = All

2. Thyrotropin-releasing hormone (TRH; Protirelin)
   1. affects only thyrotrope cells.
   2. releases TSH and prolactin from the pituitary.
   3. is made only in the hypothalamus.
   4. does not cause release of TSH in hyperthyroid patients.

3. Pituitary growth hormone
   1. has proven value in the treatment of pituitary dwarfism.
   2. induces production of somatomedin by the liver.
   3. is species specific.
   4. promotes growth characterized by increased body fat relative to other body constituents.

4. In cases of infertility in women with hypopituitarism ovulation may be induced with
   1. estrogens.
   2. oxytocin.
   3. clomiphene.
   4. human postmenopausal gonadotropins.

5. Diabetes insipidus may be treated by the use of
   1. tolbutamide.
   2. chlorothiazide.
   3. crystalline zinc insulin.
   4. desmopressin acetate (DDAVP).

6. Vasopressin
   1. is a coronary constrictor.
   2. is administered intranasally.
   3. reduces urine volume markedly.
   4. is synthesized in hypothalamic neurons.

44

Jerome M. Hershman

Pharmacology of the Thyroid Gland

THYROID HORMONE

In 1891, Murray administered an extract of sheep thyroid glands to a patient with myxedema, and within a few years thyroid therapy became commonplace. Although Kendall crystallized thyroxine in 1914, its structure was not determined until 1926 by Harington, who also synthesized it. In 1952 Gross and Pitt–Rivers discovered the second more active thyroid hormone, L-triiodothyronine (Fig. 44-1).

CHEMISTRY AND METABOLISM

The normal adult thyroid gland secretes about 100 μg of thyroxine (T_4) and about 8 μg of triiodothyronine (T_3), the two active thyroid hormones, each day. Another 32 μg of T_3 arises from peripheral (nonthyroidal) monodeiodination of the outer ring of T_4 mainly in the liver and kidneys. T_4 has a plasma T½ of 7 days; the T½ for T_3 is about 1 day. The normal extrathyroidal pools of T_3 and T_4 are 40 μg and 100 μg, respectively.

In serum, T_4 binds to a specific binding globulin, thyronine-binding globulin (TBG), and to prealbumin and albumin with only 0.03% being free. T_3 binds to TBG and albumin with 0.3% being free. The total serum level of T_4, about μg/dl (120 nM), is fiftyfold higher than the serum level of T_3, 120 ng/dl (2.2 nM).

George Redmayne Murray, 1865–1939. English physician. In 1891 reported treatment of myxedema with injections of sheep thyroid gland extract. Studied medical effects of dust in local textile mills.

Edward Calvin Kendall, 1886–1972. Minnesota biochemist. Isolated crystalline thyroxin (later, thyroxine) in 1914 and adrenal cortical hormones in 1934. Studied ACTH and cortisone effects on rheumatoid arthritis. Won Nobel prize in 1950, with P. S. Hench and R. Reichstein.

Charles Robert Harington, 1897– . London biochemist. Renamed thyroxin as thyroxine, determined molecular structure and mode of synthesis from tyrosine (1926).

Rosalind Venetia Pitt–Rivers. British biochemist. Reported, in 1952–1953, with Jack Gross, 1921– , Canadian-born Israeli endocrinologist, on the isolation, synthesis, and physiology of triiodothyronine.

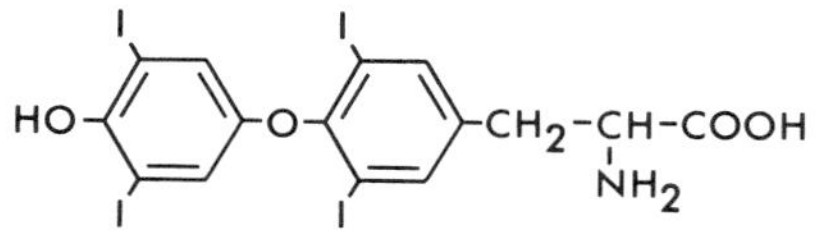

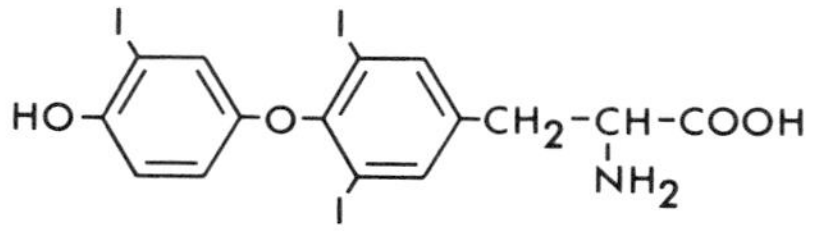

FIG. 44-1. Structures of active thyroid hormones.

ACTIONS

Thyroid hormone (the term denotes both T_4 and T_3) has many effects on nearly every organ-system. The effects may be divided into two general categories: promotion of normal growth and development; and maintenance of normal cellular metabolism. At a cellular level, thyroid hormones increase cell turnover, protein anabolism and catabolism, and lipid turnover. Additionally they increase oxygen consumption and heat production (calorigenesis) of many body tissues.

Thyroid hormones bind to specific acidic protein nuclear receptors and thus exert effects on expression of DNA. The affinity of T_3 for this receptor is about 10 to 100 times greater than that of T_4. Additionally thyroid hormones facilitate the intracellular transport of amino acids and sugars, possibly through a direct effect on the cell membrane, and increase membrane Na–K ATPase activity, which maintains the cellular-extracellular gradients of sodium and potassium. Thyroid hormones rapidly bind to a mitochondrial receptor to increase ATP production and oxidative metabolism. Thyroid hormones increase the activity of the mitochondrial enzyme α-glycerophosphate dehydrogenase. Thyroid hormones increase the number of β-adrenergic receptors in the heart and other tissues.

Although the predominant action of thyroid hormones is thought to occur on the cell nucleus, direct effects on mitochondria and the plasma membrane may be very important. The evidence favoring a single site of action has become less tenable in recent years.

BIOSYNTHESIS AND RELEASE

Dietary iodine is well absorbed from the stomach and upper intestinal tract and is actively transported as iodide from plasma into thyroid follicular cells (Fig. 44-2). Thyroid peroxidase oxidizes the iodide, which then iodinates tyrosine to form monoiodotyrosine (MIT) and diiodotyrosine (DIT), a process called organic binding of iodine. The tyrosine that is iodinated is in

FIG. 44-2. Biosynthesis of T_4 and T_3. MIT = monoiodotyrosine; DIT = diiodotyrosine.

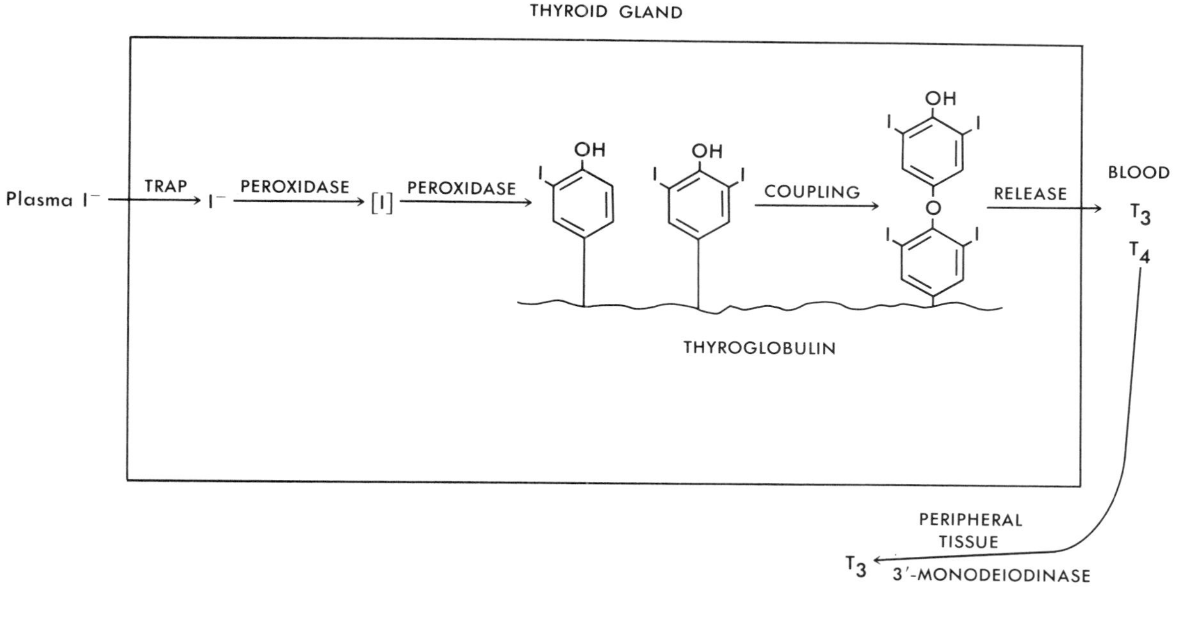

peptide linkage within the large thyroglobulin molecule. Iodinated tyrosines couple to form T_3 and T_4. Thyroid peroxidase also catalyzes the coupling reaction. Each molecule of human thyroglobulin usually contains about 1 to 3 residues of T_4, with a molar ratio of T_4/T_3 of about 10:1. Thyroglobulin is stored in the colloid of the thyroid follicles.

Secretion of thyroid hormone requires fusion of the vesicles of thyroglobulin with lysosomal enzymes, proteolysis of thyroglobulin to liberate T_4 and T_3, and then release (endocytosis) of the hormones into the blood.

Because iodine is a scarce element, the active iodide transport system can generate gradients of more than 100:1 (tissue/plasma) if plasma iodide concentration is very low, compared with the usual gradient of about 20:1. In addition, an iodotyrosine deiodinase liberates iodide from iodotyrosines. This iodide is conserved within the thyroid or retrapped if it enters the circulation from another organ. The usual American diet contains about 300 to 800 μg of iodine per day. With this high intake, only about 10% to 30% of dietary iodine is taken up by the thyroid. The rest is excreted by the kidneys, so that urinary iodine reflects dietary intake. In Western Europe, daily iodine intake is about 100 μg. In many underdeveloped areas, particularly mountainous regions, iodine intake is less than 100 μg/day. Severe iodine deficiency (<50 μg/day) causes edemic goiter.

CONTROL OF SECRETION

Thyroid-stimulating hormone (TSH) is the principal control of T_4/T_3 secretion. It binds to a thyroid follicular cell membrane receptor, activates adenyl cyclase, increases cyclic AMP, and thereby accelerates the release of thyroid hormone and concomitantly all the biosynthetic processes within the thyroid cell. In turn, there is negative (inhibitory) feedback by T_4 and T_3 on the TSH-secreting cells of the pituitary. This feedback regulates the secretion of thyroid hormone. Hypothalamic thyrotropin-releasing hormone controls release of TSH from the pituitary (*see* Chap. 43).

PREPARATIONS

The therapeutic preparations of thyroid hormone and their properties are listed in Table 44-1. Synthetic sodium L-thyroxine is preferable because its purity assures uniform potency and reliability of action (Fig. 44-3). Thyroid U.S.P. is a dried, defatted extract of the thyroid glands of animals (usually hogs and cattle) slaughtered for food. It has been used successfully for more than 80 years. The U.S.P. requirement for standardization is still based only on its iodine content, which should be between 0.17% and 0.23%; some pharmaceutical companies also bioassay the material. Because the molar ratio of T_4/T_3 is about 4.3:1, patients taking desiccated thyroid will have variable serum levels of T_3, depending on the time after ingestion of the preparation (Fig. 44-3). A refined thyroid extract, purified thyroglobulin, has also been marketed.

Sodium L-triiodothyronine (liothyronine) is about three times more potent than L-thyroxine. Its short T½ makes it ideal for special tests that take advantage of the rapid rebound (after about 10 days) of serum TSH after the withdrawal of triiodothyronine or the occurrence of very low serum T_4 levels owing to the inhibition of TSH secretion. A 4:1 mixture of synthetic T_4 and T_3 is also available (liotrix).

D-Thyroxine has about one fifth the metabolic action of L-thyroxine. It was hoped that D-thyroxine would lower serum cholesterol levels without altering metabolic rate, but this

TABLE 44-1. Therapeutic Preparations of Thyroid Hormone

Drug	Source	Average Daily Dose*	Biologic Half-Life
Sodium L-thyroxine	Synthetic	150 μg	1 wk
Sodium L-triiodothyronine	Synthetic	50 μg	1 day
Thyroid U.S.P.	Animal thyroids	150 mg	1 wk
Liotrix	Synthetic	100 μg	1 wk
	$T_4 + T_3$ (4:1)	25 μg	
Thyroglobulin†	Animal thyroids	150 mg	1 wk

* Based on equivalent biologic effects.
† Rarely prescribed.

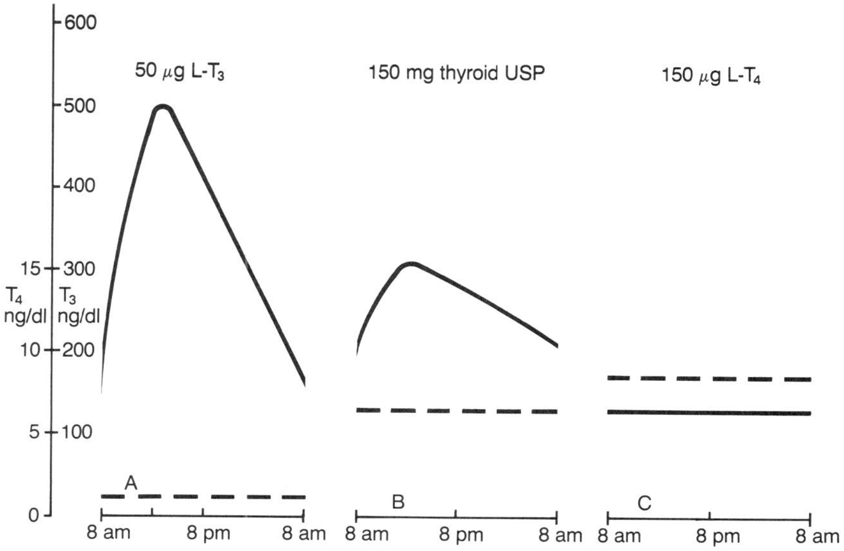

FIG. 44-3. Serum levels of T_4 and T_3 at various times after ingestion at 8 a.m. of a daily dose of 50 μg of triiodothyronine (*left*), 150 mg thyroid USP (*center*), or 150 μg of thyroxine (*right*).

relative dissociation of the effects of thyroid hormone analogues has not been proved.

USES

Hypothyroidism

Hypothyroidism affects about 1% of the population and is rectified by giving a daily replacement dose of thyroid hormone. Table 44-2 lists the usual dose of sodium L-thyroxine based on patient age. Adults who receive 2 to 2.5 μg/kg body weight have normal serum levels of T_4 and T_3 and restoration of a normal metabolic state.

Goiter

Goiter (enlargement of the thyroid gland) usually arises from compensatory hypertrophy in patients who have either normal or decreased thyroid function. Hypertrophy depends on secretion of TSH, and its suppression by full replacement doses of thyroid hormone results in shrinkage of the goiter.

TABLE 44-2. Daily Replacement Dose of Sodium L-Thyroxine Based on Age

Age	Dose
yr.	*μg/kg*
0–1	9
1–5	6
6–10	4
11–20	3
21–40	2.5
>40	2

Thyroid Carcinoma

Papillary and follicular thyroid carcinomas usually contain TSH receptors on their plasma membranes. Growth of these cancers usually depends on TSH secretion, and postoperatively thyroid hormone is prescribed in a dose sufficient to suppress its secretion completely. Such therapy also provides the replacement hormone necessary because of the thyroidectomy. The dose of thyroid hormone should totally suppress serum TSH activity, as assessed by showing that there is no TSH increment after administration of TRH.

Weight Reduction

Large doses of thyroid hormones have been prescribed for weight reduction, but this practice is hazardous because it leads to loss of lean body mass, as well as fat, and may produce adverse cardiac effects such as tachycardia.

ANTITHYROID AGENTS

HYPERTHYROIDISM

Hyperthyroidism results from the effects of excessive amounts of thyroid hormones on body tissues. Symptoms and signs include goiter, tachycardia, weight loss, nervousness, tremor, muscle wasting and weakness, fatigue, excessive perspiration, and intolerance to heat.

In Graves' disease, responsible for most cases of hyperthyroidism, an abnormal thyroid-stimulating immunoglobulin G (IgG) stimulates excessive thyroid hormone production. The cause of this immune disorder is unknown. Therapy is directed at reducing the production and metabolic effects of thyroid hormone.

Thionamides

The three clinically useful thionamide compounds (Table 44-3) contain the essential moiety (Fig. 44-4): $-\overset{\overset{\displaystyle S}{|}}{C}-NH-$. Thiourea also has an antithyroidal effect. The thyroid gland concentrates the thionamides, and carbimazole is rapidly converted to methimazole *in vivo*. The drugs are absorbed well from the gastrointestinal tract.

The thionamides bind to thyroid peroxidase, interfering more with the coupling reaction than with organic binding of iodine. They do not block the iodide trap. Propylthiouracil blocks the extrathyroidal monodeiodination of T_4 to T_3 in the liver and probably elsewhere. The thionamides suppress the immune system, which may partly explain their effectiveness in Graves' disease.

Usually the thionamides are prescribed for 6 to 18 months in a dose sufficient to normalize the serum thyroid hormone concentrations. The initial dose can be lowered to a maintenance dose in 2 to 4 months. After the thionamide is withdrawn, about one half of the patients will have a recurrence of hyperthyroidism, which is the main disadvantage of this therapy.

Toxic effects of these drugs include skin rash, hepatic dysfunction, arthralgia, serum sickness, and rarely agranulocytosis.

Iodine

Iodine blocks the release of thyroid hormone from the hyperthyroid gland and thus rapidly lowers the circulating levels of thyroid hormones. In addition, iodine may inhibit the peroxidase enzyme system. Both effects are usually transient. The effective dose is only 6 mg daily, but much larger doses are customarily prescribed.

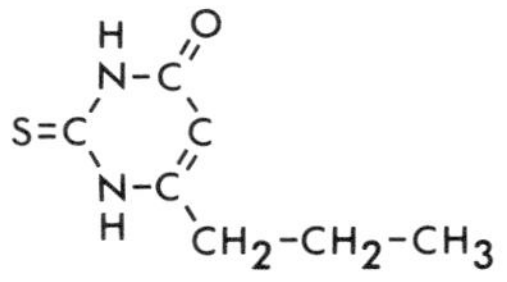

PROPYLTHIOURACIL

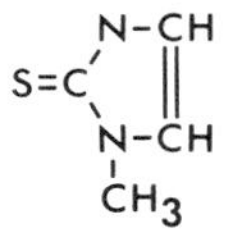

METHIMAZOLE

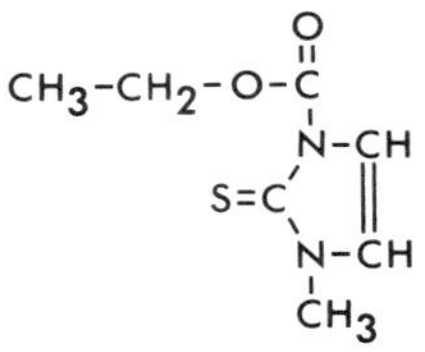

CARBIMAZOLE

FIG. 44-4. Structures of thionamide drugs used for treatment of hyperthyroidism.

The two preparations used are *saturated potassium iodide*, a colorless solution that contains 750 mg of iodine/ml; and Lugol's solution, a brown liquid mixture of potassium iodide and iodine that contains 125 mg of iodine/ml. The usual dose prescribed is 5 to 10 drops of either preparation every 8 to 12 hours.

Iodine is often given before thyroidectomy for hyperthyroidism because it causes involution of the hyperplastic thyroid and reduces gland vascularity, which aids the surgeon. The usual duration of therapy is 7 to 10 days because patients tend to "escape" from the blocking effect after this period.

Iodine has the disadvantage of increasing the total iodide pool, and thus diluting any tracer or therapeutic doses of radioiodine so that the proportion of a dose of radioiodine taken up by the thyroid would be lowered. This effect is useful, however, to protect the thyroid from radiation damage after a nuclear accident or attack that released ^{131}I. About 100 mg of io-

TABLE 44-3. Properties of Thionamide Drugs Used for Treatment of Hyperthyroidism

	Propylthiouracil	Methimazole	Carbimazole
Relative potency	1	10	10
Duration of action, *hr*	6–8	12–24	12–24
Blockade of extrathyroid $T_4 \rightarrow T_3$	Yes	No	No
Plasma T½, *hr*	1–2	6–14	6–14
Initial daily dose, *mg*	300	30	30
Maintenance dose, *mg*	25–200	5–20	5–20

dine per day for 1 week will lower the thyroid uptake of radioiodine to less than 1%.

Other Agents

The lithium ion acts similarly to iodine and has been used to treat hyperthyroidism with moderate success. The usual doses are 900 to 1200 mg of *lithium carbonate* daily to achieve serum lithium levels of about 1 mEq/liter. Lithium may be useful in manic hyperthyroid patients, but it has not been approved by the FDA for treatment of hyperthyroidism.

The *perchlorate ion* blocks the iodide trap and thus prevents hormone biosynthesis, but it is very toxic and has been abandoned in hyperthyroidism. Single doses of perchlorate, usually 1 g, are used, however, to block the iodide trap to dissociate trapping and binding of radioiodide. *Thiocyanate* is another monovalent anion that inhibits the iodide trap and is also a weak blocker of organic binding of iodine.

Several drugs, *propylthiouracil, glucocorticosteroids, propranolol, sodium ipodate,* and *iopanoic acid,* are useful for blocking the extrathyroidal production of T_3 from T_4 in hyperthyroidism. Ipodate and iopanoic acid are iodine-containing compounds concentrated in the biliary tract and used for cholecystography. Both block outer ring deiodination of T_4 very effectively and lower serum T_3 levels of hyperthyroid patients quickly. Part of their effectiveness may be due to liberation of iodine and the effect of the inorganic iodine on the thyroid gland. Sodium ipodate is especially useful for treating severe hyperthyroidism. Propranolol causes rapid improvement of the tachycardia, tremor, and nervousness of hyperthyroid patients. Recent data show that thyroid hormones increase the number of beta-adrenergic receptors (*see* above), which may explain the enhanced sympathetic activity of hyperthyroidism and the beneficial effect of beta blockers. To control hyperthyroidism, combinations of drugs are used, such as propylthiouracil and propranolol.

Radioiodine-131

Radioiodine-131 has been used to treat hyperthyroidism for more than 35 years. Hyperplastic thyroid follicular cells concentrate the ^{131}I, which destroys some cells, damages the physiologic function of others, and impairs replication. The therapy is simple because the patient merely drinks a radioactive solution or swallows a capsule. The usual therapeutic dose for hyperthyroidism delivers about 5000 to 10,000 rad to the thyroid, but larger doses (30–150 mCi) can be given to achieve total destruction of the gland in the case of papillary and follicular thyroid cancer. Beta radiation causes 90% of the destructive effect of ^{131}I and gamma radiation, 10%. Depositing 1 μCi/g thyroid gives a radiation dose of 90 rad. For a thyroid dose of 5000 rad, the administered dose in microcuries may be calculated from the following formula.

$$\text{Microcuries } (\mu\text{Ci}) = \frac{5000 \text{ rad}}{90 \text{ rad}/\mu\text{Ci}} \times \frac{\text{gland weight (g)}}{\text{24-hour uptake}}$$

For an 80-g thyroid gland with 24-hour uptake of 0.6 (60%), the administered dose would be 7400 μCi (7.4 millicuries).

The main drawback to the use of ^{131}I for therapy of hyperthyroidism is the high incidence of permanent hypothyroidism that ensues. With the usual therapeutic dose, 30% to 50% of patients become hypothyroid 10 years after therapy. Because hypothyroidism seems to be related to the dose, smaller doses of 3500 to 5000 rad may be preferable. With smaller doses, however, many patients seem to have little beneficial effect and require multiple courses of treatment. Fear of thyroid cancer, leukemia, and untoward genetic effects is unjustified because careful followup studies have not found these consequences. The radiation to the gonads and pelvic organs from a therapeutic dose of ^{131}I (most of which is excreted in the urine) is no more than that resulting from many diagnostic x-ray procedures.

FURTHER READING

1. Hershman, JM: Thyroid disease. In Hershman JM (ed): Management of Endocrine Disorders, pp. 25–51. Philadelphia, Lea & Febiger, 1980
2. Hershman, JM, Bray GA (eds): The Thyroid: Physiology and Treatment of Disease. Oxford, Pergamon Press, 1979
3. Hershman JM, Pittman JA Jr: Control of thyrotropin secretion in man. N Engl J Med 285:997, 1971
4. Oppenheimer JH, Schwartz HL, Surks MI et al: Nuclear receptors and the initiation of thyroid hormone action. Recent Prog Horm Res 32:529, 1976
5. Sawin CT, Hershman JM, Fernandez–Garcia R et al: Comparison of thyroxine and desiccated thyroid in patients with primary hypothyroidism. Metabolism 27:1518, 1978
6. Sterling K: Thyroid hormone action at the cell level. N Engl J Med 300:117, 173, 1979
7. Stock JM, Surks MI, Oppenheimer JH: Replacement dosage of L-thyroxine in hypothyroidism: A reevaluation. N Engl J Med 290:529, 1974
8. Volpé R (ed): Thyrotoxicosis. Clin Endocrinol Metab 7:1–241, 1978
9. Werner SC, Ingbar SH (eds): The Thyroid, 4th ed. New York, Harper & Row, 1978

CHAPTER 44 QUESTIONS

(*See* P. 7 for Full Instructions)

Select the One Best Answer

1. Levothyroxine may produce all of the following effects EXCEPT
   A. tachycardia.
   B. increased cardiac output.
   C. heart failure.
   D. increased peripheral resistance.
   E. angina pectoris.

2. All of the following indicate how liothyronine (T_3) differs from levothyroxine EXCEPT that
   A. it requires a smaller dose to produce the same effect.
   B. it does not have as marked an effect on oxygen consumption.
   C. it must be administered more frequently.
   D. its onset of action is more rapid.
   E. it is found in lower concentrations in the peripheral blood.

3. Each of the following statements is true EXCEPT
   A. methimazole inhibits iodination of monoiodotyrosine.
   B. propylthiouracil inhibits coupling of diiodotyrosine.
   C. perchlorate inhibits the release of thyroxine.
   D. iodide reduces the vascularity of the thyroid.
   E. iodide inhibits the release of thyroxine.

4. Propylthiouracil
   A. inhibits iodide uptake by the thyroid.
   B. has long duration of action.
   C. inhibits release of TSH.
   D. inhibits proteolysis of thyroglobulin.
   E. inhibits the conversion of thyroxine (T_4) to liothyronine (T_3).

A = 1,2,3; B = 1,3; C = 2,4; D = 4; E = All

5. The following drugs are useful in the management of hyperthyroidism for the reasons stated.
   1. Propylthiouracil—inhibits iodide concentrating mechanism in thyroid gland.
   2. Iodide—inhibits release of thyroxine.
   3. Propranolol—inhibits conversion of iodide to iodine.
   4. Methimazole—inhibits iodination of tyrosine.

6. When patients with myxedema are given levothyroxine (T_4),
   1. the euthyroid serum T_4 levels will be higher than in patients treated with liothyronine (T_3).
   2. the therapeutic effect will occur sooner than in patients treated with liothyronine (T_3).
   3. the daily dose is larger than that required for liothyronine (T_3).
   4. the drug is given several times daily because of its short half-life.

7. Propylthiouracil
   1. inhibits the thyroid coupling reaction.
   2. may cause agranulocytosis in about 0.2% of the patients.
   3. in hyperthyroidism may produce remissions that persist after drug withdrawal.
   4. is absorbed rapidly after oral administration.

8. Radioiodine (^{131}I)
   1. is useful for treating hyperthyroidism mainly because of its strong gamma radiation.
   2. can destroy the thyroid gland and cause hypothyroidism.
   3. can cause so many mutations that it has no clinical usefulness.
   4. may be concentrated in papillary and follicular thyroid carcinoma.

FREDERICK R. SINGER

45 Pharmacology of the Parathyroid Glands and Calcitonin

PARATHYROID HORMONE

CHEMISTRY

Parathyroid hormone (PTH) is an 84-amino acid polypeptide, and the complete amino acid sequence of bovine, porcine, and human varieties has been characterized (Fig. 45-1). J. B. Collip prepared the first extracts of PTH in 1925. Two precursor peptides, *preproparathyroid hormone* and *proparathyroid hormone*, have been identified. The former is the initial biosynthetic product and has an additional 31 peptides attached to its amino-terminal end. Intracellular cleavage of the 25-amino-terminal amino acids of preproparathyroid hormone generates the 90-amino acid proparathyroid hormone. The amino-terminal hexapeptide of proparathyroid hormone is highly susceptible to cleavage by trypsin, yielding PTH.

JAMES BERTRAM COLLIP, 1892–1965. Canadian physician and biochemist. First to isolate pure insulin (1921). In 1925 described isolation and physiology of parathyroid hormone and its links to calcium deficient tetany.

SECRETORY CONTROL

The dominant factor that controls PTH secretion is the concentration of blood ionized calcium perfusing the parathyroid glands. A decrease in blood ionized calcium produces an immediate rise in PTH secretion, and an increase in blood ionized calcium suppresses hormone output. Hypermagnesemia and severe magnesium deficiency also suppress PTH secretion. Beta-adrenergic agonists, histamine, dopamine, secretin, and prostaglandin E_2 stimulate and vitamin D metabolites, in some studies, suppress PTH secretion, but the physiological significance of these responses is unknown.

PHYSIOLOGICAL EFFECTS

The main physiological role of PTH is prevention of hypocalcemia. PTH maintains extracellular calcium levels by acting directly or indirectly on three organs. The most physiologically important mechanism is stimulation of osteoclastic bone resorption and osteocytic osteolysis. In addition, PTH increases

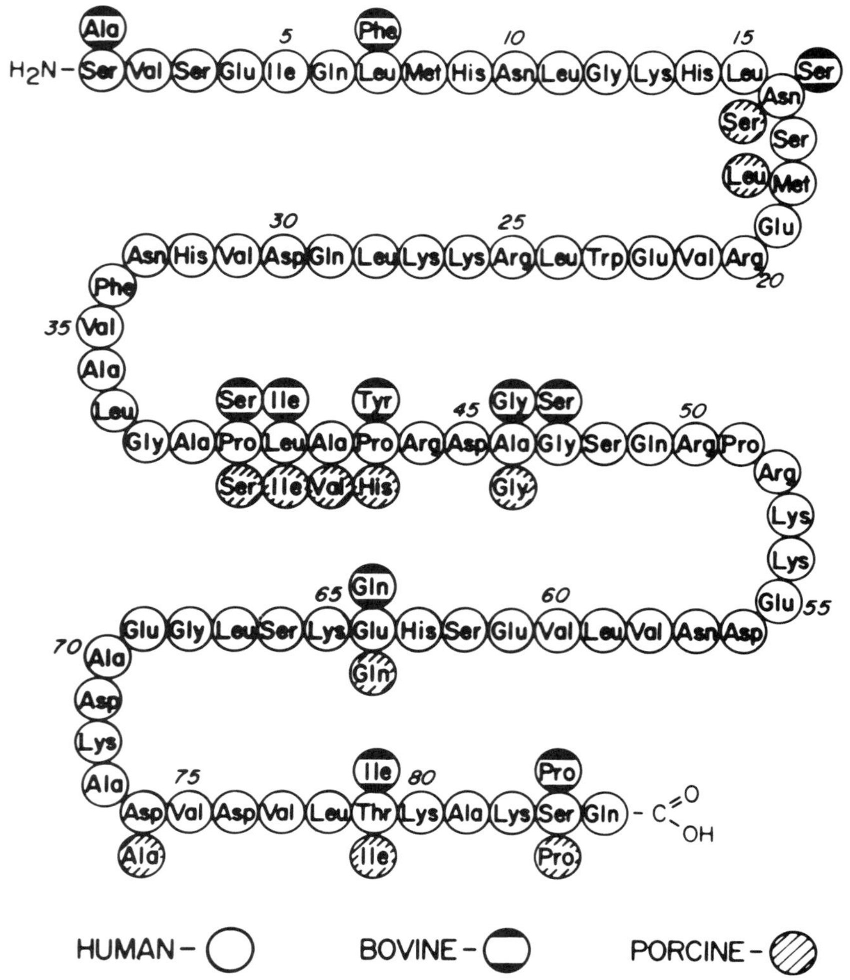

FIG. 45-1. Amino-acid sequences of human, bovine, and porcine parathyroid hormone (*PTH*). The backbone sequence depicts the human structure, and added residues indicate sequence differences found in the bovine and porcine hormones. (Keutmann HT: In De Groot L (ed): Endocrinology, Vol. 2. New York, Grune and Stratton, 1979)

renal tubular reabsorption of glomerular filtered calcium and indirectly facilitates intestinal calcium absorption. The latter effect results from PTH-induced renal metabolism of 25-hydroxyvitamin D to the more active 1α,25-dihydroxyvitamin D.

Phosphate also is released from bone along with calcium under the influence of PTH. However, PTH reduces renal tubular phoshate absorption, accounting for the common finding of hypophosphatemia in hyperparathyroid patients with normal renal function.

MECHANISM OF ACTION

The known biologic activity of PTH resides within its initial 27 amino acids; the biosynthetic PTH precursors are inactive. PTH acts, at least in part, through the stimulation of membrane-bound adenylate cyclase. Initially the amino-terminal region binds to specific high-affinity receptor sites on the surfaces of target cell membranes. Cyclic AMP is generated (*see* Chap. 50), and this key step is regulated by a membrane guanylyl nucleotide regulatory protein and by calcium and magnesium concentrations. PTH also activates a cyclic AMP-dependent kinase in bone cells, but subsequent steps remain to be elucidated.

Calcium may mediate some actions of PTH. For example, intracellular calcium transport (independent of the adenylate cyclase-cyclic AMP pathway) occurs in response to PTH.

METABOLISM AND EXCRETION

Parathyroid hormone exists in a heterogeneous state in the blood. Biologically active intact hormone is present in smaller concentrations than inactive carboxyl-terminal fragments. Amino-terminal fragments of PTH have not been found consistently. The $T^{1/2}$ of intact PTH in the circulation is less than 5 minutes, whereas that of the carboxyl-terminal fragment is up to 1 hour. PTH is metabolized during passage of the intact hormone through the liver, kidneys, and extremities (presumably removed by bone). Carboxyl-terminal fragments may also be secreted by the parathyroid glands, particularly in the presence of hypercalcemia. However, only the kidney appears to remove carboxyl-terminal fragments from the circulation, which must account for the markedly elevated concentration of these hormonal fragments in patients with renal failure. Excretion of PTH by the kidney appears to be insignificant.

ADVERSE EFFECTS

Administration of excessive amounts of bovine parathyroid extract could produce hypercalcemia, renal stones, and osteitis fibrosa, findings typical of primary hyperparathyroidism.

Antibodies to bovine PTH can develop during chronic treatment and lead to resistance to hormone action as well as to allergic manifestations (*see* Chap. 11).

CLINICAL USES AND INDICATIONS

Bovine parathyroid extract has been used to treat hypocalcemia due to hypoparathyroidism, but its suitability is limited because of its immunogenicity in humans. Intravenous or *oral calcium salts* and *vitamin D* or its analogues are more commonly used to manage acute and chronic hypoparathyroidism.

The main use of parathyroid extract has been in assessing patients suspected to be resistant to endogenous PTH. In normal subjects and in patients with hypoparathyroidism, an injection of parathyroid extract will produce an acute increase in urinary phosphate and cyclic AMP excretion. In patients with pseudohypoparathyroidism and magnesium deficiency, the response may be absent or blunted.

Current research using the synthetic biologically active 1-34 fragment of human PTH should lead to a therapeutic agent that can be used chronically as well as in acute studies of a diagnostic nature.

CALCITONIN

CHEMISTRY

Calcitonin (CT) is a 32-amino acid peptide whose structure varies considerably among different species, but all have a 7-amino acid disulfide ring at the amino-terminus and a carboxyl-terminal prolinamide (Fig. 45-2). The composition of human biosynthetic precursor peptides has not yet been elucidated. D. H. Copp discovered calcitonin in 1960.

SECRETORY CONTROL

Calcitonin is primarily synthesized in the parafollicular cells (C cells) of the mammalian thyroid and in the ultimobronchial glands of nonmammalian species. Regulation of CT secretion in all species studied appears to be mainly mediated by the level of ionized calcium in the circulation. High levels stimulate and low levels inhibit CT secretion. Gastrin and various gastrointestinal hormones are also potent secretogogues, but the physiological role of these agents is still unsettled.

PHYSIOLOGIC EFFECTS

The physiological role of CT has not been firmly established in all species. In lower mammals the hormone protects against excessive hypercalcemia after ingestion of a high calcium meal. This phenomenon has not been shown in humans. Calcitonin may protect the skeleton from calcium loss during pregnancy, lactation, and periods of low dietary calcium intake. The skeletal effects of CT are mainly directed toward the osteoclasts and the osteocytes. Injection of CT produces an immediate inhibition of bone resorption reflected by hypocalcemia or reduced urinary hydroxyproline excretion. Calcitonin may also stimulate bone formation in the growing animal.

Pharmacologic doses of CT produce extraskeletal effects in humans, namely, increased renal excretion of sodium, decreased gastric acid secretion, increased gall bladder contractility, and suppressed pancreatic secretion.

DOUGLAS HAROLD COPP, 1915– . Canadian physiologist (from British Columbia). Did research into parathyroid function, calcitonin, serum calcium, and bone and iron metabolism.

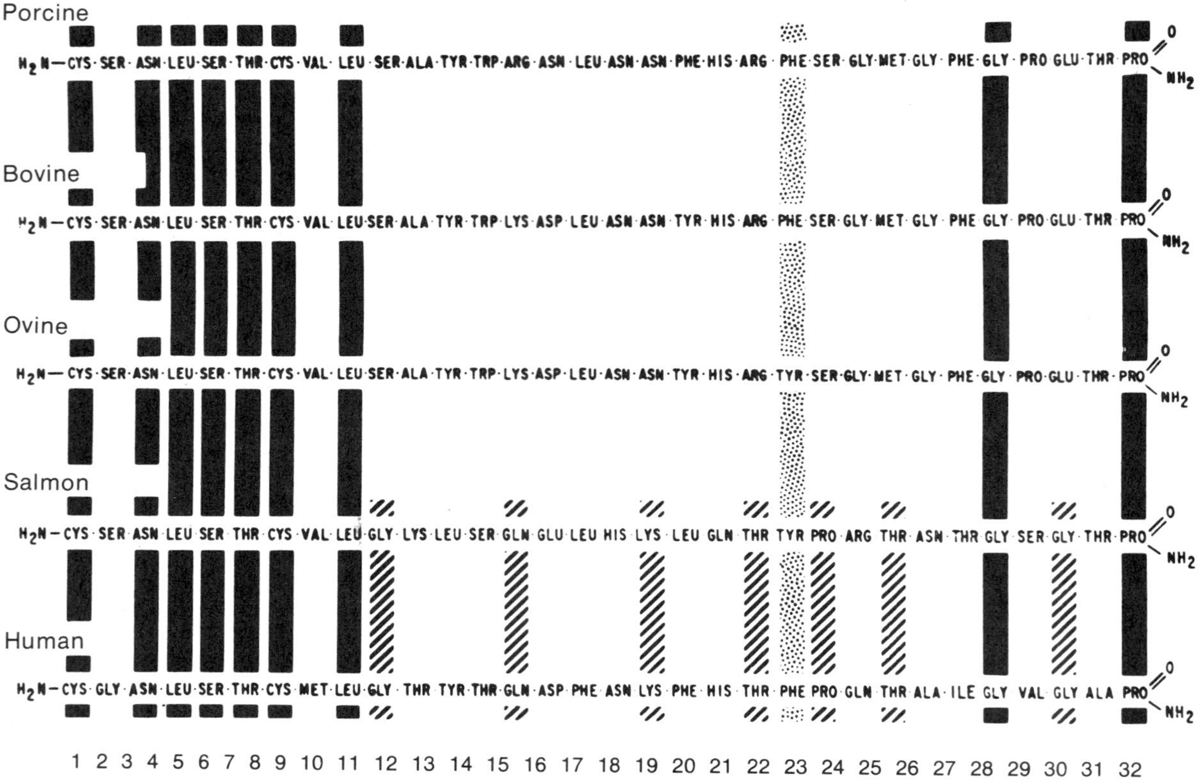

FIG. 45-2. Comparison of amino-acid sequences of porcine, bovine, ovine, salmon, and human calcitonin. Solid bars indicate sequence positions homologous among all five molecules; cross-hatched bars indicate salmon and human calcitonin. (Potts JT Jr, Niall HD, Keutmann HT et al: In Talmage RV, Munson PL (eds): Calcium, Parathyroid Hormone and the Calcitonins. Amsterdam, Excerpta Medica, 1972)

Salmon CT is more potent than the mammalian hormones in producing all the known biologic effects.

MECHANISM OF ACTION

Calcitonin binds to skeletal and renal tissue receptors and stimulates adenylate cyclase activity (*see* Chap. 50). Activation of a cyclic AMP-dependent protein kinase in renal cells has also been reported. In addition CT may also be dependent on intracellular calcium movement and shift of phosphate out of the extracellular fluid.

The greater potency of salmon CT is probably due to a greater affinity of this agent for target-organ receptors and to slower metabolism (*see* below).

METABOLISM AND EXCRETION

The metabolism of CT is species dependent. Salmon CT is cleared only by the kidney. Human CT is cleared by the kidney and liver. This accounts for the longer $T^{1/2}$ of salmon CT (about 15 minutes) than of human CT (about 5 minutes). Less than 1% of calcitonin administered to patients is excreted in urine.

ADVERSE EFFECTS

Nausea, facial flushing, a metallic taste, and polyuria may occur shortly after CT injection. Rarely hives or other allergic manifestations may develop in patients treated with nonhuman CT.

CLINICAL USES AND INDICATIONS

Calcitonin has become a standard treatment in patients with symptomatic Paget's disease of bone. Salmon CT is available for use in the United States, and porcine and human CT are also used in other countries. Chronic subcutaneous administration of these agents produces relief of bone pain and suppression of the intense metabolic activity as manifested by decreased serum alkaline phosphatase activity and urinary hydroxyproline excretion. Salmon CT therapy becomes ineffective in about 25% of patients with Paget's disease treated chronically. This is usually attributable to the presence of salmon CT-specific circulating antibodies.

Calcitonin has also been used in the acute therapy of hypercalcemia. The serum calcium concentration will acutely decrease by 1 to 2 mg/dl after CT injection, but sustained correction is seldom observed during chronic administration except in patients with hypercalcemia due to immobilization.

FURTHER READING

1. Aurbach GD (ed): Handbook of Physiology, Vol 7, Parathyroid Gland. Washington, DC, American Physiological Society, 1976
2. Austin LA, Heath H III: Calcitonin: Physiology and pathophysiology. N Engl J Med 304:269–278, 1981

CHAPTER 45 QUESTIONS

(See P. 7 for Full Instructions)

Select the One Best Answer

1. Tetany due to hypoparathyroidism may be alleviated by
   A. parathyroid hormone orally.
   B. calcitonin intravenously.
   C. a high phosphate diet.
   D. calcium gluconates intravenously.
   E. edetate calcium disodium (EDTA calcium) intravenously.
2. The origin of calcitonin (CT) used in the United States to treat Paget's disease of bone is
   A. human.
   B. beef.
   C. pork.
   D. sheep.
   E. salmon.

A = 1,2,,3; B = 1,3; C = 2,4; D = 4; E = All

3. Parathyroid hormone (PTH)
   1. decreases urinary phosphate excretion.
   2. decreases renal tubular absorption of calcium.
   3. has a long plasma half-life (6 hours).
   4. increases urinary cyclic-AMP excretion.
4. Calcitonin
   1. secretion is inhibited by hypercalcemia.
   2. is secreted by the thyroid gland.
   3. promotes the resorption of new bone.
   4. increases urinary phosphate excretion.
5. Diphosphonates, such as EHDP,
   1. retard the growth of bone mineral (hydroxyapatite) crystals.
   2. are recommended for the treatment of osteoporosis.
   3. retard the dissolution of bone mineral.
   4. cause ectopic calcification in muscle.
6. The clinical use of parathyroid hormone (PTH) is limited to
   1. treatment of rickets.
   2. treatment of vitamin D toxicity.
   3. treatment of hyperparathyroidism.
   4. patients suspected of PTH resistance.

46

HARRISON J. L. FRANK
JOSIAH BROWN

Insulin, Hypoglycemic Drugs, and Glucagon

Insulin has been available for treating diabetes mellitus since its discovery in 1922 by Banting and Best. Only in the last 5 to 10 years, however, has it become apparent that conventional methods of therapy do not prevent vascular complications in most patients. Thus there is a trend to try to regulate more closely the blood sugar concentration by using multiple injections of insulin each day or through the use of a continuous subcutaneous insulin infusion pump. To devise optimal schedules for insulin administration to diabetic patients, one must have knowledge of the normal processes of insulin synthesis, release, and actions as well as knowledge of available insulin preparations and their properties.

There are two main types of diabetes (Table 46-1). *Type I diabetics* are insulin-dependent patients, usually young people. Disease onset is often abrupt, with symptoms of thirst, polyuria, and weight loss and a tendency for the liver to produce ketone. Ketone production may be excessive and lead to ketoacidosis as the presenting clinical picture. The primary defect is insulin deficiency due to disease of the beta cells of the islets of Langerhans, and the ketoacidosis results from severe insulin deficiency.

Type II diabetes, characterized as non-insulin-dependent or insulin-resistant, may be present for months or years with few or no symptoms and is the type that occurs predominantly in middle and old age. This disorder may be diagnosed by routine testing of blood or urine for glucose, by worsening of the diabetes with infection, or by the presence of vascular complications. In some patients the cause of the insulin resistance may be removed, as in weight reduction of obesity, termination of pregnancy, or cessation of adrenal corticosteroid therapy,

---

FREDERICK GRANT BANTING, 1891–1941. Toronto physician. With C. H. Best and J. J. R. MacLeod, first reported the isolation of insulin in 1922, for which he received the Nobel prize, with MacLeod, in 1923. He was also a pioneer in aviation medicine.

CHARLES HERBERT BEST, 1899–1978. Toronto physician. Shared in the discovery of insulin, although not the Nobel prize. Also known for his discovery of histaminase (1930) and his coauthorship with N. B. Taylor of the textbook *Physiological Basis of Medical Practice*, first edition in 1937.

TABLE 46-1. Types of Diabetes Mellitus

Type I—INSULIN-DEPENDENT DIABETES MELLITUS (IDMM)
Insulinopenic and dependent on exogenous insulin for life
Ketosis-prone under basal conditions
Onset generally in youth, but may occur at any age
Islet cell antibodies frequently present at diagnosis
Associated with certain HLA types
Former Terms: Juvenile-onset; Ketosis-prone; Unstable or brittle diabetes
Type II—NON-INSULIN-DEPENDENT DIABETES MELLITUS (NIDDM)
Nonobese NIDDM
Obese NIDDM
Insulin levels ↑, ↓, or normal
Not ketosis-prone under basal conditions
Onset generally after age 40, but may occur at any age
May require insulin for control of symptoms or fasting hyperglycemia
60% to 90% are obese
Includes families with autosomal dominant inheritance of NIDDM
Former terms: Adult-onset, maturity-onset; Ketosis-resistant, stable diabetes; Maturity-onset diabetes of the young

and the glucose tolerance may return to normal.

INSULIN

SYNTHESIS, RELEASE, AND METABOLISM

Insulin is synthesized in the beta cells of the islets of Langerhans as a single long-folded polypeptide of 63 amino acids called *proinsulin* (Fig. 46-1). Proinsulin is converted to *insulin* by enzymatic cleavage of the connecting peptide (C peptide) in granules that form in the Golgi apparatus. As the granule moves out along a microtubule toward the cell membrane, maturation results in a dense central core of zinc–insulin crystals and a surrounding clear area that contains the biologically inactive C peptide (Fig. 46-2). As the granule approaches the plasma membrane, microfilaments extrude it from the cell, releasing equal molar quantities of insulin and C peptide into the venous sinusoids of the islet. A small amount of proinsulin is also released. The venous drainage from the islets empties into the pancreatic vein and then into the portal vein.

In the basal fasting state, release of insulin from the beta cells is continuous, with a regular periodicity of 13 minutes (Fig. 46-3). Increased release is stimulated within a few minutes by glucose or an unknown metabolic product of glucose metabolism, probably mediated by an effect of calcium on contraction of the microtubular–microfilament structure; c-AMP (*see* Chap. 50) also may be involved in this process. Vagal stimulation of insulin release also acts by this calcium-mediated mechanism. Other stimuli of the rapid first phase are free fatty acids, amino acids, and sulfonylurea drugs. A second phase, slower release of insulin, begins 5 to 10 minutes after an oral glucose load is superimposed on the first phase and lasts for 30 to 60 minutes (Fig. 46-3); the amount and duration of this phase are related to blood glucose concentrations. Among modulators of insulin release are gastrointestinal peptide (GIP), which enhances glucose-stimulated insulin release, and alpha- and beta-adrenergic activity. Alpha-adrenergic action inhibits insulin release, whereas beta agonists stimulate insulin release.

The liver plays a key role in regulating the blood sugar and in the metabolism of insulin. Of the insulin entering the liver, almost one half is extracted in first pass (*see* Chap. 4). Insulin binds to surface membrane receptors on hepatocytes and then is internalized, presumably for degradation. Additionally insulin is diluted in the circulation to 10% to 30% of the insulin concentration in the portal vein. The concentration of insulin in the peripheral blood of normal people is 5 to 15 μU/ml after an overnight fast, which rises to 50 to 100 μU/ml after a carbohydrate-rich meal or a glucose load.

Blood C peptide concentrations are more reliable indicators of pancreatic beta-cell function than are blood insulin levels. First, C peptide is not extracted or metabolized in the liver to any great extent, whereas there may be variations in the degree of insulin extraction; and second, the content of C peptide in commercial preparations of insulin is very low.

Proinsulin constitutes only 2% to 5% of the total insulin released, and very little is extracted or metabolized by the liver. The concentration of proinsulin in peripheral blood normally averages 15% of that of insulin, with a maximum in normal subjects of 22%. Proinsu-

PAUL LANGERHANS, 1847–1888. German pathologist. In 1869 described the insulin-producing islands of cells in the pancreas now named for him. There are also Langerhans cells and the Langerhans layer in the epidermis.

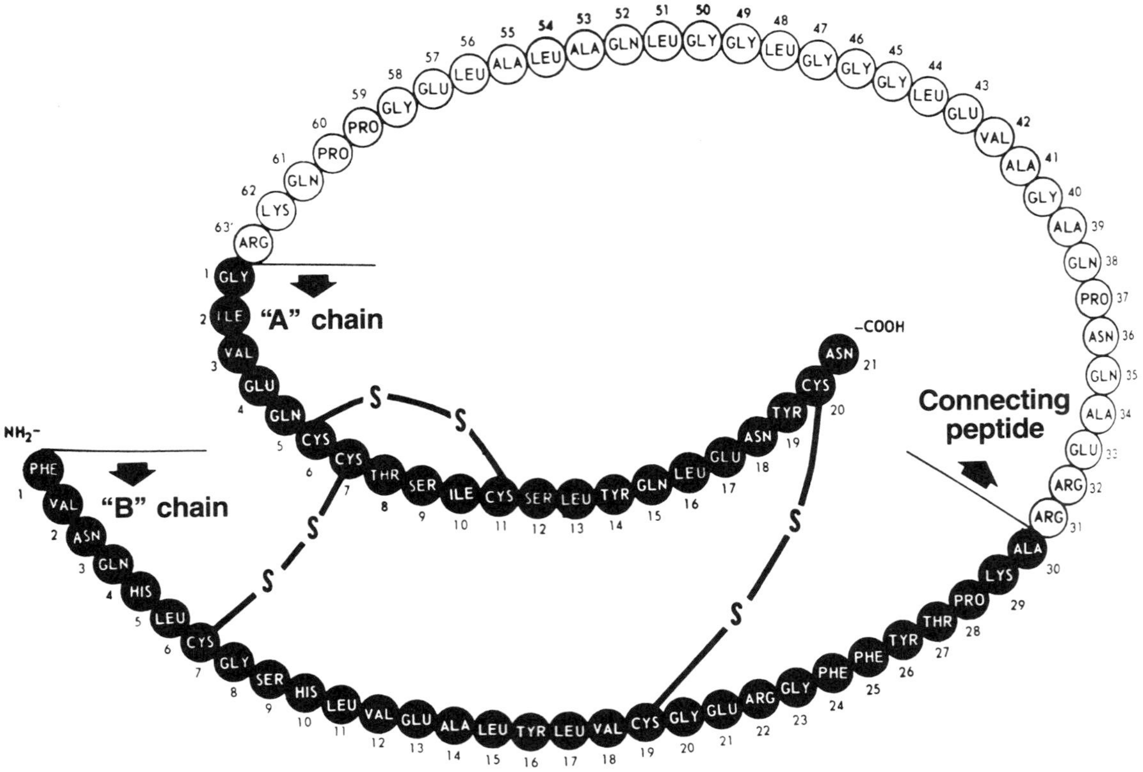

FIG. 46-1. Amino-acid sequence of porcine proinsulin. Position 35 was corrected to Glu_{35} from Gln_{35}, which was the proposed original.

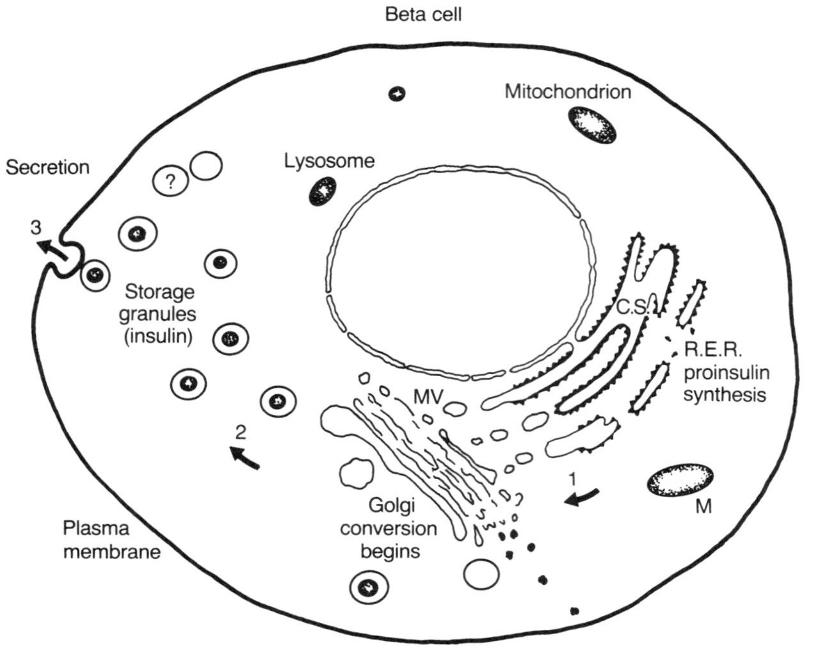

FIG. 46-2. Schematic representation of morphologic organization of biosynthetic and secretory apparatus of pancreatic beta cell.

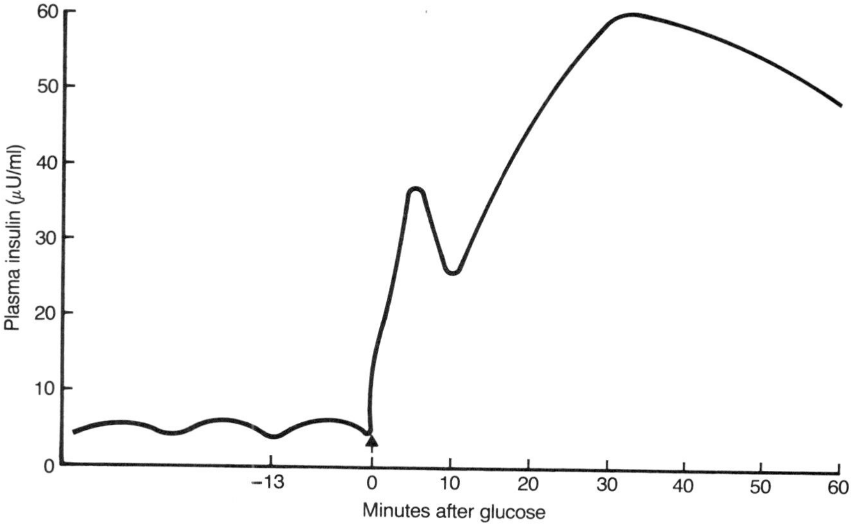

FIG. 46-3. Insulin release in the basal state and after a meal. Insulin is released regularly from the pancreas with a periodicity of 13 minutes in the fasting state. After a meal (at time 0), an initial rapid first phase of insulin release is followed by a prolonged second phase release that may last several hours.

lin has low biologic activity (5% of insulin). The ratio of proinsulin to insulin is higher in the blood of patients with functioning islet cell tumors, after glucose stimulation, and in states of severe hypokalemia.

The kidney plays a major role in metabolizing insulin, proinsulin, and C peptide, removing 36% to 50% of the amount that passes through the organ. Since the liver extracts about one half of the insulin released from the pancreas, only about 33% of the hormone ends up in the kidneys, compared to 69% of C peptide and 55% of proinsulin. In diabetic patients with kidney failure the amount of insulin required to control the blood sugar may fall, since a decreasing amount is extracted and degraded as kidney function decreases.

MECHANISM OF ACTION

Insulin exerts various metabolic effects on responsive tissues, acting as both an anabolic agent and an anticatabolic agent (Table 46-2). Thus hexose transport is enhanced into muscle and adipose tissue cells, lipolysis is inhibited in fat cells, and glycogen and protein synthesis are increased in muscle and liver.

TABLE 46-2. Effects of Insulin on Various Pathways in Liver, Adipose Tissue, and Muscle

Tissue	Anabolic Effects	Anticatabolic Effects
Liver	↑ Glycogen synthesis ↑ Amino acid uptake ↑ Protein synthesis	↓ Glycose production ↓ Gluconeogenesis ↓ Glycogenolysis ↓ Ketogenesis (also probably an indirect effect due to decreased delivery of substrate)
Adipose	↑ Glucose uptake ↑ Glycerol synthesis ↑ Fatty acid synthesis ↑ Triglyceride synthesis	↓ Lipolysis ↓ Free fatty acid and glycerol release
Muscle	↑ Glucose uptake ↑ Glucose utilization ↑ Glycogen synthesis ↑ Glucose oxidation ↑ Amino acid uptake ↑ Protein synthesis	↓ Glycogenolysis ↓ Amino acid release

INSULIN RECEPTORS

Generally, insulin action can be represented by the equation [I] + [R] $\rightleftharpoons$ I-R → "second messenger" → biologic response, where [I] is the concentration of insulin, [R] is the concentration of receptors, and [I-R] is the insulin-receptor complex.

Studies using biologically active ^{125}I-labeled insulin show hormonal binding, at least initially, to a specific cell surface plasma membrane receptor. Binding specificity can be demonstrated using chemically modified insulin or insulin isolated from different species. These studies show a good correlation between the ability of the altered insulin molecules to displace insulin from the native receptor and their biologic potency (Fig. 46-4). Receptor binding is rapid and saturable, generally reaching a maximum in less than 15 minutes under physiologic conditions, and is readily reversible when the tissues are placed in insulin-free media.

Both the number and the affinity of insulin receptors may vary. Alterations in receptor number occur over several days and reflect changes in the ambient insulin concentration; for example, states characterized by high concentrations of insulin, such as insulin-resistant (type II) diabetes or insulin-secreting islet cell tumors, will have a decreased or "down-regulated" number of receptors. In contrast, conditions that affect the affinity of the receptor for insulin occur rapidly (in several hours) and include such things as eating and ketoacidosis, which decrease affinity, or exercise, which increases affinity.

How changes in receptor number and affinity correlate with changes in insulin action is not entirely understood. However, because formation of a hormone-receptor complex is a prerequisite to insulin action, it follows (from the law of mass action) that the biologic response may be enhanced either by increasing the concentration of insulin or by increasing the concentration of receptors at a given insulin level. Therefore the sensitivity of a given tissue is proportional to the ratio of receptors to the hormone level. For example, with fat cells *in vitro*, a decreased receptor number appears to correlate with a decreased insulin sensitivity, as demonstrated by a shift to the right in the dose-response curve without changing the maximum response. This implies that the greater the relative number of insulin receptors on the cell surface, the more sensitive the cell will be to a given concentration of insulin but that the maximum ability of the cell to respond to insulin is not altered by changes in receptor number. The influence of receptor affinity on insulin action is less well understood.

FIG. 46-4. Effects of insulins and insulin derivatives on porcine ^{125}I-insulin binding to liver membranes and on glucose oxidation in fat cells. (*Left*) The inhibition of ^{125}I-insulin binding to liver membranes expressed as a percentage of maximum is plotted as a function of the concentration of unlabeled peptide. (*Right*) The stimulation of glucose oxidation in isolated fat cells expressed as a percentage of maximum is plotted as a function of the concentration of unlabeled peptide. (Freychet P, Roth J, Neville DM Jr: Insulin receptors in the liver. Specific binding of [^{125}I]insulin to the plasma membrane and its relationship to insulin bioactivity. Proc Natl Acad Sci, 68:1833–1837, 1971)

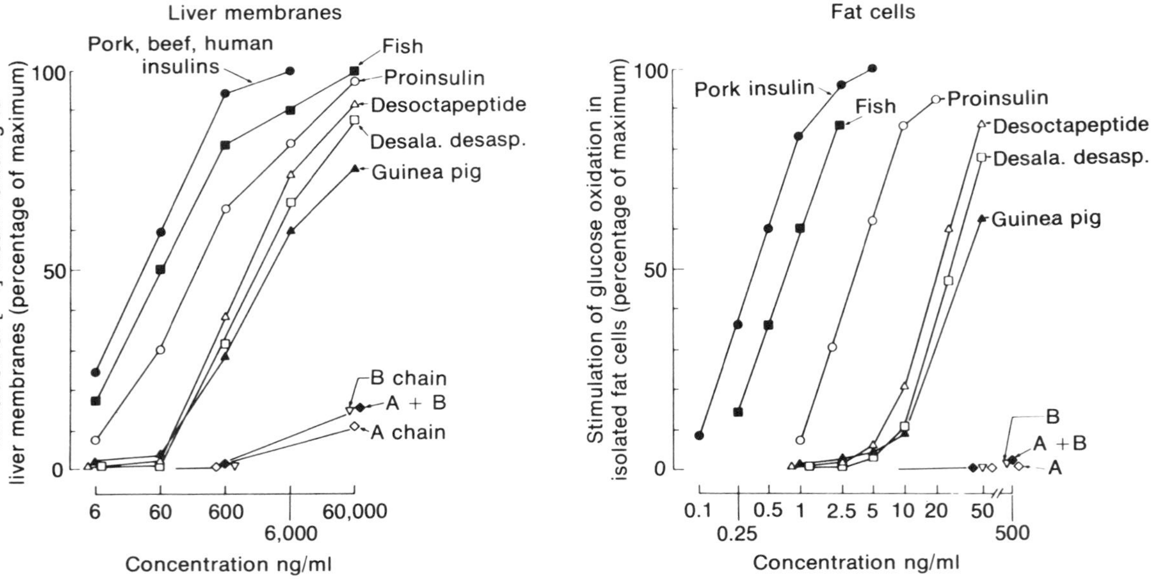

Postreceptor Events

If changes in insulin receptor number influence only the sensitivity of tissues to insulin (left and right shifts in the dose-response curve), postreceptor events must be responsible for modulating the maximum biologic response.

Recent studies have shown that insulin regulates phosphorylation and dephosphorylation of several proteins in target cells. Effects on one of these proteins, the alpha subunit of pyruvate dehydrogenase, suggests a possible mechanism for insulin regulation of glycolysis, and effects on another, a phosphoprotein phosphatase, is important in stimulating glycogen synthesis. However, even these changes in protein phosphorylation appear to be secondry events. Insulin may act at least partly by generating a 1000- to 1500-dalton polypeptide via an enzymatic cleavage step at the plasma membrane. This "second messenger" in turn activates a system of phosphatases that mediate the intracellular actions of insulin. Thus, in analogy with the cyclic AMP stimulation of protein kinases, one may speculate that insulin's second messenger may activate a cascade of phosphatases to promote its actions. Other substances, such as cyclic GMP, calcium ions, and hydrogen peroxide, have also been suggested as intracellular messengers for insulin. The exact role of these substances and their relation to the polypeptide remains to be elucidated.

Action on Specific Tissues

Biologically different tissues have differing sensitivities to insulin, and within a given tissue different pathways have different sensitivities. Tissue sensitivity is related to the number of cell surface receptors (*see* above). However, a 1:1 correlation between insulin binding and insulin action does not exist. For example in the fat cell, generally the most insulin-sensitive tissue, only 2% to 10% of receptors need to be occupied to achieve the 100% maximal biologic response. The remaining 90% to 98% of receptors are "spare receptors" that constitute a large pool of identical potentially functional receptors.

Of the major metabolic tissues, liver is probably one of the least sensitive, requiring 100 μU/ml of insulin to stimulate glycogen and fatty acid synthesis (Fig. 46-5). As expected, liver has fewer "spare receptors" than do fat cells, requiring up to 40% occupancy (60% spare receptors) to achieve maximum response. Teleologically, this relative insensitiv-

FIG. 46-5. Insulin action on liver, adipose tissue, and muscle. (Hershman JM: Endocrine Pathophysiology. A Patient Oriented Approach. Philadelphia, Lea & Febiger, 1977)

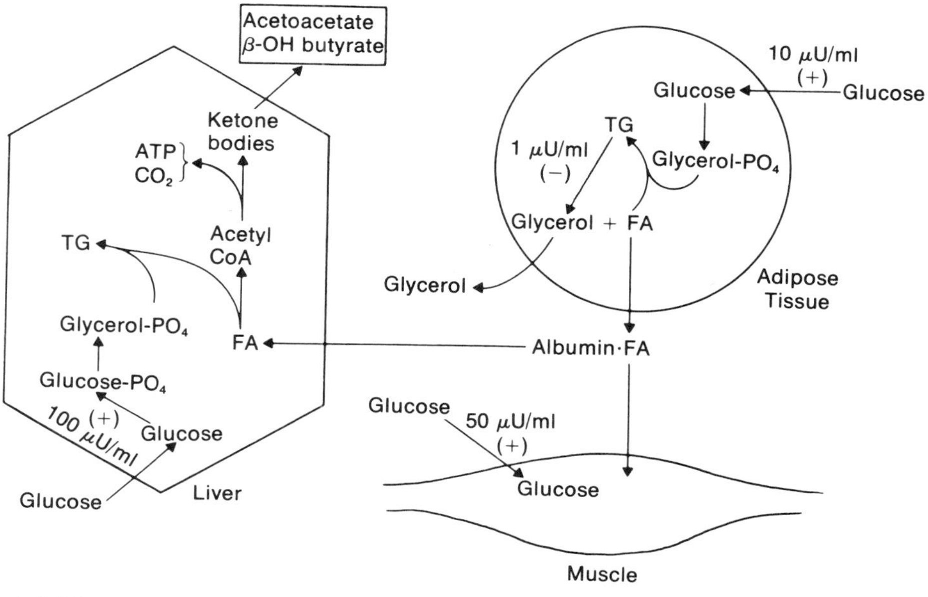

ity is plausible because the liver is exposed to the relatively high concentrations of insulin present in portal blood. Muscle also requires a relatively high concentration of insulin, about 50 μU/ml, to stimulate glucose transport. Fat, the most insulin-sensitive tissue, requires about 10 μU/ml of insulin to facilitate glucose transport but only 1 μU/ml to inhibit lipolysis by inhibiting the hormone-sensitive lipase. Thus only if insulin drops to very low levels will triglycerides be broken down to fatty acids, released into the blood stream, transported to the liver, and then used as substrates to generate ketoacids.

One of the major actions of insulin is to lower blood glucose, accomplished in two ways: A relatively low concentration of insulin inhibits gluconeogenesis and breakdown of liver glycogen; and a high concentration of insulin facilitates glucose transport through the plasma membrane into fat and muscle. Insulin does not directly affect glucose transport into liver, but, long-term, it increases the synthesis of hepatic glucokinase. This enzyme converts glucose to glucose-6-phosphate and hence allows subsequent intracellular glucose metabolism. Because muscle cells lack the enzyme glucose-6-phosphatase, they cannot release free glucose from glycogen stores. Under conditions of low blood insulin, muscle cells release lactic acid and amino acids, mainly alanine, which are transported to the liver and serve as substrates for gluconeogenesis.

USE

Insulin was first introduced clinically in 1922. Since then, insulin preparations have been improved to increase their chemical purity and vary their time-course of action. Optimal therapeutic use of insulin requires a knowledge of the various preparations and an awareness of the factors that modify their use. In general, use of insulin is mandatory for all diabetics who have type-I or juvenile-onset, ketosis-prone diabetes. Insulin is also used for type-II or adult-onset, ketosis-resistant diabetics who fail to achieve adequate glucose regulation by diet therapy alone or by diet therapy plus an oral sulfonylurea agent. The exact guidelines for insulin use and the definition of adequate control are variable, but recent information suggests that normalization of blood glucose reduces the developmental rate of diabetic microvascular complications.

Insulin may also be used in total parenteral nutrition (*see* Chap. 75), in hypoglycemic challenge to evaluate pituitary and hypothalamic function, in insulin coma to treat psychiatric conditions, and rarely, along with glucose infusion, to lower serum potassium rapidly in severe hyperkalemia.

Insulin is generally administered by s.c. injection. The site is usually "rotated" (alternated) on a daily schedule between thighs, abdomen, and arms. The advent of disposable syringes with small needles has made this an acceptable and relatively painless procedure. In emergency situations such as diabetic ketoacidosis, insulin can be delivered either by i.v. or i.m. injection. Other routes such as intraperitoneal injection in conjunction with an implantable insulin infusion pump or peritoneal dialysis or by application of modified insulin to mucosal membranes are not practical for general use at present.

PURIFICATION

In the past, insulin preparations have been packaged as U-40, U-80, or U-100, but for the sake of standardization U-100 (100 units of insulin/ml) is the only product now available in the United States. The U-40 and U-80 dilutions may still be obtained in Europe. Unless otherwise stated, insulin preparations are a mixture of beef and pork insulin (Table 46-3). Insulin is biologically assayed by lowering the blood sugar in fasted rabbits. One unit is the amount that lowers the blood sugar to 45 mg/dl. The international standard insulin contains 22 units/mg of protein. In anticipation of an increasing diabetic population, dwindling supplies of animal pancreas, and the demand for purer insulin preparations, recombinant DNA technology has been used to coax bacteria into making human insulin. These preparations are just becoming available for clinical use, but preliminary investigation shows that they are roughly equal in potency and side-effects to purified porcine preparations.

Recently new "single-peak" (they show only one peak on analysis), purer preparations of insulin have been made available (Table 46-3). Their purity is based on the amount of contaminating proinsulin. "Improved single peak" insulin contains less than 50 ppm of proinsulin and is now the industry standard, as compared to former preparations that contained 300 to 3000 ppm of proinsulin. Single component, or "purified," insulin that contains less than 10 ppm of proinsulin is commercially available and may be used in patients with insulin resistance or insulin allergy.

TABLE 46-3. History of Insulin Purification*

Time Period	1923–1972	1972–1979	1980–	1980–
Descriptive terminology	Conventional insulin	Single-peak insulin	Improved single-peak insulin	Purified or single-component insulin
Species source	Beef–pork Pork or beef	Beef–pork Pork or beef	Beef–pork	Pork or beef
Proinsulin contamination	10,000–50,000 ppm	<3000 ppm	<50 ppm	<10 ppm

* All preparations (*i.e.*, Regular, NPH, Semilente, Lente, and so forth) are available for each degree of purity mentioned in the table. In addition, the less impure preparations (conventional and single-peak insulin) are still available but are being gradually phased out. The purified or single-component insulins are generally about twice as expensive as improved single-peak preparations.

PREPARATIONS

All insulin preparations are available as regular, NPH, semilente, lente, and ultralente formulations and as pork, beef, or beef-pork mixtures (Table 46-4). The time-course of action depends on the modifying agent.

Regular insulin or crystalline zinc insulin (CZI) is the most rapid acting preparation and is the only preparation used intravenously or intramuscularly for treating diabetic ketoacidosis or in insulin infusion pumps. It can be used alone in multiple daily injections or mixed with a longer-acting preparation.

Semilente, lente, and ultralente insulin are crystalline zinc preparations that vary only in the size of their crystals, and hence in their absorption characteristics from the injection site. Semilente can safely be mixed with lente and ultralente insulins in the same syringe to achieve a combination of rapid and longer-acting insulins.

Ultralente and protamine zinc insulin (PZI) are rarely used, partly because of their long half-lives that result in frequent nocturnal hypoglycemia; however, newer trends in therapy may combine a small amount of long-acting insulin with premeal injections of regular insulin in an attempt to achieve tighter control of diabetes.

The amount of insulin and protamine in neutral protamine Hagedorn (NPH) insulin is carefully balanced so that the rapid action of regular insulin can be preserved when mixed with it. Protamine is no more allergenic than lente insulin, with its high zinc content.

STRATEGY FOR INSULIN USE

Insulin is used in various combinations to lower the plasma glucose in diabetes. The exact dose and combination must be determined for each patient, and both the physician and the patient must understand the actions of the given preparation and the factors that modify it. The information presented here is intended only as a guideline. In the past, diabetic ketoacidosis was treated with regular insulin given in a large initial s.c. or i.v. dose (about 100 units), with subsequent s.c. doses every 2 to 6 hours based on plasma glucose determina-

TABLE 46-4. Insulin Preparations

Type	Preparation	Modifying Agent	Peak Action	Duration of Action
			hr	*hr*
Rapid acting	Regular, CZI	None	½–2	4–6
	Semilente	Acetate crystals	2–4	8–12
Intermediate acting	NPH	Protamine	8–12	18–24
	Lente	Acetate crystals (3:7 mixture of semilente and ultralente)	8–12	18–24
Long acting	PZI	Protamine (excess)	12–16	36+
	Ultralente	Large acetate crystals	12–16	36+

tions. Currently popular use is i.v. insulin (bolus of 5 to 10 units) followed by about 0.1 unit insulin/kg/hr. The serum insulin level is maintained at a relatively high level during this continuous infusion, which allows normalization of glucose over 6 to 12 hours.

After the plasma glucose level is controlled, an intermediate acting preparation is begun subcutaneously. The daily morning dose, chosen empirically, is 10 to 15 units for adolescents, 15 to 20 units for thin adults, and 20 to 30 units for obese adults. The daily dose is increased in increments of 10% to 20% until the blood glucose is lowered into a reasonable range. If the 4 p.m. blood glucose level (8 to 10 hours after the morning dose) is controlled but the morning fasting blood glucose level remains elevated, a second injection of intermediate-acting NPH or lente insulin may be needed before the evening meal. The usual ratio is to give about two thirds of the total daily dose in the morning to cover the daytime meals and one third of the daily dose at 4 p.m. to 5 p.m. to obtain nocturnal coverage. If the patient continues with glycosuria before lunch or after dinner, a small amount of rapid-acting insulin may be mixed in the syringe of the morning or evening dose to cover these times.

When drawing insulin into the syringe, the short-acting preparation should always be drawn first to avoid contamination of the short-acting insulin in the vial by modifying agents in the longer-acting preparations. Only after the dose of NPH or lente insulin is adjusted should the short-acting insulin be added to the regimen. Because the different preparations of insulin peak at differing times after injection, the patient must be aware of when his insulin peaks and that the timing of his meals is an important part of the diabetic regimen.

The action of insulin is influenced by [1] the site of injection. Absorption is most rapid after abdominal injection and slowest after anterior thigh injection; [2] depth of injection. The deeper the injection, the more rapid the absorption; [3] exercise increases absorption, especially if the site of injection is in a heavily exercised area such as a thigh; [4] insulin antibodies in the blood, which bind insulin and release it slowly into the circulation; and [5] the dynamics of insulin interaction with its receptors.

ADVERSE EFFECTS

The major side-effect of insulin is hypoglycemia, which is also the therapeutic effect, but hypoglycemia may present clinically in the paradoxical setting of the Somogyi effect or posthypoglycemic hyperglycemia. Hypoglycemia, especially at night when the patient may be unaware of it, results in the release of counter regulatory hormones (*e.g.*, glucagon and catechols) that raise the blood glucose level and often produce a very high value when checked the following morning. The Somogyi effect may be suspected when the patient complains of having slept poorly, having had nightmares or nocturnal sweats, and has had negative urine tests at bedtime but awakens with positive tests for glucose and often ketones. The hypoglycemia can be verified by admitting the patient to the hospital and monitoring the nocturnal plasma glucose, or perhaps more simply by having the patient set his alarm to awaken at night so that a urine glucose or a fingerstick blood glucose can be determined at home. The treatment for the Somogyi effect is to lower the dose of insulin gradually.

Local pruritus or a wheal and flare reaction frequently occurs at the sites of the injection during the first year of insulin therapy, and probably represents delayed hypersensitivity responses to impurities in the insulin. These reactions are usually transient and treatable with H_1 blockers. If the reactions are severe, a change to a more purified insulin may relieve the symptoms. Anaphylactic reactions to insulin are rare (less than 0.1% of diabetics). The usual setting is in a middle-age patient who has started and stopped insulin therapy several times. This is an IgE-mediated process, beginning within 20 to 60 minutes after an injection, with a local reaction that spreads quickly to generalized urticaria and can progress to vascular collapse and death. Immediate supportive therapy is indicated, and it should be determined whether the patient truly needs insulin for regulation of diabetes. If the patient needs insulin, a careful series of desensitization injections is begun.

Immunologic insulin resistance due to insulin binding (IgG, IgM, IgE) antibodies is defined as insulin requirements in excess of 200 units/day in the absence of other causes for insulin resistance. Diagnosis is difficult because antibodies may be present in patients who have been on insulin therapy for more than 1 year and yet who do not possess immunologic insulin resistance. The usual treatment is to in-

Michael Somogyi, 1883– . Austrian-born American biochemist. With others, published a method for glycogen determination in 1933 and developed the analysis of serum diastase as a test for pancreatitis.

crease the amount of insulin to prevent the development of ketoacidosis. Many physicians also recommend switching to a more highly purified and less antigenic porcine preparation or adding 50 to 100 mg/day of oral prednisone or an equivalent steroid. Although the steroid itself is diabetogenic (*see* Chap. 47), the predominant effect appears to be a lessening of the immunologic resistance. About one third of patients improve by changing the type of insulin. These patients must be watched closely because they may have rapidly fluctuating insulin requirements.

Subcutaneous fat hypertrophy or atrophy (insulin lipodystrophy) may develop at the site of hormone injection. The hypertrophy is probably due to a local insulin effect, whereas the atrophy is often ascribed to impurities in the insulin. The prevalence of both conditions has decreased with the introduction of purer insulins; in fact, the treatment is to inject the area around the atrophy with a purified insulin preparation.

ORAL HYPOGLYCEMIC AGENTS

Two classes of oral hypoglycemic compounds, the *sulfonylureas* and the *biguanides* (Fig. 46-6; Table 46-5), have been used. Only the sulfonylureas are currently available in the United States; the biguanides have been discontinued because of the high incidence of lactic acidosis associated with their use.

MODE OF ACTION

Sulfonylureas are not an oral form of insulin because they do not lower plasma glucose in

FIG. 46.6. Chemical structure of the four oral hypoglycemic agents currently marketed in the United States, glyburide, and phenformin (no longer available). The active component of each drug is set off by dotted lines. The first four structures show the sulfonylurea radical, and the last two show glyburide and the biguanide radical. The other components of the molecular structures are responsible for the differing metabolic fates of the individual drugs. (Modified from Williams RH, Porte D Jr: The pancreas: In Textbook of Endocrinology, 5th ed. Philadelphia, WB Saunders, 1974)

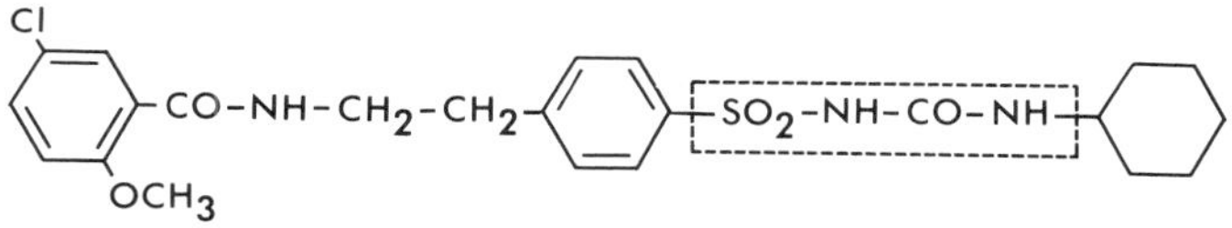

GLYBURIDE
(1-[[P-[2-(5-CHLORO-O-ANISAMIDO)ETHYL]PHENYL]SULFONYL]-3-CYCLOHEXYLUREA

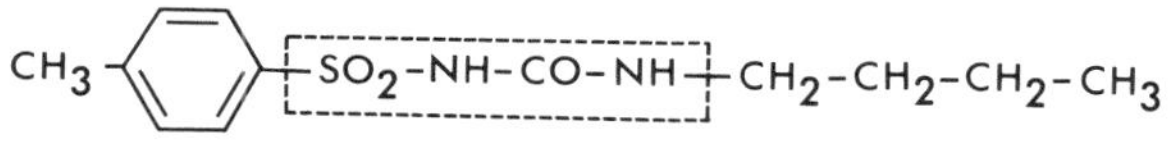

TOLBUTAMIDE
(1-BUTYL-3-P-TOLYLSULFONYLUREA)

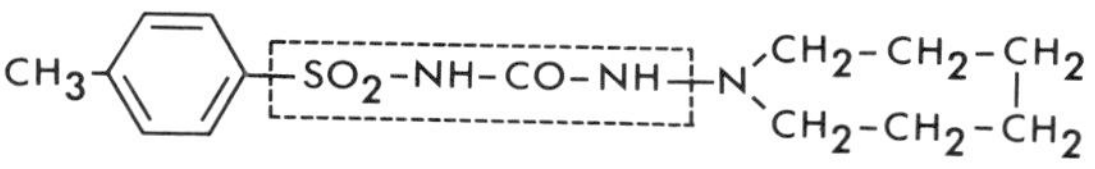

TOLAZAMIDE
(1-(HEXAHYDRO-1-AZEPINYL)-3-P-TOLYLSULFONYLUREA)

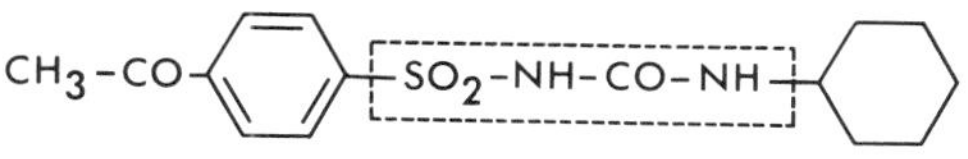

ACETOHEXAMIDE
(N-(P-ACETYLBENZENESULFONYL)-N′-CYCLOHEXYLUREA)

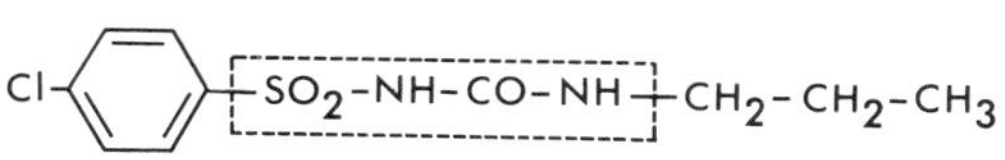

CHLORPROPAMIDE
(1-PROPYL-3-P-CHLOROBENZENESULFONYLUREA)

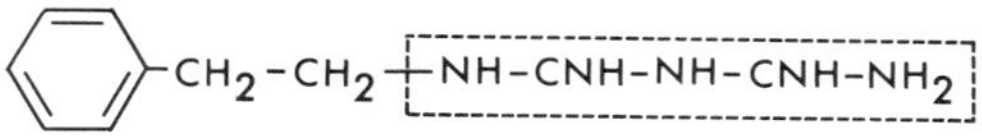

PHENFORMIN
(N′-B-PHENETHYLFORMAMIDINYLIMINOUREA OR PHENETHYLBIGUANIDE)

TABLE 46-5. Properties of the Oral Hypoglycemic Agents

Name	Duration of Action	Tablet Size	Maximum Dose	Dose Range
Sulfonylureas	*hr*	*mg*	*mg*	*mg*
Tolbutamine (Orinase)*	6–12	500	3000	500–2000 (divided)
Acetohexamide (Dymelor)*	12–24	250, 500	1500	200–1000 (single or divided)
Tolazamide (Tolinase)*	12–24	100, 250	750	100–500 (single or divided)
Chlorpropamide (Diabinese)*	Up to 36 hr	100, 250	500	100–500 (single dose)
Glyburide (Micronase, Glibenclamide)*	24	2.5	30	1.25–20 (single dose)
Phenformin† (DBI-TD)*	12–18	50, 100	150	50–150 (single or divided)

* Trade name.
† No longer available for clinical use.

pancreatectomized animals or ketosis-prone diabetics. A functioning pancreas must be present for the drugs to work, and hence their use is confined to the adult-onset type II diabetic who has failed on diet therapy alone.

In the first 2 weeks of administration, sulfonylureas enhance the release of insulin from the pancreas, especially in response to an oral glucose load, through an inhibition of beta-cell cyclic AMP phosphodiesterase (*see* Chap. 50). After 4 to 5 weeks, however, both the basal and postprandial insulin levels return to or below the pretreatment levels, even though the glucose levels remain lowered. Thus, enhanced insulin release alone cannot explain the entire action of sulfonylureas.

Sulfonylureas probably increase the number of insulin receptors per cell, making the patient more sensitive to the existing insulin concentration. This explains why glucose level remains low despite the fact that insulin concentration returns to pretreatment level.

PROPERTIES

The sulfonylureas share common chemical groups (Fig. 46-5), and the differences in their action is determined primarily by their metabolism. Tolbutamide is rapidly carboxylated in the liver and is more suitable for elderly patients who may not eat regularly and would be more susceptible to hypoglycemic reactions. Acetoheximide is also rapidly metabolized by hepatic hydroxylation, but the metabolite is more active than the parent compound, thereby extending the duration of action. Tolazamide is broken down to six major metabolites, three of which are active. Chlorproamide is excreted slowly in the urine unchanged. Its long half-life is due to avid albumin binding and allows the drug to be given only once per day. However, chlorproamide should be avoided in the elderly and in patients with renal failure. Chlorproamide therapy must be stopped at least 1 day before planned surgery since, if continued, it may result in postoperative hypoglycemia.

Glyburide and glipizide are second-generation oral agents that have been used in Europe and will soon be available in the United States. They, like chlorpropamide, are highly serum bound and are metabolized only slowly to inactive products. These drugs are much more potent than the other sulfonylureas and are effective in doses of 1.25 mg to 30 mg/day, approximately one hundredth that of tolbutamide. The peak action is in 2 to 6 hours, and they have a duration of action of about 24 hours. The reported incidence of side-effects, other than hypoglycemia, is much lower than that with the other sulfonylureas.

SIDE-EFFECTS

Drugs that interact with the sulfonylureas include dicumarol, phenylbutazone, probenicid, sulfonamides, chloramphenicol, and salicylates, which may reduce binding, especially of chlorpropamide, to serum proteins and hence predispose to transient hypoglycemia (*see* Chap. 8). Thiazides, steroids, and propranolol may block release of insulin from the pancreas or cause peripheral resistance to insulin, and hence to oral sulfonylurea agents.

Side-effects, especially hypoglycemia, anorexia, epigastric discomfort, nausea, vomiting, or diarrhea, develop in 3% to 5% of patients, Alcohol intolerance with a disulfiram-like reaction may occur, and patients should be specifically warned about this possibility. Skin rashes and photosensitivity have also been reported. Chlorpropamide and acetohexamide have been associated with a reversible cholestatic jaundice, and reversible inappropriate ADH secretion has been observed with chlorpropamide. Pancytopenia or occasionally isolated agranulocytosis is rare.

The University Group Diabetes Program (UGDP) in the 1960s reported an increased incidence of cardiovascular deaths in patients treated with oral agents, specifically tolbutamide. This study has been severely criticized on the basis of experimental design and statistical conclusions. Most diabetologists continue to use oral agents and will do so until a more definitive study is done.

"Secondary failure" is a more serious problem and presumably represents pancreatic beta-cell exhaustion with failure of the oral agents to control blood sugar. In one retrospective study at 6 to 9 years after starting therapy with sulfonylureas, 6% of patients had secondary failure.

GLUCAGON

Glucagon is a single-chain, 29-amino acid polypeptide synthesized in the alpha cells of the islets of Langerhans. It is synthesized as proglucagon, which is cleaved in the alpha-cell granules before extrusion into the venous sinusoids. Insulin and glucagon appear to act on the liver cell with opposite effects to maintain blood glucose at a normal level and to respond to eating and fasting.

Glucagon regulates glucose release from the liver by binding to a liver-cell plasma membrane receptor that stimulates the enzyme adenylate cyclase to increase intracellular cyclic AMP levels. Glucose is provided either by stimulation of gluconeogenesis from amino acids or by glycogenolysis via activation of the glycogen phosphorylase cascade. Increased formation of ketone bodies in the liver also results from glucagon stimulation.

Release of glucagon from the pancreas increases in fasting with hypoglycemia and in response to dietary amino acids, especially arginine and alanine. Plasma glucagon is elevated in diabetics, but meticulous control of the blood sugar with insulin returns the blood level of glucagon to normal and also restores the normal suppressibility of glucagon that results from glucose administration.

Glucagon is used therapeutically for emergency administration to diabetic patients who are so hypoglycemic that they cannot be given glucose by mouth. It is usually injected subcutaneously or intramuscularly in a dose of 1 mg, and the blood glucose level will begin to rise within 10 minutes and peak within 20 to 30 minutes.

Other uses of glucagon are in the diagnostic work-up for hypoglycemia and pheochromocytoma and in diagnostic radiology to inhibit motility of the gastrointestinal tract.

Glucagon is available in ampules containing 1 mg (1 unit) of dry powder; it is diluted in 1 ml of diluting solution included in the package. Side-effects are unusual and only consist of occasional nausea and vomiting.

FURTHER READING

1. Galloway JA: Insulin treatment for the early 80's: Facts and questions about old and new insulins and their usage. Diabetes Care 3:615–622, 1980
2. National Diabetes Group: Classification and diagnosis of diabetes mellitus and other categories of glucose intolerance. Diabetes 28:1039–1057, 1979
3. Proceedings, Fiftieth Anniversary Insulin Symposium. Diabetes 21(Suppl 2):385–723, 1972
4. Roth J, Grunfeld C: Endocrine systems: Mechanisms of disease, target cells, and receptors. In Williams RH (ed): Textbook of Endocrinology, 6th ed, pp 15–72. Philadelphia, WB Saunders, 1981
5. Shen SW, Brusler R: Oral hypoglycemic agents. Disease-A-Month 22:1–35, 1976

CHAPTER 46 QUESTIONS

(See P. 7 for Full Instructions)

A = 1,2,3; B = 1,3; C = 2,4; D = 4; E = All

1. Factors that can influence the action of insulin include
   1. site of injection.
   2. depth of injection.
   3. exercise.
   4. the presence of insulin antibodies.

2. Concerning the action of oral sulfonylurea agents,
   1. they increase the release of insulin from the pancreas.
   2. they have been shown to improve control in insulin-deficient type-I diabetes mellitus.

3. they increase the number of insulin receptors on target tissues in patients who respond.
4. aspirin blocks the hypoglycemic action of these agents.

3. Insulin receptors
   1. increase in number, or upregulate, in response to high ambient insulin levels.
   2. have a decreased affinity in response to ketoacidosis.
   3. can decrease the maximum responsiveness of a cell if they are down regulated.
   4. exist in excess as spare receptors to increase the sensitivity of a cell to insulin.

4. Which of the following statements about insulin preparation is (are) true?
   1. When drawing up mixed insulin preparations, the (clear) regular insulin should be drawn into the syringe before the (cloudy) NPH insulin.
   2. The peak action of intermediate-acting insulin is 8 to 12 hours after injection, but it may be prolonged by the presence of insulin antibodies.
   3. The newer purified insulin preparations can be used to treat insulin lipoatrophy by injection into the area of atrophy.
   4. It is generally acceptable to have a patient inject U-100 insulin with a U-40 syringe.

Select the One Best Answer

5. Which of the following agents are routinely administered intravenously?
   A. Lente insulin
   B. Acetoheximide
   C. Protamine zinc insulin
   D. Crystalline zinc insulin

6. All of the following statements about insulin are correct EXCEPT that
   A. it is released periodically from the pancreas even in the basal, nonstimulated mode.
   B. it works by initially combining with a specific receptor on the surface of the target cell.
   C. it is released from the pancreas in response to a rise in serum free fatty acids.
   D. it is released as proinsulin by the pancreas and converted to active insulin by an enzymatic cleavage in the liver.
   E. it increases amino acid synthesis by liver and muscle.

7. An insulin-dependent diabetic patient on a single morning injection of NPH insulin is referred with the following plasma glucose profile:

   Fasting (0700 hr) = 380 mg/dl;
   Before dinner (1700 hr) = 48 mg/dl, with symptoms of headache and sweating;
   Before bed (2200 hr) = 180 mg/dl.

   To optimize the insulin schedule, the patient should be advised to
   A. add regular insulin to the morning NPH.
   B. increase the morning NPH and add a second dose of NPH in the evening.
   C. decrease the morning NPH and add a second dose of NPH before dinner.
   D. add regular insulin to the morning NPH and a second dose of regular insulin before dinner.
   E. switch to ultralente insulin.

8. All of the following statements about oral sulfonylurea agents are true EXCEPT that
   A. one of the most common side-effects of oral hypoglycemic agents is gastrointestinal upset.
   B. it can cause a reversible cholestatic jaundice.
   C. chlorpropamide is the best agent for older debilitated patients because it has to be taken only once a day.
   D. acetoheximide is rapidly metabolized by liver to active metabolites.
   E. tolbutamide is carboxylated in the liver to inactive metabolites.

DON H. NELSON

Pharmacology of the Corticosteroids and Adrenocorticotropic Hormone

47

The pharmacology of the corticosteroids and adrenocorticotropic hormone (ACTH), the anterior pituitary hormone that stimulates the adrenal gland to secrete, is discussed herein.

PHYSIOLOGY AND BIOCHEMISTRY

CHEMISTRY

The corticosteroids have the basic cyclopentanoperhydrophenathrene structure (Fig. 47-1) found in all steroid hormones, plus the characteristic of three to five oxygen groups that gives them greater water solubility than is found with other steroids such as cholesterol, estrogens, or androgens. In addition, the corticosteroids have ketones in the 3 and 20 positions and a hydroxyl group in the 21 position, and many have a hydroxyl group at the 11 or 17 position, or both, on the molecule. *Cortisol,* the steroid secreted in largest quantity by the human adrenal cortex, has all of these ketone and hydroxyl groups (11β,17,21-trihydroxy-4-pregnene-3,20 dione). *Aldosterone* is unique in having an oxygen at the 18 position (Fig. 47-2).

Adrenal cortical hormones are commonly divided into *glucocorticoids* (cortisol and corticosterone), *mineralocorticoids* (aldosterone and 11-desoxycorticosterone), and adrenal *androgens* (dehydroepiandrosterone, androstenedione, and testosterone); small amounts of *estrogens* may also be secreted but are seldom of physiological significance.

The glucocorticoids chiefly act on carbohydrate, protein, and fat metabolism. The mineralocorticoids primarily act on absorption of sodium and chloride by the renal tubule. These classifications are broad representations of major activity when the hormones are given in physiologic doses. However, glucocorticoids have some renal sodium-retaining activity and mineralocorticoids some glucocorticoid activity. For example, cortisol (predominantly a glucocorticoid) is of major importance in maintaining a difference in the sodium and potassium concentrations of the intracellular and extracellular compartments.

Adrenal androgens are of low potency as compared with testosterone. Conversion to testosterone usually precedes significant physiological action by these compounds. The adrenal cortex is the chief source of androgens in females and prepubertal males.

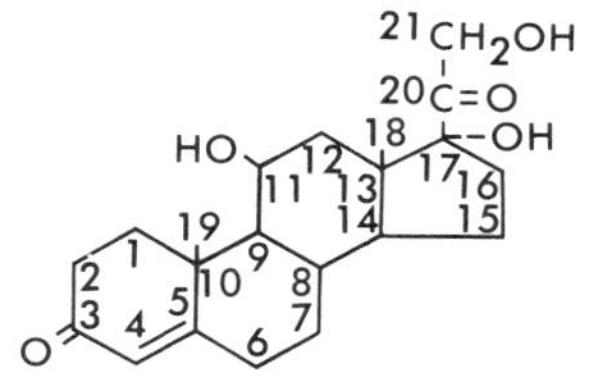

CORTISOL(11 β,17,21-TRIHYDROXY-4-PREGNENE-3,20 DIONE)

FIG. 47.1. Cortisol.

FIG. 47-2. Chemical structures of adrenocortical steroids.

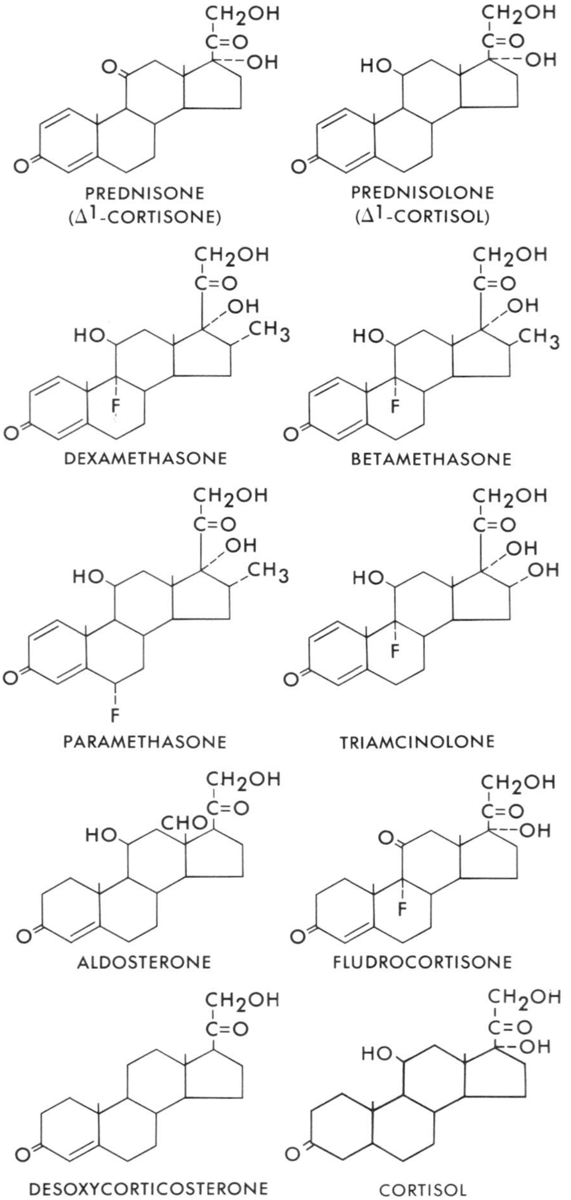

Aldosterone is secreted primarily from the zona glomerulosa, the outer of the three zones of the adrenal cortex. Glucocorticoids and androgens are secreted from the zona fasciculata (middle zone) and the inner zona reticularis. The production of the catecholamines by the adrenal medulla, which is surrounded by the cortex, is discussed in Chapter 13. The corticosteroids pass through a network of veins to the medulla and have significant effects on enzymes necessary for the synthesis of epinephrine and norepinephrine (*see* Chap. 13).

ACTH AND ADRENAL CORTICAL SECRETION

Physiologically and pharmacologically, ACTH stimulates the secretion of corticosteroids, chiefly cortisol, by the adrenal cortex. It also stimulates androgens. In the absence of ACTH, as after hypophysectomy, the adrenal cortex rapidly atrophies and becomes relatively resistant to the acute stimulatory effect of the hormone. With continuous stimulation, however, the gland hypertrophies and develops increased sensitivity to ACTH. ACTH combines with receptors on the cortical cell plasma membrane, which couple with adenylate cyclase to increase production of cyclic AMP (*see* Chap. 50). The action of the cyclic AMP on protein kinases and the phosphorylation of proteins is intimately involved in stimulating the synthesis of corticosteroids. ACTH also influences cholesterol esterase activity to make free cholesterol available and the production of polyphosphoinositides, phosphatidylglycerol, and other phospholipids that increase enzymatic hydroxylations important in corticosteroid synthesis. Most of the cholesterol used in synthesis comes from the breakdown of plasma cholesterol-containing, low-density lipoproteins (*see* Chap. 37). Increased quantities of polyphosphoinositides increase the binding of cholesterol to the cytochrome P-450 involved in its conversion to pregnenolone, the first step in steroid synthe-

CHARLES EDOUARD BROWN-SEQUARD, 1817—1894. French physician and physiologist. Best known for his work on the nervous system, especially spinal cord and sympathetic nerve function, and epilepsy. Later became an advocate of organotherapy, the use of testicular fluid for rejuvenation. In 1856 demonstrated the effect of adrenalectomy in animals.

TADEUS REICHSTEIN, 1897— . Polish-born Zurich chemist. During the 1930s synthesized several steroid hormones as well as vitamin C in 1933. Also studied cardiac glycosides and plant steroids and won the Nobel prize in 1950.

sis. A number of cytochrome P-450-related enzymes then successively hydroxylate the pregnenolone molecule, synthesizing specific corticosteroids.

Control of Adrenal Secretion

Cortisol secretion depends on the presence of anterior pituitary ACTH. ACTH is secreted in 8 to 12 pulses each 24 hours. The frequency of this episodic release increases during stress or other stimulation of pituitary hormone secretion. Cortisol secretion is responsive to these variations in ACTH release and also exhibits episodic increases and decreases in secretion. ACTH secretion also varies diurnally, characterized by high levels and more frequent spikes of secretion during the early morning and by lower levels with less frequent spikes during the late afternoon and evening.

ACTH secretion occurs in response to various "stresses" that cause release of hypothalamic CRH (corticotropin releasing hormone). CRH passes through the hypothalamic hypophyseal portal venous system to the anterior pituitary gland and stimulates release of ACTH (*see* Chap. 43). ACTH secretion is suppressed by "negative feedback": Plasma cortisol suppresses ACTH secretion directly at the pituitary and indirectly via inhibition of CRH secretion. During periods of severe stress, however, even high plasma corticosteroid levels fail to suppress ACTH secretion.

Aldosterone is secreted in response to a decrease in the effective circulating volume such as may occur after severe sodium depletion, hemorrhage, or dehydration. The significant mediator is *renin* secreted by the juxtaglomerular apparatus of the kidney to act on angiotensinogen to form angiotensin I, which is further metabolized by converting enzyme (predominantly in the lungs) to form angiotensin II. Angiotensin II has pressor effects and also stimulates the zona glomerulosa to secrete aldosterone. In addition, an elevated serum potassium level and a decreased serum sodium level directly stimulate aldosterone secretion. ACTH has some action to increase aldosterone secretion, but hypophysectomy does not completely stop production of aldosterone.

Androgenic effects in both sexes before puberty arise from adrenal steroids. These effects are chiefly controlled by ACTH, since their production is markedly reduced after hypophysectomy. Other factors are thought to be important, however, in bringing about the disproportionate increase in adrenal androgens as compared to cortisol production at the time of puberty.

ABSORPTION AND METABOLISM

These hormones are rapidly absorbed when taken by mouth. Peak levels of cortisol occur in the blood 30 to 60 minutes after ingestion. Although the chemical T½ of cortisol is only about 90 minutes, the biologic effects last for 6 to 12 hours or more. The T½ of aldosterone is 15 minutes.

Metabolism of the corticosteroids occurs chiefly in the liver, although some cortisol is converted to cortisone in peripheral tissues. Major effects of metabolism are the reduction of ketones in the 3 and 20 positions and the unsaturation at $\Delta 4-5$ (Fig. 47-1). Most of these reduced steroids are conjugated as glucuronides for excretion in the urine, although small amounts of the free compounds are also excreted. Because the amount of free steroid in the urine is proportional to the level of free "biologically active" hormone in the blood, urinary free cortisol is a good method for estimating adrenal activity. The metabolic products of the corticosteroids are measured by reactions that give values for 17-hydroxycorticosteroids, 17-ketogenic steroids, or 17-ketosteroids. 17-ketosteroids are chiefly a measure of androgens, whereas 17-ketogenic steroids and 17-hydroxycorticosteroids are chiefly metabolic products of cortisol.

MECHANISM OF ACTION

Corticosteroids (like other steroids) pass freely intracellularly and bind to cytosolic receptors present in almost all tissues. The steroid/receptor complex is modified or activated and passes into the nucleus, where it influences DNA-directed formation of messenger RNA involved in protein synthesis. Increased synthesis of specific RNA is responsible for synthesis of specific proteins. The enzymes shown to increase in response to corticosteroid administration are particularly those involved in gluconeogenesis, such as tyrosine amino transaminase and tryptophan pyrrolase.

Total RNA synthesis increases markedly after corticosteroid administration. This indicates an effect on more systems than those that have been studied in detail. In addition to those enzymes whose synthesis has been shown to be directly increased by an increase in mRNA, the synthesis of other proteins or enzymes may modify the activity of other enzymes. Cyclic AMP, through modification of protein phosphoxylation, may also influence corticosteroid activity. Corticosteroid action is not directly mediated by cyclic AMP activity, however, as is that of many peptide hormones.

The *permissive action* of the corticosteroids includes those activities that are not directly controlled by these hormones but that require their presence, including receptor-mediated activity of *glucagon, epinephrine,* and *ACTH* and enzymatic activity without increased enzyme synthesis. Some of these effects may result from modification of cellular membrane lipids (phospholipids and cholesterol).

Corticosteroids markedly influence the function of a number of specific tissues. Action on *leukocytes* is important in suppressing inflammation by suppressing chemotaxis and superoxide anion production. Suppression of phospholipase A2 and liberation of arachidonic acid from membrane phospholipids limit the substrate for prostaglandin synthesis. Long-term pharmacologic doses of corticosteroids *limit antibody production,* and, acutely, antigen/antibody reactions with cellular receptors are suppressed. Corticosteroids significantly *decrease collagen formation,* thereby limiting wound healing as well as bone matrix formation.

In large doses, the corticosteroids produce increased *sodium retention* and *hypertension* and contribute to the development of *atherosclerosis,* possibly by means of increased cholesterol synthesis. Although excessive retention of sodium results from increased aldosterone production, high levels of cortisol or corticosterone will also produce this effect. The hypertension is associated with hypervolemia. Many studies that have attempted to demonstrate a specific sodium-retaining steroid associated with essential hypertension have been unsuccessful.

CORTICOSTEROID BINDING IN THE CIRCULATION

Normally 10% to 15% of plasma cortisol (about 1 μg/dl) is free, the remainder being bound to a specific corticosteroid-binding globulin (CBG, transcortin) or to albumin. A considerable amount of plasma CBG is not associated with steroid, but, as the plasma level of the hormone rises, both CBG and albumin become increasingly saturated with cortisol, and there is increased hormone in the free state. Biologic effects result chiefly from the free fraction.

Plasma CBG increases during pregnancy or after estrogen administration. Thus at the end of the third trimester, a threefold increase in the amount of cortisol bound to CBG may occur, which means that plasma cortisol levels are more than doubled. Similar increases are seen after estrogen therapy, but there is no increase in biologic action of the corticosteroids under these circumstances. Progesterone also binds to CBG and can displace cortisol when the progesterone concentration is high, as in cord blood. Aldosterone binds poorly to CBG.

DEFICIENCY OR EXCESS OF ADRENAL SECRETION

Adrenal insufficiency results from loss of pituitary secretion of ACTH or decreased ability of the adrenal cortex to respond to ACTH.

Primary adrenal insufficiency (Addison's disease) is characterized by fatigue, hyperpigmentation (secondary to increased ACTH and β-lipotropin production by the pituitary), hypoglycemia when fasting, hyponatremia, hyperkalemia, decreased blood pressure, dehydration, and, in the late stages, shock and death. In *secondary adrenal insufficiency* due to loss of ACTH, the gland continues to produce aldosterone, and thus there are fewer electrolyte abnormalities. Stress may still, however, produce shock and death if cortisol is not administered.

Cushing's syndrome or adrenal hyperfunction may occur secondary to increased production of ACTH or autonomous production of corticosteroids by adrenal cortical tumors. More commonly Cushing's syndrome results iatrogenically from the excessive administration of corticosteroids as antiinflammatory agents. Typically patients complain of weakness and fatigue, easy bruisability, and weight gain. Increased emotional lability may also be present. Physical examination findings include plethora, hypertension, trunkal obesity, and hirsutism in females. Increased fat deposits produce the "moon face," a "buffalo hump" over the upper dorsal spine, and increased supraclavicular fat pads. In severe or long continued Cushing's syndrome demineralization of bone, increased susceptibility to infection, peptic ulcer disease, and cardiovascular complica-

---

THOMAS ADDISON, 1793—1860. London physician. First described Addison's disease in 1849, chronic adrenal insufficiency usually due to tubercular infection. Also distinguished between pernicious anemia and that caused by Addison's disease.

HARVEY WILLIAMS CUSHING, 1869—1939. American neurosurgeon and neurologist. Known for many classic studies of neurologic disease, in particular disorders of the pituitary, and for his pioneering brain surgery.

tions, including myocardial infarction and stroke, may occur.

INHIBITORS OF ADRENAL SECRETION

The most common suppressor of corticosteroid secretion is exogenous corticosteroid, which actively suppresses ACTH secretion. Chronic administration of corticosteroids results in adrenal atrophy. While the corticosteroids are being administered the patient feels fine, and after withdrawal of the hormone the adrenal gland quickly returns to normal in most cases as ACTH production returns. If such a patient is stressed, before adrenal regrowth, sufficient cortisol will not be secreted to protect against the stress, and *relative adrenal insufficiency* will result. In rare instances patients who have not received corticosteroid therapy for months and even years continue to have adrenal atrophy and less than a normal response to stress. These patients require treatment with corticosteroids when stressed.

A number of drugs reduce or inhibit ACTH release, including *cyproheptadine, metergoline, methysergide, morphine, barbiturates, reserpine,* and *chlorpromazine*. Reserpine and chlorpromazine may be either stimulatory or suppressant depending on the dose used. Bromocriptine (2-bromoergocryptine) suppresses ACTH secretion from pituitary tumors but not from the normal gland.

A number of drugs have direct effects on the adrenal gland to suppress or modify secretion, including *o, p'DDD, amphenone, metyrapone,* and *aminoglutethamide*. *Spironolactone* blocks aldosterone action by competing for receptor sites in the renal tubule (*see* Chap. 40).

Metyrapone is widely used in estimating adrenal function because it suppresses 11-hydroxylation during cortisol synthesis, causing a fall in plasma cortisol levels and an increase in 11-desoxycortisol (substance S). Since substance S has little glucocorticoid activity, plasma ACTH increases, with a subsequent ACTH-stimulated increase in substance S secretion by the adrenal cortex. A significant increase in plasma substance S and ACTH after metyrapone administration rules out either primary or secondary adrenal insufficiency.

THERAPEUTIC USES OF ADRENAL STEROIDS

Some therapeutic indications for corticosteroids are given in Table 47-1. Replacement

TABLE 47-1. Some Indications for the Corticoids

Acute and chronic adrenal insufficiency
Bronchial asthma
Hypopituitarism
Rheumatoid arthritis
Rheumatic carditis
Congenital adrenal hyperplasia
Cerebral edema
Lupus erythematosus
Nephrotic syndrome
Occular inflammations
Skin diseases
Leukemia

therapy for adrenal insufficiency is life-saving. Administration of 20 mg of cortisol in the a.m. and 10 mg in the p.m. is usually sufficient for patients with unstressed Addison's disease or hypopituitarism. In addisonian patients, 0.1 mg of flurohydrocortisone is added to increase sodium-retaining activity, but this is not necessary in patients with hypopituitarism.

Used as replacement therapy, the corticosteroids have almost no side-effects. Patients with prolonged untreated adrenal insufficiency may have increased sensitivity to the hormones, and psychotic reactions or marked sodium retention and edema may occur in response to normal amounts of hormones. This "deficiency sensitivity" may be due to increased availability of receptors; it disappears with continued therapy.

The most widely used corticosteroids are the synthetic analogues of cortisol (Fig. 47-2). These compounds have chiefly cortisol-like glucocorticoid activity, since mineralocorticoid aldosterone-like sodium-retaining activity has been largely eliminated by various chemical modifications of the steroid structure. For example, introduction of the 9α-fluorine, as in fludrocortisol, markedly increases its sodium-retaining activity. When combined with unsaturation of the 1,3 position and a methyl group in position 16, however, sodium-retaining activity decreases markedly.

All widely used synthetic corticosteroids have the 1,3 saturation seen in *prednisone* and *prednisolone*. These compounds have a half-life in the circulation of about 200 minutes and combine with aldosterone receptors less well than do aldosterone and cortisol. With the addition of 9α-fluorine and the 16 methyl group, dexamethasone or betamethasone is formed. These compounds have a long half-life (about 300 minutes) and also have reduced sodium-retaining activity and greatly increased glucocorticoid activity (Table 47-2). The Δ4-3 ketone is not significantly reduced by the liver in these steroids as it is in cortisol. Prednisone and dexamethasone are poorly bound to plasma proteins and thus produce considerable biologic effect when present in low concentration. The naturally occurring corticosteroids have the shortest half-lives, and the synthetic analogues, such as prednisone and dexamethasone, circulate for much longer periods. These compounds also have a reduced rate of reduction and conjugation for excretion in the urine. Increased potency indicates only that fewer milligrams must be given to produce a desired effect, not that the biologic activity is qualitatively different. The mechanism of action of these synthetic corticosteroids is thought to be the same as that for naturally occurring cortisol, but receptors for dexamethasone exist in some cell types that are different from the cortisol receptors.

THERAPEUTIC USES OF SYNTHETIC GLUCOCORTICOID ANALOGUES

Corticosteroids are used chiefly for their antiinflammatory effect, which probably occurs at three levels: the *suppression of leukocyte activity; immunosuppression;* and suppression of *receptor-mediated tissue response* to antigen–antibody complexes and other ligands.

Corticosteroid effects on leukocytes are multifactorial, leading to suppression of leukocyte accumulation and release of potentially tissue destructive substances (free radicals and enzymes active in the production of the inflammatory response). Pharmacologic doses suppress *leukocyte adherence, chemotaxis,* and *superoxide anion production* and block *prostaglandin* release owing to inhibition of phospholipase A2. The phospholipase A2 releases archidonic acid from phospholipids to act as a substrate for prostaglandin formation. Very large doses of corticosteroids stabilize lysosomes, preventing release of their enzymes, thus reducing the inflammatory reaction.

TABLE 47-2. Relative Antiinflammatory Activities of Corticosteroids*

Antiinflammatory Agent	
Cortisol (Cortef)	1 (1†)
Prednisone	3 (5†)
Dexamethasone (Decadron)	20 (150†)
Aldosterone	<1
Desoxycorticosterone	<1
Fludrocortisone (Florinef)	15

* Effect obtained depends on the time after dosage at which response is measured.

† These relative values are ACTH suppression 14 hours after a single oral dose.

Glucocorticoids slowly suppress antibody production. High doses of glucocorticoids given for weeks produce lower serum immunoglobulin levels and may convert a positive tuberculin skin test to a negative one. Acutely, corticoids produce a redistribution of lymphocytes to sites outside the circulation and reduce the numbers of both T and B cells; there is a preferential decrease in helper T cells.

Rheumatoid arthritis, systemic lupus erythematosus, and various vasculitides may result from local immune complex formation, leading to inflammation, destruction, and fibrosis. Glucocorticoids inhibit immune-complex cellular receptor interaction. The antiinflammatory action of the corticoids functions at all levels of immune-mediated inflammation. An effect with high doses appears to be intercalation of the steroids into lipid membranes. In more moderate doses, the hormones modify the lipid composition and fluidity of the membranes. Physiologic and moderate pharmacologic doses of the corticosteroids act on intracellular receptors to increase the synthesis of specific proteins that mediate the response.

The therapeutic dosage of corticosteroids depends on the condition being treated and the duration of action required. Thirty milligrams of cortisol given in divided doses of 20 mg in the a.m. and 10 mg in the late afternoon most nearly equals normal diurnal variation in corticosteroid secretion and produces no significant side-effects. The conditions most often treated with this drug and dosage are Addison's disease, hypopituitarism, and congenital adrenal hyperplasia. The longer-acting analogues are avoided because they are likely to produce the complications of long-term therapy and have no sodium-retaining activity to replace the loss of aldosterone seen in primary insufficiency.

Rheumatic diseases are usually treated first with salicylates and other nonsteroidal antiinflammatory agents. Failure to respond to these drugs often leads to prednisone administration in a dosage of 5 to 15 mg every 12 to 24 hours. An alternate-day regimen will usually not control these conditions. In the therapy of inflammatory manifestations (serositis, pericarditis, and pleuritis) of systemic lupus erythematosus, high dosage of 40 to 60 mg of prednisone a day in divided doses is required initially, but a single daily or every-other-day equivalent dose may be used to maintain control of the disease. It is not certain why variations in dosage and frequency of administration are required in different conditions.

The use of *"pulse" therapy* (1 g of methylprednisolone intravenously daily for 3 days followed by a rest period) is controversial. Prednisone in the range of 60 to 100 mg daily may give similar results. Glucocorticoids (1–3 g doses) may be life-saving in treating severe shock. The steroids possibly intercalate into vascular membranes, stabilize lysosomes, and prevent anoxia- and toxin-induced cellular breakdown.

Mineralocorticoids are used sparingly in therapeutics. Their chief indication is as replacement therapy for aldosterone deficiency in Addison's disease or primary adrenal insufficiency. In these cases 0.1 to 0.2 mg of fluorohydrocortisone is used daily. Excessive dosage may result in sodium retention and hypertension, whereas insufficient dosage fails to correct the pathologically increased sodium excretion and hyperkalemia. Fluorohydrocortisone (0.5–1 mg) has been used in treating severe postural hypotension, where it acts to retain sodium and water and expand the extracellular volume. Continued use in high dosage may, however, produce potassium depletion and hypertension. Hypertension may be present at night, and thus blood pressure should be checked before the patient assumes the erect position.

ADVERSE EFFECTS

Pharmacologic doses of corticosteroids (equivalent of 40 mg cortisol or greater per day) for prolonged periods lead to all of the complications associated with Cushing's syndrome. Patients may have increased appetite and weight, truncal obesity, muscular atrophy, loss of bone matrix and demineralization of bone, aseptic necrosis of bone, impaired wound healing, increased sensitivity to infections, psychotic episodes, peptic ulcer disease, a diabetogenic state, acne, hypertension, and development of posterior subcapsular cataracts or glaucoma. Patients often develop the typical cushinoid appearance of a rounded plethoric face, hirsutism, and purple stria of the abdomen.

SPECIFIC MEASURES DIRECTED TOWARD HARMFUL EFFECTS OF CORTICOSTEROIDS

Salt retention, a concomitant of high dosage of all of the naturally occurring corticosteroids, leads to overexpansion of the extracellular volume and in some cases to hypertension. Patients seldom develop edema, however, because of the "escape mechanism" that allows the kidney to excrete sodium in the presence of sodium-retaining steroids when the extracellular space becomes expanded. Patients with other conditions predisposing to edema, such as heart, liver, or kidney disease, may have sodium retention and edema accentuated by corticosteroid therapy. These steroids also produce increased potassium excretion that requires dietary potassium supplementation. Increased sodium retention is minimized or avoided by using synthetic analogues such as prednisone and dexamethasone.

Osteoporosis and demineralization of bone predisposing to fractures is one of the most severe complications of long-term therapy. Corticosteroids interfere with collagen formation and formation of bone matrix. Decreased intestinal calcium absorption and increased urinary excretion of calcium also occur. There is no known treatment for the inhibitory effect on collagen formation. The effect on vitamin D metabolism is controversial. 1,25-Dihydroxy vitamin D increases intestinal absorption of calcium in glucocorticoid-treated patients and may be useful in preventing calcium loss.

Adrenal atrophy occurs in all patients who receive pharmacologic doses of glucocorticoids. Depression of ACTH secretion leads to reduced adrenal weight and secretory capacity within a few days of initiating therapy. Considerably less atrophy occurs if corticosteroids are given in a single dose on alternate days. Adrenal atrophy causes the patient no immediate harm but must be compensated for by increased corticosteroid dosage when the patient is stressed or after therapy is stopped if normal adrenal regeneration has not occurred.

Severe muscle weakness and atrophy owing to the catabolic and antianabolic effect of the corticoids occur. Uptake of glucose and amino acids by the muscle tissue is decreased. Triamcinolone and other 9α-flourine analogues may be more harmful in producing this effect. Therapy with the anabolic androgens may compensate partially for these negative effects on muscles. Glucocorticoids prevent normal wound healing primarily because of inhibition of collagen synthesis. Inhibition of growth is seen in children, resulting partially from inhibition of growth hormone secretion as well as the general catabolic effect of the corticosteroid. It is not practical, however, to administer growth hormone as replacement to children receiving corticoids.

Corticosteroids may exacerbate or encourage a variety of *infections*, particularly certain viral infections, such as herpes simplex keratitis and chickenpox, and those associated with delayed hypersensitivity, such as tuberculosis.

Corticosteroid use should be avoided in these conditions. Action of these hormones to reduce inflammation, the immune response, and leukocyte function exacerbates most infective processes. Close observation and early antibiotic therapy are indicated in the corticoid-treated patient.

Corticosteroids have been implicated in causing *peptic ulcer disease,* although this is controversial. Adequate antacid therapy is indicated for the patient with a history of peptic ulcer placed on corticoid therapy.

Topical corticosteroids are used widely for the therapy of various dermatologic conditions. Generally they have only local effects but, when applied in large doses to inflamed areas, may be absorbed in sufficient quantity to produce systemic harmful effects. Similarly, steroids given rectally for inflammatory bowel disease may be absorbed and exert systemic effects.

FURTHER READING

1. DeGroot LJ, Cahill GF, Odell WD, Martini L, Potts JT, Nelson DH, Steinberger E, Winegrad AI (eds): Endocrinology (3 volumes). New York, Grune and Stratton, 1979
2. Nelson DH: The Adrenal Cortex: Physiologic Function and Disease. Philadelphia, W B Saunders, 1980
3. Nelson AM, Conn DL: Glucocorticoids in rheumatic disease. Mayo Clin Proc 55:758–769, 1980
4. Baxter JD, Rousseau GG (eds): Glucocorticoid Hormone Action. Berlin, Springer–Verlag, 1979

CHAPTER 47 QUESTIONS

(See P. 7 for Full Instructions)

Select the One Best Answer

1. The glucocorticoids may produce each of the following EXCEPT
   A. psychosis.
   B. myopathies.
   C. lowered seizure threshold.
   D. sodium depletion.
   E. potassium depletion.

2. Each of the following is true of ACTH EXCEPT that it
   A. may be used to test functional integrity of the adrenal cortex.
   B. is not effective by the oral route.
   C. can cause allergic manifestations.
   D. can be used in any condition that responds to adrenal steroids.
   E. may be effective therapy for certain convulsive disorders.

3. Corticosteroids are of value in the treatment of each of the following EXCEPT
   A. refractory asthma.
   B. edema of the brain.
   C. chronic lymphatic leukemia.
   D. resistance to insulin.
   E. osteoarthritis.

4. Each of the following disorders could be exacerbated by high doses of glucocorticoids EXCEPT
   A. diabetes mellitus.
   B. glaucoma.
   C. systemic lupus erythematosus.
   D. infection.
   E. hypertension.

A = 1,2,3; B = 1,3; C = 2,4; D = 4; E = All

5. Corticosteroids
   1. suppress contact dermatitis.
   2. are used in replacement therapy of Addison's disease.
   3. ameliorate the severity of the nephrotic syndrome.
   4. can be used as the sole agent in treating herpes infections of the eye.

6. Methylprednisolone
   1. has a high glucocorticoid/mineralocorticoid activity ratio.
   2. withdrawal may result in marked adrenal insufficiency.
   3. is useful in the management of rheumatic carditis.
   4. increases patient susceptibility to tuberculosis.

7. All steroidal antiinflammatory drugs
   1. have potent glucocorticoid activity.
   2. cause disturbances in the pituitary–adrenal axis.
   3. have the ability to induce a cushingoid state.
   4. can reduce resistance to infection.

8. 9-α-Flurocortisol has which of the following characteristics?
   1. High potency for promotion of sodium retention
   2. Effective in microgram (50–100) quantities
   3. Seldom produces edema in normal subjects
   4. High concentration in adrenal cortex.

9. Chronic administration of high doses of corticosteroids may result in
   1. fluid loss and dehydration.
   2. reduced glucose tolerance and hyperglycemia.
   3. increased resistance to viral infections.
   4. decreased growth.

MORTIMER B. LIPSETT

48 Pharmacology of Androgens and Estrogens

Androgen, estrogen, and *progestin* are operational definitions for compounds that have specific actions: stimulation of growth of prostate (androgens) and uterus (estrogens) are appropriate examples. In humans, the important steroids of these classes are testosterone (androgen), estradiol (estrogen), and progesterone (progestin), which are secreted primarily by testis and ovary, but adrenal cortex and placenta also can secrete them. Additionally, testosterone and estradiol can be formed in many tissues of the body from closely related precursors, but only the endocrine glands and placenta can synthesize steroids *de novo* from basic compounds such as acetate or cholesterol. Many synthetic androgens, estrogens, and progestins differ in potency and biologic properties.

BIOSYNTHESIS

Serum cholesterol is the important precursor of ovarian and testicular steroid hormones, although both glands use acetete to synthesize sterols and steroids. The testis and ovary use the same biosynthetic sequences (Fig. 48-1) except that the specific enzyme activities vary between the glands. The conversion of cholesterol to pregnenolone, the first steroid, is regulated by luteinizing hormone (LH) that acts presumably by stimulating one or more of the enzymatic processes that lead to oxidation and subsequent scission of the cholesterol side-chain between C_{21} and C_{22}. Certain drugs interfere with specific enzymatic steps, blocking cholesterol synthesis (aminoglutethimide), oxidation at C_{11} (the final step leading to cortisol) (metyrapone), and aromatization (aminoglutethimide). Aminoglutethimide has been used to treat women with breast cancer and metyrapone to test for the pituitary's ability to secrete ACTH. The placenta and the luteinized granulosa cells of the corpus luteum are deficient in the enzyme, 17 α-hydroxylase, so that steroid synthesis in these glands from early precursors stops at progesterone.

MECHANISM OF ACTION

All steroid hormones act similarly. The steroid diffuses across the plasma membrane and binds to a specific protein receptor in the cyto-

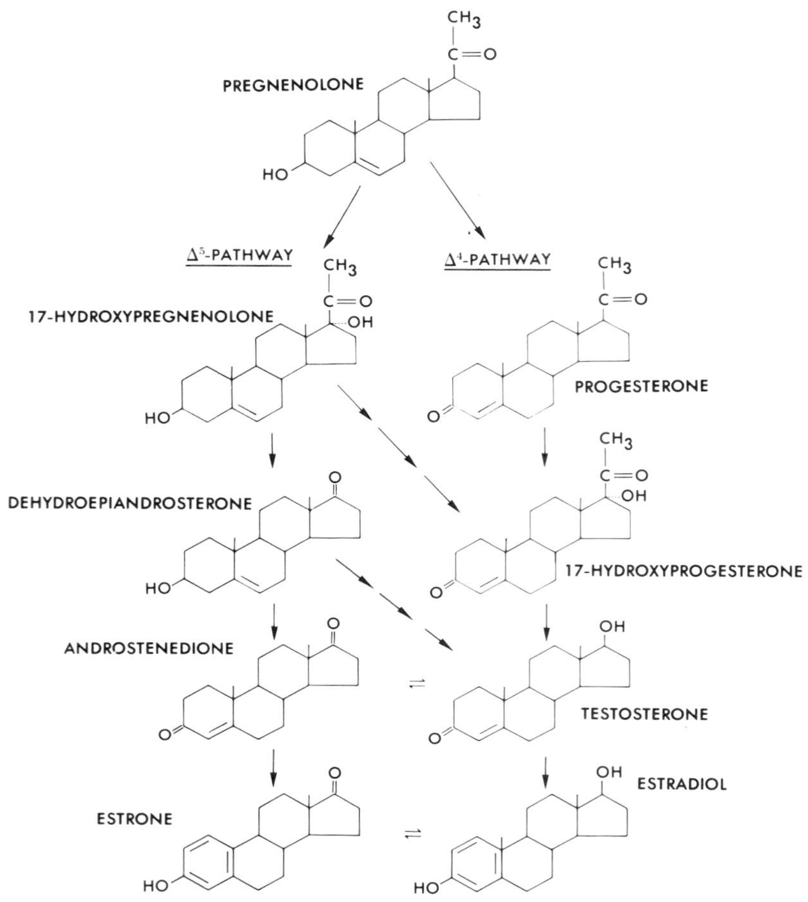

FIG. 48-1. Biosynthesis of androgens and estrogens.

sol. These receptors have the following characteristics: *high binding affinity, biologic specificity,* easily *saturable,* and *present in highest concentrations* in those cells that are targets for the specific hormone. Binding affinity is, generally proportional to biologic activity, although some antiestrogens and antiandrogens also have high binding affinities. The steroid-receptor complex undergoes a temperature-dependent conformational change and diffuses into the nucleus, where it binds to specific sites on the nonhistone proteins of chromatin, initiating transcription of RNA and new protein synthesis.

Testosterone differs from the other steroid hormones in that it is reduced by a cytosol 5 α-reductase in most androgen-responsive tissues to *dihydrotestosterone,* the active proximate androgen with receptor binding affinity about 20 times that of testosterone.

ARNOLD ADOLF BERTHOLD, 1803–1861. German physician and anatomist. In 1849 reported that comb growth (a secondary male characteristic) could be induced in castrated roosters by transplantation of testicular tissue, one of the foundation stones of hormone research.

EDGAR ALLEN, 1892–1943. American endocrinologist. With E. A. Doisy in 1924, described the induction of sexual maturity by injecting a partially purified preparation of estrogen.

EDWARD ADELBERT DOISY, 1893– . St. Louis physiologist and biochemist. With others, prepared crystalline ovarian hormones, such as estradiol, in the 1920s and 1930s. Isolated crystalline vitamin K in 1939, and in 1943 shared the Nobel Prize with H. Dam, who had discovered this coagulation factor in 1934.

ADOLF FRIEDRICH JOHANN BUTENANDT, 1903– German biochemist. Synthesized crystalline progesterone in 1931 and testosterone in 1935. Also studied insecticides, and won the Nobel Prize in 1939.

FREDERICK CONRAD KOCH, 1876–1948. Chicago biochemist. In 1929 reported the first isolation of a potent testicular extract.

ANDROGENS

MAJOR ACTIONS

Androgens act at many sites. Testosterone is necessary for spermatogenesis and for the structure and function of prostate and seminal vesicles. Function of these two exocrine glands can be assessed by measuring acid phosphatase and fructose, respectively, in semen. The pilosebaceous apparatus is sensitive to androgen, and the growth of sexual hair (ears, beard, mustache, and, to a lesser extent, chest, axillary, and pubic) depends on androgen action. Recession of the temporal hair line and male pattern baldness are also evidences of androgen effect. Androgens induce thickening of the vocal cords, relative increases in muscle size, polycythemia through enhanced secretion of erythropoeitin, rugosity of the scrotum, and increased bone growth at open epiphyseal plates.

PHYSIOLOGY

Adult men secrete 3 to 10 mg of testosterone daily, resulting in plasma concentrations of 300 to 900 ng/dl. Within this wide normal range of concentrations, no differences can be discerned in physiological or psychologic behavior. A daily production rate of as little as 2 mg of testosterone is sufficient to virilize a normal woman.

Androgen operates in a negative feedback mode in the hypothalamic–pituitary system that regulates gonadotropin secretion. These effects in men are mediated by androgen acting at androgen receptors, and in part by estradiol, secreted by the testis and synthesized, peripherally from testosterone, acting via estrogen receptors.

ABSORPTION, METABOLISM, AND EXCRETION

Blood testosterone is bound to a β-globulin (sex-steroid-binding globulin, or SSBG), with an affinity sufficiently high so that only 1% to 1.5% is free at equilibrium. Thus to evaluate testosterone levels precisely, a knowledge of the binding capacity of SSBG is necessary. SSBG is increased by estrogen, thyroxine, in cirrhosis, and idiopathically. It is decreased by androgen administration, in obesity, or when there are large protein losses from the circulation, as in the nephrotic syndrome.

The liver extracts and metabolizes more than 80% of the free testosterone in a single pass (*see* Chap. 4), thereby accounting for the ineffectiveness of orally administered hormone. Testosterone is cleared rapidly from the blood, with a T½ of about 50 minutes. The many metabolites of testosterone are usually conjugated with glucosiduronic acid or sulfate, and about 40% of these are measurable in the urine as 17-ketosteroids (17-KS), predominantly *androsterone* and *etiocholanolone*. However, only 20% of the urinary 17-KS is derived from testosterone in man, the rest originating from adrenal dehydroepiandrosterone. Thus urinary 17-KS excretion is an inadequate index of Leydig cell function.

PREPARATIONS

Many synthetic androgens (Table 48-1, Fig. 48-2) have been developed that have the advantage of being active orally, the 17 α-methyl group protecting them against first-pass hepatic inactivation. They differ somewhat in the ratio of androgenic to anabolic activity, but none of them is without androgenic effect. Mi-

FRANZ VON LEYDIG, 1821–1908. German anatomist. Described as the founder of comparative histology. In 1850 reported on the interstitial cells, the Leydig cells, of the testes.

TABLE 48-1. Preparations of Androgens

Preparation	Common Route of Administration	Common Dose Range*
Testosterone propionate	i.m.	25 mg i.m. 3 ×/wk
Testosterone enanthate (Delatestryl)	i.m.	300 mg q 3 wk
Testosterone cypionate (Depo-Testosterone cypionate)	i.m.	300 mg q 3 wk
Methyltestosterone	Sublingual	10–20 mg
Fluoxymesterone (Halotestin)	p.o.	10–20 mg
Methandrostenolone (Dianabol)	p.o.	5 mg
Ethylestrenol (Maxibolin)	p.o.	5–15 mg
Stanazalol (Winstrol)	p.o.	5–10 mg
Oxandrolone (Anavar)	p.o.	2.5–10 mg

* These doses are given as androgen replacement therapy.

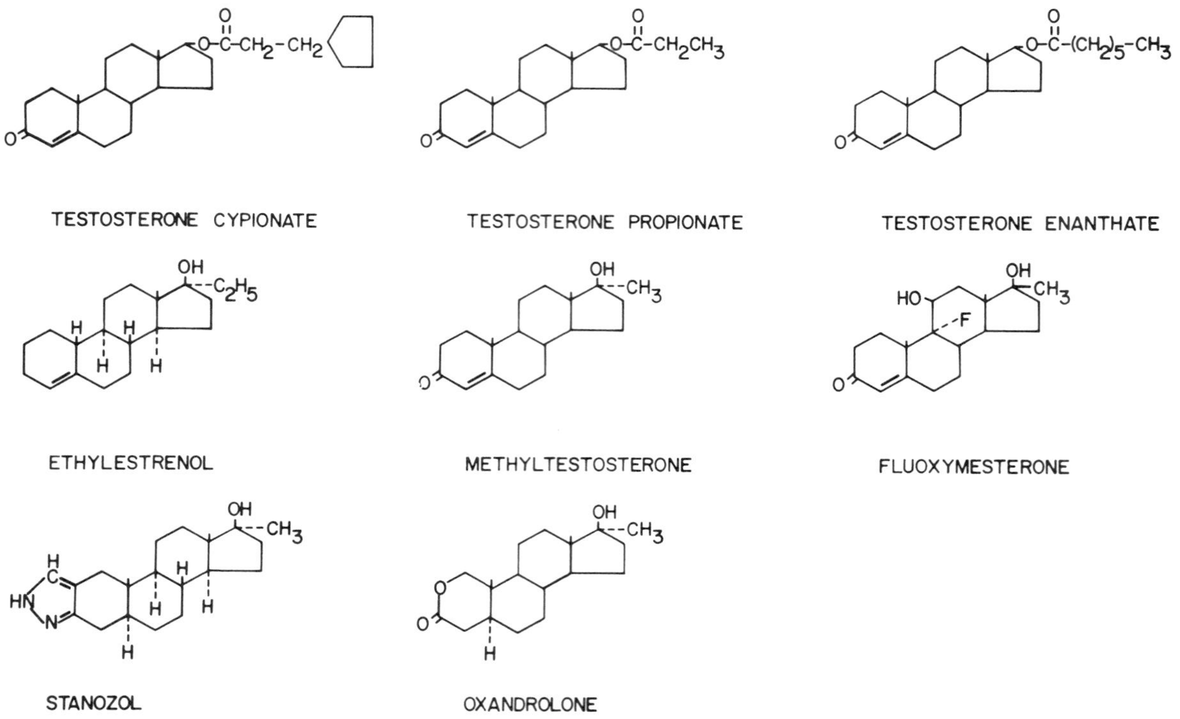

FIG. 48-2. Structural formulae of synthetic androgens.

cronized testosterone and testosterone undecanoate are undergoing clinical trials, since significant amounts are absorbed via the lacteals into the thoracic duct, thus bypassing the liver.

CLINICAL USES

Androgens are used at physiologic doses in patients with Leydig cell failure and pharmacologically in several conditions. Replacement therapy is indicated in hypogonadotropic hypogonadism, in some boys with delayed puberty, and in patients with Leydig cell failure such as Klinefelter's syndrome and the vanishing testis syndrome. The esterified androgens, testosterone cypionate or enanthate in oil, maintain effective blood testosterone levels at dosages of 200 mg intramuscularly every other week or 300 mg intramuscularly every third week. Some men will respond satisfactorily to methyl testosterone, to halotestin, or to other oral agents. Generally, however, long-acting testosterone preparations are more satisfactory as replacement therapy.

Oral androgens or testosterone propionate in oil are useful in treating women with metastatic breast cancer; the remission rate is about 20%, and the median duration of remission is 5 months. Long-acting testosterone preparations should not be used because, occasionally, androgens may accelerate the course of metastatic cancer.

Androgens in large doses have been useful in some patients with acquired or constitutional aplastic anemia (possibly by stimulating erythropoietin synthesis) and in patients with renal failure. Months of treatment may be required in aplastic anemia, but when a remission develops it is usually sustained.

Androgens in small doses have been used experimentally to increase the heights of boys and girls whose growth charts predict small stature. Such trials must be run by experienced endocrinologists because androgens both accelerate long bone growth and hasten epiphyseal closure; thus these opposing effects must be balanced by careful observation and titration of dose.

The use of androgens as anabolic agents by male and female athletes is now common. Their use is based on the obvious disparity of muscle mass between men and women. Continuous androgen administration in men will produce only limited nitrogen retention, of which most is retained by parenchymal tissue rather than by muscle. The results of trials in animals and men have been conflicting so that one cannot yet conclude that athletic performance can be improved. In several double-blind cross-over studies, anabolic agents have produced small but measurable increases in sports performance such as weight lifting, where isometric contraction is an important component of the process. Anabolic androgens reversibly suppress spermatogenesis by lowering luteinizing hormone levels, with consequent decreased Leydig cell secretion of testosterone and low concentration of testosterone at the seminiferous tubule.

Systematic studies of androgen use in female athletes have not been reported, although, in conjunction with training, they would probably confer significant advantage. Side-effects of hirsutism, virilization, and menstrual disturbances are formidable and constitute medical and ethical barriers to their use.

Since androgens are anabolic, they have been tried in situations where it was thought desirable to promote protein deposition. They have not, however, proved useful in such conditions as prematurity, postsurgical convalescence, delayed wound healing, and aging. Combinations of androgens and estrogens in small doses are still being promoted for use in geriatric patients but are theoretically unsound and have never been proved useful.

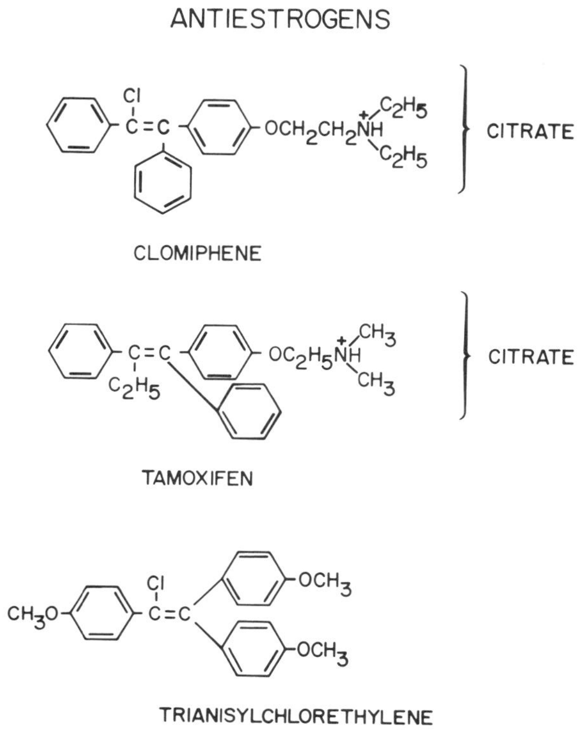

FIG. 48-3. Structural formulae of antiestrogens. Trianisylchlorethylene is a long-acting estrogen; tamoxifen and clomiphene are antiestrogens.

ADVERSE EFFECTS

Generally, adverse effects are normal responses in inappropriate situations, such as virilization and menstrual disturbances in women, decreased stature owing to premature epiphyseal closure in children, acne, and gynecomastia.

The 17 α-methylated androgens may impair bile secretion and produce reversible cholestasis. Prolonged use of high doses of synthetic androgens in aplastic anemia may produce peliosis hepatis and rarely hepatocellular carcinoma.

ANTIANDROGENS

Since sexual hair growth depends on androgens, androgenic effects on the pilosebaceous apparatus should be inhibited. Many progestins are antiandrogenic; the only one being used clinically is *cyproterone acetate,* a derivative of the 17-acetoxyprogestins (Fig. 48-3). This steroid is a potent progestational agent, suppresses gonadotropins, and inhibits androgen action. It has proved very useful in acne and moderately so in idiopathic hirsutism. Cyproterone acetate is not available in the United States because of its reputed carcinogenic potential (*see* below).

ESTROGENS

PHYSIOLOGY

In the menstruating woman, the ovarian follicles secrete *estradiol* and *estrone* during the first half of the follicular phase; with selection and growth of a dominant follicle, plasma estradiol increases rapidly, triggering the release of LH, ovulation, and corpus luteum formation (Fig. 48-4). Plasma estradiol levels are about 50 pg/ml in the early follicular phase and increase to 300 to 500 pg/ml just before ovulation. During the luteal phase, the corpus luteum maintains plasma estradiol concentrations at about 200 pg/ml.

After menopause with the disappearance of the last follicle, estrogen secretion ceases. Estrone becomes the predominant blood estrogen, being derived almost exclusively from periph-

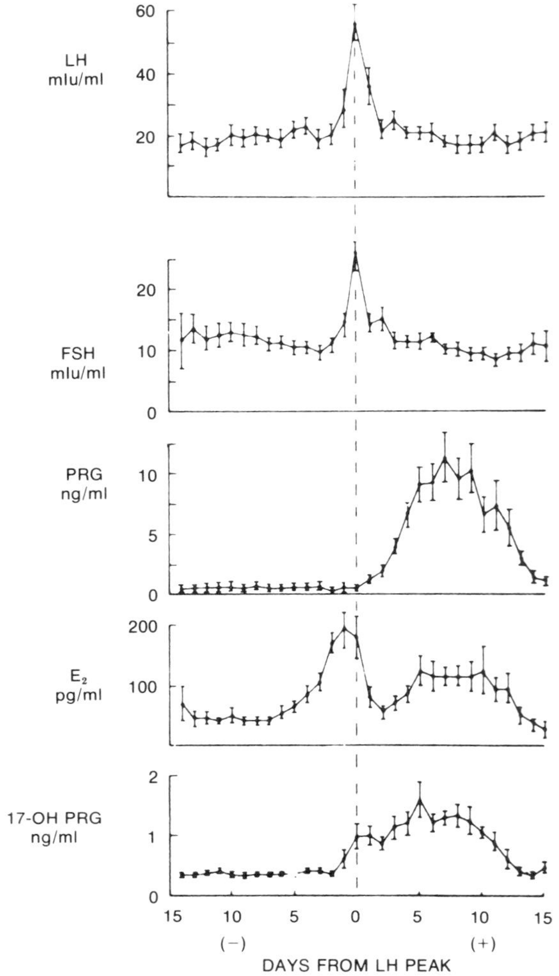

FIG. 48-4. Hormone patterns during the normal menstrual cycle. LH = luteinizing hormone; FSH = follicle-stimulating hormone; PRG = progesterone; E_2 = estradiol; 170H PRG = 17-hydroxyprogesterone.

eral aromatization of adrenal cortical androstenedione.

ABSORPTION, METABOLISM, AND EXCRETION

Estradiol and estrone are extensively metabolized, but the two main routes are by 16 α-hydroxylation and 2-hydroxylation (Fig. 48-5). Both estriol and 2-hydroxyestrone are produced in the liver and conjugated there so that little free steroid enters the plasma. The plasma concentration of both steroids is below 10 pg/ml. Estriol and 2-hydroxyestrone are weak estrogens only having about 25% and 2%, respectively, of the affinity of estradiol for estrogen receptors.

Urinary estrogen excretion is a poor guide to blood estrogen levels and is of little clinical significance except in pregnancy, where its excretion can be related to the health of the fetus. About two thirds of the urinary estrogens during pregnancy are derived from fetal adrenal secretion of dehydroepiandrosterone and its metabolism to estrogens by the placenta. In fetal hypoxia, as occurs in poorly controlled diabetes or Rh incompatibility, the adrenal secretory activity fails.

Estradiol and estrone are readily absorbed from the bowel but undergo some metabolism and conjugation by gut tissues. Additionally most of the absorbed estrogen is hydroxylated and conjugated on first pass through the liver. Thus high doses of these estrogens by mouth are needed to achieve normal blood levels; in so doing, the liver is exposed to high doses of estrogens.

Micronized estradiol, a preparation of crystalline estradiol, is metabolized to estrone by mucosal enzymes and absorbed via the lacteals, thus entering the systemic circulation by way of the thoracic duct. This bypass of the liver renders the estradiol preparation effective by mouth.

Estrogen creams and suppositories are used vaginally to treat keratosis and dyspareunia attributable to estrogen insufficiency, usually after menopause. Estrogens are well absorbed through the vaginal mucosa so that the effects noted are probably due to a systemic effect of the hormone. Similarly, estrogens produce systemic effects when used in large amounts topically due to absorption through the skin.

Modifications of the route of administration and of the estrogen itself allow the hormone to bypass the liver and reach the systemic circulation. The commonly used estrogens (Fig. 48-6) *ethinyl estradiol, estrone sulfate,* and *diethylstilbestrol* are effective orally. Differences in potency are due to differing rates of hepatic metabolism, clearance from the circulation, and binding affinity for the estrogen receptor. The mode of action of any of the strong estrogens is not fundamentally different because all of their physiologic effects are mediated by the estrogen receptor.

Blood estradiol is bound to SSBG less strongly than is testosterone. It is rapidly cleared from the blood, with a T½ of about 40 minutes. A metabolite of estradiol, *estrone sulfate,* is the most abundant estrogen in blood because it is tightly bound to albumin and cleared very slowly.

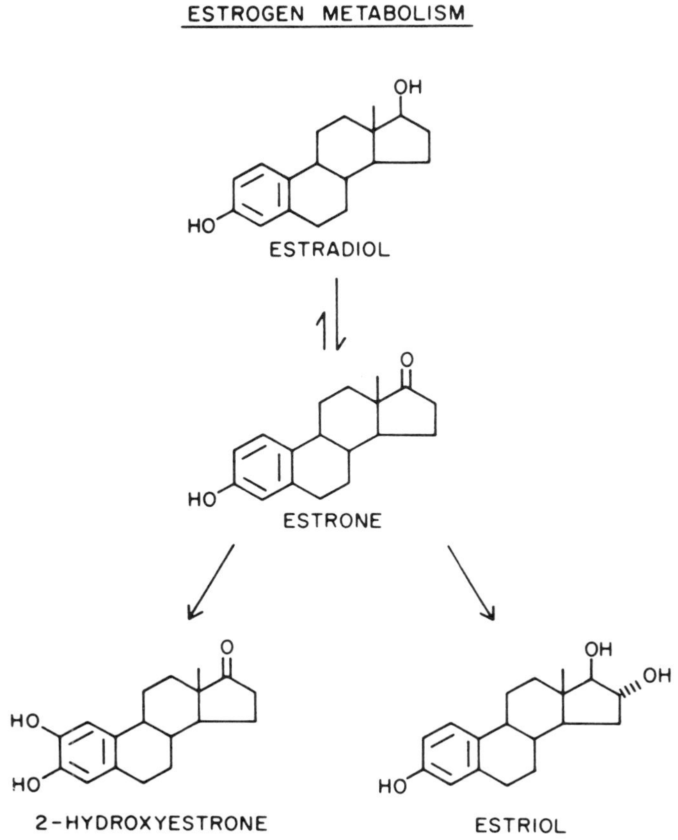

FIG. 48-5. Metabolism of estradiol.

FIG. 48-6. Formulae of estrogens.

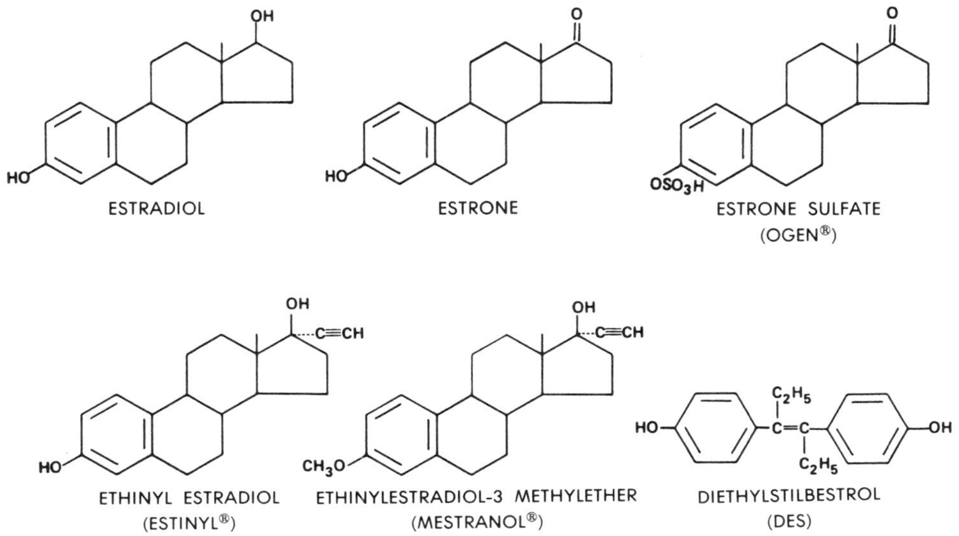

Certain weak estrogens act as both agonists and antagonists. Their estrogenic effects can be seen in the ovariectomized animal; in the presence of estrogen they are effective antagonists. The two agents that have found the greatest clinical usefulness are *clomiphene citrate* and *tamoxifen* (Fig. 48-3). Both are related to the long-acting estrogen, trianisylchlorethylene.

PREPARATIONS AND CLINICAL USE

Estrogens may be used to replace the ovarian secretions after ovariectomy or menopause. The lowest effective dose equivalent to estradiol's secretion rate of about 50 μg/24 hours during the follicular phase of the menstrual cycle should be used. Roughly equivalent doses of orally active estrogens are given in Table 48-2.

Postmenopausally estrogens may be used safely for 6 months to 2 years to treat *severe hot flashes*. Estrogens are useful in slowing the rate of bone resorption and skeletal calcium loss that apparently accelerates after menopause. Not all postmenopausal women should be given estrogens. Not only are there risks involved (*see* below), but not all women are equally susceptible to accelerated bone loss and osteoporosis.

Estrogens in large doses (1–5 mg of diethylstilbestrol or equivalent) are useful in women with metastatic breast carcinoma or in men with metastatic prostatic carcinoma. A 60% remission rate may be expected in women with estrogen-receptor-positive cancer; the median duration of remission is 9 months. The mechanism of action is unknown. In men, estrogen suppresses testosterone secretion directly by inhibiting the Leydig cell and indirectly by suppressing LH production. Results of estrogen therapy are equivalent to those of orchiectomy; in both cases there is a 70% remission rate that lasts about 9 months.

Two weak estrogen agonists have found wide therapeutic use as antagonists. *Clomiphene* competes successfully with estradiol for the estrogen receptor blocking its action. In women with adequate estradiol blood levels but anovulatory cycles, clomiphene causes a release of gonadotropins and induces ovulation. *Tamoxifen* acts as an antagonist in the presence of estradiol and is now the agent of choice for treating many women with metastatic breast cancer.

The "interceptive" effect of large doses of estrogens has been exploited to prevent unwanted pregnancy. Following rape or unprotected intercourse, 25 to 50 mg of diethylstilbestrol has been used to interrupt corpus luteum function and thereby precipitate endometrial bleeding.

TABLE 48-2. Estrogens

Chemical Classification	Example	Common Route of Administration	Common Dose Range
			mg
Naturally occurring estrogen	Estradiol-17-β		
Semisynthetic steroid estrogens	Ethynylestradiol (Esteed, Estinyl)	p.o.	0.02–0.05
	Mestranol	p.o.	05–0.1
	Quinestrol (Estrovis)	p.o.	0.05–0.1
Long-acting	Estradiol valerate (Delestrogen)	i.m.	10–20
Long-acting	Estradiol cypionate	i.m.	5–10
Nonsteroidal estrogens	Diethylstilbestrol (Stilbitin)	p.o.	0.2–1
	Hexestrol	p.o.	3–6
	Methallenestril (Vallestril)	p.o.	3–6
	Chlorotrianisene (Tace)	p.o.	10–20
Polymeric estrogen	Polyestradiol phosphate (Estradurin)	i.m.	40
Conjugated estrogen	Estrone sulfonate (Ogen) (Premarin)	p.o.	0.5–1
	Mixture of estrogen		0.6–1.2

Estrogens are not useful in preventing habitual abortion or in maintaining pregnancy in threatened abortion. The use of estrogens during the first trimester of pregnancy has resulted in an increased risk of adenocarcinoma of the cervix and vagina in women born from that pregnancy.

ADVERSE EFFECTS

Estrogens given after menopause maintain the endometrium and the ductal epithelium of the breast and thereby increase the opportunity for carcinogenesis. The risk of endometrial or breast cancer increases with the duration of estrogen use; 10 years of use increases the risk of endometrial and breast cancer about ten-fold and twofold, respectively. Thus the benefits of postmenopausal estrogens must be weighed against these risks.

Estrogen administration may produce temporary nausea and, in older persons or in patients with heart or kidney disease, may induce salt and water retention.

Estrogens stimulate hepatic synthesis of several proteins: cortisol-binding globulin, thyroxine-binding globulin, sex-steroid binding globulin, ceruloplasmin, α_1-antitrypsin, renin substrate, and certain components of the clotting system. The increase levels of hormone-binding proteins alter the kinetics of such hormones as cortisol, thyroxine, and testosterone and the interpretation of plasma levels. The increase of renin substrate is associated with hypertension in about 5% of women who use oral contraceptives.

PROGESTINS

SECRETORY CONTROL

Progesterone is secreted in small amounts by the ovary during the follicular phase of the menstrual cycle and by the adrenal cortex. With the development of the corpus luteum, the secretion rate rises from 50 μg/day to 1 to 2 mg/day. Progesterone secretion is initiated at, or even slightly before, ovulation and is enhanced by LH (Fig. 48-4). Elevations in both FSH and LH occur before the increased secretion of progesterone into the blood. If the ovum is not fertilized, progesterone secretion from the corpus luteum gradually diminishes until the end of the cycle.

ACTIONS

During the luteal phase of the cycle, progesterone acts on the estrogen-primed uterus to stimulate endometrial growth and development in preparation for implantation and growth support of the fertilized ovum. These actions of progesterone are manifest only after priming by estrogens. Thus the actions of estrogen and progesterone on the uterus are synergistic.

If fertilization does not occur, the uterine endometrium is sloughed and menstruation occurs. If fertilization occurs, the life span of the corpus luteum is maintained by chorionic (placental) gonadotropin (HCG). When conception occurs, the corpus luteum continues to secrete progesterone for about 2 months, and the uterine lining continues to grow and to proliferate. Placental synthesis of progesterone then maintains the endometrium through pregnancy. Occasionally if endogenous progesterone secretion is inadequate, pharmacologic supplementation may ensure a successful full-term pregnancy.

Progesterone depresses the contractility of the uterine myometrium. When the uterus shifts from a progesterone- to an estrogen-dominated state in late pregnancy, uterine excitability is increased, which facilitates parturition. Pharmacologic amounts of progesterone used in an estrogen-primed animal have caused a regression of the endometrium but an increased growth of the myometrium.

Progesterone transforms the estrogen-dominated cervical secretions from thin and watery to thick and mucoid. Various oral contraceptive preparations exert similar actions (*see* Chap. 49). The increased viscosity of these secretions may act to impede the migration of spermatozoa in the female genital tract.

Progesterone is thermogenic. The slight elevation in basal body temperature shortly after ovulation may be used to detect ovulation in women and is the basis of rhythm method of birth control. It is not a reliable index of ovulation.

ABSORPTION AND METABOLISM

Progesterone is removed almost quantitatively in a single pass through the liver and is therefore inactive by mouth. Its main urinary metabolite is pregnanediol glucosiduronidate, and the excretion of this substance may be used to evaluate corpus luteum function, although direct radioimmunoassay of plasma progesterone is now simpler and more economical.

Many orally active progestins have been synthesized (Fig. 48-7). They are of two main classes: the *19-nor-derivatives* related to the androgens; and the *17-acetoxy derivatives* related to 17-hydroxyprogesterone.

USES

The main use of progestins is in oral contraceptives (*see* Chap. 49), but they are also used to augment progesterone effect in women with inadequate luteal phases; to test the adequacy of estradiol secretion where, if bleeding is precipitated by progestins, there has been adequate estrogen stimulation of the endometrium; to control vaginal bleeding that results from endometrial hyperplasia; and to treat menopausal symptoms, especially hot flashes.

Progestins also constitute a unique class of chemotherapeutic agents. In high doses, they produce objective regression of metastatic endometrial carcinoma in about 40% of patients with periods of remissions lasting 6 months to several years. This treatment of metastatic cancer is unique because there are essentially no side-effects.

FURTHER READING

1. Jensen EV, DeSombre ER: Steroid hormone receptors and action. In DeGroot LJ (ed): Endocrinology pp 2055–2063. New York, Grune & Stratton, 1979
2. Lipsett MB: Physiology and pathology of the Leydig cell. N Engl J Med 303:682–688, 1980
3. Neumann F: The physiological action of progesterone and the pharmacologic effects of progestogens—a short review. Postgrad Med J 54 (Suppl 2):11–24, 1978
4. Ross GT, Cargille CM, Lipsett MB et al: Pituitary and gonadal hormones in women during spontaneous and induced ovulatory cycles. Recent Prog Horm Res 26:1–62, 1970
5. Wilson JD, Griffin JE: The use and misuse of androgens. Metabolism 29:1278–1295, 1980

FIG. 48-7. Synthetic progestins.

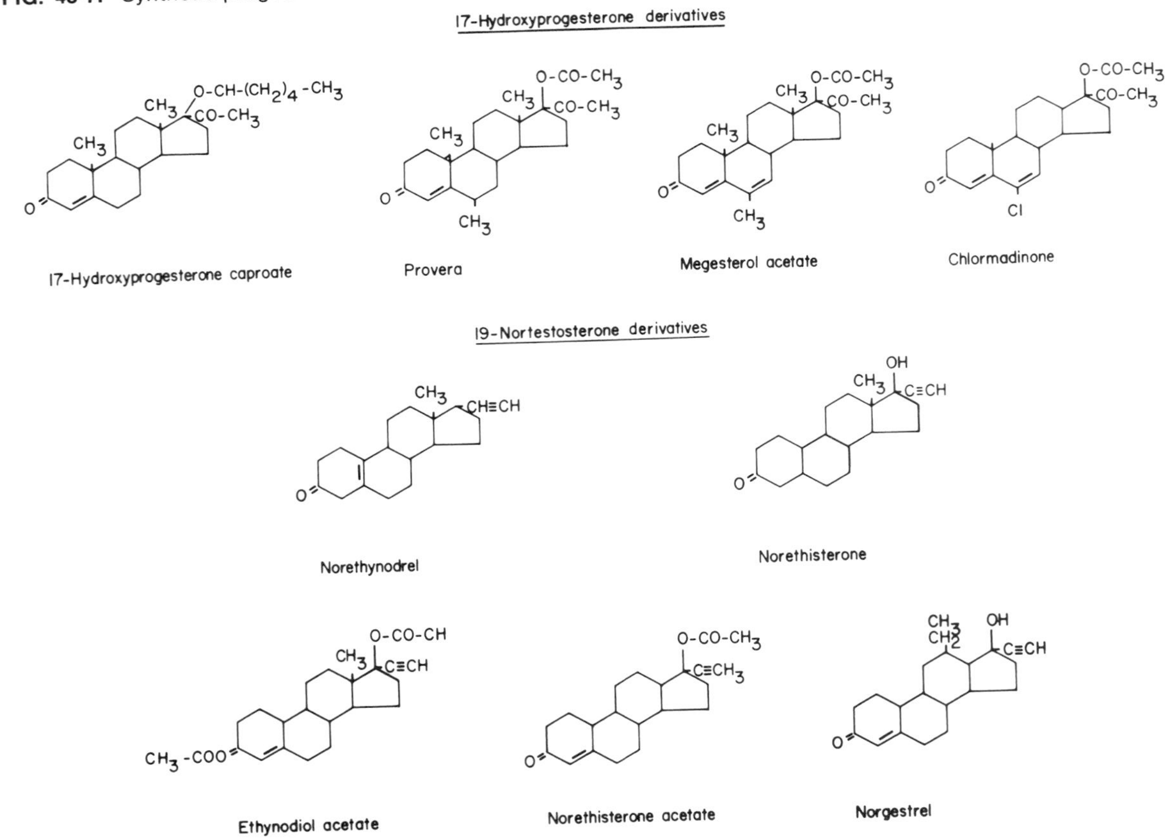

CHAPTER 48 QUESTIONS

(See P. 7 for Full Instructions)

Select the One Best Answer

1. Estrogens stimulate hepatic synthesis of each of the following EXCEPT
   A. renin substrate.
   B. albumin.
   C. cortisol-binding globulin.
   D. thyroxine-binding globulin.
   E. ceruloplasmin.
2. The source of plasma estrone in the postmenopausal woman is
   A. ovarian secretion.
   B. adrenal secretion.
   C. conversion of ovarian androstenedione.
   D. conversion of adrenal androstenedione.
   E. conversion of adrenal dehydroepiandrostenedione.
3. A nonsteroidal, antiestrogenic, orally active compound effective for the induction of ovulation is
   A. norethindrone.
   B. ethinyl estradiol.
   C. methyltestosterone.
   D. diethylstilbestrol.
   E. clomiphene.
4. Which of the following is used principally for its anabolic action?
   A. Norethindrone
   B. Methandrostenolone
   C. Dexamethasone
   D. Ethinyl estradiol
   E. Prednisone
5. Cyproterone
   A. causes acne.
   B. is an antiandrogen.
   C. is contraindicated in the treatment of prostatic carcinoma.
   D. is useful in treating infertility in females.
   E. is secreted by the placenta.

A = 1,2,3; B = 1,3; B = 2,4; D = 4; E = All

6. Estrogen therapy is indicated for treatment of
   1. menopause.
   2. acne in women.
   3. dysmenorrhea (painful menstruation).
   4. thromboembolic disease.
7. Ethinyl estradiol
   1. is more potent than diethylstilbestrol.
   2. commonly causes nausea.
   3. may cause gynecomastia.
   4. inhibits the secretion of FSH.
8. Ethinyl estradiol
   1. exerts an anabolic effect.
   2. is used to treat prostatic carcinoma.
   3. produces an effect on salt and water retention.
   4. is an ingredient of some oral contraceptive preparations.
9. Clinically useful androgens may
   1. cause osteoporosis.
   2. be valuable in treating pituitary dwarfism.
   3. alleviate bronchial asthma.
   4. produce jaundice.
10. Methyltestosterone
    1. is an orally effective androgen.
    2. may cause jaundice.
    3. is metabolized less rapidly than testosterone.
    4. may cause premature closure of the epiphyses.

49

MORTIMER B. LIPSETT

Oral Contraceptives

STEROID CONTRACEPTIVES

During the past 20 years, the oral contraceptives (OCs) developed by Rock and Pincus have brought about a social revolution in family planning and substantial changes in sexual mores. These agents are among the most biologically effective drugs ever described and are currently used by 60 million women worldwide. It is hoped that the risks ascribed to their use will be decreased appreciably by new formulations; their current risk-benefit ratio, taking into account the mortality and morbidity of pregnancy, favors their use. Recent studies show that oral contraceptive use decreases the risk of development of ovarian and uterine cancer and has no effect on the incidence of breast cancer.

GREGORY PINCUS, 1903–1967. American zoologist and physiologist. Studied nervous responses to stress, the biochemistry of hormones, and reproductive physiology. Developed an antifertility pill and conducted, with J. Rock and others, the first field trials in the late 1950s in Puerto Rico and Haiti.

JOHN ROCK, 1890– . Boston physician. With M. K. Bartlett, delineated the cyclic changes of the endometrium. Also demonstrated fertilization of human ova *in vitro* and efficacy of progestational steroids as contraceptive agents in animals and humans.

ESTROGEN-CONTAINING CONTRACEPTIVES

MECHANISMS OF ACTION

The OCs suppress ovulation. In normal women, the increasing estradiol secretion by the developing follicle before ovulation triggers the release of luteinizing hormone (LH), which causes ovulation (*see* Fig. 48-4). However, when estrogens with or without progestins are given chronically, gonadotropin levels remain in the low normal range and the ovulatory LH peak does not occur. The OC agents available in this country contain both an estrogen and a progestin at varying dosage ratios (Table 49-1). The addition of a progestin to the estrogen prevents endometrial hyperplasia and produces complete shedding of the endometrium when the hormones are withdrawn.

Progestational compounds alone are contraceptive acting by three different mechanisms:

TABLE 49-1. Heinen's Relative Potency Table for Commonly Used Combination Estrogen and Progestins

2	Norethindrone acetate 1 mg	Loestrin 1/20 Zorane 1/20	Ethinyl estradiol 20 μg	0.7–0.8
0.5	Norethindrone 0.5 mg	Modicon Brevicon	Ethinyl estradiol 35 μg	1.2–1.4
1	Norethindrone 1 mg	Ortho-Novum 1/50 Norinyl 1/50	Mestranol 50 μg	1
3	Norethindrone acetate 1.5 mg	Loestrin 1.5/30 Zorane 1.3/20	Ethinyl estradiol 30 μg	1–1.2
1	Norethindrone 1 mg	Ortho-Novum 1/8 Norinyl 1/80	Mestranol 80 μg	1.6
2	Norethindrone acetate 1 mg	Norlestrin-1	Ethinyl estradiol 50 μg	1.7–2
2	Norethindrone 2 mg	Ortho-Novum 2 mg Norinyl 2	Mestranol 100 μg	2
2.7	Norethynodrel 2.5 mg	Enovid-E	Mestranol 100 μg	2
5	Norethindrone acetate 2.5 mg	Norlestrin 2.5	Ethinyl estradiol 50 μg	1.7–2
15	Norgestrel 0.5 mg	Ovral	Ethinyl estradiol 50 μg	1.7–2
15	Ethynodiol diacetate 1 mg	Demulen	Ethinyl estradiol 50 μg	1.7–2
15	Ethynodiol diacetate 1 mg	Ovulen	Mestranol 100 μg	2
Potency (units)				Potency (units)
5 0				0 1 2

(Modified from Mishell DR Jr: Clin Obstet Gynecol 19:743–764, 1976).

In large doses they suppress gonadotropins; they reduce the endometrial estrogen receptor content, which eventually leads to an atrophic endometrium; and they change the character of the cervical mucus, converting the secretions from the thin watery type seen under estrogenic influence to a thick mucoid type that hinders sperm penetration. This last action is probably the significant one for the minipill (the small-dose oral progestin).

When the OCs were first developed, the dose of the estrogenic component, usually mestranol, was more than 100 μg. With the realization that most side-effects of the OCs were due to the estrogen, the dose has gradually been lowered (Table 49-1), but this is associated with an increased incidence of breakthrough bleeding. Thus the physician, by trial and error, must find the appropriate dosage form for each woman. Most of the serious complications of OC use have been reported with high-dose estrogen formulations; mortality and morbidity attributable to OCs have diminished considerably now that lower-dose estrogen-containing preparations are being used.

PHARMACOKINETICS

With the realization that mestranol is an active estrogen only after demethylation in the body, ethinyl estradiol has become the estrogen of choice in OCs. As with other steroids, peak plasma concentrations are reached about 1 hour after ingestion; there is then a two-component plasma disappearance curve with the half-life of the first phase being about 7 hours. Ethinyl estradiol is not metabolized extensively, and about 30% is excreted in the feces.

Even with doses of ethinyl estradiol as low as 20 μg/day, some women have an increase of one or more of the estrogen-induced alpha or beta plasma globulins. The proteins include cortisol-binding globulin, thyroxine-binding globulin, ceruloplasmin, and α_1-antitrypsin and may be used as an index of estrogen effect. The best estimate of the potency of ethinyl estradiol is about 10 times that of estradiol, but even the low-dose OC is equivalent to a slight excess of estrogen.

One cannot assume that the kinetics of the steroids will be invariant throughout the world. Intercurrent disease, nutritional status, environmental contaminants, and genetic differences have been shown to alter clearance rates of estrogens and progestins. Thus formulations of OCs may need to be tailored for a particular population. Additionally, enzyme-inducing agents accelerate steroid metabolism (*see* Chap. 8), leading to decreased effectiveness of ordinary doses of OCs.

USES

Besides their contraceptive use, OCs have proven value in about 50% to 70% of women with idiopathic hirsutism, primarily as a result of suppression of LH. The OCs that contain higher doses of progestin are probably more effective. OCs are also used to control the bleeding of endometrial hyperplasia and to treat some women with polycystic ovaries.

ADVERSE EFFECTS

Oral contraceptive use and arterial and venous thrombosis are clearly associated. The relative risk for these complications is decreasing as the amount of estrogen in the OC has decreased. OCs are contraindicated in women with migraine headache because of the increased risk of cerebrovascular thrombosis in such patients. The risk for myocardial infarction in white women under 35 who used OCs was slightly increased and was greatly further increased in cigarette smokers. The risk of gallbladder disease is about twice that of the normal population in women who take either estrogens or OCs. Estrogen increases cholesterol saturation of bile, this being the probable mechanism.

Oral contraceptives cause hypertension in up to 5% of women (*see* Chap. 48). Renin substrate is increased, but this does not adequately explain the hypertension. Estrogens and OCs produce some degree of insulin resistance, with slightly higher plasma glucose levels, and cause increased plasma triglyceride levels, usually within the normal range. Prolonged use of OCs has been associated with a number of hepatic lesions, especially *peliosis hepatica*, *hepatic adenomas*, and *benign focal nodular hyperplasia*.

Contraindications to the use of OCs include a history of thromboembolic disorders, cancer of the breast or endometrium, migraine headaches, gallbladder disease, high blood pressure, extensive varicose veins, and possibly obesity. The frequency of side-effects increases with increasing age, women over 35 years being at increased risk.

PROGESTATIONAL CONTRACEPTIVES

Continuous low-dose progestin therapy may be satisfactory for contraceptive purposes in this country for women who should not receive estrogens. Breakthrough bleeding is common, and the pregnancy rate is higher than with OCs. The use of long-acting injectable progestins is valuable in certain societies because the woman needs to be treated only once every 3 months. However, spotting, irregular bleeding, and unpredictable duration of effect make this a less satisfactory method of contraception. The two agents in use are medroxyprogesterone acetate, 150 mg intramuscularly every 3 months, and norethindrone enanthate, 200 mg every 12 weeks.

An ingenious method for using progestins is the development of an intrauterine device that releases progesterone at a rate of 65 μg/day for 1 year. The local effect prevents implantation, and the dose is in the range of progesterone secretion during the follicular phase.

FURTHER READING

1. Durand JL, Bressler R: Clinical pharmacology of the steroidal oral contraceptives. Adv Intern Med 24:97–126, 1979
2. Liggins GC: Hormonal steroid contraceptives. II. Clinical considerations. Drugs 1:461–483, 1970
3. Lipsett MB, Combs JW, Catt K et al: Problems in contraception. Ann Intern Med 74:251–263, 1971
4. McQueen EG: Hormonal steroid contraceptives. III. Adverse reactions. Drugs 2:40–44, 1971
5. McQueen EG: Hormonal steroid contraceptives. IV. Adverse reactions and management of the patient. Drugs 2:138–164, 1971
6. Seddon RJ: Hormonal steroid contraceptives. I. Physiological and clinical pharmacological considerations. Drugs 1:399–420, 1970

CHAPTER 49 QUESTIONS

(See P. 7 for Full Instructions)

Select the One Best Answer

1. Oral contraceptive preparations may contain each of the following EXCEPT
   A. mestranol.
   B. ethinylestradiol.
   C. norethynodrel.
   D. medroxyprogesterone.
   E. progesterone.

2. Adverse reactions to oral contraceptive agents include all of the following EXCEPT
   A. increased blood clotting factors.
   B. breakthrough bleeding.
   C. markedly altered ovarian function.
   D. fluid retention.
   E. thrombophlebitis.

3. Combination oral contraceptive agents may cause *clinically* evident deficiency of
   A. vitamin A (retinol).
   B. vitamin C (ascorbic acid).
   C. vitamin K.
   D. vitamin B_6 (pyridoxine).
   E. vitamin D.

A = 1,2,3; B = 1,3; C = 2,4; D = 4; E = All

4. The undesirable side-effects from use of combination estrogen–progestin oral contraceptives include
   1. decreased glucose tolerance.
   2. hypertension.
   3. nausea and headache.
   4. osteoporosis.

5. Side-effects that occur during the use of oral contraceptives include
   1. weight loss.
   2. thrombophlebitis.
   3. hypotension.
   4. headache.

6. Progestins
   1. must be combined with estrogens to inhibit ovulation effectively.
   2. are anabolic agents useful in promoting growth.
   3. may produce masculinization of the female fetus.
   4. are not absorbed after oral administration.

7. Estrogens are
   1. essential components for the antifertility effect of oral contraceptive preparations.
   2. capable of causing decreases in serum cholesterol levels.
   3. equal to androgens in anabolic potency.
   4. useful in the treatment of physiological and psychological symptoms of menopause.

AUTACOIDS AND RELATED DRUGS

50

G. ALAN ROBISON

Cyclic AMP as a Mediator of Drug Action

Cyclic AMP was discovered in 1957 by Earl W. Sutherland and colleagues as the mediator of the hepatic glycogenolytic response to epinephrine and glucagon. Cyclic AMP has become especially important in pharmacology for several reasons: historically because it led to the discovery of adenylate cyclase; and because the stimulation of adenylate cyclase by hormones was the first receptor-mediated event that could be studied in a cell-free system. Continued study of this phenomenon has led to much of our present understanding of what receptors are and how they function. Cyclic AMP is important physiologically and clinically because such a large variety of naturally occurring drugs (hormones, neurotransmitters, and a miscellaneous group sometimes referred to as autacoids) produce at least some of their effects by altering the intracellular level of cyclic AMP.

EARL WILBUR SUTHERLAND, JR., 1915–1974. American physician and pharmacologist. Worked on carbohydrate metabolism and hormonal mechanisms. Discovered cyclic AMP in 1957 and did much to elucidate its biologic significance. Received the Nobel Prize in 1971 for these and other contributions.

RECEPTORS AND ADENYLATE CYCLASE

Presented in Table 50-1 is a list of the drugs known to produce at least some of their effects by this mechanism—that is, either by stimulating or by inhibiting the activity of adenylate cyclase, thereby leading to either an increased or a decreased level of cyclic AMP. Many of the drugs produced in the body can interact with two or more different types of receptors. Most of these receptors were initially distinguished from each other in terms of their anatomical localization or surface characteristics (*e.g.*, the order of potency of the various agonists and antagonists that interact with them) and were arbitrarily named by pharmacologists before anything was known about the biochemical details of the responses that they mediate. As a result, what these receptors are called and what they do are not consistently related. With adrenergic receptors, for example, although β_1 and β_2 receptors (which may have evolved as receptors for norepinephrine and epinephrine, respectively) both can mediate the stimulation of adenylate cyclase, only α_2 receptors (as opposed to α_1 receptors) can inhibit the system. With do-

TABLE 50-1. Drugs That Can Stimulate Adenylate Cyclase and Ca^{++} Influx and Inhibit Adenylate Cyclase

Stimulatory Drugs	Type of Receptor	Inhibitory Drugs	Type of Receptor
Adenylate cyclase			
Norepinephrine	β_1 Adrenergic	Catecholamines	α_2
Epinephrine	β_2 Adrenergic	Dopamine	D_2
Dopamine	D_1	Acetylcholine	Muscarinic
Glucagon	Glucagon	Melatonin	Melatonin
Vasopressin (ADH)	Vasopressin (ADH)	Insulin	Insulin
TRH	TRH	Thromboxane A_2*	Thromboxane
TSH	TSH	Adenosine	P
ACTH	ACTH	Opiates	Opiate
Secretin	Secretin	Nicotinic acid	?
VIP	VIP		
LH (ICSH)	LH (ICSH)		
PTH	PTH		
Calcitonin	Calcitonin		
Histamine	H_2		
Serotonin (5-HT)	Serotonin 1		
Prostacyclin*	Prostacyclin		
MSH	MSH		
Adenosine	R		
Ca^{++} influx			
Catecholamines	α_1		
Acetylcholine	Muscarinic		
Histamine	H_1		
Serotonin (5-HT)	Serotonin 2		
Angiotensin	Angiotensin		

* Other derivatives of arachidonic acid, notably the prostaglandins, can also stimulate and inhibit adenylate cyclase in some cells, possibly by way of the same receptors that mediate the effects of prostacyclin and thromboxane A_2. *See* Chapter 53 for further discussion of these drugs.

pamine, one needs to remember that D_1 receptors stimulate whereas D_2 receptors do not; with histamine, H_2 receptors stimulate whereas H_1 receptors do not.

Table 50-1 is not meant to be exhaustive. Extrapolating from the example of vasoactive intestinal peptide (VIP), which was discovered only recently, one may reasonably conclude that other drugs will have to be added to this list in the future.

With drugs that stimulate adenylate cyclase, most, if not all, of the physiologically important effects of these drugs are mediated by cyclic AMP. Whether the same receptors that mediate the stimulation of adenylate cyclase might not simultaneously have another effect that could also be important is unknown. By contrast, with drugs that inhibit cyclase, there is considerable uncertainty as to how important the effect on cyclic AMP is compared to other effects that may be mediated by the same receptor. Clearly many of the effects mediated by muscarinic cholinergic receptors, for example, are not the result of a decreased level of cyclic AMP; this also seems to be true of some of the effects of insulin.

There may be a good deal of cross-reactivity between some of the agonists and receptors listed in Table 50-1, especially when supraphysiologic concentrations of the agonists are used. The tendency of epinephrine to interact with β_1 receptors, for example, and of norepinephrine to interact with β_2 receptors is sufficiently great that the distinction drawn in Table 50-1 is often not made. Similarly, as might be predicted from chemical structures, glucagon has some affinity for secretin receptors, just as secretin can interact with the receptors for glucagon. The important point is that any drug that can interact as an agonist with one of the receptors mentioned in Table 50-1 will have the predicted effect on the activity of adenylate cyclase.

Although most of the drugs in Table 50-1 are listed as interacting only with one type of receptor, this may not be true indefinitely. Vasopressin, for example, can produce many effects (including the pressor effect for which it was named) that are *not* mediated by cyclic AMP. Several possibilities may explain this observation: One is that the same receptors that have such a striking effect on adenylate cyclase in the vasopressin-sensitive cells of the kidney are somehow prevented from having this effect in other tissues. From what is known of the receptors for other drugs that have been studied more thoroughly, this seems unlikely. Another possibility is that these other effects of vasopressin are simply vasopressin cross-reacting with receptors that have evolved to mediate the effects of a different hormone, such as oxytocin. Yet another possibility is that the receptors for vasopressin are of two types, analogous to the α receptors with which the catecholamines can interact, in which event future students will probably have to remember that there are V_1 receptors that do one thing and V_2 receptors that do another. Consideration of this example provides an excuse for introducing some good advice from the late Professor Walter B. Cannon, who contributed greatly to our present understanding of the function of the autonomic nervous system.

For medical students especially, the idea that knowledge of phenomena is not fixed and static but continuously growing must be repeatedly stressed. Perhaps there is no realm of scientific enterprise in which progress is being more rapidly made than in medicine. Students should learn, therefore, that the routine curriculum of a medical school provides only the beginning of their education. If they are to be useful, efficient physicians they must always be alert to learn and apply the discoveries which are constantly being made and which may be of the utmost importance for their patients.

Those words were first published in 1945, and the rate of our progress in understanding drug action has accelerated significantly since then. The lower left-hand portion of Table 50-1 indicates that some of the drugs that can either stimulate or inhibit adenylate cyclase can also produce an effect on membrane phosphatidylinositol metabolism that leads to an influx of calcium. In some cases this effect is known to be mediated by receptors separate and distinct from those related to adenylate cyclase. The muscarinic receptors that mediate this effect in response to acetylcholine may eventually be shown to differ from the superficially similar receptors responsible for inhibiting adenylate cyclase in other cells. All drugs in the right-hand column can stimulate guanylate cyclase, and hence can increase the level of cyclic GMP in cells that possess these receptors. Cyclic GMP is the only 3,′5′-nucleotide other than cyclic AMP known to exist in mammalian cells, but neither its biologic nor its pharmacologic significance is understood at present. This list is included primarily because it illustrates another receptor-mediated event, analogous to, but different from, a change in the level of cyclic AMP that may be responsible for many of the effects produced by a number of different drugs in different tissues.

MECHANISM OF ACTION OF CYCLIC AMP

The ability of drugs to stimulate adenylate cyclase in a receptor-specific way has been known and studied for many years, and an early result of these studies was the development of the second messenger concept of hormone action. This concept, incorporating our present understanding of how cyclic AMP acts to produce its effects, is illustrated in Fig. 50-1. Briefly, the hormone or other drug interacts with its receptors on the external surface of the cell membrane, which leads to the activation of adenylate cyclase on the other side of the membrane and to an increased rate of formation of cyclic AMP. The level of cyclic AMP at any instant reflects the difference between its rate of formation by adenylate cyclase and its rate of hydrolysis by phosphodiesterase. For this reason, drugs that can inhibit phosphodiesterase tend to act synergistically with drugs that stimulate adenylate cyclase. The increased level of cyclic AMP activates a special type of protein kinase that differs from the other protein kinases found in cells in that they are completely dependent on cyclic AMP. The discovery of this important group of enzymes was made in 1968 by E. G. Krebs and his colleagues. These enzymes comprise regulatory and catalytic subunits such that in the absence of cyclic AMP (or in the presence of low concentrations of cyclic AMP) the subunits are tightly bound to each other and the enzyme is inactive. As the level of cyclic AMP increases, cyclic AMP interacts

WALTER BRADFORD CANNON, 1871–1945. American physiologist. Introduced the bismuth meal for radiographic study of digestive function and observed stomach movements with x-rays in 1898. Demonstrated the "fight–flight" reaction of the body to stress. His work on sympathetic nervous control led to the concept of "homeostasis," which he introduced.

EDWIN GERHARD KREBS, 1918– . American biochemist. Has worked especially on carbohydrate metabolism in muscle, enzyme regulation, and hormonal mechanisms.

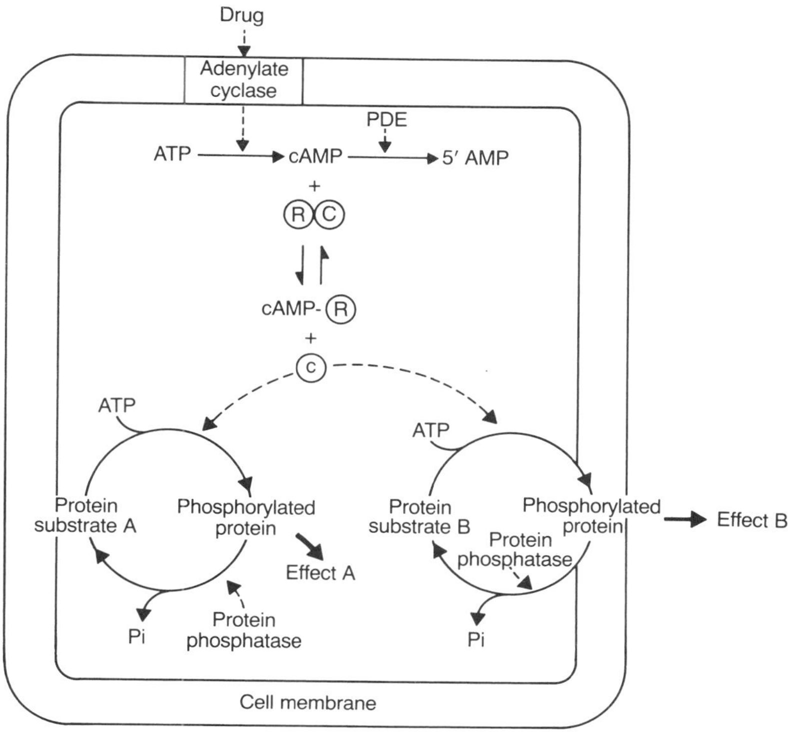

FIG. 50-1. The second messenger concept and the mechanism of action of cyclic AMP (*cAMP*). The drug-receptor interaction leads to the activation of adenylate cyclase (*see* Fig. 50-2 for details). The level of *cAMP* is also influenced by the action of phosphodiesterase (*PDE*). The regulatory (*R*) and catalytic (*C*) subunits of cyclic AMP-dependent protein kinase are shown. Different cells have different substrates for this enzyme. The function or activity of these substrates is altered by phosphorylation, leading to the various effects associated with the drug that initiated the response.

with the regulatory subunit, causing the subunits to dissociate. As a result, the catalytic subunit becomes free to act. The catalytic subunit is generally similar in all cells and can catalyze the ATP-dependent phosphorylation of many proteins such that the activity or function of the protein is altered. An example of this is the activation of glycogen phosphorylase. Another well-studied example is the activation of triglyceride lipase in adipose tissue, which is responsible for the lipolytic effect of many drugs. Different cells contain different substrates for protein kinase, and an increasing body of evidence suggests that all physiologically important effects of cyclic AMP (at least in vertebrates) are mediated by this same mechanism. In some cases the substrate has been found to be a component of the cell membrane. In all cases the phosphorylated protein becomes subject to the action of a protein phosphatase such that the activity of the protein at any given instant reflects the balance between phosphorylation and dephosphorylation.

This is, of course, an oversimplified description of what happens in a cell when the level of cyclic AMP is increased. The activated protein kinase seldom, if ever, phosphorylates only one protein, but rather may act on many substrates simultaneously, and these substrates may interact with each other in a highly complex way. Many cells contain a protein that acts to inhibit a protein phosphatase that dephosphorylates one of the substrates for protein kinase. This inhibitory protein is itself a substrate for the protein kinase and becomes active only when phosphorylated by the protein kinase. The relatively simple result in this case is to reinforce the action of the protein kinase previously described (*i.e.*, not only is the rate of phosphorylation increased, but the rate of dephosphorylation is decreased). Each protein may be influenced in different ways by other hormones, including those that act rapidly, such as the ones mentioned in Table 50-1, and those such as the steroid hormones that act to influence gene expression. Although our understanding of how cells are regulated by drugs has grown enormously in recent years, we are developing a greater appreciation of the complexity of the mechanisms involved.

MECHANISM OF CYCLASE ACTIVATION

How does the agonist–receptor interaction lead to the stimulation of adenylate cyclase? We now know, from experiments involving a myriad of techniques, including especially the use of mutant cell lines, that the adenylate cyclase system comprises at least three separate proteins, referred to in Figure 50-2 as R, C, and N. R and C are the receptor and the catalytic component, respectively, whereas N is a guanyl nucleotide binding protein that serves to transmit the influence of R to C. Each of these proteins has been separated from the other two, and each has been recombined (with components from the same or a different type of cell) to reconstitute a functional system.

Figure 50-2 illustrates the activation of adenylate cyclase in a cell-free system in which tachyphylaxis or "down regulation" does not occur, that is, in a system in which the concentrations of both the receptor and the agonist can be maintained constant. The first step in the process is the activation of R by the agonist A. The active form R* clearly interacts with N but does so much as an enzyme interacts with its substrate. The substrate in this case would be the N protein liganded with GDP, the reaction catalyzed would be the displacement of GDP by GTP, and the product would be N-GTP. This process has also been referred to as "collision coupling." The N-GTP complex then reacts stoichiometrically with the free catalytic component C to form the active enzyme. This complex also has GTPase activity, which serves to hydrolyze the GTP and thus terminate cyclase activity. Agents that inhibit GTPase activity, such as cholera toxin, tend to produce a persistent activation of adenylate cyclase, leading to very high levels of cyclic AMP in the affected cells. Under normal conditions, however, the inactive complex dissociates to C and N-GDP and the cycle is repeated. The activity of adenylate cyclase at any instant thus reflects the rate of conversion to the active form and the rate of inactivation by the GTPase. The displacement of bound GDP by GTP ordinarily takes place at a slow, but measurable, rate, which accounts for the fact that most cells contain low, but measurable, levels of cyclic AMP even without hormonal stimulation.

The mechanism by which drugs such as the catecholamines or acetylcholine act to inhibit this process is not as well understood but may involve inhibiting the reaction between N-GTP and C, possibly because the N-GTP is diverted to a different pathway. This is currently an active area of research interest.

PHOSPHODIESTERASE INHIBITORS

As noted above, drugs that inhibit cyclic nucleotide phosphodiesterase activity tend to act synergistically with drugs that stimulate adenylate cyclase, but it does not follow that all of these drugs' effects are related to changes in the level of cyclic AMP. An important principle of pharmacology (sometimes referred to as Toman's Law, after the pharmacologist who first enunciated it) is that "enough of anything will inhibit anything." This is as true of the naturally occurring drugs that stimulate cyclase as it is of the various xenobiotics that inhibit phosphodiesterase, but there is nevertheless an important difference between these two groups of drugs: The phosphodiesterase inhibitors, like most drugs that inhibit enzymes, are effective only at relatively high concentrations, and at these concentrations they may have many other effects. (An important exception to this generalization is provided by penicillin and other antibiotics, which are used to poison en-

FIG. 50-2. The mechanism by which the agonist-receptor interaction leads to the activation of adenylate cyclase (*see* text for further description).

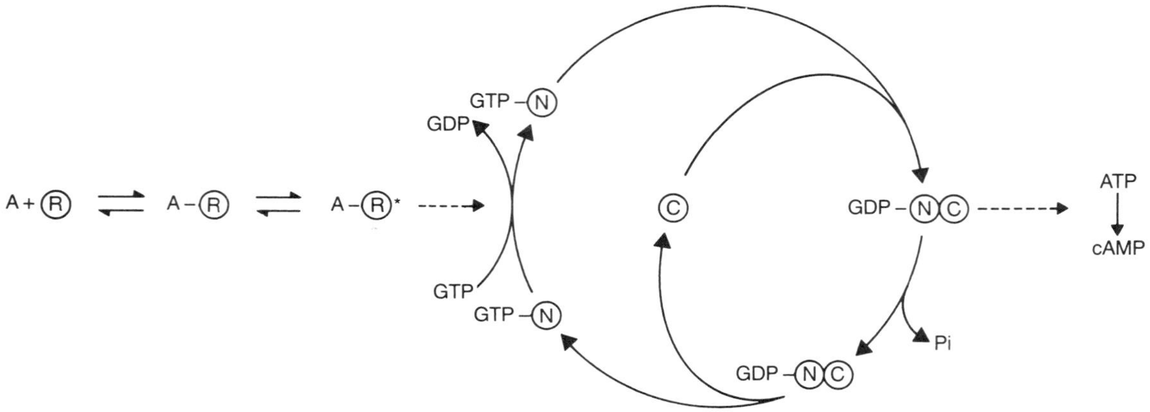

zymes that do not occur in mammalian cells; *see* Chap. 56.) The methylxanthines such as caffeine and theophylline are among the best known phosphodiesterase inhibitors because they were used by Sutherland and his colleagues in their original studies that led to the discovery of cyclic AMP. There seems little doubt that some of the effects of these drugs can be attributed to their inhibition of phosphodiesterase, but, at the concentrations needed for this, they can also exert many other actions, including inhibition of protein phosphatases (which is originally why Sutherland used them) and, perhaps more important, antagonism of adenosine by interaction with adenosine receptors, an effect that might have been predicted from their chemical similarity to adenosine. Subsequently many drugs have been found to inhibit phosphodiesterase, but all have many other effects.

Many of the drugs listed in the first column of Table 50-1 can stimulate adenylate cyclase at concentrations so low that they have no other known effect. By contrast, no known drug can inhibit phosphodiesterase without, at the same time, producing many other effects, an important point to remember when considering the mechanism of action of these drugs.

FURTHER READING

1. Robison GA, Butcher RW, Sutherland EW: Cyclic AMP. New York, Academic Press, 1971
2. Greengard P: Cyclic Nucleotides, Phosphorylated Proteins, and Neuronal Function. New York, Raven Press, 1978
3. Franklin TJ: Binding energy and the excitation of hormone receptors. Trends in Pharmacological Sciences 1:431–433, 1980
4. Dumont JE, Greengard P, Robison GA (eds): Advances in Cyclic Nucleotide Research, Vol 14. New York, Raven Press, 1981. (This volume contains most of the papers presented at the Fourth International Conference on Cyclic Nucleotides, including a number of papers on the relation of receptors to adenylate cyclase.)

51

JEREMY H. THOMPSON

Histamine and the Antihistamines

HISTAMINE

Histamine (hist = tissue), a *biogenic amine,* occurs in many tissues in nearly all forms of life. Histamine occurs naturally in an inactive (bound) form but is released in a free active state in response to tissue injury, inflammation, nerve stimulation, some drugs, or some antigen/antibody reactions.

Histamine was synthesized in 1907, and its main biologic actions were discovered in 1910, when it was identified as a uterine stimulant in extracts of ergot (*see* Chap. 39). The ubiquity of histamine, plus its potency, and, as originally described by Sir Henry Dale, the similarity of many of its effects to anaphylactic shock and other allergic phenomena suggest a fundamental role in biologic function. With few exceptions, however, there is widespread controversy over its role in physiological and pathologic functions.

Histamine is intimately involved in a number of pathologic processes and therefore represents at least a potential site of pharmacologic attack. Two groups of antihistamines (H_1- and H_2-receptor blockers) can antagonize most of the effects of histamine, and certain chemical agents and drugs may liberate histamine into the circulation from tissue storage sites, producing specific symptoms.

SYNTHESIS, DISTRIBUTION, AND STORAGE

Histamine [1-methyl-4-(β-amino-ethyl)-imidazole] is predominantly synthesized from L-histidine by L-histidine decarboxylase, pyridoxal-5-phosphate being required as cofactor (Fig. 51-1). Histidine may also be decarboxylated to histamine by nonspecific aromatic L-amino-acid decarboxylase (dopa-decarboxylase), but this enzyme has a low affinity for L-histidine. α-Methyl histidine and α-methyl dopa specifically inhibit L-histidine decarboxylase and dopa decarboxylase, respectively. In humans, using ^{14}C-L-histidine, about 5 mg of histamine are formed daily. It is unlikely that dietary histamine or histamine synthesized in the gut lumen by bacteria contributes significantly to

---

ADOLF OTTO REINHOLD WINDAUS, 1876–1959. German chemist. Worked particularly with steroids, showing ergosterol activation with ultraviolet light to yield vitamin D_2. Won Nobel prize for chemistry in 1928. With Vogt, synthesized histamine in 1907.

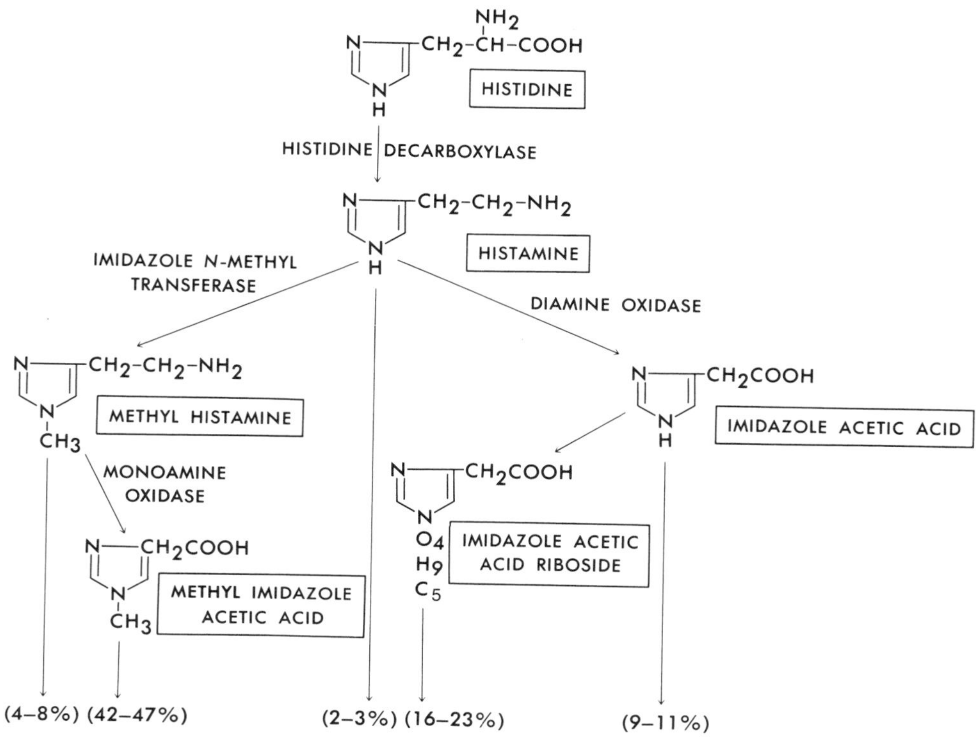

FIG. 51-1. Major routes of formation and metabolic disposition of histamine. The values in parentheses refer to percent recovery of histamine and its metabolites in the urine in the 6 hours after intradermal (approximately 1 μg/kg) ^{14}C-histamine in three normal human males. Percentage of total radioactivity collected ranged from 81 to 84. (Schayer RW, Cooper JAD): Metabolism of C^{14}histamine. J Appl Physiol 4:481–483, 1956)

the endogenous tissue histamine pool, since the amine is usually inactivated to N-acetylhistamine by intestinal bacteria or metabolized in the gastrointestinal mucosa, liver, and lungs.

Histamine occurs in varying amounts in almost all tissues of almost all mammals. In humans, the concentration is particularly high in the skin, gastrointestinal mucosa (except the pyloric gland area of the stomach), lungs, and bone marrow. In the brain, histamine has a pattern of distribution very similar to that of serotonin: a high concentration in the hypothalamus, particularly the mammillary bodies and supraoptic nucleus; and a low concentration in the white matter, cerebral cortex, medulla, and pons. The histamine content of any tissue is not indicative of the rapidity with which the amine is turning over, and there is only partial correlation between the histamine content and the "histamine-forming capacity" (decarboxylase activity) of tissues.

Histamine is stored through electrostatic forces in granules in several cell types. Mast cells universally contain high concentrations where the amine is bound along with heparin and serotonin. Gastrointestinal histamine probably occurs in at least three cell types: mast cells, cells of the APUD (amine precursor uptake and decarboxylation) system, and a nonmast cell, non-APUD cell system. Histamine is also present in the polymorphonuclear basophil and in some nerves, nerve endings, and synaptic vesicles. Histamine binding probably occurs at the primary amino group that is protonated at physiologic *p*H, allowing reaction with anionic groups.

Nonmast cell histamine has a more rapid turnover than does mast cell histamine and is probably of greater physiological importance because the associated L-histidine decarboxylase is "inducible," being subject to activation by such stimuli as gastrin, insulin-induced hypoglycemia, and nicotine. The cellular binding of histamine is not uniform, since variations occur to the releasing agent, compound 48/80 (a mixture of p-methoxy-N-methylphenyl ethylamines).

METABOLISM

The relative importance of the four routes of histamine metabolism (Fig. 51-1) varies between species. Conjugation with ribose is unique, histamine being the only known compound to be biotransformed in such a manner. Chlorpromazine (*see* Chap. 25) depresses imidazole N-methyl transferase activity, thereby augmenting tissue levels of histamine. Except for N-methylhistamine and N-demethylhistamine, which are potent gastric secretagogues, the various metabolites of histamine possess little or no pharmacologic activity and are excreted in the urine. The histaminase activity of plasma rises during pregnancy, but the significance of this is not known.

PHARMACOLOGIC ACTIONS

With a few exceptions, the degree and even the direction of histamine actions differ markedly between species. The principal actions of histamine in humans are indicated in Table 51-1.

Cardiovascular System

Hypotension, the most important effect of histamine, is primarily due to dilatation of the terminal arterioles via H_2-receptors with subse-

TABLE 51-1. Major Actions of Histamine in Humans

Organ-System	Action	Effect	Receptor
Cardiovascular system	Dilatation of arterioles, capillaries, and small veins. Constriction of large veins	Hypotension, flushing, tissue edema, tachycardia	H_1 H_2
	Triple response of Sir Thomas Lewis	Circumscribed erythema at site of injection/stimulation; irregular flare; circumscribed wheal	H_1 H_2
	Heart: direct (somewhat unimportant)	Increased rate	H_2
		Increased force of contraction and cardiac output	H_1 H_2
		Depressed A-V conduction	H_1 (some H_2)
	Heart: indirect	Tachycardia (due to hypotension and release of catecholamines)	—
	Histamine "shock"	Loss of blood volume, fall in venous return and cardiac output	H_1 H_2
Smooth muscle	Contraction of smooth muscle in gut/bronchi	Cramps/diarrhea, bronchospasm	H_1
Exocrine glands	Stomach	Secretion of acid, pepsin, and intrinsic factor	H_2
	Other exocrine glands not fully studied but relatively unimportant		
Peripheral nervous system	Direct stimulation of nerve endings	Itch/pain	H_1
	Axon reflex	Irregular flare of triple response	H_1 H_2
	Adrenal medulla	Epinephrine/norepinephrine release	H_1
Central nervous system	Actions not fully clear	?	?H_1 ?H_2
Hematopoetic system	Neutrophils	Reduced release of lysosomes on phagocytosis	H_2
	T lymphocytes	Reduction in release of lymphokines	H_2
	B lymphocytes	Reduction in release of antibody	H_2
	Mast cell	Increase in cyclic AMP and histamine concentrations	H_2

quent passive postcapillary venular dilatation, and to constriction of the large veins. All small vessels are involved, but the response after i.v. injection in humans is most obvious over the face and upper trunk ("blushing area"). Histamine-induced dilatation of the cerebral vessels produces a severe, throbbing headache probably due to stretching of dural pain sensors.

Reflex tachycardia and increased cardiac output occur secondary to the hypotension, which reverts rapidly as compensatory reflexes are activated, and the amine is destroyed. Large doses of histamine cause a severe fall in blood pressure, shock (due to pooling of blood), and tissue edema.

Histamine increases the permeability of the capillary and the postcapillary vessels by causing separation of endothelial cells and by increasing the size of their gap junctions, allowing transudation of plasma proteins and fluid and thus generating tissue edema. Histamine may variably depress A-V conduction and induce arrythmias.

When histamine is injected into the skin (or when the skin is scratched, liberating endogenous histamine), the *triple response* of Sir Thomas Lewis is seen, which comprises [1] a *circumscribed erythematous zone* that extends for several millimeters around the injection or scratch site owing to terminal arteriolar dilatation. It develops within seconds and after about 1 minute becomes bluish owing to relative deoxygenation; [2] a wider, *irregular area or erythema* or "flare" that develops over several minutes owing to local arteriolar dilatation mediated by axon reflexes; and [3] *localized edema* at the same site as the initial erythema owing to increased permeability of the capillary and postcapillary beds.

Smooth Muscle

Histamine is a powerful, direct stimulant of various smooth muscles, particularly uterine and bronchial smooth muscles in laboratory animals. Bronchoconstriction is most obvious in guinea pigs, where it usually produces death. In normal persons, histamine has little effect on extravascular smooth muscles but in asthmatic subjects may precipitate an acute attack. Stimulation of the pregnant human uterus by histamine is insignificant.

THOMAS LEWIS, 1881–1945. English pathologist and cardiologist. First to use the term "auricular fibrillation" in 1909, also named the sinoauricular node the heart's "pace-maker" (1910). Known for his work in the 1930s on cardiac pain in coronary occlusion.

Exocrine Glands

Although histamine has some stimulant effect on lacrimal, salivary, bronchial, and pancreatic exocrine gland function, its most important secretory effect is exerted on the gastric parietal cells. Doses of histamine less than those required to cause a sustained fall in arterial pressure produce a copious secretion of acid and pepsin. After vagotomy in humans, the maximal secretory response to histamine may fall by about two thirds. This permissive role of the parasympathetic nervous system may partly account for the partial antagonism of antimuscarinic agents for the secretory effects of histamine. It is not yet clear whether histamine is the "final common path" in stimulating parietal cells or whether it is one facet of multireceptor control that involves gastrin and acetylcholine.

Nerve Endings

The "flare" of the triple response (*see* above) is ascribed to excitation of cutaneous sensory nerves, eliciting an axon reflex. When histamine is introduced into the superficial layers of the skin, it induces itching (pruritus) or, more deeply, pain often accompanied by pruritus. Pain and pruritus associated with various stings and venoms may partly be due to endogenous histamine release.

A clearly defined circadian variation is observable to the s.c. injection of histamine; whereas a concentration of 1:10,000 is needed to produce pruritus at 2:00 p.m., a concentration of only 1:1,000,000 is sufficient at 2:00 a.m. There is a parallel variation in the effectiveness of H_1-blockers (*see* below) to antagonize such symptomatology.

Various smooth muscles and exocrine glands are stimulated by histamine both directly and indirectly by way of their motor nerves. Adrenal medullary chromaffin cells, for example, are stimulated by histamine directly, and through the splanchnic nerves indirectly, to secrete epinephrine and norepinephrine. In normal subjects catechol secretion in response to histamine is insignificant, but in patients with a pheochromocytoma, sufficient amines may be released to raise the blood pressure (*see* below).

MODE OF ACTION: H_1 AND H_2 RECEPTORS

Histamine acts on at least two receptors, denoted H_1 and H_2 (Table 51-1). Further refinement into effects mediated by different receptors or subtypes will require more specific agonists and antagonists than are currently available.

There is a direct analogy between histamine and adrenergic receptors: α-Adrenergic receptor blockers are structurally unrelated to norepinephrine, as H_1-receptor blockers are structurally unrelated to histamine, whereas β-adrenergic blockers are closely related to the β agonist isoproterenol, as H_2-receptor blockers are related to histamine.

Some interesting H-receptor agonists have been identified: *2-Methylhistamine* is eight times more active than histamine on H_1-receptors, and *4-methylhistamine* and *dimaprit* (*DI-M*ethyl-*A*mino-*PR*opyl-*I*so-*T*hiourea) are about 200 times more active than the autacoid on H_2-receptors. H_1- and H_2-Blockers may produce some of their effects by mechanisms other than interaction with H_1- and H_2-receptors for histamine. Histamine receptors are probably distinct from those stimulated by serotonin, acetylcholine, and the catecholamines. Clonidine and tolazoline and some antidepressants (*see* Chaps. 22 and 23) are partial H_2 agonists. Some of the effects of histamine in animals may not be mediated through H_1- or H_2-receptors.

ENDOGENOUS HISTAMINE: ROLE IN PHYSIOLOGICAL AND PATHOLOGIC PROCESSES

Gastric Secretion

Histamine is a mediator in normal gastric secretion, and, in patients with cirrhosis and portocaval shunts where absorbed histidine and histamine bypass the liver and may produce hypersecretion of gastric acid and acid/peptic disease. Stress ulcers such as those that follow burns may be mediated by histamine.

Anaphylactic Shock

The similarity between anaphylactic shock and the pharmacologic effects of histamine led Dale and Laidlaw in 1910 to suggest that histamine may serve as a mediator in that condition. Histamine is released during some antigen/antibody reactions, and the intensity of many hypersensitivity phenomena may be considerably reduced by histamine antagonists. Other autacoids and hormones, however, are also liberated or activated to varying degrees from mast cells, in particular bradykinin and other vasoactive kinins (formed on release of a Hageman factor-activating proteolytic enzyme), prostaglandins, 5-hydroxytryptamine (serotonin), an unsaturated fatty acid formed *in vivo* from arachidonic acid known as "slow-reacting substance of anaphylaxis" (SRS-A), platelet activating factor, dopamine (in some instances), and eosinophil chemotactic factor. The relative importance of these other substances in producing symptoms is in dispute. The limited effectiveness of H_1-blockers in "allergy" may be due to the mediation of these other "autacoids." SRS-A, for example, may be important in human asthma. The chemical structure of SRS-A has recently been described, and this, along with the development of a "specific" antagonist (FPL 55712), may lead to a new treatment of asthma.

Histamine Release

Histamine release from mast cells (degranulation) is a complex, poorly understood process that involves several "steps" (Fig. 51-2). Release can be induced by antigen reacting with specific membrane-bound antibody, through drugs or physical agents (Table 51-2), or *in vitro* by calcium ionophores. The calcium on entering the cell may couple with an energy source to facilitate microtubule mediation of exocytosis. Histamine is released from its heparin-protein complex by exchange with extracellular ions, particularly calcium. Normally calcium influx is prevented by cAMP and facilitated by cGMP (*see* Chap. 50).

There are about 10^5 IgE "receptor" sites per mast cell, and their affinity is high ($K_A = 10^{11}$ liters-mole^{-1}). Antigen must bridge at least two membrane-bound antibody molecules to initiate degranulation. Degranulation and possibly Ca^{++} influx initiate mast-cell mediator synthesis.

Other Physiological and Pathologic Processes

Histamine may play a role in the inflammatory reaction, in regulation of the microcirculation, in tissue repair and growth, in modulation of the immune system, and as a neuroeffector transmitter at certain synapses, particularly in the brain and spinal cord. Certainly brain tissue contains a histamine-sensitive adenylcyclase coupled to H_2-receptors, and some antipsychotic and antidepressant drugs may act by way of histaminic neurones (*see* Chaps. 21–24). Gastric carcinoid tumors (*see* Chap. 52) may secrete histamine, and, in urticaria pigmentosa and systemic mastocytosis, release of

---

PATRICK PLAYFAIR LAIDLAW, 1881–1940. British physician. Worked with H. H. Dale on histamine shock; these studies were important in medical care of the wounded in World War I. Also worked on bacteriology and virology. Showed (with others) that human epidemic influenza was viral in nature.

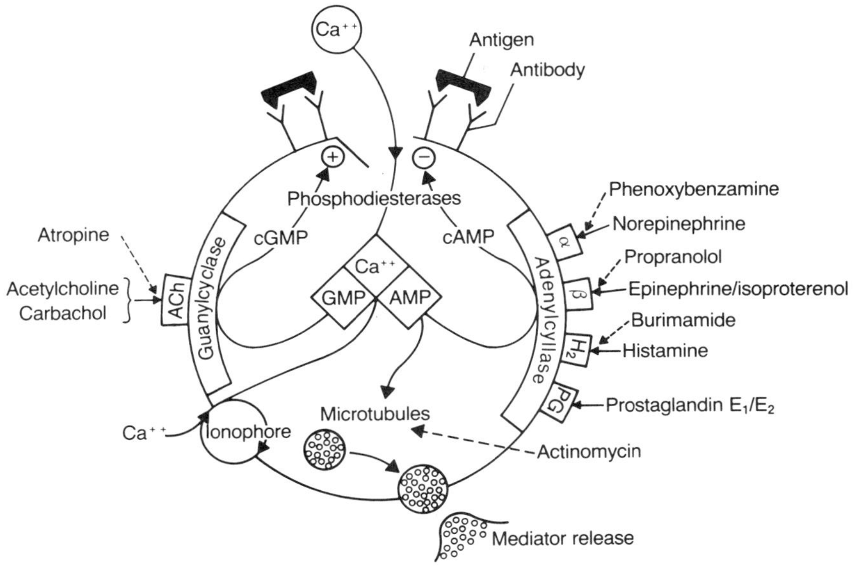

FIG. 51-2. *Diagrammatic representation of a mast cell and a summary of the hypotheses of mediator release* (*see* text for details). ACh = receptors for acetylcholine; α, β = receptors for α, β adrenergic agonists, respectively; H_2 = receptors for histamine; PG = receptors for prostaglandins. Dotted arrows represent inhibition.

mast cell histamine may produce specific symptomatology. Patients with chronic myelogenous leukemia have high blood histamine levels but surprisingly few symptoms, since the histamine is bound tightly in the basophils.

HISTAMINE RELEASE BY DRUGS AND PHYSICAL AGENTS

Endogenous histamine may be released by various physical agents and chemical substances (Table 51-2) in sufficient magnitude to produce symptoms that vary from mild effects to a full-scale anaphylactoid reaction. Rapid i.v. administration of the releaser favors discharge mainly from mast cells along with other substances (*see* above). Drugs likely to initiate histamine release generally possess two or more basic groups separated by, and carried on, an aliphatic or aromatic moiety. Release may simply depend on displacement from storage sites. There are certainly specific subsets of mast cells.

TABLE 51-2. Chemical and Physical Agents That Release Histamine

Chemical Agents		Physical Agents
Antihistamines, H_1-type	Polyvinylpyrrolidine	Mechanical trauma
Chymotrypsin	Propamidine	Radiant energy
Compound 48/80	Reserpine	Thermal energy
Detergents	Surface active agents	
Dextran	Stilbamidine	
DMSO (dimethylsulfoxide)	Toxins	
Morphine and other opioids	Tubocurarine	
Pentamidine	Venoms	
Polymyxin B	X-ray contrast media	

USES

Histamine, or its analogue betazole (*see* below), may be used as a test for gastric acid secretion. In the "augmented" (maximal histamine) test, histamine, 0.04 mg/kg, is given subcutaneously 30 minutes after 100 mg intramuscularly of pyrilamine to minimize its systemic, but not gastric, secretory effects. This test gives a measure of the total number of functional parietal cells (parietal cell "mass") present, and is useful in identifying patients with true achlorhydria (the hallmark of addisonian pernicious anemia), to lower the gastric *p*H below 6 in response to maximal histamine stimulation.

Histamine (3 μg/kg intravenously) *tyramine* (1.0 mg intravenously), *glucagon* (0.5–1.0 mg intravenously) and *phentolamine* (*see* Chap. 18) can be used as provocative tests for pheochromocytoma, but false-positive and -negative responses occur in about 30% of patients. These tests should be done only when the laboratory data are equivocal and when the blood pressure is normal or only slightly elevated. Since fatalities due to hypertensive crises and cerebrovascular accidents have been reported using these tests, they should be performed only in patients with an i.v. running and an α-adrenergic receptor blocking agent (*see* Chap. 18) available.

PREPARATIONS

Histamine phosphate, U.S.P., is available as a solution for injection in concentrations of 100 μg, 200 μg, and 1000 μg/ml. Doses of histamine are classically expressed in terms of the base: 2.75 mg of the phosphate salt are equivalent to 1 mg of histamine base.

BETAZOLE

Betazole, an isomer of histamine, possesses potent gastric secretagogue activity but little or no systemic activity. Thus it is a convenient alternative to histamine in gastric secretory function tests because premedication with an H_1-blocker is not required.

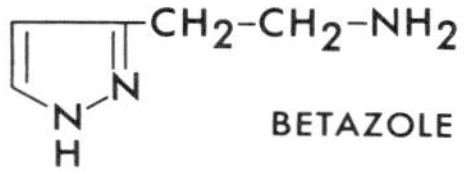

BETAZOLE

Betazole hydrochloride, U.S.P. (Histalog), is given in a dose of 0.5 mg/kg subcutaneously.

DRUGS THAT AFFECT THE RELEASE OR ACTIONS OF HISTAMINE

The pharmacologic actions or release of histamine can be countered in several ways. *Cromolyn sodium*, for example, prevents release of histamine from mast cells (*see* below); *antihistamines* block the actions of histamine at H_1- and H_2-receptors; *glucocorticosteroids* (*see* Chap. 47) suppress some of the effects of antigen/antibody reactions, particularly those of a chronic nature; and *epinephrine* (*see* below and Chap. 17) acts as a physiological antagonist.

H_1-RECEPTOR ANTAGONISTS

After the synthesis of the first compound with significant H_1-receptor blocking in 1937, dozens of H_1-blockers became available for clinical use. These agents differ from each other primarily in *antihistaminic potency*, *duration* of action, *severity of adverse effects*, *cost*, and in the possession of certain additional pharmacologic properties coincidentally associated, such as *sedation*.

Structure–Activity Relationships

Most of the important H_1-blockers contain a substituted ethylamine-CH-CH-N= that is also present in histamine (Fig. 51-3). This moiety may present as a straight chain (*e.g.*, diphenhydramine) or as part of a ring structure (*e.g.*, chlorcyclizine) but is also present in many compounds that possess no histamine-blocking ability.

Histamine Antagonism

H_1-Blockers do not influence the formation or release (It should be noted, however, that when given rapidly intravenously some H_1-blockers may liberate histamine from storage sites [Table 51-2].) of histamine but selectively and competitively antagonize its actions at specific receptor sites by exclusion of histamine, without themselves initiating a response. Generally urticaria and pruritus are well antagonized, but bronchospasm and hypotension are less well controlled. *There is considerable variation in their efficacy for blocking the different pharmacologic actions of histamine.* Thus H_1-blockers are most effective when given before the interaction of histamine with its receptor. A dramatic example occurs in guinea pigs, where death by asphyxia after severe bronchospasm occurs with quite small doses of histamine, yet a hundred lethal doses of histamine may be given with impunity if the animal is protected by an H_1-blocker.

H_1-Blockers are more effective against exogenously administered histamine than in combating symptoms of anaphylaxis and allergy, or after histamine release by chemicals (Table 51-2). This may be due to the following: [1] Other autacoids such as SRS-A, against which H_1-blockers are ineffective, may be concomitantly liberated; [2] the appropriate histamine receptor may be inaccessible to the anithistamine in sufficient concentration; and [3] antigen/antibody reactions may under certain circumstances directly evoke a response without intervention of a humoral mediator, such as in bronchial smooth muscle.

Miscellaneous Actions

H_1-Blockers possess variable parasympatholytic activity and sedative properties that may be exploited clinically.

Central Nervous System. Drowsiness is commonly produced. Rarely restlessness, nervousness, and insomnia may occur, and, in some patients with focal lesions of the cerebral cor-

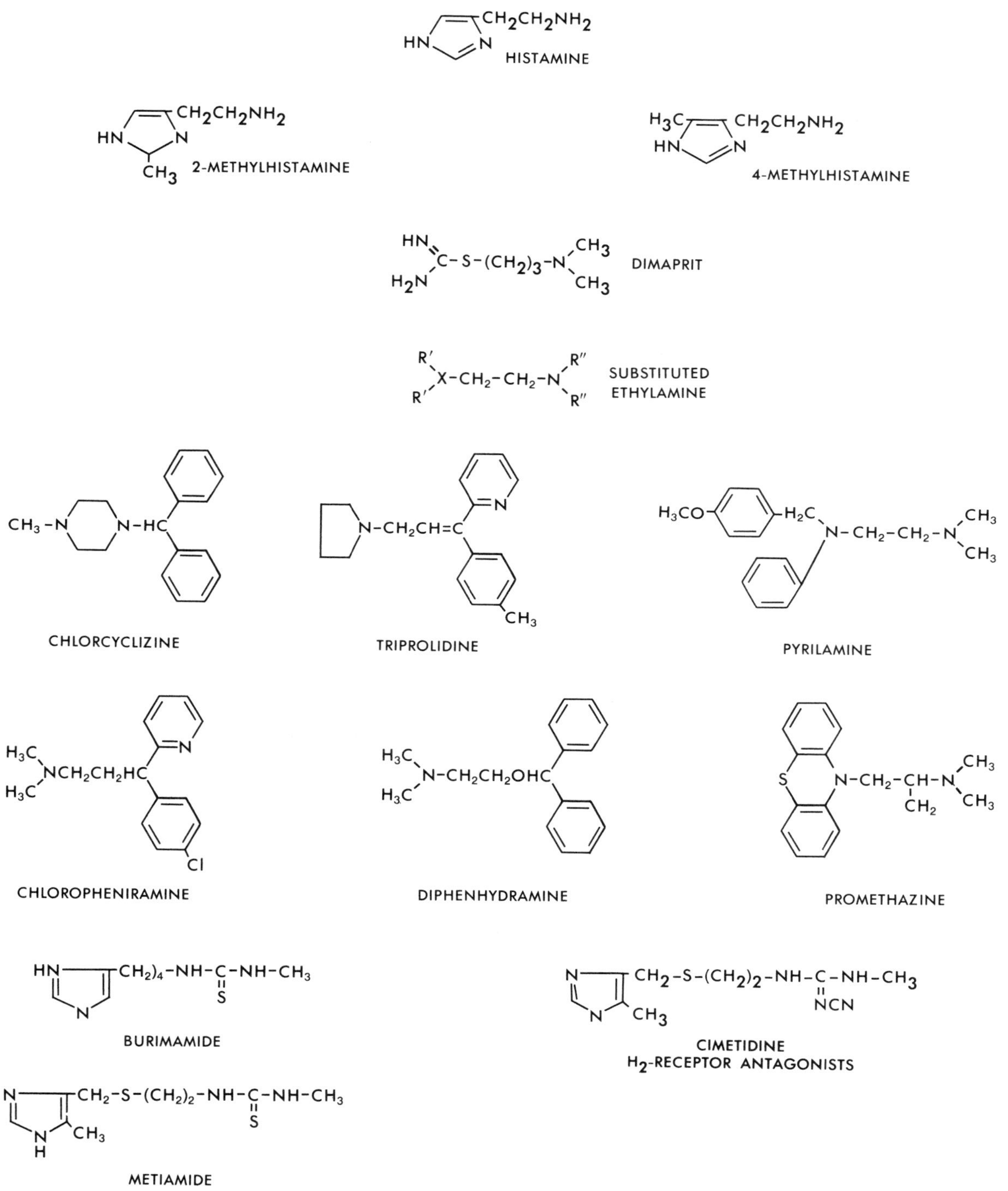

FIG. 51-3. Histamine, some histamine receptor agonists, and some important H_1 and H_2 receptor antagonists.

tex, EEG activation and epileptiform seizures may develop. Some weak H_1-blockers suppress motion sickness and the nausea and vomiting that result from labyrinthine disturbance without producing sedation. Others lessen rigidity and improve spontaneous movement and speech in drug-induced extrapyramidal disorders.

Peripheral Nervous System. A local anesthetic action contributes to the relief of pruritus after topical application. When given intravenously in sufficiently high dosage, some H_1-blockers may produce quinidine-like effects on myocardial conduction.

Absorption, Metabolism, and Excretion

H_1-Blockers are readily absorbed after oral or parenteral administration, with effects usually manifesting themselves within 30 minutes. Their duration of action varies (Table 51-3), but little is known about their metabolic fate or excretion. Being weak bases, their gastrointestinal absorption and renal excretion critically depend on *p*H (*see* Chaps. 3 and 4).

Adverse Effects

In therapeutic doses all H_1-blockers elicit adverse effects that are rarely serious but may in

TABLE 51-3. Major Groups of Official H_1-Blocking Antihistamine Preparations

	Group and Nonproprietary Name	Formulary	Trade Name	Single Adult Dose	Duration of Action	Comment
				mg	*hr*	
I	*Alkylamines*					
	Chlorpheniramine maleate	*U.S.P.*	Chlor-Trimeton maleate, Histaspar, Teldrin	2–4	4–6	Slightly sedative but may cause excitement
	Triprolidine		Actidil	2–5	8–12	Weak sedative, prolonged action
II	*Ethanolamines*					
	Dimenhydrinate	*U.S.P.*	Dramamine	50	4–6	Similar actions to diphenyhydramine because it is the 8-chlorotheophyllinate salt of that compound
	Diphenhydramine hydrochloride	*U.S.P.*	Benadryl hydrochloride	25–50	4–6	Marked sedative, parasympatholytic, local anesthetic, useful in drug-induced extrapyramidal disorders. Intravenous injection must be given very slowly
III	*Ethylenediamines*					
	Pyrilamine maleate	*N.F.*	Neo-Antergan maleate, Paraminyl maleate, Pyramal maleate, Stamine, among others	25–50	4–6	One of the most specific histamine antagonists known. Possesses no significant atropinic activity. Weak sedative
	Tripelennamine hydrochloride	*U.S.P.*	Pyribenzamine hydrochloride	50	4–6	Moderately sedative, local anesthetic, sometimes causes excitement and gastric irritation
IV	*Phenothiazines*					
	Promethazine hydrochloride	*U.S.P.*	Phenergan hydrochloride	25–50	4–6	Marked sedative, some atropinic action, effective against motion sickness. Prototype phenothiazine that led to development of tranquilizers (*see* Chap. 25)
V	*Piperazines*					
	Chlorcyclizine hydrochloride	*N.F.*	Di-Paralene hydrochloride	50	8–12	Slightly sedative, little atropinic activity
	Cyclizine hydrochloride	*U.S.P.*	Marzine hydrochloride	50–100	4–8	Little sedative or atropinic activity, used primarily for motion sickness
	Meclizine hydrochloride	*U.S.P.*	Bonine hydrochloride	25–50	8–16	Used mainly for motion sickness. Prolonged action

susceptible persons necessitate discontinuance of therapy. Importantly, *there is marked patient variation in predisposition to adverse effects.*

Depression of the CNS with sedation is common and may be a desirable phenomenon in overanxious patients or in those about to retire for the night, but during the day sedation may cause accidents. *Potentiation of H_1-blocker-induced sedation by alcohol and other CNS depressants* (Table 51-4) *is a major cause of automobile and other accidents.* Dizziness, tinnitus, incoordination, impaired judgment, ataxia, hyporeflexia, diplopia, dilated pupils, and fatigue may develop. Very rarely central excitement may occur with development of euphoria, insomnia, nervousness, tremor, hyperreflexia, and paresthesias.

Some H_1-blockers possess antimuscarinic properties that produce dry mouth, nose, and throat (cough) and dysuria or urinary retention, blurring of vision, impotence, and gastrointestinal symptoms. Very rarely, loss of teeth or loosening of dentures may occur with chronic therapy. Anorexia, nausea, vomiting, and alteration in bowel habit are not unusual and can generally be controlled by administering the drug with meals. Bone marrow depression (leukopenia or agranulocytosis), hemolytic anemia, or hepatitis may rarely develop, usually with phenothiazine H_1-blockers. Because some H_1-blockers are teratogenic in animals, the use of these agents is generally contraindicated during pregnancy; most antihistamines are excreted in milk. The topical administration of H_1-blockers may result in hypersensitivity, and systemic therapy particularly with phenothiazine derivatives may result in photosensitivity reactions (*see* Chaps. 11 and 22). H_1-Blockers commonly suppress the immediate cutaneous response to allergens.

Accidental acute poisoning is not uncommon with over-the-counter (OTC) H_1-blockers, particularly in children. Generally, two to three dozen capsules or tablets of most commercially available H_1-blockers constitute a near lethal or fatal dose in children. Whereas central depression with sedation usually accompanies therapeutic doses of pure antihistamines, toxic doses (particularly with OTC sleeping tablets that contain atropinic agents) may produce stimulation with hallucinations, excitement, involuntary movements, convulsions, fixed dilated pupils, and hyperpyrexia. Terminally, deepening cardiorespiratory collapse develops. Treatment is symptomatic and supportive. Mechanical support of ventilation and a short-acting barbiturate to control convulsions are important adjuncts in therapy.

Preparations and Dosage

Numerous H_1-blockers are available (Table 51-3) either singly or in combination with other pharmacologic agents, and "new" H_1-blockers are constantly being introduced, usually with exaggerated therapeutic claims.

Except for individual specific properties (Table 51-3), *the most important factor that governs the use of H_1-blockers is variation in patient response.* Desirably, therapy should be started with a well-tried agent and additional agents should be substituted only if the first proves unsatisfactory. Tolerance may appear with chronic therapy; switching to a second H_1-

TABLE 51-4. Drug Interactions with Antihistamines

Antihistamine	Second Drug	Comment
Antihistamines, H_1-blocking type	Alcohol, sedatives, tranquillizers, hypnotics, or other CNS depressants	Enhanced sedation
Diphenhydramine and other agents with anticholinergic effects (Table 51-3)	Anticholinergic agents	Anticholinergic side-effects more likely
Antihistamines, H_1-blocking type	Tricyclic antidepressants	Anticholinergic side-effects more likely
Antihistamines, H_1-blocking type	Guanethidine	Reduced effectiveness of the antihypertensive agent
Cimetidine	Antacids	Absorption of cimetidine may be reduced
Cimetidine	Warfarin, phenindione, diazepam, chlordiazepoxide	Cimetidine retards the metabolism of the second drug
Cimetidine	Iron and vitamin B_{12} (in the diet)	Cimetidine in chronic therapy may be associated with decreased absorption of the dietary nutrients

blocker, possibly from a different chemical class, is usually effective.

Uses

Hypersensitivity States. In the symptomatic treatment of *acute and chronic urticaria and pruritus* (*e.g.*, atopic and contact dermatitis, allergic drug reactions, insect bites, and reactions to plants such as poison ivy or poison oak), H_1-blockers serve as adjuncts to removal of the allergen and to specific desensitization or suppression of the antigen/antibody reaction with glucocorticoids. They are most valuable in the acute situation and may be given either systemically or topically. Topical administration may have the additional advantage of a local anesthetic action but is often followed by the development of contact hypersensitivity. Additionally H_1-blockers are valuable in *hay fever* and *vasomotor rhinitis* (often accompanied by decongestants). In serum sickness, H_1-blockers reduce pruritus and urticaria but have no effect on fever or arthralgia.

H_1-Blockers play a secondary role in the therapy of anaphylactic shock, angioneurotic edema, and bronchial asthma, where physiological antagonists to histamine are of prime importance, namely, epinephrine to treat anaphylactic shock and angioneurotic edema, and epinephrine, theophylline, and isoproterenol to treat asthma. Physiological antagonists are desirable over H_1-blockers because they act more rapidly than do the antihistamines; they produce an opposing effect rather than an agonist blockade; and autacoids unaffected by H_1-blockers are presumably involved in symptomatology. Epinephrine, for example, produces vasoconstriction in the presence of histamine, but in a similar situation H_1-blockers antagonize the vasodilation produced by histamine but do not in themselves produce vasoconstriction.

H_1-Blockers are usually contraindicated in the treatment of asthma because they antagonize bronchoconstriction poorly and they dry bronchial secretions. Occasionally H_1-blockers are indicated, for example, in the relief of upper respiratory symptoms of allergy that may precipitate bronchospasm.

Sedation, Motion Sickness, Nausea, Vomiting, and Miscellaneous Uses. Some H_1-blockers are marketed specifically as *sedatives*, often combined with atropinic agents—for example, methapyrilene plus scopolamine. Piperazine class H_1-blockers and promethazine and diphenhydramine are particularly useful in the *symptomatic treatment of motion sickness* or the *nausea and vomiting* that occur postoperatively or after radiation exposure. H_1-Blockers have been used to treat nausea and vomiting of pregnancy, but it is preferable to minimize drug use during pregnancy. Some H_1-blockers have been used to treat *drug-induced extrapyramidal reactions*.

Despite extravagant advertising claims, there is no evidence that H_1-blockers influence the course of the common cold, although some symptomatic benefit may be obtained, particularly if there is a superimposed allergic component.

H_2-RECEPTOR ANTAGONISTS

Burimamide, the first H_2-blocker, had low potency, was inactive orally, and was toxic in animals. The second agent, *metiamide,* was withdrawn after a few cases of agranulocytosis had developed, probably due to its thiourea moiety. *Cimetidine* is the only H_2-blocker now clinically available. It is closely related to metiamide with a cyanoguanidine substitution for the thiourea radical (Fig. 51-3). It is estimated that more than 20% of the British population has received an H_2-blocker. Several more potent congeners of cimetidine are under clinical trial, especially ranitidine.

Chemistry

H_2-Blockers are hydrophilic, bear a close structural similarity to histamine, and have a side-chain which, although polar, is uncharged. Thus they differ from H_1-blockers, which possess a side-chain that is positively charged at physiologic *p*H. Lacking a side-chain charge, H_2-blockers cannot act as agonists mimicking histamine.

Actions and Receptor Location

The tissue location of H_2-receptors is indicated in Table 51-1. In humans, cimetidine reduces basal and nearly all forms of stimulated and nocturnal gastric acid secretion in both normal subjects and those with duodenal ulcer disease. Secretory depression is dose related, and a 50% reduction is obtained by a dose of cimetidine yielding a blood level of 1 to 2 μmol/liter (0.25–0.50 μg/ml). Cimetidine has no direct effect on blood gastrin levels, but pepsin secretion and intrinsic factor output are variably depressed. Cimetidine reduces the absorption of protein-bound vitamin B_{12}. It has no major effect on the rate of gastric emptying (presumably the reduced duodenal acid load reduces, in turn, the secretin response) or on esophageal motility or pressure changes in normal subjects or in those with various esophagogastric disorders. A peripheral antiandrogen effect (a diminution of testicular, prostatic, and seminal vesicular size and hypospermia) is seen in humans and several animals, but no interference is observed with reproduction. In humans, cimetidine depresses sebum production.

The presence of H_2-receptors on mast cells suggests that histamine released locally could, through simple feedback, limit its own release. In clinical use of H_2-blockers, however, no evidence suggests that exaggerated release of histamine occurs. Further, no evidence suggests that the use of H_2-blockers is followed by an exaggerated cell-mediated immune response. Cimetidine inhibits (within a couple of days) the rate of metabolism of warfarin and phenindione (increasing the prothrombin time) and chlordiazepoxide and diazapam. After 1 month of standard therapy with cimetidine, the gastric flora becomes significantly changed with the presence of some "fecal" organisms.

Absorption, Distribution, Metabolism, and Excretion

Cimetidine is well absorbed (bioavailability 65–75%) by the small bowel after oral administration. In the fasting state, peak absorption occurs within 60 to 120 minutes and is dose related between 100 and 800 mg; in fasting subjects a second unexplained plasma peak occurs at about 3 hours. When given with food, cimetidine has lower peak concentrations and they occur later than when given in the fasting state, but the area under the serum concentration/time curve (AUC) (*see* Chap. 5) for 6 hours is about the same. Thus clinically, cimetidine should be given with meals because more sustained gastric secretory inhibition is produced. Net absorption may be depressed by antacids.

Cimetidine has a large apparent volume of distribution (~25 liters), but little reaches the brain because of the drug's low lipophilicity. Cimetidine crosses the placental barrier and is excreted by the kidney, with a half-life of about 2 hours. Excretion is inversely proportional to creatinine clearance, and at a value of less than 1 to 2 ml/min cimetidine has a half-life of about 5 hours. About 70% of cimetidine is excreted unchanged within 2 hours; about 5% appears in the urine as a 5-hydroxymethyl derivative, and about 10% as a sulfoxide. Cimetidine is cleared by hemodialysis.

Adverse Effects

About 5% to 20% of patients develop symptoms of headache, tiredness, myalgia, skin rashes, dizziness, fever, constipation, and diarrhea. These symptoms have also been reported by placebo-treated patients in clinical trials of treatment for ulcer disease. Mastodynia with or without unilateral or bilateral gynecomastia has been reported, particularly in patients with the Zollinger–Ellison syndrome or in those taking very high doses of cimetidine. Gynecomastia may be due to a blockade of an androgen-responsive receptor in breast tissue, and it usually regresses during, or promptly after, discontinuation of therapy. Galactorrhea has been reported in a few women taking high doses of cimetidine. Cimetidine raises serum prolactin levels without affecting serum testosterone, LH, FSH, GH, T_3, T_4, or TSH. Bromocriptine, a dopamine agonist, blocks cimetidine-induced hyperprolactinemia in humans. (Dopamine is considered to be the inhibitor of prolactin release by the anterior pituitary; *see* Chap. 43.)

Rare side-effects reported with cimetidine therapy include cholestasis, loss of libido, impotence, iron-deficiency anemia, hypertension, ileus, pancreatitis, bradycardia, A-V dissociation, Stevens–Johnson syndrome, autoimmune hemolytic anemia, and thrombocytopenia. Central nervous system toxicity may also develop rarely, and agitation, belligerence, slurred speech, carphologia, dysarthria, diplopia, mental confusion, visual hallucinations, myoclonus, and coma have been described. Some of these side-effects have appeared in patients with raised trough concentrations of cimetidine usually in response to renal or, rarely, hepatic dysfunction.

Parietal cell hyperplasia, hypergastrinemia, and megaloblastic anemia are theoretical consequences of chronic therapy but have not been reported.

Bone Marrow. Leukopenia has been reported in association with cimetidine therapy. Cimetidine blocks 4-methylhistamine-induced stimulation of mouse-marrow stem cells from the G_0 state into the DNA synthetic phase and histamine-induced DNA synthesis. Thus there remains the remote possibility that cimetidine may produce bone marrow depression. Additionally, there is still concern about the possible immunologic consequences of acute or chronic H_2-blockade.

ROBERT MILTON ZOLLINGER, 1903– . American physician. Described with E. H. Ellison the Zollinger–Ellison syndrome in 1955, involving gastric hypersecretion, recurrent peptic ulceration, and pancreatic tumors.

EDWIN HOMER ELLISON, 1918–1970. American surgeon. Specialized in pancreatic secretion and the pathogenesis of ulcers. Coauthor of the first paper, in 1955, to describe the Zollinger–Ellison syndrome.

Biochemical Changes. Plasma creatinine values rise (usually within the normal range) in about 40% to 60% of patients, but, in 3% to 5% of patients, values of greater than 2 mg/dl occur. This elevation is unexplained, since plasma BUN and uric acid levels remain unchanged. Plasma levels of SGOT and SGPT may rise during cimetidine therapy.

Uses

In the United States, cimetidine is approved for control of gastric secretion in duodenal ulceration and recurrent ulceration after surgery, including the Zollinger–Ellison syndrome and hypergastrinemic states such as the short-bowel syndrome, multiple endocrine adenomatosis, and systemic mastocytosis. In countries other than the United States, cimetidine has been used in gastric and esophageal ulceration to prevent stress-induced gastrointestinal bleeding/ulceration, as prophylaxis against gastrointestinal side-effects of certain ulcerogenic drugs, to treat reflux esophagitis, gastritis, and duodenitis, to lessen the gastric destruction of oral enzyme replacement therapy in patients with pancreatitis, and as prophylaxis in Mendelson's syndrome.

The precise role of cimetidine in relation to the use of other drugs for ulcer disease is not yet established (*see* Chap. 38). Similarly, it is not clear as to what type of patient needs chronic therapy, what dose should be used, and for how long therapy should continue. *Some malignant ulcers will heal temporarily with cimetidine,* and most peptic ulcers will promptly relapse after withdrawal of the drug. Some ulcers have perforated during "adequate" cimetidine therapy.

Preparations and Dosage

Cimetidine (Tagamet) is available in the United States as 300-mg tablets or ampoules. In duodenal ulcer and ulceration in hypersecretory states, the dose is 300 mg every 6 hours (with meals and at bedtime). For duodenal ulcer disease, treatment should be continued until the ulcer heals or, if reassessment is not possible, for up to 8 weeks. In the Zollinger–Ellison syndrome, doses up to 2 to 4 g daily may be given. If parenteral administration is required, the drug should be diluted in physiologic saline and infused intravenously over 20 minutes.

CROMOLYN SODIUM

Cromolyn sodium is available as a dry powder for inhalation as an adjunct in the management of patients with severe perennial bronchial asthma.

Chemistry

Cromolyn sodium is a highly water-soluble synthetic analogue of khellin, the active spasmolytic ingredient extracted from the seeds of *Ammi visnaga,* an herb long used in eastern Mediterranean areas to prepare a tea found effective in treating colic in children. Chemically, cromolyn is the disodium salt of 1,3-bis-(2-carboxychromone-5-yloxy)-2-hydropropane.

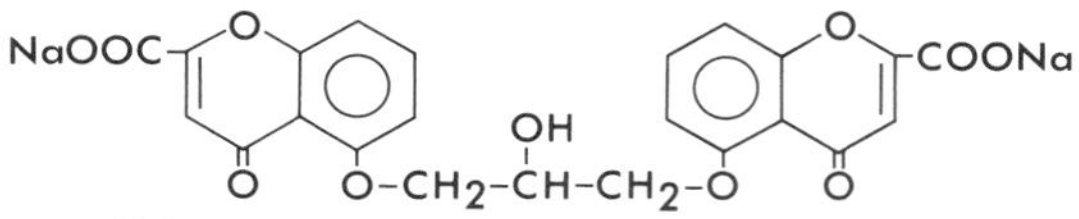

Mode of Action

Cromolyn sodium "stabilizes" the membrane of sensitized animal mast cells, possibly by inhibiting the action of phosphodiesterase, thus preventing the influx of Ca^{++} with subsequent release of histamine and other substances.

Absorption, Metabolism, and Excretion

Cromolyn sodium is inhaled by means of a special device known as the spinhaler. Only about 10% of the total inhaled dose is absorbed, and cromolyn sodium is rapidly excreted unchanged in the bile and urine, with a half-life of about 80 minutes. That portion of the inhaled dose not absorbed is either exhaled or swallowed, and cleared through the gastrointestinal tract. Cromolyn sodium is very poorly absorbed after oral administration.

Adverse Effects

The incidence of serious adverse effects is about 2%. Maculopapular and urticarial skin rashes and urethral burning may develop, but these usually clear on cessation of therapy. Cough, bronchospasm, nasal congestion, and rarely an eosinophilic pneumonia have also been reported, as have dizziness, joint pains and swelling, nausea, and headaches. Allergic dermatoses and anaphylactic shock may develop rarely.

Preparations and Dosage

Cromolyn sodium is most useful in preventing exercise-induced and "extrinsic" asthma as opposed to "intrinsic" asthma. It is not effective in treating an acute attack of asthma or in treating *status asthmaticus.* Children usually respond better than do adults, and patients treated prophylactically may need lesser amounts of other drugs. Cromolyn sodium therapy should be attempted in patients who cannot be managed without glucocorticosteriods.

Cromolyn sodium has been used to treat systemic mastocytosis, food allergies, and ulcerative colitis.

FURTHER READING

1. Ahmad S: Side effects of cimetidine. South Med J 72:509–513, 1979
2. Ash ASF, Schild HO: Receptors mediating some actions of histamine. Br J Pharmacol 27:427–439, 1966
3. Beaven MA: Histamine. N Engl J Med Part 1: 30–36, January 1976, Part 2:320–325, February 1976
4. Brimblecoombe RW, Parsons ME: Histamine H_2-receptor antagonists. In Goldberg ME (ed): Pharmacological and Biochemical Properties of Drug Substances, Vol 1, pp 329–352. Washington, DC, Pharmaceutical Manufacturers Association, 1977
5. Burland WL, Duncan WAM, Hesselbo T et al: Pharmacological evaluation of cimetidine, a new histamine H_2-receptor antagonist, in healthy man. Br J Clin Pharmacol 2:481–486, 1975
6. Chand N, Eyre P: Classification and biological distribution of histamine receptor subtypes. Agents Actions 5:277–295, 1975.
7. Fordtran JS, Grossman MI: Third symposium on histamine H_2 receptor antagonists: Clinical results with cimetidine. Gastroenterology 74, No. 2:338–488, February 1978
8. Hirschowitz BI: H_2 receptors. Ann Rev Pharmacol Toxicol 19:203–244, 1979
9. Pearlman DS: Antihistamines: Pharmacology and clinical use. Drugs 12:258–273, 1976
10. Reite OB: Comparative physiology of histamine. Physiol Rev 52:778–819, 1972
11. Roche E, Silva M (eds): Histamine and Antihistamine. Handbook of Experimental Pharmacology, Vol 18, Part 1, pp 1–991. New York, Springer, 1965

CHAPTER 51 QUESTIONS

(See P. 7 for Full Instructions)

Select the One Best Answer

1. Each of the following is true for histamine EXCEPT that
   - *A.* biosynthesis requires adequate vitamin B_6.
   - *B.* inactivation occurs principally through N-methylation.
   - *C.* storage is in mast cell granules.
   - *D.* it produces the "triple response" in the skin.
   - *E.* it generally causes bradycardia.

2. Each of the following has a marked effect on gastric secretion EXCEPT
   - *A.* betazole hydrochloride.
   - *B.* pentagastrin.
   - *C.* cimetidine.
   - *D.* tripelennamine.
   - *E.* 4-Methyl histamine.

3. What agent should be administered parenterally to relieve the laryngeal edema and bronchial constriction caused by an acute allergic reaction to penicillin?
   - *A.* Diphenhydramine
   - *B.* Epinephrine
   - *C.* Prednisolone
   - *D.* Atropine
   - *E.* Cromolyn sodium

4. An antihistamine characterized by its usefulness in treating drug-induced extra-pyramidal disorders and motion sickness is
   - *A.* chlorpheniramine.
   - *B.* diphenhydramine.
   - *C.* tripelennamine.
   - *D.* promethazine.
   - *E.* meclizine.

5. Known effects of cimetidine include each of the following EXCEPT
   - *A.* reduction of muscarinic stimulation of gastric acid secretion.
   - *B.* protection against gastric ulceration in the Zollinger–Ellison Syndrome.
   - *C.* production of pernicious anemia.
   - *D.* gonadotropic side-effects.
   - *E.* healing of duodenal ulcers.

A = 1,2,3; B = 1,3; C = 2,4; D = 4; E = All

6. Drugs that can release histamine include
   - *1.* codeine.
   - *2.* diphenhydramine.
   - *3.* *d*-tubocurarine.
   - *4.* DMSO (dimethylsulfoxide).

7. Histamine
   - *1.* -induced gastric acid secretion may be prevented by diphenhydramine.
   - *2.* is a pressor agent in the presence of pheochromocytoma.
   - *3.* inhibits intrinsic factor secretion.
   - *4.* is released during anaphylactic shock.

8. H_1-Blockers are not "pure" drugs in a pharmacologic sense. In addition to the

antagonism of histamine action, they may produce
1. sedation.
2. local anesthesia.
3. anticholinergic effects.
4. sympathomimetic effects.

9. Chlorpheniramine
1. will ameliorate the symptoms of seasonal allergic rhinitis.
2. inhibits histamine-induced secretion of gastric acid.
3. produces less drowsiness than does diphenhydramine.
4. is widely used in treating motion sickness.

10. Cimetidine
1. inhibits the cardiovascular effects of histamine.
2. reduces gastrointestinal motility.
3. antagonizes the gastric secretory effect of histamine.
4. reduces the symptoms of hay fever.

11. Cromolyn sodium
1. may cause anaphylactic shock.
2. is the drug of choice for treating anaphylactic shock.
3. inhibits the release of histamine and SRS-A.
4. inhibits the contraction of bronchioles in response to autacoids.

JEREMY H. THOMPSON

52 Serotonin and Serotonin Antagonists

The discovery of serotonin as a naturally occurring amine resulted from independent investigations on two substances: *enteramine* (by Erspamer), present in the enterochromaffin (argentaffin) cells of the gastrointestinal tract; and *vasotonin* (by Page), a vasoconstrictor present in serum. Both substances have been shown to be *serotonin* (5-hydroxytryptamine), first synthesized in 1951. Like histamine, serotonin is ubiquitous in nature, being found in almost all vertebrates and invertebrates and in many fruits (avocados, bananas, eggplant, passion fruit, pineapples, plantain, plums, tomatoes), nuts (walnuts), stings (cowhage, the source of "itching powder," nettle), and venoms (bee, scorpion, and wasp).

The wide distribution of serotonin and its potent pharmacologic actions have prompted speculation on the functions of the amine in health and disease. Despite an enormous quantity of research, however, the precise role of serotonin in the mammalian organism is far from clear.

IRVINE HEINLY PAGE, 1901– . American physician. In 1930s and 1940s worked on determination methods, for example, for plasma proteins and lipids. Also known for studies on hypertension, Page synthesized angiotensin in 1956 with F. M. Bumpus and H. Schwartz. Suggested that hypertension and arteriosclerosis have similar causes.

VITTORIO ERSPAMER, 1909– . Italian pharmacologist. Extensive research on serotonin and other biogenic amines. First to describe octopamine, leptodactyline, murexine, and several polypeptides active on smooth muscle.

CHEMISTRY AND BIOCHEMISTRY

Serotonin (Fig. 52-1) is 3(β-aminoethyl)-5-hydroxyindole and is usually prepared as the creatinine sulfate salt.

SYNTHESIS, DISTRIBUTION, AND STORAGE

The major pathway of serotonin synthesis is from dietary tryptophan (Fig. 52-1). Local synthesis accounts for the serotonin content of mammalian tissues except for platelets, that are devoid of 5-hydroxytryptophan decarboxylase. During passage through the splanchnic

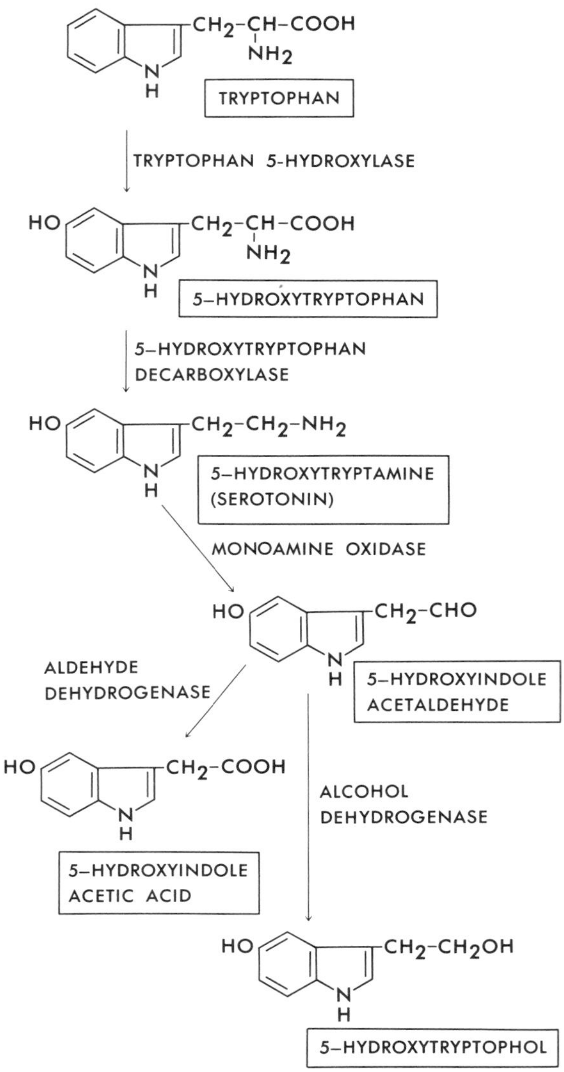

FIG. 52-1. Major pathways of serotonin synthesis and degradation in humans.

area, platelets avidly take up the amine released from enterochromaffin cells and store it in an inactive form. Greater than 99% of the serotonin released from the gastrointestinal tract and not taken up by platelets is inactivated by uptake or catabolic processes in the hepatic and pulmonary vascular beds, thus "protecting" the systemic circulation. Many central neurons that normally synthesize and store serotonin also have the capacity to take up preformed serotonin from the cerebrospinal fluid; little serotonin passes the blood–brain barrier. Brain serotonin levels can be raised, however, by diets rich in tryptophan.

About 1% to 2% of dietary tryptophan is converted into serotonin in normal subjects, but greater than 60% may be converted in patients with the carcinoid syndrome (*see* below).

The distribution and content of serotonin within the body vary widely in different species. The amount in humans is about 10 mg, of which about 90% is present in the gastrointestinal tract. Of the remainder, most is present in platelets, lungs, bone marrow, and brain, although most tissues can be shown to contain some serotonin. Quantitative data on the serotonin concentration within any given tissue are only of limited value because the single measurement gives no indication of the rapidity of turnover, that is, the degree of amine synthesis and storage, or of release and metabolism. The gastrointestinal tract, for example, contains about 90% of the total body serotonin, whereas the brain contains about 3%; yet the turnover times for gastrointestinal serotonin and brain serotonin are about 12 to 16 hours and 1 hour, respectively. In platelets, serotonin is strongly bound but liberated on platelet destruction.

Gastrointestinal serotonin is present in the enterochromaffin (argentaffin) cells, cells of the APUD (Amine Precursor Uptake and Decarboxylation) series, and in the myenteric plexus. Mast cells of many species, particularly rodents, contain serotonin, but the amine has been identified only in human mast cells from patients with the carcinoid syndrome. In studies of animals (particularly rodents), serotonin-containing neurones have been found in the raphé nucleus of the lower brain stem, from which tracts innervate many diverse areas of the CNS. For a further discussion of central serotoninergic mechanisms, *see* Chapter 21.

The mechanisms of serotonin uptake and storage have been mainly studied using platelets. Serotonin is taken up by an active process into the cytoplasm, and from there incorporated by an energy-dependent process into storage granules. Within the storage granules, serotonin is complexed with ATP and possibly other substances. Reserpine has similar actions on the storage of catecholamines and serotonin (*see* Chap. 36). Reserpine blocks the energy-dependent uptake of serotonin and promotes its release. Storage of serotonin in enterochromaffin granules and neuronal vesicles may involve a similar energy-dependent storage process.

METABOLISM

The metabolism of serotonin is subject to wide species variation, but in humans two routes predominate (Fig. 52-1). In these two pathways, serotonin is initially oxidatively deaminated by nonspecific monoamine oxidase to 5-hydroxyindoleacetaldehyde, which is then further oxidized to predominately 5-hydroxyindoleacetic acid (5-HIAA) or reduced to the corresponding alcohol, 5-hydroxytryptophol (5-HTOL). Both 5-HIAA and 5-HTOL, mainly as glucuronides or sulfates are excreted in the urine. About 2 to 10 mg of 5-HIAA are excreted daily, but higher values are found in some patients with the carcinoid syndrome or in those eating serotonin-containing foods. Ethyl alcohol ingestion greatly increases 5-HTOL excretion at the expense of 5-HIAA. Several other minor pathways of serotonin metabolism have been described, particularly oxygenation, conjugation, *O*-methylation, *N*-methylation, and *N*-acetylation. These may assume importance when monoamine oxidase inhibitors are used.

PHARMACOLOGIC ACTIONS

Serotonin has numerous pharmacologic effects on various types of smooth muscle, nerves, and exocrine glands in animals and humans. Because serotonin causes direct, as well as indirect, and reflex effects and because tachyphylaxis is common, the ultimate pharmacologic responses are invariably complex. Effects of serotonin show not only wide species variation but also wide variation within a given species, and even variation between consecutive experiments in the same animal. The following description generally applies to humans. Responses characteristic of a given animal species are identified.

CARDIOVASCULAR SYSTEM

Constriction or dilation of the arterial tree may be produced depending on the dose of serotonin administered and the vascular bed under study. Direct vasoconstriction is the classic response to 5-hydroxytryptamine and is the effect responsible for its names *vasotonin* and *serotonin*. Vasodilation occurs in skeletal muscles and cutaneous vessels, and in the latter bed it is responsible for the "flush" of the carcinoid syndrome. The flush, initially red, becomes bluish owing to stagnation (probably as a result of distal venoconstriction) and subsequent deoxygenation.

In rodents, serotonin is more potent than histamine in producing increased capillary permeability and edema, but these effects are not prominent in humans. Serotonin causes positive inotropic and chronotropic responses on the myocardium, but these may be overshadowed by actions of the amine on afferent nerve endings initiating reflex cardiorespiratory changes (Bezold-like reflex). Most veins are strongly constricted by serotonin.

EXTRAVASCULAR SMOOTH MUSCLE

Low doses of serotonin (insufficient to alter arterial blood pressure) produce small intestinal motility and colonic relaxation. Responses in animals are exceedingly complex due to various elements, both neuronal and muscular, that respond to the amine. Serotonin produces bronchoconstriction in patients with bronchial asthma but rarely in normal subjects. The human pregnant uterus is relatively insensitive to serotonin.

EXOCRINE GLANDS

Serotonin is generally inhibitory toward most exocrine glands. The amine depresses gastric acid and pepsin secretion but increases the output of mucosubstances by the gastric mucosa.

MISCELLANEOUS ACTIONS

Serotonin can stimulate many nerve endings, and many of its actions on the cardiovascular, respiratory, and gastrointestinal systems are mediated by local nerve reflexes. The injection of serotonin into human skin is associated with pain and pruritus.

Serotonin increases the ventilatory minute volume, probably owing to stimulation of aortic and carotid chemoreceptors. In animals, other actions can be demonstrated, particularly those associated with stimulation of various autonomic ganglia. In humans, insulin hypoglycemia is followed by a rise in the serotonin levels of the hypothalamus and by growth hormone secretion. Cyproheptadine and methysergide (*see* below) prevent insulin hypoglycemia-induced growth hormone secretion.

ALBERT VON BEZOLD, 1836–1868. German physiologist. Discovered the accelerator nerves of the heart in 1862 and demonstrated their spinal cord origin. Also showed that, after spinal nerve and vagal section, pressure could stimulate the heart to beat. Bezold's ganglion lies in the interauricular septum.

MODE OF ACTION

Evidence from animal experiments suggests that there are two types of serotonin receptors: *M* receptors (blocked by morphine; *see* Chap. 32) in nerve elements; and *D* receptors (blocked by phenoxybenazmine; *see* Chap. 18) in smooth muscle. However, the complexity of the pharmacologic responses to serotonin and the unavailability of potent and specific serotonin antagonists have made receptor characterization difficult. Serotonin receptors probably reside in the cell membrane.

ENDOGENOUS SEROTONIN: ROLE IN PHYSIOLOGY AND PATHOLOGY

The wide distribution of serotonin, its potent pharmacologic actions, and its rapid turnover, particularly in the CNS, have generated numerous hypotheses on the possible role of this autacoid in physiologic and pathologic states. A few of the more probable hypotheses are mentioned briefly.

CENTRAL NERVOUS SYSTEM

Much evidence has been accumulated in recent years from animal experiments to suggest that serotonin is involved as a neurotransmitter at various synapses, but what role it serves is far from clear. Participation of serotonin in thought, perception, and mood has been suggested because many hallucinogens (Fig. 52-2) are chemically similar to serotonin, and drugs such as morphine, reserpine, phenothiazines, imipramine, and monoamine oxidase inhibitors interfere with serotonin (and catecholamine) metabolism and may induce psychoses. Alterations in serotonin metabolism have been identified in patients with schizophrenia and endogenous depression, but at present it is impossible to separate cause from effect. Serotonin may be involved in sleep and thermoregulatory mechanisms, and low levels of the amine have been reported in patients with phenylketonuria. In rats, a brisk circadian rhythm in pineal gland serotonin is present, where the amine is a precursor for melatonin (5-methoxy, *N*-acetyltryptamine).

PERIPHERAL NERVOUS SYSTEM

Based on experiments in animals, there is evidence for the presence of "serotonin" transmission in the peripheral nervous system. Serotonin appears to be involved as a neurotransmitter in various cardiovascular and gastrointestinal reflexes.

GASTROINTESTINAL TRACT

Despite the fact that about 90% of the total body serotonin is present in the gastrointestinal tract, its role in that tissue is not understood. Bowel serotonin may be involved in peristalsis, control of gastric secretion, intestinal absorption, epithelial cell renewal, or release of polypeptide hormones. There is little doubt that platelet serotonin stores derive from the gut, but the role of platelet serotonin is unknown; it may be involved in hemostasis and blood coagulation. Substance P and serotonin may be involved in the pharmacologic actions of capsaicin (8-methyl-N-vanillyl-6-nonenamide), the active principal ingredient in various peppers and paprika.

The Dumping Syndrome

The dumping syndrome occurs in 10% of patients following operations that alter the normal gastroduodenal emptying mechanisms. Typically, there is a variable combination of intestinal (epigastric discomfort, fullness, cramps, hyperperistalsis, diarrhea) and vasomotor (weakness, dizziness, pallor, palpitations, sweating, tachycardia) symptoms. Both components may be reproduced by the i.v. administration of serotonin. Since blood levels of serotonin have been shown to be elevated during a glucose test meal in most patients with established dumping syndrome, this autacoid may be involved in its etiology.

If serotonin is in fact the humoral agent responsible for many of the symptoms of dumping, the question remains as to how the amine reaches the peripheral circulation in view of the avid catabolic activity of the liver and lung. Perhaps serotonin is not directly involved in the symptomatology of the dumping syndrome but is released incidently by the "dumping" stimulus from APUD or other cells in conjunction with polypeptide hormones or other humoral agents.

The Carcinoid Syndrome

The important manifestations of the carcinoid syndrome are cutaneous flushing, bronchospasm, diarrhea, malabsorption, swings in blood pressure, and occasionally mental symptoms. In chronic cases, a pellagra-like skin rash

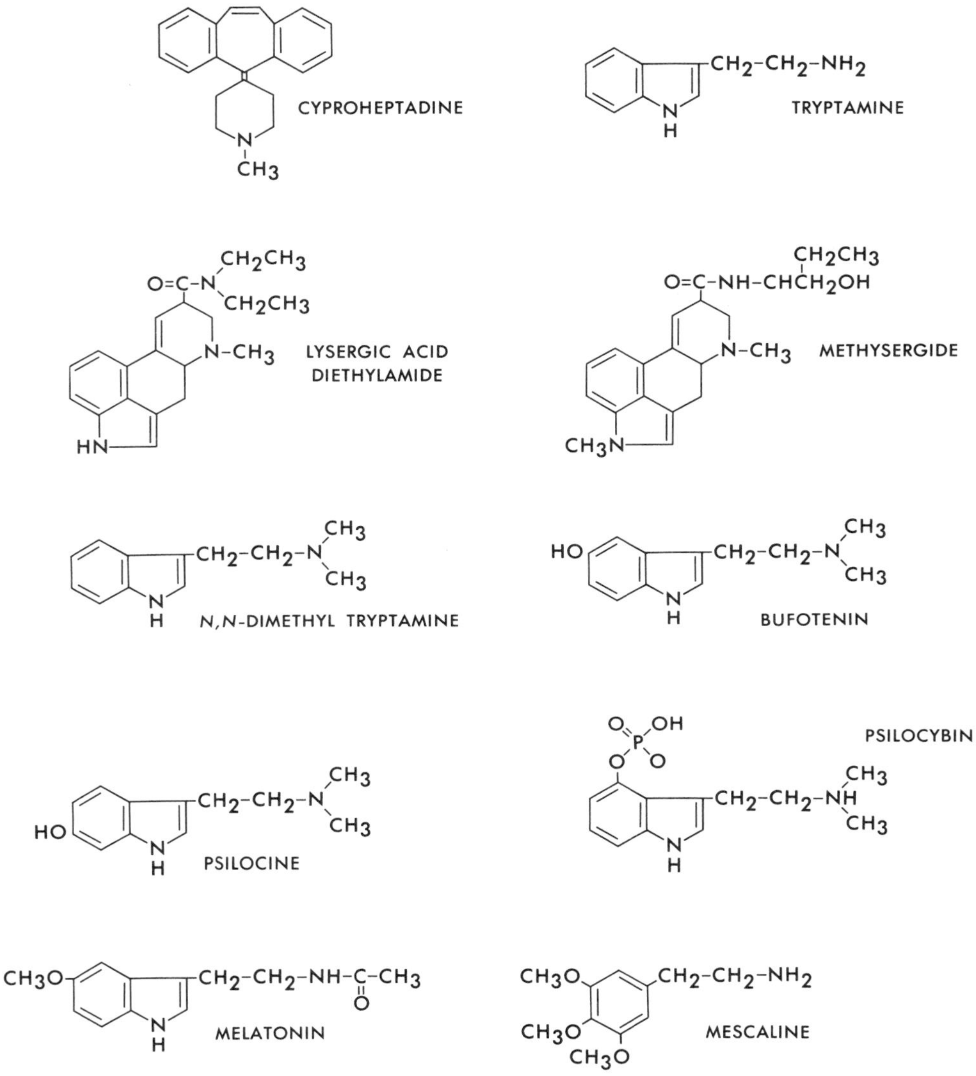

FIG. 52-2. Some potent serotonin antagonists and serotonin-like drugs.

and right-sided heart lesions of endocardial fibrosis with valvular stenosis or incompetence may also be seen. The carcinoid syndrome was originally believed to occur only as a result of serotonin overproduction by malignant carcinoid tumors of the bowel with hepatic metastases, but clearly the spectrum of symptoms produced by a carcinoid tumor depends on many factors, including the *cell of origin* (enterochromaffin, APUD) the *site of origin* (derivation from foregut, midgut, or hindgut), *the size of the tumor*, the *presence or absence of hepatic metastases*, and *the mediator produced.*

Besides serotonin, 5-hydroxytryptophan, histamine, kallikrein, bradykinin, prostaglandins, tyramine, dopamine, norepinephrine, and epinephrine have been implicated as mediators in some cases, but the role of thyrocalcitonin, growth hormone, and other substances normally associated with APUD cells is not clear. A diversity of hormonal secretory patterns and tumor enzymes have been reported.

Inappropriate hormone secretion from many tumors has been recognized in recent years, indicating the varying hormonal potential of such lesions. In view of the origin of carcinoid tumors, they may fall into a similar category, and different carcinoids may be either occasionally or continually unihormonal or multihormonal with regard to their "endocrine secretion." Thus, because of the wide variations in symptoms, the term *carcinoid spectrum* is preferred by some for this condition.

Four types of cutaneous flushing have been described in the carcinoid syndrome, and serotonin, histamine, and kallikrein may all be etiologically involved. Ethanol, epinephrine, isoproterenol, food (release of gastrin), pentagastrin, and prostaglandins may precipitate flushing in patients with carcinoid tumors. Ethanol and catecholamine administration are the basis of diagnostic tests. Temporary palliation of *flushing* may be obtained using *phenoxybenzamine*. In patients in whom histamine is secreted, combination therapy with *H_1- and H_2-blockers* may give symptomatic relief. *Bronchospasm* in the carcinoid syndrome may depend on serotonin or histamine release, but it does not respond well to either serotonin antagonists or H_1-blockers. The precise cause of *malabsorption* seen in patients with the carcinoid syndrome is not clear, but diarrhea undoubtedly exacerbates the defect; *methysergide, Diphenoxylate,* or *codeine* may be palliative.

The *swings in blood pressure* are unpredictable and probably depend on the proportion of autacoids produced and on the tone of the different vascular beds. The excessive diversion of tryptophan by the tumor leaves less available for the synthesis of protein and niacin. Consequently, *protein deficiency* and a *pellagra-like state* may develop in severe cases. One of the more intriguing manifestations of the carcinoid syndrome is the occurrence of *fibrotic lesions*. These take the form of fibrotic deposits in many parts of the body, particularly the endocardium and cardiac valves, but also in the pericardium, lungs, pleura, retroperitoneal area, and skin. A related phenomenon may be the fibrosis that develops with methysergide therapy and in patients with endomyocardial fibrosis and schistosomiasis. *In vitro*, serotonin increases the rate of growth of fibroblasts by shortening their lag phase, but it is unclear whether this effect can be extrapolated to the genesis of fibrotic lesions in humans. In the carcinoid syndrome, significantly more serotonin is contained in the platelets that show a dilated cannalicular system and bizarre shapes and exhibit unusual serotonin-containing hyaloplasmic organelles not seen in normal platelets. There appear to be two separate absorption mechanisms for serotonin in platelets from patients with the carcinoid syndrome, and altered platelet or pulmonary function may encourage cardiac fibrosis.

MIGRAINE

Some forms of migraine appear to be associated with altered serotonin metabolism. Attacks are frequently shown to be associated with a rapid release of bound serotonin in blood. Serotonin antagonists are not uniformly successful in treatment.

MENTAL DISEASE

The possible association of serotonin in various mental disorders is discussed in Chapter 21.

SEROTONIN ANTAGONISTS

Antiserotonin drugs are either *direct, indirect,* or *physiologic antagonists*. Direct antagonists block the effects of serotonin on the end-organ involved; indirect antagonists interrupt serotonin-induced ganglionic transmission; and physiologic antagonists exert balancing counteractions. Only the directly acting antagonists are considered below. A great variety of chemicals have been tested in animals with respect to serotonin receptor agonist properties (5-methoxy-N,N-dimethyltryptamine), blocking activity on central or peripheral serotonin storage or uptake systems (fluoxetine, femoxetine, nitalapram, zimelidine), or direct neuronal destruction (p-chloroamphetamine). None of these is considered further here.

ERGOT ALKALOID DERIVATIVES

Lysergic Acid Diethylamide (LSD)

LSD was first shown by Gaddum to be a competitive antagonist of serotonin on uterine smooth muscle. It is more widely known as a hallucinogen (*see* Chap. 26).

2-Bromolysergic Acid Diethylamide (BOL)

BOL has no hallucinatory properties but retains the antagonism of LSD for serotonin on smooth muscle. It has been used mainly in animals.

JOHN HENRY GADDUM, 1900– British pharmacologist. Developed a sensitive test for adrenaline in 1933 and, with Wilhelm Feldberg, showed in 1933 that acetylcholine is the chemical transmitter in sympathetic ganglia.

1-Methyl-D-Lysergic Acid Butanolamide (Methysergide)

Methysergide (Fig. 51-2) inhibits the effects of serotonin on smooth muscle and possesses only minimal ergot-like direct spasmogenic activity. Adverse reactions comprise gastrointestinal irritation (heartburn, anorexia, dyspepsia, cramps, diarrhea) and central nervous effects (insomnia, restlessness, nervousness, euphoria, unsteadiness). Retroperitoneal, pleuropulmonary, or endocardial fibrosis may occasionally be seen in patients taking methysergide chronically. The fibrosis may regress when drug therapy is stopped, but not always. The occurrence of fibrosis is intriguing because of the structural similarities of methysergide to serotonin and the development of fibrotic lesions in the carcinoid syndrome.

Methysergide is of some value in the prophylaxis of migraine and in "cluster headaches." The beneficial effect of methysergide takes 1 or 2 days to develop, and "rebound" headaches may occur when therapy is stopped. Methysergide is of no benefit when given during an acute attack but of occasional benefit in reducing diarrhea and malabsorption of the carcinoid syndrome and in reducing symptoms in the postgastrectomy dumping syndrome. Contraindications to its use are pregnancy, thromboembolic disease, peripheral vascular disease, renal disease, or coronary artery disease.

Methysergide bimaleate (Sansert) and methysergide base (Deseril) are available as tablets of 2 and 4 mg. The usual dose is 2 to 4 mg two or three times daily.

CYPROHEPTADINE

Cyproheptadine is related to the phenothiazine antihistamines. Like ergot derivatives, it possesses an *N*-substituted heterocyclic ring. Cyproheptadine is unique in that it is a potent antagonist of many of the peripheral actions of both serotonin and histamine and possesses some parasympatholytic and antidopaminergic activity.

Adverse reactions are usually minimal. Drowsiness and dry mouth are most common and may disappear with chronic therapy. Skin rashes, dizziness, ataxia, anorexia, and gastrointestinal irritation may also develop.

Cyproheptadine is used mainly to treat pruritic dermatoses. It may be of some value in the postgastrectomy dumping syndrome and the carcinoid syndrome.

Cyproheptadine hydrochloride (Periactin) is available as 4 mg tablets and as a syrup containing 0.4 mg/ml. The usual dose is 4 mg three times daily.

PARACHLOROPHENYLALANINE (PCPA)

An experimental agent, PCPA depresses tryptophan hydroxylase. After its administration of 3 to 4 g daily in humans, the urinary excretion of 5-HIAA falls rapidly. In a few patients with the carcinoid syndrome, PCPA has improved the intestinal symptoms but has had no effect on flushing. Mild gastrointestinal irritation, ataxia, and dyskinesia occasionally develop. In some animal species, PCPA has been shown to increase sexual behavior.

FURTHER READING

1. Essman WB (ed): Serotonin in Health and Disease, Volumes I–V. New York, Spectrum, 1977/1978
2. Gaddum JH, Picarelli ZP: Two kinds of tryptamine receptor. Br J Pharmacol 12:323–328, 1957
3. Gyermek L: 5-Hydroxytryptamine antagonists. Pharmacol Rev 13:339–439, 1961

CHAPTER 52 QUESTIONS

(See P. 7 for Full Instructions)

Select the One Best Answer

1. Each of the following is a characteristic effect of serotonin (5-HT) EXCEPT
   A. dyspnea.
   B. histamine release.
   C. inhibition of intestinal motility.
   D. cyanotic flush.
   E. variable blood pressure response.
2. Each of the following is true for bradykinin, serotonin, and histamine EXCEPT
   A. potent vasoactive agents.
   B. produce pain on intradermal injection.
   C. implicated in anaphylactic reactions.
   D. decarboxylated amino acids.
   E. involved in inflammatory responses.

A = 1,2,3; B = 1,3; C = 2,4; D = 4; E = All

3. Both serotonin and histamine
   1. produce effects that are antagonized by cyproheptadine.
   2. are derived from essential amino acids.

3. are metabolized in the body by monoamine oxidase.
4. are produced and stored in argentaffin cells.

4. Mast cell tumors release a substance that can produce
   1. hypotension.
   2. bronchoconstriction.
   3. flushing.
   4. itching.

5. Methysergide
   1. has structural similarities to serotonin.
   2. is useful primarily for the prevention rather than for the treatment of migraine headaches.
   3. has been associated with cardiac, pulmonary, and renal complications secondary to inflammatory fibrosis.
   4. is an effective, useful antihistamine.

6. Intestinal hypermotility in the carcinoid and postgastrectomy dumping syndromes may be inhibited by
   1. methysergide.
   2. phentolamine.
   3. cyproheptadine.
   4. chlorpheniramine.

A. 5-Hydroxytryptamine (Serotonin)
B. 5-Hydroxyindoleacetic acid (5-HIAA)
C. Both
D. Neither

7. produce(s) marked cutaneous vasoconstriction.
8. high concentrations present in walnuts, avocados, and bananas.
9. is (are) substrate(s) for monoamineoxidase.
10. is (are) commonly secreted by gastric carcinoid tumors.

JOHN C. MCGIFF

53 Prostaglandins, Prostacyclin, and Thromboxanes

HISTORY

Almost 50 years ago, semen was shown to contain material that contracted smooth muscle and lowered blood pressure, effects that could not be ascribed to any of the then-known naturally occurring compounds. The active substances in semen were tentatively identified as fatty acids, and, because they were thought to arise primarily from the prostate gland, they were named prostaglandins. In 1960, the Swedish scientist Bergström announced the structures of prostaglandins of the E and F series, which led, within a few years, to their synthesis. Von Euler, the Swedish Nobel Laureate and codiscoverer of prostaglandins, was the first to predict the importance of these autacoids.

We have indeed in prostaglandin a unique hormone. . . . Its scope of action is still wider, however, and it may well be that the prostaglandins represent a group of compounds which are involved in a variety of actions ranging from effects on the central nervous system to intricate metabolic actions, thus justifying their very special chemical configuration.[4]

This work was supported by USPHS grant HL-26394-02.

Sune Bergström, 1916– . Swedish biochemist. Extensive research on heparin, cholesterol, bile acids, and the prostaglandins. In 1960 announced the structures of the E and F series of prostaglandins. Bergström was a recipient of the Nobel Prize in 1982.

Ulf Svante Von Euler, 1905–1983. Swedish physiologist. With J. H. Gaddum, identified substance P in 1930–1931, discovered prostaglandin in 1935, and identified noradrenaline as the adrenergic nervous system transmitter in 1946. Von Euler received the Nobel Prize in 1970, as had his father in 1929.

This prediction was fulfilled within a decade. The magnitude of prostaglandins' impact on all fields of biology is evident in reviewing the Proceedings of the Fourth International Prostaglandin Conference, held in Washington, D.C., in 1979: three volumes that run to 2000 pages and 900 contributing authors.[3]

CHEMISTRY

Primary prostaglandins are unsaturated fatty acids that contain 20 carbon atoms disposed in a cyclopentane ring; they originate from common intermediates, the cyclic endoperoxides (Fig. 53-1). The nature of the substitution on the ring is denoted by a capital letter (*e.g.*, D, E, F). Prostacyclin (PGI_2), the most recently discovered member of the prostaglandin family, is bicyclic and also arises from the endoperoxides; it is unstable at physiologic *p*H. Thromboxanes, distinguishable by a six-membered oxane ring in place of the cyclopentane ring, are unstable products of the prostaglandin endoperoxides. They were so named because thromboxane A_2 (TxA_2) was identified as a metabolite of arachidonic acid in platelets (thrombocytes). All of these products—thromboxanes, prostaglandins, and prostacyclin—are derived from unsaturated essential fatty acids, primarily arachidonic acid, a major component of membrane phospholipids. Prostaglandins and TxA_2, derived from arachidonic acid (also called eicosatetraenoic acid), retain two double bonds in their alkyl side-chains, denoted by subscript 2 (Fig. 53-1). Prostaglandins and thromboxanes derived from eicosatrienoic and eicosapentaenoic acids have either one or three double bonds, respectively, designated by subscripts 1 and 3. The number of double bonds in the side-chains usually does not fundamentally alter the biologic properties of prostaglandins; for example, prostaglandins E_1, E_2, and E_3 have similar effects on smooth muscle.

FIG. 53-1. Metabolism of arachidonic acid to form prostaglandins and thromboxanes. The more unstable products are indicated by shading. Eicosatrienoic and eicosapentaenoic acids, bracketed at the top of the figure, give rise to products (not shown) having one and three double bonds, respectively.

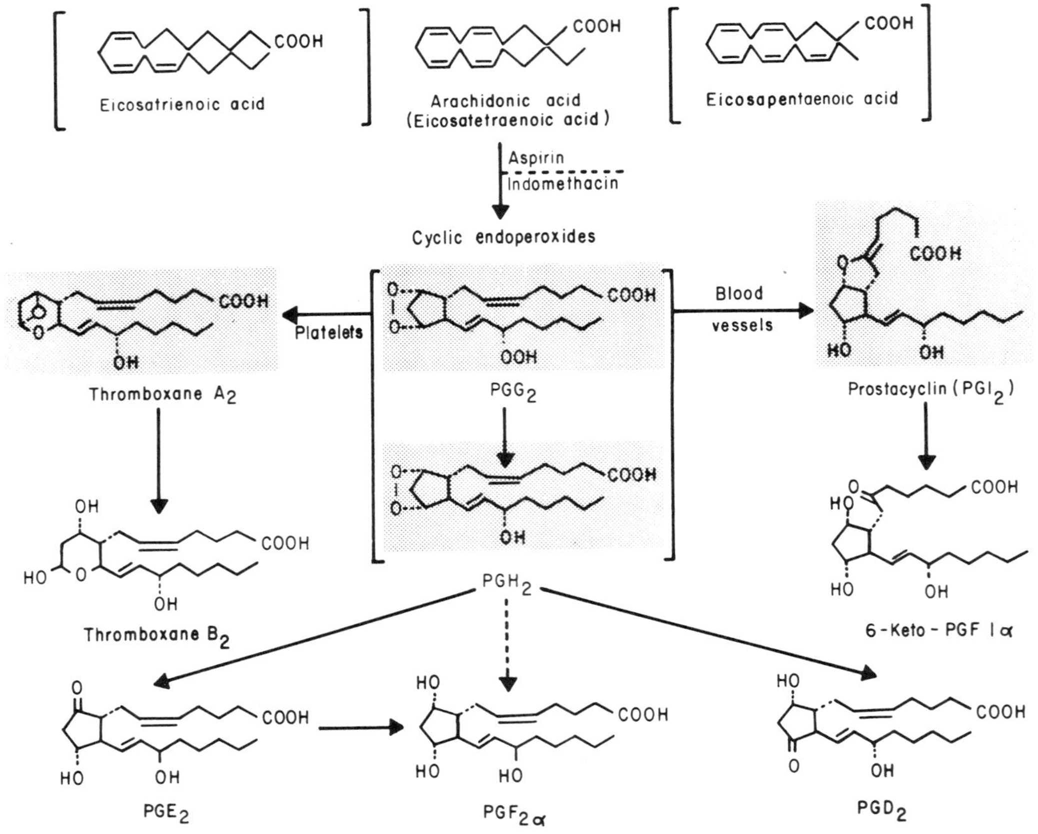

BIOSYNTHESIS OF PROSTAGLANDINS

Prostaglandins are derived from 20-carbon polyunsaturated essential fatty acids of which arachidonic acid is the most abundant (Fig. 53-1). The precursor is released from storage in bound form, chiefly phospholipids, by a group of enzymes, acylhydrolases, that includes phospholipases. Glucocorticoids are thought to derive their antiinflammatory effects by promoting formation of a naturally occurring inhibitor of phospholipases, which thereby decreases prostaglandin synthesis. Hormonal and other stimuli, including antigen challenge, thrombin, and collagen, which induce prostaglandin synthesis, cause release of arachidonic acid from stored forms by stimulating acylhydrolases. The activity of acylhydrolases appears to be under hormonal control; for example, the potent vasoactive hormones—kinins and angiotensins—promote prostaglandin synthesis by stimulation of tissue phospholipases. This results in changes in the intensity and range of activities of angiotensin and bradykinin, as the released prostaglandins can inhibit or augment the action of these hormones; that is, prostaglandins modulate the activity of vasoactive polypeptides. The modulator action of PGE_2 is the basis for its antihypertensive effect: inhibition of pressor hormones and augmentation of depressor hormones.

After arachidonic acid is released from tissue stores, its conversion into prostacyclin, prostaglandins, and thromboxanes occurs in two steps. The first step is catalysis by cyclooxygenase, which is found in nearly all mammalian cells and can be inhibited by aspirinlike drugs. The cyclooxygenase catalyzes oxygenation and cyclization of the fatty acid, forming the unstable intermediates, the cyclic endoperoxides (Fig. 53-1). The second step involves enzymes that are tissue specific and results in the formation of products characteristic of a tissue, such as thromboxane in platelets and prostacyclin in blood vessels. Thus the pivotal intermediates PGG_2 and PGH_2 that arise from the initial transformation of arachidonic acid are enzymically transformed to end-products in a manner characteristic for a tissue.

Disease or physical stress may cause expression of pathways of arachidonic acid metabolism not normally active within a tissue, for example, the production of TxA_2 by the kidney when urine flow is obstructed. Because TxA_2, PGI_2, PGE_2, and $PGF_{2\alpha}$ differ greatly in their biologic properties, the principal product of prostaglandin endoperoxide metabolism is very important to tissue function. For example, PGE_2 dilates bronchial and vascular smooth muscle, whereas $PGF_{2\alpha}$ constricts bronchi and blood vessels. In addition, prostaglandins may have similar actions on some tissues but differ substantially in their major effects. Although PGE_2 and PGI_2 are vasodilators, PGE_2 inhibits release of the adrenergic neurotransmitter, attenuates the vasoconstrictor action of angiotensin II, and affects salt and water transport, properties not shared with PGI_2, which, unlike PGE_2, is a potent inhibitor of platelet aggregation. Prostacyclin, unstable in body fluids, may be metabolized by platelets, the kidney, and other tissues to a biologically active and stable material, 6-keto-PGE_1, which may also arise from oxidation of 6-keto-$PGF_{1\alpha}$, the unstable hydrolysis product of prostacyclin. Transformation of PGI_2 to 6-keto-PGE_1 may explain the unexpectedly prolonged cardiovascular effects of infused PGI_2 in man. The major end-products of prostaglandin endoperoxides may be restricted to an anatomical compartment; for example, within the lung, the predominant prostaglandin of the respiratory tree is the bronchodilator PGE_2, whereas pulmonary blood vessels form primarily PGI_2. In like manner, zones and structures within the kidney vary quantitatively and qualitatively in their capacity to synthesize prostaglandins, which is finally translated into alterations of renal function.[1] Synthesis of PGI_2 by the renal vasculature and PGE_2 by the urinary compartment has particular significance for renal function because of the different properties of PGI_2 and PGE_2. PGA_2, once thought to be the principal antihypertensive prostaglandin formed by the kidney, is not a naturally occurring prostaglandin. PGE_2 may degrade spontaneously to PGA_2 during processing of blood for assay.

With the exception of seminal fluid, prostaglandins are not stored. In response to diverse stimuli, prostaglandins enter the extracellular space upon synthesis, which is reflected in elevated levels in plasma, urine, and other biologic fluids. After removal of the stimulus, prostaglandin levels rapidly subside as a result of metabolism, diffusion, and removal in blood, lymph, and urine. Concentrations of PGE_2 and $PGF_{2\alpha}$ in arterial blood are very low because of pulmonary degradation, which normally removes more than 90% of these prostaglandins from the venous blood as it passes through the lungs. Prostacyclin escapes pulmonary metabolism and therefore may act as a circulating hormone. The initial and most important step in the catabolism of prostaglandins results in their rapid inactivation through oxidation of the 15-OH group to a ketone by prostaglandin dehydrogenases, which are widely distributed in the body.

Recently, a new group of arachidonic acid metabolites, the leukotrienes, has been discovered. These substances, which arise from lipoxygenase pathways of arachidonic acid transformation, have changed the way we view the biology of health and disease, just as the prostaglandins did 20 years ago.

PHYSIOLOGY AND PHARMACOLOGY

In addition to their varied effects on body function, prostaglandins and thromboxanes have opposing effects in many tissues. PGE_2, for example, dilates and $PGF_{2\alpha}$ constricts bronchioles. TxA_2 is a vasoconstrictor and aggregates platelets, effects that can be antagonized by PGI_2. Prostaglandins may function as secretagogues, modulators of nervous activity and hormones, and as mediators of hormone effects. Under basal conditions, the levels of prostaglandins in tissues are low and rise with activity or in response to stress. Some of the most important biologic actions on organ-systems are indicated below primarily for PGE_2, PGI_2, $PGF_{2\alpha}$, and TxA_2, which arise from arachidonic acid, the most abundant precursor.

NERVOUS SYSTEM

Prostaglandins of the E series have anticonvulsant and sedative properties. Prostaglandin-dependent mechanisms are involved in regulating food and water intake, blood pressure, and body temperature and may cause fever in response to pyrogens. They also participate in regulating pituitary hormone release and modulating the central effects of peptide hormones and transmitters.

PGE_2 and PGI_2 sensitize pain receptors to chemical mediators and mechanical stimuli. Prostaglandins, primarily PGE_2, modulate autonomic nervous transmission centrally and peripherally through prejunctional effects on neurotransmitter release. PGI_2 has been shown to have postjunctional effects on the neuroeffector response to nerve stimulation.

CARDIOVASCULAR SYSTEM

PGE_2 and PGI_2 decrease blood pressure, dilate blood vessels, and prevent vasoconstriction induced by pressor hormones and excitation of adrenergic nerves. $PGF_{2\alpha}$ elevates blood pressure, constricts veins, and potentiates the vasoconstrictor response to adrenergic stimuli. TxA_2, the most labile arachidonic acid metabolite, has local vasoconstrictor effects.

Prostaglandin-induced changes in cardiac output are usually related to reflex nervous changes induced by alterations in blood pressure, although a positive inotropic effect has been shown for prostaglandins of the E series. PGI_2, when given intravenously, produces bradycardia induced by reflexly mediated vagal stimulation. The cardiovascular effects of prostaglandins are either blunted or prevented by intravenous administration because of rapid pulmonary degradation, except for PGI_2 and its active metabolite 6-keto-PGE_1, which are not removed by the lungs.

RESPIRATORY SYSTEM

PGE_2 is a bronchodilator, whereas $PGF_{2\alpha}$ constricts bronchi. The constriction may be exaggerated in some asthmatic patients. PGE_2 can inhibit the bronchoconstrictor effects of histamine, acetylcholine, serotonin, and bradykinin. PGI_2, a weak bronchodilator, dilates pulmonary blood vessels, whereas the other prostaglandins and TxA_2 constrict pulmonary blood vessels. Changes in the responses of the pulmonary circulation occur with age; for example, PGE_2 dilates pulmonary blood vessels of the neonate and constricts those of the adult.

KIDNEY

PGE_2, PGA_2, and PGI_2, when infused into the renal artery of dogs, increase renal blood flow and promote salt and water excretion. In contrast, $PGF_{2\alpha}$ has little effect on renal function. Diuresis and natriuresis produced by administered prostaglandins are caused primarily by changes in renal blood flow, although PGE_2 has a direct effect on tubular function and inhibits the effects of ADH. Either prostacyclin or its active metabolite, 6-keto-PGE_1, mediates the prostaglandin-dependent mechanism that regulates renin release.

BLOOD

The most prominant action of arachidonic acid metabolites is their effect on platelet aggregation: TxA_2 is proaggregatory, whereas PGI_2 inhibits aggregation and may disaggregate clumped platelets. In man, *in vitro*, the antiaggregatory potency of PGI_2 is at least 15 times that of 6-keto-PGE_1 and more than 20 times that of PGE_1 or PGD_2. PGE_2 and PGI_2 promote erythropoiesis by stimulating erythropoietin release. Prostaglandins of the E series may cause deformation of red cells, and thereby affect red cell fragility.

GASTROINTESTINAL TRACT

Gastrointestinal motility is enhanced by PGE_2 and $PGF_{2\alpha}$, which limit their use when given intravenously, as to induce labor. Diarrhea and abdominal cramps are common side-effects in patients given intravenous prostaglandins. In contrast to prostaglandins of the E and F series, those of the A and D series have little effect on gastrointestinal motility. PGE_2 and PGI_2 inhibit gastric acid secretion, reducing volume and acidity as well as pepsin content in gastric fluid. PGE_2 and PGI_2 are thought to participate in the local regulation of gastric and intestinal blood flow. PGE_2 inhibits pancreatic secretion when stimulated. PGE_2 and prostacyclin are cytoprotective, preventing mucosal injury induced by noxious agents.

REPRODUCTIVE SYSTEM

Prostaglandin-related mechanisms are involved in implantation. Prostaglandins also participate in the regulation of cyclic events in the ovary and uterus. Prostaglandin-dependent mechanisms are involved in luteinizing hormone (LH) release, ovulation, and termination of corpus luteum function (luteolysis), although species differences must be recognized; for example, $PGF_{2\alpha}$ functions as the leuteolytic hormone in many species but not in man.

Most prostaglandins increase uterine motility, a property that has led to their use in inducing labor and terminating pregnancy.

The importance of prostaglandins to the normal birth process, as in the initiation of parturition, is well recognized. An additional physiologic role has been suggested for uterine prostaglandins in the endometrial changes that lead to menstruation.

ENDOCRINE SYSTEMS

Prostaglandin-dependent mechanisms have been implicated in the regulation of endocrine activity at all levels, from that of the central nervous system and the events leading to release of trophic hormones from the anterior pituitary gland to the peripheral regulation of insulin and glucagon secretion and response of target-organs to hormones. Prostaglandin-related mechanisms acting locally, for example, affect not only TSH secretion but also can influence the response of the thyroid to TSH. Steroidogenesis may be affected by local prostaglandin-related mechanisms in the adrenal gland, testes, and ovaries.

MECHANISM OF ACTION

One of the first demonstrations of an important action of prostaglandins—one suggesting an effect on cyclic nucleotides—was the observation that prostaglandins of the E series inhibit lipolysis in response to various hormonal stimuli. This effect of prostaglandins was related to prevention of hormone-induced elevation of cyclic AMP levels in fat cells and generated a large number of studies that examined the mechanism of action of prostaglandins in terms of changes in cyclic nucleotide levels.

Prostaglandin-cyclic nucleotide interactions have been studied most intensively in platelets. The affinity of prostaglandins for platelet-receptors has been correlated with the relative ability of prostaglandins to stimulate membrane-associated adenylate cyclase of platelets. Inhibition of platelet aggregation is associated with elevated levels of cyclic AMP; the capacity of prostacyclin and other prostaglandins to increase levels of cyclic AMP has been correlated with their antiaggregatory activity. Contrariwise, TxA_2, which promotes platelet aggregation, reduces cyclic AMP levels in platelets. Drugs such as aspirin and dipyridamole that are known to affect aggregability of platelets do so either by preventing TxA_2 generation by platelets or by promoting prostacyclin generation by blood vessels, effects finally translated into elevations in cyclic AMP levels within platelets and inhibition of aggregation. These interactions of cyclic nucleotides, PGI_2, and TxA_2 may ultimately affect calcium mobilization, the final determinant of whether platelets aggregate. In this regard, TxA_2 acts as a calcium ionophore, mobilizing calcium from storage sites probably through effects on calmodulin, the versatile intracellular calcium-binding protein. Some of the effects of $PGF_{2\alpha}$ have been associated with changes in tissue levels of cyclic GMP.

Prostaglandins of the E series have also

been suggested to act on calcium movement in some tissues, preventing the accession of calcium to intracellular sites. For example, PGE_2-induced inhibition of norepinephrine release from adrenergic nerve endings can be overridden by increasing the calcium content of the extracellular fluid.

THE ROLE OF PROSTAGLANDINS IN HEALTH AND DISEASE

Most of the important actions of prostaglandins result from their local effects at very low concentrations, whereby they act as tissue or local hormones. The potency of prostaglandins is evident from studies that indicate effects of PGE_1 at concentrations less than 10 pg/ml (10^{-11} M), a level that approaches one molecule per cell. At these concentrations, PGE_1 has been reported to affect the shape of red blood cells and stimulate formation of cyclic AMP.

Prostaglandins have important roles in defensive mechanisms that protect organ function and the integrity of the organism. This is most evident in response to acute injury when prostaglandins, in concert with amines and peptides, act as mediators of the acute inflammatory response. The contribution of prostaglandin-dependent mechanisms to homeostasis is evident in the cytoprotective function of prostaglandins in the heart and gastrointestinal tract, the adaptation of the fetal and maternal circulations during gestation, and the support of the renal circulation in response to disease or when affected by drug-induced changes, such as acute depletion of extracellular fluid volume induced by a diuretic agent. These studies indicate the importance of prostaglandins in maintaining organ function when the *milieu interieur* is altered. In this regard, it is useful to consider prostaglandins as modulators of the activity of hormones and nerves. The concept of prostaglandins as modulators has been extended to the renin–angiotensin, the kallikrein–kinin, and the autonomic nervous systems and has led to a better understanding of the complex network of interacting hormonal and nervous factors that determines the integration of bodily function, as in the respiratory, circulatory, and digestive systems.

The pathophysiology of diseases can also be better understood in terms of abnormalities of prostaglandin metabolism—for example, deficiencies of prostaglandin formation, as has been found in atherosclerosis, ischemic disease of the heart and the extremities, and in hypertension. Excessive prostaglandin formation may also explain some inflammatory diseases such as arthritis and the tissue response to neoplasia. In addition, Bartter's syndrome, characterized by excessive potassium loss and low or normal blood pressure despite increased plasma renin activity, is associated with increased prostaglandin excretion. These patients benefit from treatment with inhibitors of cyclooxygenase such as indomethacin.

Prostaglandin-dependent mechanisms are evoked locally in an attempt to reestablish normal function through regulation of blood flow and metabolism. Prostaglandins, when they act as agents of defense, are released by various stimuli that alter the basal or resting-state of the animal, such as a surge of local prostaglandins in response to tissue hypoxia that contributes to reactive hyperemia in skeletal muscle. The importance of prostaglandin-dependent mechanisms in facilitating the transition from the basal state to a condition of stress can be viewed at several levels in terms of their participation in the circulatory adjustments evoked. Some of the most important roles of prostaglandins are in those intrinsic mechanisms that regulate the microcirculation, particularly adjustment of local blood flow to changing metabolic requirements of the tissue, as well as to local autoregulatory mechanisms that stabilize blood flow to a tissue. Prostaglandin-dependent mechanisms not only contribute to the microcirculation's response to the requirements for increased nutrient delivery by increasing blood flow and vascular permeability, but also participate in local metabolic processes, such as glucose uptake. As in many of the circulatory actions of prostaglandins, their effects on tissue metabolism and vascular permeability are related to the kallikrein–kinin system. The nephropathy of analgesic abuse has been suggested to be due to ischemia of the renal medulla secondary to reduced synthesis of a vasodilator prostaglandin induced by phenacetin or other analgesic drugs, which favors the unopposed activity of local vasoconstrictor substances.

The study of platelet aggregation and subsequent adhesion to the blood vessel wall as affected by PGI_2–TxA_2 interactions (Fig. 53-2) holds great promise, already partially realized, for designing novel measures for preventing and treating vascular diseases. These studies have resulted in new insights into atherosclerosis and thromboembolism in terms of a dynamic interaction between the endothelium and platelet, one largely determined by the outcome of thromboxane–prostacyclin interac-

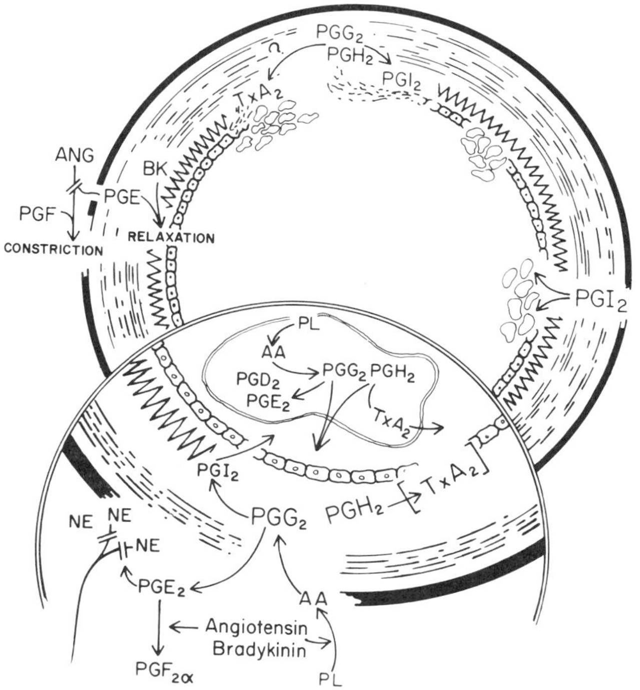

FIG. 53-2. Schema of cross-section of a blood vessel with enlargement of the vascular wall showing possible platelet–endothelial surface interactions. Thromboxane (*TxA_2*) generated by platelets is related to aggregation and subsequent deposits of platelets at the blood endothelial interface (11 o'clock), which can be prevented by prostacyclin (*PGI_2*) synthesized by the vascular wall (3 o'clock). TxA_2 may be formed by diseased blood vessels. PGE_2, also formed by blood vessels, blunts the vasoconstrictor action of angiotensin (*ANG*) and augments the vasodilator action of bradykinin (*BK*), whereas $PGF_{2\alpha}$ may augment angiotensin-induced vasoconstriction. In the enlargement, arachidonic acid (*AA*) may be released from tissue stores, such as phospholipids (*PL*), in response to either angiotensin or bradykinin, which may also accelerate enzymic conversion of PGE_2 to $PGF_{2\alpha}$. PGE_2, but not $PGF_{2\alpha}$, may inhibit release of norepinephrine (*NE*) from nerve endings in the vascular wall.

tions. The ability of blood vessels to generate prostacyclin seems to be essential to prevention of platelet aggregation and deposits on endothelial surfaces, events that can lead to alterations of the vascular wall, predispose to thromboembolism, and perhaps initiate atherosclerosis. Ischemic disease of the heart and the extremities, as indicated, are thought to arise from prostacyclin deficiency. Infusion of PGI_2 has led to healing of ischemic ulcers in patients with advanced peripheral arterial disease.

CLINICAL APPLICATIONS

Agents analogous to adrenergic blocking drugs that inhibit the response of cells selectively to prostaglandins and thromboxanes are not available. Moreover, traditional approaches based on studies intended to characterize prostaglandin receptors probably will not identify compounds such as those that effectively block the endogenous amines. Thus it has yet to be shown that the traditional receptor theory will accommodate the actions and interactions of the multiple products of arachidonic acid metabolism found in most tissues, products with a wide range of action, many of which are dissimilar.

From recent studies on prostaglandins has come the recognition that many drugs whose modes of action were poorly understood owe their therapeutic efficacy to their effect on prostaglandin-related mechanisms. Nitroglycerin, for example, used to manage angina pectoris, hydralazine, used to treat hypertension, and dipyridamole, used to prevent thrombosis, have important effects on prostaglandin metabolism. Awareness of these drugs' interactions with prostaglandin-related mechanisms will lead to a more rational approach to the development of new drugs that have greater selectivity and fewer side-effects.

PREVENTION OF THROMBOSIS

The clinical usefulness of a selective inhibitor of thromboxane synthesis to prevent thrombosis is evident. Effective antagonists of TxA_2 are, however, not available. Another therapeutic approach, inhibition of the enzyme that converts prostaglandin endoperoxides to thromboxanes, has been attempted but thus far has not resulted in a clinically useful selective inhibitor of thromboxane synthesis for use *in vivo*. Thromboxane synthesis may be inhibited, however, by administration of aspirinlike drugs. These effects are usually nonselective, although at low dose the cyclooxygenase of platelets, which initiates formation of TxA_2, is more susceptible to inhibition than that of the vascular wall where prostacyclin is primarily formed. This serves as the basis for aspirin and related drug use in patients with thrombotic diseases.

The ideal antithrombotic agent should inhibit platelet aggregation while stimulating prostacyclin production by blood vessels. Dipyridamole may have these properties, since it has been reported to reduce synthesis of TxA_2 and to enhance prostacyclin production in man. The combination of aspirin and dipyridamole has been thought to be particularly effective in preventing thrombosis (*see* Chap. 31). The addition of dipyridamole to low doses of aspirin contributes to maintenance of prostacyclin-induced elevation in platelet levels of cyclic AMP.

DIETARY LIPIDS AND VASCULAR DISEASE

An intriguing therapeutic approach has been suggested from studies of Eskimos.[2] In contrast to Western man in industrialized societies, the Eskimo demonstrates delayed atherosclerosis and low incidence of myocardial infarction. An important difference between the Eskimo and Western man, one perhaps accounting for the resistance of the Eskimo to vascular disease, is the principal polyunsaturated fatty acid found in the lipid fractions of blood: eicosapentaenoic acid in the Eskimo and arachidonic acid in Western man. Eicosapentaenoic acid differs from arachidonic acid (eicosatetraenoic acid) in the degree of unsaturation, five versus four double bonds (Fig. 53-1). Thus eicosapentaenoic acid gives rise to products with three double bonds as designated by the subscript in TxA_3 and PGI_3. TxA_3 is a less potent aggregator of platelets than is TxA_2, whereas PGI_3 possesses similar antiaggregatory activity to that of PGI_2. In addition, eicosapentaenoic acid is a poor substrate for the cyclooxygenase and competes with arachidonic acid for metabolism by this enzyme, resulting in reduced formation of TxA_2 by platelets and thereby suppressing platelet aggregation. These studies offer the remarkable prospect of reducing vascular disease through enrichment of the diet with either eicosapentaenoic acid or its precursor fatty acid, linolenic acid.

PROSTACYCLIN INFUSION

Because prostacyclin deficiency is thought to contribute to the initiation and progression of some diseases, such as peripheral vascular disease, preliminary studies in man suggest a longlasting increase in muscle blood flow, subsidence of pain, and healing of trophic ulcers after intraarterial infusions of prostacyclin into the affected limb for several days.

Infusions of PGI_2 are beneficial during extracorporeal circulation of blood in such procedures as cardiopulmonary bypass and hemodialysis. PGI_2 infusion, under these conditions, reduces the loss of platelets and prevents formation of microemboli. Infusions of prostaglandins of the E series have been used in infants to maintain patency of the ductus arteriosus in those with severe congenital abnormalities of the heart in which closure, before surgery can be performed, would be life-threatening.

PROSTAGLANDIN ANALOGUES

Because of the cytoprotective action of prostaglandins, the development of analogues of these prostaglandins may be useful in managing peptic ulcer, and perhaps ischemic heart disease. The clinical usefulness of prostaglandin analogues, however, has been limited by their relatively short-lived effects because of rapid metabolism, as well as unwanted side-effects. A methyl analogue of PGE_2, when taken orally, has been shown to prevent blood loss due to oral treatment with aspirin and indomethacin.

OBSTETRICS AND GYNECOLOGY

Primary dysmenorrhea is the most common gynecologic disorder. Until recently, treatment has been nonspecific with analgesics. Dysmenorrhea has been shown to be related to a high menstrual release of prostaglandins, a finding that led to the use of aspirinlike drugs in its treatment. Nonsteroidal antiinflammatory drugs are also effective in suppressing abnormal uterine bleeding whether dysfunctional or induced by intrauterine devices. Indomethacin and related drugs also have a role in arresting premature labor, since activation of a prostaglandin-dependent mechanism will lead to spontaneous abortion.

Prostaglandins and their analogues have been used to induce labor and to terminate pregnancy. To circumvent the gastrointestinal side-effects induced by oral or intravenous administration of prostaglandins, the use of intravaginal gels that contain analogues have been substituted for systemic administration of these drugs.

FURTHER READING

1. McGiff JC: Thromboxane and prostacyclin: Implications for function and disease of the vasculature. Adv Intern Med 25:199–216, 1980
2. Moncada S, Vane JR: Pharmacology and endogenous roles of prostaglandin endoperoxides, thromboxane A_2, and prostacyclin. Pharmacol Rev 30:293–331, 1979
3. Samuelsson B, Ramwell P, Paoletti R (eds): Advances in Prostaglandin and Thromboxane Research, Volume 6. New York, Raven Press, 1980
4. von Euler US: Welcoming address. In Bergström S, Samuelsson B (eds): Nobel Symposium 2—Prostaglandins, pp. 17–20. New York, Interscience, 1966

CHAPTER 53 QUESTIONS

(*See* P. 7 for Full Instructions)

Select the One Best Answer

1. The administration of prostaglandins E_1 or E_2 may be effective for producing each of the following EXCEPT
   A. bronchoconstriction.
   B. inhibition of norepinephrine release from adrenergic nerves.
   C. diuresis.
   D. induction of labor.
   E. dilatation of the ductus arteriosus.

2. Some of the therapeutic effects of the drugs listed below are thought to be related to modification of a prostaglandin or thromboxane-dependent mechanism EXCEPT
   A. nitroglycerin.
   B. dipyridamole.
   C. hydralazine.
   D. aspirin.
   E. guanethidine.

3. Arachidonic acid is the precursor for the biosynthesis of each of the following EXCEPT
   A. prostacyclin.
   B. SRS-A.
   C. substance P.
   D. thromboxane.
   E. prostaglandin $F_{2\alpha}$.

A = 1,2,3; B = 1,3; C = 2,4; D = 4; E = All

4. PGI_2 (prostacyclin)
   1. is a peripheral vasodilator.
   2. relaxes bronchial smooth muscle.
   3. antagonizes thromboxane A_2-induced platelet aggregation.
   4. inhibits renin release.

5. Prostaglandin synthesis may be suppressed by inhibiting
   1. cyclooxygenase.
   2. lipoxygenase.
   3. phospholipase.
   4. prostaglandin dehydrogenase.

6. Inhibition of prostaglandin synthesis with indomethacin can cause
   1. gastric ulcer.
   2. uterine relaxation.
   3. elevated blood pressure.
   4. closure of the ductus arteriosus.

7. Pain due to inflammation may be relieved by inhibiting prostaglandin formation with
   1. cortisone.
   2. indomethacin.
   3. aspirin.
   4. codeine.

54

JOHN H. WALSH AND I. L. TAYLOR

Pharmacology of Gastrointestinal Hormones

Numerous biologically active peptides are present in endocrine cells and nerves throughout the gastrointestinal tract, including the pancreas (Table 54-1). The chemical structures of many of these peptides have been delineated, but only a few have been established as true hormones that act physiologically on target cells using endocrine, neurocrine, or paracrine modes of delivery. A comprehensive description of these peptides is beyond the scope of this chapter but can be obtained elsewhere (*see* Walsh JH, in Further Reading list at the end of this chapter).

The pathologic effects of gut peptides become clinically apparent when the peptides are secreted by hormone-producing tumors. Several clinically distinct syndromes are now recognized (Table 54-2).

When released into the blood in response to a physiological stimulus or when administered intravenously, these peptides have a short half-life, usually only a few minutes. They appear to be metabolized by peptidases present in many organ-systems and are not usually found in high concentrations in urine. These peptides do not appear to cross the blood–brain barrier in large amounts.

The actions of these peptides appear to depend on their binding to high-affinity receptors on effector cell plasma membranes. Such receptors appear to be specific for each peptide or family of closely related peptides. Intracellular second messenger systems have been delineated for some, but not all—for example, secretin, vasoactive intestinal peptide (VIP), and glucagon stimulate adenylate cyclase activity in target cells. Cholecystokinin (CCK) causes calcium influx and stimulates the formation of intracellular inositol phosphate. Several neuropeptides influence calcium fluxes in nerves and alter depolarization and repolarization patterns.

The clinical use of gut peptides and their biologically active synthetic analogues has been limited.

PENTAGASTRIN

CLINICAL PHARMACOLOGY

Pentagastrin (N-t-butyloxycarbonyl-B-alanyl-L-tryptophyl-L-methionyl-L-aspartyl-L-phenylalanyl amide) is a synthetic pentapeptide that

TABLE 54-1. Gastrointestinal Peptides

Major Location	Most Potent Biologic Actions
Endocrine cells in gut	
Gastrin	Stimulates gastric acid
Somatostatin	Inhibits multiple hormone release and function
Secretin	Stimulates pancreatic bicarbonate
Cholecystokinin (CCK)	Stimulates pancreatic enzymes and gallbladder
Gastric inhibitory peptide (GIP)	Enhances glucose-stimulated insulin release
Motilin	Initiates small intestine motility
Substance P	Contracts smooth muscle
Enteroglucagon	Unknown
Neurotensin	Unknown
Endocrine cells of pancreas	
Insulin	Increases cellular glucose uptake (*see* Chap. 46)
Glucagon	Causes glycogenolysis and gluconeogenesis (*see* Chap. 46)
Pancreatic polypeptide (PP)	Inhibits pancreatic secretion
Somatostatin	Inhibits pancreatic secretion
Gut nerves	
Vasoactive intestinal peptide (VIP)	Relaxes smooth muscle and arterioles
Enkephalins	Unknown (*see* Chap. 32)
Substance P	Unknown
Somatostatin	Unknown
Bombesin	Releases gastrin
Cholecystokinin (CCK)	Unknown
Thyrotropin releasing hormone (TRH)	Unknown (*see* Chap. 43)

shares the carboxyl-terminal four amino acids with the antral hormone gastrin. Gastrin was isolated and sequenced by Gregory and Tracy, and a physiological role for the peptide in the control of acid secretion was established by Grossman and his colleagues. Natural gastrin is heterogeneous (Tables 54-3, 54-4, and 54-5). The carboxyl terminal tetrapeptide amide is the minimal fragment required for biologic activity, and molecular forms that contain this fragment all exhibit the same spectrum of biologic activities; substitution or deamidation of the phenylalanyl amide results in loss of bio-

TABLE 54-2. Pancreatic Islet Cell Tumor Syndromes

Product	Major Manifestations
Insulin	Fasting hypoglycemia
Glucagon	Hyperglycemia, skin lesions
Gastrin (Zollinger–Ellison syndrome)	Acid hypersecretion, duodenal ulcer, diarrhea
VIP (Pancreatic cholera, watery diarrhea syndrome	Diarrhea, hypokalemia
Somatostatin	Steatorrhea, mild hyperglycemia, gallstones
PP	None known

logic activity. Stimulation of hydrochloric acid secretion by parietal cells in the body of the stomach is the action of gastrin that has the lowest dose requirement and appears to be a physiologic action of the hormone. Gastrin, acetylcholine, and histamine all stimulate parietal cell secretion in mammals. The responses to all three stimulants can be inhibited *in vivo* by anticholinergic drugs (*see* Chap. 16) or by histamine H_2 antagonists (*see* Chap. 51). *In vitro,* however, studies using isolated parietal cells show separate receptors for gastrin, histamine, and acetylcholine that must all be stimulated for maximal parietal cell function. A three-way potentiation exists among these agents so that a combination of submaximal doses of each agent produces a maximal response and inhibition of a single receptor inhibits total response to a combination of stimulants. The parietal cell *in vivo* normally is "primed" by natural release of acetylcholine from nerve fibers, histamine from mucosal histaminocytes, and gastrin from blood. A maximal gastric acid secretory response can be produced by injecting either exogenous gastrin or histamine.

CLINICAL USES

Petagastrin has now largely replaced other drugs as the stimulant for acid secretory studies (Table 54-6). The recommended dose (6 μg/kg of body weight subcutaneously) produces peak acid output equivalent to that produced by 40 μg/kg of histamine acid phosphate or 1500 μg/kg of betazole hydrochloride. This response is reproducible in that a similar rate of acid secretion is achieved when repeated doses are given to the same person. Pentagastrin acts within 10 minutes, with a maximal response occurring in most patients within 20 to 30 min-

---

RODERIC ALFRED GREGORY, 1913– . British physiologist. Wrote numerous papers on gastroenterology. In 1959 published a method for obtaining pure gastrin, a gastric secretion-stimulating hormone first postulated by J. S. Edkins in 1905–1906.

TABLE 54-3. Structures of Some Gut Peptides

Peptide	Structure*
Cholecystokinin	
CCK39	YIQQARKAPSGRVSMIKNLQSLDPSHRISDRDYMGWMDF#
CCK33	--
CCK8	--------------------
Enkephalins:	
Leu	YGGFL
Met	-------M
Gastric inhibitory peptide (GIP)	YAEGTFISDYSIAMDKIRQQDFVNWLLAQQKGKKSDWKHNITQ
Gastrin releasing peptide (GRP)	APVSVGGGTVLAKMYPRGNHWAVGHLM#
Bombesin (frog)	† QQRL----Q-----------------
Gastrin:	
hG34	† QLGPQGPPHLVADPSKKQGPWLEEEEEAYGWMDF#
hG17	--------------------------------------
hG14	--------------------------------
Glucagon	HSQGTFTSDYSKYLDSRRAQDFVQWLMDT
Motilin	FVPIFTYGELQRMQEKERNKGQ
Neurotensin (hNT)	† QLYENKPRRPYIL
Pancreatic polypeptide:	
pPP	ASLEPVYPGDDATPEQMAQYAAE LRRYINMLTRPRY#
hPP	--P-------------BB----------------------D--------------------------
Somatostatin	AGCKNFFWKTFTSC
Secretin	HSDGTFTSELSRLRDSARLQRLLQFLV#
Substance P (equine)	RPKPQQFFGLM#
Thyrotropin-releasing hormone (TRH)	† QHP#
Vasoactive intestinal peptide (VIP)	HSDAVFTDNYTRLRKQMAVKKYLNSILN#

* Symbols used: † Q = PCA (proglutamyl); # = carboxyl terminal amide; Y = tyrosine sulfate; h = human; ----- = identical to line above.

TABLE 54-4. Abbreviations of Amino Acids

Amino Acid	Abbreviation	
	3-Letter	*1-Letter*
Alanine	Ala	A
Arginine	Arg	R
Asparagine	Asn	N
Aspartic acid	Asp	D
Asn or Asp	Asx	B
Cysteine	Cys	C
Glutamic acid	Glu	E
Glutamine	Gln	Q
Gln or Glu	Glx	Z
Pyroglutamyl	pGlu	pE
Glycine	Gly	G
Histidine	His	H
Isoleucine	Ile	I
Leucine	Leu	L
Lysine	Lys	K
Methionine	Met	M
Phenylalanine	Phe	F
Proline	Pro	P
Serine	Ser	S
Threonine	Thr	T
Tryptophan	Trp	W
Tyrosine	Tyr	Y
Valine	Val	V

utes (Table 54-6). Its activity usually lasts from 60 to 80 minutes. The plasma half-life after i.v. injection is thought to be less than 5 minutes, but the effects are more prolonged after s.c. injection. No biochemical abnormality that might indicate specific organ toxicity has been encountered. This test has little use in diagnosing uncomplicated duodenal ulcer disease because of the marked degree of overlap of secretory rates with normal subjects (Table 54-7). An acid secretory study is indicated in hypergastrinemic patients to exclude an "appropriate" hypergastrinemia secondary to a loss of acid inhibition of gastrin release from the antrum in diseases such as atrophic gastritis and pernicious anemia. The role of acid secretory studies in diagnosing a gastric ulcer is not well established. Thus, although the association of a gastric ulcer with achlorhydria highly suggests gastric carcinoma, it is not absolutely diagnostic. Conversely, most patients with ulcerating carcinoma of the stomach (malignant ulcer) retain the ability to secrete acid.

The injection of pentagastrin may be as reliable as calcium infusion as a provocative test to diagnose medullary cell carcinoma of the thyroid, where it stimulates an increase in

TABLE 54-5. Structures of Gastrins of Various Species

Gastrin	Species	Abbreviation	Structure*
Gastrin-34	Human	hG34	pELGPQGPPHLVADPSKKQGPWLEEEEEAYGWMDF#
("Big")	Porcine	pG34	pELGLQGPPHLVADLAKKQGPWMEEEEEAYGWMDF#
Gastrin precursor	Porcine		----HRRQLGLQGPPHLVADLAKKQGPWMEE------
Gastrin-17	Human	hG17	pEGPWLEEEEEAYGWMDF#
("Little")	Porcine	pG17	pEGPWMEEEEEAYGWMDF#
	Feline	fG17	pEGPWLEEEEAAYGWMDF#
	Canine	cG17	pEGPWMEEAEEAYGWMDF#
	Bovine	bG17	pEGPWVEEEEAAYGWMDF#
	Ovine	oG17	pEGPWVEEEEAAYGWMDF#
Gastrin-14	Human	hG14	WLEEEEEAYGWMDF#
("Mini")	Porcine	pG14	WMEEEEEAYGWMDF#
1-13 pG17 ("N-terminal fragment")			pEGPWMEEEEEAYG
C-Terminal tetrapeptide G/CCK4			WMDF#

* Symbols used: X = residue different from column above; pE = pyroglutamyl; Y* = tyrosine residue either sulfated or nonsulfated; # = carboxyl terminal amide; ---- = amino acid extensions; underlined letters = species differences.

serum calcitonin levels. The response to pentagastrin, however, may be markedly less than that to calcium, and *vice versa,* suggesting that no single provocative test can as yet be recommended.

PREPARATION

Pentagastrin (Pentavalon) is the ammonium salt of the peptide that is soluble in water in concentrations of 1 mg/ml. Each 2-ml vial contains 500 μg of pentagastrin.

ADVERSE EFFECTS

Pentagastrin causes fewer and less severe cardiovascular and systemic effects than does histamine or betazole hydrochloride. Adverse effects that may occur include abdominal pain, a desire to defecate, nausea, vomiting, bor-

TABLE 54-6. Dose, Route, and Timing of Peak Acid Secretory Responses to Various Stimuli

Drug	Dose	Route	Timing of Peak Response
			min
Histamine	40 μg/kg	s.c.	20–60
	40 μg/kg/kr	i.v.	30–45
Betazole	1.5 μg/kg	s.c.	30–90
Gastrin	2 μg/kg	s.c., i.m.	30–40
	0.8 μg/kg/hr	i.v.	20–60
Pentagastrin	6 μg/kg	s.c.	15–45
	6 μg/kg	i.m.	10–30
	6 μg/kg/hr	i.v. infusion	5–20
Insulin	0.2 unit/kg	i.v.	30–90

(Isenberg JI: Gastric secretory testing. In Sleisenger M, Fordtran S (eds): Gastrointestinal Disease, pp 714–732. Philadelphia, WB Saunders, 1978)

TABLE 54-7. Basal and Maximal Stimulated Gastric Acid Secretion in Normal Male Subjects and Patients with Duodenal Ulcer

	Acid Output			
	Normal		*Duodenal Ulcer*	
	Mean	*ULN**	*Mean*	*LV–DU*†
	mEq/hr			
Basal	2.4	6.6	5.3	0.1
Histamine	21.6	49.2	42.0	15
Betazole	21.8	45.8	35.0	14.4
Pentagastrin	25.0	45.0	43.0	15.0

(Isenberg JI: Gastric secretory testing. In Sleisenger M, Fordtran S (eds): Gastrointestinal Disease, pp 714–732. Philadelphia, WB Saunders, 1978)

* ULN = upper limit of normal (mean + 2 SD).

† LV–DU = lowest value duodenal ulcer.

borygmi, flushing, tachycardia, dizziness, faintness, lightheadedness, drowsiness, a sinking feeling, amblyopia, tiredness, and headache. Allergic and hypersensitivity reactions may theoretically occur but have not been well documented; a history of hypersensitivity or an allergic response to the drug is a contraindication to its use. The use of pentagastrin in pregnant patients has not been evaluated. Cautious use is advised in patients with pancreatic, hepatic, or biliary disorders. As with gastrin, the drug could in some instances stimulate secretion of pancreatic enzyme and bicarbonate output as well as biliary flow.

GLUCAGON

CLINICAL PHARMACOLOGY

Glucagon produced by the alpha cells of the pancreas (*see* Chap. 46) exhibits structural similarities with secretin and is a member of the same family whose other members include VIP and GIP (Table 54-1). Glucagon is also a potent inhibitor of gastrointestinal motility. When administered parenterally, glucagon produces a prompt increase in blood glucose concentration by stimulating the conversion of hepatic glycogen to glucose. Like epinephrine, it activates liver phosphorylase and thereby increases glycogenolysis; it differs in that its glycogenolytic action is not blocked by adrenergic blocking agents (*see* Chap. 18).

CLINICAL USES

Glucagon is used to counteract severe hypoglycemic reactions in diabetic patients and to terminate insulin stress tests (*see* Chap. 46). Glucagon's ability to relax gastrointestinal musculature and to minimize spasm is increasingly utilized by gastroenterologists; for example, during endoscopy of the gastric mucosa; in performing endoscopic retrograde catheterization of the pancreatic duct (ERCP), aiding passage of the endoscope through the pylorus into the duodenum; and in radiology when hypotonic studies of the stomach, duodenum, or colon are needed.

PREPARATION AND DOSAGE

Glucagon for injection is supplied in ampules of 1 and 10 mg with 1- and 10-ml vials of diluent. The commercially available preparation is a naturally occurring porcine-derived straight-chain peptide that contains 29 amino-acid residues and has a molecular weight of 3485. Glucagon can be injected intramuscularly, intravenously, or subcutaneously and may be added to dextrose solutions, but it will precipitate when added to solutions that contain chlorides of sodium, potassium, or calcium.

ADVERSE EFFECTS

Glucagon is relatively free of adverse effects but may occasionally cause nausea and vomiting. Because it is a foreign protein, hypersensitivity reactions may occur.

SECRETIN

Secretin is released from the duodenum and upper jejunum in response to the entry of acid and is a potent stimulant of pancreatic fluid and bicarbonate secretion from the denervated pancreas. This demonstration by Bayliss and Starling established secretin as the first hormone and was the foundation of endocrinology as we know it today. The bicarbonate secreted in response to secretin serves to buffer acid that enters the small intestine from the stomach. Secretin also inhibits gastric acid secretion.

CLINICAL USES AND INDICATIONS

Secretin (Kabi Diagnostica) has recently been approved by the FDA because of its proven usefulness in diagnosing several disorders.

Pancreatic Function Test

After a submaximal dose of secretin (1 unit/kg intravenously), the duodenal contents are aspirated and the total volume and bicarbonate content of the juice measured. A diagnosis of

---

WILLIAM MADDOCK BAYLISS, 1860–1924. Physiologist at University College, London. Worked with E. H. Starling on gastrointestinal tract physiology, including the neural control of peristalsis (1899–1900) and the mechanism of pancreatic secretion (1902). They introduced their chemical (hormonal) control theory of the body in 1904. Bayliss introduced saline injections for treating wound shock in World War I.

ERNEST HENRY STARLING, 1866–1927. Physiologist at University College, London. Introduced the word "hormone" in 1905. Worked on lymph production and the functions of serum proteins, and in 1925 showed water reabsorption to occur in the kidney tubules. His law of the heart (1915) relates the energy of contraction to the length of the muscle fibers.

chronic pancreatitis is suggested by a low bicarbonate concentration (less than 90 mEq/liter) in combination with a low secretory volume (less than 2 ml/kg/80 min). Pancreatic carcinoma is suggested if volume is low but bicarbonate concentration normal (90–130 mEq/liter). As an additional benefit, many pancreatic tumors can be diagnosed by cytologic examination of secretin-stimulated pancreatic juice.

Gastrinoma Provocative Test

A gastrinoma is the most common cause of inappropriate hypergastrinemia (*i.e.*, increased basal serum gastrin concentrations in the face of high rates of acid secretion). Patients with this disease need to be distinguished from those with G-cell hyperfunction, retained isolated antrum, and, rarely, uncomplicated duodenal ulcer disease. Fortunately, the chance finding that secretin and calcium were both potent stimulants of gastrin release from tumor cells, but not antral G cells, led to the introduction of provocative tests.

A gastrinoma is suggested when secretin (2 clinical units/kg rapidly intravenously) produces an elevated serum gastrin greater than 110 pg/ml. Normal subjects and patients with G-cell hyperfunction or an isolated antrum have responses indistinguishable from those seen in uncomplicated duodenal ulcer disease where gastrin concentrations either do not change or fall. In patients with positive responses, peak gastrin response to a bolus injection of secretin occurs within 10 minutes. False-positive responses have been described with some secretin preparations extracted from animal tissues and contaminated with CCK-like peptides (*e.g.*, Boot's secretin), emphasizing the need to use pure, natural, or synthetic secretin.

Radiology

Secretin is used during angiographic studies of the pancreas. An injection into the celiac trunk or the superior mesenteric artery before the injection of angiographic dyes enhances pancreatic blood flow and, in so doing, aids angiographic visualization of the small pancreatic blood vessels.

Duodenal Ulcer Disease

Secretin inhibits acid secretion and gastrin release and stimulates a pancreatic secretion rich in bicarbonate. Because it must be given parenterally, however, secretin is not likely to replace other drugs currently used to treat duodenal ulcers. Repeated injections of secretin may be associated with asymptomatic hyperamylasemia in humans. Continuous i.v. infusions of secretin has been proposed as a treatment for acute upper gastrointestinal hemorrhage, but large controlled trials will be needed to prove effectiveness.

PREPARATIONS

Two commercial preparations of secretin are available. The purer of these is extracted from hog intestine by the Gastrointestinal Hormone Research Laboratories, Karolinski Institute, Stockholm, Sweden, and is marketed by Kabi Diagnostica, Stockholm, Sweden. Each vial contains 75 clinical units, a reducing agent *l*-cysteine hydrochloride (1 mg) to prevent oxidation of the methionine residue, and 20 mg of manitol. The activity is ⩾3000 clinical units/mg of secretin. The contents of each vial are dissolved in 7.5 ml of sterile physiologic saline and given by i.v. injection.

The second preparation, Boot's secretin, is marketed by Warren–Teed Laboratories in the United States. This preparation exhibits greater contamination with other gastrointestinal peptides, including CCK-like peptides. It is supplied as a sterile powder containing about 100 clinical units in a 10-ml vial.

ADVERSE EFFECTS

Hog secretin, as a foreign protein, can induce hypersensitivity reactions. The use of secretin is contraindicated in patients with acute pancreatitis because the stimulation of pancreatic exocrine secretion may exacerbate the inflammatory process. Asymptomatic hyperamylasemia may follow the prolonged use of systemic secretin.

OTHER USES OF GASTROINTESTINAL PEPTIDES

CHOLECYSTOKININ (CCK)

The synthetic octapeptide of CCK has been used to stimulate contraction of the gallbladder in patients undergoing cholecystography. Inability of the gallbladder to contract under these circumstances may indicate pathology.

BOMBESIN

Bombesin was initially extracted from the skin of the European frog *Bombina bombina*. A similar peptide is found in the gastrointestinal tract of humans. Synthetic bombesin has been infused to distinguish patients with gastrinoma from those with a postsurgical retained gastric antrum. Bombesin is thought to be a specific stimulant of gastrin release from the antral G cell with little effect on tumor tissue.

PANCREATIC POLYPEPTIDE

Pancreatic polypeptides' (PP) release mechanisms exhibit unique vagal–cholinergic dependence, and PP concentrations in blood may reflect vagal tone on the pancreas. The PP response to insulin hypoglycemia has been used to assess the damage to the autonomic nervous system in diabetic subjects and in patients with idiopathic autonomic neuropathy. An elevated basal PP concentration (>300 pM) may be a useful marker for pancreatic endocrine tumors.

SOMATOSTATIN

Somatostatin is a potent inhibitor of acid secretion and also decreases mesenteric blood flow. These features suggest a possible use for this peptide in treating gastrointestinal hemorrhage. Somatostatin is a potent inhibitor of pancreatic secretion, an observation that has led to its use in treating acute pancreatitis. Further studies are, however, needed. Somatostatin has been used to treat acromegaly, where it presumably reduces the secretion of growth hormone (*see* Chap. 43).

FURTHER READING

1. Isenberg JI: Gastric secretory testing. In Sleisenger MH, Fordtran JS (eds): Gastrointestinal Disease, pp 714–732. Philadelphia, WB Saunders, 1978
2. Walsh JH, Lam SK: Physiology and pathology of gastrin. Clin Gastroenterol 9:567–591, 1980
3. Lamers CBH, Ruland CM, Joosten HJM et al: Hypergastrinemia of antral origin in duodenal ulcer. Am J Dig Dis 23:998–1002, 1978
4. Lamers CBH, van Tongeren JHM: Comparative study of the value of the calcium, secretin, and meal stimulated increase in serum gastrin to the diagnosis of the Zollinger–Ellison syndrome. Gut 18:128–135, 1977
5. Brady CE, Johnson RC, Williams JR et al: False positive serum gastrin stimulation due to impure secretin. Gastroenterology 76:1106, 1979
6. Walsh JH: Gastrointestinal hormones and peptides. In Johnston LR (ed): Textbook of Physiology, 1981

CHAPTER 54 QUESTIONS

(*See* P. 7 for Full Instructions)

Select the One Best Answer

1. Each of the following associates a gastrointestinal peptide with its correct action EXCEPT
   A. cholecystokinin—increases pancreatic enzyme secretion.
   B. somatostatin—inhibits pancreatic secretion of insulin and glucagon.
   C. enteroglucagon—increases hepatic glycogen storage.
   D. vasoactive intestinal peptide—relaxes smooth muscle and arterioles.
   E. secretin—stimulates gastrin secretion from gastrinomas.
2. Gastric secretion commonly increases after oral administration of
   A. secretin.
   B. cimetidine.
   C. pentagastrin.
   D. caffeine.
   E. cholecystokinin.

A = 1,2,3; B = 1,3: C = 2,4; D = 4; E = All

3. Gastrin is
   1. the vasoactive intestinal peptide.
   2. a stimulant of gastric acid secretion.
   3. used clinically more than is pentagastrin.
   4. inhibited by cimetidine from stimulating gastric acid secretion.
4. Glucagon is effective for
   1. producing hyperglycemia.
   2. relaxing the gastrointestinal tract.
   3. cardiac stimulation in the presence of β-adrenoceptor blockade.
   4. activating skeletal muscle glycogenolysis.
5. Accepted clinical uses for secretin include
   1. treatment of watery diarrhea syndrome.
   2. provocative test for diagnosing gastrinoma.
   3. treatment of pancreatitis.
   4. pancreatic function tests.
6. Pancreatic glucagon
   1. may be effective for increasing blood glucose in a hypoglycemic patient.
   2. is a term synonymous with enteroglucagon.
   3. relaxes intestinal smooth muscle.
   4. inhibits the release of insulin.

MICHAEL J. PEACH

55

Vasoactive Peptides

The physiological or pathologic roles of most vasoactive polypeptides remain unknown. None of these peptides are used therapeutically, but agents that block their synthesis or interaction with receptors in effector organs may have therapeutic value.

THE RENIN–ANGIOTENSIN SYSTEM

RENIN

The proteolytic enzyme renin (molecular weight 42,000) is secreted by the renal juxtaglomerular apparatus (JGA), which comprises the juxtaglomerular segment of the afferent arteriole and the macula densa (granular epithelial cells situated between the distal tubule and glomerulus in the angle formed by the afferent and efferent arterioles). Renin has also been isolated from several other organs; it is not clear, however, whether these tissues release the enzyme. The storage form of renin in the JGA may be a zymogen with a higher molecular weight (63,000) and lower activity than renin, and the term "prorenin" has been proposed. Few studies have addressed control of renin synthesis and storage, and controversy abounds on the mechanism to mediate conversion of prorenin to renin. At present, three mechanisms that mediate stimulus–secretion of renin are accepted: Baroreceptors in the afferent arteriole (JG cells) that respond to pressure/volume in the arteriole; chemoreceptors in the macula densa that monitor NaCl load in tubular urine; and B_1-adrenergic receptors in JG cells that respond to sympathetic nerve stimulation or plasma-borne catecholamines (Fig. 55-1).

Vasodilators stimulate renin release by means of the baroreceptor JGA mechanism and probably by an action on the secretory mechanism for renin release. Prostacyclin appears to be an important endogenous vasodilator that mediates renin release and accounts for the suppression of plasma renin activity (PRA) by indomethacin. Diuretics lead to activation of the chemoreceptor mechanism in the macula densa. Antiadrenergic agents that act either by decreasing the nerve activity or by blocking the β_1 adrenoceptors inhibit the release of renin. Angiotensin II appears to exert negative feedback on the JGA to suppress renin release. Plasma renin is cleared metabolically

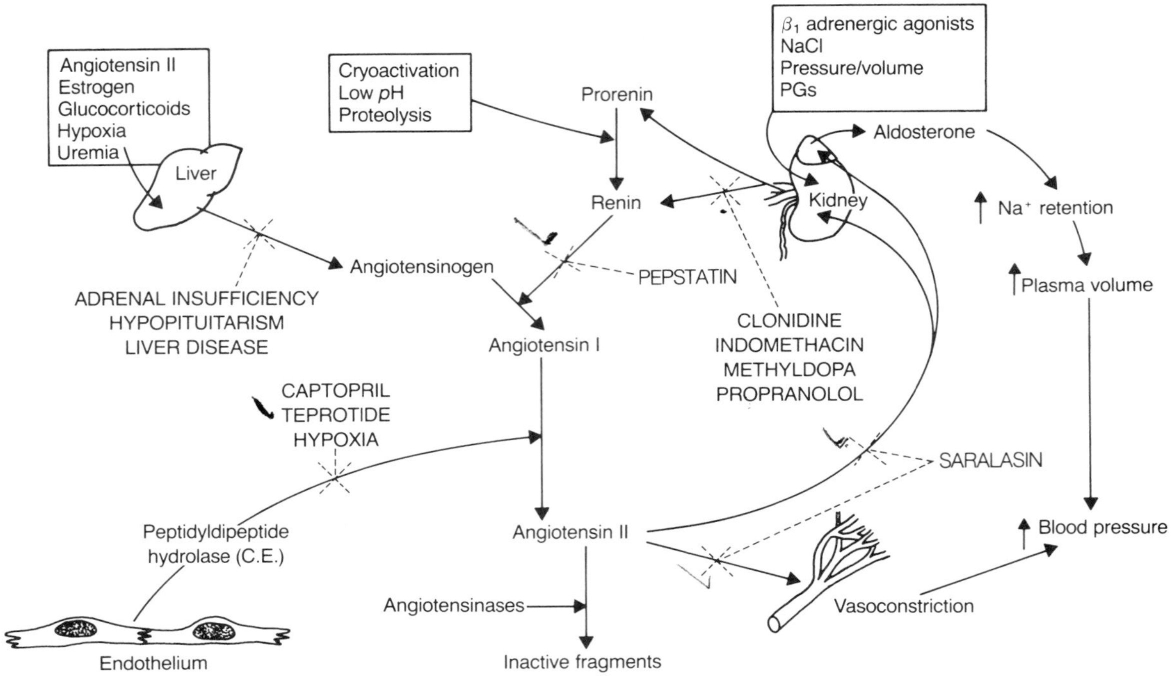

FIG. 55-1. The renin–angiotensin system. Large boxes represent stimuli of various steps in the renin–angiotensin cascade. ----X represent inhibitors at various steps in the renin–angiotensin cascade.

by the liver and has a half-life of about 15 minutes.

RENIN SUBSTRATE

Once released from the JGA, renin hydrolyzes a plasma (and ECF) glycoprotein (α_2-globulin, molecular weight ≈58,000) to form the decapeptide angiotensin I. Renin substrate (angiotensinogen) is synthesized by the liver and exported to plasma. The hepatic rate of synthesis is increased by estrogens, glucocorticoids, angiotensin II, uremia, and hypoxia. Recent studies suggest that multiple substrates for renin may exist; however, their importance is not known.

Angiotensin I, elaborated by the hydrolysis of substrate by renin, has minimal biologic activity. It is rapidly hydrolyzed by a peptidyldipeptide hydrolase (converting enzyme) located on the plasma membrane of vascular endothelial cells and epithelial cells of the proximal tubule and small intestine. This enzyme is a metalloenzyme (Zn^{++}) that requires chloride ion and is inhibited by hypoxia. The biologically active product generated from angiotensin I by converting enzyme is angiotensin II.

ANGIOTENSIN II

Angiotensin II is an octapeptide and a potent vasoconstrictor and modulator of central and peripheral sympathetic nervous system activity. Most evidence suggests that angiotensin is the dominant control mechanism for adrenal cortical aldosterone biosynthesis and release. This peptide stimulates sodium transport by epithelial cells in gut and kidney independent of aldosterone. (Biochemistry of this system is reviewed in Figure 55-1). This peptide has little value as a therapeutic agent.

INHIBITORS OF THE RENIN–ANGIOTENSIN SYSTEM

Pharmacologic agents such as angiotensin antagonists and converting enzyme inhibitors

---

Leonard Tucker Skeggs, 1918– . American biochemist. Has worked especially on hypertension and automatic chemical analysis.

James William McCubbin, 1921–1981. American physician. Has done research into hypertension and other cardiovascular diseases.

have been relied on heavily to identify contributions of the renin–angiotensin system in the regulation of arterial pressure. Although responses to such agents suggest interruption of angiotensin-mediated response, their pharmacology is complex, and precise mechanisms of action remain unknown.

SARALASIN

SAR-Arg-Val-Tyr-Val-His-Pro-ALA is a substituted analogue of angiotensin II and a competitive receptor antagonist.

Absorption, Metabolism, and Excretion

Saralasin may be administered by i.v. bolus or infusion. In hypertensive patients with high renin levels, saralasin has a plasma half-life of 3 minutes and a pharmacologic half-life of 8 minutes. The peptide is metabolized by plasma and tissue peptidases to inactive fragments. Saralasin does not cross the blood–brain barrier and is distributed in the vascular and extracellular fluid compartments. In a bolus dose, saralasin is administered at 10 mg, whereas the maximum effective dosage by i.v. infusion is 10 μg/kg/min.

Actions and Mechanism of Action

Saralasin is a competitive inhibitor of angiotensin receptors in various tissues and species and decreases blood pressure in patients with renovascular hypertension, end-stage renal disease, and malignant hypertension. The peptide has little hypotensive action in patients with essential hypertension (except patients with high renin concentrations) unless the patients are pretreated with a diuretic or are placed on a diet deficient in sodium. Hemodynamic studies indicate that the depressor response to saralasin is due to decreased total peripheral resistance. The response to saralasin is potentiated by directly acting vasodilators (hydralazine and minoxidil), which is related to the increased plasma renin activity induced by vasodilator therapy. The drug may cause increased blood pressure initially (partial agonist), followed by decreased blood pressure. The pressor response is minimized by pretreatment with a diuretic except in low renin forms of hypertension—patients in whom the pressor response is most pronounced. A rare sustained or rebounded pressor response is observed after termination of saralasin infusion. This hypertensive response may be related to the dramatic increase in plasma renin activity induced by saralasin.

Clinical Uses

Saralasin has been proposed as a diagnostic agent for angiotensin-dependent hypertension and the selection of surgical candidates with renovascular hypertension. It has been advocated for outpatient screening to detect functionally significant renovascular disease. Saralasin may also be valuable in the hospital management of malignant hypertension.

Adverse Effects

Major side-effects are severe hypotension; rebound hypertension, seen most often in patients with accelerated or malignant hypertension; and acute hypertension, which may be dramatic in patients with low renin forms of hypertension. No additional adverse effects have been reported.

INHIBITORS OF PEPTIDYLDIPEPTIDE HYDROLASE (CONVERTING ENZYME)

One of the first agents to be studied was *teprotide* (SQ 20,881), a peptide inhibitor of converting enzyme. This agent is an experimental compound, and its pharmacologic effects are similar to those of captopril.

Teprotide has an immediate onset of action and a biologic half-life of about 90 minutes. This nonapeptide does not enter the central nervous system and is distributed in the extracellular fluid. Teprotide is metabolized and excreted by the kidney. It is administered intravenously in doses of 0.25 to 1 mg/kg.

Studies with this inhibitor have generated renewed interest in the role of the renin–angiotensin system in cardiovascular and salt/water homeostasis. Severe hypotension is the only adverse effect or toxicity reported with teprotide.

CAPTOPRIL

Captopril, an orally effective inhibitor of peptidyldipeptide hydrolase, was first reported in

---

George White Pickering, 1904–1981. English physician. With Thomas Lewis described evidence for sympathetic vasodilation in humans in 1931. Has written many works on hypertension, headache, and peptic ulcer, for example.

Harry Goldblatt, 1891–1977. American pathologist. Invented the autotechnicon (for tissue specimen preservation) in 1929 with L. Gross. Did extensive research into experimental hypertension from the early 1930s, and worked on the purification and standardization of renin.

1977. It was designed rationally from a model of the active site of peptidyldipeptide hydrolase derived from the numerous studies on this enzyme and its parallels with carboxypeptidase A. Captopril was approved for human use in severe hypertension in late July 1980.

Clinical Uses

Treatment with captopril reduces blood pressure in patients with renovascular and essential hypertension. Captopril has been found to be effective in severe forms of hypertension. In essential hypertension, the hypotensive response to captopril is potentiated by concomitant therapy with a diuretic. In severe hypertension the combination of captopril and a diuretic is more efficacious than is maximum triple-drug therapy with vasodilator, beta-adrenergic blocker, and diuretic (*see* Chap. 36). Captopril is administered at 25 to 125 mg three or four times daily, and some patients do well on 200 to 250 mg twice daily. The hypotensive response to captopril is concomitant with a decreased plasma aldosterone concentration and an increase in renin release. There is an excellent correlation acutely among these variables and inhibition of peptidyldipeptide hydrolase activity or responses to angiotensin I. Captopril enhances cardiac output in patients with acute and chronic congestive heart failure by decreasing ventricular afterload and preload.

Absorption, Metabolism, and Excretion

The onset of action after oral administration is about 15 minutes, and peak blood level occurs in 30 to 60 minutes. The biologic half-life is 2 to 4 hours, and renal function is important for eliminating captopril.

Adverse Effects

A maculopapular rash has been reported in about 10% of the treated patient population. The rash is dose-related and often disappears when the dosage of captopril is reduced. Since the rash occurs most often with doses in excess of 400 mg/day and remissions are associated with decreased dosages instead of discontinuation of therapy, it is unlikely that this reflects a hypersensitive (allergic) response. Other common adverse effects are fever, loss of taste, and severe hypotension. A 1% incidence of proteinurea with renal biopsy evidence of glomerulonephritis and, rarely, leukopenia and agranulocytosis have been reported.

THE KALLIKREIN–KININ SYSTEMS

The kallikrein–kinin system is thought to represent an enzymatic–peptide cascade that assists the body in mediating the vascular and cellular responses needed for tissue defense and repair.

Two enzymes (kallikreins) catalyze the formation of the plasma kinins kallidin and bradykinin: [1] *Plasma kallikrein* (molecular weight ≈100,000) is formed from a precursor (prekallikrein, molecular weight 130,000) by an activator that is initiated by the Hageman factor, plasmin, and kallikrein. Plasma prekallikrein is complexed with high molecular α_2-plasma globulin (molecular weight 100 to 200,000) known as kininogens or kallikrein substrates. On activation of prekallikrein, plasma kallikrein rapidly hydrolyzes the complexed high molecular weight kininogens to form bradykinin; [2] *tissue or glandular kallikrein* (molecular weight 27 to 43,000) is generated from tissue prekallikrein and catalyzes the formation of kallidin (Lys-bradykinin) from low (48,000) and high molecular weight plasma kininogens. Kallikrein has been suggested as a mediator of conversion of prorenin to renin. A plasma and tissue aminopeptidase converts kallidin to bradykinin by hydrolysis of the NH_2-terminal lysyl residue from kallidin (Fig. 55-2).

PLASMA KININS

Plasma kinins (kallidin and bradykinin) are inactivated by COOH-terminal degradation by the catalytic actions of a plasma and tissue carboxypeptidase (kininase I) and peptidyldipeptide hydrolase (kininase II or angiotensin I converting enzyme). Kininase I is the primary degradative enzyme for these peptides, which have biologic half-lives of 3 to 4 minutes. Several other kinins occur naturally in animal phyla (Schlachter and Barton in Further Reading list at the end of this chapter). Numerous analogues of the plasma kinins have been synthesized and assayed for agonist/antagonist activities, and, to date, primarily agonist peptides have been identified (for review, *see* Regoli and

---

Emil Karl Frey, 1888–1961. German surgeon. Author of many works on the cardiovascular system.

Mauricio Rocha e Silva, 1910– . Brazilian pharmacologist. Has done extensive research on shock mechanisms, hormones, active polypeptides, and receptor theory.

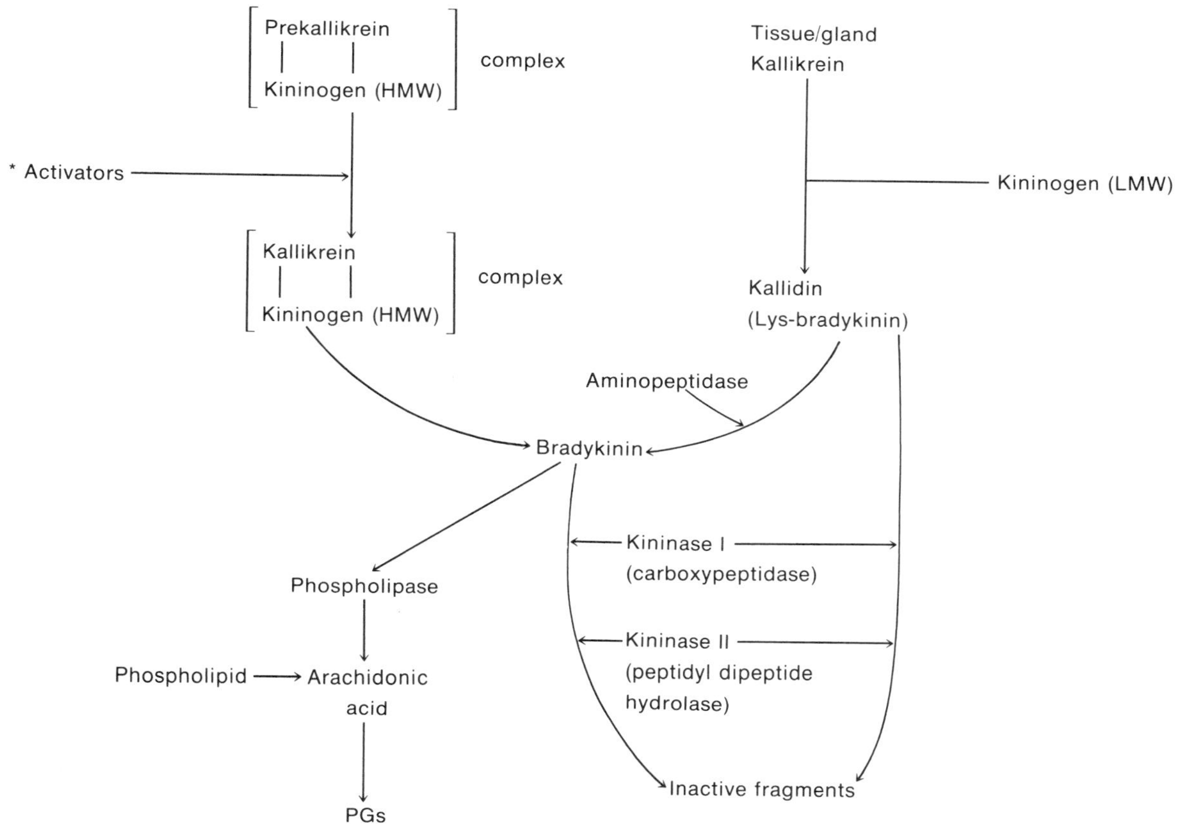

* Activators = Hageman factor, plasmin, kallikrein

FIG. 55-2. The kallikrein–kinin system. HMW = high molecular weight; LMW = low molecular weight.

Barabe in Further Reading list at the end of this chapter).

PHARMACOLOGIC ACTIONS

Kinins are very potent vasodilators and exert a direct effect on resistance vessels in most vascular beds. The plasma kinins increase intraendothelial junctions in small venules, resulting in edema formation. Bradykinin induces a contractile response in nonvascular smooth muscle. The kinins cause intense pain on application to the base of a blister, and pain is also induced when these peptides are administered intraarterially or intraperitoneally. The plasma kallikrein–kinin system is involved in hemeostasis, particularly coagulation and fibrinolysis. Complement activation, inflammatory responses, blood pressure regulation, control of organ blood flow, and tubular sodium reabsorption are suggested functions of the plasma kallikrein–kinin system. Kinin-induced vasodilatation, pain, and inflammatory responses are attenuated by pretreatment with indomethacin and other inhibitors of prostaglandin synthesis. In various tissues (lung, kidney, endothelium), the kinins appear to activate phospholipase A_2, which releases arachidonic acid from membrane phospolipids. However, the full functional significance of plasma and tissue kallikrein–kinin systems remains uncertain. These polypeptides have no use as therapeutic agents. Responses to the kinins are potentiated by captopril and teprotide. The effects of these agents depend on inhibition of kininase II, which results in slower metabolic inactivation of the kinins.

INHIBITORS OF THE KALLIKREIN–KININ SYSTEM

At present, there are no specific kinin receptor antagonists. Many responses to the kinins are blocked by inhibitors of prostaglandin biosynthesis. Although no protease inhibitors have proved very useful *in vivo*, several have been beneficial in *in vitro* studies of the kallikrein–kinin system. Trasylol is a commercially available endogenous inhibitor of plasma and tissue kallikrein, which is isolated from bovine lung. In addition, kallikreins are susceptible to several protease inhibitors. The soya bean trypsin inhibitor blocks plasma kallikrein but has little effect on glandular kallikrein. There are probably several unidentified endogenous mammalian inhibitors of kallikrein and perhaps prekallikrein activator.

OTHER PEPTIDES

In 1931 substance P, an undecapeptide, was isolated from extracts of brain and gut. This was the first of many peptides isolated from the gastrointestinal tract that was believed to be associated with endocrine and neurogenic control of gastrointestinal function. In recent years, most of these gut peptides have been identified in brain and are thought to function as neuroendocrine or neurotransmitter substances. Peptides believed to exert regulatory effects in brain and gut include bombesin, cholecystokinin, endorphins, enkephalins, gastrin, neurotensin, secretin, somatostatin, substance P, and vasoactive intestinal polypeptide. Although each of these peptides is a potent pharmacologic agent, the physiologic (or pathologic) roles subserved by each are not clear.

FURTHER READING

1. Kotchen TA, Guthrie GP Jr: Renin-angiotensin-aldosterone and hypertension. Endocr Rev 1:78–99, 1980
2. Mini-symposium on captopril. Hypertension 2:551–593, 1980
3. Peach MJ: Renin-angiotensin system: Biochemistry and mechanisms of action. Physiol Rev 57: 313–370, 1977
4. Regoli D, Barabě J: Pharmacology of bradykinin and related kinins. Pharmacol Rev 32:1–46, 1980
5. Schlachter M, Barton S: Kallikreins (kininogenases) and kinins. In Cahill G Jr, deGroot LJ (eds): Endocrinology: Metabolic Basis of Clinical practice pp 1716–1727. New York, Grune & Stratton, 1979
6. Vaughan ED Jr, Peach MJ (eds): Saralasin. Kidney Int (Suppl 9), 15: 1–122, 1979
7. Zimmerman EG (ed): Symposium—Peptides of the brain and gut. Fed Proc 38:2286–2354, 1979

CHAPTER 55 QUESTIONS

(See P. 7 for Full Instructions)

Select the One Best Answer

1. Which of the following substances produces a rise in blood pressure that is not antagonized by hexamethonium or by phentolamine?
   A. Norepinephrine
   B. Angiotensin
   C. Nicotine
   D. Tyramine
   E. Isoproterenol

2. The most common effect of an elevated blood concentration of angiotensin on the cardiovascular system is
   A. direct peripheral vasoconstriction.
   B. coronary insufficiency.
   C. a positive inotropic effect.
   D. cardiac arrhythmias during anesthesia.
   E. hypervolemia.

3. In treating cardiogenic shock complicated by heart block and poor renal perfusion, the most appropriate drug would be
   A. metaraminol.
   B. hydralazine.
   C. isoproterenol.
   D. digitoxin.
   E. angiotensin.

A = 1,2,3; B = 1,3; C = 2,4; D = 4; E = All

4. Bradykinin
   1. causes hypotension.
   2. decreases capillary permeability.
   3. is a naturally occurring polypeptide.
   4. relaxes bronchial smooth muscle.

5. The renin–angiotensin system may be enhanced by
   1. furosemide.
   2. hydralazine.
   3. oral contraceptives.
   4. levodopa.

JEREMY H. THOMPSON

56 Introduction to Antimicrobial Agents

Drugs used in treating infectious diseases are either *antiseptics* (*see* Chap. 66), *antibiotics*, or *chemotherapeutic agents*. *Antibiotics* (derived from the word *antibiosis*), are antiinfective substances of natural origin metabolically produced by, for example, *fungi* (penicillin), *bacteria* (polymyxin B), *streptomyces* (streptomycin), and *micromonospora* (gentamicin), whereas *chemotherapeutic* agents are synthetic antimicrobial drugs (for example, sulfonamides). The terms antibiotic, chemotherapeutic agent, and antimicrobial agent are often used interchangeably to refer to either natural or synthetic drugs. Additionally, the term chemotherapeutic agent is often used to describe individual *anticancer* drugs. Paul Ehrlich coined the word "chemotherapy" in 1913 to mean "injury of an invading organism without injury to the host."

Although nearly all antibiotics, at least initially, were obtained from living organisms, there are certain disadvantages in relying entirely on natural sources for commercial purposes, and synthetic (*e.g.*, chloramphenicol) or semisynthetic (*e.g.*, the newer penicillins) production is becoming more common.

HISTORY OF ANTIMICROBIAL THERAPY

Ehrlich stressed that drugs should be sought that demonstrate greater effects on the pathogen than on the host. This concept, which crystallized as the chemotherapeutic index, attempts to relate drug potency and toxicity and to measure antimicrobial effectiveness. As defined by Ehrlich, the chemotherapeutic index is

$$\frac{\text{maximal tolerated dose}}{\text{minimum curative dose}}.$$

PAUL EHRLICH—born in Silesia in 1854, may very appropriately be called the father of chemotherapy, since he coined the term and defined it as the use of drugs to injure an invading organism without injury to the host. The year 1899 is generally considered the start of Ehrlich's specific interest in chemotherapy, but unquestionably his previous interests in immunity were of fundamental importance. Interestingly, Ehrlich did not receive a great deal of initial encouragement in his pursuit of chemotherapy either from his colleagues or from the government. He received the Nobel prize in 1908 for his work on immunity.

Thus no real therapeutic advantage is gained if a new drug is half as toxic as an old one and not more than half as active.

The unwitting application of "antibacterial" therapy is very old. Medical lore abounds with tales of the use of soil, plants, and moldy ferments for the treatment of various skin lesions, the reported beneficial effects undoubtedly resulting from antibiotics produced by associated bacteria, fungi, and actinomycetes. Several antiinfective drugs were available before Ehrlich's time; for example, malaria and dysentery were widely treated with the alkaloids of cinchona and ipecacuanha, mercury had been used in treating syphilis, and carbolic acid had been introduced as an antiseptic by 1865. Moreover, that bacteria could produce substances antagonistic to other bacterial species had been noted by Pasteur in 1877 while working with *Bacillus anthracis*. Ehrlich, however, established the major principles that govern the investigation of experimental infections and pioneered the idea (in 1906) of *therapia sterilisans magna*, the total control of pathogenic bacteria with a single dose of a nontoxic chemical (a magic bullet).

Before the development of sulfonamides, several antiseptic and disinfectant arsenic, antimony, bismuth, and dye compounds were introduced into therapy. Because of their systemic toxicity, these compounds mainly were used topically. Some antimony compounds are still used (*see* Chap. 67). The overwhelming therapeutic success of the sulfonamides and penicillin (introduced into therapy in 1935 and 1941, respectively) initiated systematic investigations into distribution of antibacterial drugs in nature. Over the past 35 to 40 years, thousands of new antimicrobial agents have been discovered and tested. Most of these drugs have proved too toxic for use in humans, but a sizable number have been retained. Despite the introduction of many potent drugs, the elimination of all infections has not been realized, nor is it likely to be. Indeed, the indiscriminate use of antibiotics has frequently resulted in the development of a more serious infection than might otherwise have occurred. Many antimicrobial drugs have been useful in the investigation of cellular biochemistry and in laboratory bacteriology.

Louis Pasteur, 1822–1895. French chemist and microbiologist. The first to demonstrate optical isomerism and a pioneer of industrial microbiology. Discredited spontaneous generation theory for microorganisms, revealed microbial cause of fermentation and putrefaction. Developed first immune therapy for rabies.

Antibiotics are widely used (15–20% of all prescriptions) and account for about 70% to 80% of hospital drug costs. Epidemiologic studies have shown that greater than 50% of antibiotics used in certain situations are not needed, an inappropriate agent is often chosen, or the dose used is incorrect. To facilitate an understanding of the correct use of antibacterial drugs, some basic principles governing their action are presented.

BASIC PRINCIPLES OF ANTIMICROBIAL CHEMOTHERAPY

BACTERICIDAL AND BACTERIOSTATIC DRUGS

On *in vitro* testing, antimicrobial drugs are often categorized as *bactericidal* or *bacteriostatic*. Bactericidal drugs kill organisms and are usually more effective during logarithmic growth, since the increased metabolic activity provides appropriate targets (*see* Chap. 57) and maximum susceptibility. Bacteriostatic agents only prevent bacterial growth and thus clinically are less desirable; other terms such as *fungistatic* and *amebecidal* are self-explanatory. This categorization is partly dose dependent. Thus bactericidal drugs may produce bacteriostasis if present in suboptimum concentrations, and typical bacteriostatic agents such as erythromycin may become bactericidal at high concentrations, for example, in the urine.

If body defense mechanisms are impaired (Table 56-1), the antibiotic may be unable to do more than slow the spread of infection, and a relapse occurs when therapy is discontinued. Although bactericidal drugs can eradicate an infection in theory, this rarely, if ever, occurs, and *intact host defense mechanisms and anatomical barriers are needed for full recovery.*

ANTIMICROBIAL SYNERGISM AND ANTAGONISM

When used concurrently, antimicrobial drugs may exhibit *additive, antagonistic,* or *synergistic* effects; an *additive* effect is the usual response, for example, when two bacteriostatic antibiotics are combined. Alternatively, most bactericidal drugs act maximally on multiplying bacteria, and, because bacteriostatic drugs depress bacterial cell multiplication and growth, a mixture of the two types may result in *antagonism* (*e.g.*, with penicillin plus a tet-

TABLE 56-1. Some Major Factors That Predispose to Local or Systemic Infections

Level of Defense	Predisposing Factor
Anatomic barriers and secretions	Foreign body (*e.g.*, calculus, sequestrum, implant)
	Congenital anomaly (*e.g.*, ectopic ureter)
	Burns, trauma, or surgery
	Catheters (*e.g.*, urinary, i.v., intraarterial, tracheal)
	Therapeutic procedures or use of diagnostic apparatuses (*e.g.*, dental prophylaxis, ultrasonic nebulizers, IPPB apparatuses)
	Bacterial proliferation in large-volume parenteral or hyperalimentation fluids
	Increased secretions (*e.g.*, pulmonary edema reduces the activity of alveolar macrophages)
	Reduced secretions (*e.g.*, achlorhydria, Sjögrens syndrome)
	Poor diet, alcoholism, major systemic metabolic disease
Normal bacterial flora	Cross-infection with drug-resistant pathogens
	Suprainfections
White blood cells	Disorders of granulocyte production (*e.g.*, neutropenia, agranulocytosis, aplastic anemia)
	Depression of chemotaxis (*e.g.*, glucocorticosteroids and ethyl alcohol)
	Depression of opsonization (*e.g.*, glucocorticosteroids)
	Depression of intracellular bacterial killing (*e.g.*, glucocorticoids stabilize lysosomal membranes, and colchicine and vinblastine inhibit microtubule formation and stabilize lysosomal membranes)
Immunologic mechanisms	Antibody, cellular or combined immunodeficiencies
	Defects of complement or the phagocytic system

racycline in the treatment of pneumococcal meningitis). *Synergism* is rare, but two important examples are penicillin plus streptomycin in the treatment of enterococcal endocarditis, where penicillin probably facilitates the intracellular passage of the aminoglycoside; and sequential blockade of folic acid synthesis by cotrimoxazole (*see* Figs. 57-5, 57-6). Synergism may allow either a reduced dosage of one or both of the drugs without loss of antibacterial activity, or achievement of a more pronounced antibacterial effect.

ANTIBACTERIAL SPECTRUM

Antibiotics can be classified as broad or narrow spectrum, depending on the range of organisms they affect. Thus penicillin G has a *narrow spectrum* because it primarily affects only gram-positive organisms and neisseriae, whereas the tetracyclines have a *broad antibacterial spectrum* because they depress not only gram-positive and gram-negative bacteria, but also the rickettsiae and the chlamydiae. Separation into broad- and narrow-spectrum categories is often blurred, since overuse of broad-spectrum agents (particularly ampicillin and the tetracyclines) has resulted in the emergence of many resistant strains. Thus the current *clinically effective spectrum* of broad-spectrum antibiotics may be narrower than that of some narrow-spectrum antibiotics. Broad-spectrum antibiotics should be restricted to treatment of specific infections caused by a few organisms or even a single species of organism. *The property of broad spectrum should not be confused with a license for broad nonspecific use.*

DETERMINATION OF BACTERIAL SENSITIVITY *IN VITRO*

Two standard microbiologic methods are used to determine bacterial sensitivity to antibiotics, but neither reflects precisely the factors operating *in vivo*. In the first method the isolated organism is inoculated into tubes or onto plates of solid culture medium that contain sequentially diminishing drug concentrations. After incubation for 18 to 24 hours, the lowest concentration of the drug that inhibits bacterial growth

TAGE ANTON ULTIMUS SJÖGREN, 1859–1939. Swedish surgeon. As well as describing Sjögren's syndrome, a drying of the mucous membranes, he is believed to have been the first to use x-rays successfully against cancer, an epithelioma, in 1899.

HANS CHRISTIAN JOACHIM GRAM, 1853–1938. Copenhagen physician and bacteriologist. In 1884 published differential stain method for bacteria. Also worked on the physiology of anemia.

(the minimum inhibitory concentration; MIC) can be determined. Additionally, the lowest concentration that sterilizes the culture medium or that results in a 99.9% decline in the bacterial count is the minimal bactericidal concentration (MBC). Bacteria are usually considered sensitive when the MIC is lower than concentrations routinely achieved in blood, and bactericidal activity usually occurs at drug concentrations 2 to 10 times greater than MIC. How long antibiotic levels must remain at the MIC *in vivo* to achieve optimum results is unknown for most organisms.

Antibacterial potency varies depending on the test organism used, the size of the inoculum, and the conditions (*p*H, temperature, presence of oxygen, tissue fluid, pus, drugs) of the *in vitro* test system.

The second method (the Kirby–Bauer technique) is even less precise and consists of the application of standardized, antibacterial, drug-impregnated filter paper disks onto the surface of a uniformly seeded agar plate. An approximate indication of bacterial sensitivity may be obtained by measuring the zone of inhibition of colony growth. This technique is cheap and rapid and is widely used to give an indication of which antibiotic to use and the approximate dosage level required to produce a therapeutic effect.

Two specific infections in which routine sensitivity testing may be misleading are subacute bacterial endocarditis and urinary tract infections. Subacute bacterial endocarditis has only rarely, if ever, been cured with bacteriostatic drugs. Therefore bactericidal agents should be used in preference to bacteriostatic agents.

Two important considerations apply to urinary tract infections: First, some antibacterial agents excreted in the urine achieve higher concentrations there than in the blood and thus may be useful in treatment, even though *in vitro* sensitivity testing (performed with antibiotic-containing disks relating to commonly achieved blood levels) indicates that the organism is "resistant." Second, *in vitro* sensitivity testing is usually performed at *p*H 7.2 to 7.4, whereas urine is usually more acidic at *p*H 5 to 6. Therefore antibiotics such as streptomycin that possess greater antibacterial activity at an alkaline *p*H will appear more effective *in vitro* than *in vivo* unless the urine is concomitantly alkalinized. On the other hand, antimicrobial agents such as nalidixic acid, which is more effective at an acid *p*H, may appear ineffective when studied *in vitro*, whereas in acid urine *in vivo* they might be clinically valuable. The rate of drug excretion may be influenced by the urine *p*H (*see* Chap. 3); for example, the tetracycline antibiotics are more effective and more slowly excreted at an acid *p*H.

Rarely, antibiotic sensitivity tests need not be performed, since experience has indicated with a few species that sensitivity is predictable (*e.g.*, use of pencillin G in treating group A β-hemolytic streptococci).

WILLIAM MURRAY MAURICE KIRBY, 1914– . American physician. Has done extensive research on infectious diseases and the testing of new antibiotics. Developed *in vitro* testing methods for antibiotics.

ALFRED W. BAUER, 1923– . German-born American pediatrician.

ANTIBIOTIC LEVELS IN TISSUE FLUID AND BLOOD

The distribution of antibiotics is important because most infectious processes are not limited to the blood or urine. Interstitial antibiotic concentrations are usually lower and occur later than those observed in the serum, but there is no simple association between the two. Distribution of antibiotics follows the general principles outlined earlier (*see* Chaps. 3, 5), and drug concentrations at the site of an infection and bacterial antibiotic uptake will thus depend on the drug's physiochemical properties (pK_a, protein binding, $T\frac{1}{2}$, and so forth) as well as the causative organism, the location of the infection, the presence of tissue fluid, pus, or an abscess cavitiy, and the route of drug administration and dose. Penicillin G, for example, which produces an effective blood level for 2 to 4 after a standard i.m. dose, may persist in pus for 8 to 12 hours, and rifampin, because of its lipophilicity, is rapidly taken up into *M. tuberculosis*.

Little is known about tissue levels of antimicrobial drugs or the importance of protein binding in tissue fluids. Experimental and clinical evidence has shown that some drugs pass poorly into certain "compartments," for example, cephalosporins as a class diffuse poorly into the central nervous system, but for most antibiotics the question "Is it better to achieve periodic high peak serum levels or a sustained level?" cannot be answered. Similarly, for most infections, it is not clear how long the tissue "drug free" (level below the MIC) interval can be or how long a given course of antimicrobial therapy should last. Many drugs used to treat urinary tract infections are effective despite low plasma levels because they are concentrated in the urine.

Blood antibiotic levels (*see* Chap. 79) can be a useful measurement in patients with nonresponding infections, in those with symptoms that suggest toxicity, or in treating infections in patients with hepatic or renal disease to minimize inadequate dosage and toxicity. Obviously, blood samples must be drawn at the appropriate time, they must be handled, transported, and processed correctly, and the assay should be accurate, reproducible, and reasonably rapid (*see* Chap. 79). Most assays report on total quantity of drug (free plus bound) present in the serum.

BACTERIAL RESISTANCE TO ANTIMICROBIAL DRUGS

Considered by species, bacteria are susceptible to some antibacterial drugs and resistant to others, but strains may develop that are resistant to drugs normally effective against that species. This is particularly true of staphylococci, gram-negative bacilli, and *M. tuberculosis* but may occur with any organism; bacterial strains are known that are resistant to every antibiotic in current use. Bacterial resistance is a major medical problem because it severely limits the usefulness of many antibiotics and often necessitates the substitution of costly, toxic, and less potent drugs where the more acceptable agents are found to be ineffective.

Development of bacterial resistance makes it essential to revise periodically the drugs of choice for different bacterial infections and to determine the antibacterial sensitivity of the invading organism in all infections whenever possible. Failure to do this wastes time and money and needlessly exposes the patient to potentially harmful drugs. If antibiotics have to be administered before results of sensitivity testing are available, it is useful to know the probable sensitivity pattern (antibiogram) of a given bacterial species based on the recent experience of the individual clinical laboratory or on the hospital environment.

Patterns of drug resistance may change abruptly when new antibiotics are introduced or when there are changes in the customary use of antibiotics within a hospital community. Thus patterns of drug resistance may vary considerably from hospital to hospital. Organisms that become resistant to one antibacterial drug usually exhibit *cross-resistance* to related drugs; for example, bacteria developing resistance to sulfadiazine are resistant to equipotent concentrations of all other sulfonamides.

TYPES OF BACTERIAL RESISTANCE

Bacterial resistance to antimicrobial drugs is either *natural* or *acquired; dependence,* a related phenomenon, is rare. The development of bacterial resistance is simply an expression of bacterial evolution, with survival of the fittest. Bacterial multiplication is so rapid that within 3½ years an average strain of organism may have passed through as many generations as man has gone through in 1 million years.

Natural Resistance

Natural resistance is genetically determined and depends on the absence of the metabolic process affected by the antibiotic in question. Naturally resistant organisms proliferate as sensitive ones are killed. Natural resistance may be characteristic of an entire species but sometimes, as with penicillin-resistant staphylococci, is confined to particular strains within that species.

Acquired Resistance

Acquired resistance is resistance that develops in a previously sensitive bacterial species. It can arise through *mutation* (spontaneous, induced), *adaptation,* or *infectious (multiple) drug resistance.*

By *spontaneous mutation* (about once per 10^5–10^{10} cells), a bacterial species produces *de novo* some members that differ from the parent strain. If the mutation is favorable, the bacteria will survive. If susceptible bacteria are exposed to subinhibitory concentrations of antibacterial drugs, drug-resistant mutants may develop (induced mutation) either in one step or in a series of steps. A stepwise increase in resistance is probably due to mutations that occur in a number of different genes, each of which is responsible for a slightly increased resistance. A one-step increase in bacterial resistance is due to mutations that occur in more powerful genes conferring a considerable degree of resistance.

Adaptation presupposes that an organism contains the potential for resisting or countering the antibiotic and that the mechanism is "triggered" through enzyme induction after antibiotic exposure, for example, pencillinase induction after semisynthetic penicillin exposure in some strains of staphyloccocci (*see* Chap. 59).

Infectious (multiple) drug resistance refers to the inheritance (from a resistant to a sensitive bacterium *in vivo* or *in vitro*) of new genetic material (R factors) coding for resistance. R factors are carried on plasmids (extrachromosomal DNA) and code for a variety of enzymes (*e.g.*, β-lactamases).

Plasmids replicate independent of host chromosomes and can be either *conjugative* (initiate and mediate DNA transfer through conjugation) or *nonconjugative* (cannot mediate DNA transfer by themselves but are transferred by transformation, transduction, or a conjugative plasmid). Plasmids that contain R factors may increase (or decrease) their level of resistance by acquiring (or loosing) additional genes from various sources, such as bacteriophages, other plasmids, or chromosomes.

R factors (to four different classes of antibiotics) were first reported in Japan in 1959–1960 during an epidemic of *Shigella flexneri* dysentery; subsequently they have been identified worldwide. The origin of R factors remains unknown. Their development, as distinct from their spread, is probably not directly related to antimicrobial chemotherapy. Why they have not spread throughout the entire bacterial population is unclear. Plasmids may affect bacterial properties (phage typing, toxin production, fermentation reactions), confusing their identification.

Gram-negative bacteria possess, in addition to R factors, a resistance transfer factor (RTF: sex factor) that determines replication and transfer (*see* below)—that is, they code for self-transmission and are thus conjugative (*see* above). R factors in gram-positive bacteria are considered nonconjugative. R factors transfer in one of three ways: *Transformation* (incorporation by a sensitive bacterium of free genes from a drug-resistant cell) occurs rarely (about $1/10^8$ cells) and is probably of little clinical importance. *Transduction* (the transfer of an R-factor-carrying-plasmid by a temperate bacterial virus, a bacteriophage vector, along with its own genes) occurs mainly in gram-positive cocci and rarely in gram-negative bacilli, and usually resistance to only one or two antibiotics is transferred. Transduction occurs approximately once for every 10^3–10^6 exposed cells and is more readily accomplished if both the donor and recipient strains belong to the same group than if they belong to different groups.

Conjugation, the most important, depends on a plasmid-containing, drug-resistant "male"-type bacterial cell that passes R factor and RTF to a drug-sensitive "female" cell by way of a "sex pilus." Formation of the sex pilus is induced by RTF. The infected female cell then becomes a male cell. Transfer factors have thus far been determined in *E. coli, Shigellae spp., Salmonella typhimurium, Klebsiella-Enterobacter spp., Vibrio cholerae, Pasturella spp., Proteus spp., Serratia marcescens,* and *Pseudomonas aeruginosa.* R-factor transfer encoding for resistance to one or as many as seven drugs (chloramphenicol, erythromycin, penicillin, tetracyclines, aminoglycosides, sulfonamides, and fusidic acid) at one time has been identified. Donor and recipient strains may belong to different species or even to different genera, and, more important, transfer can develop between pathogenic and nonpathogenic organisms indiscriminately. Studies of penicillin-resistant gonococci from the Orient and from England have shown that they both contain similarly sized plasmids (4,4Mdal and 3,2Mdal, respectively) coding for the same β-lactamase produced normally by *H. influenza.*

SIMON FLEXNER, 1863–1946. New York pathologist and bacteriologist. One of the pioneers of American microbiology. In 1900 discovered *Bacillus dysenteriae,* named after him, and led research that identified poliomyelitis as a viral disease (1909–1910).

Dependence

Organisms may become dependent on an antibacterial drug. Clinically this may be seen occasionally in the treatment of tuberculosis with streptomycin (*see* Chap. 60).

MECHANISMS OF RESISTANCE TO ANTIMICROBIAL DRUGS

When an organism has developed means for countering the antiinfective drug, it is said to be *resistant;* several general mechanisms are known (Table 56-2). Bacteria may exhibit more than one mechanism of resistance, and not all resistant organisms of any particular group possess the same mechanism of resistance. Resistance that arises through alteration of the organism (such that a drug either does not reach or does not interact normally with its bacterial target site) generally occurs through mutational alteration of the cellular components. Resistance that arises through enzymatic destruction of an antibiotic generally is associated with plasmids.

Antimicrobial agents for which no plasmid-mediated resistance has been described include bacitracin, cycloserine, methicillin, nalidixic acid, nitrofurantoin, polymyxin B, and vancomycin.

FACTORS THAT INFLUENCE DEVELOPMENT OF BACTERIAL RESISTANCE

Bacterial resistance to antibiotics is a major therapeutic problem because many pathogenic

TABLE 56-2. General Mechanisms of Resistance to Antimicrobial Agents

General Mechanism	Antimicrobial Drug	Remarks
Alteration of bacterial target (binding) site, reducing binding	Aminoglycosides	Single amino-acid change on the 30S ribosome to which aminoglycoside normally binds causes misreading of genetic code
	Clindamycin/lincomycin	Methylation of a nucleotide sequence of the 23S subunit of bacterial RNA by a plasmid-coded RNA methylase, resulting in failure of antibiotic binding to the 50S ribosome
	Erythromycin	As for clindamycin/lincomycin
	Fusidic acid	Presence of altered bacterial G factor, resulting in failure of antibiotic binding
	Rifampin	Bacterial RNA polymerase possesses an altered B1 subunit, resulting in failure of antibiotic binding
Altered bacterial cell permeability to antibiotic	Aminoglycosides	Acetylation of amino groups, or phosphorylation or adenylation of hydroxyl groups, by appropriate bacterial enzymes, leading to poor affinity with transport systems. Interference with energy requirements for antibiotic transport systems
	Chloramphenicol	Reduced uptake
	Clindamycin/lincomycin	Reduced cell uptake?
	Sulfonamides	Reduced cell uptake?
	Methicillin	Bacterial cells impermeable to the drug. Methicillin binds to penicillinases but is not destroyed by the enzymes
	Tetracyclines (other than minocycline)	Bacterial cells do not bind the antibiotic and may produce an inhibitor of tetracycline transport
	Polymyxin B	Genesis of a permeability barrier blocking access of the antibiotic to critical phospholipids
Antibiotic inactivation	Penicillin G and other penicillinase-sensitive penicillins	Cleavage (hydrolysis) of penicillin β-lactam ring by plasmid-coded (usually) bacterial β-lactamases (penicillinases) (*see* Chap. 59)
	Cephalosporins	Cleavage (hydrolysis) of the cephalosporin β-lactam ring by (usually chromosomally mediated) bacterial β-lactamases (cephalosporinases) (*see* Chap. 59)
	Chloramphenicol	Acetylation of the antibiotic's hydroxyl groups by plasmid-coded, or chromosomally coded, bacterial chloramphenicol acetyltransferases
Bypassing the reaction blocked by the antibiotic	Cycloserine	Increased production of alanine racemase and D-alanyl:D-alanine synthetase by bacteria. Increased production of D-alanine by bacteria (*see* Chap. 59)
	Sulfonamides	Bacterial production of para-aminobenzoic acid, a direct sulfonamide antagonist. Development of alternate pathway of folic acid synthesis through plasmid-coded dihydropteroate synthetase
	Trimethoprim	Development of alternate pathway of folic acid metabolism through plasmid-coded dihydrofolate reductase

species that were highly sensitive are now resistant to the formerly effective drugs. Precautions to decrease the rate of emergence of resistant strains include avoiding unnecessary, promiscuous use of antibiotics, selection of antibiotics on the basis of *in vitro* bacteriologic investigation, when possible, and cycling the use of specific agents to reduce selective pressures. Additionally, antibiotics that usually demonstrate a wide spectrum of cross-resistance or that are likely to induce resistance should be avoided, if possible. The combination of two or more antibacterial drugs reduces the development of resistance in the treatment of tuberculosis (*see* Chap. 60) and in the use of a second drug with rifampin, and possibly with cotrimoxazole.

CLINICAL IMPLICATIONS OF DRUG RESISTANCE

The spectrum of resistance conveyed by R factors drastically curtails the antibacterial spectrum of many drugs. Thus each hospital should develop an antibiotic policy whereby certain drugs are reserved for specific use in critically ill patients infected with dangerous pathogenic organisms (*e.g.*, *Staphylococcus aureus* and *Pseudomonas aeruginosa*. In addition, cross-infection within the hospital environment should be controlled by careful attention to environmental hygiene, the treatment of carriers, and the strict use of isolation procedures. Clinical and veterinary use of antibiotics may not lead inexorably to increased bacterial resistance, since the frequency of resistance to some antibiotics falls if the use of those agents is abandoned or at least greatly curtailed. Tetracycline resistance is exceptional since the gene that determines resistance is closely linked to, or possibly part of, the genes that govern transfer. Thus selection for tetracycline resistance automatically selects for ability to transfer resistance from strain to strain, a special consideration when tetracyclines are used prophylactically or for other purposes, for example, in subtherapeutic doses in agriculture to increase the rate of weight gain in livestock. Mutational changes leading to resistance may also alter pathogenicity by increasing (*Staph. aureus*), or decreasing (*N. gonorrhoeae*) virulence.

ANTIBACTERIAL DRUG COMBINATIONS

ANTIBIOTIC COMBINATIONS

Fixed dosage combinations of antibiotics should not be used. However, the simultaneous administration of two or more separate antibiotics may be justified in *mixed bacterial infections* (gram-positive and gram-negative pathogens) such as occur in peritonitis, where the infecting organisms do not share antimicrobial sensitivity; in *gram-negative bacteremic shock* (gentamicin plus a cephalosporin); in *severe infections of doubtful etiology* until results of culture and sensitivity testing are known; *to produce synergism* (*see* above); and *to delay the emergence of resistant strains* in tuberculosis (*see* Chap. 60) and in severe *Ps. aeruginosa* infections (carbenicillin plus gentamicin). The disadvantages of dual treatment are increased incidence of side-effects, increased cost, obscured diagnosis, and a wider antibacterial spectrum with greater chance of suprainfection. Some antibiotics with similar modes of action may antagonize each other and therefore should not be used; for example, erythromycin may antagonize chloramphenicol (*see* Chap. 57). Bactericidal and bacteriostatic drugs may show antagonism when combined (*see* above).

CHEMOTHERAPEUTIC DRUG COMBINATIONS

There is ample justification for combining several sulfonamides to minimize crystalluria (*see* Chap. 64) or for combining antitubercular drugs to minimize emergence of mycobacterial resistance (*see* Chap. 60).

ANTIBIOTIC AND CHEMOTHERAPEUTIC DRUG COMBINATIONS WITH NONANTIBACTERIAL SUBSTANCES

Many fixed dosage preparations of antibiotics and chemotherapeutic agents plus analgesics, antihistamines, antipyetics, and glucocorticosteroids, among others, are on the market. Physicians are advised against using these preparations.

EXPERIMENTAL DRUG COMBINATIONS

Several agents under study possess little or no inherent antimicrobial activity yet potentiate *in vitro* the activity of some antibiotics. Such agents include clavulanic acid (an inhibitor of β-lactamase) and alaphosphin (which blocks peptidoglycan synthesis; *see* Chap. 57). Clavulanic acid, obtained from *Streptomyces* organisms, is a chemical analogue of penicillin; an oxygen-containing ring has replaced the antibiotic's sulfur-containing ring.

GENERAL USE OF ANTIBACTERIAL DRUGS

In the clinical management of parasitic disease, the selection of the most suitable antimicrobial drug is only one aspect of therapy; adequate supporting measures must be undertaken because *final recovery depends on host defense mechanisms.*

BACTERIOLOGIC DIAGNOSIS

Generally, the selection of an antibiotic should be based on an etiologic diagnosis. Culture of infected material (*e.g.*, pus) will, in most instances, enable the pathogen to be isolated and identified with subsequent determination of its sensitivity (or resistance) to antimicrobial drugs. Although sensitivity determinations are desirable, particularly in infections caused by *E. coli*, *Proteus spp.*, *Ps. aeruginosa*, and *Staphylococcus spp.*, they are not absolutely necessary in infections caused by some organisms (*T. pallidum*, pneumococci, β-hemolytic streptococci) usually sensitive to drugs, like penicillin.

Because many common pathogenic microorganisms have different antibacterial resistance, a hit-or-miss philosophy in treatment can lead to delayed administration of the correct drug and to diagnostic confusion. In some instances bacteriologic diagnosis and sensitivity determination are difficult. In the acutely ill patient, for example, delay before the start of therapy may not be justified clinically, and treatment can be begun after appropriate culture material has been taken. Additionally, appropriate material may not be readily available for culturing, and in these instances a Gram stain may be invaluable. The occasional necessity for administering a combination of antibiotics to febrile patients who are seriously ill and who are suspected of having an unknown bacterial infection cannot be denied. The initiation of an antibiotic program, however, should not commit the physician to its continuance if a change is suggested by the culture and sensitivity report. Thus, as soon as the pathogen is isolated, an antibiotic should be selected that has the most narrow spectrum against that organism in order to minimize suprainfection (*see* below).

Major factors that influence the choice and dose of an antibacterial drug in the absence of sensitivity testing are the location of the infection, a "statistical" guess as to the causative organisms, the presence of concomitant illness, knowledge of previous drug therapy, and a history of drug reactions.

DRUG RESPONSE AND DOSAGE

An antibacterial drug usually causes significant clinical improvement within 12 to 24 hours. If no clinical improvement is obvious after 48 to 72 hours of full therapy, the organisms are probably resistant to that drug or some other problem such as an undrained abscess is preventing a favorable response. However, a knowledge of the natural history of a particular infection is exceedingly helpful. The patient with pneumococcal pneumonia, for example, usually shows prompt inprovement, whereas the patient with typhoid fever typically remains ill for several days after the start of optimal antibiotic treatment. If symptoms and fever redevelop after a period of amelioration, *suprainfection* with resistant organisms, *abscess formation*, or an *adverse drug reaction* (*i.e.*, agranulocytosis) may be responsible.

PROPHYLACTIC USE

Antimicrobial drugs have drastically altered the natural history of bacterial disease by reducing the morbidity and mortality from infections. Not surprisingly, these same antimicrobial agents have been used to *prevent* rather than to *treat* infections (Table 56-3). Specific disadvantages to prophylactic therapy in any given patient are, the risk of masking a serious infection (*i.e.*, penicillin prophylaxis of gonorrhea masking syphilis); the cost and inconvenience of therapy; and the development of adverse effects. The major hazard of prophylactic antibiotics for the biosphere is that their use provides a strong selective environment that favors the appearance and maintenance of resistant bacteria, particularly through R-factor transfer. When antibiotics are used appropriately as treatment or to prevent potentially life-threatening infections, we accept the ecologic risk and the potential long-term medical hazards to the community. However, we must question whether the prophylactic use of antibiotics is acceptable when they are used for more "trivial" reasons—*economic* reasons (growth promotors in animal feeds), *prevention of mild illness* (vacation diarrhea), or *a disease for which alternatives are available* (venereal disease).

TABLE 56-3. Some Indications for Prophylactic Antibiotics

Disease	Drug
1. Protection of a healthy person exposed to a pathogen:	
Ophthalmia neonatorum	Silver nitrate
Siblings and close contacts of patients with *N. meningitidis* infection	Minocycline, rifampin, sulfadiazine
Prevention of gonorrhea or syphilis after exposure	A penicillin
Household contacts of patients with cholera	A tetracycline
Household contacts of patients with bacillary dysentery	A sulfonamide
Clostridial prophylaxis in hip joint implant surgery	A penicillin
Prophylaxis of general uterine infection in prolonged labor after rupture of membranes	A penicillin
Heavily contaminated surgical sites or sites likely to become infected	Various antibiotics depending on the circumstances
Bacteroides infection in large bowel or gynecologic surgery	Erythromycin, gentamicin metronidazole, tobramycin plus kanamycin, or clindamycin
2. Prevention of recurrent disease in "hypersensitive" patients:	
Group A streptococcal infection in patients with rheumatic fever	A penicillin or a sulfonamide
3. Prevention or modification of acute infectious episodes in patients with specific diseases:	
Bacterial endocarditis in persons with rheumatic endocarditis, prosthetic valves, or congenital cardiac lesions who are undergoing oral surgery, dental scaling or dental prophylaxis, or genitourinary manipulations/instrumentation.	A penicillin (plus streptomycin for those with prosthetic valves). A cephalosporin or vancomycin in penicillin allergy
Urinary tract infection prophylaxis in children or adults with vesicoureteric reflux, unoperable obstructive uropathy, or chronic pyelonephritis	Ampicillin, cephalexin, cotrimoxazole, nalidixic acid or nitrofurantoin
Respiratory tract infection prophylaxis during the winter months in patients with chronic bronchitis	Ampicillin, methacycline or another tetracycline
Clostridial prophylaxis after midthigh amputation in a diabetic	A penicillin
4. Protection of the compromised patient:	*See* Table 56-6.

Prophylaxis cannot prevent colonization or infection with all potential invaders; generally, there is no place for prophylaxis unless therapy is directed against one particular microorganism or a small group of microorganisms. Some make a distinction between *primary prophylaxis* (prevention of colonization) and *secondary prophylaxis* (treatment of bacteria only recently becoming established). Since it is impossible to determine (in any bacterial invasion) at what stage *infection*, as distinct from *colonization*, is present, some would consider the terms synonymous. Antimicrobial agents are not substitutes during surgery for meticulous technique, preservation of vascularity, hemostasis, débridement, removal of foreign particles, and anatomic closure without tension or dead space.

CONCOMITANT DRUG THERAPY

Gamma globulin and *antitoxic sera* are required as adjunct agents in specific circumstances (*see* Table 58-1). Glucocorticosteroids produce both beneficial and deleterious effects, and which effect will be dominant is often impossible to predict. Glucocorticosteroids mask the symptoms of infection and alter the host–parasite relationship in favor of the parasite by inhibiting the inflammatory response; enhancing tissue invasion and dissemination of pathogens; depressing polymorphonuclear production, migration, phagocytosis, and intracellular digestive mechanisms; and reducing interferon production. On the other hand, they possess beneficial antitoxic, antiallergic, and antiinflammatory effects (*See* Chap. 47).

Their antitoxic property may be life-saving in patients with septic shock caused by, for example, gram-negative bacilli, where the steroid restores endotoxin-damaged vessel sensitivity to sympathomimetic amines, and in Herxheimer reactions (typhoid fever, leprosy, syphilis, and filariasis) and viral hepatitis. Their "antiallergic" and antiinflammatory properties are of value countering severe or life-threatening hypersensitivity reactions, re-

TABLE 56-4. Some Important Drug Interactions with Antibiotics

Drug	Antibiotics	Interaction
Antacids, iron, calcium, bismuth, zinc sulfate	Oral tetracyclines	Tetracycline not absorbed. Insoluble chelate formed
Antacids	Oral penicillin G	Increased bioavailability of the penicillin because less destroyed
Coumarin anticoagulants	Tetracyclines and other broad-spectrum antibiotics	Reduced production and availability of vitamin K by gut flora
Coumarin anticoagulants	Rifampin	Rifampin, an enzyme inducer, shortens T½ of the anticoagulant
Coumarin anticoagulants	Griseofulvin	As for rifampin (above), plus reduced absorption of the anticoagulant
Coumarin anticoagulants	Chloramphenicol	Reduced metabolism of the anticoagulant
Coumarin anticoagulants	INAH	As for chloramphenicol (*see above*)
Coumarin anticoagulants	Metronidazole	Reduced metabolism of S warfarin but no effect on R warfarin (*see* Chap. 42)
Coumarin anticoagulants	Nalidixic acid	May displace anticoagulants from plasma protein binding sites
Coumarin anticoagulants	Cotrimoxazole	As for chloramphenicol (*see* above)
Ethacrynic acid and furosemide	Aminoglycosides	Increased aminoglycoside nephrotoxicity, and ototoxicity
Gentamicin	Carbenicillin	Interact to destroy each other
Phenobarbital	Chloramphenicol	Increased rate of chloramphenicol metabolism through enzyme induction
Probenecid	Penicillins and cephalosporins (not cephaloridine)	Prolonged antibiotic T½ because renal tubular secretion reduced
Oral contraceptive steroids	Rifampin	Increased rate of metabolism of the steroid (intermenstrual bleeding, pregnancy)
Oral contraceptive steroids	Broad-spectrum antibiotics	Failure of oral contraception, possibly due to depletion of gut flora (β-glucuronidase activity) interrupting enterohepatic cycle of steroid

spectively, to an antibiotic (*e.g.*, penicillin) that must be used or as an adjunct agent in treating tubercular meningitis (*see* Chap. 60). Glucocorticosteroid therapy is mandatory in the Waterhouse–Friderichsen syndrome, and additional glucocorticosteroids are mandatory in patients on long-term steroid therapy who develop infections. Except for isoniazid (*see* Chap. 65), prophylactic antibiotics need not be given to patients on long-term glucocorticosteroid therapy.

CONDITIONS OF THE HOST THAT MODIFY THE RESPONSE TO ANTIMICROBIAL DRUGS

Although the causative organism and the site of infection largely determine the antibiotic to be used, consideration of host factors is also important (*see* Chap. 11). Significant interactions may develop between antibiotics and other drugs or dietary constituents (Table 56-4).

Rupert Waterhouse, 1873–1958. English physician. In 1911 described malignant form of meningococcal meningitis with bilateral adrenal hemorrhage known as Waterhouse–Friderichsen syndrome. Also described in 1918 by Carl Friderichsen, a Copenhagen physician.

FAILURE OF ANTIBACTERIAL THERAPY

Some important reasons for difficulty with, and the clinical failure of, antimicrobial therapy are listed in Table 56-5. Antimicrobial drugs may mask abscess formation by reducing the spread of microorganisms. Abscesses are never cured by antibiotics and must be drained. Drainage reduces the number of bacteria, increases antibiotic penetration, removes drug antagonists, and may reduce the development of bacterial resistance.

ADVERSE DRUG EFFECTS

No antibacterial drug is totally devoid of toxicity, and specific adverse effects are described in the following chapters. Suprainfection and hy-

TABLE 56-5. Some Reasons for Difficulty with and Failure of Antimicrobial Drug Therapy

I. Incorrect clinical diagnosis or procedures
- Failure to recognize mixed infections
- Treatment of "fever" or an undiagnosed condition, or valueless prophylaxis
- Treatment of untreatable infections (*e.g.*, measles, mumps, upper respiratory tract viral disease)
- Inappropriate antibiotic selection (*e.g.*, ampicillin for staphylococcal disease)
- Complete reliance on culture and sensitivity reports
- Improper dose (too large, too small), duration (too long, too short), or route of antibiotic administration
- Concomitant administration of other drugs or foods that interfere with antibacterial drugs (*see* Table 56-4)
- Failure to control urinary *p*H (*e.g.*, aminoglycosides are more active at an acid *p*H)
- Inappropriate combination of bacteriostatic and bactericidal drugs

II. Incorrect bacteriologic diagnosis
- Badly collected, stored, or transported specimens
- Failure to recognize mixed infections (frequently anaerobic bacteria are missed)
- Incorrect determination of sensitivity
- Identification of "wrong" organism in mixed cultures (*e.g.*, sputum)
- Organism tested at incorrect *p*H (pertains particularly to organisms causing urinary tract infections)
- Transfer of (contaminated by) R factors

III. Bacterial factors
- Development of bacterial resistance
- Organism present in host in altered metabolic state (*e.g.*, protoplasts, spheroplasts, L-forms)
- Development of bacterial persisters (development of forms other than L-forms)

IV. Host factors
- Failure of host defense mechanisms because of debility (malnutrition), disease (*e.g.*, agammaglobulinemia, lymphoma), drugs (*e.g.*, anticancer agents, corticosteroids), or radiation therapy (*see* Table 56-1)
- Inaccessibility of infection to drug (*e.g.*, in meninges, bone, or skin or in the urinary tract in patients with renal insufficiency)
- Abscess formation. Failure to perform surgical drainage or débridement
- Incurability of infection owing to presence of foreign body, kidney stone, sequestrum, prosthetic device, malignancy, congenital anomaly, bronchiectasis, abnormal mucus (cystic fibrosis)
- Presence of inadequately controlled or undiagnosed systemic disease such as diabetes mellitus, sarcoidosis, hypoparathyroidism
- Presence of pus ("neutralization" of sulfonamides)
- Inactivation of antibiotic by nonpathogenic host flora (*e.g.*, penicillinase production)
- Presence of nonantibacterial drugs that possess antibacterial activity and that contaminate collection of pus, for instance, for *in vitro* study (*e.g.*, by damaging the cytoplasmic membrane, lidocaine and procaine and preservatives in normal saline may be bactericidal)
- Patient noncompliance

V. Drug effects
- Drug overdosage (*e.g.*, failure to decrease the dose in renal or hepatic disease) or underdosage
- Drug removed by hemodialysis or peritoneal dialysis
- Development of suprainfections
- Development of some drug reaction
- Problems associated with generic inequivalency

persensitivity, common reactions to many antibiotics, are mentioned briefly here.

Suprainfection

Suprainfection (superinfection; replacement infection) is the appearance of both microbiologic and clinical evidence of a new infection with pathogenic microorganisms or fungi (either a new strain or a new species) during antimicrobial treatment of a primary disease. It occurs in about 5% of patients and is more common following broad-spectrum antibiotic therapy or when host resistance is impaired. Not all suprainfections are the result of antibiotic use. Other important factors are conditions that alter anatomical barriers (catheterization, intubation, instrumentation), allowing entry and colonization (Table 56-1).

More than 300 different species of organisms normally inhabit the body. They are varyingly depressed on exposure to antibacterial drugs, broad-spectrum antibiotics producing a greater depression because of their wider range of antimicrobial activity. With depression of the normal nonpathogenic bacterial flora, drug-resistant noncommensal or commensal pathogenic organisms or fungi (usually *Candida albicans*) can more easily initiate suprainfection, especially in the gastrointestinal and genital tracts. Pseudomembranous (clindamycin-associated, antibiotic-associated) colitis is an important example (*see* Chap. 63). Symptoms of gastrointestinal suprainfection usually include oral burning, xerostomia, stomatitis, glossitis, cheilosis, black hairy tongue, diarrhea, signs of intestinal infection (enteritis, colitis), and pruritus ani. Infection transmitted from one patient to another patient or from a doctor or a nurse is called *cross-infection*. *Nos-*

TABLE 56-6. Principal Opportunistic Pathogens and Their Treatment

Organism	Drug	Status on Availability
Bacteria		
Bacteriodes spp.	Clindamycin Chloramphenicol (*see* Table 58-1)	
Listeria monocytogenes†	*See* Table 58-1	
M. tuberculosis†	*See* Table 58-1	
Pseudomonas aeruginosa	Carbenicillin, gentamicin	
Serratia marcessens	Carbenicillin, gentamicin	
Viruses (DNA)		
Cytomegalovirus	Cytarabine	Drugs classified as experimental for treating these viruses, but of doubtful value
Herpes simplex	Idoxuridine	
Varicella-zoster	Zoster immune globulin	Available only at specific authorized centers
Fungi		
Asperigillus fumigatus	Amphotericin B	
Candida albicans	Amphotericin B	
Cryptococcus neoformans	5-flucytosine	5-Flucytosine classified as experimental for treating these infections. Most effective in *C. albicans* infection of the urinary tract. Available only at specific authorized centers
Mucor	Amphotericin B	
Protozoa		
Pneumocystis carinii	Pentamidine isethionate	Available only from Parasitic Disease Drug Service, National Center for Disease Control, Atlanta (Table 58-2)
	Sulfadiazine and pyrimethamine	Useful if pentamidine isethionate unavailable
	Cotrimoxazole	
Toxoplasma gondii (obligate intercellular pathogen)	Sulfadiazine and pyrimethamine Cotrimoxazole	
Other		
*Nocardia asteroides**	Sulfonamides, ampicillin	

* Intracellular pathogen.
† *See* also Table 58-2.

ocomial infections refer to cross-infections acquired in a hospital environment.

Patient's with impaired cellular immune and phagocytic defense mechanisms due to disease or drugs (the compromised host) may suffer a specific type of suprainfection, *opportunistic infection*. This refers to diseases produced by ubiquitous parasites (Table 56-6) which in normal persons either live symbiotically or produce minimal illness, and which are controlled by cellular immune and phagocytic systems rather than by immunoglobulins. *Opportunistic pathogens are not in themselves rare, but their pathogenicity in compromised hosts takes a form far different from, and far more serious than, that usually encountered.*

Hypersensitivity

Hypersensitivity reactions may develop to most antibacterial drugs, particularly in atopic persons and in those who have had allergic drug reactions (*see* Chap. 11). Generally, allergy to an antibacterial drug precludes its future use or the use of related drugs. Patients who develop a sulfonamide allergy should not, for example, be exposed to any sulfonamide or to the chemically related drugs, the sulfones, acetazolamide, sulfonylurea compounds, dapsone, or thiazide diuretics. Penicillin allergy is discussed in Chapter 59.

FURTHER READING

1. Craig WA, Welling PG: Protein binding of antimicrobials: Clinical pharmacokinetics and therapeutic implications. Clin Pharmacokinet 2:252–268, 1977
2. Davies J: General mechanisms of antimicrobial resistance. Rev Infect Dis 1:23–29, 1979
3. Hewitt WL, McHenry MC: Blood level determinations of antimicrobial drugs. Med Clin North Am 62:1119–1140, 1978
4. Jacoby I, Mandell LA, Weinstein L: The chemo-

prophylaxis of infection. Med Clin North Am 62:1083–1098, 1978
5. Matthew M: Plasmid-mediated β-lactamase of gram-negative bacteria: Properties and distribution. J Antimicrob Chemother 5:349–358, 1979
6. Stiehm ER, Fulginiti VA: Immunologic Disorders in Infants and Children. Philadelphia, WB Saunders, 1980
7. Von Graevenitz A: The role of opportunistic bacteria in human disease. Ann Rev Microbiol 31:447–471, 1977
8. Watanabe T: The origin of R factors. Ann NY Acad Sci 182:126–140, 1971

CHAPTER 56 QUESTIONS

(*See* P. 7 for Full Instructions)

Select the One Best Answer

1. The simultaneous administration of two antibiotics (not in fixed dosage combination) is indicated in each of the following situations EXCEPT
   A. treatment of tuberculosis.
   B. treatment of mixed bacterial infections where the organisms may not share antimicrobial sensitivities.
   C. treatment of gram-negative bacteremic shock.
   D. in the presence of cross-resistance between the two drugs.
   E. to treat severe infections before obtaining the results of a culture and sensitivity report.

2. Each of the following are common suprainfecting organisms EXCEPT
   A. *Staphylococcus aureus.*
   B. *Pseudomonas aeruginosa.*
   C. *Candida albicans.*
   D. *Escherichia coli.*
   E. *Clostridium difficile.*

3. Patients with allergy to sulfonamides should not receive any of the following drugs EXCEPT
   A. nalidixic acid.
   B. diaminodiphenylsulfone.
   C. thiazide diuretics.
   D. acetazolamide.
   E. sulfonylureas.

A = 1,2,3; B = 1,3; C = 2,4; D = 4; E = All

4. The simultaneous use of two or more sulfonamides is associated with each of the following EXCEPT
   1. greater antimicrobial potency.
   2. reduced incidence of drug allergy.
   3. reduced incidence of crystalluria.
   4. reduced drug cost.

5. Important factors predisposing to local infections are
   1. loss of epithelium, as in severe burns.
   2. an indwelling urinary catheter.
   3. neutropenia.
   4. diabetes mellitus.

6. Important factors governing the development of bacterial resistance to erythromycin are
   1. reduced antibiotic uptake by bacteria.
   2. R-factor mediation of destructive enzyme synthesis.
   3. development by the bacteria of an alternate energy source.
   4. failure of antibiotic binding to ribosomal subunits.

7. Principal opportunistic pathogens are
   1. *Bacteroides spp.*
   2. *Serratia marcescens.*
   3. *Pneumocystis carinii.*
   4. *S. aureus.*

8. Measurement of blood antibiotic levels is of value in
   1. evaluating nonresponding infections.
   2. monitoring antibacterial treatment in patients with renal disease.
   3. those patients suspected of having drug toxicity.
   4. routine evaluation of suprainfections.

A. Bactericidal antibiotic
B. Bacteriostatic antibiotic
C. Both
D. Neither

9. is (are) most effective against growing organisms.

10. usually eradicate(s) a sensitive organism even if host defense mechanisms are not intact.

11. is (are) never associated with suprainfection.

12. commonly produce(s) bacterial dependence.

A. Broad-spectrum antibiotic
B. Narrow-spectrum antibiotic
C. Both
D. Neither

13. is (are) likely to result in suprainfection.

14. is (are) commonly "abused" by physicians through being prescribed without full categorization of infecting organisms.

15. commonly potentiate(s) coumarin anticoagulants.

16. has (have) a clinical usefulness that usually parallels *in vitro* spectrum.

JEREMY H. THOMPSON

57 Mode of Action of Antibiotic Agents

Antibiotics exhibit selective toxicity because host and bacterial cells differ structurally and functionally in many ways. They act directly on microorganisms and do not increase host defense mechanisms. Occasionally the opposite is true, as in β-hemolytic streptococcal infections when large doses of penicillin given early, by killing off all the bacteria, prevent adequate antibody production. Drugs that can bolster host defense mechanisms, such as levamisole (Tramisol), a veterinary anthelmintic, may be developed in the future.

Antimicrobial drugs can be classified on the basis of their general mode of action (Fig. 57-1). Many of them, particularly those that inhibit protein and nucleic acid synthesis, have more than one biochemical site of action so that secondary effects often confuse the picture. Further, drugs given in combination may possess different patterns of action than when given individually—for example, erythromycin plus chloramphenicol.

Little is known about the importance for antibiotic action of local conditions (*p*H, ionic and chemical environment) at the site of infection *in vivo*. Aminoglycosides, for example, are less active but metronidazole is more active in an anaerobic environment.

INHIBITORS OF BACTERIAL CELL WALL FORMATION

The unique, rigid bacterial cell wall, a 100- to 200-Å thick coat external to the cytoplasmic membrane (bacterial cell membrane: cell envelope), represents a logical target for therapeutic attack. The wall serves primarily to maintain the organism's characteristic shape and to prevent cell rupture, since bacteria sustain a high internal osmotic pressure—about 5 and 20 atm, for gram-negative and gram-positive bacteria, respectively. During cell division and growth, enzymes (peptidoglycan hydrolases: murein hydrolases) must break open strategic peptide links in the wall to allow interpolation of new building units. If wall synthesis is blocked by antibiotics (Fig. 57-1), the bacterium grows with gaps in its coat through which the cell membrane extrudes (owing to osmotic imbibement of water), forming a protoplast (spheroplast) that eventually lyses (bacte-

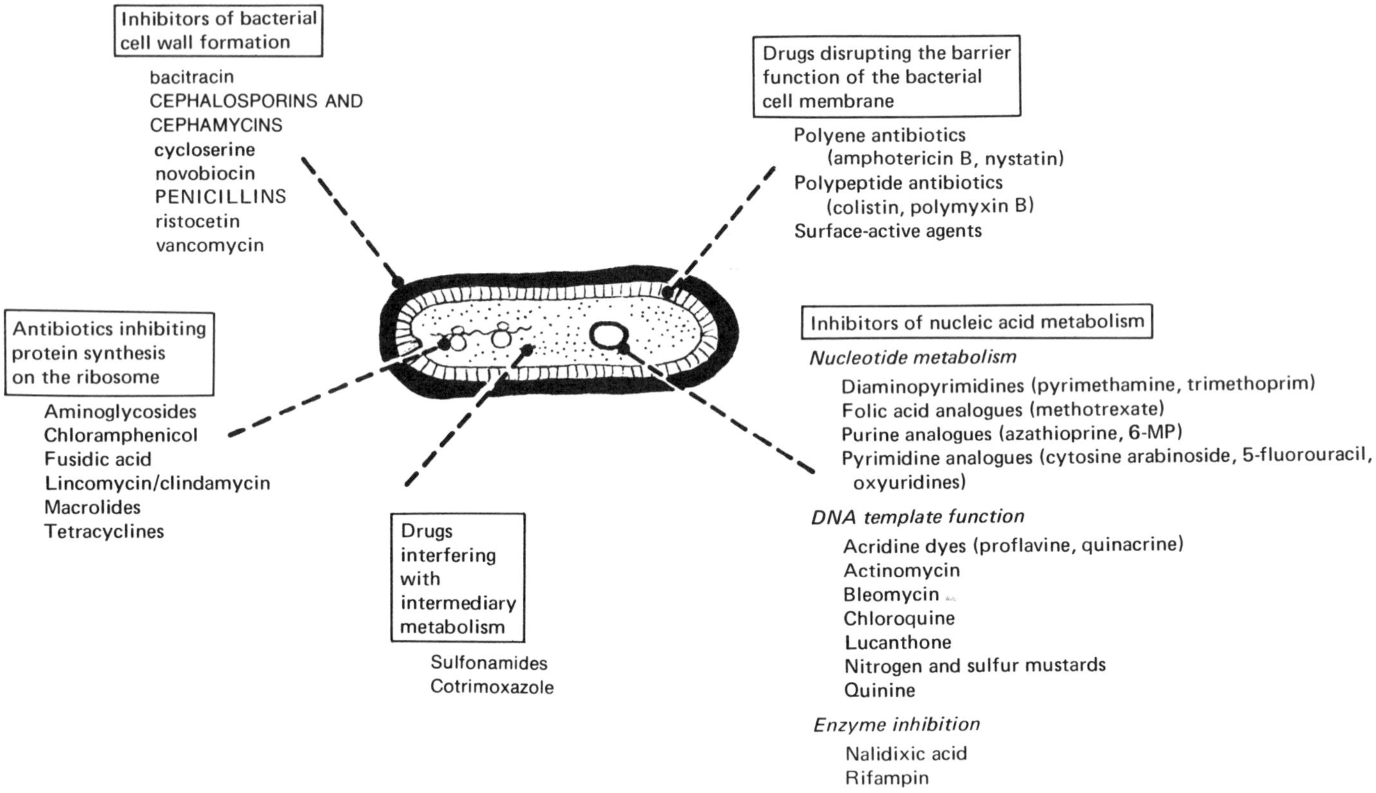
Inhibitors of bacterial cell wall formation
bacitracin
CEPHALOSPORINS AND CEPHAMYCINS
cycloserine
novobiocin
PENICILLINS
ristocetin
vancomycin
Drugs disrupting the barrier function of the bacterial cell membrane
Polyene antibiotics (amphotericin B, nystatin)
Polypeptide antibiotics (colistin, polymyxin B)
Surface-active agents
Antibiotics inhibiting protein synthesis on the ribosome
Aminoglycosides
Chloramphenicol
Fusidic acid
Lincomycin/clindamycin
Macrolides
Tetracyclines
Inhibitors of nucleic acid metabolism
Nucleotide metabolism
Diaminopyrimidines (pyrimethamine, trimethoprim)
Folic acid analogues (methotrexate)
Purine analogues (azathioprine, 6-MP)
Pyrimidine analogues (cytosine arabinoside, 5-fluorouracil, oxyuridines)
DNA template function
Acridine dyes (proflavine, quinacrine)
Actinomycin
Bleomycin
Chloroquine
Lucanthone
Nitrogen and sulfur mustards
Quinine
Enzyme inhibition
Nalidixic acid
Rifampin
Drugs interfering with intermediary metabolism
Sulfonamides
Cotrimoxazole

FIG. 57-1. Mode of action of some antimicrobial and anticancer drugs.

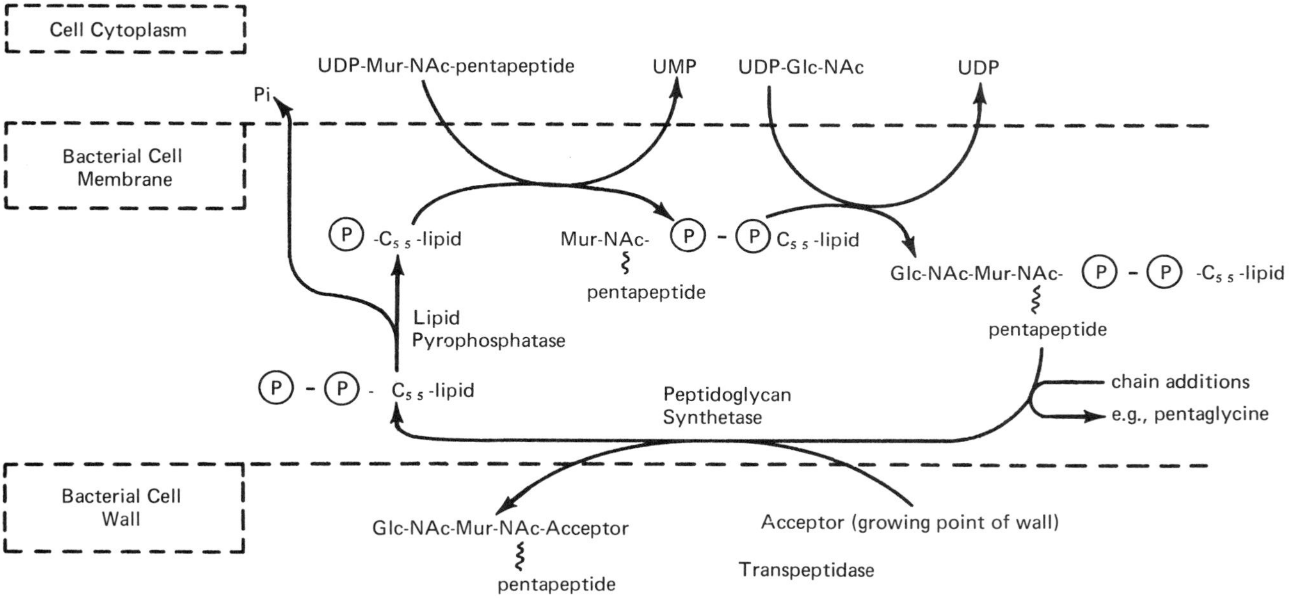

FIG. 57-2. Transport of peptidoglycan subunits in *Staphylococcus aureus.* The precise location of the enzymes within the membrane is not known.

ricidal effect). To facilitate an understanding of the mode of action of antibiotics that prevent cell wall formation, the structure and biosynthesis of cell wall peptidoglycans (mucopeptide: murein) in *Staph. aureus* and *E. coli* are noted briefly. Much of our information derives from the work of Strominger and associates.

INTRACELLULAR BIOSYNTHESIS OF SUBUNITS

Peptidoglycan subunits are oligosaccharide chains of two alternating amino sugars: *N*-acetylglucosamine (Glu-NAc); and its 3-O-*D*-lactic acid derivative, *N*-acetylmuramic acid (Mur-NAc) linked β-1,4 (Fig. 57-2). Attached to carboxyl groups of the lactic acid side-chain of the Mur-NAc moiety is a species-dependent pentapeptide chain, which in *Staph. aureus* is *L*-ala-*D*-glu-*L*-lys-*D*-ala-*D*-ala.

TRANSPORT OF SUBUNITS

The highly polar nonnucleotide portions of the peptidoglycans are transported across the cell membrane by a lipid soluble carrier (C_{55} isoprenoid alcohol pyrophosphate) (Fig. 57-2). During translocation, modifications to the pentapeptide moiety may be made, as in *Staph. aureus,* where a pentaglycine chain is added to the R_3 amino acid *L*-lys. This precursor is frequently named a "Park nucleotide." Finally, under the influence of peptidoglycan synthetase, the subunit transfers to an acceptor that *in vivo* is the growing point of a backbone glycan chain, releasing the carrier that is dephosphorylated by lipid pyrophosphatase to complete the cycle.

ASSEMBLY OF SUBUNITS

After translocation, three-dimensional cross-linkages occur between polypeptide chains of adjacent peptidoglycans, imparting stability to the wall. The pentapeptide of nascent peptidoglycans binds to a membrane-bound transpeptidase, forming an acyl-enzyme intermediate. The enzyme cleaves the terminal *D*-ala-*D*-ala bond, conserves the bond energy, and uses it to form a new bond between the carboxyl group of the penultimate *D*-ala and the free amino group of either the diamino acid or the penta-

---

JACK LEONARD STROMINGER, 1925– . American physican and microbiologist. His special interests are in antibiotic mechanisms and chemotherapy. Has worked extensively on understanding bacterial cell wall synthesis and the mode of actions of penicillins.

JAMES THEODORE PARK, 1922– . American microbiologist. Has worked particularly on the biosynthesis of bacterial cell walls and the mechanism of action of penicillin.

glycine bridge in an adjacent peptidoglycan; the terminal *D*-ala is lost. In *E. coli*, the pentapeptide chains are joined together directly by means of peptide bonds, whereas in *Staph. aureus* cross-links are formed between the penultimate *D*-ala and an adjacent pentaglycine bridge. Some peptide substituents do not form cross-links and have their terminal *D*-ala cleaved by a carboxypeptidase. Thus, although a *pentapeptide* is formed initially in *Staph. aureus* as part of the basic subunit, a *tetrapeptide* is the structure finally incorporated into the bacterial cell wall. Cross-linkage imparts unity and rigidity so that the final product resembles a wire netting (chain-link) fence. By virtue of the multiple cross-linkages, the bacterial cell wall can become one molecule comprising up to 12 or more peptidoglycan layers with, in some instances, a molecular weight of greater than 10^{12}.

ANTIMICROBIAL DRUGS THAT INHIBIT BACTERIAL CELL WALL FORMATION

As the first, and probably still the most clinically important, antibiotic, penicillin G provided the impetus that led to exploration of the reactions involved in bacterial cell wall biosynthesis. However, the mechanisms whereby interference with bacterial cell wall synthesis leads to death of the organism, and its lysis, appear far more complex than originally thought. Initial models of the action of β-lactam antibiotics, for example, assumed that they all acted similarly, but such appears not to be the case.

PENICILLINS, CEPHALOSPORINS, AND CEPHAMYCINS

Early observations of the effects of penicillin G on sensitive bacteria demonstrated a primary effect on cell wall integrity. It was believed that penicillin could assume a configuration similar to the acyl D-ala-D-ala terminus of the nascent peptidoglycan. Thus penicillin probably linked covalently to the membrane transpeptidase, producing an inactive peniciloylated enzyme that resulted in the accumulation of uncross-linked peptidoglycan chains, and the genesis of a "chain-linked fence" without the links; with an imperfect cell wall, bacteria would then rupture because of their high internal osmotic pressure.

This was, of course, an overly simplistic view. β-Lactam antibiotics certainly bind to membrane transpeptidase, but they bind also to several other bacterial proteins, for example, a total of four in *Staph. aureus*, five in *B. subtilis*, and seven to nine in *E. coli*. Some or part of these binding proteins are enzymes (such as the membrane transpeptidase) involved in multiple essential functions such as septation, maintenance of shape, and cell wall integrity. Thus current views hold that cell lysis is not primarily due to osmotic drive but results from the activation of autolysin (endogeneous peptidoglycan hydrolases: murein hydrolyses) as a direct result of β-lactam inactivation of membrane transpeptidase and other enzymes. How the activation of autolysin comes about is not clear, but presumably several mechanisms are involved, since bacterial species may respond (biochemically) quite differently on exposure to different β-lactam antibiotics. Additionally, structurally different β-lactam antibiotics may produce different morphological, biochemical, and antibacterial effects even within the same bacterial species. The penicillins may decrease the availability of an inhibitor of peptidoglycan hydrolase.

In vitro penicillin-sensitive microorganisms grown in the presence of penicillin in a hypertonic (sucrose or sodium chloride) medium form protoplasts, which do not lyse; reconversion to normal shape and development occur rapidly if the penicillin is washed out. This may be clinically important, since bacteria may survive as viable protoplasts during therapy in sites where the medium is hypertonic, as in abscesses, osteomyelitis cavities, or renal parenchyma. Thus antibiotic inhibition of cell wall synthesis is not itself lethal.

Bacterial persisters are cells that survive exposure to ostensibly lethal concentrations of bactericidal antibiotics, yet whose progeny remain fully sensitive to the agent; they occur about once per 10^6 cells. The occurrence of persisters may explain recurrence of infection after "effective" antimicrobial therapy. Thus if a small percentage of bacteria in a certain population have a peptidoglycan coat unbroken by peptidoglycan hydrolase, these cells cannot undergo growth and development until appropriate interpolation gaps are made. Penicillin and antibiotics that depress protein synthesis may inhibit hydrolase activity, thus selecting persisters.

CYCLOSERINE

By its similarity to *D*-ala (*see* Chap. 59), cycloserine competitively inhibits alanine racemase and *D*-alanyl: *D*-alanine synthetase, the enzymes required for the formation of the terminal *D*-ala-*D*-ala dipeptide of the peptidoglycan subunits. Since cycloserine acts through true competitive inhibition, its effect may be overcome by increasing the concentration of *D*-ala in the surrounding medium. Resistant mutants to cycloserine have been isolated that overcome inhibition through increased production of *D*-ala.

BACITRACIN, VANCOMYCIN, RISTOCETIN, AND NOVOBIOCIN

Bacitracin is a specific inhibitor of membrane lipid pyrophosphatase (Fig. 57-2), probably by complexing with the lipid pyrophosphate portion of the peptidoglycan. It therefore deprives the growing cell of a needed carrier and stops cell wall formation. Bacitracin also disrupts the bacterial cell membrane.

Vancomycin and *ristocetin* act similarly by inhibiting the action of the membrane polymerase, peptidoglycan synthetase (Fig. 57-2). They form stable 1:1 complexes with the moiety acyl-*D*-ala-*D*-ala, presumably blocking peptidoglycan synthetase activity by altering the substrate. *Novobiocin* has been studied infrequently, but *in vitro* peptidoglycan residues accumulate in the presence of the drug, and it may also chelate magnesium cofactors. The role of autolysins (*see* above) and other enzymes in the mode of action of these "lesser" cell wall inhibitors is not known.

ANTIBIOTICS THAT AFFECT THE BACTERIAL CELL MEMBRANE

The bacterial cell membrane (cytoplasmic membrane:cell envelope) is a semipermeable, triple-layered, lipoprotein structure located between the cytoplasm and the cell wall. It is a dynamic structure, constantly undergoing modification, particularly during repair, growth, and cell division, and possessing several vital functions. The bacterial cell membrane poses an *osmotic barrier* between the interior and the exterior of the cell; it contains *enzymes* needed for intermediary metabolism and cell wall formation and contains various "binding proteins" and lipids responsible for the *transportation of amino acids and sugars* into the cell, and for transporting cell wall subunits out of the cell. Antibiotics may *disorganize membrane function, inhibit specific enzymes* involved in transport or growth, or *alter ion permeability.*

DISORGANIZATION OF MEMBRANE FUNCTION

Drugs (surface active agents and polypeptide and polyene antibiotics) that disorganize membrane function are usually bactericidal. They possess well-defined, but distinctly separated, hydrophobic and hydrophilic moieties that bind to complimentary portions in the membrane. Binding results in interference with the membrane's semipermeable properties, and essential substances such as purines, pyrimidines, sugars, amino acids, and various ions are "leaked" (lost) from the cell.

Cationic surface active agents (*e.g.*, CTAB; *see* Chap. 66) possess a hydrophobic group such as a hydrocarbon chain or alkyl substituted benzene ring along with a positively charged hydrophilic moiety such as a quaternary ammonium group. The activity of such agents increases with increasing *p*H, and substances of opposite charge may negate the effect. *Anionic surface active agents* (*e.g.*, fatty acids, phenols) possess a hydrophobic group (as described above) in addition to a negatively charged hydrophilic group (carboxyl, sulfate, sulfonate, phosphate).

Polypeptide antibiotics (polymyxin B, colistin, tyrocidine) contain lipophilic and lipophobic groups and act like surface active agents. Sensitive bacteria bind and take up more antibiotic strains than resistant ones, and with polymyxin B there is a stoichiometric relation between the quantity of drug present and the number of cells killed. Polymyxin B appears to bind to phospholipids on the cell surface, and its activity can be reduced by soaps.

Polyene antibiotics contain a lactone ring (macrolides) that has a rigid hydrophobic polyene section and a flexible hydrophilic hydroxylated section. Polyenes complex with membrane sterols (primarily ergosterol), inducing breakdown of function; disorganization is proportional to the ratio of sterol:phospholipid rather than to the presence of sterol *per se*. Polyenes may also produce specific blockade of nutrient uptake; for example, nystatin blocks uptake of glycine at concentrations lower than those that cause leakage of cell contents.

INHIBITION OF SPECIFIC ENZYMES AND ALTERATION IN PERMEABILITY

Chlorhexidine, a potent inhibitor of bacterial cell membrane ATPase, inhibits growth, since ATPase is required for energy conversion and ion transport. Many other substances produce similar effects but are too toxic for human use. The *gramicidins,* along with several experimental antibiotics such as the *macrotetralideactins,* are cation conductors or "ionophores," comprising cyclic molecules with lipophilic side-chains oriented to the exterior of the molecule. Thus by complexing cations in the center of the molecule, they render them lipid soluble, enabling them to pass across membranes and be lost from the cell.

INTERFERENCE WITH PROTEIN SYNTHESIS

Antibiotics that affect protein synthesis inhibit ribosomal function. Little is known, however, about the molecular basis of their action, since the structure, functions, and interactions of ribosomes are still (often with the help of antibiotics) being elucidated. A brief review of protein synthesis (translation) will facilitate an appreciation of how important antibiotics may act (Fig. 57-3).

INITIATION

A 30S ribosomal subunit combines with mRNA and formylmethionyl-tRNA (f-met-tRNA), the latter at the A (amino acyl acceptor) site; a 50S subunit complexes to complete the 70S ribosome. The f-met-tRNA translocates to a second position, the P (peptidyl donor) site. Under some circumstances the f-met-tRNA may bind directly onto site P. At least three separate protein factors (F1, F2, and F3), not normally part of ribosomes are necessary for initiation.

ELONGATION

The amino acyl-tRNA called for by the first mRNA codon binds to site A. Binding depends on the formation of an amino acyl-tRNA-GTP complex with a "transfer factor" (TF1). The complex delivers the amino-acyl-tRNA to site A with release of TF 1-GTP and Pi. Each binding step requires the splitting of one of GTP's high-energy bonds. Then the f-met is transferred back to site A from site P under the influence of peptidyl transferase. Peptidyl transferase is a 50S ribosomal enzyme that catalyzes peptide bond formation between the nascent peptide on site P and the amino acyl-tRNA on site A. This reaction results in polypeptide chain lengthening at its carboxy terminus by one amino acid residue. After peptide bond formation, the f-met-amino acyl-tRNA translocates to site P, displacing the discharged methionyl-tRNA and freeing site A for the next codon-directed amino acyl-tRNA. Translocation after peptide bond formation requires the $G(S_2)$ factor, and GTP is hydrolyzed to GDP and Pi in the process. *The puromycin reaction* (release of peptide from site A) is often referred to in analyzing drug effects on protein synthesis. Puromycin, an experimental anticancer drug, acts as an analogue of amino acyl-tRNA. It binds to site A and takes part in peptide bond formation, accepting the nascent polypeptide chain from site P, but because puromycin binds only weakly to ribosomes the resultant peptidyl-puromycin moiety usually "falls off" the ribosome readily and can be measured.

TERMINATION

Release of completed protein occurs when all the codons have been read; peptidyl transferase may be involved in the release mechanism. On termination, the 30S and 50S subunits dissociate, joining a pool of free subunits before combining with new mRNA.

ANTIBIOTICS THAT AFFECT PROTEIN SYNTHESIS

Chloramphenicol binds to the 50S subunit (approximately one molecule is bound per ribosome), inhibiting peptide bond formation. It may also inhibit mRNA:30S ribosome attachment and binding of amino acyl-tRNA moieties. The antibiotic blocks the puromycin reaction, possibly by inhibiting peptidyl transferase activity. In some *in vitro* systems, chloramphenicol reduces the binding of erythromycin and the lincosamides, but the clinical significance of this response is not known.

Streptomycin and other aminoglycosides interact with site A on the 30S bacterial ribosomal subunit, causing chain elongation to cease by preventing adequate binding; additionally, they may prevent binding of amino acyl-tRNA to mRNA. Early studies suggested that the aminoglycosides caused misreading of the genetic code of the RNA template, but this is now considered artifactual. It is not clear why the aminoglycosides are bactericidal agents whereas other antibiotics that also cause inhibition of protein synthesis through binding to the 30S or 50S ribosomal subunits are only bacteriostatic.

Spectinomycin binds to the 30S subunit of

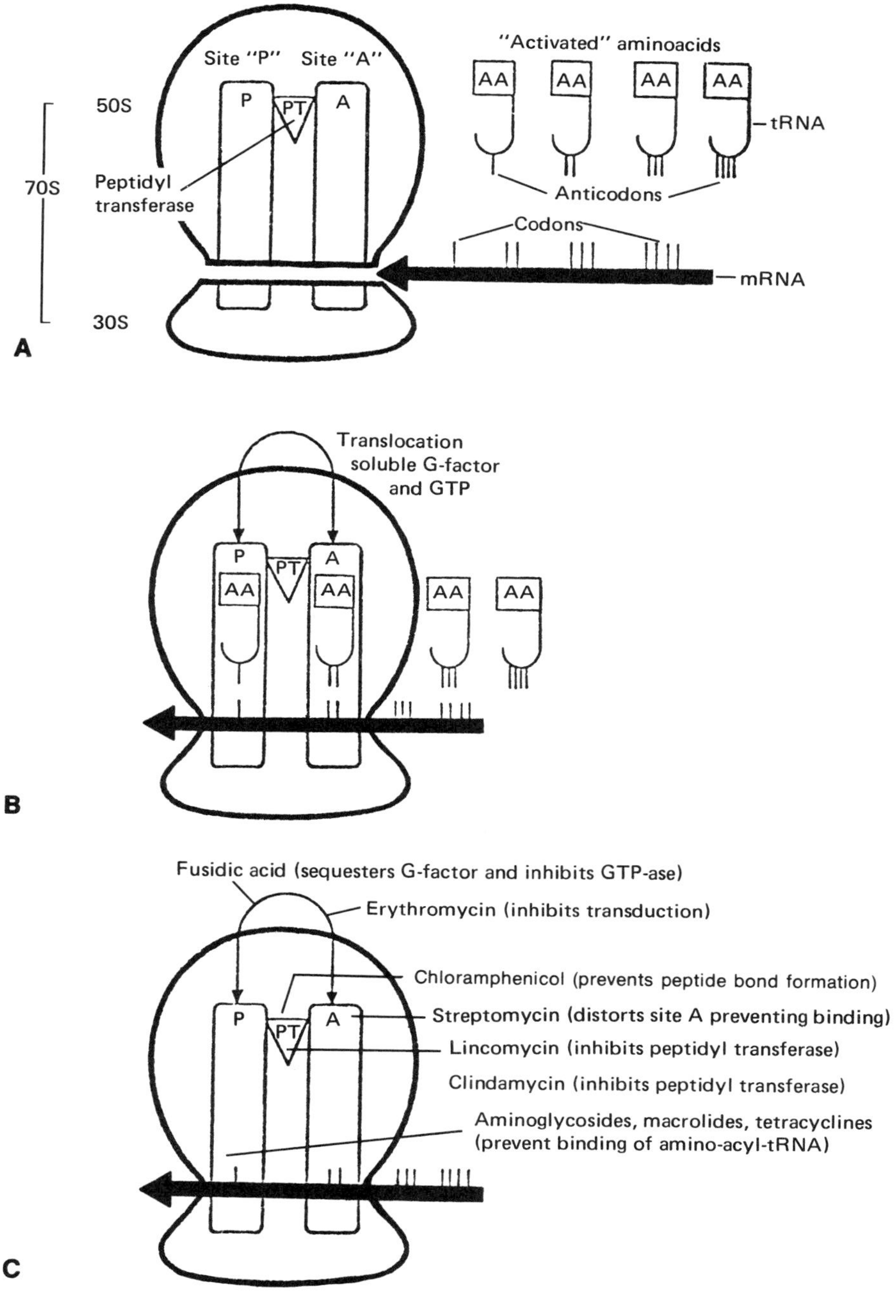

FIG. 57-3. Diagrammatic view of protein synthesis and mode of action of antibiotics interfering with protein synthesis. (*A*) Exploded diagrammatic view of the ribosomal components. (*B*) Diagrammatic view of an operational ribosome. (*C*) Antimicrobial drug targets.

the bacterial ribosome, terminating protein synthesis. It may act in similar fashion to the aminoglycosides; however, it is a bacteriostatic antibiotic only.

Erythromycin and related macrolides bind to the 50S subunit inhibiting translocation between sites A and P. Additionally, they may block amino acyl-tRNA binding to mRNA. *In vitro*, erythromycin prevents the attachment of chloramphenicol to the 50S subunit; the clinical importance of this interaction is unknown. *Lincomycin* and *clindamycin* bind exclusively to the 50S subunit of bacterial ribosomes, inhibiting peptidyl transferase activity and thus blocking protein synthesis. They may also prevent chloramphenicol binding.

The *tetracyclines* produce many effects, and it is impossible at present to separate primary from secondary sites of action. Two separate processes are involved in transporting tetracyclines into susceptible bacteria: passive diffusion through the outer bacterial cell membrane; and an energy-dependent active transport system at the inner cell membrane. Tetracyclines bind to the 30S ribosome and block the binding of amino acyl-tRNA to mRNA and to site A. In addition, because they are excellent *chelating agents* (*see* Chap. 61), they may bind necessary cofactors such as calcium, iron, or magnesium.

Fusidic acid sequesters G factor and depresses GTPase activity, thus interfering with translocation.

INHIBITORS OF NUCLEIC ACID METABOLISM

Several antimicrobial and anticancer drugs interfere with nucleic acid synthesis in three general areas (Fig. 57-1 and 57-4). For further details on anticancer drugs, *see* Chapter 71.

FIG. 57-4. Diagrammatic representation of the mode of action of drugs inhibiting nucleic acid metabolism.

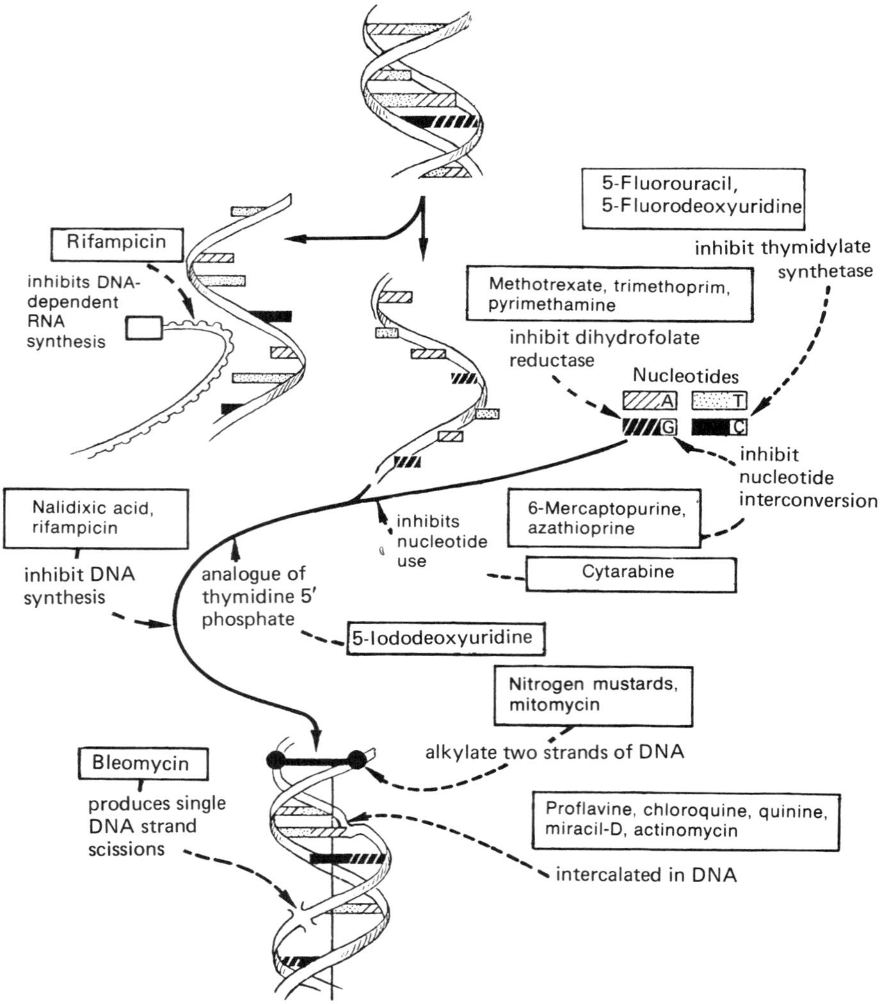

INHIBITION OF NUCLEOTIDE METABOLISM

Inhibition of *de Novo* Purine and Pyrimidine Synthesis

Drugs that inhibit dihydrofolate reductase, an enzyme needed for the synthesis of tetrahydrofolic acid, are of two classes: the anticancer folic acid analogues *methotrexate* and *aminopterin* (the "antifols"); and the antibacterial and antiprotozoal diaminopyrimines *trimethoprim* and *pyrimethamine,* respectively. Tetrahydrofolic acid is required as a donor of one carbon unit at several stages in purine, pyrimidine, and methionine synthesis and in the initiation of protein synthesis. Although the antifols inhibit dihydrofolate reductase from any source (mammalian or parasitic) *in vitro,* these agents possess no antibacterial or antiprotozoal properties *in vivo.* Conversely, the diaminopyrimidines possess no anticancer properties.

There is a ready explanation for this apparent paradox. Cells that require exogenous dihydrofolic acid (mammalian cells and most cancer cells) possess an active energy-requiring enzymic process for dihydrofolic acid uptake. The antifols, by virtue of their close structural similarity to the natural substrate, are readily taken up by the same system and inhibit dihydrofolate reductase intracellularly. The diaminopyrimidines, however, have no important inhibitory properties on mammalian dihydrofolate reductase because they penetrate poorly into mammalian and cancer cells and their affinity for the enzyme is low. Bacteria and protozoa do not possess the active energy-requiring process developed in mammalian cells for dihydrofolic acid uptake and must therefore synthesize their own *de novo;* thus antifols have no significant antimicrobial properties. Trimethoprim and pyrimethamine, however, readily penetrate parasitic cells, and because of their higher affinity for parasitic dihydrofolate reductase than for the mammalian enzyme, they exhibit selective toxicity.

Pyrimethamine is primarily of value in treating protozoal diseases such as malaria (*see* Chap. 67), since the affinity of this agent is far greater for protozoal than for bacterial dihydrofolate reductase. Conversely, trimethoprim possesses significant affinity for both bacterial and protozoal dihydrofolate reductase and thus is effective as an antibacterial (*see* Chap. 64) and as an antiprotozoal agent (*see* Chap. 67).

Inhibitors of Nucleotide Interconversion

6-Mercaptopurine (6-MP) and *azathioprine* (which converts *in vivo* to 6-MP by nonenzyme thiolysis) are metabolized to a nucleotide analogue 6-thioinnosinic acid (Thio-IMP) that inhibits purine metabolism at a number of sites. *5-Fluorouracil* and *5-fluorodeoxyuridine* are metabolized to 5-fluorodeoxy-UMP, which inhibits thymidylate synthetase (*see* Fig. 70-2), resulting in deprivation of thymine nucleotides and impairment of DNA synthesis.

Inhibition of Nucleotide Utilization

Cytarabine (*see* Chap. 70) inhibits nucleotide use, but its precise mode of action is not clear.

Analogues that Become Incorporated into Polynucleotides

Many naturally occurring and synthetic analogues of nucleic acid components possess the normal sugars ribose and 2′-deoxyribose attached to purine and pyrimidine bases. These agents can become phosphorylated intercellulary to the triphosphate level and serve as unnatural substrates for DNA and RNA polymerization reactions, distorting the structure and properties of nucleic acid. For example, *5-bromodeoxyuridine* (BDuR) and *5-iododeoxyuridine* (IDuR) replace thymidine 5′ phosphate in DNA (*see* Fig. 70-2), presumably leading to base-paring errors during replication and transcription of viral DNA, with resulting impairment of the fidelity of gene expression.

INHIBITION OF DNA TEMPLATE FUNCTION

Drugs may interfere nonspecifically with the role of DNA as a template in replication and transcription by reacting directly to form a complex or by reacting indirectly to cause structural alterations. Such interference inhibits DNA and RNA polymerase activity.

Drugs that Complex with DNA

Drugs can complex covalently, noncovalently, or through electrostatic binding (insertion–intercalation). For example, the *acridine dyes* (proflavine, quinacrine, neutral red), *chloroquine, quinine, lucanthone* (Miracil-D), and *actinomycin* intercalate between adjacent base pairs of the double helix.

Drugs that Cause Structural Alterations in DNA

Mitomycin C and the bifunctional *nitrogen* and *sulfur mustards* covalently bind as bifunctional alkylating agents to two sites of DNA (one on each strand), inhibiting its function as a template. Binding is accompanied by massive degradation of preexisting DNA but no alteration in RNA and protein synthesis. *Bleomy-*

cin causes formation of single-strand scissions (breaks) in the sugar phosphate backbone of DNA.

INHIBITORS OF ENZYMIC PROCESSES IN NUCLEIC ACID SYNTHESIS

Inhibitors of RNA Polymerase

Rifampin is the most potent inhibitor known for DNA-dependent RNA polymerase in bacteria; DNA-dependent polymerase from eukaryotic cells is however, not effected. Rifampin binds to RNA polymerase and blocks initiation of RNA synthesis. Rifampin-resistant bacteria produce DNA-dependent RNA polymerase, which does not bind the antibiotic.

Inhibitors of DNA Replication

Nalidixic acid inhibits DNA synthesis probably by interfering with specific enzymes. It is surprising that nalidixic acid possesses such activity, since it is a negatively charged compound and thus would not be expected to bind to the strongly negatively charged DNA.

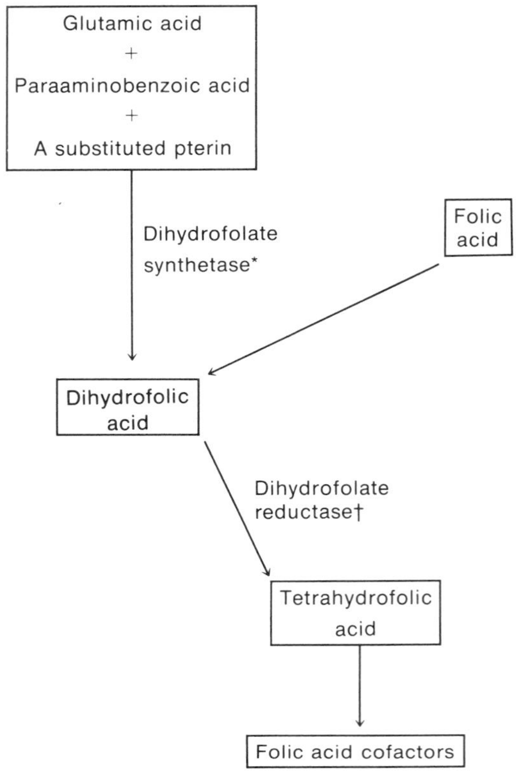

* Enzyme inhibited by sulfonamides.

† Enzyme inhibited by trimethoprim and pyrimethamine.

FIG. 57-5. Simplified scheme of synthesis of tetrahydrofolic acid, and the sites of action of sulfonamides, trimethoprim, and pyrimethamine.

DRUGS THAT INTERFERE WITH INTERMEDIARY METABOLISM

Numerous drugs interfere with microbial intermediary metabolism, but little is known of their precise mode of action; only the sulfonamides are considered here.

SULFONAMIDES

All bacteria require dihydrofolic acid for the synthesis of folic acid cofactors. Sulfonamide-sensitive bacteria cannot assimilate preformed dihydrofolic acid from the environment but must synthesize it *de novo* from precursors. Humans require preformed dihydrofolic acid, which is synthesized by dihydrofolate synthetase from glutamic acid, para-aminobenzoic acid, and a substituted pterin (*see* Fig. 57-5) to form a dihydropteroate, which subsequently combines with glutamic acid to form dihydrofolic acid (*see* Fig. 57-5). Because of the close structural similarity between sulfonamides (as typified in Fig. 57-6 by sulfanilamide) and para-aminobenzoic acid (PABA), the sulfas reduce the synthesis of dihydrofolic acid either by *inhibiting dihydrofolate synthetase* or by becoming incorporated by dihydrofolate synthetase into a *nonfunctional dihydropteroate* (dihydrofolic acid).

Although sulfonamides inhibit the synthesis of dihydrofolic acid in sensitive organisms immediately on exposure, there is a lag phase of several cell cycles during which growth continues normally. Presumably this growth depends on stored cofactors. *In vitro* studies have shown that one molecule of PABA can competitively antagonize the bacteriostatic activity of 5,000 to 25,000 molecules of sulfanilamide, and *in vivo* bacteriostasis induced by sulfonamides is reversed by PABA and PABA-containing drugs competitively.

A combination of a sulfonamide with trimethoprim or pyrimethamine (inhibitors of dihydrofolate reductase) results in a double sequential attack on folic acid metabolism (Fig. 57-5) (*see* Chap. 64).

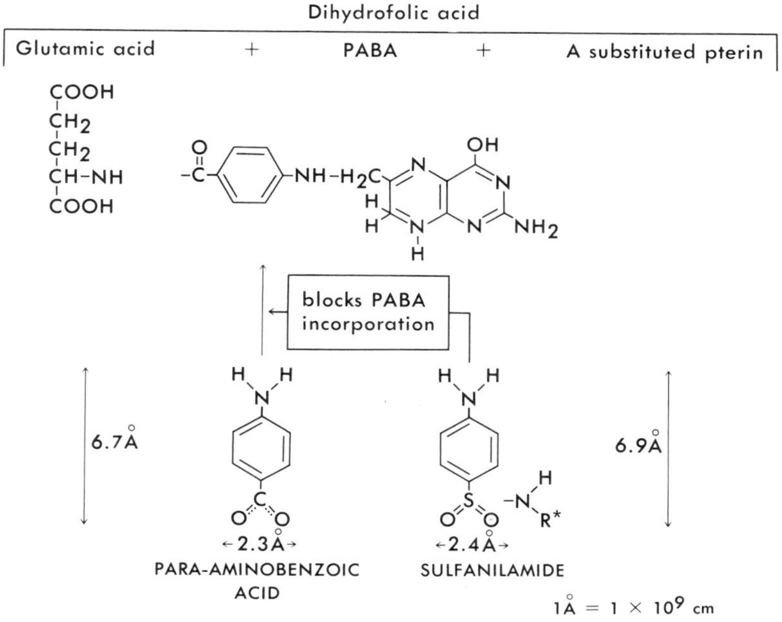

FIG. 57-6. The dimensions of para-aminobenzoic acid and sulfanilamide and the mode of action of the sulfa drugs. Asterisk indicates the R in sulfanilamide, the site of N^1 substitutions, which is out of the plane of the main drug molecule and therefore does not prevent attachment of the sulfa onto the appropriate receptor. (Part of this figure is from Albert A: Selective Toxicity p 103. New York, John Wiley & Sons, 1960)

FURTHER READING

1. Gale EF, Cundliffe E, Reynolds PE et al: The Molecular Basis of Antibiotic Action. New York, John Wiley & Sons, 1972
2. Hash JJ: Antibiotic mechanisms. Ann Rev Pharmacol 12:35–56, 1972
3. Tipper DJ: Mode of action of B-lactam antibiotics. Rev Infect Dis 1:39–54, 1979
4. Tomasz A: From penicillin-binding proteins to the lysis and death of bacteria: A 1979 view. Rev Infect Dis 1:434–467, 1979

CHAPTER 57 QUESTIONS

(*See* P. 7 for Full Instructions)

Select the One Best Answer

1. Interference with microbial cell wall synthesis is the mechanism of action of each of the following EXCEPT
   A. bacitracin.
   B. cycloserine.
   C. cephalothin.
   D. polymyxin B.
   E. vancomycin.

2. Penicillins
   A. are more active against growing organisms than resting organisms.
   B. are more active against resting organisms than growing organisms.
   C. inhibit protein synthesis.
   D. disrupt the bacterial cell membrane.
   E. are none of the above.

3. An agent that interferes with nucleic acid formation by binding to DNA and inhibiting RNA polymerase is
   A. penicillin G.
   B. erythromycin.
   C. actinomycin D.
   D. cycloserine.
   E. streptomycin.

4. Disorganization of microbial membrane function is the mechanism of action of each of the following EXCEPT
   A. gentamicin.
   B. colistin.
   C. nystatin.
   D. polymyxin B.
   E. benzalkonium chloride.

5. Sulfonamides act synergistically with trimethoprim because
   A. sulfonamides inhibit the metabolism of trimethoprim.
   B. trimethoprim inhibits the metabolism of sulfonamides.
   C. both drugs act at the same step in inhibiting folic acid synthesis.
   D. both drugs act at different steps in inhibiting folic acid synthesis.
   E. none of the above.

6. Nystatin acts by
   A. blocking cell wall synthesis.
   B. blocking synthesis of the cytoplasmic cell membrane.
   C. depressing protein synthesis.
   D. increasing the permeability of the cytoplasmic cell membrane.
   E. interfering with intermediary metabolism.

A = 1,2,3; B = 1,3; C = 2,4; D = 4; E = All

7. Which of the following competes with para-aminobenzoic acid (PABA) for incorporation into dihydrofolic acid?
   1. Diaminodiphenylsulfone
   2. Mafenide
   3. Para-aminosalicylic acid (PAS)
   4. Pyrimethamine
8. Antibiotic agents that act by interfering with protein synthesis include
   1. tetracycline hydrochloride.
   2. streptomycin hydrochloride.
   3. chloramphenicol.
   4. ampicillin.
9. A deficiency of tetrahydrofolic acid (folinic acid) in humans may be produced by therapy with
   1. sulfadiazine.
   2. diaminodiphenylsulfone.
   3. para-aminosalicylic acid (PAS).
   4. trimethoprim.
10. A drug that inhibits protein synthesis at the 30S ribosomal subunit is
   1. polymyxin B.
   2. chloramphenicol.
   3. vancomycin.
   4. lincomycin.
11. A drug that disrupts bacterial cell membrane function in sensitive organisms is
   1. polymyxin B.
   2. nystatin.
   3. amphotericin B.
   4. carbenicillin.
12. A drug that blocks protein synthesis in sensitive organisms is
   1. kanamycin.
   2. clindamycin.
   3. gentamicin.
   4. lincomycin.
13. An important consequence of penicillin action in sensitive organisms is
   1. depression of cell wall formation.
   2. depression of bacterial septation.
   3. osmotic-induced lysis.
   4. activation of peptidoglycan hydrolase.
14. Chloramphenicol
   1. inhibits peptide bond formation.
   2. increases lincomycin binding *in vitro*.
   3. binds primarily to the 50S ribosome.
   4. binds primarily to the 30S ribosome.
15. Streptomycin
   1. inhibits peptide bond formation.
   2. increases lincomycin binding *in vitro*.
   3. binds primarily to the 50S ribosome.
   4. binds primarily to the 30S ribosome.

JEREMY H. THOMPSON

58

Drugs of Choice for Common Infections

Chapters 56 through 70 describe the important antiparasitic agents and their properties. Since their classification and description bear little relation to current therapeutic use, a summary table (Table 58-1) is presented in an attempt to place each drug in the perspective of its clinical usefulness. *Table 58-1 should be used as a rough guide to therapy based on current opinions.* Further, with the introduction of new agents and the development of changes in bacterial sensitivity, recommendations (in a table such as this) must be continually revised. A drug of choice for any parasite implies that the agent will reach the site of infection in a high enough concentration to be effective. Practically, a drug of choice is either the most active agent against a given parasite or the least toxic alternative among several approximately equal chemicals.

Drugs of choice for the following groups of diseases are listed elsewhere: for tuberculosis, Tables 60-3 and 60-4; for protozoal disease, Table 67-1; and for mycotic infections, Tables 69-1, 69-2, and 69-3.

The recommendation of a drug or drugs of choice for any specific infection is frequently debatable, since for some infections the physician may have available several drugs of approximately equal value. For the rational treatment of infections caused by bacterial species with variable antibiotic sensitivity patterns—for example, *Klebsiella, Enterobacter, Bacteroides, Proteus spp., Escherichia coli, Staphylococcus aureus,* and *Pseudomonas aeruginosa*—antibiotic susceptibility tests are mandatory. Further, the selection of an antibiotic in other infections should also be based, if possible, on the results of a culture and sensitivity determination. Sensitivity patterns of many bacteria vary between communities, reflecting primarily the degree of use of specific antibiotics. A drug active in sensitivity testing may, nonetheless, be ineffective clinically if the wrong route of administration is used, the dose or absorption is inadequate, the antibiotic

(*Text continues on p. 575*)

THEODOR ALBRECHT EDWIN KLEBS, 1834–1913. German pathologist and bacteriologist. Introduced paraffin impregnation to microscopy in 1869. Was the first experimentally to infect cows with tuberculosis by feeding them infected milk (1873). Described the *Corynebacterium diphtheriae* in 1883, later isolated and proved to be the diphtheria-causing agent by F. Löffler.

TABLE 58-1. Drugs of Choice for Some Microbial Diseases (drugs are listed alphabetically)

Organism	Illness	Drugs of First Choice	Alternative Drugs[1]
Gram-positive Cocci			
Staphylococcus aureus[2]	Various tissue and wound infections, abscesses, bacteremia, endocarditis, pneumonia, meningitis, osteomyelitis	Nonpenicillinase producing: Penicillin G[3], penicillin V	A cephalosporin[4], clindamycin[4], vancomycin
		Penicillinase producing: A penicillinase-resistant penicillin[5]	A cephalosporin[4], clindamycin[4], vancomycin
		Resistant to penicillinase-resistant penicillins: Vancomycin ± rifampin[6] or gentamicin	Erythromycin + rifampin[6]
Streptococcus pyogenes[2] (A, C, G)	Various tissue and wound infections, including bacteremia, cellulitis, erysipelas, otitis media, pharyngitis, acute pneumonia, scarlet fever	Penicillin G[3], penicillin V	A cephalosporin, erythromycin, vancomycin
Streptococcus viridans[2]	Bacteremia, endocarditis	Penicillin G[3] ± streptomycin	A cephalosporin, vancomycin
Streptococcus bovis	Bacteremia, endocarditis[7]	Penicillin G[3]	A cephalosporin, vancomycin
Streptococcus faecalis[2] (Enterococcus)	Endocarditis[7] or other serious infection	Penicillin G[3] + streptomycin, or gentamicin	Vancomycin + streptomycin or gentamicin
Strep. faecalis[2]	Urinary tract infection (acute)	Amoxicillin	Ampicillin, nitrofurantoin, vancomycin
Streptococcus agalactiae (Group B)	Bacteremia, meningitis	Ampicillin or penicillin G[3] ± an aminoglycoside	A cephalosporin[4], chloramphenicol, erythromycin
Streptococcus[2] (anaerobic spp.)	Various tissue infections, including bacteremia, endocarditis, and localized abscesses	Penicillin G[8]	A cephalosporin[4], chloramphenicol, clindamycin[4], erythromycin, a tetracycline[9]
Streptococcus pneumoniae[2]	Various tissue infections, including arthritis, endocarditis, otitis media, pneumonia, meningitis	Penicillin G[3], penicillin V	A cephalosporin[4], chloramphenicol[10], clindamycin[4], erythromycin[2,11], vancomycin
Gram-negative Cocci			
Neisseria gonorrhoeae[12]	Infections of the genitalia: Nonpenicillinase producing	Penicillin G[3], or amoxicillin ± probenecid, a tetracycline[9]	Cefoxitin, erythromycin, spectinomycin
	Infections of the genitalia: Penicillinase producing	Spectinomycin	Cefoxitin, co-trimoxazole
	Arthritis–dermatitis syndrome	Amoxicillin, ampicillin, or penicillin G[3] ± probenecid	A tetracycline[9]
Neisseria meningitidis[13]	Bacteremia, meningitis	Penicillin G[3]	Chloramphenicol, a sulfonamide[2]
Gram-positive Bacilli			
Bacillus anthracis[2]	Anthrax	Penicillin G	A cephalosporin, chloramphenicol, erythromycin, a tetracycline[9]

(*continued*)

KARL FRIEDLÄNDER, 1847–1887. German physician. Described the pneumococcus of lobar pneumonia in 1882–1883 while working with C. H. J. Gram, who developed the Gram stain at this time.

TABLE 58-1. (*Continued*)

Organism	Illness	Drugs of First Choice	Alternative Drugs[1]
Clostridium perfringens (welchii)	Gas gangrene[14]	Penicillin G	A cephalosporin, chloramphenicol, clindamycin, a tetracycline[9]
Clostridium tetani	Tetanus[15]	Penicillin G	A cephalosporin, erythromycin, a tetracycline[9]
Corynebacterium diphtheriae	Diphtheria[16]	Penicillin G, erythromycin	A cephalosporin, rifampin
Corynebacterium spp. (diphtheroids)	Various tissue infections	Penicillin G ± an aminoglycoside or ± rifampin	Vancomycin
Erysipelothrix rhusiopathiae	Erysipeloid	Penicillin G	Chloramphenicol, erythromycin, a tetracycline[9]
Listeria monocytogenes	Various tissue infections, including bacteremia, endocarditis, meningitis	Amoxicillin, or penicillin G ± an aminoglycoside	Chloramphenicol, erythromycin, a tetracycline[9]
Gram-negative Bacilli			
Acinetobacter[2] (*Mima, Herellea*)	Various tissue infections, including bacteremia	An aminoglycoside (usually gentamicin)	Amikacin, cefoxitin, co-trimoxazole, a tetracycline (usually minocycline)
Bacteroides fragilis[2]	Various tissue and wound infections, including bacteremia, endocarditis, tissue abscesses	Chloramphenicol[17], clindamycin	Carbenicillin (or ticarcillin), cefoxitin[4], metronidazole[18], penicillin G, a tetracycline[9]
Bacteroides spp.[2]	Various tissue and wound infections, including otitis, sinusitis, oral disease	Penicillin G[3]	Chloramphenicol, clindamycin, erythromycin, a tetracycline
Bordetella pertussis	Whooping cough	Erythromycin	
Brucella abortus[2]	Brucellosis	A tetracycline[9] ± streptomycin	Chloramphenicol ± streptomycin, co-trimoxazole
Calymmatobacterium granulomatis	Granuloma inguinale	A tetracycline[9]	An aminoglycoside (usually streptomycin)
Campylobacter fetus[2] (*Vibrio fetus*)	Bacteremia	Chloramphenicol or an aminoglycoside (usually gentamicin)	A tetracycline[9]
	Enteritis	Erythromycin	A tetracycline[9]
Enterobacter aerogenes[2]	Various tissue infections, including those of the urinary tract	A cephalosporin (usually cephamandole), an aminoglycoside[19] (usually gentamicin)	Carbenicillin, chloramphenicol, ticarcillin, a tetracycline[9]
Escherichia coli[2]	Various infections, including bacteremia	Ampicillin, gentamicin	A cephalosporin, chloramphenicol
	Urinary tract infections (acute, uncomplicated)	A sulfonamide (usually sulfisoxazole), co-trimoxazole, nalidixic acid[20], nitrofurantoin[20]	
	Urinary tract infections (complicated)	Ampicillin, amoxicillin, carbenicillin[21], ticarcillin[21]	A cephalosporin, a tetracycline[9]

(*continued*)

WILLIAM HENRY WELCH, 1850–1934. Baltimore pathologist and bacteriologist. Often credited with founding modern medical education in America. Described *Clostridium welchii*, the agent of gas gangrene, in 1892, and during the same period discovered *Staphylococcus epidermidis albus* in wound infections.

FRIEDRICH AUGUST JOHANNES LÖFFLER, 1852–1915. German bacteriologist. Introduced the methylene blue stain for bacteria and a method for staining flagella. Discovered the causative agent of glanders in 1883 and completed Klebs' work on the Klebs–Löffler diphtheria bacillus in 1884. In 1897 showed that foot-and-mouth disease was caused by a filterable virus.

TABLE 58-1. (*Continued*)

Organism	Illness	Drugs of First Choice	Alternative Drugs[1]
Flavobacterium meningosepticum	Meningitis	Erythromycin	Rifampin
Francisella tularensis[2]	Tularemia	Streptomycin	Chloramphenicol, a tetracycline[9]
Haemophilus ducreyi[2]	Chancroid	A tetracycline[9]	A sulfonamide (usually a triple sulfonamide); streptomycin
Haemophilus influenzae[2]	Various tissue infections, including otitis media	Amoxicillin, ampicillin	A cephalosporin (usually cefaclor[4] or cephamandole[4]), co-trimoxazole, streptomycin, a sulfonamide, a tetracycline[9]
	Respiratory tract infections, including epiglottitis, meningitis	Ampicillin[22] ± chloramphenicol	Cephamandole[4]
Haemophilus vaginalis	Vaginal infection	Metronidazole	
Klebsiella pneumoniae[2]	Pneumonia	A cephalosporin[23] ± an aminoglycoside (usually gentamicin or tobramycin)	Amikacin, chloramphenicol, co-trimoxazole, kanamycin, a tetracycline[9]
	Urinary tract infections	A cephalosporin[23]	Chloramphenicol, co-trimoxazole, gentamicin, tobramycin
Legionella pneumophila	Legionnaires' disease	Erythromycin ± rifampin[24]	A tetracycline[9]
Leptotrichia buccalis	Various infections, including Vincent's angina	Penicillin G[3]	A cephalosporin, chloramphenicol, clindamycin, erythromycin, a tetracycline
Pasteurella multocida	Various tissue and wound infections, including bacteremia, meningitis	Penicillin G[3]	A cephalosporin[4], a tetracycline[9]
Proteus mirabilis[2]	Various tissue infections[25], particularly those in the urinary tract[26]	Ampicillin or amoxicillin ± an aminoglycoside (usually gentamicin or tobramycin), sulfisoxazole[26]	A cephalosporin, chloramphenicol, co-trimoxazole
Proteus spp.[2]	Various tissue infections	An aminoglycoside (usually gentamicin or tobramycin) ± carbenicillin or ticarcillin	Cefoxitin, chloramphenicol, co-trimoxazole, a tetracycline[9]
Providencia[2] (*Proteus inconstans*)	Various tissue infections	Amikacin	Carbenicillin, a cephalosporin[4] (usually cefamandole or cefoxitin), chloramphenicol, co-trimoxazole, gentamicin, ticarcillin, tobramycin

(*continued*)

JOHN ELMER WEEKS, 1853–1949. American ophthalmologist. In 1904 published his method for the insertion of artificial eyes, but is perhaps best known for his discovery of *Hemophilus influenzae*, the causative agent of "pink eye," acute contagious conjunctivitis.

TABLE 58-1. (*Continued*)

Organism	Illness	Drugs of First Choice	Alternative Drugs[1]
Pseudomonas aeruginosa[2]	Various wound and tissue infections, including bacteremia and respiratory tract infections	An aminoglycoside[27] (usually gentamicin or tobramycin) ± carbenicillin or ticarcillin	Amikacin + carbenicillin, or tobramycin
	Urinary tract infections	Carbenicillin or ticarcillin	An aminoglycoside (usually amikacin, gentamicin, or tobramycin), colistimethate, polymyxin B
Pseudomonas mallei	Glanders	An aminoglycoside (usually streptomycin) + a tetracycline[9]	Chloramphenicol + an aminoglycoside (usually streptomycin)
Pseudomonas pseudomallei	Melioidosis	A tetracycline ± chloramphenicol[28]	Co-trimoxazole
Salmonella typhi[2]	Typhoid fever	Chloramphenicol	Amoxicillin[29], ampicillin, co-trimoxazole
Salmonella spp.[2]	Gastroenteric infections[30]	Amoxicillin, ampicillin	Chloramphenicol, co-trimoxazole
Serratia marcessens[2]	Various nosocomial and opportunistic infections	Gentamicin ± carbenicillin or ticarcillin	Amikacin + carbenicillin or ticarcillin, cefoxitin[4], co-trimoxazole
Shigella spp.[2]	Gastroenteric infections[31]	Amoxicillin, ampicillin, chloramphenicol, Co-trimoxazole	A tetracycline[9]
Spirillum minor	Rat bite fever	Penicillin G[3]	Streptomycin, a tetracycline[9]
Streptobacillus moniliformis	Various wound and tissue infections, including bacteremia, endocarditis	Penicillin G[3]	Streptomycin, a tetracycline[9]
Vibrio cholerae	Cholera[32]	A tetracycline[9]	Chloramphenicol, co-trimoxazole
Yersinia pestis	Plague	Streptomycin ± a tetracycline[9]	Chloramphenicol, a tetracycline[9]
Spirochetes			
Borrelia recurrentis	Relapsing fever	A tetracycline[9]	Penicillin G[3]
Leptospira canicola	Similar to Weil's disease	Penicillin G[3]	Clindamycin, a tetracycline[9]
Leptospira icterohaemorrhagiae	Weil's disease	Penicillin G[3]	Clindamycin, a tetracycline[9]
Treponema pallidum	Syphilis	Penicillin G[3]	Erythromycin, a tetracycline[9]
Treponema pertenue	Yaws	Penicillin G[3]	A tetracycline[9]
Acid-fast Bacilli			
Mycobacterium leprae	Leprosy	Dapsone ± rifampin	Acedapsone[33], clofazimine, rifampin[34]. *See also Table 65–3*

(*continued*)

ALFRED WHITMORE, 1876–1946. British physician in the Indian Medical Service. Was the first to describe melioidosis in 1912. The causative agent was later shown to be *Pseudomonas pseudomallei*, originally named *Pfeifferella Whitmori*.

GERHARD HENRIK ARMAUER HANSEN, 1841–1912. Norwegian physician and bacteriologist. Director of the Leprosy Hospital in Bergen, he discovered Hansen's bacillus, *Mycobacterium leprae*, in 1869 and insisted, against opposition, that the disease was contagious. A. L. S. Neisser first accurately described the organism in 1879.

TABLE 58-1. (*Continued*)

Organism	Illness	Drugs of First Choice	Alternative Drugs[1]
Mycobacterium tuberculosis	Various tissue infections of tuberculosis	Isoniazid + ethambutol ± rifampin[34] Isoniazid ± rifampin[34] + streptomycin	*See* Table 65-2
Chlamydiae			
Chlamydia psittaci	Psittacosis, ornithosis	A tetracycline[9]	Chloramphenicol
Chlamydia trachomatis	Various infections, including trachoma[35], inclusion conjuctivitis[35], urethritis, pneumonia	A sulfonamide + a tetracycline[9]	Chloramphenicol[36], erythromycin, a sulfonamide, a tetracycline[9]
Lymphogranuloma venereum	Lymphogranuloma venereum	A tetracycline[9]	Chloramphenicol, erythromycin, a sulfonamide
Mycoplasma			
Mycoplasma pneumoniae (Eaton agent)	"Atypical" pneumonia	Erythromycin	A tetracycline[9]
Rickettsia			
Rickettsia spp.[2]	Various diseases, including Brill's disease, murine typhus, Q fever, rickettsial pox, Rocky Mountain spotted fever, typhus fever	Chloramphenicol, a tetracycline[9]	

MONROE DAVIS EATON, 1904– . American microbiologist. Especially interested in viral diseases, including viral pneumonia, and virally induced tumors, including murine leukemia.

NATHAN EDWIN BRILL, 1860–1925. New York physician. Was the first to describe Brill's disease, a form of typhus, in 1910. Is also eponymously remembered by Brill–Symmers disease, a giant follicular hyperplasia of the lymph nodes and spleen (1925).

"Q" fever was not named for Queensland, Australia, where it was first identified in 1935; rather the "Q" stands for "Query," because the causative agent was initially unidentified. The fever was described by E. H. Derrick in 1937, and in the same year F. M. Burnet and M. Freeman wrote on the viral causative agent *Coxiella burneti.*

[1] Drugs in this category are useful in patients hypersensitive to equally effective or more potent agents.
[2] Susceptibility tests must be performed because of the high probability of bacterial resistance.
[3] Oral therapy cannot be relied on for serious infections.
[4] Therapeutic levels are not reached in the cerebrospinal fluid.
[5] Cloxacillin or dicloxacillin is preferred for oral use. In severe infections nafcillin or oxacillin should be used parenterally. Methicillin can be used parenterally but is more toxic than oxacillin or nafcillin.
[6] Resistance develops rapidly (single-step mutation) to rifampin when used alone.
[7] Tube-dilution tests should be performed to assess bactericidal antibiotic levels required.
[8] Large doses of penicillin G parenterally are needed.
[9] Tetracycline hydrochloride is the preferred tetracycline.
[10] Recommended for CNS infections in penicillin-allergic patients.
[11] Preferred for respiratory infections in penicillin-allergic patients.
[12] Many strains are resistant to the penicillins and may also be resistant to tetracycline.
[13] A sulfonamide, orally, is recommended for prophylaxis in contacts of patients with sulfonamide-sensitive strains; rifampin or minocycline can be used in cases of sulfonamide resistance.
[14] Surgical débridement mandatory; hyperbaric O_2 may be a useful adjunct to very large doses of penicillin G.
[15] Tetanus toxoid and tetanus immune globulin (human) should be used in prophylaxis. Débridement is necessary.
[16] Antitoxin is mandatory. Antibiotics are used to limit toxin production and to treat the carrier state.
[17] Of particular importance in CNS infections.
[18] Possesses bactericidal activity against *B. fragilis.*
[19] Carbenicillin or ticarcillin can be added in serious infections.
[20] Can be used in prophylaxis or for suppressive therapy in recurrent infection.
[21] For very serious infection.
[22] Since ampicillin resistance is common, therapy for serious infections should combine this agent with chloramphenicol before the determination of bacterial sensitivity.
[23] Because of increasing cephalosporin resistance, it may be wise to add an aminoglycoside.
[24] Rifampin should be reserved for those who do not respond to erythromycin therapy alone.
[25] For systemic infections, doses of penicillin should be at least 6 g/day, and consideration should be given to adding an aminoglycoside. Carbenicillin or ticarcillin can replace ampicillin/amoxicillin in seriously ill patients.

TABLE 58-2. Non-FDA-Approved Drugs (distributed by Bureau of Epidemiology for Parasitic Disease)* for Specific Disease Entities

Chemical Name	Proprietary Name	Indication
Bayer 2502	Lampit	*Trypanosoma cruzi* infection (Chagas' disease)
Bithionol N.F.	Lorothidol	Paragonimiasis, fascioliasis
Dehydroemetine	—	Amebiasis, severe
Diloxanide furoate	Furamide	Amebiasis
Melarsoprol	Arsobal, Mel B	*Trypanosoma gambiense* and *T. rhodesiense* infections of the CNS (African sleeping sickness)
Niclosamide	Yomesan	Various helmintic infections
Niridazole	Ambilhar	Schistosomiasis
Pentamidine isethionate	Lomidine	*Pneumocystis carinii* pneumonia, *Trypanosoma gambiense* infection (sleeping sickness)
Sodium antimony dimercaptosuccinate	Astiban	Schistosomiasis
Sodium antimony gluconate	Pentostam	Leishmaniasis
Suramin (Bayer 205)	Antrypol	Early *Trypanosoma rhodesiense* infection, onchocerciasis

* Drugs obtained as Investigational New Drugs (IND) from the Parasitic Disease Division, Bureau of Epidemiology (404) 329-3670 (day), or (404) 329-3644 (night, holidays, and weekends).

William Boog Leishman, 1865–1926. British Army surgeon. Best remembered for his identification in 1903 of the trypanosome (*Leishmania donovani*) that causes kala-azar, visceral leishmaniasis. Was also the first to cultivate gonococcus successfully and, with Almroth Wright (Fleming's mentor), developed a typhoid vaccine in 1901.

cannot reach the site of infection, an abscess is not drained properly, or host resistance is poor. These and other factors have been summarized in Chapter 56.

The selection of an antimicrobial agent involves several factors: the type of organism causing the infection and its degree of sensitivity; the need for single or multiple agents; the site of infection; host determinants that may govern adverse reactions; and the pharmacokinetics of the antibiotic (and its breakdown products); and its toxicity, cost, and potential for drug interactions.

A number of drugs with proven therapeutic efficacy and safety are used widely outside the United States but are not available in this country through over-the-counter sales or through prescription. Because the demand for these drugs is small, no American pharmaceutical firm has sought FDA approval for these agents, but some are nonetheless available (Table 58-2).

FURTHER READING

1. The choice of antimicrobial drugs. Med Lett 22, No. 2:5–12, January 25, 1980

[26] For acute uncomplicated urinary tract infection, a soluble sulfa drug may be sufficient.
[27] Single-agent therapy with either an aminoglycoside or a penicillin should not be relied on for serious *Pseudomonas aeruginosa* infection, particularly in the compromised host.
[28] Chloramphenicol should be added to tetracycline in severe illness.
[29] Drug of choice for treating the carrier state.
[30] Mild infections do not require antibiotic therapy.
[31] Many strains are now both penicillin- and chloramphenicol-resistant.
[32] Fluid and electrolyte therapy is mandatory.
[33] Investigational drug in the United States.
[34] Rifampin should always be used in isoniazid resistance. It may be of particular value with isoniazid in cavitary pulmonary tuberculosis.
[35] For trachoma and inclusion conjuctivitis, oral plus topical sulfonamides and tetracyclines can be used.
[36] Topical application in inclusion conjuctivitis.

CHAPTER 58 QUESTIONS

(*See* P. 7 for Full Instructions)

Select the One Best Answer

1. A staphylococcal septicemia in a patient allergic to ampicillin and cephalothin and whose organisms are resistant to methacycline and erythromycin could be treated with
   A. carbenicillin.
   B. vancomycin.
   C. colistin.
   D. polymyxin B.
   E. cephaloridine.
2. Ampicillin is the preferred drug in infections due to each of the following susceptible microorganisms EXCEPT
   A. *H. influenzae.*
   B. *E. coli.*
   C. *Proteus mirabilis.*
   D. *Shigella* spp.
   E. *Streptococcus pyogenes.*
3. Which of the following antibiotics should be used to treat acute streptococcal pharyngitis in a child known to be allergic to penicillin?
   A. Carbenicillin
   B. Ampicillin
   C. Erythromycin
   D. Amoxicillin
   E. Vancomycin
4. In ampicillin-resistant meningitis (*H. influenzae*), a preferred substitute would be
   A. chloramphenicol.
   B. a tetracycline.
   C. erythromycin.
   D. carbenicillin.
   E. streptomycin.
5. The drug indicated for beginning therapy in *E. coli* sepsis if no other complications exist is
   A. trimethoprim.
   B. ampicillin.
   C. a tetracycline.
   D. chloroquine.
   E. chloramphenicol.

A = 1,2,3; B = 1,3; C = 2,4; D = 4; E = All

6. Penicillin G can be used effectively to treat
   1. pneumococcal pneumonia.
   2. streptococcal pharyngitis.
   3. gonorrhea.
   4. klebsiella pneumonia.
7. Drugs effective against *Pseudomonas aeruginosa* include
   1. carbenicillin.
   2. gentamicin.
   3. polymyxin B.
   4. kanamycin.
8. Chemotherapeutic agents effective in the treatment of *Mycobacterium leprae* infections include
   1. streptomycin.
   2. dapsone.
   3. aminosalicylic acid (PAS).
   4. rifampin.
9. Sulfonamides used solely as intestinal chemotherapeutic agents include
   1. sulfacetamide.
   2. phthalylsulfathiazole.
   3. sulfisoxazole.
   4. succinylsulfathiazole.

JEREMY H. THOMPSON

59

Antibiotics That Interfere with the Bacterial Cell Wall

Several antimicrobial agents interfere with the biosynthesis of bacterial cell walls, acting maximally during the logarithmic phase of growth and having little or no effect on nongrowing organisms. Of these, the most widely used are the *penicillins*, the *cephalosporins*, and the *cephamycin* cefoxitin; bacitracin, cycloserine, and vancomycin (Table 59-1) are of lesser importance.

THE PENICILLINS

HISTORY

At St. Mary's Hospital, London, in 1928, Alexander Fleming (later Sir Alexander Fleming) observed that a contaminating mold on a staphylococcal culture plate caused the adjacent bacterial colonies to undergo lysis. This mold (*Penicillium notatum*), grown in broth culture, was bactericidal *in vitro* against a variety of organisms; Fleming named the antibacterial principle *penicillin*. Desultory research continued on penicillin until 1939, when, under the stimulus of World War II, Howard Walter Florey (later Sir Howard Florey) and Ernst Boris Chain, at the Sir William Dunn School of Pathology, Oxford University, England, began intensive work on this problem. Crude penicillin G became available for limited therapeutic trials in 1941; supplies were at first so scanty that the antibiotic was recovered from patients' urine. In 1942 various

ALEXANDER FLEMING, 1881–1955. London physician and bacteriologist. In 1928 discovered the antibacterial action of penicillin, for which he received the Nobel Prize, with H. W. Florey and E. B. Chain, in 1945. Fleming also conducted extensive research on lysozyme, which he discovered in 1921.

HOWARD WALTER FLOREY, 1898–1968. Australian-born Oxford pathologist. With E. B. Chain made a systematic investigation of antibacterial natural substances, resulting in the rediscovery and production of penicillin (1938–1939), for which he shared the Nobel Prize in 1945.

ERNST BORIS CHAIN, 1906–   . German-born biochemist. With H. W. Florey prepared a very concentrated, active form of penicillin and shared in the Nobel Prize in 1945. Other fields of interest include bacterial fermentation technology and nervous tissue metabolism.

TABLE 59-1. Miscellaneous Bacterial Cell Wall Inhibitors

Drug	Source and Properties	Adverse Effects	Preparations, Dosage, and Usage
Bacitracin	Bacitracin is the generic name for a group of at least four separate bactericidal polypeptide antibiotics, originally isolated from *Bacillus subtilis* that contaminated a compound fracture in a young girl named Margaret Tracy (hence its name). About 80% of most commercial preparations are bacitracin A, a cyclic decapeptide with a molecular weight of about 1500 and containing a thiazolidine ring structure. Bacitracin has a gram-positive antibacterial spectrum resembling that of penicillin G and some activity against neisseriae, *H. influenzae, T. pallidum,* and clostridiae, but because of its nephrotoxic potential (tubular necrosis) bacitracin is used only topically, or rarely for a local effect in the bowel lumen, since it is poorly absorbed. Bacterial resistance is rare and develops slowly. Antibacterial cross-resistance has not been described.	Bacitracin is usually safe topically, but after oral administration suprainfections and gastrointestinal upsets may occur. Cutaneous hypersensitivity reactions may show cross-reactivity to kanamycin and neomycin.	Bacitracin, U.S.P. (Baciguent), is available in a wide range of topical preparations, usually in a concentration of 500 units/g; 1 unit is equivalent to the activity of 26 μg of the U.S.P. standard. Preparations for ophthalmic and dermatologic use usually contain, in addition, neomycin, polymyxin B, or tyrothricin; cutaneous hypersensitivity rarely results from continued topical use. The usual oral dose (rarely prescribed) is 20,000 to 30,000 units q 8 hr.
Cycloserine	A broad-spectrum, bactericidal antibiotic, produced by *Streptomyces orchidaceus.* Its use should ordinarily be restricted to the treatment of tuberculosis. Mycobacterial resistance develops slowly, but cross-resistance has not yet been described. Following oral administration, rapid and almost total absorption occurs, mainly from the stomach and upper small bowel. Cycloserine passes freely to most tissues and to the cerebrospinal fluid, and it is so diffusible that growth of bacilli inside macrophages may be inhibited. After conventional dosage, blood levels usually average 15 to 35 μg/ml. In prolonged therapy, plasma drug levels should be checked periodically because cumulation may occur. Cycloserine is partially degraded in	Adverse reactions are dose-dependent and are more likely with blood levels greater than 50 μg/ml. With doses of 1 g or more daily, they can be expected in more than 25% of patients, but this figure falls to about 2% to 5% with doses of 500 mg daily. Reactions may occur at any time but most commonly appear within the first 2 or 3 weeks of therapy. Headaches, tremors, hyperreflexia, dysarthria, petit or grand mal seizures (in 5–10%), vertigo, sleepiness or excitement, acute psychotic episodes (in 2–3%), and allergic dermatitis have been reported. Seizures and psychotic episodes are more likely in persons with a history of epilepsy and mood disturbances, such as depression or anxiety, and in those taking	Initial dosage of cycloserine (Oxamycin, Seromycin) should be low (250 mg daily); this should be increased over a 2-week period to 250 to 500 mg twice daily.

(continued)

TABLE 59-1. (Continued)

Drug	Source and Properties	Adverse Effects	Preparations, Dosage, and Usage
Cycloserine (continued)	the body, but 60% to 70% of an oral dose is excreted unchanged by glomerular filtration. Because the drug reaches high concentrations in the urine and is more effective at an acid *p*H, cycloserine is especially valuable in treating renal tuberculosis. Cycloserine inhibits the metabolism of phenytoin.	alcohol. Pyridoxine (100 mg daily), sedatives, tranquilizers, or anticonvulsants may be administered with cycloserine in an attempt to reduce the CNS symptoms.	
Vancomycin	A bactericidal antibiotic obtained from *Streptomyces orientalis*, vancomycin is primarily effective against gram-positive organisms; bacterial resistance is rare, and cross-resistance has not been described. Minimal absorption follows oral administration, and, because i.m. administration is painful, the antibiotic is usually given i.v. The distribution and metabolic fate of vancomycin are unknown, but therapeutically effective cerebrospinal fluid levels do not occur despite only 10% protein binding. Vancomycin is excreted by the kidney, 80% of an i.v. dose being cleared within 12 to 16 hours. Thus patients with poor renal function rapidly achieve seriously high serum drug levels with conventional therapy. It is not removed by hemodialysis.	A relatively dangerous drug: chills, fever, allergic skin rashes, thrombophlebitis, and anaphylactoid reactions occur, and suprainfections with gram-negative bacteria and fungi may appear. Vancomycin is highly nephrotoxic and cochleotoxic, and lesions may progress despite drug withdrawal if renal function is inadequate, impairing excretion. Vancomycin commonly produces sterile abcesses and thrombophlebitis on parenteral administration despite alteration of muscle sites and appropriate drug dilution, respectively.	Sterile vancomycin hydrochloride, U.S.P. (Vancocin), in doses of 1 g i.v., is given to adults q 12 hr. The usual dose for children is 10 mg/kg q 6 hr. Vancomycin should not be used indiscriminately but rather reserved for the treatment of seriously ill patients with gram-positive (particularly staphylococcal) infections resistant to less toxic antibiotics. It is widely used in hemodialysis patients to suppress staphylococcal shunt infections since it is not dialyzable. It is a valuable alternative to metronidazole (*see* Chap. 67) in the treatment of pseudomembranous colitis.

centers in the United States undertook mass production of penicillin, since facilities were not available in England owing to the pressures of World War II. By 1943, sufficient quantities of the antibiotic were being produced to serve the allied forces, and in 1944 the antibiotic became available for limited civilian use.

The biosynthesis of penicillins up to 1958–1959 depended on the growth of *Penicillium notatum* and *P. chrysogenum* in deep vat culture. It was fortuitously found that by adding various chemicals to this fermentation process a variety of new penicillins could be produced by the mold (*e.g.*, phenylacetic acid to induce penicillin G), and by international agreement these antibiotics were designated with letters of the alphabet: B, F, G, K, O, and so forth. However, the capacity of the molds to add new side-chains was limited, and of all the early penicillins only penicillin G has survived. Penicillin G (sodium penicillin G, sodium benzylpenicillinate, sodium benzylpenicillin) is the penicillin prototype, and on a weight basis, provided an organism is susceptible, it is still the most potent.

Unfortunately, penicillin G is acid labile and therefore variably destroyed following oral administration; is destroyed by bacterial β-lactamase (penicillinase); has a relatively narrow antibacterial spectrum; is excreted rapidly from the body; penetrates poorly into tissue compartments, for example, the cerebrospinal fluid; and is antigenic. When, in 1958, the basic penicillin nucleus, 6-aminopenicillanic acid (6-APA), was isolated, it became possible to produce a range of semisynthetic penicillins that collectively surmount some of the shortcomings of penicillin G. Although there are many differences among the various types of penicillin, a single and unified description of these drugs is presented here, followed by a description of the more important penicillins and their properties; the generic term penicillin is used throughout to include the natural, the synthetic, and the semisynthetic penicillins. New penicillins are continually being introduced, necessitating a full understanding of the properties of the older agents.

SOURCE

Commercial penicillin has been prepared from *P. notatum* and *P. chrysogenum*. Current production uses the 6-APA nucleus (obtained through the action of bacterial amidases [Fig. 59-1] on regular penicillin), with subsequent chemical manipulations. The 6-APA nucleus is also produced by *P. notatum* if no amino acids are available in deep vat culture, but the yield is small and the method complex and usually impractical. Total *in vitro* chemical synthesis of penicillin has been achieved, but the process has no commercial usefulness.

Natural penicillin is probably synthesized by fungi from residues of valine, cysteine, and L-aminoadipic acid.

CHEMISTRY

All penicillins possess (Figure 59-1) a sulfur-containing thiazolidine ring (1), fused to a β-lactam ring (2), upon which antibacterial activity depends, and a side-chain (R″) that determines the individual penicillin characteristics (*see* Table 59-5); the moiety R′ is the site of salt formation, typically sodium or potassium. Bacterial β-lactamases (penicillinases), acids such as gastric acid, dilute bases, and primary or secondary amines hydrolyze penicillin to penicilloic acid by breaking the β-lactam ring (3). Penicilloic acid has no antibacterial activity but is potentially allergenic.

Penicillin salts are stable for many months in powder form but rapidly decompose to penicilloic acid and other metabolites after reconstitution. Thus solutions must be freshly prepared to ensure adequate antibacterial therapy and to minimize the infusion of potentially allergenic compounds.

Penicillin G and other acid-labile penicillins are rapidly inactivated at an acid *p*H. Additionally, all penicillins are rapidly inactivated at an alkaline *p*H in the presence of carbohydrate by an unknown mechanism. Aqueous suspensions of procaine and benzathine penicillin G are stable for many months.

FIG. 59-1. Penicillin and various derivatives. (*1*) thiazolidine ring; (*2*) β-lactam ring; (*3*) site of cleavage of the β-lactam ring by acid and penicillinase; (*4*) site of cleavage by bacterial amidases. R′ = site of salt formation; R″ = site of side chain conferring individual penicillin characteristics.

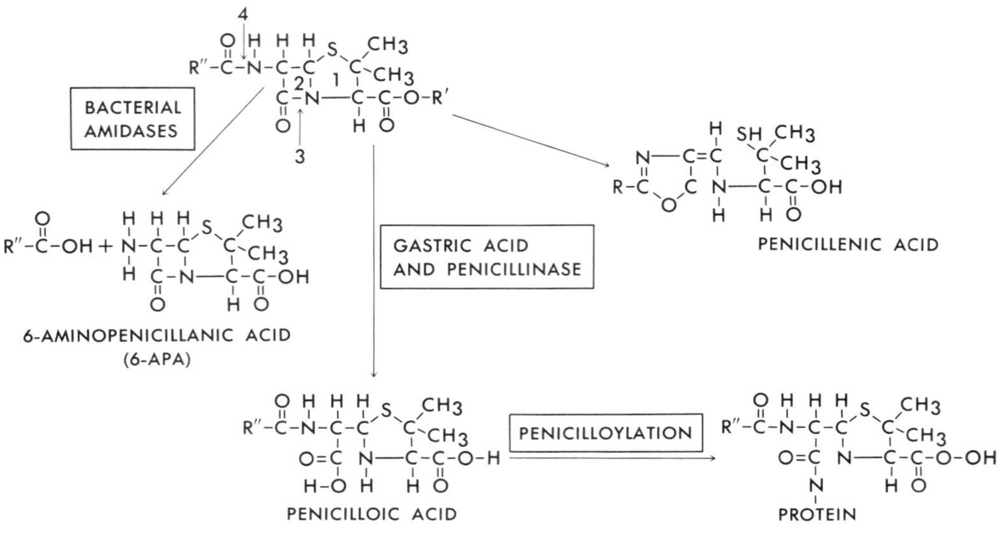

The semisynthetic penicillins, especially methicillin, the isoxazole derivatives, carbenicillin, and ticarcillin react with aminoglycoside antibiotics (other than streptomycin) with resulting loss of antibacterial activity.

MEASUREMENT

The early natural penicillins were impure substances, and consequently measurement in international units by microbiologic assay (*see* Chap. 9) was required. The *international unit of penicillin* is the specific penicillin activity contained in 0.6 μg of the International Penicillin Master Standard, a sample of crystalline sodium penicillin G. The semisynthetic penicillins derived from 6-APA are measured in milligrams, and 1 mg of crystalline sodium penicillin G equals 1667 units. Because of the difference in atomic weight between sodium and potassium, the equivalent penicillin salts have slightly different unit values. In clinical practice penicillin is usually measured either in milligrams or in megaunits (1,000,000 international units).

ANTIBACTERIAL SPECTRUM

Apart from the "broad-spectrum" penicillins, penicillin has a relatively narrow range of activity (Table 59-2). It is highly effective against most gram-positive and gram-negative cocci, although many strains of staphylococcus are now resistant.

TABLE 59-2. Common Organisms Affected by Penicillin G

Organism	Sensitivity*
Actinomyces israelii	++
Alcaligenes faecalis	+
Bacillus anthracis	++R
Bacillus subtilis	++R
Bacteroides spp	++
Bordetella pertussis	++
Borrelia	++
Clostridia	++
Corynebacterium diphtheriae	++R
Diplococcus pneumoniae	+++
Enterobacter aerogenes	+R
Erysipelothrix rhusiopathiae	+++
Escherichia coli	++R
Haemophilus ducreyi	++
Haemophilus influenzae	++
Klebsiella pneumoniae	+R
Leptospira icterohaemorrhagiae	++
Listeria monocytogenes	++
Neisseria gonorrhoeae	+++
Neisseria meningitidis	+++
Pasturella multocida	++
Pasturella pestis	+
Proteus mirabilis	++
Proteus vulgaris	R
Salmonellae	++R
Shigellae	++R
Spirillum minor	++
Staphlococci	+++R
Streptobacillus moniliformis	++
Streptococci (groups A, C, G, H, L)	+++
Streptococci (groups B, E, F, K, N)	++R
Streptococci (group D)	+R
Treponema pallidum	+++
Treponema pertenue	++

* R = *in vitro* testing is essential because many strains are penicillin resistant.
+++ = high sensitivity.
++ = moderate sensitivity.
+ = some sensitivity (penicillin G not recommended for therapy).

MODE OF ACTION

The exact mechanism of action of penicillin is not known. The concept that it inhibits only the final step in cell wall synthesis is almost certainly incorrect (*see* Chap. 57). Penicillin is a bactericidal antibiotic that acts maximally during the logarithmic phase of cell growth. In some gram-negative bacteria, penicillin may be more effective near the stationary growth phase rather than during logarithmic growth.

BACTERIAL RESISTANCE

Bacterial resistance is a major therapeutic problem, especially with staphylococci carried by medical and paramedical personnel in hospital environments. For example, during 1944–1946, 10% to 20% of isolates of *Staph. aureus* were resistant to penicillin G, but by 1950 and 1960 the resistance rates were 50% and 80%, respectively, and today resistance is greater than 90%.

Organisms that develop resistance *in vivo* seldom revert to a sensitive strain, although their pathogenic and antigenic activity usually remain unimpaired. *Acquired penicillin resistance develops in a stepwise manner and may be delayed by a dose sufficiently large to overcome the emergence of first-step mutants.* Some strains of microorganisms such as pneumococci and *Strep. pyogenes* rarely develop penicillin resistance despite the frequency with which infections caused by these organisms have been treated with the antibiotic.

Three main mechanisms of penicillin resistance—*enzymatic destruction*, *failure of antibiotic penetration*, and *failure of antibiotic binding*—are known. The first is the most important.

Enzymatic Destruction

Several penicillinases (β-lactamases) variably (because of differing kinetics) inactivate the individual penicillins through rupture of the β-lactam ring (Figure 59-1). For example, in *Staph. aureus* the penicillinase is plasmid mediated and exocellular, whereas in many gram-negative bacteria the enzyme is cell bound and may be either chromosomally or plasmid mediated, and may be either constitutive or inducible (*see* Chap. 56). *Nutrapen* penicillinase purified from Bacillus spp.) can be used *in vitro* to inactivate penicillins, for example, during bacterial culture. Clavulanic acid and similar compounds that inhibit penicillinase (*see* Chap. 56) may become important clinically.

Resistance to penicillinase in penicillinase-resistant penicillins depends on side-chain R″ additions (*see* Table 59-5) that greatly diminish the affinity between β-lactamase and the antibiotic at therapeutic concentrations. For example the K_m (concentration at $1/2$ V_{max}) for methicillin is about 7000 μg/ml, and yet therapeutic drug levels are about 10 μg/ml, at which point the degree of penicillinase activity is diminished about 1000-fold. Bacterial resistance to methicillin has become a severe therapeutic problem since about 50% of the strains are also resistant to cephalosporins.

β-lactamases are neither exclusively a penicillinase nor a cephalosporinase. Some microorganisms produce more than one type. Typically, β-lactamases from different microorganisms possess varying activities against the different β-lactam antibiotics because of differing kinetics. Penicillinase produced by host flora, for example, in the gut lumen, is not absorbed into the general circulation to inactivate systemically administered penicillin.

Failure of Antibiotic Penetration

Permeability block is particularly seen in resistant gram-negative organisms that possess a complex outer layer. Bacterial resistance to penicillinase-resistant penicillins is frequently associated with failure of antibiotic penetration since the antibiotic modification that increases enzyme stability also diminishes its intracellular passage.

Failure of Antibiotic Binding to Active Sites

Failure of binding to active sites may explain natural or acquired (by mutation) resistance but is not of particular clinical importance.

ADVERSE REACTIONS

About 10% of courses with penicillins result in some adverse effect, but only about 0.01% are serious and only about 0.001% are fatal. Adverse effects to penicillin are either toxic or sensitivity reactions (Table 59-3).

Toxic Reactions

Penicillins are remarkably nontoxic, and, provided that renal function is normal, doses of up to 200 mega units of penicillin G/day intravenously have been tolerated without the appearance of toxic effects. With semisynthetic penicillins, however, particularly methicillin, bone marrow depression (neutropenia, elevation of the serum iron, and saturation of the iron binding capacity) and renal damage may appear with excessive dosage.

When renal tubular function is impaired or in the presence of hyponatremia, penicillin may induce cerebral irritation with hyperreflexia and myotonic seizures. Penicillin produces partial depolarization and increased excitability of neural cells in tissue culture, suggesting that this may be the mechanism of penicillin-induced seizures in humans. In addition, encephalopathy will follow conventional penicillin therapy in patients with renal failure if cerebrospinal fluid drug levels rise above 10 units/ml. Similarly, too concentrated intrathecal penicillin injections may result in chemical meningitis or transverse myelitis.

A breakdown (as yet unexplained) of the blood–brain barrier occurs during cardiopulmonary bypass operations, and penicillin therapy in such situations may be followed by CNS toxicity. Injection near a large mixed nerve, such as the sciatic, may be followed by severe and persistent pain in the peripheral nerve distribution and some residual loss of function, both motor and sensory. Procaine penicillin should be injected with extreme care, since pulmonary embolism and acute psychotic episodes (pseudoanaphylaxis) have followed accidental intravascular injection.

Suprainfection occurs in about 1% of patients. Oral therapy is frequently followed by intestinal upsets, nausea, and vomiting. Local oral penicillin (lozenges or aerosol) is prone to produce cheilosis, buccal ulceration, black hairy tongue, and glossitis—symptoms not

TABLE 59-3. Some Important Sensitivity Reactions to Penicillin

Type of Allergy	Antigen*	Antibody	Clinical Response	Comment
Type I	PCN, PC, and PI; occasionally PO	IgE	Anaphylaxis, laryngeal edema, early onset (<72 h) urticaria	Symptoms (Table 59-4) of anaphylaxis usually develop within 0 to 20 minutes of exposure
Type II	PO	IgG	Coombs' positive hemolytic anemia	Specific IgG binds to the PO/red blood cell complex and activates complement. Hemolysis subsequently occurs in the reticuloendothelial system
Type III	PO (probably soluble)	IgG and IgM	Serum sickness	Site of injury is nonspecific, reflecting the intravascular lodgement of antigen/antibody immune complexes. Complement is activated.
Type IV		T cell	Contact dermatitis	Rarely seen today because topical penicillin therapy no longer used. May be seen in those persons exposed accidentally to topical penicillin (pharmaceutical employees, pharmacists, nurses, patients in whom back leakage of the antibiotic occurs after an i.m. injection)
Unknown but strongly suspected	?	?	Drug fever, maculopapular (excluding "ampicillin rash"; *see* text) and other skin rashes, including erythema nodosa, erythema multiforme, Stevens–Johnson syndrome, late onset urticaria, eosinophilia, hepatitis/nephritis, neutropenia	Negative prospective testing for IgE or other parameters of "allergy" does not provide evidence for or against the development of these reactions

* PCN = penicillin G; PC = penicilloate; PI = penilloate; PO = penicilloyl.

necessarily due to suprainfection. Patients with diminished renal reserve being given large doses of penicillin should be checked carefully for the development of cation intoxication: for example, 3 megaunits of potassium penicillin G contains approximately 5 mEq of ionic potassium, and 4 g of sodium methicillin contains approximately 10 mEq of ionic sodium. Cardiac arrest due to transient hyperkalemia has been reported following the too rapid i.v. administration of potassium penicillins. Methicillin, oxacillin, nafcillin, cloxacillin, dicloxacillin and carbenicillin have been reported occasionally to cause evidence of liver damage (increase of serum glutamic oxalacetic transaminase, alkaline phosphatase, lactic acid dehydrogenase, and sulfobromophthalein retention). Carbenicillin and ticarcillin occasionally induce a bleeding diathesis through binding to adenosine diphosphate in platelets; they may also produce thrombocytopenia, inhibit platelet aggregation, and prolong the bleeding time.

Jarisch-Herxheimer reactions may develop within a few hours of primary penicillin exposure in most patients with secondary syphilis, the syphilitic lesions becoming edematous and hyperemic. Serious symptoms occur if the granulomata are present at the coronary artery ostia or larynx.

Sensitivity Reactions

Hypersensitivity to the penicillins is of practical significance in that it causes potentially fatal reactions and thus limits the use of these antibiotics. Hypersensitivity to the penicillins is of theoretical significance in that it indicates how a simple nontoxic molecule can be altered into an extremely powerful immunizing and sensitizing antigen.

The penicillins are the most common drug causes of allergy, and reactions ranging from mild to fatal have been reported to follow the administration of nearly all pencillins by almost all routes of administration. Although the incidence of allergic reactions is difficult to assess, the risk seems greater with the use of procaine and benzathine penicillin G than with other preparations. This difference may be partly due to occurrence of allergy to procaine or benzathine or to the fact that these preparations may act as adjuvants (*see* Chap. 11) and as depôts of antigen.

The incidence of penicillin sensitivity increases with prolonged therapy and high total dosage. *Topical application is most likely to produce sensitization;* oral administration is the least hazardous. Many persons who manifest penicillin hypersensitivity have no history of penicillin exposure. They may, however, have been exposed unknowingly to the antibiotic from agricultural (milk, food), industrial (drug manufacture), or medical (ointments, vaccines) contamination or from skin fungi.

Penicillin Antigens. When penicillin G is metabolized and the products combine with tissue proteins and other macromolecules, about 95% forms the *penicilloyl* (*PO*) *group;* this constitutes the *major antigenic determinant.* The remaining 5% constitutes the *minor antigenic determinants* and primarily consists of penicillin G (PCN) reacting via its sulfur moiety, *penicilloate* (PC) and *penilloate* (PI); other potential antigens, probably clinically insignificant, are fermentation contaminants such as mycelial fragments or moieties derived from bacterial amidases linked with penicillin or its degradation products, and nonprotein polymers of penicillin or its degradation products. The terms *major* and *minor antigenic determinants* are somewhat confusing because they refer to the *frequency of their formation* rather than to *the severity of reactions* they produce. Thus antibodies to the minor antigenic determinants are more serious because they typically mediate most anaphylactic reactions. Cross-reactivity must be considered the rule; hence a subject sensitized to one penicillin usually reacts with varying severity to all other penicillins.

Antibodies Produced. Various antibodies are produced (Table 59-3). Atopic persons reportedly have a threefold to fourfold increased risk of developing IgE antibodies compared to normal subjects, but this has been challenged. Between 60% and 100% of patients who have received penicillin, and many persons who have never knowingly received the antibiotic, possess hemagglutinating IgM antibodies to the major determinant. The concentration of antibodies is higher in those patients who have experienced some reaction to penicillin, and titers tend to be higher just after reactions and fall with time.

Penicillin Reactions

The outstanding clinical feature of penicillin hypersensitivity is its unpredictability. Severe allergic reactions (Table 59-4) may develop in subjects with no history of atopic disease, in patients who have never knowingly received the antibiotic before, or in patients who have received penicillins without incident for days, months, or years. Further, having occurred once, a reaction may recur and persist for variable periods, or it may never reappear.

Ampicillin Skin Rash

Therapy with ampicillin or with ampicillin esters may be associated with an erythematous, maculopapular (exanthematous, morbilliform) lesion over the exterior aspects of the extremities and trunk developing within 5 to 8 days of the start of therapy. It is three times more common in women than men and is particularly associated with acute viral infections, especially those of the respiratory tract. In patients with infectious mononucleosis, cytomegalovirus infections, and lymphatic leukemia, the incidence rate approaches 90%. The rash is dose related, unaffected by glucocorticosteroids, and IgE antibodies are not present. It may be a "toxic" effect of ampicillin associated with the presence of abnormal lymphocytes or due to the presence of drug impurities. Patients may not respond similarly when challenged with the drug a second time. Of therapeutic importance, *the occurrence of the rash is not in itself a contraindication to future treatment with any penicillin, but it is prudent to skin-test such persons beforehand.*

TABLE 59-4. Outline of Treatment for Anaphylaxis

Symptom/Sign	Immediate Treatment	General Supportive Treatment as Required
Minor		
Erythema Pruritus Urticaria Conjunctivitis Rhinitis Patient complains of feeling "funny"	Epinephrine hydrochloride, 0.3 ml of 1:1000 solution i.m./i.v.,* plus H_1-antagonist† p.o./i.m./i.v.*	Repeat epinephrine and H_1-antagonist*
Major		
Bronchospasm	Epinephrine hydrochloride, 0.3 ml of 1:1000 i.m./i.v.* plus H_1-antagonist† i.m./i.v.* Oxygen	Repeat epinephrine* Oxygen Aminophylline, 250 to 500 mg i.v. q 4 to 6 hr Glucocorticosteroid*,‡
Laryngeal edema	Epinephrine hydrochloride, 0.3 ml of 1:1000 i.m./i.v.* plus H_1-antagonist† i.v.*	Repeat epinephrine* or substitute ephedrine sulfate,* 25 to 50 mg q 6 hr Oxygen Glucocorticosteroid*,‡ H_1-antagonist*,†
Cardiac arrhythmia	Oxygen Antiarrhythmics and vasopressors as dictated by clinical picture	Continue drugs for immediate treatment
Hypotension	Epinephrine hydrochloride, 0.3 ml i.m./i.v.* plus H_1-antagonist† i.v. Oxygen	Sympathomimetic amine to control blood pressure Oxygen Intravenous fluids*

* Dose or route depend on severity of symptoms/signs.
† Usually diphenhydramine hydrochloride, 50 mg.
‡ Usually hydrocortisone or equivalent.

PHARMACOLOGY OF PENICILLIN G

Absorption

Oral. Penicillin G is erratically absorbed (usually 15–40%) from the gastrointestinal tract, primarily the duodenum, and *no reliance should be placed on this form of therapy in severe infections*. Nonabsorbed penicillin is variably destroyed by gastric acid or by colonic flora. Since absorption is influenced by the degree of gastric acidity, greater absorption is seen in neonates, elderly patients, and those taking antacids due to the presence of relative achlorhydria. To minimize inactivation by gastric acid and food, penicillin G should be given no later than ½ hour before meals or no earlier than 3 hours after meals.

Parenteral. Parenteral administration preferably by i.m. injection is the route of choice for serious infections; i.v. injection may occasionally be needed. Following i.m. injection, peak serum levels develop within about 20 minutes but fall rapidly to therapeutically ineffective concentrations over the next 3 to 4 hours because of renal excretion. Blood antibiotic levels in ambulatory patients 2 hours after i.m. penicillin administration are about twice as high as those that occur in patients confined to bed. Absorption of penicillin following i.m. administration may be reduced in patients with diabetes mellitus.

Several procedures can be adopted to prolong blood penicillin levels: The renal tubular excretion of penicillin can be blocked through the concomitant administration of probenecid, and repository preparations of procaine or benzathine penicillin may be used. Recent controlled studies suggest, however, that for many infections in humans it is not mandatory to maintain a plateau of penicillin activity in the blood, but that peak levels for 6 to 8 hr/24 hr will suffice.

Intrathecal. Penicillin G passes slowly and erratically into the cerebrospinal fluid under normal circumstances. When the meninges are inflamed, antibiotic levels are higher but are still inconstant and unreliable. Intrathecal penicillin as an adjunct to systemic therapy is recommended by some authorities for pneumococcal meningitis or sensitive gram-negative meningitis in neonates. *Intrathecal penicillin administration is dangerous.* The maximal dose should never exceed 5000 units at a concentration of not more than 1000 units/ml.

Topical. Although penicillin G is still available in creams, ointments, and some deodorants, *these preparations should never be used.* They are very likely to produce hypersensitivity.

Local. Penicillin G is available in suppository form, as an aerosol, or for local instillation into the pleural, peritoneal, or joint cavities. There is rarely any justification for their use.

DISTRIBUTION, METABOLISM, AND EXCRETION

Penicillin G is distributed widely in the body, tissue concentrations usually being about 20% of simultaneous plasma levels. Antibiotic concentrations in the kidney and urinary tract are high. (Cerebrospinal fluid passage is discussed above.) Penetration of penicillin G into joint fluid is usually excellent.

Penicillin G is partially broken down in the body by unknown mechanisms. About 90% of the drug is excreted unchanged by the kidney; some is excreted in the bile, from where it may undergo an enterohepatic recirculation, and in the milk. Urinary excretion of penicillin is rapid and approximates total renal plasma flow. Thus, following the i.m. administration of aqueous penicillin G, 90% can be recovered from the urine after 2 hours. Excretion is by both glomerular filtration (10–15%) and tubular secretion (85–90%). The tubular secretion of penicillin is reduced by the excretion of natural organic acids (pantothenic acid, uric acid) and by certain drugs such as probenecid (*see* below), aspirin, indomethacin, phenylbutazone, and some sulfonamides. Penicillin clearance is diminished in elderly patients and is relatively slow in infants (*see* Chap. 7).

Renal insufficiency may increase the plasma half-life from about 30 minutes to 10 to 15 hours. Under these circumstances, biliary excretion of the antibiotic increases. Patients with renal failure can be treated with penicillin G with reasonable safety as long as dosage is reduced; after a loading dose, maintenance doses can be given 10 to 12 hourly, but cation intoxication may be a problem in these circumstances.

Some penicillins are cleared by hemodialysis (penicillin G, ampicillin, amoxicillin, carbenicillin, ticarcillin) and peritoneal dialysis (carbenicillin, ticarcillin).

PREPARATIONS

Three main types of penicillin G are available: penicillin G for oral use; aqueous penicillin G for parenteral use; and depôt (repository, "slow release") preparations for parenteral use.

Sodium penicillin G, *N.F.*, and potassium penicillin G, *U.S.P.*, are available as tablets. Penicillin G is available as a sterile powder for s.c., i.v., or intrathecal administration; the calcium, aluminum, and sodium salts are not as effective as the potassium salts. Penicillin G should be reconstituted with sterile distilled water or normal saline; 5% dextrose is not recommended, because it may have a *p*H of 4.5 to 5.5, which destroys the antibiotic. Potassium penicillin G, *U.S.P.*, is a popular preparation. The usual i.m. dose is 500,000 units every 6 hours; i.v. doses may be considerably higher.

Depôt penicillin G was developed for deep i.m. injection to provide a prolonged release of the active drug over hours or days. Slow release from a muscle depôt avoids the wide fluctuations in plasma drug concentrations seen with multiple injections of aqueous penicillin G. These preparations should never be injected intravenously, subcutaneously, or intrathecally. Commonly used preparations are sterile procaine penicillin G suspension, *U.S.P.*, and sterile benzathine penicillin G suspension, *U.S.P.*

Following 600,000 units of procaine penicillin G, intramuscularly, peak serum levels are achieved in 2 to 4 hours, and measurable blood levels may persist for up to 1 week. This dose of procaine penicillin contains about 240 mg of procaine. Usually no adverse effects are seen due to the procaine, and it may, by its local anesthetic action, reduce the pain of the i.m. injection. Some patients, however, may develop a hypersensitivity reaction to the local anesthetic, and severe toxic reactions—for example, cardiac arrhythmias and psychotic behavior—frequently develop if the preparation is accidently injected intravascularly. To minimize rapid intravascular passage of procaine, subjects receiving procaine penicillin should not engage in any strenuous physical activity for about an hour after receiving an injection. Benzathine penicillin G is even more slowly absorbed following i.m. administration than are procaine preparations. Therapeutic serum levels may persist for 10 to 20 days following an injection of 600,000 units of benzathine penicillin G. This preparation should be used only for prophylaxis, for example, against streptococcal throat infections in patients who have had an episode of rheumatic fever.

USE OF PROBENECID

Probenecid was specifically developed to block the renal tubular secretion of penicillin. It also blocks the renal tubular transport of other or-

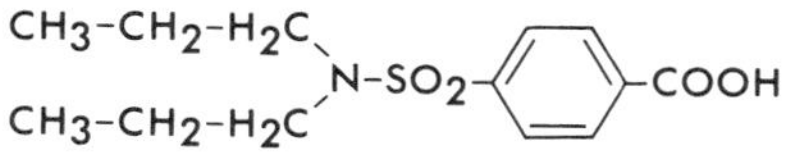

PROBENECID

ganic acids (uric acid, pathothenic acid, the cephalosporins) and reduces organic acid transport into the cerebrospinal fluid. When used concomitantly with penicillin, plasma levels of the antibiotic are increased about twofold and maintained for about twice as long as when penicillin is given alone.

Probenecid is almost totally absorbed following oral administration. Peak levels develop within 2 to 4 hours. The drug is bound to plasma proteins about 80% to 90%, and its half-life is between 6 to 12 hours.

Probenecid, *U.S.P.* (Benemid), is costly. It causes gastrointestinal upsets and thus should be used with care in patients with peptic ulcer disease. Rarely hypersensitivity skin rashes may develop. The usual dose to augment serum penicillin levels is 0.5 g every 6 hours. Because probenecid is costly and potentially toxic, it is rarely used in conventional infections; larger and more frequent doses of penicillin are considered easier, safer, and cheaper. Probenecid is valuable, however, in single-dose treatment of gonorrhea and in the rare patient who refuses parenteral therapy or who has poor veins. Probenecid is also used in the treatment of gout (*see* Chap. 31).

PHARMACOLOGY OF SOME PENICILLIN PREPARATIONS

More than 100 penicillin preparations are available on the market. Some are combinations of penicillin with other antimicrobial drugs or with probenecid, and they often carry misleading proprietary names. Thus confusion is often apparent about the relative merits of any particular compound. In selecting a penicillin, the physician should base his choice on its potency and antibacterial spectrum, its optimum route of administration and protein binding, its susceptibility or resistance to penicillinase, and its cost and intended use (therapeutic or prophylactic). The clinically useful penicillins can be readily classified into natural penicillin G preparations and semisynthetic penicillins (Table 59-5).

CLASSIFICATION OF PENICILLINS

More than 3000 different drugs have been developed, but only a handful are important therapeutically. They can be divided into several specific groups (Table 59-5)

The penicillin G group is orally active, narrow spectrum, and penicillinase sensitive; *the penicillinase-resistant group* is variably acid labile, resistant to bacterial penicillinase, and narrow spectrum; *the broad-spectrum group* contains ampicillin and amoxicillin and various esters that degrade *in vivo* to ampicillin (*e.g.*, hetacillin, pivampicillin, bacampicillin, talampicillin) or amoxicillin (*e.g.*, epicillin and cyclacillin), and thus offer little or no advantage over the parent drug; and *the special group,* which although comprising drugs that possess a wide antibacterial spectrum, should be restricted to treatment of a few specific infections such as those caused by *Ps. aeruginosa*, *Enterobacter* spp., *Proteus* spp., and *B. fragilis* (ticarcillin). Several additional penicillins and penicillin-like agents (*e.g.*, azlocillin, mezlocillin, and piperacillin) are being evaluated experimentally.

CEPHALOSPORINS AND CEPHAMYCINS

CEPHALOSPORINS

The "cephalosporins" P, N, and C were isolated from the fungus *Cephalosporium acremonium*, obtained by Guiseppe Brotzu in 1945 from a sewage outlet off the coast of Sardinia. "Cephalosporins" P (a steroid related to fusidic acid) and N (a penicillin-like agent) have not achieved medical importance. Cephalosporin C possesses a D-α-aminoadipic acid-derived side-chain attached to 7-amino-cephalosporanic acid (7-ACA), the cephalosporin building block.

7-ACA (Fig. 59-2) is composed of a β-lactam ring (2) fused to a dihydrothiazine ring (1) (in distinction to the thiazolidine ring of the penicillins). 7-ACA is readily isolated by dilute acid

(*Text continues on p. 593*)

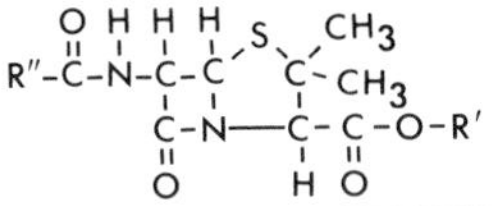

TABLE 59-5. Major Penicillins

R″ Substitutions	Nonproprietary or Generic Name	General	Properties: Penicillinase Resistance	Properties: Broad Spectrum	Properties: Route of Administration	Properties: Plasma Protein Binding %	Properties: Liver Failure Increases T½	Preparations and Dosage
Penicillin G group								
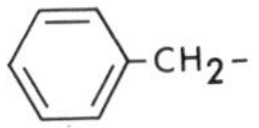	Penicillin G	*See* text	No	No	Parenteral (oral)	35–65	+	*See* text
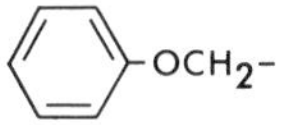	Penicillin V	Similar to penicillin G but less potent. Following equivalent doses, blood levels are 3 to 5 times higher than with penicillin G, but sericidal activity is similar. The potassium salt is better absorbed than is the free acid	No	No	Oral	55–88	+	Potassium phenoxymethyl penicillin, *U.S.P.*, 250–500 mg q 8 hr. Should be taken not earlier than 3 hours after food
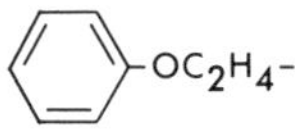	Phenethicillin	Similar to penicillin V	No	No	Oral	50–60	+	Potassium phenethicillin, *N.F.*, 250–500 mg q 8 hr
Penicillinase-resistant group								
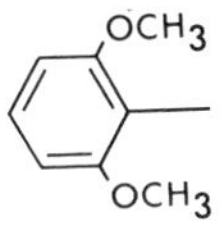	Methicillin	The first penicillinase-resistant penicillin. Resistance due to the R″-substituted-CH_3 group that blocks hydrolysis by β-lactamase but not by acids Antibacterial spectrum about equal to that of penicillin G but *much less potent against nonpenicillinase producers.* Following i.m. injection, plasma	Yes, but variable	No	Parenteral	20–50	+	Sodium methicillin, *U.S.P.*, 3 to 6 g, q 4 to 6 hr, because of its acid lability should not be dissolved in large volumes of acidic i.v. fluids, e.g., 5% dextrose. Methicillin and other penicillinase-resistant penicillins or a cephalosporin should be reserved for treatment of infections due to

		levels peak at about 40 min. Excreted rapidly in bile and urine. Methicillin resistance probably due to failure of antibiotic uptake by bacteria. May produce hepatic or renal damage. Many bacteria now resistant.						penicillin G-resistant staphylococci and for initial treatment of all new staphylococcal infections until their sensitivity is determined
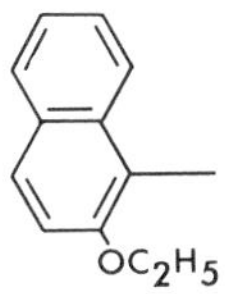	Nafcillin	Partially acid stable, but absorption following oral administration erratic and unreliable. Bile levels may reach 100 times plasma levels, and T½ is prolonged due to an enterohepatic recirculation. Highly irritating on parenteral administration	Yes	No	Parenteral (oral)	70–90	+++	Sodium nafcillin, *U.S.P.*, 0.5 to 1.0 g q 4 to 6 hr
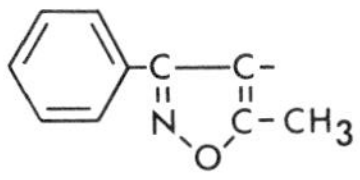	Oxacillin	The first isoxazole penicillin to be developed. Less potent than penicillin G but 6 times more potent than methicillin. About 60% of an oral dose is absorbed. Cleared in urine and bile	Yes	No	Oral parenteral	80–90	+	Sodium oxacillin *U.S.P.*, 250 mg to 1 g q 4 to 6 hr
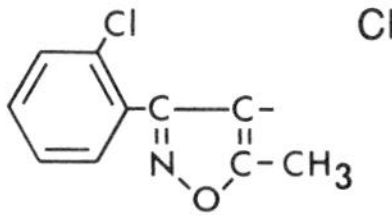	Cloxacillin	Similar to oxacillin but more readily absorbed after oral administration. Following i.m. administration, blood levels are about twice those following oral administration	Yes	No	Oral parenteral	80–95	++	Sodium cloxacillin *U.S.P.*, 250 to 500 mg q 4 to 6 hr

(*continued*)

TABLE 59-5. (Continued)

R″ Substitutions	Nonproprietary or Generic Name	General	Properties: *Penicillinase Resistance*	*Broad Spectrum*	*Route of Administration*	*Plasma Protein Binding %*	*Liver Failure Increases T½*	Preparations and Dosage
Penicillinase-resistant group								
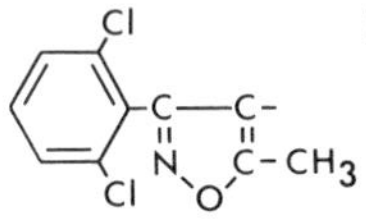	Dicloxacillin	More potent than oxacillin or cloxacillin than against penicillinase-producing staphylococci. Rapid absorption following oral administration, with blood levels about twice those seen with cloxacillin. Half-life longer than most other penicillins due to high plasma protein binding	Yes	No	Oral	80–95	++	Dicloxacillin sodium 250 to 500 mg q 4 to 6 hr
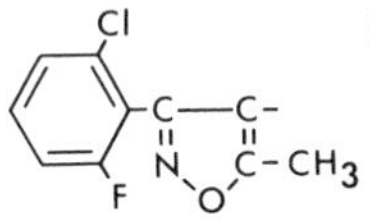	Flucloxacillin	Similar to dicloxacillin except less protein bound	Yes	No	Oral	60–80	++	Flucloxacillin, 250 to 500 mg q 4 to 6 hr
Broad-spectrum group								
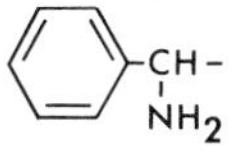	Ampicillin	Gram-positive spectrum similar to that of penicillin G. Gram-negative spectrum against many strains of *E. coli, H. influenzae, Enterobacter aerogenes, Klebsiella, Proteus mirabilis, Salmonella, Shigella,* and *Enterococci.* Readily absorbed following oral and i.m. administration, but rate delayed by food. May reach 20 to 40	No	Yes	Oral, parenteral	15–25	++	Sodium ampicillin *U.S.P.*, 500 mg orally q 6 hr in severe infections, 3 to 5 g q 6 hr

		times simultaneous plasma levels and can be increased still further by probenecid. Sometimes useful in the treatment of biliary tract disease, including the typhoid carrier state						
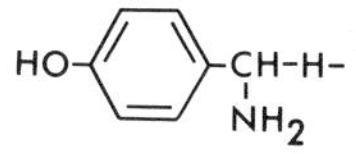	Amoxicillin	Similar *in vitro* spectrum to ampicillin but twofold to threefold better absorption. Food does not affect absorption. May eventually replace ampicillin and its esters	No	Yes	Oral	15–25	+	Amoxicillin, U.S.P. 25 to 50 mg/kg/day
Special group								
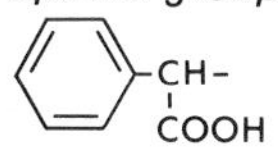	Carbenicillin	Similar antibacterial spectrum to ampicillin *plus* activity against *Ps. aeruginosa* and indole positive *Proteus.* Very high serum levels (40–200 μg/ml) are required to treat susceptible gram-negative organisms, levels only obtainable with parenteral therapy. CSF passage is poor, and the drug is cleared 80% to 100% in 4 hours by the kidney. One gram i.m. gives peak serum levels of 20 μg/ml. Serum levels of 150 to 200 μg/ml achieved only with doses of 70 to 100 mg/kg q 2 to 4 hr	No	Yes	Parenteral	50	++	Carbenicillin sodium. Additive effects or synergism produced against *Ps. aeruginosa* with concomitant aminoglycoside therapy. These antibiotics should not be mixed in the same container because they inactivate each other. Usual dosage is 50 to 100 mg/kg/day

(continued)

TABLE 59-5. ***(Continued)***

R″ Substitutions	Nonproprietary or Generic Name	General	Properties: *Penicillinase Resistance*	*Broad Spectrum*	*Route of Administration*	*Plasma Protein Binding %*	*Liver Failure Increases T½*	Preparations and Dosage
Special group								
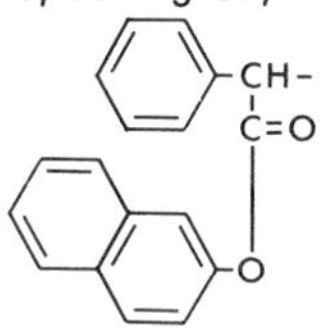	Indanyl carbenicillin	Only about 40% absorbed. Converted by plasma and tissue esterases to carbenicillin. The indanyl moiety excreted as glucuronide conjugates or sulfate esters in the urine. *Very low plasma levels* (10 μg/ml) are produced with doses of 1 g orally, and it should be reserved for treating mild urinary tract infections due to *Ps. aeruginosa* or indole positive Proteus.	No	Yes	Oral	50	++	Carindacillin, 50 to 60 mg/kg/day
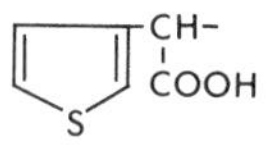	Ticarcillin	Spectrum identical to that of carbenicillin, but 2 to 4 times as active against *Ps. aeruginosa*. Some activity against *B. fragilis*.	No	Yes	Parenteral	50	++	Ticarcillin, 50 to 100 mg/kg/day

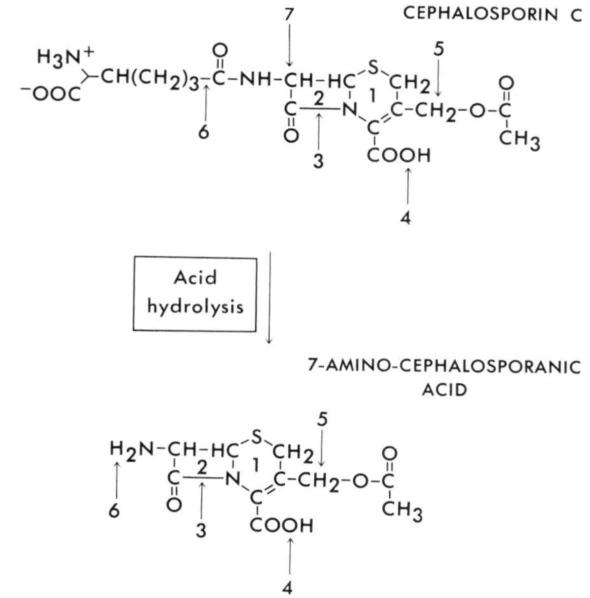

FIG. 59-2. Cephalosporin C and 7-aminocephalosporinic acid. (*1*) dihydrothiazine ring; (*2*) β-lactam ring; (*3*) site of action of cephalosporinase; (*4*) site of salt formation; (*5*) site for deacetylation and subsequent substitutions (Table 59-8); (*6*) site of acetylation and substitutions (Table 59-8); (*7*) carbon 7 of the β-lactam ring, site of methoxy moiety ($-OCH_3$) of cephamycins.

hydrolysis of cephalosporin C and can be considered as the 6-APA ring system of the penicillins (*see* above). The basic cephalosporin structure differs from that of the penicillins in that cephalosporin possesses only two asymmetric points compared to the three in 6-APA and has three instead of two sites at which chemical modifications may be made. Numerous semisynthetic cephalosporins have been produced from 7-ACA that possess greater antibacterial activity than the original cephalosporin C (*see* Table 59-8) but differ among themselves primarily in pharmacokinetic properties and cost. The cephalosporins are widely used; for example, $160 million was spent on these agents in 1974, and they represent about 30% of the average American hospital pharmacy budget.

CEPHAMYCINS

The cephamycins are similar to the cephalosporins but are derived from *Streptomyces* spp. (*S. lactamdurans* for cefoxitin). Chemically they differ from "true" cephalosporins in that they have a methoxy group at position 7 of the β-lactam ring of the 7-ACA nucleus (Figs. 59-2, 59-3). Cephalosporin is used usually generically to refer to both cephalosporins and cephamycins.

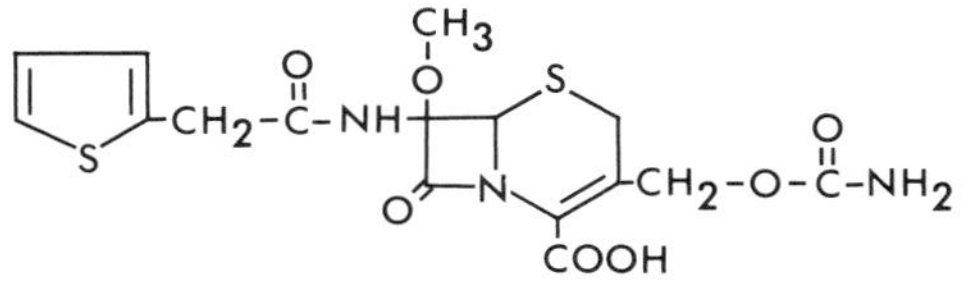

FIG. 59-3. The cephamycin cefoxitin.

Classification of Cephalosporins

The first-generation cephalosporins (cephalothin, cephaloridine, cephaloglycine, cephalexin, cephazolin, cephapirin, cephradine, and cephadroxil) have many similar properties (*see* Table 59-8). Second-generation cephalosporins (cephamandol, cefaclor, cefuroxime (available only in Europe), and cefoxitin) differ from first-generation drugs primarily in possessing variable resistance to gram-negative β-lactamases and in having a small but important extension of antibacterial spectrum (Tables 59-6, 59-7). Third-generation cephalosporins (moxalactam, cefotaxime, cefoperazone, ceforane, ceforanide, ceftizoxime, cefsulodin) have a further extension of antibacterial spectrum and, especially with moxalactam (*see* below), the ability to penetrate the CNS.

TABLE 59-6. Common Microorganisms Affected by the First-Generation Cephalosporins

Organism	Sensitivity*
Actinomyces israelii	+++
Bacillus subtilis	+++
Diplococcus pneumoniae	+++
E. coli	++R
Haemophilus influenzae	+R
Cl. welchii	+++
Corynebacterium diphtheriae	+++
Listeria monocytogenase	+++
Klebsiella spp.	+++
Neisseria gonorrhoeae	++R
Neisseria meningitidis	+++R†
Proteus mirabilis	++
Salmonella	++R
Shigella	++R
Staph. aureus	+++R
Staph. epidermidis	+++
Strep. faecalis	+R
Strep. pyogens	+++
Strep. viridans	+++

* R = *in vitro* testing essential because many strains are resistant; +++ = highly sensitive; ++ = moderately sensitive; + = some sensitivity.

† Not recommended for therapy because the cephalosporins pass poorly into the CSF.

TABLE 59-7. Important Organisms Affected by Second Generation Cephalosporins

Cephalosporin	Bacterial Species
Cefamandol	*Enterobacter* spp. *H. influenzae* (extra CNS infections only) Indole-positive *Proteus* spp.
Cefaclor	*H. influenzae*, including β-lactamase-producing strains
Cefoxitin	*B. fragilis* Indole-positive *Proteus* spp. *N. gonorrhoeae*, *Providencia* spp. *Serratia marcescens*

Antibacterial Spectrum

The antibacterial spectra of the first-generation cephalosporins are similar (Table 59-6); organisms invariably resistant are *Enterobacter*, *Serratia marcescens*, *Citrobacter*, indole-positive *Proteus*, *Bacteroides* spp., and *Ps. aeruginosa*.

Second-generation cephalosporins have an extended spectrum because they are variably resistant to gram-negative bacterial β-lactamases. Thus they possess the same general activity seen with the earlier cephalosporins against aerobic and anaerobic bacteria (Table 59-6), plus the important extensions in spectrum given in Table 59-7. Third-generation agents are discussed below (under Moxalactam).

Mode of Action and Bacterial Resistance

The cephalosporins are bactericidal and probably act similarly to the penicillins (*see* Chap. 57). Activity primarily depends on the integrity of the β-lactam ring and on the three-dimensional structure of the antibiotic. Bacterial resistance may be due to *failure of antibiotic penetration* (mainly in gram-negative organisms), *failure of antibiotic binding*, or *production of β-lactamase* (cephalosporinase); cephalosporins are usually not destroyed by penicillinase and may actually absorb it.

Cephalosporinases are different from penicillinases. In gram-positive organisms they are usually secreted exocellularly, whereas in gram-negative bacteria they are located in the periplasmic space. In addition to chromosomally mediated cephalosporinases, the enzyme may be mediated by R factors (*see* Chap. 56). The cephalosporins are not reliably synergistic when combined with aminoglycosides against enterococci.

General Properties of First- and Second-Generation Cephalosporins

The bioavailability of orally administered cephalosporins is delayed by food. Generally, all cephalosporins pass well to most tissues and tissue spaces such as the synovial fluid and serosal sacs, to the fetus, and into milk and bile; penetration into the eye, prostatic gland, and (*see* below) the CSF is poor. Of the first-generation cephalosporins, cefazolin achieves highest concentrations in bile; cefamandol may achieve fourfold to eightfold higher levels than cefazolin, but the clinical importance of this phenomenon for biliary infections is not yet clear. *Passage of cephalosporins into the CSF is poor*, and except in special situations these drugs should not be used to treat infections of the CNS.

Some cephalosporins (cephalothin, cephapirin, cephaloglycin, cephacetile) are metabolized (Table 59-8) to the desacetyl metabolite, which is about fourfold and eightfold to sixteenfold less antibacterially active against gram-positive and negative bacteria, respectively.

Cephalosporins are excreted by glomerular filtration and renal tubular secretion (except for cephaloridine). Probenecid therefore prolongs the half-life of all cephalosporins except cephaloridine. Properties of individual cephalosporins are noted in Table 59-8.

Adverse Reactions

All cephalosporins have a similar spectrum of adverse effects. Locally they produce *tissue irritation*. Thus gastrointestinal upsets (nausea, dyspepsia, vomiting, diarrhea) may follow oral therapy, and thrombophlebitis commonly occurs with i.v. administration even after careful drug dilution; cefazolin and cephapirin may be less irritating to endothelia than are other agents. Cephalothin is the most painful of the cephalosporins when given intramuscularly, and sterile abcesses and sloughing have been occasionally reported with this drug; cefazolin and cephaloridine are less painful than cephalothin. Intrathecal cephalosporins are highly toxic, causing similar damage to that of penicillin.

Suprainfection, including pseudomembranous colitis, may develop, and, in the presence of diminished renal function, cation (sodium) loading may pose a problem. A positive reaction for urinary sugar develops with the "Clinitest" tablets, or with Benedicts and Fehlings reagents, but not with specific tests that use glucose oxidase, such as Clinistix or "Tes-Tape."

Elevation of SGOT, SGPT, LDH, and alkaline phosphatase activity may be seen, and rarely cephalosporins reduce platelet function (producing a bleeding tendency) and cause renal tubular damage.

A positive Coombs' test develops in 3% of courses, but this is only rarely associated with hemolytic anemia; cephaloridine and cephalothin cause this reaction most frequently and cefazolin least frequently. The reaction is not immunologic but results from coating of the erythrocytes nonspecifically by a cephalosporin globulin complex; it may be more likely in the presence of hypoalbuminemia and impaired renal function. Nail shedding may occur following high doses of cephalosporins in patients with renal failure.

Cephaloridine-Induced Renal Damage. Apart from causing the general adverse effects discussed above, cephaloridine is highly nephrotoxic and may produce acute proximal tubular necrosis, particularly in doses of greater than 4 g/day in adults or 30 to 50 mg/kg/day in children. The pathogenesis of this reaction is not known, but its severity seems to parallel the accumulation of cephaloridine within renal tissue. Such toxicity is more common in patients with preexisting renal disease and in those taking other nephrotoxic drugs concomitantly; it may be minimized by probenecid.

Cephalosporin Allergy. Types I to IV allergic reactions may occur, but types III and IV are rare. The risk of an allergic reaction to a cephalosporin (other than acute anaphylaxis) in penicillin-allergic patients is about 10%. Whether this increased sensitivity is due to true cross-sensitivity or to an increased reactivity of penicillin-allergic patients is unclear.

It is not known which determinants of the cephalosporin nucleus are antigenic, but probably the side-chain substitutions are more important than the cephalosporoyl group. Since the putative antigens are unknown, no skin tests can reliably predict cephalosporin allergy. Other than anaphylactic shock, many adverse effects of the cephalosporins are believed to be "allergic" in nature, but exact proof is lacking. Thus drug fever, chills, urticaria, morbilliform skin rashes, pruritus, eosinophilia, serum sickness, isolated lymphadenopathy, thrombocytopenia, leukopenia, and renal damage (nephritis and acute tubular necrosis) may be seen. Renal damage may be more likely when other nephrotoxic drugs are given concomitantly, especially diuretics and aminoglycoside antibiotics, and in the presence of diminished renal function. To date, the balance of clinical experience suggests that clinically significant cross-sensitivity for anaphylactic shock is rare between penicillins and cephalosporins. This is not surprising since, unlike the penicillins, hydrolysis of the β-lactam ring of the cephalosporins is unusual, and when it does occur the resulting compounds are highly unstable and do not readily form haptenes. Several instances of possible cross-sensitivity have, however, been reported.

HERMANN CHRISTIAN VON FEHLING, 1812–1885. German chemist. Did much research into qualitative analysis, including his test for the presence of sugar reported in 1848. Isolated benzonitrile and discovered succino-succinic ester.

Properties of Third-Generation Cephalosporins

Of the drugs mentioned above, only *moxalactam* has been approved. Moxalactam is a semisynthetic, broad-spectrum cephalosporin whose sulfur atom of the basic nucleus has been replaced with an oxygen atom. It is not as active against common pathogenic gram-positive cocci (*S. aureus, S. epidermidis, Strep. pneumoniae*) as first- and second-generation drugs. However, it is highly effective against enterobacteriaceae—especially *E. coli, Proteus mirabilis,* indole-positive *Proteus* spp., *Enterobacter* spp., *Citrobacter* spp., *Serratia marcescens, Klebsiella* spp., and *Pseudomonas aeruginosa*—and against *Hemophilus influenzae* and anaerobes, including *B. fragilis.* Like all cephalosporins, it is inactive against enterococci.

Moxalactam is given intravenously or by deep i.m. injection. It is bound about 50% to plasma proteins and excreted predominantly by glomerular filtration. Its half-life is between 2 and 3 hours following i.v. administration to normal volunteers and about 19 hours in patients with severe renal impairment (creatinine clearance less than 10 ml/min). *Unlike other cephalosporins, moxalactam penetrates well into the CSF.* It also penetrates well into bile, the eye, and most tissue fluids.

In addition to the usual cephalosporin side-effects (*see* above), moxalactam produces, in

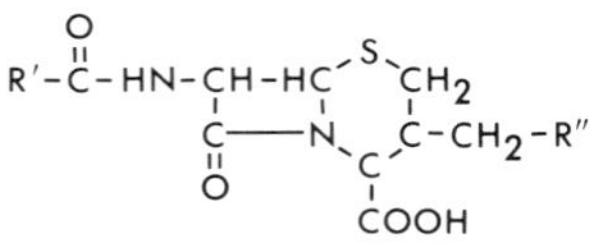

TABLE 59-8. Major Cephalosporins and the Cephamycin Cefoxitin

R′ Substitutions	R″ Substitutions	Date Intro-duced	Nonproprietary or Generic Name	General Properties	Route of Admini-stration	Half-Life
						min
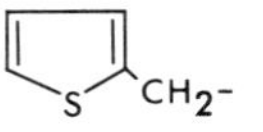	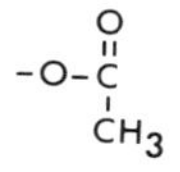	1964	Cephalothin	Not measurably destroyed by gastric acid, but absorption following oral administration is poor. Best given i.v. since i.m. painful. Fetal blood levels usually reach 20% of maternal levels. About 30% converted in the liver to the O-desacetyl metabolite. Almost completely removed during hemodialysis and peritoneal dialysis. Least susceptible to staphylococcal penicillinase.	i.m. i.v.	30–60
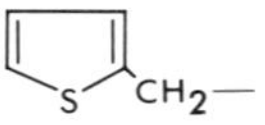	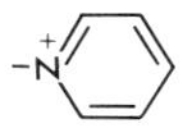	1966	Cephaloridine	May possess greater activity against some staphylococci, pneumococci, and hemolytic streptococci and less activity against the neisseriae and *H. influenzae* than does cephalothin. Cephaloridine is a zwitterion and relatively nonpolar, and clearance is equivalent to the glomerular filtration rate. Thus probenecid has little effect on its excretion.	i.m. i.v.	60–90
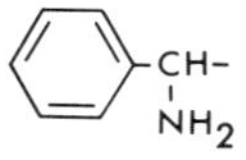	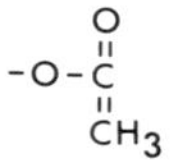	1970	Cephaloglycine	Hydrolyzed to cephalothin *in vivo.* Slowly and incompletely (30%) absorbed following oral administration, resulting in low plasma levels. Metabolized to an O-desacetyl metabolite. Because of prompt renal clearance of free drug cephaloglycine, may have place in treating urinary tract infections. Usually produces diarrhea.	Oral	90–100
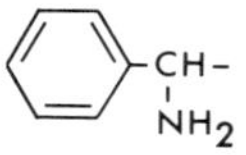	-H	1971	Cephalexin	Acid stable. Less potent than cephalothin or cephaloridine. About 80% absorbed following oral administration. Removed by hemodialysis and peritoneal dialysis	Oral	30–70

(*continued*)

TABLE 59-8. ***(Continued)***

Plasma Protein Binding	Resistance (R) or Susceptibility (S) to G-β-Lactamase	Vd	Peak Serum Level After 500 mg p.o. or 1.0 g i.m.	Percentage Metabolized	Percentage Excreted by Kidney at 6 Hours	Preparations and Dosage
%		*liter/1.73 m²*	*μg/ml*			
50–80	S	18	18	33	50	Cephalothin sodium, U.S.P., is available in sterile ampules for reconstitution with normal saline or 5% dextrose. Usual adult dose is 1 g q 6 hr. In serious infections or life-threatening infections, 1 g q 3 hr or 1 g q 2 hr i.v. is recommended. The usual dose in children is 40 to 80 mg/kg day in divided doses.
20–30	S	20	30–40	0	80	Cephaloridine, U.S.P., is available as powder for reconstitution. The usual dose is 0.5 to 1 g q 6 hr. A total daily dose of 4 g or 50 mg/kg should not be exceeded in adults and children, respectively
15–25	—	?	1–2	90	20	Cephaloglycine, 250 to 500 mg q 6 hr. Should be used only for treatment of urinary tract infections due to highly sensitive organisms. Otherwise obsolete.
15–25	R*	16	15	0	80	Cephalexin, U.S.P. The usual dose in adults is 250 mg to 1 g q 6 hr. In children the usual dose is 25 to 50 mg/kg daily.

(continued)

TABLE 59-8. *(Continued)*

R′ Substitutions	R″ Substitutions	Date Introduced	Nonproprietary or Generic Name	General Properties	Route of Administration	Half-Life
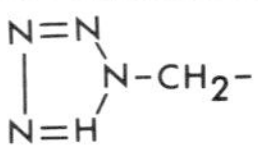	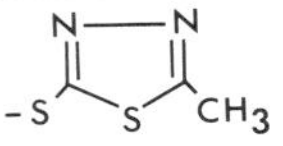	1973	Cefazolin	Less painful and may possess greater activity against *Enterobacter* species than cephalothin. Not removed by hemodialysis	i.m. i.v.	90–120
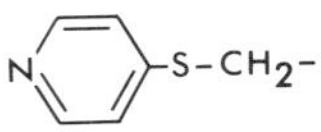	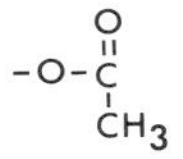	1974	Cephapirin	Metabolized to desacetyl metabolite. Best given i.v. since painful on i.m. injection	i.m. i.v.	30–40
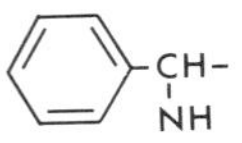	-H	1974	Cephradine	Chemically similar to cephalexin but may be more potent against enterococci	Oral (i.m.) (i.v.)	40–100
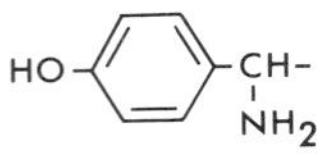	-H	1979	Cefadroxil	Not destroyed by gastric acid and thus reliably absorbed after oral administration. Its relatively long T½ allows q 12 hr dosage.	Oral	80–90
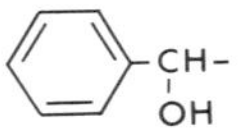	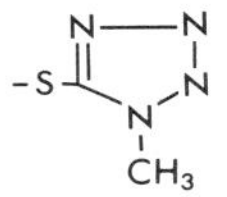	1979	Cefamandol	*See* text and Table 59-7.	i.m. i.v.	50–60
—	—	Investigational	Cefaclor	*See* text and Table 59-7.	Oral	40–50
See Figure 59-3.		1979	Cefoxitin	A cephamycin; *see* Table 59-7. A small fraction metabolized to descarbamyl form	i.m. i.v.	40–50

* Resistance shown to some β-lactamases from gram-negative bacteria.

about 5% of patients, hematopoietic abnormalities (especially eosinophilia, thrombocytopenia, hypoprothrombinemia, and reversible leukopenia), transient elevations in SGOT, and colonization and suprainfection with enterococci. An antabuse-type reaction may appear when ingested with alcohol. It is very expensive.

Uses

The cephalosporins are rarely drugs of first choice unless other antibiotics are unsuitable because of *toxicity* or *allergy*. Because of their relatively broad antibacterial spectrum, however, they are frequently misused, particularly in place of less costly agents with a narrower spectrum. Of particular importance is their action against staphylococcal spp., *Clostridium welchii*, most streptococci, pneumococci, and some strains of *Klebsiella*, *Proteus*, and *E. coli*.

Cephalosporins are unsuitable as sole agents in gram-negative septicemia, particularly in the neutropenic patient, but may be combined with carbenicillin (or ticarcillin) or an aminoglycoside. A parenteral cephalosporin is usually the drug of choice in treating penicillin-resistant *Staph. epidermidis* infection in a prosthetic joint. Additionally, penicillinase-producing gonococci resistant to spectinomycin may respond to cefoxitin (2 g intramuscularly plus probenicid, 1 g orally). Since the cephalosporins pass poorly into cerebrospinal fluid, their use in treating bacterial meningitis

TABLE 59-8. *(Continued)*

Plasma Protein Binding	Resistance (R) or Susceptibility (S) to G-β-Lactamase	Vd	Peak Serum Level After 500 mg p.o. or 1.0 g I.m.	Percentage Metabolized	Percentage Excreted by Kidney at 6 Hours	Preparations and Dosage
70–90	S	10	60	0	80–90	Cefazolin sodium, U.S.P., 250 to 500 mg q 8 hr for mild infections, or 1 g q 6 hr for severe infections. The dose in children is 25 to 50 mg/kg/day.
40–50	S	15	20	40	50	Cephapirin sodium, U.S.P., is given in doses of 500 mg to 1 g q 4 hr for adults or 40 to 80 mg/kg/day for children.
15–20	R′	16	20	0	80	Cephradine, U.S.P. In adults the oral dose is 250 mg to 1 g q 6 hr. In children the dose is 50 to 100 mg/kg/day.
15–25	—	?	15	0	70	Cefadroxil, U.S.P. The usual dose is 500 mg q 12 hr.
70–80	R*	15	25	0	80	Cephamandol naftate; 1 to 2 g q 4 or 6 hr up to 12 g/day in adults. For children, 50 to 150 mg/kg/day.
20–50	R*	15	10–12	0	60	Cefaclor, 250 mg to 500 mg q 4 to 6 hr daily in adults. Daily dose should not exceed 4 g.
70–80	R	14	20	5	85	Cefoxitin, 1 to 2 g q 4 or 6 hr up to 12 g daily in adults.

is unreliable. In fact, cephalosporin-sensitive bacteria have initiated meningitis during treatment of systemic infection with these antibiotics. Cephalosporins may be valuable for preventing infections in prosthetic devices or in vascular grafts or during vaginal hysterectomy. Cephalexin and cephradine are the preferred oral agents, but cefadroxil, which is of established efficacy for urinary tract infections only, has the advantage of twice daily dosage. Based on pharmacokinetic grounds and on cost, cefazolin is the preferred parenteral cephalosporin. Cephaloridine probably should not be used. Cefaclor may become useful in treating *H. influenzae* infections, including those caused by ampicillin-resistant strains. Third-generation cephalosporins should be reserved for treating serious mixed infections. Moxalactam should not be used alone in treating *Ps. aeruginosa* infections.

FURTHER READING

1. Cook FV, Farrar WE: Vancomycin revisited. Ann Intern Med 88:813–818, 1978
2. Neu HC: Amoxicillin. Ann Intern Med 90:356–360, 1979
3. Saxon A: Immediate hypersensitivity reactions to beta-lactam antibiotics. Rev Infect Dis (in press)
4. Simberkoff MS, Thomas L, McGregor D et al: Inactivation of penicillins by carbohydrate solutions at alkaline pH. N Engl J Med 283:116–119, 1970
5. Weinstein AJ: The cephalosporins—Activity and clinical use. Drugs 19:137–154, 1980
6. Winston DJ, Young LS: The cephalosporins. In Kagan BM (ed): *Antimicrobial Therapy*, 3rd ed, pp 35–55. Philadelphia, WB Saunders, 1980

CHAPTER 59 QUESTIONS

(See P. 7 for Full Instructions)

Select the One Best Answer

1. Penicillinase-sensitive, a broad antibacterial spectrum, and oral and parenteral effectiveness characterizes best
   - *A.* penicillin G.
   - *B.* ampicillin.
   - *C.* benzathine penicillin.
   - *D.* cloxacillin.
   - *E.* methicillin.
2. An analogue of penicillin G particularly effective against urinary tract infections due to *Pseudomonas* or resistant strains of *Proteus* is
   - *A.* ampicillin.
   - *B.* carbenicillin.
   - *C.* phenoxymethyl penicillin.
   - *D.* cloxacillin.
   - *E.* phenethicillin.
3. An antibacterial agent related to penicillin G in structure and mode of action but which has significant nephrotoxicity is
   - *A.* erythromycin.
   - *B.* cycloserine.
   - *C.* ampicillin.
   - *D.* moxalactam.
   - *E.* cephaloridine.
4. Which of the following agents is least likely to produce an allergic response in a patient with documented anaphylaxis to benzyl penicillin G?
   - *A.* Procaine penicillin G
   - *B.* Cephalothin
   - *C.* Carbenicillin
   - *D.* Ampicillin
   - *E.* Dicloxacillin
5. All of the following statements about first-generation cephalosporins are true EXCEPT that
   - *A.* they are generally resistant to penicillinase.
   - *B.* they have a longer plasma half-life than penicillin G.
   - *C.* they are effective in treating enterococcal endocarditis.
   - *D.* they diffuse poorly into the CSF.
   - *E.* they may cause thrombophlebitis when administered intravenously.
6. Which of the following antibiotics is not effective orally for systemic infections?
   - *A.* Oxacillin
   - *B.* Erythromycin
   - *C.* Clindamycin
   - *D.* Cephalexin
   - *E.* Vancomycin

A = 1,2,3; B = 1,3; C = 2,4; D = 4; E = All

7. Penicillin G can be used effectively to treat
   1. pneumococcal pneumonia.
   2. streptococcal pharyngitis.
   3. gonorrhea.
   4. klebsiella pneumonia.
8. Ampicillin is
   1. acid stable.
   2. resistant to pencillinase.
   3. effective against both gram-positive and gram-negative organisms.
   4. effective against *Pseudomonas aeruginosa*.
9. Ampicillin
   1. is resistant to penicillinase.
   2. is effective against gram-negative organisms.
   3. formed on hydrolysis of amoxicillin.
   4. demonstrates cross-hypersensitivity with penicillin G.
10. Penicillin G
    1. is bactericidal in high concentrations.
    2. is secreted by the renal tubules.
    3. is acid labile.
    4. action on gram-positive bacteria is potentiated by tetracycline.
11. Mechanisms of bacterial resistance to penicillins include
    1. elaboration of destructive enzymes.
    2. failure of antibiotic penetration.
    3. failure of antibiotic binding.
    4. elaboration of clavulanic acid.

JEREMY H. THOMPSON

60

Antibiotics That Interfere with Protein Synthesis: I

THE AMINOCYCLITOL AMINOGLYCOSIDES

The aminocyclitol aminoglycosides, usually called *aminoglycosides*, are highly polar polycations (*see* Chap. 3). Thus enteral absorption is poor, whereas absorption after parenteral injection is rapid. Additionally, aminoglycosides bind poorly to plasma proteins, are not metabolized *in vivo*, and depend on glomerular filtration for their elimination. Regretfully, these drugs have a very narrow therapeutic index, commonly producing severe ototoxicity and nephrotoxicity. Because of wide abuse, increasing resistance in both staphylococci and gram-negative bacteria has appeared in recent years. Several promising agents (sisomicin, 5-episisomicin, netilmicin, dibekacin, and UK 18-82) are undergoing evaluation.

CHEMISTRY AND NOMENCLATURE

The aminoglycosides contain either a nonamino hexose (streptose) as in *streptomycin*, or a diamino hexose (2-deoxystreptamine), with two or three additional amino sugars linked by single glycosidic bonds (Figure 60-1). Individual drugs are spelled with "mycin" if obtained from *Streptomyces* spp, or with "micin" if obtained from *Micromonospora* spp or semisynthetically. Based on their structure and properties, they can be divided into four groups (Table 60-1). All aminoglycosides have exposed hydroxyl and amino groups susceptible to attack by bacterial enzymes with loss of activity (*see* below).

The characteristics of the amino sugars confer important properties. Thus tobramycin is kanamycin B with an O at position 3′, and Amikacin is a semisynthetic derivative of kanamycin A where the L-amino group of 2-deoxystreptine is acylated with 2-hydroxy 4-aminobutyric acid; this minor change results in less susceptibility to destructive enzymes. Sisomicin is gen-

(*Text continues on p. 608*)

Selman Abraham Waksman, 1888–1973. Russian-born New Jersey microbiologist. In 1944 introduced streptomycin and went on to isolate many other antibiotics, including actinomycin, neomycin, and candicidin, work for which he won the Nobel Prize in 1952.

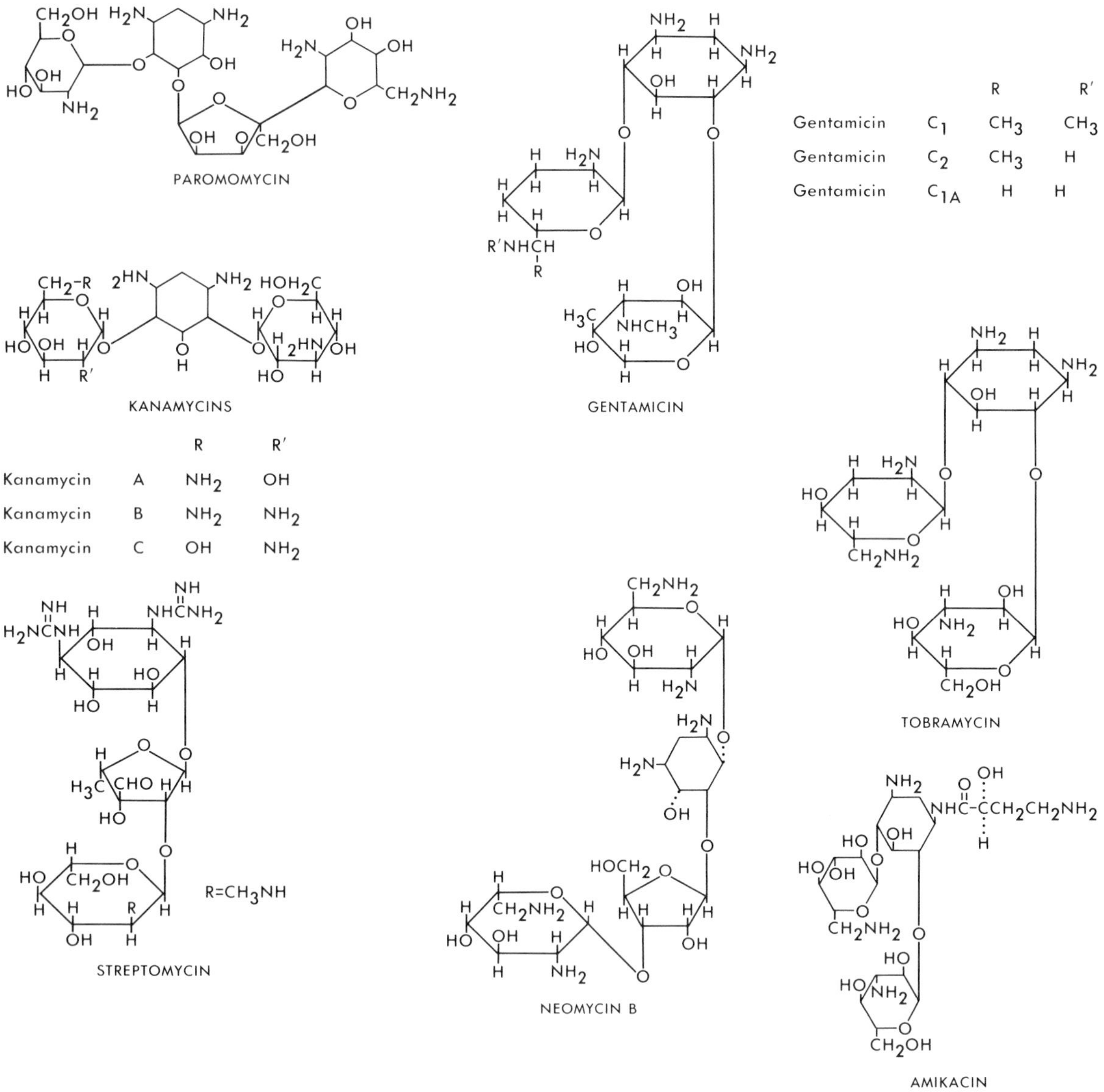

		R	R′
Kanamycin	A	NH_2	OH
Kanamycin	B	NH_2	NH_2
Kanamycin	C	OH	NH_2

		R	R′
Gentamicin	C_1	CH_3	CH_3
Gentamicin	C_2	CH_3	H
Gentamicin	C_{1A}	H	H

FIG. 60-1 Some important aminoglycosides.

TABLE 60-1. Some Important Aminoglycoside Antibiotics

Group/Drug	Source and Chemistry	Properties	Preparation/Uses
Streptomycin Group			
Streptomycin	Isolated in 1944 from *Streptomyces griseus* following a carefully planned screening of soil *actinomycetes.* A highly polar and complex glycosidic base usually prepared as the freely water-soluble sulfate or hydrochloride.	*See* text. Approximately 20% is degraded by unknown pathways. The remainder is excreted unchanged by glomerular filtration (70%) and by biliary excretion (10%). Resistance may develop so explosively that within two or three generations organisms are over 1000 times less sensitive. Development of mycobacterial resistance is delayed by the simultaneous use of one or more other antitubercular agents, but this is not necessarily true for other organisms. On exposure of sensitive bacteria to subinhibitory concentrations of streptomycin *in vitro,* a paradoxical stimulation of bacterial cell growth may be seen. Additionally, a state of dependence may develop with bacteria *requiring* the antibiotic for growth (*see* Chap. 57). Dependence is usually not permanent, since growth of organisms in subdependence-inducing concentrations usually results in a reversion to sensitive or resistant bacteria. The clinical importance of dependence is not clear.	Streptomycin sulfate, U.S.P., is available for use by various routes, the most important being i.m. Dosage depends on the infection, but it is seldom desirable (except in the treatment of tuberculosis or subacute bacterial endocarditis) to exceed the average adult dose of 0.5 to 1.0 g q 12 hr for 7 to 14 days, best given by deep i.m. injection. Sufficiently large doses must be given to prevent the development of bacterial resistance. Other limitations to its use are the risk of VIIIth cranial nerve damage and the preferred mode of administration (i.m.). Streptomycin is still an important drug for treating tuberculosis and for treating infections in patients hypersensitive to other drugs. Streptomycin is highly effective in tularemia, plague, severe brucellosis, granuloma inguinale, and, combined with penicillin, in *Strep. viridans* and enterococcal endocarditis. Oral preparations for the treatment of diarrheal diseases (some of which may be of viral origin) contain streptomycin, but the efficacy of this antibiotic for this purpose is unproved and may even be dangerous because of the generation of multiple antibiotic resistance (*see* Chap. 56). The many proprietary preparations containing fixed dosage ratios of penicillin and streptomycin should not be used.
Kanamycin Group			
Kanamycin	Three polybasic water-soluble antibiotics (Kanamycins A, B, C) are obtained from *Streptomyces kanamyceticus.*	The use of kanamycin has declined due to the emergence of bacterial resistance and with the introduction of more potent	Kanamycin sulfate, U.S.P. (Kantrex), is available for oral, i.m., and i.v. use. Kanamycin is occasionally used to treat infections

(continued)

TABLE 60-1. ***(Continued)***

Group/Drug	Source and Chemistry	Properties	Preparation/Uses
Kanamycin Group (continued)	In the U.S., less than 5% of commercial preparations are kanamycin B, whereas almost 95% are kanamycin A.	aminoglycosides. *See* text.	due to *E. coli, Klebsiella* spp., *Enterobacter,* atypical mycobacteria, *Proteus rettgeri,* and *Providencia* spp. and in tuberculosis. It is a toxic drug that should be reserved for infections resistant to less dangerous antibiotics or for use in patients allergic to other drugs. It is inactive against *Ps. aeruginosa.* Orally it is occasionally used to treat hepatic coma and in preoperative bowel "sterilization" (*see* neomycin). Intramuscular therapy (10–15 mg/kg daily in two or three divided doses for 7–14 days) should be carefully monitored by frequent determinations of renal function. Typically 1 g i.m. gives peak levels of 20 to 25 μg/ml within 60 minutes. A total daily dose of 1.5 g should not be exceeded irrespective of patient age, and a total dose of 15 g should not be exceeded for a single course of therapy. Optimum blood levels are probably in the range of 20 to 30 μg/ml. If VIIIth cranial nerve symptoms occur, kanamycin should be withdrawn immediately. Intravenous kanamycin should be reserved for the critically ill patient with a life-threatening infection. *It should be given in reduced dosage in the presence of renal failure.* The usual dose is 10 to 15 mg/kg daily in divided increments, given by slow infusion as a 0.25% solution.
Amikacin	Semisynthetically derived from kanamycin A by acylation of the 1-amino group of the hexose with	*See* text. Generally less potent than tobramycin or gentamicin but less susceptible to inactivating	Amikacin sulfate, U.S.P. (Amikin), is available in vials of 100, 500, and 1000 mg. Dosage must be carefully

(continued)

TABLE 60-1. *(Continued)*

Group/Drug	Source and Chemistry	Properties	Preparation/Uses
Kanamycin Group (continued)	2-hydroxy-4 amino-butyric acid.	enzymes. Serum levels are four-fold or five-fold higher than those obtained with tobramycin or gentamicin. Amikacin is concentrated in adipose tissue more avidly than are other aminoglycosides. Possesses activity against *Mycobacterium tuberculosis* and against atypical mycobacteria.	regulated based on renal function but is in the area of 5 mg/kg q 8 hr. Because of its relative resistance to inactivation by bacterial enzymes, amikacin should probably be reserved for treatment of infections (primarily gram-negative in nature) caused by gentamicin- or tobramycin-resistant strains.
Tobramycin	Derived from fermentation of *Streptomyces tenebrarius.*	*See* text. Following a dose of 1.5 mg/kg i.m., plasma levels of 4 to 8 μg/ml develop within about 90 minutes.	Tobramycin sulfate, U.S.P. (Nebcin), is available for i.m. and i.v. use. Doses are generally similar to those given for gentamicin. Aside from its range of uses as an aminoglycoside, tobramycin combined with a penicillin is effective in treating *Ps. aeruginosa.*
Gentamicin Group			
Gentamicin	A broad-spectrum, bactericidal antibiotic obtained from *Micromonospora purpurea* composed of three loosely related fractions: gentamicins C_1, C_2, and C_{1a}. All fractions have similar molecular weights and are highly water-soluble and stable in solution. Commercial preparations contain varying mixtures of the three fractions.	Gentamicin is probably the most widely used aminoglycoside. Following i.m. doses of 1 mg/kg, peak levels of 4 μg/ml develop within 60 minutes, but absorption can be variable, necessitating the determination of serum levels to monitor therapy in severe infections. Gentamicin is bound about 30% to plasma proteins and in normal persons has a half-life of 2 to 4 hours, with an apparent volume of distribution of 25% to 30% of body weight. Gentamicin is primarily excreted unchanged by glomerular filtration and, in patients with uremia, may have a half-life of 40 to 50 hours or longer. Either the tube dilution or agar diffusion tests are satisfactory for evaluating *in vitro* sensitivity to gentamicin. The Kirby/Bauer disk method yields irregular results.	Gentamicin sulfate, U.S.P. (Garamycin sulfate), is available in solutions of 40 mg/ml and as a 0.1% ointment and cream for topical use and 0.3% opthalmic formulations. The usual dose for parenteral administration is 5 mg/kg in three divided doses on Day 1 followed by 3 mg/kg from the 2nd day. For severe infections, 2 mg/kg q 8 hr may be given the 1st day irrespective of renal function. Thereafter, therapy should be monitored preferably by serum assays, attempting to maintain peak serum levels between 4 and 8 μg/ml. For severe bacterial meningitis, intrathecal gentamicin (4 mg) should be combined with i.m. therapy. Dosage must be drastically reduced in patients with renal insufficiency. Gentamicin is used topically in primary skin infections (*e.g.*, impetigo,

(continued)

TABLE 60-1. *(Continued)*

Group/Drug	Source and Chemistry	Properties	Preparation/Uses
Gentamicin Group (continued)		Slow stepwise resistance has been demonstrated *in vitro* for various organisms, an occurrence that has reduced its effectiveness for many infections. Explosive resistance as seen with streptomycin therapy apparently does not occur. Gentamicin may be active against bacteria resistant to streptomycin, kanamycin, and neomycin, but, if organisms are resistant to gentamicin, cross-resistance is invariably shown toward the other aminoglycosides, except possibly amikacin. VIIIth cranial nerve toxicity is commonly observed if trough/peak serum levels of gentamicin continually exceed 3 and 10 μg/ml, respectively.	ecthyma, pyoderma gangrenosum, sycosis barbae) and secondary skin infections (*e.g.*, pustular acne, pustular psoriasis). Gentamicin has no antifungal activity but is occasionally useful in treating the secondary bacterial infections superimposed on such conditions (*see* Chap. 69). The cream is preferable for moist areas and the ointment for dry locations. Topical gentamicin should be reserved for use in burn units and only in critically ill patients with *Pseudomonas, E. coli,* or *Klebsiella/Enterobacter* infections. It may, on occasion, be combined successfully with mafenide or silver nitrate. Parenteral gentamicin may be life-saving in patients with serious infections due to gram-negative bacilli such as *Pseudomonas aeruginosa, E. coli,* and *Klebsiella/Enterobacter* spp. resistant to less dangerous antibiotics. Carbenicillin may be given concomitantly to treat *Pseudomonas* infections; however, the two antibiotics must not be mixed in the same syringe because they interact and mutually destroy one another. Cephalosporins, heparin, and amphotericin B also inactivate gentamicin *in vitro.* When gram-negative meningeal infections resistant to chloramphenicol are suspected, for example, in neonates, subjects with meningomyelocoel, or postoperative neurosurgical patients, intrathecal gentamicin may be life-saving.

(*continued*)

TABLE 60-1. *(Continued)*

Group/Drug	Source and Chemistry	Properties	Preparation/Uses
Gentamicin Group (continued)			
Sisomicin	Semisynthetic	Demonstrates cross-resistance with gentamicin. May be more active than gentamicin against *Ps. aeruginosa*. Highly toxic.	Not yet released in U.S.
Netilmicin	Semisynthetic	Active against some gentamicin- and tobramycin-resistant strains. May be less ototoxic and nephrotoxic than other agents.	Not yet released in U.S.
Neomycin Group			
Neomycin	Neomycins A, B, and C are closely related, water-soluble, polybasic antibiotics obtained from *Streptomyces fradiae*. Neomycins B and C are isomers. Commercial preparations contain about 90% of neomycin B, the remainder being neomycin C.	Never given parenterally because of its high nephrotoxicity. Topical use occasionally produces sensitivity reactions and cross-sensitivity with other aminoglycosides. Sufficient absorption occurs with oral therapy to produce nephrotoxicity in patients with diminished renal function. Oral neomycin commonly produces gastrointestinal upsets and suprainfection with staphylococci or fungi. Rarely, a patchy or generalized malabsorption syndrome resembling nontropical sprue may develop; normal bowel function returns when therapy is stopped, but a gluten-free diet or glucocorticosteroids have no effect. Oral neomycin may depress intestinal disaccharidase activity through direct damage to the small-intestinal brush border. Neomycin precipitates bile acids and may produce temporary hypocholesterolemia due to decreased sterol absorption.	Neomycin sulfate, U.S.P. (Mycifradin), is available for topical and oral administration and for local instillation into closed cavities such as the bladder. Topically (0.5% creams or ointments, q 8 hr) neomycin is highly effective for a variety of skin, external ear, and conjunctival infections, and preparations are often combined with other antibiotics, sulfonamides, and cortisone. Neomycin (2–4 g q 8 hr) is used mainly to reduce urease- and ammonia-producing organisms such as *Proteus* and *Klebsiella* sp in patients with cirrhosis and in *E. coli* gastroenteritis. Additionally, neomycin with other drugs, such as erythromycin or tetracyclines, is advocated for preoperative bowel "preparation" since there is some evidence that its use is associated with a reduced incidence of septic complications following colonic surgery.
Paromomycin	*See* Chap. 67.		
Lividomycin	Experimental use only		
Ribostamycin	Experimental use only		

tamicin with an unsaturated bond in the diamino sugar between 4′ and 5′, and this minor change yields in sensitive organisms more efficient drug uptake, greater *in vitro* sensitivity, and a greater bactericidal effect. In netilmicin the substitution of an ethyl group yields stability to three of five enzymes commonly associated with resistance in *Ps. aeruginosa,* and enterobacteriaceae.

MODE OF ACTION

Aminoglycosides are bactericidal, but their exact mechanism of action is not known. They bind to the 30 S ribosome and cause interference with protein synthesis through a misreading of the genetic code. Additionally, they alter the bacterial cell membrane, either secondary to inhibition of protein synthesis or directly by combining with membrane anionic groups (*see* Chap. 57). They also block energy production at the pyruvate-oxalacetic acid step of the Krebs' cycle.

Transport of aminoglycosides intracellularly in bacteria depends on a passive step and two energy-dependent steps. Sensitive bacteria possess all three and can concentrate the antibiotics up to 250-fold; many resistant bacteria lack the second energy-dependent step. The rate and degree of antibiotic concentration generally parallels *in vitro* sensitivity. Importantly, uptake kinetics can be significantly influenced by osmolality, oxygen tension, the presence of cations, and *p*H. For example, *in vitro* there is approximately, (depending on the antibiotic) a tenfold to eightyfold increase in potency in going from *p*H 5.5 to 8.0. Consequently, in the treatment of urinary tract infections, the concomitant administration of urinary alkalinizers is usually advised. Low (subinhibitory) concentrations of streptomycin rarely produce dependence.

ANTIBACTERIAL SPECTRUM

The aminoglycosides are broad-spectrum antibiotics (Table 60-2) but the use of some agents should be restricted. Generally, gentamicin, amikacin, and tobramycin are highly effective against aerobic gram-negative microorganisms. *Providencia* spp. *Ps. cepacia, Ps. maltophilia,* and many gram-positive cocci are usually resistant. Tobramycin is the most active against *Ps. aeruginosa,* whereas kanamycin is inactive. Streptomycin and occasionally kanamycin are used in tuberculosis, and kanamycin is effective in atypical mycobacterial infections particularly due to *Myco. kansasii.* Aminoglycosides commonly exhibit a synergistic effect against some organisms when supplemented with a penicillin or vancomycin. This was demonstrated originally with Penicillin G + streptomycin against *Strep. fecalis.*

Chloramphenicol, by preventing release of proteins from the ribosome, may diminish the activity of tobramycin and gentamicin.

TABLE 60-2. Organisms Affected by Aminoglycosides

Acinetobacter spp.	*L. monocytogenase*
Aeromonas spp.	*Moraxella* spp.
Alcaligenes spp.	*M. tuberculosis*
Brucella spp.	*Mycoplasma* spp.
Citrobacter	*N. gonorrhoeae*
Diplococcus pneumoniae	*N. meningitidis*
E. coli	*Pr. mirabilis*
Enterobacter spp.	*Pr. vulgaris*
Erysipelothrix	*Ps. aeruginosa*
Herellea spp.	*Salmonella* spp.
H. ducreyi	*Serratia* spp.
H. influenzae	*Shigella* spp.
K. granulomatis	*Staph. aureus*
K. pneumoniae	*Staph. epidermidis*

RESISTANCE

Three main mechanisms of natural or acquired resistance have been identified. The most important is *elaboration of destructive enzymes.* Resistant bacteria possess 1 or more of 11 enzymes outside their cell membrane (periplasmic space) at or near sites of drug transport. These enzymes *adenylate, acetylate,* or *phosphorylate* up to six exposed amino or hydroxyl groups on the glycosidic rings, thereby modifying the antibiotic so that it cannot bind to ribosomes. Gentamicin and tobramycin possess several amino or hydroxyl groups, whereas amikacin possesses only two. Enzymes can be constitutive or acquired through plasmids (*see* Chap. 56). Because enzyme kinetics differ for various aminoglycosides, many bacteria that possess inactivating enzymes are still susceptible to these antibiotics.

Reduction in intracellular transport (per-

HANS ADOLF KREBS, 1900–1981. German-born English biochemist, once assistant to Otto Warburg. As well as the tricarboxylic acid cycle (Krebs' cycle), he discovered the ornithine cycle of urea synthesis in mammalian liver. Won the Nobel Prize, with F. A. Lipmann, in 1953.

meability block) is the second most important mechanism; for example, streptomycin fails to penetrate *Ps. aeruginosa*, and some resistant organisms exclude amikacin. Permeability block may be overcome *in vitro* by increasing the concentration of the antibiotic. *In vivo* permeability block may be transferred by R factors.

Finally, bacterial *ribosomes may undergo mutation* so that they do not bind the aminoglycoside. For example, single-step mutants have been isolated that involve a single amino acid. This mechanism is not too important, and, if present, no synergistic effects can be seen with the penicillins.

Bacteria frequently develop permanent resistance to aminoglycosides. In any large population of microorganisms, naturally occurring, single-step, high-level resistant mutants appear and are rapidly selected. Resistance is more common with multiple exposure or prolonged therapy and is one of the most common reasons for therapeutic failure.

Cross-resistance is variable within the group, but gentamicin and tobramycin frequently show cross-resistance. Resistance to amikacin is least common.

ABSORPTION

Since the aminoglycosides are polar cations, absorption following oral administration is insignificant (less than 3%). Additionally, since little is destroyed in the bowel lumen, streptomycin, neomycin, kanamycin, and paromomycin may be given orally for a local effect in the gastrointestinal tract. However, sufficient neomycin is absorbed following oral administration to produce toxicity in patients with renal insufficiency. If systemic activity is required, streptomycin, kanamycin, gentamicin, tobramicin, and amikacin must be given intramuscularly or intravenously (or rarely subcutaneously), where peak absorption develops within 30 to 90 minutes. Neomycin and gentamicin may be applied topically, but streptomycin commonly induces hypersensitivity reactions by this route. Neomycin is occasionally instilled into closed cavities such as the bladder.

DISTRIBUTION AND METABOLISM

Because of their polar nature, the aminoglycosides are essentially distributed in extracellular fluid. However, they are concentrated in the renal cortex, and in the aural endolymph and perilymph, often up to 20 times simultaneous plasma levels; even with chronic therapy and local inflammation, levels in other tissues are poor. Penetration into the cerebrospinal fluid should not be relied upon. Aminoglycosides are bound to plasma proteins about 0 to 20% and to red blood cells about 5% to 10%. Unless aminoglycoside dosage is calculated on lean body weight, plasma drug levels will be higher in obese patients. Additionally, plasma aminoglycoside levels will be reduced in the presence of an expanded extracellular fluid volume (anasarca, edema) and increased in states of dehydration. Since the aminoglycosides bind to red cells, plasma drug levels are inversely proportional to the hematocrit. The aminoglycosides are not metabolized *in vivo*.

EXCRETION

The aminoglycosides are cleared by glomerular filtration (with some tubular reabsorption), and urine levels may reach 200 μg/ml. Clearance is about two thirds that of creatinine. Aminoglycosides have a biologic T½ of 2 to 4 hours in adults (except in the renal cortex and inner ear, where it may be 8 to 28 hours) and 5 to 12 hours in neonates. The biologic T½ may be reduced in patients with cystic fibrosis. Between 60% and 90% of any given dose is excreted unchanged within 24 hours. Aminoglycosides are slowly removed by hemodialysis or peritoneal dialysis.

Because of the dependence of these agents on renal excretion, dosage must be critically controlled to maintain adequate therapeutic levels with minimum toxicity. Various nomograms of posology have been delineated but are too complex to discuss here. Therapy is often difficult to control in ill patients with rapidly altering fluid and electrolyte balance and renal function.

Generally, peak and trough blood aminoglycoside levels should be checked after three to five doses and again after 5 days of therapy. Thereafter they should be checked as clinically indicated but usually twice per week, and always within 24 hours of changing the dose. Therapy should be calculated on lean body weight because any alteration in extracellular fluid volume will affect blood levels (*see* above).

ADVERSE EFFECTS

The major limiting factor in the use of aminoglycosides is their propensity to damage the kidney and the middle ear. Toxicity is dose dependent other than for hypersensitivity reactions.

Central and Peripheral Nervous System

Both divisions of the VIIIth cranial nerve may be damaged by all aminoglycosides (3–30% of courses); however amikacin, tobramycin, kanamycin, and neomycin are predominantly cochleotoxic, whereas streptomycin and gentamicin, are predominantly vestibulotoxic. The exact mechanism of toxicity is not known, but the antibiotics are concentrated in the inner ear and have a long T½ in this tissue (*see* above). Single doses of aminoglycosides can be shown to depress the VIII cranial nerve function in animal models, and in humans streptomycin in daily doses of 2 g produces acute labyrinthine dysfunction within 1 month. Cochleotoxic aminoglycosides result in loss of high-frequency sounds (outside the conversation range) initially, a loss detected only by careful audiometric examination. With continuing therapy lower frequency sounds are gradually affected, and deafness may ensue rapidly. To monitor aminoglycoside therapy a pretherapeutic audiogram is desirable, particularly in those over 40 years old. Severe toxicity is irreversible; once sensory cells have been destroyed, they cannot regenerate. Detection of early signs and symptoms of toxicity, and termination of antibiotic therapy (where clinically possible) may result in some restoration of function. Children are less susceptible to ototoxicity than are adults.

Early symptoms of cochleotoxicity are *tinnitus* and *pressure or fullness* in the ears. Early symptoms of vestibulotoxicity are *nausea, vomiting, vertigo*, and *Ménières-like* disease; *nystagmus* is invariably seen.

Aminoglycoside-induced ototoxicity probably predisposes to later hearing loss. Predisposing factors for ototoxicity are previous aminoglycoside or other ototoxic drug use such as ethacrynic acid, furosemide, or mannitol, ear disease, particularly infections, high aminoglycoside peak and trough blood levels, renal disease, intrathecal therapy (rare today), dehydration, older age (age loss of hair cells), and possibly exposure to excessive noise.

Aminoglycosides may rarely cause peripheral neuritis, facial and peripheral paresthesia, and optic neuritis. Intrathecal therapy may be followed by chemical meningitis, radiculitis, transverse or patchy myelitis, seizures, and encephalopathy.

Neuromuscular Blockade

All aminoglycosides inhibit the prejunctional release of acetylcholine and depress postsynaptic sensitivity to this hormone. Thus they may induce a curare-like neuromuscular block (*see* Chap. 19), particularly when given intraperitoneally in large doses postoperatively to patients who have received neuromuscular blocking agents. The paralysis is partially reversed by i.v. calcium salts or cholinesterase inhibitors (*see* Chap. 15). Death may, however, result from ventilatory paralysis. In patients with myasthenia gravis, aminoglycosides may induce a dramatic increase in skeletal muscle weakness.

Nephrotoxicity

The concentration of aminoglycosides in the renal cortex parallels their ability to produce nephrotoxicity. Neomycin is the most toxic, and, even though only trace quantities of this agent are absorbed after oral, topical, or intravesical administration, nephrotoxicity may develop in the presence of diminished renal function. Other aminoglycosides ranked in order of decreasing nephrotoxicity (from animal experiments) are tobramycin, kanamycin, gentamicin, and amikacin.

Predisposing factors to nephrotoxicity are high trough concentrations (there is poor correlation with peak aminoglycoside plasma levels), length of therapy, preexisting renal disease, concomitant use of other nephrotoxic drugs, particularly diuretics (ethacrynic acid, furosemide, and mannitol) and antibiotics, shock, dehydration, and oliguria. Symptoms and signs of nephrotoxicity are an inability to concentrate urine, proteinurea, the appearance of casts, and a rising serum BUN level.

Miscellaneous Effects and Drug Interactions

Intravenous administration may produce transient hypotension. Pain occurs on i.m. injection, and injection sites should be alternated to minimize the development of sterile abscesses. Gastrointestinal irritation usually follows oral therapy. Suprainfection, primarily with staphylococci and fungi, occurs in about 5% of cases. Rarely aminoglycosides may produce a consumption coagulopathy.

Aminoglycosides potentiate skeletal muscle relaxants (*see* above and Chap. 19). Heparin, amphotericin B, and some penicillins (especially carbenicillin and ticarcillin) and cephalosporins inactivate aminoglycosides (gentamicin, tobramycin, and amikacin) *in vitro*.

HYPERSENSITIVITY

The most important hypersensitivity reactions are various skin rashes (in about 7% of patients), particularly maculopapular, erythematous, and urticarial lesions; contact dermatitis (particularly to streptomycin) in pharmacists, nurses, and physicians who handle the drugs frequently; exfoliative dermatitis; stomatitis; drug fever; eosinophilia; angioneurotic edema; serum sickness; lymphadenopathy; and anaphylactic shock. Granulocytopenia may progress to agranulocytosis; aplastic anemia, thrombocytopenic purpura, and hypoprothrombinemia occur rarely. Hypersensitivity reactions usually occur together but may appear individually.

TREATMENT OF TUBERCULOSIS

Treatment of tuberculosis is a complex, long-term procedure primarily because of the characteristics of the causative organism, the nature and course of the disease process, and the unpredictability of host defense mechanisms. Drug treatment is the cornerstone of therapy, surgical intervention being required only rarely, but many factors must be considered in treatment, since the disease is frequently associated with poverty, malnutrition, inadequate housing, or other disease states.

Drug treatment of tuberculosis is twofold: therapy of active disease and prophylaxis.

TREATMENT OF ACTIVE DISEASE

Antitubercular drugs effectively treat active disease and control infectiousness. They are clinically divided into first-line (primary) and second-line (secondary) drugs (Table 60-3), depending on their efficacy and degree of toxicity.

Between 5% and 10% of patients with primary tuberculosis yield cultures resistant to one first-line drug. Therefore, it may be best to initiate therapy with three primary drugs, thus ensuring that at least two drugs to which the mycobacteria are susceptible are given. However, the use of three or two first-line drugs is controversial. Initial therapy should be continued in the dosage given in Table 60-4 for between 6 weeks to 6 months, depending on the location and severity of the disease. Long-term continuation therapy can then be initiated for 1 to 2 years, again depending on the location and severity of the infection.

The use of two or three first-line drugs in the treatment of active disease is paramount, first to reduce the development of mycobacterial resistance and second to produce a potentiated tuberculostatic effect. Mycobacterial sensitivity should be determined in fresh cases and periodically in chronic cases, but results of testing are often unreliable, and greater weight should be placed on clinical response and radiologic findings.

The simultaneous use of the three primary drugs is justified in severe overwhelming infections and in new cases of active disease before the results of sensitivity tests or when there is some indication that resistance to one of the primary drugs may be present.

Isoniazid, streptomycin, and PAS are time-honored first-line drugs, but because of the difficulties of administering streptomycin and the problems associated with the use of PAS, these last two agents are being replaced by rifampin

TABLE 60-3. First- and Second-Line Antitubercular Drugs

First Line	Second Line
Isoniazid (INAH)	Pyrazinamide
Streptomycin	Ethionamide
Para-aminosalicylic acid (PAS)	Cycloserine
Ethambutol	Kanamycin
Rifampin	Viomycin
	Capreomycin

TABLE 60-4. Dosage of Antitubercular Drugs

Drug	Total Dose	Details of Administration
Streptomycin	1 g	Patients < 40 yr, daily for 1st mo, then 3/wk
	0.75 g	Patients > 40 yr, daily for 1st mo, then 3/wk
	1 g	2 or 3/wk with high dose isoniazid
Sodium PAS	12–16 g	In 2–4 divided doses daily
Isoniazid*	300 mg	In 1 or 3 divided doses daily
	15 mg/kg	2 or 3/wk with streptomycin
Ethambutol	25 mg/kg	Single dose daily for first 2 mo
	15 mg/kg	Single dose daily after 2 mo
Rifampin	600 mg	Single dose daily

(Modified from Citron KM: Tuberculosis. Br Med J 2:296–298, 1973)

* Pyridoxine 10 mg/100 mg isoniazid/day should be added to minimize nerve toxicity.

and ethambutol. Both rifampin and ethambutol are expensive.

Secondary drugs are used after mycobacterial resistance to primary drugs develops or in the presence of allergy to the primary drugs. All secondary drugs exhibit low potency, and most are considerably more toxic than primary ones and must be withdrawn after several months. It is usually advantageous to combine three secondary drugs, but in practice various combinations of primary and secondary drugs are used. Secondary drugs may be valuable in giving short-term chemotherapeutic cover during the surgical removal of tubercular tissue.

Drug Resistance

Resistance to antitubercular drugs is a major therapeutic problem. Patterns of drug resistance show striking differences in different populations. For example, the higher incidence of drug resistance in India and the Near East may reflect the added hazards of poor housing and nutrition as well as (possibly) irregular and inconstant self-medication. In the United States, resistant organisms are reportedly more common in blacks than in whites. As indicated above, the use of a second drug tends only to reduce the likelihood of emergence of drug resistance; *it will not prevent its occurrence.* Mycobacteria resistant to isoniazid may be less pathogenic than isoniazid susceptible organisms. *Uncontrolled intermittent therapy and failure to take both or all antitubercular drugs favor the development of resistant strains and are the principal causes of therapeutic failure.*

Use of Corticosteroid Drugs

Adrenocorticosteroid drugs are frequently advocated as adjunctive agents to treat tuberculosis, to reduce symptoms and inflammatory adhesions, and to facilitate healing of caseous foci. Aside from their indispensability in adrenal insufficiency, their value is debatable. Many authorities believe that if mycobacteria are highly sensitive to primary drugs, a short concomitant course of corticosteroids is valuable in tuberculous meningitis with intraspinal or intracisternal block, in tuberculous pneumonia, or in miliary tuberculosis. Corticosteroids depress the tuberculin reaction.

If glucocorticosteroids are required for nontuberculous disease in a patient with either inactive tuberculosis or a positive skin test, these agents need not be withheld provided adequate prophylactic therapy with isoniazid (300 mg/day for the duration of steroid therapy and continued for an additional 6 months) is undertaken. Glucocorticosteroids may be of symptomatic benefit in the treatment of allergies to antitubercular drugs.

PROPHYLAXIS

Prophylaxis with isoniazid or isoniazid plus PAS is often undertaken to prevent the development of active tuberculosis in persons at high risk. Prophylaxis can either be primary (prevention of infection) or secondary (prevention of disease in an infected patient) and should usually be continued for at least 1 year. There is some debate as to who should receive prophylactic therapy and as to the dosage and time sequence of therapy.

A strong case can be made for prophylaxis in the following situations: recent skin test converters; contacts, especially young children, and all subjects with positive skin tests in the following categories: adolescent females, children with measles or who receive measles vaccine, pregnant women (treatment is started in the last trimester and continued for 1 year), patients with silicosis, lymphoma, or unstable diabetes mellitus, and postgastrectomy patients or those taking glucocorticosteroids.

Conventionally, isoniazid alone, 100 mg q 8 hr is used; PAS 4 g q 8 hr is added by some authorities. However, since patient compliance on daily therapy is far from 100%, it has been suggested that large doses of two antitubercular drugs be given twice or three times a week (preferably supervised by a physician or a Public Health employee) to minimize the development of mycobacterial resistance. Recommended twice weekly therapy has been either isoniazid, 15 mg/kg plus PAS 12 g, or isoniazid, 15 mg/kg plus streptomycin 1 g (Table 60-4). The intermittent nature of twice weekly therapy is apparently not followed by a higher incidence of drug resistance, since there is a delay of several days in the establishment of logarithmic growth in mycobacteria after clearance of antitubercular drugs.

TREATMENT OF ATYPICAL MYCOBACTERIA

Atypical mycobacterial infections are difficult to treat. *In vitro* testing and clinical effectiveness frequently correlate poorly, particularly with infections caused by the Battey strain. The five primary drugs are usually administered concomitantly. Pyrazinamide or cycloserine may replace PAS. Treatment is complicated by the high degree of mycobacterial resistance, the need for surgical intervention in localized disease, and even with sensitive strains the need for a prolonged course of drug exposure.

FURTHER READING

1. Appel GB, Neu HC: Gentamicin in 1978. Ann Intern Med 89:528–538, 1978
2. Barza M, Laurermann M: Why monitor serum levels of gentamicin? Clin Pharmacokinet 3:202–215, 1978
3. Citron KM: Tuberculosis. Br Med J 2:296–298, 1973
4. Jackson GG: Present status of aminoglycoside antibiotics and their safe, effective use. Clin Ther 1:200–215, 1977
5. Pechere JC, Dugal R: Clinical pharmacokinetics of aminoglycoside antibiotics. Clin Pharmacokinet 4:170–199, 1979

CHAPTER 60 QUESTIONS

(See P. 7 for Full Instructions)

Select the One Best Answer

1. Systemic action of streptomycin is terminated mainly by
   A. inactivation by resistant bacteria.
   B. glomerular filtration.
   C. inactivation by the liver.
   D. biliary excretion.
   E. renal tubular secretion.

2. Characteristics of aminoglycoside antibiotics include all of the following EXCEPT
   A. poor absorption after oral administration.
   B. extensive metabolism *in vivo*.
   C. dependence on glomerular filtration for their elimination.
   D. commonly produce severe ototoxicity.
   E. commonly produce severe nephrotoxicity.

3. The major limiting factor in the use of aminoglycosides is
   A. cost.
   B. rapid emergence of resistant bacteria.
   C. their narrow antibacterial spectrum.
   D. propensity to damage the kidney and middle ear.
   E. rapid urinary secretion.

4. Which of the following statement pertaining to the use of aminoglycosides is false?
   A. Plasma aminoglycoside levels will be reduced in the presence of an expanded extracellular fluid volume.
   B. Plasma drug levels are inversely proportional to the hematocrit.
   C. Peak and trough blood aminoglycoside levels should be checked after three to five doses and again after 5 days of therapy.
   D. Dosage should be calculated on lean body weight.
   E. The drugs are primarily cleared by hepatic metabolism.

A = 1,2,3; B = 1,3; C = 2,4; D = 4; E = All

5. Prolonged therapy with streptomycin alone increases the probability of
   1. developing vertigo and ataxia.
   2. renal failure.
   3. the emergence of resistant strains of *M. tuberculosis*.
   4. hemolytic anemia.

6. Neomycin
   1. is a secondary drug for treating diarrhea caused by *E. coli*.
   2. is commonly used parenterally.
   3. produces vestibular toxicity after oral administration.
   4. may produce respiratory paralysis when used postoperatively to irrigate the peritoneal cavity.

7. Gentamicin is
   1. rapidly absorbed orally.
   2. inactivated when mixed in the same bottle with carbenicillin.
   3. more potent than tobramycin against *Pseudomonas aeruginosa*.
   4. nephrotoxic.

8. Drugs that may cause deafness include
   1. kanamycin.
   2. streptomycin.
   3. gentamicin.
   4. furosemide.

9. Renal damage may be produced by parenteral therapy with
   1. polymyxin B.
   2. neomycin.
   3. streptomycin.
   4. kanamycin.

10. Aminoglycoside antibiotics are bactericidal. Proposed mechanisms of action include

1. binding to the 30S ribosome.
2. alteration in bacterial cell membrane function.
3. blockade of cellular energy production.
4. interference with bacterial cell wall formation.

11. Bacterial resistance to aminoglycosides has been shown to be due to
    1. elaboration of destructive enzymes.
    2. reduction in intracellular antibiotic transport.
    3. ribosomal mutational change.
    4. enzymatic adaption so that the organism uses the antibiotic.

12. First-line drugs to be used in the treatment of tuberculosis include
    1. isoniazid.
    2. streptomycin.
    3. rifampin.
    4. cycloserine.

JEREMY H. THOMPSON

61

Antibiotics That Interfere with Protein Synthesis: II

Several important antibiotics that inhibit protein synthesis are presented herein. Some specific drug interactions are given in Table 61-1.

THE TETRACYCLINES

Tetracyclines were originally isolated from various species of *Streptomyces* (Fig. 61-1). Several semisynthetic derivatives were then developed (some of which were subsequently identified from natural sources) and introduced into therapy. There are seven major tetracycline antibiotics (Table 61-2), and the generic term tetracycline is used to describe the group. A single, unified description of this class of compounds is possible since there are only minor differences in properties among the individual members; these are discussed in the text and in Fig. 61-1 and Tables 61-2 and 61-3.

CHEMISTRY

Tetracycline crystalline bases are yellowish, odorless, and slightly bitter compounds. They are poorly water soluble but readily form highly soluble sodium and hydrochloride salts. Dry powders are highly stable, but aqueous solutions usually show appreciable loss of activity within 24 to 48 hours, particularly at an elevated *p*H.

ANTIBACTERIAL SPECTRUM AND RESISTANCE

The tetracyclines are *broad-spectrum antibiotics* with an antibacterial spectrum that overlaps those of the penicillins and cephalosporins, the aminoglycosides, and chloramphenicol (Table 61-3). Gram-positive bacteria are usually more affected by lower concentrations of the antibiotics than are gram-negative species. *Broad spectrum* must not be confused with *license* for broad nonspecific use (*see* Chap. 56).

The incidence of bacterial resistance is increasing. Typically resistant are *E. coli, Shigella spp.*, *β-Hemolytic strep.*, *D. pneumoniae*, *N. gonorrhoeae*, and *Bacteroides spp*. The abuse of tetracyclines (primarily because of their broad antibacterial spectrum) and their indiscriminant use in animals and animal feeds (*see* Chap. 56) may be partly responsible for increasing resistance.

Bacterial resistance develops in a slow, stepwise manner, as with penicillin. (Mechanisms of resistance are discussed in Chapter 56.) Organisms resistant to one tetracycline are almost invariably resistant to equipotent concentrations of other tetracyclines. Very rarely, organisms that depend on chlortetracycline have been isolated from humans but are of no clinical import. Bacteria may show varying susceptibility to the different tetracyclines on *in vitro* testing, but how important these differences are in clinical infections is uncertain.

TABLE 61-1. Potential Drug Interactions with Tetracyclines, Macrolides, and Chloramphenicol

Antibiotic	Second Drug	Comment
Oral tetracyclines	Oral hematinics containing iron	Nonabsorbable iron-tetracycline chelate formed
Oral tetracyclines	Aluminum, magnesium, and calcium-containing antacids	Nonabsorbable metal–tetracycline chelate formed
Oral tetracyclines	Sodium bicarbonate	Reduced disintegration, dissolution of tetracycline, and therefore reduced antibiotic bioavailability
Doxycycline	Enzyme inducers, *i.e.*, chronic ethanol ingestion	Shortened T½ of the tetracycline
A tetracycline	A penicillin or other bactericidal antibiotic	Reduced *in vivo* activity of the bactericidal antibiotic
Oral tetracyclines	Hypoprothrombinemic anticoagulants	Potentiation of hypothrombinemic effect due to antibiotic inactivation of bowel flora
Chloramphenicol	Dicoumarol, phenytoin, tolbutamide, tricyclic antidepressants	Prolongation of T½ of second drug due to chloramphenicol-induced inhibition of of its metabolism
Chloramphenicol	Enzyme inducers	Shortened T½ of chloramphenicol
Triacetyloleandomycin (TAO) and erythromycin	Theophylline	Prolonged T½ of theophylline possibly due to reduced metabolism

TABLE 61-2. Popular Oral and Parenteral Tetracycline Preparations

	Doses for Oral Administration		Doses for Parenteral Administration*	
Drug	***Loading***	***Maintenance***	***i.v.***	***i.m.***
	←	mg		→
Chlortetracycline hydrochloride, *N.F.*	500	250–500, 6 hourly	Must be freshly prepared since relatively unstable; 250–500, 12 hourly	100, 8 hourly
Demeclocycline hydrochloride, *N.F.*	600	150–300, 6–12 hourly	—	—
Doxycycline	100–200	100 mg, 12–24 hourly	—	—
Methacycline hydrochloride, *N.F.*	300	150, 6 hourly	—	—
Minocycline	200	100 mg, 12 hourly	—	—
Oxytetracycline hydrochloride *U.S.P.*	500	250–500, 6 hourly	250–500, 12 hourly	100, 8 hourly
Tetracycline hydrochloride, *U.S.P.*	500	250–500, 6 hourly	250–500, 12 hourly	100, 8 hourly
Tetracycline phosphate complex	500	250–500, 6 hourly	—	—

* Do not give more than 2 g of tetracycline/day parenterally, since this is likely to produce hepatic damage.

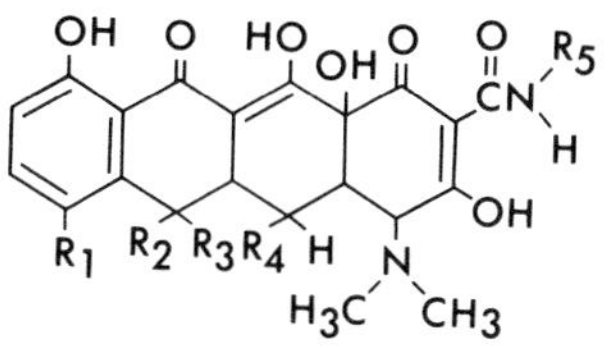

Drug	Source	Plasma protein binding (%)	Renal clearance (ml/min)	Half-life (hr)	R_1	R_2	R_3	R_4	R_5
					SUBSTITUTIONS				
Chlortetracycline (1948)	*Streptomyces aureofaciens*	40–70	30	4–6	Cl	CH_3	OH	H	H
Oxytetracycline (1950)	*Streptomyces rimosus*	20–35	85	8–10	H	CH_3	OH	OH	H
Tetracycline (1952)	Semisynthetically derived from chlor-tetracycline	25–60	60	8– 9	H	CH_3	OH	H	H
Demeclocycline (1959)	*Streptomyces aureofaciens*	40–90	25–35	10–17	Cl	H	OH	H	H
Methacycline (1961)	Semisynthetically derived from oxytetracycline	75–90	30	10–16	H	CH_2	H	OH	H
Doxycycline (1966)	Hydrogenation of methacycline	25–90	20–30	12–20	H	CH_3	H	OH	H
Minocycline (1970)	Semisynthetically derived from tetracycline	70–75	10	12–19	N $(CH_3)_2$	H	H	H	H

FIG. 61-1. The major tetracycline antibiotics. The year of introduction into therapeutics is indicated in parenthesis.

TABLE 61-3. Common Organisms Affected by the Tetracyclines

Organism	Sensitivity*	Organism	Sensitivity*
Actinobacillus malleii	++	*Leptospira icterohemorrhagiae*	+
Actinomyces israelii	+++	*Listeria monocytogenes*	++
Enterobacter aerogenes	++R	*Lymphogranuloma venereum*	+++
Bacillus anthracis	++	*Mima–Herellae*	++
Bacteroides spp.	++R	*Mycoplasma pneumoniae*	+++
Balantidium coli	++	*Neisseria gonorrhoeae*†	++R
Borrelia recurrentis	+++	*Neisseria meningitidis*‡	++
Brucella spp.	+++R	*Nocardia asteroides*§	+++
Chlamydia (Bedsonia)	+++	*Pasturella pestis*	++
Cholera vibrio	+++	*Pasturella tularensis*	+++
Calymmatobacterium granulomatis	+++	*Pseudomonas pseudomallei*	+++
Clostridium perfringens	++	*Psittacosis/ornithosis*	+++
Clostridium tetani	++	*Rickettsia*	+++
Escherichia coli	++R	*Salmonella*	++R
Entameba histolytica	++	*Shigella*	++R
Hemophilus duceyi	++	*Straphylococcus aureus*	+R
Hemophilus influenzae	+++R	*Streptococcus*	++R
Inclusion conjunctivitis	+++	*Treponema pallidum*	+
Klebsiella pneumoniae	++R	*Treponema pertenue*	+

* R = in vitro testing essential because many strains are resistant.
+++ = high sensitivity.
++ = moderate sensitivity.
+ = some sensitivity, but tetracyclines not recommended for therapy.
† Minocycline in penicillin-allergic patient.
‡ Minocycline for the carrier state.
§ Minocycline.

For example, on a weight basis minocycline is more active than other tetracyclines against many strains of staphylococci, most other gram-positive cocci (except enterococci), and many gram-negative bacilli, except *Proteus* spp.

MODE OF ACTION

The tetracyclines variably disrupt protein synthesis by blocking the binding of tRNA: amino acid complexes to the ribosome (*see* Chap. 57) and may additionally disrupt the bacterial cell membrane by complexing essential divalent metals. They are usually bacteriostatic but under exceptional circumstances may be bactericidal.

ABSORPTION, METABOLISM, DISTRIBUTION, AND EXCRETION

Generally the tetracyclines are incompletely and irregularly absorbed after oral administration, with as much as 30% being excreted unchanged. Absorption, however, is usually adequate to treat most infections. Absorption is depressed by food (least for doxycycline), calcium, magnesium, iron, zinc, and aluminum salts and slightly by milk, since the tetracyclines form nonabsorbable chelates with heavy metals. The addition of phosphate (as in tetracycline phosphate complex) may partially neutralize this chelating effect. In order of decreasing absorbability are doxycycline, minocycline, methacycline, demeclocycline, tetracycline, chlortetracycline, and oxytetracycline.

A single oral dose of 100 mg of doxycycline produces plasma levels similar to 300 mg twice daily of demeclocycline and 250 mg four times daily of chlortetracycline, tetracycline, and oxytetracycline. The prolonged plasma levels seen with doxycycline and demeclocycline are primarily due to slow renal excretion (Fig. 61-1), making these agents effective for outpatient use. Methacycline has a long half-life that results from high plasma protein binding.

For i.v. administration the tetracycline solution should be less than 5 mg/ml to minimize thrombophlebitis. Intramuscular tetracycline is effective but painful; the antibiotic can be detected in plasma within about 15 minutes, and peak levels develop within 60 minutes. Chlortetracycline is poorly absorbed from i.m. sites.

Generally the tetracyclines have a slightly larger volume of distribution than that of total body water, and doxycycline and minocycline are significantly distributed in fat. Tetracyclines are cleared by the liver (minocycline most effectively); thus high antibiotic concentrations occur in both hepatic parenchyma and bile, reaching one to three times simultaneous plasma levels. Biliary excretion results in a diminishing enterohepatic recirculation. Tetracycline levels in the cerebrospinal fluid primarily depend on duration of therapy rather than on actual dosages and usually average about one fifth of simultaneous plasma levels. Tetracycline passes most readily into the cerebrospinal fluid and demeclocycline least readily. Tetracycline and oxytetracycline readily cross the placenta (demeclocycline and chlortetracycline do so poorly) to the fetus, and antibiotic concentrations in milk during lactation may be one-third to one-half simultaneous plasma levels (*see* below). Minocycline penetrates well into salivary gland tissue, a property that may explain its effectiveness in treating the *N. meningitidis* carrier state.

The tetracyclines are minimally metabolized to inactive compounds. Of clinical importance, however, is that the rate of doxycycline metabolism may be doubled by enzyme-inducing drugs such as phenytoin and by chronic alcohol ingestion, so that plasma antibiotic levels may fall below the required minimum inhibitory concentration.

Tetracyclines are excreted in the urine (Fig. 61-1) by glomerular filtration and to a lesser extent in the bile, and in the milk during lactation. Oxytetracycline is preferentially excreted in the urine and chlortetracycline, doxycycline, and minocycline in the bile. Most of the tetracyclines are cleared by peritoneal dialysis (not doxycycline) or hemodialysis.

ADVERSE EFFECTS

Numerous adverse effects may be seen.

Suprainfection

Because of their broad spectrum, tetracyclines rapidly depress the normal body flora, particularly those of the gastrointestinal and genital tracts. After a couple of days of therapy, the feces become soft, unformed, and odorless, and suprainfection (*see* Chap. 56) is likely. Common suprainfecting organisms are penicillinase-producing staphylococci, various strains of *Proteus* and *Pseudomonas*, and *Candida albicans*. Clinically, cheilosis, black hairy tongue, glossitis and anogenital pruritus, burning, pain, or tenesmus occur in about 20% to 30% of patients. These may be partly hypersensitivity or toxic reactions rather than solely due to suprainfection; vitamin deficiencies probably are rarely involved. Necrotizing (pseudomembranous) enterocolitis (*see* Chap. 63) may also develop.

Biologic and Toxic Reactions: Tissue Irritation

When taken orally, the tetracyclines (especially oxytetracycline) produce dose-dependent gastrointestinal irritation, particularly nausea, vomiting, anorexia, and diarrhea. Consequently, they should be given with care to patients who have peptic ulcer disease. The diarrhea of irritation must be differentiated from the diarrhea of suprainfection, since the latter demands prompt cessation of tetracycline therapy, the institution of supportive measures, and a new antibiotic. Milk and calcium and aluminum antacids reduce the gastrointestinal symptoms of oral tetracycline therapy but also depress both the rate of its absorption and the quantity absorbed. Intramuscular administration of tetracyclines is painful. Injection sites should be alternated. Intravenous therapy can induce thrombophlebitis, a reaction minimized by keeping the tetracycline concentration less than 0.5%.

Hypersensitivity Reactions

Skin lesions of all types may occur, particularly morbiliform rashes and urticaria and, in severe cases, exfoliative dermatitis. Skin rashes may be accompanied by fever, eosinophilia angioedema, or anaphylactic shock, which is supposedly more common after demeclocycline therapy. Lightheadedness, Jarisch–Herxheimer-like reactions, pancreatitis, burning of the eyes and periorbital areas, and blood dyscrasias (thrombocytopenia, lymphocytosis, and "toxic" granulation of the leukocytes) are rare.

Demeclocycline and doxycycline may cause photodermatitis; other tetracyclines produce the reaction rarely. The reaction is more common with doses of demeclocycline that exceed 100 mg/day. Usually phototoxicity is accompanied by high fever, eosinophilia, and, in severe cases, shedding of the hair and nails and residual nailbed pigmentation.

Damage to Teeth, Bones, and Nails

Tetracyclines readily bind to unerupted teeth at the time of their development and calcification, with the formation of tetracycline–calcium orthophosphate complexes. The degree of binding depends on the specific tetracycline and the total dose; oxytetracycline and doxycycline appear to be the least likely to bind. Binding results in tooth staining and, with high exposure, partial or complete enamel hypoplasia, probably due to interference with the presecretory and secretory ameloblasts. Tooth staining is seen initially as yellowish bands that fluoresce under ultraviolet light. The depth of color and the width of the band are proportional to the dose absorbed. Fluorescence is gradually lost with oxidization of the drug to gray–brown metabolites. Stained and hypoplastic teeth pose a cosmetic problem and may be more inclined to carious degeneration.

Damage to deciduous or permanent teeth depends on the time of exposure in relation to tooth development. Thus exposure of the fetus from about the third month of gestation, or of the neonate and baby up to about 12 months of age, may result in staining and or enamel hypoplasia of the deciduous teeth. Similar effects may be seen in the permanent dentition if antibiotic exposure occurs from about 6 months of gestation up to 8 to 10 years of age.

Osseous deposits of tetracyclines may cause a reversible depression of linear bone growth in premature infants. Yellow, brown, or gray discoloration and pitting of the nails may appear with therapy in any age group.

Metabolic Effects

The tetracyclines may depress liver function, particularly when given parenterally in doses of 2 g or more per day. Oxytetracycline and tetracycline are the least hepatotoxic. Hepatocytes show vacuolation and fatty infiltration, and progression to massive hepatic necrosis may occur rarely. Contributing factors are renal insufficiency (resulting in higher plasma levels), pregnancy, severe sepsis, and shock; the increased demand for protein anabolism during pregnancy may make the liver more susceptible to drugs, such as the tetracyclines, which depress this function. Tetracyclines produce weight loss and a negative nitrogen balance, presumably due to a direct depression of host protein synthesis.

Tetracyclines may prolong blood coagulation either indirectly by depressing prothrombin synthesis (depression of colonic bacterial flora) or directly by chelating serum calcium or interfering with plasma lipoproteins. Increased urinary bilirubin and decreased urobilinogen may result from depression of the colonic flora. Tetracyclines increase loss of folic acid and riboflavin and may produce increased intracranial pressure (pseudotumor cerebrii) in children. In advanced renal failure, if the dose of tetracycline is not adjusted downward, progressive azotemia, acidosis, hyperphosphatemia, negative nitrogen balance, potassium loss in the urine, anorexia, and nausea and vomiting will develop.

Renal Damage

Up until the 1960s tetracyclines were buffered with citric acid, which loses its buffering capacity under extremes of temperature and humidity with the production of (among others) anhydrotetracycline and 4-epianhydrotetracycline. These compounds frequently produced reversible facial lesions that resembled systemic lupus erythematosus and a Fanconi-like syndrome (nausea, vomiting, polyuria, glycosuria, phosphaturia, aminoaciduria, proteinuria, and acidosis). Parenteral tetracyclines are currently buffered with lactose, which is more stable than citric acid. However, lactose-buffered tetracyclines usually contain small quantities of anhydrotetracycline and 4-epianhydrotetracycline, and although these levels increase only slightly during conditions of proper storage they may increase under extremes of storage.

Demeclocycline may induce nephrogenic diabetes insipidus, and tetracyclines, when given in association with methoxyfluorane anesthesia, may produce acute renal tubular necrosis.

PREPARATIONS AND DOSAGE

Many preparations (Table 61-2) are available for oral, parenteral, and topical administration either singly, in combination, or with other drugs such as antifungal agents. Tetracyclines with antifungal agents have been suggested for use in patients with malignant or metabolic disease to prevent *C. albicans* suprainfection (*see* Chap. 69); their value is questionable.

Oral administration of tetracyclines is safest. Parenteral administration seldom needs to be continued more than a few days, but more prolonged treatment may be needed for the unconscious patient and for those who do not respond promptly or who cannot ingest or absorb oral preparations. Slow i.v. infusion (5 mg/ml or less) is preferred to i.m. injection, which should be combined with a local anesthetic. Tetracyclines should *never* be given intrathecally. Apart from the conjunctival sac in solu-

Guido Fanconi, 1892–1979. Zurich physician. Described Fanconi's anemia in 1927 and Fanconi's renal dysfunction syndrome in 1936.

tions or ointments of 0.5% to 1.0%, topical application is not recommended. Generally the newer tetracyclines offer no advantage over the older preparations but tend to be considerably more expensive.

USES

Antibacterial Uses

Tetracyclines are usually contraindicated during pregnancy and lactation and in patients with peptic ulcer disease and hepatic disease; in hepatic disease, administration is especially dangerous. Doses larger than 1 g/day are seldom required, and *doses greater than 2 g/day parenterally should not be given.*

Because of their broad antibacterial spectrum, the tetracyclines enjoy wide popularity, but other drugs may be more potent and desirable, particularly if a bactericidal effect is wanted. The tetracyclines are effective in treating many infections, notably those due to the rickettsiae, the chlamydia, *Mycoplasma* (pleuropneumonia-like organisms), bacteroides, hemolytic streptococci, and staphylococci. They are also effective in cholera, granuloma inguinale, syphilis, yaws, gonorrhea, relapsing fever, tularemia, chancroid, leptospirosis, actinomycosis, and nocardiosis. In the treatment of melioidosis, brucellosis, and glanders, streptomycin may be added with advantage. Some gram-negative bacteria that cause urinary tract infections may be susceptible to tetracyclines. The mode of action of tetracyclines in treating *Balantidium coli* and *Entamoeba histolytica* infections is probably indirect (*see* Chap. 67). Tetracyclines are the drugs of choice for Whipple's disease, some "blind loop" syndromes, and tropical sprue. In penicillin-allergic patients, the tetracyclines or chloramphenicol are of value for *H. influenzae*, pneumococcal, and meningococcal meningitis. Doxycycline and minocycline may possess greater activity against some anaerobic bacteria and some staphylococci, respectively, than other tetracyclines. In addition, minocycline may be superior to other related agents and the sulfonamides in the prophylaxis of meningococcal infections and in meningococcal carriers.

Chronic tetracycline therapy with topical desquamating agents is used for severe inflammatory, recalcitrant acne; noninflammatory acne (comedones) does not respond to antibacterial therapy. The lesions in inflammatory acne may result from a disorganization of follicular epithelium, with subsequent blockade of the sebum gland duct. Follicular contents then rupture into the dermis, where free fatty acids liberated from sebum triglycerides by lipases from *Propionibacterium acnes* and other organisms cause inflammation. Antibiotics kill lipase-producing microorganisms. Tetracycline dosage is empirical—500 to 1000 mg/day and adjusted downward to about 250 mg every 2 days. Full antilipolytic effect may not be seen for several weeks. Tetracyclines are also effective in the long-term treatment of some patients with chronic bronchitis and cystic fibrosis.

Because the bacterial flora in the colon is depressed by the tetracyclines, 5 mg of vitamin K orally is a useful adjunct to therapy. Riboflavin and folic acid deficiency are theoretically possible, and with chronic tetracycline therapy a multivitamin preparation is desirable.

Nonantibacterial Uses

All tetracyclines (particularly demeclocycline) have the property of binding to rapidly growing tissues (the liver, new bone, and various cancers) and exhibiting a golden yellow fluorescence when exposed to ultraviolet light. This property has been used as the basis of several diagnostic tests for the cytologic detection of certain cancers (stomach, colon, bladder, pleura), and to determine the rate of bone turnover.

GEORGE HOYT WHIPPLE, 1878–1976. American pathologist. Described Whipple's disease, intestinal lipodystrophy, in 1907. His work on liver function, hemoglobin, and erythrocyte synthesis led to the Nobel Prize in 1934, shared with G. R. Minot and W. P. Murphy for their combined work that led to the use of liver therapy for pernicious anemia.

CHLORAMPHENICOL

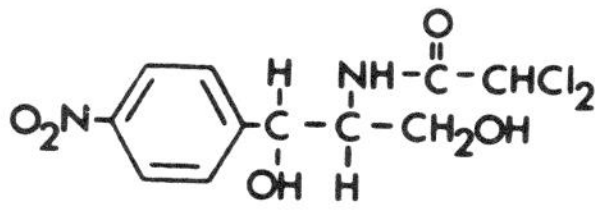

CHLORAMPHENICOL

Chloramphenicol is a broad-spectrum bacteriostatic antibiotic originally isolated from *Streptomyces venezuelae* but now produced synthetically. Its clinical use probably should be restricted because of the dangers of bone marrow toxicity. Only the L-form is biologically active. Chloramphenicol is unique in having a nitrobenzene radical; the dichloracetamide side-chain is essential for antibacterial activity.

Thiamphenicol (available in Europe) has the nitro (NO_2) group of chloramphenicol replaced by a sulfomethyl (CH_2SO_2) group. Thiamphenicol possesses several important differences over chloramphenicol: It is minimally glucuronated, therefore more is excreted unchanged in the urine, and its metabolism depends less on hepatic function; it is minimally (10%) bound to plasma proteins; and, even though it is more likely than chloramphenicol to produce "reversible" bone marrow depression (*see* below), no case of aplastic anemia has been reported with its use.

ANTIBACTERIAL SPECTRUM

Chloramphenicol has a broad spectrum of activity, almost equivalent to that of the tetracyclines. It is effective against many gram-positive and gram-negative organisms and nearly all anaerobes and demonstrates activity against the chlamydiae and rickettsiae. Because of its toxicity, chloramphenicol should be restricted to treating salmonelloses and infections due to rickettsiae, *Hemophilus influenzae*, gram-positive organisms resistant to less toxic antibiotics, the chlamydiae, and anaerobic infections, particularly due to *Bacteroides fragilis*.

Resistance

Two mechanisms of resistance to chloramphenicol have been described: R-factor coding for an acetylase (which is the most important); and the development of a permeability block (for example, in *Pseudomonas spp.*) to the antibiotic. In gram-positive bacteria the acetylase is inducible, whereas in gram-negative bacteria it is constitutive. In some bacteria slow enzymatic reduction of the nitro group takes place, but this is probably of little clinical significance. R-factor-mediated bacterial resistance is of increasing clinical consequence, however. Resistance is not seen in rickettsial organisms nor in *Bacteroides fragilis*. Para-aminosalicyclic acid therapy may favor the resistance of *Escherichia coli* to chloramphenicol, and some enteric bacteria may demonstrate cross-resistance with the tetracyclines or erythromycin.

Mode of Action and Properties

Chloramphenicol inhibits protein syntheses in bacteria by binding to the 50 S subunit of the 70 S ribosome, thereby suppressing peptidyl transferase activity (*see* Chap. 57). Chloramphenicol binding is competitively inhibited by clindamycin, lincomycin, and the macrolides. Most protein synthesis in humans takes place on 80 S ribosomes, which are "poor binders" for chloramphenicol. However, human mitochondrial ribosomes are more similar to bacterial 70 S ribosomes. Consequently, chloramphenicol-induced inhibition of mitochondrial protein synthesis in the bone marrow may explain the antibiotic's hematologic toxicity. Chloramphenicol is primarily bacteriostatic but with some organisms under certain conditions it may be bactericidal. Its important properties are indicated in Table 61-4.

ADVERSE EFFECTS

Hematopoietic Toxicity

Chloramphenicol may produce two distinctive patterns of hematopoietic toxicity: a *"benign" dose-dependent reversible depression* of marrow function; and *aplasia*.

In every patient, if the antibiotic is given long enough and in high enough dosage (particularly with blood levels of greater than 25 μg/ml), "benign" bone marrow depression may be seen, probably due to inhibition of marrow protein synthesis. This "benign" marrow depression (reticulocytopenia, an elevated serum iron level, prolonged plasma iron clearance, evidence of cellularity with vacuolation of both the red and white cell series on marrow examination) is dose dependent, reversible, and usually not an indication to stop therapy; it usually reverts promptly (1–3 weeks) on cessation of therapy but rarely may persist for several months. It may be detected by monitoring the hemoglobin level, the reticulocyte count, and the serum iron level every 24 to 72 hours.

Chloramphenicol may rarely (1:25,000 to 1:50,000 doses) cause aplastic anemia presumably as an idiosyncratic or hypersensitivity response. The reaction may appear during therapy or up to several months after the drug has been withdrawn. Since white cells turn over more rapidly than do red cells, toxicity usually appears as neutropenia (infection) or thrombocytopenia (bleeding) rather than as anemia. *Danger signs that necessitate immediate cessation of chloramphenicol therapy are neutropenia below 3000/mm^3; less than 40% polymorphonuclear leukocytes in a peripheral differential white cell count; or thrombocytopenia (less than 100,000 platelets/mm^3).* Aplasia is often irreversible.

TABLE 61-4. Antibiotics That Inhibit Protein Synthesis

Drug	Properties	Preparations
Chloramphenicol	Chloramphenicol is rapidly absorbed after oral administration, with peak plasma levels of 30 μg/ml developing within 2 hours following a 2-g dose. The i.m. preparation probably should not be used because the succinate ester hydrolyzes poorly to the active drug. Chloramphenicol is highly diffusable and appears in most body tissues and secretions and in the fetus. It is bound about 40% to 50% to plasma proteins and has a half-life of 2 to 3 hours. Chloramphenicol is primarily degraded (90%) by hepatic glucuronyl transferase, which is inducible (*see* Chap. 8). The glucuronyl metabolite is nontoxic and not antibacterially active. Free chloramphenicol is cleared by glomerular filtration and the glucuronated metabolite by tubular secretion. Chloramphenicol is cleared by hemodialysis and peritoneal dialysis.	Oral: Chloramphenicol, *U.S.P.* (Chloromycetin), capsules, and chloramphenicol palmitate oral suspension, *U.S.P.*, which is hydrolyzed in the bowel lumen to chloramphenicol Parenteral: Sterile chloramphenicol for suspension, *N.F.*, is for i.v. or i.m. use. Sterile chloramphenicol sodium succinate, *U.S.P.*, is a water-soluble preparation for i.v. use only. Topical: Chloramphenicol ophthalmic ointment, *U.S.P.*, contains 1% of the antibiotic.
Erythromycin	Erythromycin base has a pK_a of 8.6 and is variably destroyed by gastric acid; food, by delaying gastric emptying, reduces its absorption. Despite being 80% to 90% bound to plasma protein, erythromycin diffuses well into most tissue compartments except CSF; fetal levels are usually about 10% of maternal plasma levels. Erythromycin is concentrated in liver and bile, and concentrations there may reach 20 to 50 times simultaneous plasma levels. The antibiotic is demethylated by hepatic microsomal enzymes to des-N-methyl erythromycin, which is antibacterially inactive. Erythromycin has a $T\frac{1}{2}$ of 1 to 3 hours and 3 to 4 hours in adults and children, respectively. After a single oral or i.v. dose, only about 5% to 15%, respectively, of the antibiotic appears as active drug in the urine. It is cleared by glomerular filtration. Absorption of erythromycin from enteric-coated tablets is usually more uniform than that from the free base. *Erythromycin sterate* rapidly dissociates in the intestinal lumen to the base after oral administration. *Erythromycin succinate* (an ester) is somewhat acid labile, predominantly being hydrolyzed to the base after absorption. It is more rapidly hydrolyzed than the estolate. *Erythromycin estolate* (a salt of an ester) is acid stable and well absorbed after oral administration. It is hydrolyzed slowly to the base after absorption. Food does not measurably affect its rate or degree of absorption. Plasma levels are highest, more reproducible, and more prolonged (for any given dose) with this preparation. Reported plasma "antibiotic" levels resulting from its use have not distinguished between the percentage present as the parent drug and that present as the antibacterially active free base. *Erythromycin estolate possesses specific hepatic toxicity* (see adverse effects).	Oral: Erythromycin base, *U.S.P.*, and erythromycin stearate, *U.S.P.*, are available in tablets and enteric-coated tablets of 125, 150, 250, and 500 mg. Erythromycin estolate, *N.F.* (the lauryl sulfate salt of the propionic acid ester of erythromycin), is available as tablets and capsules of 125, 250, and 500 mg and as a liquid of 25 and 50 mg/ml. Erythromycin stearate and erythromycin ethyl carbonate, *U.S.P.*, are available as dry powders for reconstitution or as oral suspensions. Parenteral: Erythromycin ethylsuccinate (50 mg/ml) contains the local anesthetic 2% butyl amino benzoate for i.v. administration. Erythromycin lactobionate, *U.S.P.*, and erythromycin gluceptate, *U.S.P.*, are available in doses of 0.25, 0.50, and 1.0 g for i.v. administration. Topical: Erythromycin base, *U.S.P.*, is available as a 0.5% or 1.0% ointment.

Aplastic anemia with pancytopenia has accounted for about 75% of all blood dycrasias after chloramphenicol therapy. Other rare dyscrasias include selective depression of each cellular component and various combinations. Aplastic anemia is three times more common in females and more common in adults; it has not been reported in children less than 2 or 3 years of age. It may be more common after repeated courses of the antibiotic, particularly following oral therapy for viral infections, and it may not appear until several weeks or months after therapy has been discontinued.

There may be a genetic predisposition to aplasia (occurrence in twins), and the para NO_2 group may be necessary for its development. (It has never been reported with thiamphenicol.) Aplasia is very rare after parenteral chloramphenicol, but this may reflect greater use of the oral route of administration rather than mediation of some novel metabolite generated in the bowel lumen. Phenylalanine does not protect against aplastic anemia.

Hypersensitivity Reactions

In addition to blood dyscrasias, fever, various skin rashes (macular, papular, vesicular), angioedema, and Jarisch–Herxheimer reactions in the treatment of brucellosis and typhoid fever may develop. Glossitis, stomatitis, cheilosis, and pruritus ani may not only be due to hypersensitivity but also to suprainfections.

Nonhypersensitivity Reactions

Chloramphenicol has a bitter taste, and oral therapy may induce nausea, vomiting, and gastric irritation. Therapy may be followed by suprainfection with a wide range of organisms, in particular, *Staph. aureus*, *Ps. aeruginosa*, *Proteus* spp., and *Candida* spp.; necrotizing (pseudomembranous) entercolitis may also be seen. Diarrhea may be severe enough to produce the low salt syndrome. Purpura, excessive bleeding from mucosal surfaces (accentuated by reduced prothrombin levels; *see* below), hemolytic anemia in patients with glucose-6-phosphate dehydrogenase deficiency, optic and peripheral neuritis, "glove and stocking" paresthesias, headaches, mood disturbances, myalgia, renal glomerular and tubular damage, and chromcsomal breakages may also be seen. Chloramphenicol therapy may reduce plasma prothrombin levels owing to a sterilizing effect on the bowel microflora and possibly owing to a reduction in hepatic prothrombin synthesis. Chloramphenicol interferes with other aspects of protein synthesis; histocompatibility antigen formation in lymphocytes and antibody production; and prevention of the response to hematinics such as vitamin B_{12} or iron. Depression of the bowel microflora is associated with a lower urine urobilinogen excretion. In humans, the biotransformation of tolbutamide, phenytoin, and dicoumarol is retarded, leading to prolonged plasma half-lives with resulting toxicity (*see* Chap. 8).

Adverse Effects in the Neonate

The neonate may develop the gray (blue) baby syndrome if the dose of chloramphenicol is greater than the capacity of the immature glucuronyl transferase to metabolize the antibiotic load. The more premature the baby, the less glucuronyl transferase activity will be present. The syndrome is caused by chloramphenicol and is characterized by progressive abdominal distension, vomiting, refusal to suck, cyanosis, and loose greenish stools. Within a day or so the baby develops a grayish color and peripheral vascular collapse; death occurs in about 50% of cases within 4 or 5 days. The syndrome is accentuated by immaturity of renal clearing mechanisms (*see* Chap. 11). If chloramphenicol is needed in a neonate, the dose should not exceed 25 mg/kg/day.

PREPARATIONS, USES, AND DOSAGE

Chloramphenicol preparations are available for oral, i.v., topical, and i.m. (usually not recommended) administration (Table 61-4). Chloramphenicol should be reserved for the treatment of typhoid fever and other salmonelloses, meliodosis, some rickettsial diseases, *Hemophilus influenzae* meningitis, staphylococcal infections resistant to the semisynthetic penicillins or cephalosporins, anaerobic infections, particularly with *Bacteroides fragilis*, and urinary tract infections resistant to other antibiotics. Therapy should be monitored with hemoglobin determinations and a white cell count and differential every 24 to 48 hours.

There are several dosage regimens for typhoid fever. One popular regime is 50 mg/kg/day for 2 weeks. Parenteral administration may be initially necessary. A loading dose should probably not be given, since Jarisch–Herxheimer-like reactions can be serious in a

---

Samuel Phillips Bedson, 1886–1969. British physician and bacteriologist. One of the first virologists, he worked especially with herpes and rickettsial diseases. Discovered the causative agent of psittacosis, *Chlamydia psittaci,* also known as Bedsonia.

debilitated patient. Some physicians add corticosteroids in serious cases. Ampicillin (and its congeners), amoxicillin, and cotrimoxazole are valuable alternatives, particularly in treating infections resistant to chloramphenicol. Because of the emergence of resistant salmonellae, sensitivity testing is necessary in treating infections with such organisms.

For rickettsial disease and melioidosis, the usual dose is 50 to 75 mg/kg of body weight in four divided doses daily until 48 hours *after* the temperature has returned to normal; tetracyclines may be preferable. For *H. influenzae* meningitis, the usual dose is 50 to 75 mg/kg daily in four divided doses for 2 weeks.

THE MACROLIDE ANTIBIOTICS

The macrolide antibiotics (lactone ring-containing) comprise *erythromycin, josamycin, oleandomycin, troleandomycin, spiramycin,* and *carbomycin*. Erythromycin and josamycin are, in general, the only agents currently used because the others are either too toxic or not sufficiently potent.

Josamycin, produced by *Streptomyces narboneosis var josamyceticus,* is an investigational antibiotic similar to erythromycin stearate. It has been widely used in Japan. Compared to erythromycin, josamycin may be less irritating to the gastrointestinal tract and less likely to generate bacterial resistance.

ERYTHROMYCIN

Erythromycin, isolated in 1952 from *Streptomyces erythreus,* enjoyed wide popularity for several years in treating infections caused by many common pathogenic organisms. Its clinical effectiveness has somewhat diminished because of the development of bacterial resistance. Erythromycin depresses protein synthesis by blocking peptide bond formation (*see* Chap. 57). Depending on the organism, the dose, and the duration of exposure, it is either bacteriostatic or bactericidal.

Antibacterial Spectrum

Erythromycin has an antibacterial spectrum between that of penicillin G and the tetracyclines. It is primarily effective against some gram-positive cocci (staphylococci, streptococci, enterococci and pneumococci), neisseriae, listeriae, *Bacteroides fragilis, Legionella pneumophila, Corynebacterium diphtheriae, Hemophilus influenzae,* brucellae, some rickettsiae, the large viruses, spirochetes, and *Entamoeba histolytica*. It is also highly effective against Mycoplasma pneumoniae but not against yeasts and fungi.

Resistance. Antibacterial resistance develops fairly rapidly and is becoming more widespread. The predominant mechanism for resistance is an alteration in the microbial ribosome so that it fails to bind erythromycin. Cross-resistance is usually complete between the macrolides but rarely develops with penicillin. Erythromycin may block the antibacterial actions of clindamycin and chloramphenicol (*see* Chap. 57).

Preparations

Erythromycin base has a bitter taste, is relatively unstable in gastric juice, and, particularly because of its poor bioavailability when taken with meals, may not be sufficiently absorbed to treat most infections.

Several salts and formulations of the base have been developed to improve blood levels following oral administration, but there is no consensus with respect to their effectiveness. Enteric-coated formulations (*see* Chap. 78), for example, delay drug disintegration and dissolution until it reaches the relatively alkaline small bowel, but such preparations generally do not yield predictable blood levels. Additionally, three derivates of the base—*erythromycin stearate, succinate,* and *estolate*—possess some important properties (Table 61-4 and below), but there is still some doubt as to their clinical superiority.

The succinate and estolate erythromycin esters have several advantages over the base and its stearate salt: they are tasteless and less acid labile and possess greater stability in aqueous solutions. However, since the succinate and estolate are bound to a greater degree (96–98%) than is the base (80–90%) to plasma proteins, and since they slowly hydrolyze to the antibacterially active free base after absorption, the higher plasma levels achieved with these agents may not be clinically significant.

Several specific erythromycin salts have been developed for parenteral administration (Table 61-4); their pharmacologic properties are similar to erythromycin base.

Adverse Effects

Erythromycin has low (less than 5%) toxicity. With oral therapy, nausea, anorexia, diarrhea, glossitis, stomatitis, cheilosis, and suprainfection occur most commonly. Erythromycin is rarely given intramuscularly or intravenously since severe pain with local induration or thrombophlebitis, respectively, usually develops. Hypersensitivity reactions with fever, eosinophilia, lymphocytosis, headaches, and a variety of skin rashes are sometimes seen and are more common in patients who have received the drug repeatedly.

Erythromycin estolate (approximately 1:300,000 courses in adults) may produce either silent elevation of liver function tests, particularly the transaminases, or a syndrome of acute intrahepatic cholestasis that resembles viral hepatitis or acute cholecystitis; abdominal pain is usually severe. The syndrome is more common in atopic persons and is reported uncommon in children (approximately 1:1,500,000 courses). Symptoms typically develop 10 to 20 days after starting therapy (unless the patient has had previous erythromycin estolate exposure; the reaction may then develop within 12–48 hours) and may be accompanied by fever and eosinophilia; it usually regresses rapidly when therapy is stopped. The offending agent may not be erythromycin but the associated lauryl sulfate salt. Whether other erythromycin preparations are safe in these patients is not yet clear.

Preparations and Dosage

A variety of oral, parenteral, and topical preparations of erythromycin are available (Table 61-4). The usual oral dose of erythromycin is 500 mg every 4 to 6 hours for 10 days. The base must be taken while the stomach is empty. Intramuscular injections should never be more concentrated than 50 mg/ml and are often poorly tolerated because of excessive pain. The usual i.v. dose is 1.0 to 1.5 g every 6 hours.

Uses

Erythromycin is useful for treating upper respiratory tract infections, including streptococcal tonsillitis and pharyngitis, sinusitus, otitis media, and acute bronchitis. It is also of some value in treating penicillin-resistant gram-positive infections and infections such as syphilis in patients allergic to penicillin. The gradual emergence of erythromycin-resistant strains is, however, becoming a problem. If both penicillin and the sulfonamides are contraindicated, erythromycin may be used to prophylactically treat rheumatic fever. Erythromycin is effective in the diphtheria carrier state in Legionnaire's disease (often plus rifampin), in mycoplasma pneumonia, and in amebiasis (*see* Chap. 67). It has been used widely to treat acne as an alternative to tetracyclines, but there are no controlled trials that compare the two agents.

FURTHER READING

1. Gorbach SL, Bartlett JG: Anaerobic infections. N Engl J Med 290:1177–1184; 1237–1245; 1289–1294, 1974
2. Meyer RD, Finegold SM: Legionnaires' disease. Annu Rev Med 31:219–232, 1980
3. Scott JL, Finegold SM, Belkin GA et al: A controlled double-blind study of the hematologic toxicity of chloramphenicol. N Engl J Med 272:1137–1142, 1965
4. Suhrland LG, Weisberger AS: Delayed clearance of chloramphenicol from serum in patients with hemotologic toxicity. Blood 34:466–471, 1969
5. Wallerstein RO, Condit PK, Kasper CK et al: Statewide study of chloramphenicol therapy and fatal aplastic anemia. JAMA 208:2045–2050, 1969

CHAPTER 61 QUESTIONS

(*See* P. 7 for Full Instructions)

Select the One Best Answer

1. Each of the following statements is true about tetracycline EXCEPT that it
   - *A.* may be deposited in bones.
   - *B.* chelates with calcium and other ions.
   - *C.* is contraindicated during pregnancy.
   - *D.* is completely absorbed from the intestines.
   - *E.* may discolor teeth of young children.
2. Chloramphenicol is primarily metabolized by
   - *A.* glucuronidation.
   - *B.* acetylation.
   - *C.* oxidation.
   - *D.* demethylation.
   - *E.* hydrolysis.
3. Erythromycin estolate
   - *A.* is acid labile.
   - *B.* may cause cholestatic jaundice.
   - *C.* may be inactivated by penicillinase.
   - *D.* is primarily cleared by renal excretion.
   - *E.* is effective against *Ps. aeruginosa*.
4. Tetracyclines
   - *A.* are effective only against bacteria.
   - *B.* are more effective than the penicillins against gram-positive cocci.

C. are effective in protecting against sunburn.
D. are excreted more slowly than most penicillins.
E. are effective against most *Proteus vulgaris* infections.

5. Organisms typically resistant to tetracyclines include all of the following EXCEPT
   A. *E. coli.*
   B. *Shigellae spp.*
   C. *Hemolytic streptococci.*
   D. *Bacteroides spp.*
   E. gram-positive cocci.

6. All of the following statements about doxycycline are true EXCEPT that
   A. it is preferentially excreted in the bile.
   B. it is not cleared by peritoneal dialysis.
   C. its rate of metabolism is increased by enzyme-inducing drugs.
   D. it has a short half-life in comparison to other tetracyclines.
   E. its absorption is minimally affected by food.

7. An antibacterial drug characterized by its effectiveness against severe infections with *Salmonella* and its propensity to cause blood dyscrasias is
   A. streptomycin.
   B. cephalothin.
   C. chloramphenicol.
   D. ampicillin.
   E. erythromycin.

A = 1,2,3; B = 1,3; C = 2,4; D = 4; E = All

8. Undesirable effects of tetracycline include
   1. loose stools.
   2. fungal suprainfections.
   3. hepatic damage.
   4. discoloration of teeth in infants.

9. Erythromycin
   1. is minimally metabolized.
   2. has a spectrum of antibacterial activity similar to that of penicillin.
   3. is bactericidal in high doses.
   4. inhibits protein synthesis.

10. Tetracycline is effective in the treatment of
   1. acute trachoma.
   2. acute lymphogranuloma venereum.
   3. inclusion conjunctivitis (inclusion blennorrhea).
   4. psittacosis.

11. Common suprainfecting organisms with chronic tetracycline therapy include
   1. penicillinase-producing staphylococci.
   2. *Proteus spp.*
   3. *Pseudomonas aeruginosa.*
   4. *Candida albicans.*

12. Side-effects that may be seen following chronic therapy with demeclocycline include
   1. photodermatitis.
   2. loss of nails.
   3. iron-deficiency anemia.
   4. nephrogenic diabetes insipidus.

62

JEREMY H. THOMPSON

Antibiotics That Interfere with the Bacterial Cell Membrane

The bacterial cytoplasmic membrane is the *site of cell wall synthesis* in many organisms (*see* Chap. 57). Further, it serves as a *protective barrier* to osmotic forces, as an organ for the *selective intracellular transport* and concentration of essential cell nutrients, and as an *organ of cell "excretion."* The "surface active" antibiotics described herein and some antifungal drugs (*see* Chap. 69) damage bacterial cell membranes, increasing their permeability (*see* Chap. 57). The antibiotics described in this chapter are polypeptides derived from species of *Bacillus;* they have poor sensitizing capacity after topical application but are highly nephrotoxic when administered systemically. *Nephrotoxicity is usually dose dependent and is increased in the presence of underlying renal disease and other nephrotoxic drugs.*

TYROTHRICIN

Tyrothricin is mainly of historical interest, since chronologically it was the first antibiotic to be introduced into therapeutics. Dubos, who isolated tyrothricin from the gram-positive, aerobic, spore-bearing soil microbe *Bacillus brevis,* was impressed by the fact that soil contains very few viable bacteria despite the numbers added to it each day. He proposed that chemicals such as tyrothricin cleared the soil by the phenomenon of *antibiosis* (*see* Chap. 56). Some formulations of tyrothricin are still available in Canada and other countries. Tyrothricin has a gram-positive antibacterial spectrum and acts like a surface-active agent (*see* Chap. 57).

POLYMYXIN B

Polymyxin is the generic name for six strongly basic cyclic polypeptides (polymyxins A, B, C,

---

RENÉ JULES DUBOS, 1901– . French-born New York pathologist and bacteriologist. In 1939 introduced gramicidin, extracted from *Bacillus brevis* of soil and effective against gram-positive bacteria. One of the founders of modern chemotherapy.

D, E, and M), all differing in amino acid content and elaborated by various strains of *Bacillus polymyxa*, an aerobic spore-forming bacillus found in soil. Polymyxin E is the same as colistin (*see* below). Polymyxin B is the only other antibiotic of this group with therapeutic usefulness; the remainder are more toxic and less potent. Polymyxin B has a molecular weight of about 1000, readily forms water-soluble salts with mineral acids, and has a pK_a of 8.9. The usual preparation is polymyxin B sulfate, which is unstable in alkaline solutions.

ANTIBACTERIAL SPECTRUM

Polymyxin B has a gram-negative spectrum. Microorganisms generally susceptible are *Enterobater aerogenes, E. coli, Hemophilus influenzae, Bordetella pertussis*, and *Klebsiella pneumoniae. Pseudomonas aeruginosa, Salmonella*, and *Shigella* are variably sensitive. *Proteus* spp., *Serratia marcescens*, and *Providentia* are highly resistant and often produce suprainfections during therapy. Antibacterial synergism has, however, been reported against *Ps. aeruginosa* when polymyxin B has been supplemented with tetracyclines, chloramphenicol, carbenicillin, or co-trimoxazole. Similarly, some bacteria resistant to polymyxin B, such as *Serratia marcescens* and *Proteus* spp., may be susceptible to a mixture of the polypeptide with co-trimoxazole.

MODE OF ACTION AND BACTERIAL RESISTANCE

Polymyxin B is bactericidal even in hypertonic media, and sensitive organisms bind the drug. It complexes with phospholipid components of the cell membrane and, by its lipophilic and lipophobic groups, becomes oriented between lipid and protein membrane components, impairing their functions (*see* Chap. 57). *The bactericidal effect of polymyxin B is reduced by serum and tissue fluid and by soaps and other substances that antagonize surface active agents.* Bacterial resistance develops slowly and is rare; it is due to failure of antibiotic penetration or to the absence of a membrane phospholipid receptor. Cross-resistance is demonstrated with colistin. Some bacteria resistant to the tetracyclines and chloramphenicol show cross-resistance to polymyxin B, although the reverse is uncommon.

ABSORPTION, METABOLISM, AND EXCRETION

Polymyxin B is usually administered topically or by local irrigation; systemic absorption may result if a large granulating surface is present. Occasionally oral, or very rarely, i.v. administration is warranted. Intrathecal administration is required if polymyxin B is being used to treat meningitis. Intestinal absorption of the antibiotic reaches significant proportions in young children but is absent in adults because of mucosal maturation. After parenteral administration, peak blood levels develop within about 1 hour. Polymyxin B passes poorly into most tissues, including the cerebrospinal fluid.

Polymyxin B is primarily cleared through the kidneys, with a T½ of 3 to 6 hours; little is known about its metabolism. Renal excretion is slightly delayed, and elimination may persist for up to 2 days after cessation of therapy. In the presence of renal insufficiency, toxic plasma levels develop rapidly with conventional doses; the T½ for polymyxin in anuria is 20 to 40 hours.

ADVERSE EFFECTS

Adverse effects are minimal after topical application because the drug is not measurably absorbed. Nausea, vomiting, and diarrhea and the development of suprainfections with gram-positive bacteria, *Proteus* spp., or fungi may follow oral therapy. Serious adverse effects are seen after parenteral therapy. Pain at the injection site is common. Facial flushing, paranasal, circumoral, lingual, "glove and stocking" paresthesiae, and slurred speech may occur, as can drug fever, malaise, headaches, mental disturbances, and skin rashes, including urticaria and other manifestations of hypersensitivity. General skeletal muscle weakness, vertigo, ataxia, diplopia, ptosis, and a depression of reflexes are less common.

Proximal renal tubular dysfunction (15% of patients) with the development of proteinuria, cylinduria, and hematuria is the most important adverse reaction following parenteral drug administration, that can develop and patients receiving the drug systemically should be hospitalized for this reason. Polymyxin B is more nephrotoxic than colistin. Damage is dose dependent and easily induced in patients already suffering from diminished renal function or taking other nephrotoxic drugs; it is usually reversible in the early stages but may progress to renal tubular necrosis. Polymyxin B can potentiate neuromuscular paralysis produced by both depolarizing and nondepolarizing muscle relaxants (Table 62-1); neostigmine and calcium gluconate are usually ineffective in reversing the paralysis. Polymyxin B usually aggravates skeletal muscle weakness in patients with myasthenia gravis. Chemical meningitis, with headache, fever, and increased CSF cell and protein content, may follow intrathecal therapy of doses greater than 5 mg. Acute overdosage may occur in children because of diminished renal function. Polymyxin B lyses mast cells, releasing histamine; symptoms attributable to acute histamine release (anaphylactoid reaction) may develop (*see* Chap. 51).

PREPARATIONS AND DOSAGE

Polymyxin B sulfate, U.S.P. (Aerosporin), is available in many preparations for local, oral, and systemic administration. For topical administration a 0.25% cream or ointment, frequently combined with other antibiotics (neomycin and bacitracin) and with hydrocortisone, is popular.

The average oral dose of polymyxin B is 4.0 mg/kg daily. Intramuscularly or, preferably, intravenously, the daily dose is 1.5 to 2.5 mg/kg in three or four divided doses. A daily parenteral dose of 200 mg should not be exceeded. Procaine hydrochloride is often added to the i.m. preparation. Intrathecally, a dose of 5 mg/day with a concentration of 0.5 mg/ml should not be exceeded. Procaine hydrochloride should never be given intrathecally. Doses of polymyxin B are occasionally expressed in units of activity, with 10,000 units being equivalent to 1 mg of the base.

TABLE 62-1. Some Important Drug Interactions with the Polymyxins

Primary Drug	Second Drug	Comment
Systemic polymyxin B and colistin therapy	Muscle relaxants, for example, alcuronium, curare, gallamine, pancuronium, suxamethonium	Prolonged skeletal muscle relaxation
Systemic polymyxin B and colistin therapy	Other nephrotoxic drugs, for example, aminoglycosides cephalosporins, diuretics	Increased risk of renal damage

USES

Polymyxin B is valuable in topically treating various infections of the skin, aural canal, and conjunctivae, often combined with other agents. Oral administration is used to treat bacteria resistant to less toxic antibiotics, such as in enteropathogenic *E. coli* disease in children and in severe *Salmonella, Shigella,* and *Pseudomonas* infections. Polymyxin B may rarely be given to patients with septicemia when other drugs such as carbenicillin and gentamicin are ineffective or when a patient has developed a severe adverse reaction to one of these agents. Polymyxin B should be used with caution systemically in patients with myasthenia gravis. Antibacterial synergism with co-trimoxazole and other agents has been discussed above.

COLISTIN

Colistin, a bactericidal polypeptide antibiotic obtained from *Bacillus colistinus,* is identical with polymyxin E and differs from polymyxin B in the substitution of a D-leucine residue for D-phenylalanine. It is available as colistin sulfate for oral administration and sodium colistimethate, the methanesulfonate derivative, for i.m. administration. Sodium colistimethate is antibacterially inactive but slowly hydrolyzes *in vivo* to generate colistin.

ANTIBACTERIAL SPECTRUM AND RESISTANCE

Colistin has an antibacterial spectrum and mode of action similar to that of polymyxin B, but it is less potent. Colistin is not antagonized by serum. Resistance develops rarely. Cross-resistance is present with polymyxin B.

ABSORPTION, METABOLISM, AND EXCRETION

In children under 5 years of age, colistin sulfate is absorbed following oral administration. Little or no absorption occurs in the adult. Sodium colistimethate releases colistin slowly by hydrolysis from the i.m. injection site, and, after an injection of 150 mg, peak plasma levels of about 10 to 20 μg/ml develop within 2 hours. Release of colistin from the muscle site maintains fairly uniform blood and urinary drug levels. Colistin is excreted by glomerular filtration, and dangerous serum drug levels develop rapidly in patients with diminished renal function. Colistin passes readily across the placenta but not into the cerebrospinal fluid. Colistin is about 50% plasma protein bound and has a T½ of 4 to 5 hours. In uremia colistin has a T½ of 20 to 40 hours but is removed by peritoneal dialysis.

ADVERSE EFFECTS

Colistin demonstrates a pattern of toxicity similar to that of polymyxin B. Proximal tubular necrosis is more common when other nephrotoxic antibiotics, particularly a cephalosporin, are given concomitantly (Table 62-1). CNS toxicity may develop more readily in uremia, possibly due to an alteration in the blood–brain barrier. Colistin is contraindicated in patients with myasthenia gravis.

PREPARATIONS AND DOSAGE

Colistin sulfate, *N.F.* (Coly-Mycin Oral Suspension), is suspended in distilled water (5 mg/ml) immediately before use. The usual dose for children is 3 to 5 mg/kg daily in divided doses. Colistin sulfate is present in some topical preparations that contain neomycin and hydrocortisone. Solutions of colistin salts are unstable at a pH of 6.0 or higher.

Sodium colistimethate, *U.S.P.* (Coly-Mycin Injectable), is available for i.m. administration in doses of 150 mg. The usual i.m. dose is 2.5 to 5.0 mg/kg daily in divided doses. A total daily dose of 10 mg/kg may rarely be given for severe infections but should not be exceeded. For i.v. therapy the drug should be diluted with dextrose or sodium chloride solution and injected over a 30-minute period twice daily. The maximum intrathecal dose per day in children and adults is 5 and 20 mg, respectively. Parenteral therapy must be drastically reduced in the presence of renal insufficiency.

USES

Colistin has therapeutic applications similar to those of polymyxin B. Parenteral colistin and polymyxin B perhaps should be reserved for treating systemic *Pseudomonas aeruginosa* infections in patients in whom other more potent, but less toxic, antibiotics such as gentamicin and carbenicillin are ineffective, and in treating neomycin-resistant enteropathogenic *E. coli* infection in children. Colistin irrigation of the ear may be valuable in perichrondritis of the pinna.

FURTHER READING

1. Flacke W: Drug therapy: Treatment of myasthenia gravis. N Engl J Med 288:27–31, 1973
2. Koch–Wesser J, Sidel VW, Federman EB et al: Adverse effects of sodium colistimethate. Ann Intern Med 72:857–868, 1970
3. Wilkinson S: Identity of colistin and polymyxin E. Lancet 1:922–923, 1963

CHAPTER 62 QUESTIONS

(See P. 7 for Full Instructions)

Select the One Best Answer

1. Each of the following is true for tyrothricin EXCEPT that
   A. it is a cyclic, neutral polypeptide.
   B. it is active primarily against gram-negative organisms.
   C. it was historically the first therapeutic antibiotic.
   D. it has poor antigenicity.
   E. it is toxic parenterally.

2. Polymyxin B is
   A. to be used only parenterally.
   B. active against gram-positive organisms.
   C. markedly nephrotoxic.
   D. a drug of choice for *Proteus* infections.
   E. an inhibitor of cell wall synthesis.

3. The following statements about polymyxin B are all true EXCEPT that
   A. the bactericidal effect of polymyxin B is reduced by serum and soaps.
   B. bacterial resistance is slow in onset.
   C. bacterial resistance is commonly due to the absence of a specific membrane phospholipid receptor.
   D. cross-resistance is rarely demonstrated with colistin.
   E. *Serratia marcescens* is usually highly resistant.

4. All of the following statements about colistin are true EXCEPT that
   A. it is identical with polymyxin E.
   B. it is less potent than polymyxin B.
   C. resistance develops rarely.
   D. cross-resistance is present with polymyxin B.
   E. it is safe to use in patients with myasthenia gravis.

A = 1,2,3; B = 1,3; C = 2,4; D = 4; E = All

5. Colistin is
   1. usually found to be cross-resistant with polymyxin B.
   2. markedly nephrotoxic.
   3. well absorbed in the intestines of young children.
   4. recommended as the drug of choice for treating systemic pseudomonal infections.

6. Desirable therapeutic properties of polymyxin B include
   1. rapid intestinal absorption.
   2. activity against *Pseudomonas aeruginosa.*
   3. that it is well tolerated parenterally.
   4. that it is effective orally against *Shigella* infections.

7. Side-effects of polymyxin B when given systemically include
   1. facial flushing.
   2. potentiation of neuromuscular paralysis induced by nondepolarizing muscle relaxants.
   3. urticaria.
   4. proximal renal tubular damage.

JEREMY H. THOMPSON

63

Miscellaneous Antibiotics

Several antibiotics whose precise classification is unclear are considered herein.

LINCOMYCIN AND CLINDAMYCIN

Lincomycin, a water-soluble, acid-stable, bactericidal antibiotic produced by *Streptomyces lincolnensis var. lincolnensis*, is unrelated chemically to any known antibacterial agent other than clindamycin. Because of its toxicity, especially liver damage and cardiovascular collapse that develop after too rapid i.v. injection, lincomycin has been replaced by *clindamycin* (7-chloro-7-deoxylincomycin). Compared to lincomycin, clindamycin is more potent and bactericidal for more strains, more readily absorbed after oral administration, and less toxic.

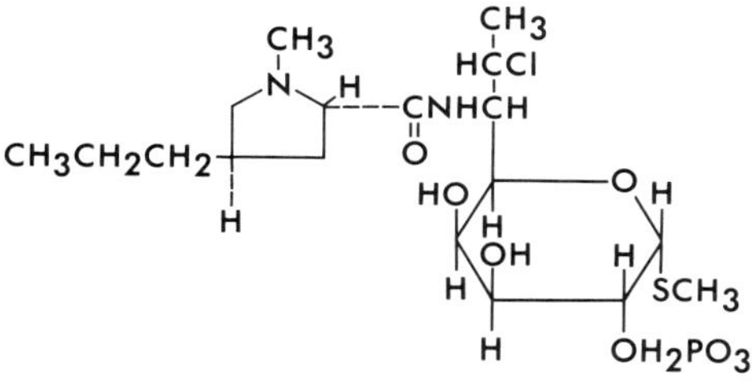

CLINDAMYCIN PHOSPHATE

CLINDAMYCIN PHOSPHATE

ANTIBACTERIAL SPECTRUM

Clindamycin possesses a semibroad antibacterial spectrum. In particular, it is effective against most pathogenic streptococci (not *Strep. faecalis*), staphylococci, pneumococci, corynebacteria, some strains of *Neisseria gonorrhoeae*, *H. influenzae*, and nocardia, and most, if not all, anaerobes, especially *Bacteroides fragilis*. Metronidazole (*see* Chap. 67) plus clindamycin, and gentamicin plus clindamycin may show synergism against some strains of *B. fragilis* and *Strep. viridans*, respectively.

MODE OF ACTION AND BACTERIAL RESISTANCE

Lincomycin and clindamycin inhibit protein synthesis (*see* Chap. 57). Erythromycin may

---

Albert Ludwig Siegmund Neisser, 1855–1916. German dermatologist. In 1879 reported discovery of bacillus that caused gonorrhea, and in 1882 named it gonococcus. Worked with August von Wassermann on the Wassermann test (1906). Also did research on leprosy.

block this effect by preventing antibiotic binding to, or by displacing bound antibiotic from, the ribosome. Thus in bacteria that bind macrolide antibiotics but are resistant to them, the activity of lincomycin and clindamycin may be blocked even though the organisms are highly sensitive to these two agents. Bacterial resistance is of slow, stepwise onset: Clinically, it is usually one component of multiple resistance. Cross-resistance is complete between lincomycin and clindamycin. Cross-resistance has been demonstrated *in vitro* with erythromycin, but this may not occur *in vivo*.

ABSORPTION, METABOLISM, AND EXCRETION

In adults, *clindamycin hydrochloride* is rapidly and almost completely absorbed after oral administration, with doses of 300 mg yielding plasma levels of 3 to 6 μg/ml within 1 to 2 hours; the presence of food has no measurable influence on absorption. For any given dose, peak serum levels are about twice as high with clindamycin as with lincomycin. Clindamycin has a T½ of about 3 hours. In children given a dose of 2 mg/kg, peak serum levels of 2 μg/ml develop at 30 to 60 minutes, and the drug has a T½ of 1 to 3 hours.

Clindamycin palmitate gives slightly lower plasma levels than does the hydrochloride salt. *Clindamycin phosphate* is well absorbed following parenteral administration, with blood levels of 12 μg/ml being achieved after doses of 300 mg. Because the phosphate ester hydrolyzes slowly, peak plasma levels are somewhat delayed, and this salt has a T½ of 4 to 6 hours. Clindamycin passes readily into most tissues and tissue fluids, including saliva, but poorly into cerebrospinal fluid, even in the presence of meningitis. The metabolism of clindamycin is complex: It is partially metabolized in the liver to the antibacterially active N-demethylated and sulfated (particularly sulfoxide) metabolites. The parent antibiotic and its metabolites are excreted in the free form and as glucuronides in the urine and bile. The antibiotic is unaffected by hemodialysis or peritoneal dialysis. Liver and kidney disease predictably delay the metabolism and excretion of clindamycin.

ADVERSE EFFECTS

Gastric irritation (nausea and vomiting) is commonly seen, and suprainfection with gram-negative bacilli or *Candida albicans* may be a problem. Pseudomembranous colitis (*see* below) is a very serious potential side-effect of therapy. Rarely granulocytopenia, thrombocytopenia, abnormal liver function tests or overt jaundice, hypersensitivity skin rashes, drug fever, the Stevens–Johnson syndrome, generalized pruritus, photosensitivity, headaches, myalgia, dizziness, and urticaria may develop. Postoperative neuromuscular block (*see* Chap. 19), probably caused by a direct effect of the antibiotic on skeletal muscle, since it is not reversed by anticholinesterases, is very rare. The too rapid i.v. injection of clindamycin may result in a "bad taste" in the mouth due to the rapid penetration of the antibiotic into saliva.

Pseudomembranous Colitis

The pathogenesis of this condition is not fully understood, but most cases are due to suprainfection with clindamycin-resistant toxigenic strains of *Cl. difficile*. Vancomycin (*see* Chap. 59), bacitracin (*see* Chap. 59), metronidazole (*see* Chap. 67), rifampin, and cholestyramine (*see* Chap. 38) have all been used in its treatment.

PREPARATIONS AND USES

Clindamycin is available in several formulations, doses being expressed as milligrams of clindamycin base. Clindamycin hydrochloride capsules of 75 and 150 mg and clindamycin palmitate granules for reconstitution of 15 mg/ml are available for oral administration. Clindamycin phosphate, 150 mg/ml, is available for parenteral administration.

Clindamycin has been used for tissue and wound infections caused by gram-positive cocci (other than enterococci) and anaerobic organisms, including *B. fragilis*. It is often combined with an aminoglycoside. Clindamycin has been used to treat *H. influenzae* respiratory tract infections in adults but is not recommended for such in children. Topically it has been used to treat acne, but the benefit of this approach is not clear.

SPECTINOMYCIN

Spectinomycin dihydrochloride is obtained from *Streptomyces spectabilis*, and some classify it with the aminoglycosides (*see* Chap. 60). It is used to treat acute genital and rectal gonorrhea but has no activity against extragenital or extrarectal gonorrhea or against syphilitic infections. Cross-resistance of gonococci between penicillin and spectinomycin has not been reported. Spectinomycin inhibits protein synthesis at the level of the 30s subunit of the ribosome, but its exact mode of action is unknown.

Spectinomycin is given by i.m. injection. Absorption is rapid, with peak serum levels of 100 μg/ml developing within 1 hour after the administration of 2 g. Protein binding of spectinomycin is low, but little is known about its metabolism and excretion.

Spectinomycin may cause pain following injection, and drug fever, skin rashes, including urticaria, nausea, insomnia, and dizziness have been reported. Rarely, evidence of hematologic, renal, and hepatic damage may appear, with falls in the hemoglobin and hematocrit, elevation of the BUN, and decreased creatinine clearance or elevation of liver function tests. Penicillin-sensitive patients appear to tolerate spectinomycin readily.

Spectinomycin (Trobicin) is indicated only in the treatment of acute gonococcal urethritis, proctitis, and cervicitis when due to susceptible strains of *Neisseria gonorrhoeae*. It is ineffective in extragenital and extrarectal gonorrhea and in syphilis. The usual dose in males is 2 g/day and in females 4 g/day.

CAPREOMYCIN

Capreomycin, a water-soluble, cyclic peptide, bacteriostatic antibiotic isolated from *Streptomyces capreolus*, is used as a second-line drug in tuberculosis (*see* Chap. 60). Capreomycin has four active components: capreomycins 1A, 11A, 1B, and 11B. The commercial preparation contains about 80% capreomycin 1A and 1B, with the remainder being a mixture of capreomycins 11A and 11B. Mycobacterial resistance is of the streptomycin type (*see* Chap. 60). Occasionally, antibacterial cross-resistance is shown with viomycin and kanamycin. One strange phenomenon reported with capreomycin is that mycobacteria resistant to streptomycin and para-aminosalicylic acid may be more susceptible to capreomycin than are normal strains. Capreomycin has produced eosinophilia, some degree of deafness and tinnitus, and, rarely, elevation of the blood nonprotein nitrogen levels and proteinuria. It is given by i.m. injection in doses of 1 g daily. Excretion is by way of the urine. The precise clinical usefulness of this antibiotic has not yet been determined, but capreomycin must be given with at least one other antitubercular drug (*see* Chap. 60). It is relatively expensive.

VIOMYCIN

Viomycin, a highly water-soluble, strongly basic cyclic polypeptide produced by *Streptomyces puniceus*, is used as a second-line drug to treat tuberculosis (*see* Chap. 60). It is weakly tuberculostatic, and mycobacterial resistance develops rapidly. As with other antitubercular drugs, the emergence of resistant strains may be delayed by the addition of one or more tuberculostatic drugs.

Viomycin is not absorbed after oral administration and must be given intramuscularly. Adverse reactions are more common with viomycin than with streptomycin. Hypersensitivity reactions (drug fever, eosinophilia, and erythematous, maculopapular, and pruritic skin rashes) and renal and VIIIth cranial nerve damage are common. Renal damage develops in more than 50% of patients treated. Skeletal muscle weakness and tetany may follow hypokalemia and hypocalcemia.

Viomycin sulfate, U.S.P. (Viocin Sulfate), is usually given in doses of 1 g every 12 hours every 3 days. More frequent therapy increases the prevalence of renal damage and ototoxicity. Viomycin should not be used to treat primary tuberculosis unless the causative organism is resistant to more potent chemotherapeutic agents or unless patients cannot tolerate more potent drugs. When viomycin is used to treat renal tuberculosis, concomitant urinary alkalinization potentiates its antitubercular effect.

FUSIDIC ACID

Fucidin is the sodium salt of fusidic acid, a steroid antibiotic obtained from *Fusidium coccineum* and related structurally to cephalosporin P. Fusidic acid contains the steroid cyclopentenoperhydrophenanthrene ring system (*see* Chap. 47) but is essentially devoid of any steroid biologic activity. It is available only in Europe. Indications for its use have decreased

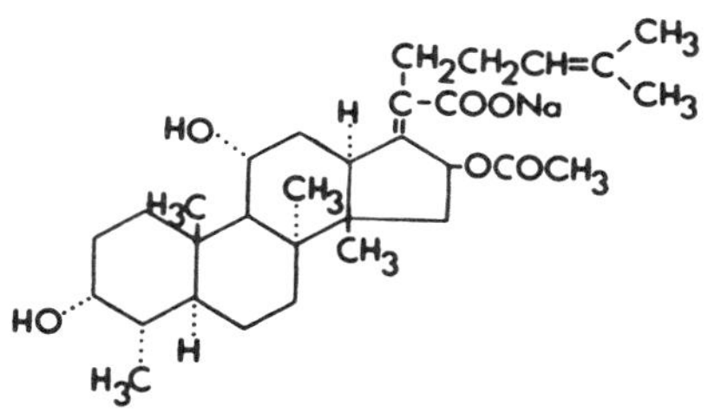

FUCIDIN

with the introduction of the newer semisynthetic penicillins.

Fucidin has a gram-positive spectrum similar to that of penicillin G and, when combined with that antibiotic, demonstrates an additive bactericidal effect. Its mode of action has been discussed (*see* Chap. 57). Fucidin is absorbed following oral administration and passes to most tissue compartments except the cerebrospinal fluid. Protein binding is high. Renal excretion amounts to less than 5% of the administered dose, elimination being primarily by way of the bile. Thus an enterohepatic circulation may develop. Fucidin should not be given intramuscularly because it may cause necrosis; i.v. administration may lead to hypotension, hemolysis, or thrombophlebitis.

Except for minor gastrointestinal upsets, dizziness, and mild skin rashes, fucidin has been shown to be relatively nontoxic. Patterns of long-range toxicity are not known.

Fucidin has been used mainly to treat *Staphylococcus aureus* infections resistant to penicillin, since it is not destroyed by penicillinase. Generally, staphylococci are inhibited by concentrations of about 0.01 μg/ml, levels readily achieved by conventional therapy. Resistance may develop rapidly, and cross-resistance is observed with cephalosporin P. Some evidence suggests that fucidin resistance develops less rapidly with concomitant penicillin or erythromycin therapy. The suggested dose is 500 mg three or four times daily.

FURTHER READING

1. Antibiotic-associated colitis—A bacterial disease. Br Med J 2:349, 1979
2. Chang TW, Gorbach SL, Bartlett JG et al: Bacitracin treatment of antibiotic-associated colitis and diarrhea caused by *Clostridium difficile* toxin. Gastroenterology 78:1584, 1980
3. Larson HE: Pseudomembranous colitis is an infection. J Infect 1:221, 1979
4. Prince AS, Neu HC: Antibiotic-associated pseudomembranous colitis in children. Pediatr Clin North Am 26:261, 1979

CHAPTER 63 QUESTIONS

(*See* P. 7 for Full Instructions)

Select the One Best Answer

1. Lincomycin is
   - *A.* less toxic than clindamycin.
   - *B.* distributed mainly in extracellular water.
   - *C.* less completely absorbed than clindamycin after oral administration.
   - *D.* especially effective against gram-negative organisms.
   - *E.* damaging to bacterial plasma membranes.

2. Which of the following statements about clindamycin is false?
   - *A.* It is excreted by the kidney, mainly in unchanged form.
   - *B.* Bacterial resistance is usually of slow onset.
   - *C.* Cross-resistance is invariably complete with lincomycin.
   - *D.* Food does not reduce its bioavailability.
   - *E.* Clindamycin passes poorly into the CSF.

3. All of the following statements about spectinomycin are true EXCEPT that
   - *A.* it possesses no activity against syphilitic infections.
   - *B.* it is valuable in treating acute genital and rectal gonorrhea.
   - *C.* it is effective against extragenital gonorrheal infections.
   - *D.* it inhibits protein synthesis at the level of the 30S subunit of the ribosome.
   - *E.* cross-resistance in gonococci between penicillin and spectinomycin is rare.

A = 1,2,3; B = 1,3; C = 2,4; D = 4; E = All

4. Clindamycin
   1. may interfere with action of erythromycin.
   2. is the drug of choice for treating bacterial abscesses in the brain.
   3. can cause fatal enterocolitis.
   4. is administered only by the parenteral route.

5. Undesirable effects of lincomycin include
   1. hypersensitivity reactions.
   2. cardiovascular depression.
   3. gastrointestinal irritation.
   4. hepatic dysfunction.

6. Inhibition of ribosomal synthesis of proteins is the proposed mechanism of action of
   1. spectinomycin.
   2. streptomycin.
   3. clindamycin.
   4. polymyxin B.

7. Pseudomembranous colitis may be treated with
   1. vancomycin.
   2. bacitracin.
   3. metronidazole.
   4. rifampin.

JEREMY H. THOMPSON

64

Chemotherapeutic Agents: I

THE SULFONAMIDES

HISTORY

In 1908, Gelmo synthesized the intermediary dye sulfanilamide for use in the dye industry. Subsequently sulfanilamide and other diazo dyes were used as urinary antiseptics after the demonstration that these chemicals had *in vitro* antimicrobial activity. Not until 1932–1935, however, did Domagk report the *in vivo* effectiveness of *Prontosil* in preventing hemolytic streptococcal infections in mice, a discovery for which he was awarded the Nobel Prize in Medicine. Soon after the introduction of Prontosil, it was shown that its action depended on rupture of the azo (—N=N—) linkage in the host, with production (Fig. 64-1) of the active sulfonamide sulfanilamide (para-aminobenzenesulfonamide). The term sulfonamide (sulfa drug) is commonly used generically to describe all derivatives of sulfanilamide.

Thousands of sulfonamides have been developed, but few have had sufficient advantages to render them effective therapeutic agents. Unfortunately, the sulfonamides were introduced into therapy before many of the general principles of antimicrobial use had been established. Although there are many differences among the individual sulfa drugs, they have enough common features to warrant a single, unified description. Individual therapeutically useful antibacterial sulfonamides, and the clinically important sulfonamide mixture with trimethoprim (co-trimoxazole), are evaluated later in this chapter and the sulfones in Chapter 65. Antidiabetic "sulfonamides" and diuretic "sulfonamides" are discussed in Chapters 46 and 40, respectively.

PAUL JOSEF JAKOB GELMO, 1879– . Viennese chemist. Synthesized sulfanilamide in 1908.

GERHARD DOMAGK, 1895–1964. German physician. His report on the effectiveness of prontosil in hemolytic streptococcal infections was published in 1935, and he was awarded the Nobel Prize in 1939. The Nazis arrested Domagk and forced him to decline the prize, which he eventually received in 1947.

CHEMISTRY

The sulfonamides can be considered as substituted derivatives of sulfanilamide. They are all white crystalline powders, mostly poorly soluble in water. Soluble sodium salts are easily prepared. The minimal basic chemical requirements for sulfa antibacterial action are

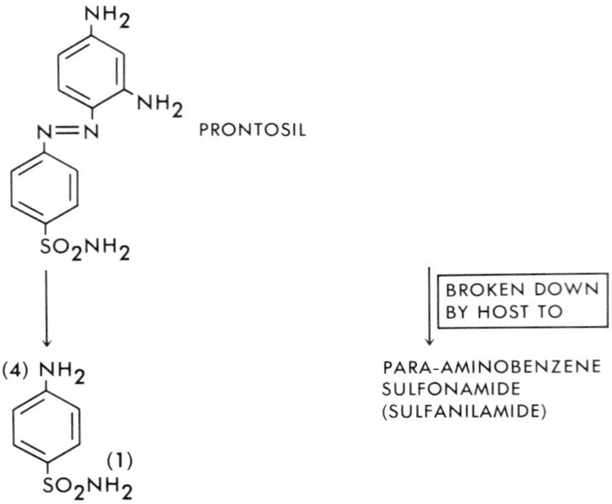

FIG. 64-1. The N of the amide NH_2 in all sulfonamides is designated as N^1, and the N of the para NH_2 as N^4.

contained in sulfanilamide (Fig. 64-1). The para-NH_2 group is essential for maximal antibacterial activity and can be replaced only by chemical groupings converted to a free amino group in the host, as in Prontosil. Ortho- and meta-NH_2 substitutions are almost devoid of antibacterial activity. The sulfamyl ($-SO_2NH_2$) group is not essential for antibacterial activity as such, but the sulfur atom is, and should be linked directly to the benzene ring. Because the sulfamyl group is the most important moiety of sulfanilamide antibacterially, the N of its amide NH_2 is designated N^1; the N of the para-NH_2 is then designated N^4. Most of the effective substituted sulfonamides are N^1 sulfanilamide derivatives (Fig. 64-2). Of these, sulfas with an additional heterocyclic ring are generally the most potent. Sulfonamides that contain a single benzene ring are considerably more toxic than are heterocyclic ring N^1 substitutions. Direct benzene ring substitution yields totally inactive compounds.

ANTIBACTERIAL SPECTRUM

The antibacterial spectrum of the early sulfa drugs is not as wide as that of the newer agents. Most currently popular sulfonamides have approximately equal spectra, but *in vitro* sensitivity testing is often unreliable, the reporting of sensitive strains as resistant being a frequent error. Highly sensitive organisms *in vitro* are most group A streptococci, *Hemophilus influenzae*, *Hemophilus ducreyi*, pneumococci, *E. coli*, *Klebsiella–Enterobacter* spp., *Proteus mirabilis*, *Brucella*, *Pasteurella pestis*, *Bacillus anthracis*, *Corynebacterium diphtheriae*, *Cholera vibrio*, nocardiae, actinomycetes, and the large viruses (agents that produce inclusion conjunctivitis, psittacosis/ornithosis, lymphogranuloma inguinale, and trachoma). Gonococci, meningococci, and shigellae are variably sensitive.

Many staphlococci, enterococci, clostridia, and pseudomonas spp. and *Serratia marcescens* are highly resistant. Some differences in activity may be useful clinically in situations where sulfa concentrations are marginal. Thus sulfadiazine is about eight times more active than is sulfamethazine against *N. meningitidis*, but the agents are equivalent against the pneumococcus. Additionally, sulfamethoxazole is about six times more active against *E. coli* than is sulfamethazine.

MODE OF ACTION

Sulfa drugs are primarily bacteriostatic agents that prevent the synthesis of folic acid (*see* Chap. 57). *In vivo*, intact host cellular and humoral defense mechanisms are essential requirements for satisfactory clinical improvement. Exceptionally, some sulfonamides may reach bactericidal concentrations *in vivo*, as in the urinary tract following therapy with soluble sulfa drugs, and in the ocular tissues following topical application of sulfacetamide. N^4-Acetylated metabolites are antibacterially inactive.

INTERFERENCE WITH THE ACTION OF SULFONAMIDES

Weight for weight, the sulfonamides are less potent than most antibiotics because their activity is reduced by pus, tissue fluids, including blood, and some drugs, for example, procaine, all of which contain para-amino benzoic acid (PABA). *In vitro* studies have shown that one molecule of PABA can competitively antago-

AUGUSTO DUCREY, 1860–1940. Italian dermatologist. Best known for his discovery of the chancroid-causing bacterium *Hemophilus ducreyi* in 1889.

MARK WINTON WOODS, 1908– . American biologist. Worked on the mechanism of action of chemotherapeutic agents, especially sulfonamides, in normal and cancer cells, genetics and biochemistry of mitochondria, and plant viral diseases.

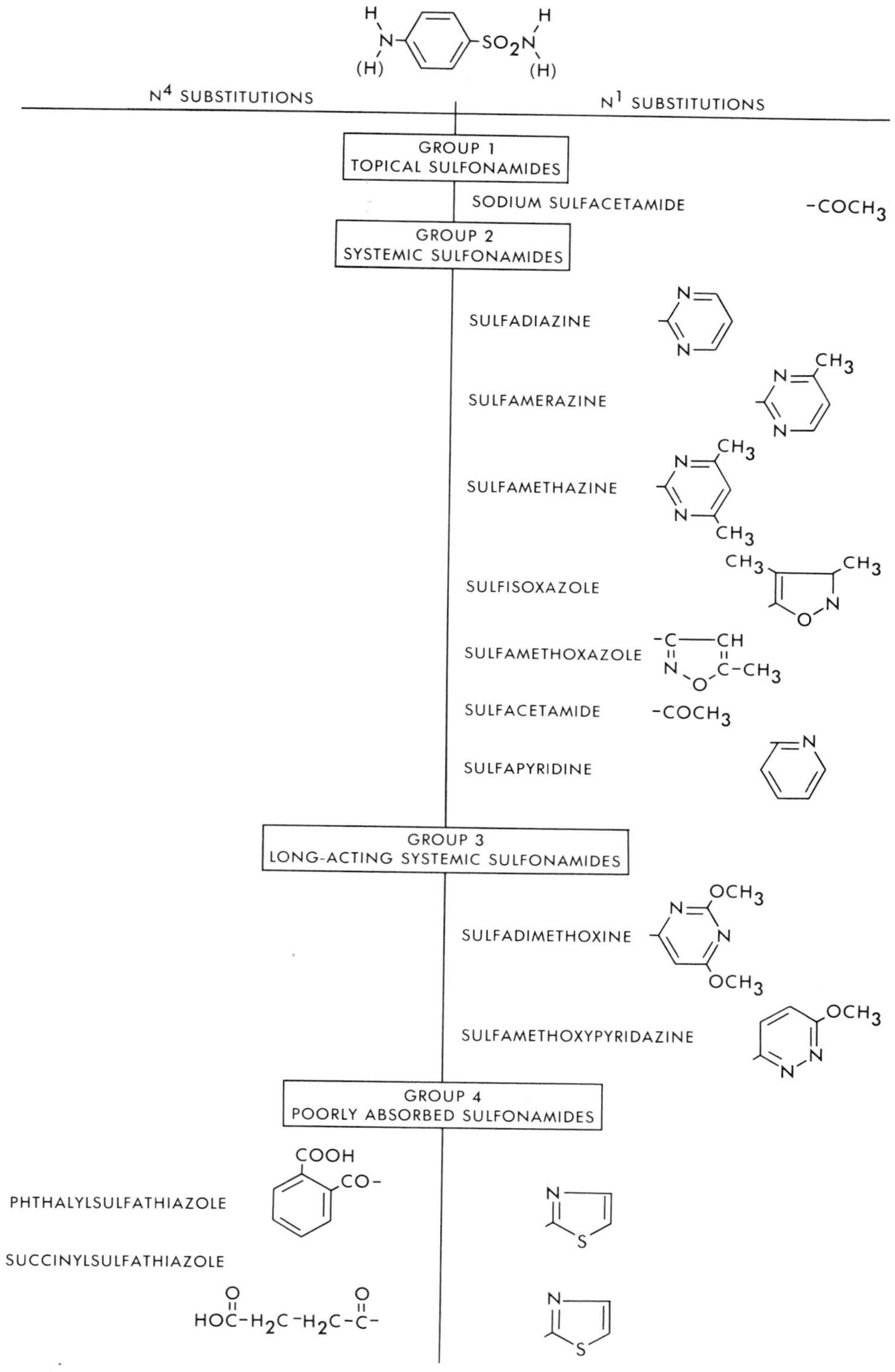

FIG. 64-2. Some important sulfonamides.

nize the bacteriostatic activity of 5000 to 25,000 molecules of sulfanilamide.

BACTERIAL RESISTANCE

Acquired bacterial resistance to sulfa drugs, first seen in *N. gonorrhoeae*, has subsequently developed in a variety of meningococci, staphylococci, hemolytic streptococci, pneumococci, and shigellae. *In vitro*, resistant organisms may reconvert to sensitive bacteria on repeated subculture, whereas *in vivo* acquired resistance is usually permanent. Bacteria resistant to one sulfonamide are usually equally resistant to equipotent concentrations of other sulfonamides. In most cases the mechanism of acquired resistance is unknown. However, some organisms may produce excessive quantities of para-aminobenzoic acid, whereas others adapt enzymatically to utilize the drug or to reduce its intracellular intake/uptake binding (*see* Table 56-2).

Acquired bacterial resistance is one of the most important causes of sulfonamide therapeutic failure. It may be minimized or delayed by avoiding promiscuous use of sulfonamides, by using sulfonamides only if they are the most satisfactory agents available, by beginning adequate therapy promptly, and by giving an adequate dose sufficiently long to eradicate the infection (*see* Chap. 56).

The use of trimethoprim with sulfamethoxazole may reduce the development of resistance to the sulfa, and *vice versa*.

ADMINISTRATION

Oral Administration

The easiest, safest, and most economical method of sulfonamide therapy is oral. "Systemic" sulfonamides (*see* below) are rapidly and almost totally absorbed, with peak blood levels developing within 2 to 4 hours. Oral administration of the poorly absorbed sulfonamides allows these drugs to act locally in the intestinal lumen.

Parenteral Administration

If oral administration is impossible or impractical, the soluble salts may be injected parenterally. Intravenous infusion (taking up to 10 minutes) is preferable to either s.c. or i.m. injection because sodium sulfonamides are intensely irritating to the tissues. Intravenous administration is rarely needed for longer than 36 to 48 hours, the incidence of crystalluria (*see* below) is approximately *doubled* with this route of therapy. Because of their irritating properties, sulfa drugs should never be injected intrathecally.

Topical Application

Topical sulfa products should be used only in the conjunctival sac, the otic canal, and the vagina. Topical application of the sulfas elsewhere should be avoided because their use entails considerable risk of generating sensitivity (allergic) reactions, and antibacterially they are inefficient. One exception, however, appears to be mafenide (*see* below).

ABSORPTION

Except for the sulfonamides designed to be used for their antibacterial effects in the bowel lumen, sulfa drugs, as a class, are rapidly absorbed from the gastrointestinal tract, principally the small bowel. Sodium bicarbonate may increase the rate but not the total amount of sulfonamide absorbed.

BLOOD LEVELS

Serum sulfonamide levels and clinical response correlate poorly, but, generally, therapeutically effective levels lie between 5 and 15 mg/dl. These levels are easily obtained with standard loading and maintenance doses.

Protein Binding

The protein binding of all sulfonamides is almost directly proportional to the plasma albumin concentration and varies considerably among members of the class (Table 64-1). Generally, acetylated sulfonamide metabolites are more highly bound to plasma albumin than is the parent drug.

Sulfonamides occupy type 1 (warfarin) binding sites and thus may lead to displacement drug interactions (*see* Chap. 8, Table 64-2). Displacement of the second agent may be followed by a transient enhanced therapeutic or toxic effect to that drug. Sulfonamide protein binding is decreased in uremia. Renal side effects are more commonly seen with sulfonamide therapy in the presence of hypoalbumenemia possibly due to reduced drug binding.

Distribution

Sulfa drugs are widely distributed (Table 64-1) throughout the body and readily pass the placental barrier. Equilibrium with most tissues

TABLE 64-1. Properties of Important Sulfonamides

Drug	pK_a	Protein Binding		T½	Apparent Vd	
		Neonate	*Adult*	*Adult*	*Neonate*	*Adult*
		%		*hr*	*liter/kg*	
Sulfadiazine	6.4	—	45–60	10–15	—	0.36
Sulfamerazine	6.7	—	75–85	25–35	—	0.36
Sulfamethazine	7.4	—	80	7–8	—	—
Sulfisoxazole	4.9	65–70	85–90	3–7	0.35–0.43	0.16
Sulfamethoxazole	5.7	—	60–70	8–12	—	0.17
Sulfadimethoxine	5.9	—	97–99	20–40	—	0.15
Sulfamethoxypyridazine	6.1	50–55	70–90	35–60	0.36–0.47	0.18–0.20

occurs within 2 to 4 hours. With standard systemic dosage, sulfas cross the blood–brain barrier to varying degrees. Cerebrospinal fluid levels of sulfadiazine, for example, may reach up to 80% of simultaneous plasma levels. Drug levels are even greater in pleural, peritoneal, and articular fluids, and, since these fluids usually contain a minimal protein concentration, most of the drug in these compartments is in the free active form.

METABOLISM

Sulfonamides vary in the degree to which they are metabolized. They are mainly degraded in the liver by N^4 acetylation and by oxidation. A small percentage may be conjugated with glucuronic acid, and some may be sulfated or sulfamated. The percentage of sulfonamide acetylated is proportional to the duration of time the sulfa remains in the body. Acetylsulfonamides have no antibacterial activity, are potentially toxic, and are usually less soluble than the parent drug.

Most sulfonamides are acetylated monomorphically, whereas others, such as salicylazosulfapyridine and sulfamethazine, are acetylated polymorphically, as are hydralazine, phenelzine, dapsone, procainamide, and isoniazid (*see* Chaps. 6, 65). Thus patients with a slow acetylator phenotype tend to suffer a higher incidence of adverse reactions (other than crystalluria) to many sulfonamides compared to patients with a rapid acetylator phenotype.

The T½ of some common sulfonamides is listed in Table 64-1. The T½ of most sulfas is prolonged during the first 2 weeks of extrauterine life, reaching an "adult" level by about 4 weeks of age.

EXCRETION

Sulfa drugs are excreted in both free and inactive forms; circadian variations in urinary excretion have been described but are of no obvious clinical importance. Elimination is principally in the urine, but some loss occurs in the sweat, tears, saliva, milk, and feces and can be therapeutically important. The sulfas are handled by the kidney similarly to urea. Free drug is filtered by the glomerulus and may be partially reabsorbed. Sulfacetamide, how-

TABLE 64-2. Potential Drug Interactions with Sulfonamides

Sulfonamide	Second Drug	Comment
Plasma protein displacement		
Highly plasma protein-bound sulfas, and co-trimoxazole	Methotrexate	Possibly increased methotrexate toxicity
	Chlorpropamide and tolbutamide	Hypoglycemia has been described with tolbutamide displacement. It may also occur with chlorpropamide
	Warfarin	Hypoprothrombinemia may be more severe
Reduced metabolism		
Sulfaphenoxazole, co-trimoxazole, and some other sulfas	Phenytoin	Phenytoin toxicity
	Tolbutamide	Hypoglycemia
	Warfarin	More severe hypoprothrombinemic response
Reduced renal tubular excretion		
Some sulfas	Methotrexate	Possibly increased methotrexate toxicity

ever, is not absorbed to any significant extent. Some tubular secretion of sulfa drugs may also occur. Acetylated derivatives are filtered through the glomerulus, and, because no tubular reabsorption occurs, a greater concentration of acetylated drug compared with free drug develops. Free sulfa drug levels in the renal tubules may be 15 to 25 times simultaneous plasma levels, explaining the effectiveness of these agents in some urinary tract infections.

ADVERSE EFFECTS

Despite their simple chemical structure, the sulfonamides are potentially dangerous drugs. The overall incidence of their varied adverse effects, which may involve almost every body-system, is probably about 5% to 10%. Many adverse reactions are minor, yet if they remain unrecognized and untreated they may progress to potentially lethal disturbances. If a patient has had a hypersensitivity reaction to any sulfonamide, subsequent exposure to sulfa drugs, including the related thiazide diuretics (*see* Chap. 40), the sulfones (*see* Chap. 65), acetazolamide (*see* Chap. 40), and the oral sulfonylurea hypoglycemic agents (*see* Chap. 46), may be hazardous.

The incidence of reactions depends on the sulfonamide used, the dose and duration of exposure, and the route of administration. Cross-sensitivity even between systemic and topically applied sulfonamides occurs. Although adverse effects are described separately, hypersensitivity reactions often occur together. Repeated exposure to sulfa drugs increases the likelihood of sensitization.

Kidney Damage

Sulfonamide crystals may precipitate anywhere in the urinary excretory ducts but particularly in the renal tubules, renal pelvis, or ureter, resulting in crystalluria. Depending on their size, crystals may cause epithelial irritation, with bleeding, or complete obstruction. Tissue damage produced by crystal formation may act as a site for infection. The development of crystalluria depends on the concentration and the solubility properties of the individual sulfonamide and its metabolites in the urine, and is more common after parenteral than oral administration. Urinary solubility of the sulfa drugs and their acetylated metabolites varies widely but with few exceptions is increased by urinary alkalinization. The measures taken to reduce crystalluria are described below (*see* Double and Triple Sulfonamide Preparations).

Toxic nephrosis and local or generalized nephritis may rarely be seen. They are probably hypersensitivity reactions. The nephritis may be either an isolated local reaction or part of a general hypersensitivity response.

Blood Disorders

Blood dyscrasias are rare but potentially fatal. Hemolytic anemia may be either acute or chronic and in some cases may represent a hypersensitivity reaction. Anemia can also develop in patients with red blood cell glucose-6-phosphate dehydrogenase deficiency (*see* Chap. 11) and in subjects with hemoglobin Zurich. Acute hemolytic anemia usually develops within the first 2 to 7 days of drug exposure and is commonly associated with fever. Acute renal tubular necrosis may follow the associated hemoglobinuria. Mild chronic hemolytic anemia may occur in patients exposed to prolonged low-dosage therapy.

Agranulocytosis (0.1%) usually appears between the 2nd and 6th week of therapy. Bone marrow examination frequently shows maturation arrest at the myeloblastic stage. Agranulocytosis is almost certainly a sensitization phenomenon, since its incidence is independent of either total drug dosage or duration of exposure. Agranulocytosis usually develops abruptly but may be preceded by progressive neutropenia. *All patients taking sulfonamides should be instructed to watch for symptoms of early agranulocytosis and, if these develop, to stop all drug therapy immediately and consult their physician.* Periodic blood counts may detect the development of neutropenia, but greater reliance should be placed on recognizing specific symptoms.

Thrombocytopenis purpura, eosinophilia, and aplastic anemia are encountered rarely. They probably have an allergic basis, although marrow aplasia may result from a myelotoxic effect of the drugs. Eosinophilia may complicate hypersensitivity reactions.

Hypersensitivity Reactions

Hypersensitivity reactions may be seen; some have already been mentioned above.

Numerous reactions in the skin and mucous membranes may develop. Seen within 7 to 20 days of the start of therapy are generalized skin rashes (morbilliform, purpuric, petechial, papular, vesicular, scarlatiniform), urticaria, and photodermatitis. In patients with a history of sulfonamide sensitivity, the lesions develop in a matter of hours and may progress rapidly to exfoliative dermatitis. Contact dermatitis and fixed drug eruptions are becoming less common because of the reduced use of topical sulfonamide drugs. Behçets syndrome, erythema nodosum, erythema multiforme, the Stevens–Johnson syndrome, and epidermolysis bullosa may rarely be seen. The Stevens–Johnson syndrome may be more common after the use of long-acting sulfonamides (*see* below).

Drug fever (3%) is almost certainly a hypersensitivity reaction. It usually develops within 10 days of the start of therapy and is often accompanied by systemic features, thus resembling serum sickness. Drug fever must be distinguished from fever due to a recurrence of the original infection or to suprainfection, or fever associated with the onset of acute hemolytic anemia or agranulocytosis. In previously nonsensitive persons, a typical serum sickness syndrome may appear within 10 to 20 days. In previously sensitized patients, a syndrome of anaphylactic shock may develop abruptly. Lesions similar to local or generalized polyarteritis nodosa, to temporal arteritis, or to lupus erythematosus are rare (1%).

Patients with lupus erythematosus should avoid taking sulfonamides and the chemically related drugs acetazolamide (*see* Chap. 40), the sulfonylureas (*see* Chap. 46), and the thiazides (*see* Chap. 40).

Gastrointestinal Disturbances

About 2% of patients taking sulfa drugs experience nausea, anorexia, and vomiting. These symptoms are probably of CNS origin, since they may also occur with parenteral therapy. Suprainfection and diarrhea do not occur often.

Miscellaneous Effects

Other rare adverse reactions include headache, peripheral neuritis (motor and sensory neuropathy), optic neuritis, changes in mood (fatigue, depression, anxiety, drowsiness, insomnia, nightmares, and psychotic episodes), ataxia, vertigo, tinnitus, hepatitis (rarely associated with antinuclear antibodies), goiter with or without hypothyroidism, arthralgia, conjunctivitis, hypersensitivity myocarditis, pulmonary eosinophilia, porphyria, and "cyanosis" (from methemoglobinemia and sulfonamide oxidation products). Sulfacetamide may produce systemic acidosis with a lowered carbon-dioxide-combining power of the blood. Sulfonamides may depress the rate of metabolism of some drugs such as phenytoin, tolbutamide, and chlorpropamide.

Sulfa therapy may result in a false-positive lupus erythematosus cell test and false-positive Benedict's test for urinary sugar.

Effects in the Fetus and Neonate. In addition to the adverse reactions described above, sulfonamides may produce kernicterus in the fetus and neonate due to the displacement of unconjugated bilirubin (*see* Chap. 11). Sulfonamides are teratogenic in some laboratory animals but thus far have not been shown to cause such lesions in humans. Because of this potential risk, however, their use should be avoided during pregnancy.

PHARMACOLOGY OF SOME COMMON SULFONAMIDES

The sulfa drugs may be classified into four main groups (Fig. 64-2 and Table 64-3). *Sulfonamides of group 1 are used topically,* but the risk of inducing sensitization is high; the only apparently safe products for use on the skin are mafenide and silver sulfadiazine. Other products may be introduced safely into the conjunctival sac, the otic canal, and the vagina. *Group 2* (systemic sulfonamides) comprises most sulfa drugs. These are rapidly absorbed after oral or parenteral administration and are rapidly metabolized and excreted. Some physicians separate systemic sulfonamides into two groups: short-acting and intermediate-acting drugs. Sulfonamides of *group 3* (long-acting sulfonamides) are absorbed rapidly following oral or parenteral administration but are excreted slowly. *Because of serious toxicity, these agents are generally obsolete* (*see* below). Sulfonamides in *group 4* are poorly absorbed after oral administration and are used only for a local effect in the bowel lumen to treat specific intestinal diseases such as shigellae infections and occasionally to reduce the lumenal bacterial population before bowel surgery. Their value in preoperative patients is being questioned, and their place in treating bacillary dysentery is gradually becoming obsolete because of the emergence of resistant organisms and the introduction of more potent specific antibiotics. Because sulfonamides suppress the normal bacterial flora, the synthesis of vitamin K may be depressed below that required to maintain adequate host synthesis of prothrombin. Consequently, patients taking

(*Text continues on p. 646*)

HALUSHI BEHÇET, 1889–1948. Although the syndrome had previously been observed by others, Behçet was the first to identify what is now known as Behçet's syndrome in 1937. It has been suggested that Behçet's syndrome has a viral etiology.

TABLE 64-3. Popular Sulfonamides

Drug	Properties	Preparations and Dose
Group 1. Sulfas for topical use		
Sodium sulfacetamide	Highly water soluble (100 times that of sulfadiazine). A 30% solution has a *p*H of 7.5 that is nonirritating. Bacteriostatic or bactericidal concentrations rapidly develop in ocular tissues following conjunctival application. Sulfa of choice for infections of the conjunctival sac. Should not be applied if a large open wound is present.	Sodium sulfacetamide, U.S.P. (Sodium Sulamyd), as an ophthalmic ointment (10%) and as an ophthalmic solution (10%, 15%, and 30%). Applied every 2 to 8 hours.
Mafenide (α-amino-para toluenesulfonamide	Differs from other sulfas in that it may not act by PABA inhibition. Contains a methyl group between the amino radical and the benzene ring. Used topically, particularly on burns, to prevent *Pseudomonas* infections. Rapidly absorbed and metabolized to paracarboxybenzenesulfonamide. Inhibits carbonic anhydrase, resulting in an alkaline urine. Rarely produces a maculopapular eruption, and local pain and burning due to hypertonicity. Mafenide hydrochloride may produce hyperchloremic acidosis in patients with reduced pulmonary function.	Mafenide acetate, U.S.P. (Sulfamylon), available as a 5% solution and a 10% cream. The burned surface should be carefully cleaned before application. Adequate bacteriostatic concentrations usually maintained for 12 hours with use of nonocclusive dressings. Cream is more effective, and therapy should be continued for 2 to 3 weeks.
Silver sulfadiazine	Equal antibacterial spectrum to mafenide. Painless on topical administration, does not produce hyperchloremic acidosis, and is less rapidly metabolized than mafenide. Mainly used to reduce or prevent colonization in skin wounds. Silver is released locally.	Silver sulfadiazine, U.S.P. (Silvadene)
Sulfisoxazole	Primarily a group-2 sulfa but used topically in the eye, nose, ear, and vagina.	Sulfisoxazole diethanolamine, 4% for general application. Sulfisoxazole, U.S.P. (Gantrisin), 10% cream, for vaginal application.
Group 2. Systemic sulfas		
Sulfadiazine	Rapidly and almost completely absorbed following oral or parenteral administration, with peak serum levels obtained between 2 and 4 hours. At serum levels of 10 mg/dl, the drug is 50% bound to plasma proteins. It is about 30% acetylated, and acetyl sulfadiazine is more soluble than the parent drug. About 200 mg/dl and 20 mg/dl of free sulfa are soluble in urine at *p*H 7.0 and 5.5, respectively. Free sulfa is absorbed about 70% by renal tubules.	Sulfadiazine, U.S.P., 2 to 4 g initially followed by 0.5 to 1.0 g q 4 to 6 hours for systemic infections. For urinary tract infections, 1 g q 4 to 6 hours. Sodium sulfadiazine injection, U.S.P., 25 to 50 mg/kg q 8 hours diluted in normal sodium chloride, $^{1}/_{6}$ molar sodium lactate, or Ringer's solution. Concentrations should not exceed 2.5% to 5.0% for s.c. and i.v. administration, respectively, to minimize sloughing or thrombophlebitis. Rarely used.
Sulfamerazine	Similar to sulfadiazine. About 50% acetylated and about 80% reabsorbed by the renal tubules.	Usually used as a component of triple sulfonamides. *See* text.
Sulfamethazine	Similar to sulfadiazine. About 70% acetylated and about 85% absorbed by the renal tubules.	Usually used as a component of triple sulfonamides. *See* text.
Double or triple sulfas	*See* text.	Trisulfapyrimidines, U.S.P. (sulfadiazine, sulfamerazine, sulfamethazine) Sulfadiazine and sulfamerazine, N.F. Sulfacetamide, sulfadiazine, and sulfamerazine, N.F.

(continued)

TABLE 64-3. *(Continued)*

Drug	Properties	Preparations and Dose
Double or triple sulfas *(continued)*		The loading dose for each preparation is 2 to 4 g followed by 1 g q 6 to 8 hours.
Sulfisoxazole	After similar dosage, blood levels are twice those of sulfadiazine, possibly because the drug is distributed only extracellularly. About 30% is acetylated, and urinary solubility of both free and acetylated sulfisoxazole is greater then that of sulfadiazine. The incidence of serious adverse reactions is about 0.1% to 0.2%.	Sulfisoxazole, U.S.P. (Gantrisin), is available in tablets of 500 mg and in several other formulations such as preparations for parenteral, topical, and vaginal use. The initial oral dose of 2 to 4 g is followed by 0.5 to 2.0 g q 6 hours. *See* above for topical preparations.
Sulfamethoxazole	Closely related to sulfisozazole but more slowly absorbed and less rapidly excreted than that compound, allowing twice daily administration; *see* text under trimethoprim : sulfamethoxazole.	Sulfamethoxazole, U.S.P. (Gantanol), 1 to 2 g initially, followed by 1 g q 8 to 12 hours. Sulfamethoxazole, 500 mg, plus phenazopyridine, 50 mg, as a fixed dosage preparation AzoGantanol. *See* sulfisoxazole.
Sulfacetamide	High urine solubility (2%) and rapid renal excretion allow treatment of urinary tract infections. Adverse reactions other than crystalluria develop in about 2% of patients. "Cyanosis" due to production of methemoglobin and oxidation products appears in about 5% of patients.	Sulfacetamide N.F. (Sulamyd), 1 to 3 g initially followed by 1 g q 8 hours.
Sulfapyridine	An early sulfa. Far more toxic than newer agents but the drug of choice for dermatitis herpetiformis.	Sulfapyridine, U.S.P., is given in doses of 500 mg q 4 to 12 hours.
Group 3. Long-acting systemic sulfas		
Sulfadimethoxine	Rapidly absorbed and excreted mainly (80%) as the glucuronide. Free drug absorbed about 95% by the renal tubules. Following an oral dose of 2 g, peak plasma levels of 10 mg/dl to 20 mg/dl develop within 4 to 6 hours, and 24 hours later are still 5 mg/dl and 15 mg/dl.	Sulfadimethoxine, N.F. (Madribon), 1 to 2 g initially followed by 0.5 to 1 g daily. *Rarely used because of high incidence of side-effects. See* text.
Sulfamethoxypyridazine	Rapidly absorbed but poorly excreted due to 80% to 90% plasma protein binding and avid renal tubular reabsorption of free sulfa. Following an oral dose of 2 g, peak plasma levels of 10 mg/dl to 20 mg/dl develop within 3 to 5 hours and after 4 days are still in the range of 1 to 3 mg/dl. About 10% is acetylated.	Sulfamethoxypyridazine, U.S.P. (Kynex, Midicel), 1 g initially followed by 0.5 to 1 g daily. *Rarely used because of high incidence of side-effects. See* text.
Group 4. Poorly absorbed sulfas		
Succinylsulfathiazole	Hydrolyzed in the bowel with release of active principle sulfathiazole. The small quantity of sulfa absorbed (3–5%) can initiate hypersensitivity in sensitized persons. Not effective in diarrhea.	Succinylsulfathiazole, U.S.P. (Sulfasuxidine), 250 mg/kg/day in 4 to 6 divided doses.
Phthalylsulfathiazole	Superior to succinylsulfathiazole in that it is effective in the presence of diarrhea. Inactive until hydrolyzed in the bowel lumen with release of sulfathiazole.	Phthalysulfathiazole, N.F. (Sulfathalidine), 50 to 125 mg/kg/day in 3 to 4 divided doses.
Salicylazosulfapyridine	Insoluble derivative of sulfapyridine used in ulcerative colitis, regional enteritis, and granulomatous colitis. Salicylazosulfapyridine is metabolized in the bowel lumen to sulfapyridine, which is readily absorbed, and 5-amino salicylate.	Salicylazosulfapyridine, U.S.P. (Azulfidine), 4 to 8 g daily in 4 to 8 divided doses.

the poorly absorbed sulfa drugs continuously over prolonged periods should receive vitamin K.

DOUBLE AND TRIPLE SULFONAMIDE PREPARATIONS

One of the common and yet avoidable adverse effects of the sulfonamides is crystalluria. Crystals are primarily composed of acetylsulfonamide metabolites but may contain free drug. The more effective sulfonamides unfortunately are usually less soluble in acidic urine, and thus crystalluria may readily result. Measures to reduce crystal formation (adequate hydration and urinary alkalinizers) are not always practical or desirable. An adequate fluid intake, for example, may be impossible to achieve in a dehydrated patient who also has diarrhea and vomiting. Alkalinizing drugs (sodium bicarbonate, lactate, acetate, and citrate), although they raise urinary *p*H, also lower blood sulfa drug levels by enhancing renal excretion. Further, large doses of alkali may be contraindicated in patients with renal failure, and soluble sodium sulfonamides may be contraindicated in patients with edema and congestive heart failure to minimize cation lode.

The solubility of most free and acetylated sulfonamides is not interfered with by addition of a second or a third sulfonamide to the solution. By using a double or triple sulfonamide mixture, additive antibacterial activity is produced with retention of independent solubility. Thus a higher total concentration of sulfonamide may be obtained in the urine (without the likelihood of drug precipitation) than would be possible if a single sulfa was used.

Triple sulfa preparations do not have a broader antibacterial spectrum, nor is the overall incidence of adverse reactions (with the exception of crystalluria) less than that of single drugs. The reduction in crystalluria is greater with a triple sulfa mixture than with full dosage of sulfadiazine plus an alkali. Combination of a triple sulfonamide and an alkali is even safer but rarely warranted clinically.

ADVERSE EFFECTS OF LONG-ACTING SULFAS

The clinical use of long-acting sulfas is obsolete except possibly in suppressive therapy of malaria. The incidence of adverse reactions to these drugs is about 10% to 20%. Hypersensitivity skin rashes are more common with these sulfonamides than with other members of the class, particularly the Stevens–Johnson syndrome. In neonates, severe kernicterus may be induced (*see* Chap. 11). Adverse drug reactions that develop in a patient receiving long-acting sulfonamides are more serious because of delayed drug excretion, and a number of deaths have followed their use.

USE OF SULFONAMIDES

The indications for the use of sulfonamides became fewer as more potent antibiotics were made available. However, sulfas are easy to administer, relatively cheap, and rarely followed by suprainfection. Sulfonamides should be given only if there is a reasonable chance of their being effective, and then only under careful supervision. All patients should be instructed to watch for signs and symptoms of toxicity (particularly fever, headaches, sore throat, diarrhea, jaundice, hematuria, loin pain) and to contact their physician immediately and discontinue therapy at the first suspicious sign. Many severe adverse reactions develop within a few days to weeks of the start of treatment, and careful monitoring of the peripheral blood count should be considered. With systemic sulfonamide therapy, an adequate fluid intake (sufficient to produce at least 1.5 liters of urine per day) is paramount. Urinary alkalinizing agents may also be prescribed.

Determination of bacterial sensitivity to the sulfas *in vitro* is desirable, but the test results are frequently misleading. Measurement of blood levels of the sulfonamides may be valuable in monitoring treatment in patients with renal insufficiency who must be given sulfonamides. Generally, the choice of a sulfonamide is based primarily on pharmacologic and toxicologic factors because *in vivo* comparisons are unreliable.

Topical Sulfonamides

Sodium sulfacetamide is valuable for some cases of blepharitis and conjunctivitis as prophylaxis against infection following penetrating eye injuries in the newborn and in the treatment of trachoma and inclusion conjunctivitis. The 30% solution is probably more useful than the 10% cream. For the treatment of trachoma and inclusion conjunctivitis, topical therapy should be combined with full doses of a short-acting sulfonamide by mouth.

Mafenide is finding wide favor in the treatment of burns, particularly those infected with *Pseudomonas aeruginosa;* silver sulfadiazine is probably equally effective.

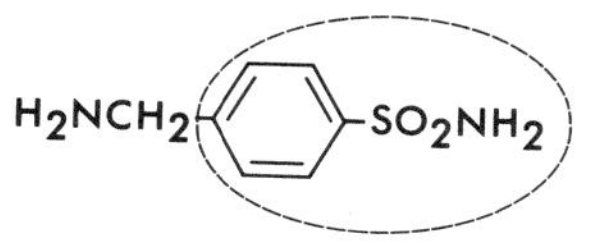

MAFENIDE

Sulfisoxazole preparations can be used, as can sulfacetamide, and are also valuable in treating some vaginal infections and infections in the nose and otic canal.

Systemic Sulfonamides

Systemic sulfonamides are bacteriostatic for a variety of organisms. However, antibiotics are currently preferred in most instances, although the low cost of sulfonamides is an important advantage.

Bacterial Infections. Many organisms that cause acute or chronic pyelonephritis or acute cystitis, such as *E. coli, Proteus* spp., and *Klebsiella* spp., may still be sensitive to sulfonamides, particularly if the infection is community-acquired. In many instances, however, the responsible organism shows multiple drug resistance (*see* Chap. 56). Sulfonamides are usually not effective in renal infections if there is extensive parenchymal involvement.

Sulfonamides are the drugs of choice for chancroid and nocardiosis. In nocardiosis, high doses of 4 to 6 g/day are required, and ampicillin or a tetracycline may be added with advantage. Sulfonamides plus streptomycin or chloramphenicol may rarely be considered for *Hemophilus influenzae* meningitis in those patients allergic to the penicillins. Sulfonamides have also been replaced in the treatment of most cases of shigellosis where ampicillin, tetracyclines, or chloramphenicol may be more active. The problem of multiple drug resistance (*see* Chap. 56) applies particularly with this species. The sulfonamides may, however, be of some value for prophylactic treatment in epidemics of shigellosis caused by sensitive strains. With meningococcal meningitis, ampicillin, penicillin G, and chloramphenicol are probably the agents of choice, since many strains of *N. meningitidis* are sulfonamide-resistant; a sulfonamide plus trimethoprim may be valuable in treating the carrier state, although either rifampin or minocycline is probably more effective. Most strains of gonococci are now resistant to sulfonamides, but recent clinical experience suggests that a sulfonamide plus trimethoprim is highly effective in many newly acquired infections. Several studies have shown the value of sulfonamides in the long-term prophylaxis of group A β-hemolytic streptococcal infections in patients allergic to the penicillins or the cephalosporins. Sulfa drugs have virtually no place in treating streptococcal pneumonia, erysipelas, or septicemia.

Protozoal Infections. Sulfonamides are of some value in chloroquine-resistant malaria (*see* Chap. 67) and, in combination with pyrimethamine, are of value in toxoplasmosis and *Pneumocytis carinii* infection. In the latter condition, pentamadine isethionate is also valuable.

Large Viruses (Chlamydia) Infections. Sulfonamides are the drugs of choice for many infections caused by the large viruses. Tetracyclines are valuable alternative agents. In trachoma and inclusion conjunctivitis, combined topical and oral sulfonamide therapy is desirable.

Fungus Infections. Sulfonamides are the drugs of choice combined with penicillin in the treatment of some cases of actinomycosis. South American blastomycosis, histoplasmosis, and maduromycosis may also respond to sulfa therapy, although amphotericin B is a more desirable drug.

Other Uses. Sulfapyridine (0.5 g–1.0 g every 4 hours) is the sulfa of choice for dermatitis herpetiformis. Dapsone (*see* Chap. 65) is an alternative agent.

Long-Acting Systemic Sulfonamides

The only theoretical advantage of the long-acting sulfonamides is in prophylactic or suppressive therapy. Most physicians agree, however, that it is safer to give a short-acting sulfa drug more frequently than to rely on a small dose of a longer-acting preparation. Recently long-acting sulfa drugs have achieved some success in treating chloroquine-resistant malaria infections (*see* Chap. 67).

Poorly Absorbed Sulfonamides

Phthalylsulfathiazole has been used to reduce the bowel flora before colonic surgery. The drug is of no value in bacillary dysentery. Succinylsulfathiazole is as effective as the systemic sulfonamides in treating acute bacillary dysentery, but its use may reduce the incidence of the carrier state. Salicylazosulfapyridine may be useful in the long-term management of

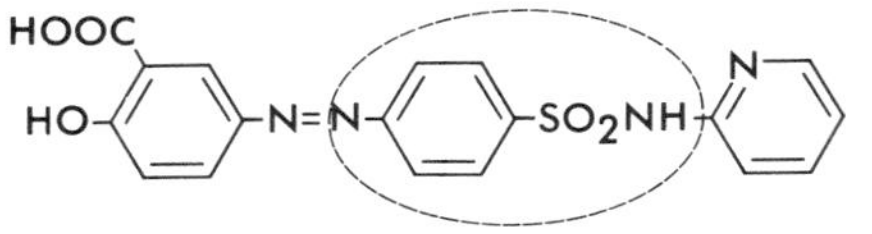

SALICYLAZOSULFAPYRIDINE

ulcerative colitis and is sometimes helpful in regional enteritis. Although the poorly absorbed sulfonamides diminish the colonic fecal flora, there is little clinical evidence to show that such an effect yields a lower incidence of postoperative infections than does no prophylactic treatment. On the contrary, preoperative bowel "sterilization" may be followed by a *higher* incidence of postoperative infections.

Sulfonamide–Antibiotic Mixtures

An additive effect may be produced when sulfonamides are combined with bacteriostatic antibiotics, for example, with chloramphenicol or streptomycin in the treatment of *Hemophilus influenzae* meningitis and *Klebsiella pneumoniae* infections, or with tetracyclines for nocardiosis. There is, however, a theoretical objection to combining a bactericidal antibiotic with the bacteriostatic sulfonamides (*see* Chap. 56). Few investigations have compared possible sulfonamide antibiotic combinations, and until any combination has been conclusively shown to be superior to either agent used separately, these mixtures should be avoided. Exceptions to this categorical statement are the combinations of sulfadiazine and streptomycin or chloramphenicol in the treatment of *Hemophilus influenzae* and the combination of sulfadiazine and penicillin in actinomycosis and anthrax. However, in the latter diseases, penicillin alone may be preferable. The concomitant use of sulfamethoxazole and trimethoprim (co-trimoxazole) is discussed below.

SULFAMETHOXAZOLE: TRIMETHOPRIM (CO-TRIMOXAZOLE)

Trimethoprim, an antimalarial agent (*see* Chap. 67), has achieved popularity in fixed dosage combination with sulfamethoxazole (co-trimoxazole). The mixture may possess a wider antibacterial spectrum than does those of its separate components. Additionally, co-trimoxazole may exhibit bactericidal properties, and may exhibit a synergistic antimicrobial effect owing to its double sequential attack on bacterial metabolism (*see* Chap. 57). The concomitant use of the sulfa reduces the emergence of bacterial resistance to trimethoprim. Sulfonamides other than sulfamethoxazole have been combined, but not as fixed dosage preparations, with trimethoprim and related drugs in the treatment of malaria and other infections (*see* Chap. 67). Sulfamethoxazole was selected over other short-acting sulfonamides for fixed dosage combination with trimethoprim because both agents are absorbed and excreted at about the same rate, thus yielding a fairly constant 20:1 concentration ratio *in vivo*. Such a ratio is optimum for the development of synergism. Other fixed dosage preparations that combine a different sulfonamide, for example, sulfadiazine, with trimethoprim, are available in Europe. These agents offer specific individual advantages, such as differing ratios of free to acetylated sulfa excreted in the urine. Some important properties of co-trimoxazole are discussed herein: The other pharmacologic properties of the mixture are discussed above (*see* under Sulfonamides) and in Chapter 67 (for trimethoprim).

ANTIMICROBIAL SPECTRUM

Most gram-positive cocci are susceptible, particularly *Staph. aureus* and *Staph. epidermidis*, *Strep. viridans*, group A β-hemolytic streptococci, and *Strep. pneumoniae*. *Neisseria meningitidis* and gonococci are variably sensitive. Many gram-negative bacteria, including *E. coli*, *Klebsiella/Enterobacter* spp., *Salmonella*, *Shigella*, and *H. influenzae* are also susceptible. Some sensitivity is observed against *Serratia marcescens*, *C. diphtheriae*, *Providencia*, *Proteus* spp., and *Nocardia*. *Pseudomonas* spp. are resistant. Co-trimoxazole is effective against *Pneumocystis carinii*.

The degree of synergism between sulfamethoxazole and trimethoprim is readily apparent in the susceptibility of *E. coli*; the minimum inhibitory concentration for co-trimoxazole against *E. coli* is 0.05 μg/ml and 1.0 μg/ml for trimethoprim and sulfamethoxazole, respectively, but individually the minimum inhibitory concentrations are 0.3 μg/ml and 4.0 μg/ml, respectively.

MODE OF ACTION

Co-trimoxazole produces a double sequential attack on bacterial metabolism (*see* Chap. 57), blocking the production of tetrahydrofolate cofactors. Such cofactors are important carriers of single carbon fragments vital in the synthesis of purines, thymine, methionine, and serine. Co-trimoxazole may possess other actions, such as interfering with the immune response.

ABSORPTION, METABOLISM, AND EXCRETION

Alone or in combination, trimethoprim and sulfamethoxazole are well absorbed after oral administration. Following a single dose of 160 mg of trimethoprim plus 800 mg of sulfamethoxazole (the optimum ratio), plasma levels peak between 1 to 2 μg/ml and 40 to 60 μg/ml, respectively, within 2 to 4 hours; trimethoprim, however, is more rapidly absorbed than is sulfamethoxazole. Steady-state plasma levels are achieved after 2 to 3 days of similar doses twice a day. Sulfamethoxazole and trimethoprim are bound about 60% to 70% and 40% to 65%, respectively, to plasma proteins; the binding of sulfamethoxazole to plasma proteins is reduced in uremic plasma.

Trimethoprim has a volume of distribution of about 100 liters, and its concentration in tissues exceeds that of plasma; sulfamethoxazole concentrations in plasma, however, exceed those achieved in most tissues. Trimethoprim and sulfamethoxazole have half-lives of 8 to 17 hours and 8 to 12 hours, respectively. After a single maternal dose, peak amniotic fluid levels develop at 10 hours and 14 hours for sulfamethoxazole and trimethoprim, respectively.

The two agents are principally excreted in the urine both in free and metabolized forms. With normal renal function, urine levels are approximately threefold and 100-fold higher than in plasma for sulfamethoxazole and trimethoprim, respectively. Sulfamethoxazole and trimethoprim have pK_a's of 5.7 and 7.3, respectively, and their renal excretion is influenced by the *p*H of the urine (*see* Chap. 3). The clearance of both agents falls rapidly in renal insufficiency, and both are removed by hemodialysis.

ADVERSE REACTIONS

The adverse reactions of co-trimoxazole are the reactions seen with either compound individually. Evidence suggests that trimethoprim may increase the gastrointestinal, cutaneous, and hematologic toxicity of sulfamethoxazole. Gastrointestinal side-effects occur in about 5% of patients, with nausea, vomiting, glossitis, and diarrhea being common; pseudomembranous colitis (*see* Chap. 63), may develop. Skin reactions are common, being reported in 5% to 10% of patients; such reactions are similar to those discussed under sulfonamides.

Co-trimoxazole (trimethoprim) may be teratogenic, and it occasionally produces a macrocytic anemia. Co-trimoxazole may also interfere with the chemical estimation of serum bilirubin and alkaline phosphatase, resulting in spuriously high values.

PREPARATIONS AND DOSAGE

Sulfamethoxazole and trimethoprim are available in two fixed-dosage tablet preparations of 400 mg plus 80 mg, and 800 mg plus 160 mg, respectively (Bactrim, Septra). A ratio of five parts sulfa to one part trimethoprim appears optimum because this yields on absorption a blood ratio of about 20:1 (sulfa:trimethoprim). A solution of 200 mg of sulfamethoxazole plus 40 mg of trimethoprim per 5 ml for oral administration is also available. Co-trimoxazole is more expensive than are sulfonamides alone.

USES

Co-trimoxazole has a potentiated antibacterial effect against many organisms. Its many uses may be summarized as follows: *recurrent* urinary tract infections; *Pneumocystis carinii* pneumonia; otitis media in children, particularly when caused by penicillinase-producing *H. influenzae;* acute exacerbations of chronic bronchitis; gonorrhea due to penicillinase-producing strains; brucellosis; nocardiosis; and antibiotic-resistant salmonellae, shigellae, and cholera vibrio infections. Other uses have been reported. The combination is not recommended for use in children under 12 years of age or during pregnancy.

FURTHER READING

1. Finland M, Kass EH: Trimethoprim–Sulfamethoxazole. J Infect Dis (Suppl) 128:5433–5816, November 1973
2. Kremers P, Duvivier J, Heusghem C: Pharmacokinetic studies of co-trimoxazole in man after single and repeated doses. J Clin Pharmacol 14:112–117, 1974
3. Lau WK, Young LS: Trimethoprim–Sulfamethoxazole treatment of pneumocystis carinii pneumonia in adults. N Engl J Med 295:716–718, 1976
4. Shuck JM, Moncrief JA: Safeguards in the use of topical mafenide (sulfamylon) in burned patients. Am J Surg 118:864–870, 1969

5. Woods DD: The biochemical mode of action of the sulfonamide drugs. J Gen Microbiol 29:687–702, 1962
6. Wust J, Wilkins TD: Susceptibility of anaerobic bacteria to sulfamethoxazole–Trimethoprim and routine susceptibility testing. Antimicrob Agents Chemother 14:384–390, 1978

CHAPTER 64 QUESTIONS

(*See* P. 7 for Full Instructions)

Select the One Best Answer

1. An agent used only for the suppression of intestinal flora is
   A. sulfamylon.
   B. succinylsulfathiazole.
   C. sulfisoxazole.
   D. sulfamethoxypyridazine.
   E. sulfacetamide.

2. Crystalluria is most likely with the oral administration of
   A. sulfadiazine.
   B. trisulfapyrimidines.
   C. sulfisoxazole.
   D. phthalylsulfathiazine.
   E. sulfacetamide.

3. Each of the following is an adverse reaction to sulfonamides EXCEPT
   A. kernicterus.
   B. agranulocytosis.
   C. "gray baby" syndrome.
   D. crystalluria.
   E. skin eruptions.

4. Sulfonamides are metabolized by each of the following EXCEPT
   A. oxidation.
   B. reduction.
   C. acetylation.
   D. sulfation.
   E. glucuronide formation.

5. Sulfamethoxazole is combined with trimethoprim as co-trimoxazole because
   A. the sulfonamide retards the metabolism of trimethoprim.
   B. trimethoprim retards the metabolism of the sulfonamide.
   C. both drugs act at the same enzymatic step in inhibiting folic acid synthesis.
   D. both drugs have similar pharmacokinetics.
   E. the required dose of the sulfonamide is reduced.

A = 1,2,3; B = 1,3; C = 2,4; D = 4; E = All

6. Antibacterial sulfonamides
   1. reduce the synthesis of folic acid.
   2. are antagonized by PABA.
   3. are bacteriostatic.
   4. inhibit dihydrofolate reductase.

7. Toxic effects of sulfadiazine include
   1. allergic reactions.
   2. hemolytic anemia.
   3. kernicterus in newborn.
   4. optic neuritis.

8. Which of the following produces its therapeutic effect by lowering the intracellular ratio of tetrahydrofolic (folinic) acid to folic acid?
   1. Sulfadiazine
   2. Co-trimoxazole
   3. Para-aminosalicylic acid
   4. Pyrimethamine

9. To minimize crystalluria induced by an antibacterial sulfonamide, a physician should
   1. increase the patient's water intake.
   2. combine different sulfonamides.
   3. alkalinize the patient's urine.
   4. acidify the patient's urine.

10. Antibacterial agents that readily diffuse across the normal blood–brain barrier include
   1. sulfadiazine.
   2. penicillin G.
   3. chloramphenicol.
   4. streptomycin.

11. Mechanisms of bacterial resistance to sulfonamides include
   1. reduced uptake/binding.
   2. development of adaptive enzymes that use the drug.
   3. production of para-aminobenzoic acid.
   4. elaboration of destructive enzymes.

12. Drugs acetylated polymorphically include
   1. hydrallazine.
   2. phenylzine.
   3. procaine amide.
   4. sulfamethazine.

13. Which of the following is contraindicated when a patient is taking sulfamethazine?
   1. Ammonium chloride
   2. Sulfamerazine
   3. Nalidixic acid
   4. Sulfadiazine

JEREMY H. THOMPSON

65

Chemotherapeutic Agents: II

Some important antimicrobial chemotherapeutic agents other than the sulfonamides (*see* Chap. 64) and the antiseptics (*see* Chap. 66) are discussed below under drugs for *tuberculosis* (isoniazid, rifampin, the aminosalicylates, ethambutol, pyrazinamide, and ethionamide); *leprosy* (the thiosemicarbazones and the sulfones); and *urinary tract infections* (the methenamines, nalidixic acid, oxolinic acid, and the nitrofurans).

DRUGS FOR TUBERCULOSIS

ISONIAZID: (ISONICOTINIC ACID HYDRAZIDE: INAH: INH)

Isoniazid is widely used in all types of tuberculosis and occasionally in atypical mycobacterial infections. It is related to the thiosemicarbazones, the monoamine oxidase inhibitor iproniazid, and nicotinic acid.

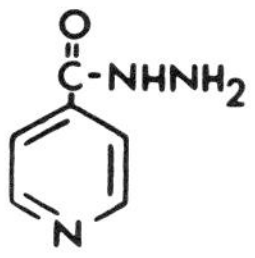

ISONIAZID

Bacterial Resistance and Mode of Action

Resistance develops rapidly and is a function of inoculum size. Isoniazid-resistant mutants are often deficient in catalases and peroxidases (*see* below) and have diminished virulence for guinea pigs. Isoniazid resistance is significant if there are large foci of persistent infection but less significant if there is minimal disease. The concomitant use of a second or a third antitubercular drug retards the development of resistance. Cross-resistance is rare.

Isoniazid is tuberculocidal or tuberculostatic *in vitro*, depending on various factors, including the inoculum size and the drug concentration. The minimum tuberculostatic concentration for most strains is about 0.05 μg/ml. Isoniazid is probably catabolized to a more active compound by mycobacterial catalases and peroxidases; many resistant bacteria are deficient in these enzymes.

Isoniazid may depress DNA synthesis but acts more effectively against dividing organisms. A lag phase of up to several days occurs after drug exposure, during which time sensitive mycobacteria do not reenter logarithmic growth. The slow growth rate of *M. tuberculosis* and its propensity to generate dormant forms have been main arguments for chronic treatment.

Absorption

Isoniazid is rapidly absorbed following oral administration, with peak levels developing within 2 hours. The drug diffuses freely to most tissues and tissue fluids, with a Vd of about 0.6 liters/kg. Isoniazid is minimally bound to plasma proteins and has significant first-pass loss (*see* Chaps. 3, 4). Active therapeutic levels may still be present in "slow" inactivators (*see* below) after 24 hours. Cerebrospinal fluid concentrations are usually at least half simultaneous blood levels, and tuberculostatic levels may be achieved in caseous foci and inside macrophages. Intramuscular, i.v. or intrarectal (suppository) administration is possible but rarely used. Because of first-pass loss, reduced absorption of the drug by food (give 30 minutes before eating) and antacids (give 60 minutes before use of aluminum antacids) should be minimized.

Metabolism

Isoniazid is primarily N-acetylated to acetyl isoniazid, which is therapeutically inactive and almost devoid of central and peripheral nervous system toxicity. N-Acetylation depends on the transfer of acetyl groups from coenzyme A by an N-acetyltransferase. The rate of acetylation is under genetic control and may be "slow" or "rapid" depending on the quantity of enzyme present (*see* Chap. 6).

Family studies show that after a standard dose of isoniazid (9.8 mg/kg) blood levels 6 hours later show a bimodal distribution with the antimode at 2.5 μg/ml. Thus "slow" acetylators have plasma levels greater than 2.5 μg/ml and "rapid" acetylators, levels less than 2.5 μg/ml. Slow acetylators are autosomal homozygous recessive, whereas rapid acetylators are either homozygous dominants or heterozygotes. The major gene operates against a background provided by other genes.

The distribution of phenotypes varies considerably. Rapid acetylators are roughly found in 20% to 30% of Middle Easterners, 30% to 50% of Europeans and black and white Americans, 80% to 90% of Orientals, and 95% to 100% of Eskimos.

Other Drugs Metabolized by Acetylation. Hydralazine, procainamide, dapsone, sulfasalazine, sulfamethazine, phenelzine, and the amine metabolite of nitrazepam are all acetylated polymorphically, whereas most sulfonamides, para-aminosalicylic acid (PAS), and ethionamide are acetylated monomorphically. Steric factors probably determine by which system drugs are acetylated. Even though they are metabolized by a different enzyme, PAS and ethionamide delay the acetylation of isoniazid, since these two agents preferentially combine with and utilize coenzyme A.

Clinical Significance of Isoniazid Polymorphism. Slow acetylators have more prolonged plasma levels of isoniazid (and other drugs acetylated polymorphically) after a standard dose than do rapid acetylators, and are more likely to develop adverse reactions (Table 65-1). There is no relation between the rate of isoniazid acetylation and the development of mycobacterial resistance, but the clinical response is poorer in rapid acetylators treated with twice weekly or less frequent (intermittent therapy) dosage regimens.

Excretion

About 3% and 30% of a single dose of INAH is excreted unchanged within 24 hours in rapid and slow acetylators, respectively; the balance is made up predominately of acetylisoniazid and isonicotinic acid, with trace quantities of isonicotinyl glycine, isonicotinyl hydrazone, and N-methyl isoniazid. All metabolites are therapeutically inactive and with one possible

TABLE 65-1. Drugs Acetylated Polymorphically, and Some of Their Important Adverse Effects in Slow Acetylators of Isoniazid

Drugs	Adverse Effects
Dapsone	More severe hematologic toxicity
Hydralazine	Systemic lupus erythematosus-like disorder. Other adverse effects are more common than in rapid acetylators (*see* Chap. 36)
Isoniazid	Peripheral neuropathy and systemic lupus erythematous-like disorder more likely. Possible increased risk of hepatitis if combined with alcohol, rifampin, or hepatotoxins such as carbon tetrachloride
Phenelzine	Higher incidence of central nervous system toxicity (*see* Chap. 24)
Procainamide	Systemic lupus erthematosus-like syndrome more common and develops earlier (*see* Chap. 34)
Sulfasalazine	Higher incidence of drug toxicity (*see* Chap. 64)

exception (*see* Liver Toxicity below) are almost devoid of toxicity.

INAH has a T½ of 40 to 80 minutes and 140 to 200 minutes in rapid and slow acetylators, respectively. In uremia the T½ may be 17 to 20 hours. INAH is excreted in milk and is removed by hemodialysis and peritoneal dialysis.

Adverse Reactions

Adverse reaction with conventional therapy occur in 5% to 10% of patients, but with daily doses above 10 mg/kg the incidence increases to 25% to 30%. With oral therapy, xerostomia, headaches, and mild gastrointestinal upsets are common. Peripheral neuritis develops in up to 25% of patients taking 6 mg/kg/day. It is more common in slow acetylators, alcoholics, malnourished persons, and those over 35 years of age and is probably due to the drug competing with vitamin B_6 for neural apotryptophanase. Peripheral neuropathy and some central toxicity (*see* below) are usually preventable by the concomitant use of vitamin B_6, 10 mg/50 to 100 mg of INAH dialy. Pyridoxine does not antagonise antitubercular activity or influence isoniazid pharmacokinetics.

Less common reactions are vertigo, ataxia, tinnitus, monoamine oxidase inhibitor-like mood changes, hallucinations, psychotic episodes, optic neuritis and atrophy, hyperreflexia, nystagmus, muscle twitching, increased appetite, hesitancy of micturition, urinary retention, and increased libido. Convulsive episodes may be produced, particularly in epileptic patients, and may reflect subclinical pyridoxine deficiency. Diabetic patients may require more insulin during high-dosage therapy because the drug is mildly diabetogenic, and pellagra may be precipitated in malnourished patients.

Rare side-effects are gynecomastia (possibly due to INAH-induced inhibition of estrogen metabolism), toxic encephalopathy, coma, metabolic acidosis, various arthrithides, sideroblastic anemia, red cell aplasia, hemolytic anemia, thrombocytopenia, agranulocytosis, methemoglobinemia and hypersensitivity reactions (pruritic skin rashes, bronchoconstriction, eosinophilia, polyarteritis nodosa, and a lupus-like syndrome with auto antibodies).

Liver Toxicity. Liver toxicity may vary from biochemical evidence alone (*e.g.*, elevation of SGOT/SGPT) to fatal necrosis. Serious toxicity is more common in those over 35 years of age, in people exposed to other hepatotoxic substances, including alcohol, or with evidence of liver disease, and in rapid acetylators. Pathogenesis may depend on the formation of a highly reactive metabolic product, *acetylhydrazine* from acetylisoniazid. The concomitant use of enzyme inducers may increase acetylhydrazine formation. Acetylhydrazine may covalently bind to vital cellular components if detoxification mechanisms are not operating optimally (*see* Chap. 4). However, other mechanisms may also be important since acetylhydrazine itself is also rapidly inactivated, particularly in rapid acetylators. Pyrazinamide and ethionamide may exacerbate INAH-induced liver damage. Hepatic necrosis tends to be preceded by a prodromal period of fatigue, malaise, weakness, anorexia, fever, and arthralgias. It may appear as late as after 8 months of therapy.

Preparations and Uses

Isoniazid, U.S.P., is available in many preparations (Table 65-2). The usual dose in adults and children is 300 mg/day and 10 to 30 mg/kg/day, respectively. In severe life-threatening disease in adults, doses as high as 30 mg/kg/day may be given for a short time. Serious adverse reactions, however, are dose dependent. In mild tuberculosis in slow acetylators, isoniazid may be given twice weekly instead of daily.

Isoniazid is highly effective against mycobacteria and in some atypical mycobacterial infections. Experimentally (10–20 mg/kg, plus pyridoxine) it has been tried in Huntington's chorea, where it may inhibit brain γ-aminotransferase, thereby elevating cerebral levels of γ-aminobutyric acid.

RIFAMPIN (RIFAMPICIN IN EUROPE)

Properties

Rifampin, 3-(4-methylpiperazinyliminomethyl) rifamycin SV, is a semisynthetic derivative of rifamycin B, one of a group of complex macrocyclic antibiotics produced by *Streptomyces mediterranei*. It is a zwitterion and is soluble in water at an acid *p*H. Rifampin's macrocyclic ring stoichiometrically binds to and inhibits DNA-dependent RNA polymerase (*see* Chap. 57). RNA polymerase from resistant bacteria does not complex with the antibiotic and thus is not inhibited. Mammalian RNA polymerase does not bind rifampin significantly.

Antibacterial Spectrum

Rifampin is a broad-spectrum antibiotic that possesses activity against many gram-positive cocci (*e.g.*, gonococci and meningococci) and gram-negative bacteria (*e.g.*, some strains of

TABLE 65-2. Chemotherapeutic Drugs Used in Tuberculosis

Drug	Preparations and Dosage
Isoniazid	Isoniazid, *U.S.P.*, available in many proprietary preparations, usually tablets of 50 to 200 mg, an injectable preparation of 100 mg/ml, and a flavored syrup of 10 mg/ml. For dosage, *see* text.
Aminosalicylates	Aminosalicylic acid, *U.S.P.* (para-aminosalicylic acid), and its salts are available in numerous dosage forms in uncoated, enteric-coated, and powder form. Many fixed dosage preparations with other antitubercular drugs and antacids are available, but physicians are advised against using these preparations (*see* Chap. 78). The usual dose of PAS is 8 to 20 g daily in divided doses.
Ethambutol	Ethambutol (Myambutol) is available in tablets of 100 mg and 400 mg of the *d*-isomer, which is about 200 times more active than the L-form. The usual dose is 15 mg/kg/day in a single oral dose.
Pyrazinamide	Pyrazinamide, *U.S.P.* (Aldinamide), is available in tablets of 500 mg. The usual dose is 20 to 25 mg/kg in divided doses; a daily dose of 3 g should not be exceeded.
Ethionamide	Ethionamide, *U.S.P.* (Trecator), is available in tablets of 125 mg and 250 mg with or without enteric coating. Suppository preparations are available for children. The usual adult dose is 250 mg twice daily increased by 125 mg/wk to a maximum dose of 500 mg twice daily.
Thiacetazone	Thiacetazone (Tibione) is given in doses of 200 mg/day.

E. coli, Ps. aeruginosa, indole positive and negative *Proteus* and *B. fragilis*). It is also highly effective against most strains of tuberculosis (minimum inhibitory concentration, 0.01–0.1 μg/ml) and many atypical mycobacteria.

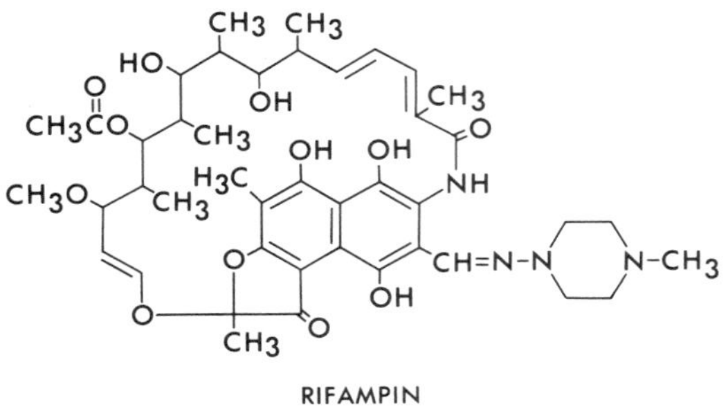

RIFAMPIN

Rifampin's gram-positive potency lies between penicillin G, which is more potent, and the cephalosporins, erythromycin, and clindamycin, but it is far less potent than the aminoglycosides, colistin, or the tetracyclines against gram-negative bacteria. Its activity against *Klebsiella* spp. and *Strep. faecalis* may be antagonized by the concomitant use of trimethoprim. The potential usefulness of rifampin is hampered by bacterial resistance that develops rapidly. Thus *in the treatment of tuberculosis, the addition of a second drug is essential* (*see* Chap. 60). However, most wild strains of *M. tuberculosis* have a remarkably small proportion of rifampin-resistant mutants, about one tenth that encountered with isoniazid. An unsettled question is, what is the potential danger of using rifampin alone in the treatment of gram-positive infections insofar as this may lead to mycobacterial resistance in concomitant but unrecognized tubercular disease? Cross-resistance is rare.

Absorption, Metabolism, and Excretion

Rifampin is well absorbed in the fasting state following oral administration, but food reduces its absorption. Peak serum levels develop within 2 to 4 hours, and measurable antitubercular activity persists for 12 to 18 hours. Rifampin is subject to significant first-pass extraction (*see* Chaps. 3, 4) with oral doses less than 300 to 450 mg. It is metabolized to a weakly active desacetylated derivative. Rifampin is bound about 80% to plasma proteins and has a T½ of 2 to 5 hours. Free rifampin undergoes an enterohepatic circulation (*see* Chap. 4), but the desacetylated metabolite is poorly absorbed. About 30% of any given dose is excreted in the urine; about one half of this is free rifampin, the remainder being the desacetylated metabolite. Probenecid depresses the hepatic uptake of rifampin, thus prolonging its half-life.

Adverse Effects

Except for the occurrence of gastrointestinal upsets and liver toxicity, rifampin is relatively nontoxic. Liver toxicity may be more common in patients with underlying liver disease or in those concomitantly ingesting other hepatotoxic drugs such as alcohol or INAH, particularly in slow acetylators. About 1% of persons taking doses of rifampin greater than 600 mg/kg/day develop biochemical evidence of liver toxicity. Liver damage may be fatal.

Headache, drowsiness, fatigue, blurred vision, dizziness, a Coombs'-positive hemolytic anemia, leukopenia, thrombocytopenia, eosinophilia, drug fever, an elevated BUN, light-chain-proteinuria, and hyperuricemia may occur. Repeated irregular courses of treatment may be followed by a "flu-like" syndrome, associated rarely with severe renal or liver damage. Body secretions may be colored orange/red and interfere with various colorimetric laboratory tests. Bromsulphthalein (BSP) retention may occur, but this may not reflect the development of liver damage, since the antibiotic competes with BSP at its site of excretion. Various skin rashes, including urticaria, are not uncommon, but generalized hypersensitivity is rare. Rifampin is a strong enzyme inducer and may have partial or reversible immune suppressive effects in humans. It interferes with bioassay of vitamin B_{12} and folate.

Rifampin and various orally administered x-ray contrast media interact in the bowel lumen, resulting in reduced rifampin absorption.

Preparations and Uses

Rifampin (Rifadin, Rimactane) is available in capsules of 300 mg. The usual adult dose is 600 to 900 mg/day 30 minutes before meals. In children, the dosage is 10 to 20 mg/kg/day, not to exceed 600 mg/day. The drug is expensive.

Rifampin plus at least one other antitubercular drug is valuable in tuberculosis, where it approaches or even surpasses isoniazid therapy both in efficacy and safety. It should not be used for single drug therapy for tuberculosis or for long-term prophylaxis.

A 4- to 7-day course of treatment has been recommended for meningococcal carriers. Rifampin should not be used, however, to treat meningococcal meningitis or the carrier with sulfonamide- or minocycline-sensitive bacteria. Other uses have not been approved; rifampin plus clindamycin in nocardiosis, leprosy, leishmaniasis, and trypanosomiasis (*see* Chap. 67) and in the treatment of pseudomembranous colitis (*see* Chap. 63).

THE AMINOSALICYLATES

The aminosalicylates, used only to treat tuberculosis, primarily as second-line drugs, include PAS; its sodium, potassium, and calcium salts; the phenyl ester; and calcium benzoylpas. In equivalent amounts, all are therapeutically similar, but the salts are more stable, are less irritating to the gastrointestinal mucosa, and have higher urinary solubilities than does the free acid. The aminosalicylates possess slightly some of the classic pharmacodynamic actions of the salicylates (*see* Chap. 31). The following description applies to PAS.

Para-aminosalicylic acid has a sour taste and a bitter aftertaste. Its weak tuberculostatic activity against human and bovine tuberculosis is potentiated by isoniazid or streptomycin.

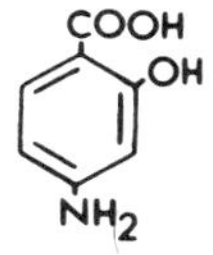

PAS

Although mycobacterial resistance is of slow onset, not appearing until after 3 or 4 months of therapy, PAS should be given only in combination with other antitubercular drugs in an attempt to delay resistance further. Cross-resistance has not been described.

Mode of Action

The exact mode of action is unknown, but the closely related compound para-aminobenzoic acid can antagonize the effect of PAS *in vitro* but appears to act differently from that involved in sulfonamide antagonism (*see* Chap. 57). Large doses of PAS are required for the treatment of disease; high, continuous blood levels may be necessary.

Absorption, Metabolism, and Excretion

The absorption of PAS after oral administration is rapid and almost complete, the sodium salt being absorbed more rapidly than the free acid. To minimize its unpleasant gastrointestinal side-effects, the drug should be given after meals.

After the patient receives a 4-g dose, peak blood levels of about 6 to 8 mg/ml develop within 1 to 2 hours. PAS has a pK_a of 3.2, has a Vd of about 0.23 liters/kg, and is protein bound about 60%. The drug distributes poorly into the cerebrospinal fluid, where drug concentrations are only one-tenth simultaneous plasma levels. Penetration into caseous material is usually satisfactory.

PAS is degraded by acetylation (monomorphically) and competes successfully with isoniazid for cofactors (*see* above). Both free PAS and its acetylated derivative are promptly excreted (over 90% in 12 hours) by renal glomerular filtration and tubular secretion. About 40% of PAS is excreted unchanged, and the drug has a $T\frac{1}{2}$ of $\frac{1}{2}$ to 2 hours. Probenecid prevents its tubular secretion. Free PAS is poorly soluble in acid urine, and the acetylated derivative is even less soluble. Thus crystalluria may develop (*see* Chap. 64). Crystalluria can be minimized by urinary alkalinization. The various salts of PAS and their acetylated metabolites have higher solubilities in urine than does PAS itself. PAS is removed by hemodialysis.

Adverse Reactions

Gastrointestinal symptoms occur in most patients who diligently take the prescribed number of tablets. Commonly seen are nausea, epigastric pain or heartburn, anorexia, and diarrhea. Symptoms are reduced by giving the drug with meals or antacids and by starting therapy with low doses (2–3 g/day) and gradually increasing the dose to optimum levels. A malabsorption syndrome and gastric bleeding are rare. Hypersensitivity reactions (5% of courses) usually develop between the 2nd and 8th week of therapy. Fever, headache, general malaise, skin rashes (especially photosensitivity), and myalgias, arthralgias, and eosinophilia may be seen. Anaphylactic shock and chemical and clinical evidence of pancreatitis, hepatitis, myocarditis, pericarditis, and nephritis are rare, as are agranulocytosis, lymphocytosis, thrombocytopenia, eosinophilic pneumonitis, a lupus-like syndrome, and an infectious mononucleosis-like illness. Hemolytic anemia may occur in patients with glucose-6-phosphate dehydrogenase deficiency. Since PAS is a strong organic acid, acidosis may develop, particularly in children. Cation intoxication may be a problem in the face of diminished renal function. Bentonite, a former excipient in some formulations of PAS, chelates rifampin, reducing its absorption. PAS depresses the absorption of digoxin.

Preparations, Dosage, and Uses

Amino salicylic acid, U.S.P. (para-aminosalicylic acid), the sodium, potassium, and calcium salts of PAS, and calcium benzoylpas are available in many preparations (Table 65-2). The various salts of PAS and calcium benzoylpas cause less gastrointestinal irritation and are more stable and more soluble in acid urine than PAS itself. *Because of its sour taste and irritant properties, patients often do not take PAS as prescribed. Thus if a patient is prescribed PAS and a second antitubercular agent but does not take the PAS, mycobacterial resistance develops more rapidly than it otherwise would to the second agent.*

ETHAMBUTOL

Ethambutol (ethylene diamino-di-1-butanol dihydrochloride), an odorless, white chrystalline base, is a first-line drug for tuberculosis, often combined with INAH. It is tuberculostatic, depressing RNA synthesis. About 70% to 80% of strains of human *M. tuberculosis* are sensitive to 1 μg/ml. Resistance develops slowly, and cross-resistance has not been described.

Ethambutol (Table 65-2) is almost completely absorbed following oral administration, with peak plasma levels developing within 2 to 4 hours. Absorption is not measurably affected by food. Ethambutol passes poorly into the various body compartments (Vd~0.8 liters/kg) except for the cerebrospinal fluid. About 90% is excreted unchanged in the urine. The remainder comprises a butyric acid metabolite and an intermediary aldehyde. Ethambutol has a T½ of 6 to 8 hours and is removed by both hemodialysis and peritoneal dialysis.

Adverse Effects

Adverse reactions are uncommon with doses less than 20 mg/kg/day, but fairly common with doses greater than 50 mg/kg/day. The most serious side-effects are ataxia, retrobulbar neuritis (with a concomitant loss in ability to perceive the color green), and peripheral neuritis. Optic neuritis is dose related, and some damage is seen in 1% of patients given doses greater than 25 mg/kg/day. All patients require monthly ophthalmoscopic examinations to monitor visual acuity and color perception/discrimination. Gastrointestinal upsets, skin rashes, pruritus, headache, confusional states, arthralgias, hyperuricemia, leukopenia, thrombocytopenia, and anaphylactic shock are rare. Ethambutol dosage must be reduced drastically in the presence of renal insufficiency.

PYRAZINAMIDE

Pyrazinamide, related to nicotinamide, is used only in tuberculosis, where it is more tuberculostatic than PAS, viomycin, or cycloserine but less active than isoniazid, rifampin, or streptomycin. It may depress protein synthesis. If pyrazinamide is given alone *in vivo*, mycobacterial resistance develops within 6 to 8 weeks. Resistance is delayed by combining a second antitubercular drug. Cross-resistance may rarely occur with isoniazid.

Pyrazinamide (pK_a 0.5) is readily absorbed after oral administration and widely distributed. A dose of 1 g produces peak plasma levels of 40 to 50 μg/ml in 2 hours. The drug is bound 40% to 60% to plasma proteins. Tuberculostatic levels occur both in caseous foci and in macrophages. Pyrazinamide has a T½ of 10 to

16 hours and is excreted by glomerular filtration and tubular secretion.

Adverse Reactions

Toxicity is dose dependent. Biochemical evidence of hepatic damage develops in 5% to 15% of patients. These effects are usually reversible by reducing the dosage or temporarily discontinuing the agent, but death from hepatic necrosis can occur. All patients should be hospitalized and have careful and continued evaluation of liver function during therapy.

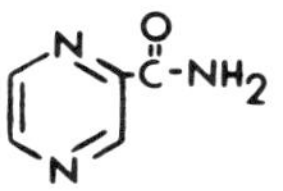

PYRAZINAMIDE

Liver damage is particularly likely when doses are greater than 40 mg/kg/day or in those patients with underlying liver disease or concomitantly exposed to other hepatotoxins such as alcohol. Nausea, vomiting, arthralgias, spiking temperature, general malaise, lymphadenopathy, anemia, photosensitivity, and dysuria may occur. Pyrazinamide decreases the renal tubular excretion of urate and may produce hyperuricemia and acute gouty arthritis; thiazide diuretics and furosemide potentiate this response. Diabetic patients may be difficult to control since their insulin requirements may change.

Uses

Because of its toxicity, pyrazinamide is usually reserved for the treatment of tuberculosis resistant to the primary drugs, especially in short courses as an adjunct to minimize the spread of local infection. The dosage of pyrazinamide in adults is 1.5 g/day.

ETHIONAMIDE

Ethionamide, related to nicotinic acid, is a second-line drug for tuberculosis. Its mode of action is unknown. It is more effective against human than against bovine strains and may be converted *in vivo* into a more active form. Resistance develops rapidly when ethionamide is given alone but can be delayed by the addition of other drugs. Cross-resistance is rare.

Ethionamide (Table 65-2) is usually given in enteric-coated capsules to minimize mucosal irritation but may rarely be given in suppository form or intravenously. Absorption following the use of suppositories or enteric-coated capsules is slower and more irregular than that following oral administration of the uncoated tablets, but blood levels persist for longer periods. The drug is poorly absorbed after partial gastrectomy.

Ethionamide is bound 10% to plasma proteins and thus widely distributed, tuberculostatic concentrations developing in most tissues and tissue fluids, including the CSF. It has a $T\frac{1}{2}$ of 2 to 3 hours.

Ethionamide is as effective as PAS in reducing the acetylation of isoniazid *in vitro* (*see* above). Ethionamide is cleared primarily in the urine. However, only about 1% to 5% of free drug is excreted, the balance being made up with numerous metabolites.

The dose of ethionamide for children is 5 to 10 mg/kg every 12 hours and for adults, 0.5 to 1 g daily in three divided doses.

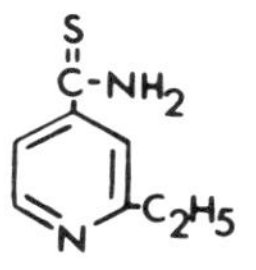

ETHIONAMIDE

Adverse Reactions

Anorexia, nausea, vomiting, stomatitis, sialorrhea, and a metallic aftertaste develop in most patients; these may be minimized by using enteric-coated tablets or by taking the uncoated tablets after meals. Headaches, mental depression, convulsions, sleepiness, postural hypotension (ganglionic blockade), allergic skin rashes, acne, alopecia, purpura, menorrhagia, amenorrhea, gynecomastia, impotence, peripheral neuritis, optic neuritis, hyperuricemia, arthralgias, and hepatitis occur rarely with prolonged therapy. Fetal abnormalities have been described, and some diabetic patients require increased insulin dosage.

DRUGS FOR LEPROSY

THIOSEMICARBAZONES

Other than methisazone (*see* Chap. 70) and thiacetazone, used rarely to treat pulmonary tuberculosis and tuberculoid leprosy, the thiosemicarbazones are obsolete. Thiacetazone is less tuberculostatic than is PAS, and its mode of action is unknown. *M. leprae* becomes resistant more readily than does *M. tuberculosis*.

Thiacetazone (Table 65-2) is well absorbed following oral administration, with excretion occurring primarily in the urine. Anorexia, nausea, vomiting, and various skin rashes are common. More serious reactions are blood dyscrasias (leukopenia, hemolytic anemia, and thrombocytopenia). If the drug is not withdrawn promptly at the first sign of a falling white blood cell count, irreversible agranulocytosis may develop. Thiacetazone may also produce hepatic and renal damage.

SULFONES

Several sulfones (Table 65-3) are derived from 4,4′-diamino-diphenyl sulfone (dapsone, DADPS, DDS) related to the sulfonamides. Many sulfones break down to dapsone *in vivo*, but in which form these agents exert their antimicrobial effects is unclear. The following description applies to dapsone, the drug of choice for leprosy. Important pharmacologic properties of other sulfones occasionally used to treat leprosy will be identified.

DAPSONE

Dapsone is primarily bacteriostatic, but its mechanism of action is unknown; some antagonism is produced by para-aminobenzoic acid (*see* Chap. 57). Dapsone is weakly tuberculostatic but is too toxic to be used in tuberculosis.

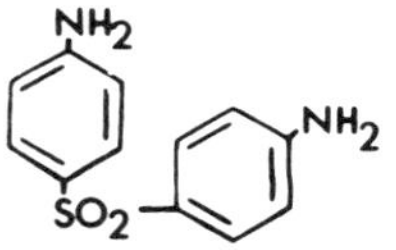

DIAMINODIPHENYL SULFONE (DAPSONE)

Dapsone is slowly but completely absorbed following oral administration. It is about 50% bound to plasma proteins and is distributed in total body water. Dapsone is concentrated in the liver, muscles, kidney, and skin, but passage into the cerebrospinal fluid is poor. Concentration may be 10 to 15 times greater in inflamed than in normal skin. Dapsone is conjugated with glucuronic acid and excreted in the urine and bile. It undergoes an enterohepatic circulation, a single dose being detected in the plasma for up to 12 days. Accumulation develops in long-term therapy. Bacterial resistance develops in 2% to 5% of patients, particularly those on low dosage or in those who comply irregularly.

Adverse Reactions

Adverse reactions are nearly all dose dependent. Gastrointestinal upsets occur in about 10% of patients. Hemolytic anemia commonly occurs in patients with glucose-6-phosphate dehydrogenase deficiency (*see* Chaps. 6, 11). Headaches, excitement, nervousness, insomnia, cholestatic jaundice, amblyopia, psychotic episodes, skin rashes (particularly erythema nodosum and erythema multiforme), pruritus, drug fever, goiter, and an infectious mononucleosis-like syndrome develop rarely. In high doses (200–300 mg/day) dapsone causes methemoglobinemia and Heinz-body formation. The "sulfone syndrome," a Jarisch–Herxheimer like reaction with fever, exfoliative dermatitis, hepatitis, methemoglobinemia, progressive anemia, and lymphadenopathy, may develop after 4 to 6 weeks of therapy in lepromatous leprosy.

Uses

Dapsone (Table 65-3) is the drug of choice for leprosy and some cases of dermatitis herpetiformis. Although not approved by the FDA, rifampin may be added to dapsone in the treatment of leprosy. Long courses of therapy (up to 5 years) may be required in leprosy, and dosage should be tailored individually. Adjunct therapy with corticosteroids, aminoglycosides, or "antimalarial" agents may be helpful. Dapsone may also be valuable in some cases of recalcitrant eczematous dermatitis and in malaria.

Acedapsone (DADDA) and *clofazimine* are under investigation as antileprotic drugs.

DRUGS FOR URINARY TRACT INFECTIONS

METHENAMINE MANDELATE, HIPPURATE, AND SULFOSALICYLATE

Methenamine mandelate (Mandelic acid, Mandelamine), *methenamine hippurate* (hippuric acid, Hiprex, Urex), and methenamine sulfosalicylate (sulfosalicylic acid, Hexalet) are three urinary antiseptic salts of methenamine, an agent obsolete when used alone.

Karl Herxheimer, 1861–1944. German dermatologist in Frankfurt. The Herxheimer (or Jarisch–Herxheimer) reaction, Salvarsan-induced inflammation in syphilitic tissues, was reported in 1902. Also independently described chronic atrophic acrodermatitis in 1902.

TABLE 65-3. Chemotherapeutic Sulfones Used in Leprosy

Drug	Properties, Preparations, and Dosage
Dapsone (4,4′-diaminodiphenyl sulfone)	Dapsone, *U.S.P.* (Avlosulfon), is available in tablets of 10, 25, 50, and 100 mg. Initial dose is 25 mg twice weekly. At intervals of 4 to 6 weeks, the dose is increased to 50, 100, 200, and 300 mg twice weekly.
4,4′-diacetyl-diaminodiphenyl sulfone	Long-acting, experimental sulfone under clinical trial in Africa. Releases dapsone or its monoacetylated derivative through action of tissue enzymes. Dose is 225 mg i.m. every 11 weeks.
Glucosulfone sodium (Promin)	A highly toxic agent of mainly historical interest, since it was the first sulfone used in therapy. Highly water soluble. Administered i.v. to minimize toxicity; oral and topical preparations also available.
Sulfoxone sodium (Diasone sodium)	A water-soluble derivative of dapsone for oral use
Thiazolsulfone (Promizole)	A poorly water-soluble preparation for oral use
Sulfetrone sodium (Cimedone)	A complex diamino-substituted derivative of dapsone for oral administration

Methenamine is a condensation of formaldehyde and ammonia (Fig. 65-1) from which, at a *p*H of 5.0 to 6.0 and below the active bactericidal protein precipitant, *formaldehyde* is increasingly liberated by decomposition. Mandelic, hippuric, and sulfosalicylic acids are simple aromatic compounds weakly bactericidal in an acid medium.

The methenamines are primarily effective against the gram-negative bacteria that commonly cause urinary tract infections. Especially important is *E. coli*. Bacterial resistance and cross-resistance develop rarely.

Following oral administration, methenamine hippurate is rapidly absorbed and concentrated in the urine, where within 2 hours levels of 10 to 80 μg/ml are achieved; almost no drug can be detected in the serum. To be bactericidal, urinary formaldehyde levels must achieve a concentration of 20 to 30 μg/ml.

To minimize gastric irritation from prematurely liberated formaldehyde, methenamine

$$N_4(CH_2)_6 + 6H_2O \xrightarrow{(H^+)} 4\ NH_0 + 6HCHO$$

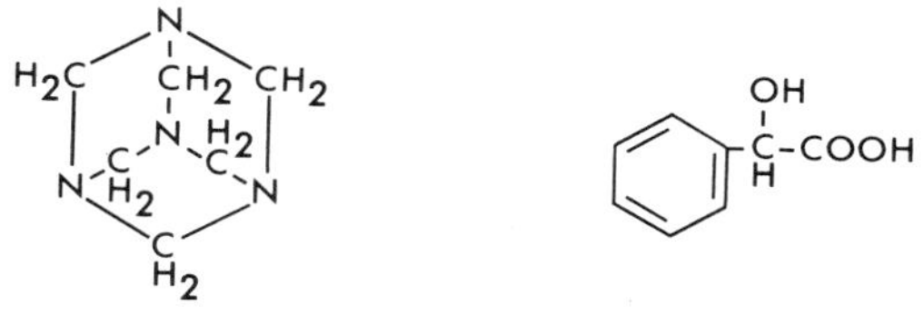

METHANAMINE MANDELIC ACID

FIG. 65-1. Methenamine mandelate.

mandelate is usually given in enteric-coated capsules. However, enteric coating delays peak urinary excretion of formaldehyde by 3 to 8 hours and may reduce the dose absorbed. Steady-state formaldehyde excretion is reached after 2 to 3 days of full therapy.

The concomitant administration of an urinary acidifying agent (*e.g.*, ammonium chloride, sodium-acid phosphate, methionine, ascorbic acid, or cranberry juice) is mandatory when using mandelic acid but not necessary for the other two salts. The antibacterial effect of the methenamines decreases rapidly as the urinary *p*H increases above 4.5—for example, during and after meals when the urinary *p*H usually becomes alkaline. Urine acidifying drugs are mandatory in treating infections caused by ammonia-producing (urease-producing) organisms such as *P. vulgaris;* some authorities recommend that the methenamines not be used to treat such infections.

Adverse Reactions

Adverse reactions are usually mild and reversible but occur in 5% to 10% of patients. Skin rashes (erythematous lesions and urticaria) and headaches may occur. Formaldehyde liberated by gastric acid may produce unpleasant intestinal symptoms and lead to poor compliance. Similarly formaldehyde-induced bladder irritation (urinary frequency, urgency, burning pain) may be troublesome, and, with large doses, mild proteinuria or hematuria may develop. The drugs are contraindicated in patients with renal insufficiency and, because of the ammonia produced, in patients with hepatic failure. Sulfonamides should not be given simultaneously because they crystalize in acid urine. Further, some sulfonamides are precipitated directly by formaldehyde, and sulfamethizole is inactivated through direct combination with methenamine. Infrequently, reversible VIIIth cranial nerve damage has been reported. Systemic acidosis may develop because of the acidifying drugs. Urinary estriol levels may be spuriously lowered since the hormone is destroyed by formaldehyde.

Preparations and Uses

Methenamine mandelate (Mandelamine) is available as methenamine mandelate tablets, U.S.P., and methenamine mandelate oral suspension, U.S.P. The usual dose for adults is 1 g every 6 hours and for children, 2 g/m^2/day in three divided doses. Methenamine hippurate and methenamine sulfosalicylate are given in an adult dose of 1 g every 12 hours and 1 g every 6 hours, respectively. Mandelamine usually clears the urine within 1 week if the organisms are susceptible and if an acid urinary *p*H is maintained. The drug enjoys wide popularity because of its relative lack of systemic toxicity and because bacterial resistance does not develop, except by *Enterobacter* spp. Methenamine should be used primarily to treat recurrent urinary tract infections, particularly those caused by *E. coli*. It cannot be used for systemic infections or for acute urinary tract infections.

NALIDIXIC ACID

Nalidixic acid (1-ethyl-7-methyl-4-oxo-1, 8-naphthyridine-3-carboxylic acid) is an expensive bactericidal urinary antiseptic related to oxolinic acid (*see* below). It is particularly valuable against some strains of *E. coli, Enterobacter aerogenes, Klebsiella* spp., *Providencia, Citrobacter* spp., and *Proteus* (particularly indole positive) spp.; *Ps. aeruginosa* and most common anaerobes are highly resistant. Nalidixic acid's gram-positive antibacterial spectrum is of little clinical importance; its activity is reduced by tissue fluid and nitrofurantoin.

Nalidixic acid interferes with DNA polymerization in late-stage chromosomal replication (*see* Chap. 57). Bacterial resistance develops rapidly, but antibacterial cross-resistance has not been described.

Absorption, Metabolism, and Excretion

Nalidixic acid is well and rapidly absorbed following oral administration; absorption is reduced in diarrheal states. After standard dosing, peak plasma levels occur within 2 to 4 hours. The drug has a pK_a of 6.5, a Vd of ~0.3 liters/kg, and is bound about 95% to warfarin type-1 plasma protein binding sites (*see* Chap. 8). Steady-state is achieved after 2 to 3 days. The drug has a T½ in neonates of 4 to 6 hours, in adults of 1 to 2 hours, and in anuria of 20 to 40 hours. Nalidixic acid is extensively metabolized. Hydroxynalidixic acid (HNA), the chief metabolite, also possesses antibacterial activity and is bound 63% to plasma proteins.

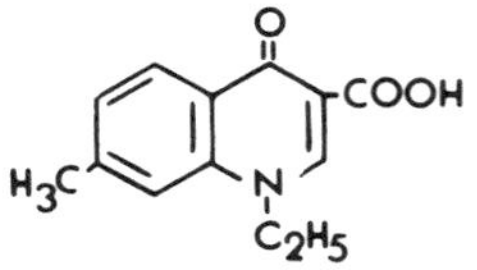

NALIDIXIC ACID

Nalidixic acid and HNA are rapidly concentrated in renal tissue and urine and also biodegraded to antibacterially inactive glucuronide and carboxylic acid metabolites. Alkalinization of the urine predictably increases the excretion of nalidixic acid but also favorably influences the ratio of active drug to inactive metabolites. Crystalluria does not occur. Nalidixic acid is concentrated in seminal fluid and excreted in milk.

Adverse Reactions

Adverse reactions are common and can be serious. Gastrointestinal upsets are usually minimized by administering the drug after meals. Transient fever, sleepiness, vertigo, myalgia, polyarthritis, headache, eosinophilia, hemolytic anemia (especially in patients with glucose-6-phosphate dehydrogenase deficiency), leukopenia, thrombocytopenia, and anaphylactic shock may develop. Confusion, nervousness, hemeralopia, amblyopia, photophobia, diplopia, alteration in perception of the color green, a toxic psychosis, and convulsions may develop rarely. Allergic skin reactions, including urticaria, purpuric and maculopapular eruptions, erythema multiforme, and photodermatitis, are not infrequent. Plasma protein displacement interactions (*see* Chap. 8) may develop.

The glucuronide conjugate of nalidixic acid gives a false-positive reaction with Benedict's reagent or Clinitest tablets; Clinistix or Testape yields valid results. Occasionally abnormal liver function test findings and false-positive elevations of urinary 17-ketogenic and 17-ke-

---

STANLEY ROSSITER BENEDICT, 1884–1936. American chemist at Cornell. Developed many tests and reagents, for example, for determination of blood sugars and phosphate, creatinine, acetate, uric acid, and urinary sulfur. Was one of the first to study tumor regression induced by metabolic disruption.

tosteroids may be seen. In neonates, because of a reduced capacity to glucuronate drugs (*see* Chap. 7), nalidixic acid may produce an acute elevation of intracranial pressure.

Preparations and Uses

Nalidixic acid, U.S.P. (NegGram), is available in tablets of 250, 500, and 1000 mg and in an oral preparation of 50 mg/ml. The usual adult dose is 1 g every 6 hours for 2 weeks, followed by 1 g every 12 hours for 2 more weeks. The usual dose for children is 15 mg/kg every 6 hours. Nalidixic acid is occasionally used to treat acute and chronic urinary tract infections not complicated by bacteremia, for long-term suppressive therapy, or for prophylaxis following genitourinary manipulations. In the last instance, therapy can be either systemic or by bladder instillation. No control of urinary *p*H is required, but, because of the rapidity with which bacterial resistance develops, bacterial culture and sensitivity tests are essential before the start of therapy.

OXOLINIC ACID

Oxolinic acid (Utibid, Prodoxol) is structurally and pharmacologically similar to nalidixic acid. It is available in tablets of 750 mg, the usual dose being 1 tablet every 12 hours. Although oxolinic acid is two to ten times more potent than nalidixic acid *in vitro* against common urinary pathogens, it has a higher incidence of adverse effects. Oxolinic acid is more extensively metabolized than nalidixic acid, and, unusually, one of its glucuronide metabolites, accounting for up to 40% of any dose, is antibacterially active.

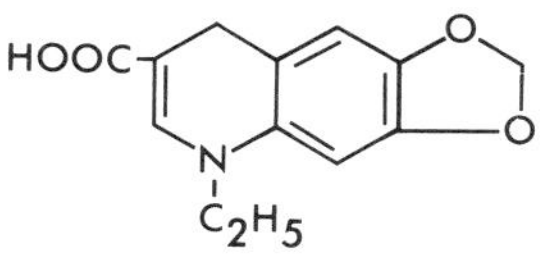

OXOLINIC ACID

Several other related drugs are under investigation: *cinoxacin, pipemidic acid, piromidic acid,* and *flumequine.*

THE 5-NITROFURANS

Several derivatives of 5-nitro-2-furaldehyde (Table 65-4) exhibit mild antibacterial, anticandidal, or antiprotozoal activity probably by depressing acetyl coenzyme A formation. The 5-position nitrogroup in the furan ring is essential for activity. Antibacterial resistance is of limited therapeutic importance. Cross-resistance is complete within the group.

TABLE 65-4. 5-Nitrofurans

Drug	Properties, Preparations, and Dosage
Nitrofurantoin (Furadantin)	Nitrofurantoin oral suspension, *U.S.P.*, 0.5%, and nitrofurantoin tablets, *U.S.P.*, are the official preparations. The usual adult dose is 5 to 10 mg/kg/day in divided doses for 2 weeks. If a further course of treatment is necessary, a 1- to 2-week rest period should be observed. Not more than 360 mg of the soluble sodium salt should be injected i.v. per day.
Nitrofurazone	Used primarily for topical treatment of mixed bacterial skin infections and rarely to treat *T. gambiense* sleeping sickness (*see* Chap. 67). Its antibacterial activity not reduced by pus, blood, or tissue fluids, and it does not depress wound healing. Topically it induces hypersensitivity in about 5% of patients. In a 0.2% concentration, it is available in many proprietary dressings, suppositories, and powders as nitrofurazone solution, *N.F.*, nitrofurazone ointment, *N.F.*, and nitrofurazone cream, *N.F.*
Nifuroxime	Occasionally effective in topical treatment of vaginal candidiasis. Often combined with furazolidone (*see* below).
Furazolidone (Furoxone)	Furazolidone usually available in combination with nifuroxime (*see* above) as a powder (furazolidone and nifuroxime powder, *N.F.*), or as suppositories (furazolidine and nifuroxime suppositories, *N.F.*). Usual adult dose is 100 mg every 6 hours.

The nitrofurans produce hemolytic anemia in patients with glucose-6-phosphate dehydrogenase, enolase, or glutathione peroxidase deficiency. In several strains of animals, high doses of nitrofurazone and furazolidone depress spermatogenesis, but this has not been reported in humans.

NITROFURANTOIN

Nitrofurantoin (1-(5-nitrofurfurylideneamino)-hydantoin), is a bacteriostatic, urinary antiseptic effective against many gram-positive and gram-negative bacteria, including some strains of *Proteus, E. coli, Enterobacter, niesseriae, staphylococci, streptococci,* and *Citrobacter* spp. Invariably resistant are *Pseudomonas, Serratia,* and *Providentia* spp. *In vitro* testing of bacterial sensitivity is often unreliable because blood plasma reduces its activity. Nitrofurantoin depresses the initiation of translation in protein synthesis *in vivo.* Nitrofurantoin is converted intracellularly by a bacterial reductase to a more active form. Some resistant organisms lack this reductase, others exhibit an R-factor-mediated decrease in drug penetration. Nitrofurantoin antagonizes nalidixic and oxolinic acids.

This agent is usually given orally. Very rarely it is given intravenously as the highly soluble sodium salt. Following oral administration absorption is rapid and almost complete by the small bowel. The drug's bioavailability is increased by food, and the microcrystalline form is more readily absorbed than is the macrocrystalline preparation. Nitrofurantoin is bound 20% to 60% to plasma proteins, but plasma and tissue levels rarely achieve bacteriostatic concentrations partly because of rapid renal excretion and partly because of enzymatic metabolism. The drug has a $T\frac{1}{2}$ of 0.3 to 1.0 hours. Nitrofurantoin readily passes the placental barrier, but the concentration achieved is too low to be either toxic or antibacterially effective. Between 30% and 50% of a dose is cleared by the kidney within 6 hours, excretion being proportional to the creatinine clearance; most of the remainder is excreted in the urine as inactive metabolites that color the urine brown. There is some tubular reabsorption of nitrofurantoin, but the drug does not usually achieve satisfactory tissue levels to be bactericidal in renal parenchyma. Nitrofurantoin has a pK_a of 7.2 and is more soluble in alkaline urine but more antibacterially active in acid urine; crystalluria does not occur. With standard doses, urine levels of 50 to 250 μg/ml are achieved. Nitrofurantoin may impart a yellowish fluorescence to the urine. It is removed by hemodialysis.

Adverse Reactions

Except for "hypersensitivity" reactions, including polyneuropathy and allergic pneumonitis, adverse reactions are probably dose dependent. Gastrointestinal upsets (15% of courses) can be reduced by administering the drug with meals, milk, or antacids. The macrocrystalline form is less irritating than the microcrystalline preparation. Hemolytic anemia (*see* above) and a folic acid-dependent megaloblastic anemia may develop in patients who receive several courses of therapy. This anemia may depend on the "hydantoin" moiety of the drug and may be akin to that occasionally seen with phenytoin therapy (*see* Chap. 29). Nitrofurantoin may produce a false-positive Benedict's test for urine sugar.

Agranulocytosis, thrombocytopenia, aplastic anemia, myalgia, fever, skin rashes, anaphylactic shock, a lupus-like disorder, and chronic active hepatitis are rare. An allergic infiltrative pneumonitis that resembles either multiple pulmonary emboli or pneumonic consolidation associated with fever, cough, dyspnea, and eosinophilia may develop but usually resolves rapidly on cessation of therapy. Physiological testing in patients with this reaction demonstrates various ventillation/perfusion abnormalities and A-V shunting in association with hypoxemia and hypocapnia.

Nitrofurantoin may rarely cause an ascending symmetric sensorimotor polyneuropathy, which begins insidiously, usually within 6 weeks of the start of therapy, and is more likely in the presence of renal insufficiency, possibly associated with reduced plasma protein drug binding. In 20% of patients an accompanying increase in cerebrospinal fluid protein occurs. Legs are more commonly affected than arms, and parasthesias and dysasthesias usually precede paralysis. Recovery is inversely related to the severity of the symptoms, but symptoms may progress even after therapy has been stopped. The neuropathy may be a toxic effect of the drug due to a metabolite or due to interference with intermediary metabolism. In normal volunteers, nitrofurantoin produces changes in sensory motor nerve conduction velocity and electromyographic changes in muscle function.

FURAZOLIDONE

This derivative demonstrates some activity against *Giardia lamblia* and *Trichomonas vaginalis.* The combination of furazolidone and nifuroxime is effective in treating vaginal trichomoniasis and candidiasis (*see* Chap. 67).

FURTHER READING

1. Acocella G: Clinical pharmacokinetics of rifampicin. Clin Pharmacokinet 3:108–127, 1978
2. De Gowin RR: A review of therapeutic and hemolytic effects of dapsone. Arch Intern Med 120:242–248, 1967

3. Goldman AL, Broman SS: Isoniazid: A review with emphasis on adverse effects. Chest 62:71–77, 1972
4. Hoeprick PD: New antimicrobials for the treatment of infections caused by gram-negative bacilli. Med Clin North Am 51:1127–1152, 1967
5. Katul J, Frank IN: Antibacterial activity of methenamine hippurate. J Urol 104:320–324, 1970
6. Lunde PKM, Frislid K, Hansteen V: Disease and acetylation polymorphism. Clin Pharmacokinet 2:182–197, 1977
7. Mitchell JR, Thorgeirsson UP, Black M et al: Increased incidence of isoniazid hepatitis in rapid acetylators: Possible relation to hydrazine metabolites. Clin Pharmacol Ther 18:70–79, 1975
8. Musher DM, Griffith DP: Generation of formaldehyde from methionine: Effect of pH and concentration and antibacterial effect. Antimicrob Agents Chemother 6:708–711, 1974
9. Ronald RR, Turck M, Petersdorf RG: A critical evaluation of nalidixic acid in urinary tract infections. N Engl J Med 275:1081–1089, 1966
10. Rossouw JE, Saunders SJ: Hepatic complications of antituberculous therapy. Q J Med 44:1–16, 1975
11. Shepard CC: Chemotherapy of leprosy. Annu Rev Pharmacol 9:37–50, 1969
12. Sovijärvi Anesi RA, Markku L, Stenius B et al: Subacute and chronic nitrofurantoin-induced acute pulmonary reactions. Scand J Resp Dis 58:41–50, 1977
13. Toole JF, Parrish ML: Nitrofurantoin Polyuropathy. Neurology 23:554–559, 1973
14. Youatt J: A review of the action of isoniazid. Am Rev Resp Dis 99:729–749, 1969

CHAPTER 65 QUESTIONS

(See P. 7 for Full Instructions)

Select the One Best Answer

1. Each of the following statements is true of isoniazid EXCEPT that
   A. most of the absorbed drug appears unchanged in the urine.
   B. it increases susceptibility to epileptiform seizures.
   C. it may produce severe hepatic injury.
   D. it may be used alone for prophylaxis of tuberculosis.
   E. it is bactericidal against actively growing tubercule bacilli.

2. An antitubercular agent whose rate of metabolism is altered in patients with a specific pharmacogenetic abnormality is
   A. rifampin.
   B. isoniazid.
   C. cycloserine.
   D. ethambutol.
   E. ethionamide.

3. The drug that acts by the release of formaldehyde in the urinary tract is
   A. nitrofurantoin.
   B. ammonium chloride.
   C. methenamine mandelate.
   D. nalidixic acid.
   E. ascorbic acid.

4. Each of the following drugs is useful in the treatment of tuberculosis EXCEPT
   A. ethambutol.
   B. streptomycin.
   C. clindamycin.
   D. rifampin.
   E. cycloserine.

5. Promin and other sulfone agents are used mainly to treat
   A. myelogenous leukemia.
   B. leprosy.
   C. trachoma.
   D. cellulitis.
   E. urinary tract infections.

6. Each of the following statements is true of isoniazid (INH) EXCEPT that
   A. gastrointestinal absorption is depressed by aluminum antacids.
   B. there is significant "first-pass" loss.
   C. cross-resistance with other antitubercular drugs is common.
   D. use of a second antitubercular drug retards development of mycobacterial resistance.
   E. it is related chemically to nicotinic acid.

7. Factors that possibly contribute to isoniazid-induced liver damage are all of the following EXCEPT
   A. patients' ages less than 35 years.
   B. patients exposed to other hepatotoxic drugs.
   C. patients with evidence of liver disease.
   D. rapid acetylators.
   E. patients taking enzyme-inducing drugs.

8. Each of the following statements is true of rifampin EXCEPT that
   A. it binds to bacterial RNA polymerase.
   B. it binds to mammalian RNA polymerase.
   C. it possesses a broad antibacterial spectrum.
   D. bacterial resistance develops rapidly when the drug is used alone.
   E. it is a potent enzyme-inducing agent.

9. Each of the following statements is true of para-aminosalicylic acid EXCEPT that
   A. it retards the emergence of mycobacterial resistance to INAH.
   B. it commonly causes hemolytic anemia in persons with glucose 6-phosphate dehydrogenase deficiency.
   C. it may produce a malabsorption syndrome.
   D. crystalluria is minimized by urinary acidification.
   E. it may cause gastric bleeding.

10. Each of the following statements is true of pyrazinamide EXCEPT that
    A. it is likely to cause liver damage in doses greater than 40 mg/kg/day.
    B. it decreases renal tubular excretion of urate.
    C. it may produce photosensitivity dermatitis.
    D. it is well absorbed after oral administration.
    E. it may cause alteration in color perception.

11. Each of the following statements about ethionamide is true EXCEPT that
    A. it is more effective against human than bovine strains of *M. tuberculosis*.
    B. mycobacterial resistance develops rapidly when used alone.
    C. it may produce sialorrhea.
    D. it may produce hyperuricemia.
    E. it is a primary drug in the treatment of tuberculosis.

12. Each of the following statements is true about methenamine mandelate EXCEPT that
    A. it is a condensation product of ammonia and formaldehyde.
    B. it acts by precipitating bacterial proteins.
    C. bacterial resistance is common.
    D. gastric irritation frequently develops.
    E. it is antibacterially effective in the urinary tract only when the *p*H remains below 4.5.

13. Each of the following statements is true of nalidixic acid EXCEPT that
    A. acidification of the urine increases nalidixic acid's renal excretion.
    B. crystalluria does not develop.
    C. it causes hemolytic anemia in patients with glucose-6-phosphate dehydrogenase deficiency.
    D. it may produce changes in visual acuity and visual perception.
    E. it is well and rapidly absorbed following oral administration.

14. Each of the following is true of nitrofurantoin EXCEPT that
    A. it is converted intracellularly by sensitive bacteria to a more active drug.
    B. it produces hemolytic anemia in patients with glucose-6-phosphate dehydrogenase deficiency.
    C. the furan ring is essential for antimicrobial activity.
    D. microcrystalline formulations of the drug are less readily absorbed than are macrocrystalline preparations.
    E. it may impart a yellowish fluorescence to the urine.

A = 1,2,3; B = 1,3; C = 2,4; D = 4; E = All

15. Chemotherapeutic agents effective in the treatment of *Mycobacterium leprae* infections include
    1. streptomycin.
    2. dapsone.
    3. aminosalicylic acid.
    4. thiacetazone.

16. Ethambutol
    1. is extensively metabolized.
    2. may decrease visual acuity.
    3. must be administered in large doses because it is not well absorbed.
    4. -resistant mycobacteria commonly emerge when the drug is administered alone.

17. Factors important to consider in treating tuberculosis include
    1. host defense mechanisms.
    2. initial determination of mycobacterial sensitivity.
    3. determining mycobacterial sensitivity periodically in chronic cases.
    4. combinations of primary drugs with secondary drugs.

PETER LOMAX

66

Antiseptics and Disinfectants

Antiseptics and disinfectants are some of the most widely used drugs. They have been used for centuries, long before the germ theory of disease was accepted (*e.g.*, Egyptian embalmers; Semmelweiss). Although the concept that all infectious diseases are the result of the spread of microorganisms was accepted only slowly by the medical profession toward the end of the 19th century, layman, aided and abetted by all the forces of the mass advertising media, grasped the idea with alacrity and enthusiasm. Antiseptics are now freely applied to almost all tissues of the body—by eye and mouth washes, throat and nasal sprays, vaginal douches, and antiseptic deodorants and soaps, among other products. In addition to the phobia that they induce in some people, these products are actually harmful to the tissues in many instances.

Although the importance of antiseptics in clinical practice has declined somewhat since the introduction of antimicrobial agents, the former still have an important place in the treatment of some local infections. Disinfectants are widely used for home and hospital sanitation.

The current terminology is rather imprecise, and common usage does not entirely reflect the original derivations. Although both antiseptics and disinfectants kill or prevent the growth of microorganisms, the terms have become more restricted in medical parlance. Today *antiseptic* is used in reference to substances applied to the tissues, whereas *disinfectant* connotes a chemical applied to inanimate objects. The term *germicide* is frequently used to cover both antiseptics and disinfectants.

An ideal germicide would have high efficacy and a wide antimicrobial spectrum. It should be lethal to bacteria, bacterial spores, fungi, viruses, and protozoa. In the case of an antiseptic, the compound should not be damaging to the tissues; it should be active in the presence of body fluids, yet not discolor the tissues or clothes unduly or have an offensive odor. Disinfectants should penetrate into organic matter

---

IGNAZ PHILIPP SEMMELWEISS, 1818–1865. Hungarian obstetrician practicing in Vienna. Reported, in 1849, that puerperal fever was contagious and, in hospitals, was spread by physicians themselves. Instituted antiseptic procedures, for example, using phenol, resulting in a dramatic fall in the maternal death rate.

and into "nooks and crannies," retain activity in the presence of organic matter (blood, sputum, feces), and be compatible with soaps. Additionally, disinfectants should be stable in solution and not be corrosive to surgical instruments and other materials.

MECHANISMS OF ACTION

Germicidal activity depends on three basic mechanisms of action: *Coagulation of protein* is frequently adduced as the means by which microorganisms are destroyed, and this may be the major effect of moist-heat sterilization; many of the new agents, the surfactants, act by *destroying the normal permeability* characteristics of the cell membrane (*see* Chap. 57). Most germicides, however, probably act directly by *poisoning bacterial enzyme systems*. For many germicides, their precise mechanism of action cannot be stated.

The classification of such a varied group of compounds as the antiseptics and disinfectants is difficult because too rigid a regimen is liable to confuse rather than to elucidate. Except for physical agents, it is generally most useful (or least objectionable) to discuss the germicides according to their chemical structure.

PHYSICAL AGENTS

HEAT

Saturated steam at 2 atmospheres pressure (120°C) is the most important single method of destroying microorganisms in general clinical use. Both the vegetative and spore forms of most bacteria are killed after exposure for 20 minutes. Dry heat is much less efficacious: 3 hours at 140°C may be needed. Simple boiling at normal atmospheric pressure may be inadequate to destroy organisms such as those of infectious hepatitis, and in office practice it is advisable to use disposable syringes and needles.

ULTRAVIOLET LIGHT

The maximum antibacterial effect of light energy is manifest around a wave length of 2700 Å. Organisms vary considerably in resistance to ultraviolet light, gram-negative, nonsporing organisms being most susceptible. Staphylococci, streptococci, and most viruses are resistant. Although not convenient and too expensive for general use, light sterilization is being employed to prevent airborne cross-infection in special hospital units such as burn wards and premature baby units by creating a light screen between patients.

CHEMICAL AGENTS

ACIDS

Boric Acid

Boric acid forms a 5% solution at room temperature. Only mildly antiseptic, it does not irritate the skin or delicate surfaces (*e.g.*, the cornea), which may account for its wide use. Also available is a 10% ointment.

Benzoic Acid

A weak, tasteless, nontoxic bacteriostatic agent, benzoic acid is used extensively as a preservative in food and drink in a concentration of 0.1%. High concentrations can be applied to the skin. It is used to treat ringworm and other skin infections (*see* Chap. 69).

Mandelic Acid

Mandelic acid is used for urinary tract infections (*see* Chap. 65). For maximum effect the urine *p*H should be maintained at less than 5.5 by the coadministration of ammonium chloride. The oral dose of mandelic acid as the sodium salt is 8 to 12 g daily.

Salicylic Acid

A weak antiseptic and fungicidal agent, salicylic acid is also used as a keratolytic (*see* Chap. 69).

ALKALIES

Strong alkalies (*e.g.*, sodium hydroxide, potassium hydroxide) are occasionally used for disinfecting excreta, particularly from patients with virus infections such as poliomyelitis. Sodium borate solution is sometimes used as a skin antiseptic.

SURFACE-ACTIVE AGENTS (SURFACTANTS)

In recent years a large number of surface-active agents have been synthesized. They all act, as does soap, by lowering the surface tension of solutions. Surfactants can be classified according to the nature of the ionic charge on the hydrophobic group.

Anionic Surfactants

Anionic surfactants include the common soaps. Soaps are active against gram-positive, but not gram-negative, organisms. However, the soaps probably owe their antiseptic action primarily to the dislodging, during the physical process of scrubbing, of bacteria embedded in the skin. Sometimes other antiseptics, such as mercuric iodide and phenols, are incorporated in the soap. Of the new anionic surfactants, octylphenoxyethoxyethyl ether sulfonate (pHisoderm) has been most widely used. When combined with hexachlorophene (*see* below), the mixture is named pHisoHex. This preparation has replaced soap for preoperative scrubbing in many hospitals, since the mechanical effect of handwashing is augmented by the additional action of the surfactant and the antibacterial properties of hexachlorophene.

Cationic Surfactants

Cationic surfactants have positively charged hydrophobic groups. Many are dimethyl ammonium compounds of the general structure shown in Figure 66-1. These agents are generally more effective than the anionic compounds; they can be used in more dilute solutions (1:20,000 range) and have broader antibacterial spectrum. In dilute solutions (0.1–1.0%) they are used for preoperative skin preparation. Common formulations include benzalkonium chloride, *U.S.P.* (Zephiran); benzethonium chloride, *U.S.P.* (Phemerol); and cetylpyridinium chloride, *U.S.P.* (Ceepryn). These are generally used as 10% solutions or as 0.1% tinctures.

PHENOLIC COMPOUNDS

The introduction of phenol by Lister in the 1860s marked the beginning of modern antiseptic techniques. Subsequently phenol became the standard against which other compounds were measured—hence the term "phenol coefficient." Such comparisons are now rarely made. A large number of phenolic derivatives have been prepared and used as germicides. These are all effective against nonsporing pathogens but are inactive against bacterial spores.

JOSEPH LISTER, 1827–1912. English surgeon. The founder of aseptic surgical technique, published in 1867. Also introduced absorbable ligatures and drainage tubes and gave the first correct account of pupil dilation in 1853.

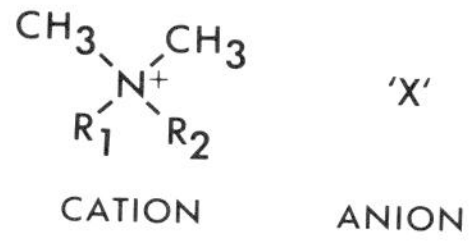

FIG. 66-1. The dimethyl ammonium cationic surfactants.

Phenol

Phenol exhibits relatively weak activity and high tissue toxicity.

Cresol

About 10 times more active than phenol with about the same toxicity, cresol is poorly soluble in water and is used as a soapy emulsion, referred to as *Lysol*.

Thymol

Thymol has been used as an anthelmintic agent. A mixture of the iodides of thymol (mainly consisting of thymol diiodide) has been used as a dusting powder.

Hexyresorcinol

Its broad anthelmintic spectrum renders hexylresorcinol a useful agent in helmintic infestations when administered orally (*see* Chap. 68). It is frequently used in throat lozenges because of its spreading and penetrating properties.

Hexachlorophene

Hexachlorophene, a new phenolic derivative, is active against gram-positive and some gram-negative organisms in a concentration of 2% to 5%. It is incorporated in various soaps for scrubbing-up, including Dial and pHisoHex. Hexachlorophene has an affinity for the skin and becomes incorporated in the deeper layers so that scrubbing time may be reduced after repeated use. Sensitivity occurs in some people, and keratitis may follow introduction into the eye.

ALCOHOLS

Ethyl Alcohol

Used extensively for cleaning the skin before parenteral injections, ethyl alcohol is most effective in a concentration of 70% by weight (78% by volume). Solutions of greater or lesser dilutions reputedly have less antiseptic action.

Isopropyl Alcohol

Rubbing alcohol has a lower volatility and higher activity than ethyl alcohol. Isopropyl alcohol is active in solutions ranging from 30% to 90%, and the effectiveness is not as sensitive to dilution as is the case with ethyl alcohol.

HALOGENS

Iodine

Effective in the elemental form only, iodine possesses high fungicidal, virucidal, and bactericidal activity. Iodine stains and is locally toxic to the tissues. Severe iodiosyncrasy may occur. The 2% aqueous solution stabilized with sodium iodide appears to be the best preparation. Tinctures of ethyl alcohol are common.

Iodophores

Iodophores are large, organic molecules that carry loosely bound iodine, which is liberated slowly. They are expensive and little more effective than elemental iodine solutions.

Chlorine

Chlorine is an effective germicide at very low concentrations (2:100,000) due to its action in suppressing enzymes associated with glucose metabolism. Hypochlorous acid is formed on reaction with water; this is the basis for chlorine use in the sterilization of drinking water and swimming pools. A 5% sodium hypochlorite solution (Dakin's solution) is used for cleaning wounds, since the liberated chlorine sterilizes the tissue and dissolves fibrinous tissues. Several organic chlorides (chloramines) release chlorine but are not much used. Examples are chloramine-T, halazone, and chloroazodin.

OXIDIZING AGENTS

Hydrogen Peroxide

As a 3% solution, hydrogen peroxide has been used extensively for cleaning wounds. The compound is unstable, and nascent oxygen is released, particularly on contact with organic matter. The evolution of oxygen mechanically loosens pus and tissue debris and kills bacteria.

Potassium Permanganate

Potassium permanganate acts in the same way as hydrogen peroxide. It has the disadvantage of staining skin and clothing and is irritating to mucous membranes. Strong solutions such as Condy's fluid have been used for sterilizing feces.

Sodium Perborate

Sodium perborate releases oxygen on contact with tissues. As a 2% solution, it is used as a mouthwash. Chronic changes in the oral mucous membranes may follow prolonged use of strong pastes.

HEAVY METALS

Dyes and vital stains used in the treatment of superficial mycoses are discussed in Chapter 69.

Mercuric Chloride

Although highly toxic, mercuric chloride is used as a hand sterilizing agent on the unbroken skin as a 1:2000 solution.

Thimerosal (Merthiolate)

Thimerosal is an organic complex that contains about 50% mercury. Solutions of 1:1000 are used for sterlizing the skin and mucous membranes but may lead to sensitivity reactions.

Silver Nitrate

Silver nitrate is used extensively as a 1% solution for instilling into the conjunctival sac of infants as prophylaxis against gonorrheal ophthalmia neonatorum.

Chlorhexidine

The biguanide chlorhexidine has been used extensively in other countries but has only recently been approved for use in the United States, where it is available as a 4% aqueous emulsion and as a tincture, 0.5% in 70% isopropyl alcohol. Chlorhexidine is effective against gram-positive and gram-negative organisms, disrupting their cell membrane. It is used primarily for preoperative skin preparation in patients and preoperative skin preparation of the surgeon's hands. Mouthwashes that contain chlorhexidine have been used in treating aphthous ulcers and in the prophylaxis of dental caries.

Henry Drysdale Dakin, 1880–1952. English-born New York chemist. First described his antiseptic solution in 1915, working with Nobel Prize winner Alexis Carrel. It was used in World War I.

Henry Bollmann Condy. English physician. His antiseptic solution (1862) was composed of sodium and potassium permanganates.

FURTHER READING

1. Lawrence CA, Block SS (eds): Disinfection, Sterilization, and Preservation. Philadelphia, Lea & Febiger, 1968

CHAPTER 66 QUESTIONS

(See P. 7 for Full Instructions)

Select the One Best Answer

1. The agent of choice for disinfection of the hands is
   - A. hexachlorophene.
   - B. ethyl alcohol.
   - C. tincture of iodine.
   - D. merbromin.
   - E. thimerosal.
2. Desirable properties of germicides include all of the following EXCEPT
   - A. nonstaining.
   - B. sporicidal.
   - C. noncorrosive.
   - D. high surface tension.
   - E. nonsensitizing.
3. An effective preoperative skin antiseptic that does not stain the skin is
   - A. boric acid.
   - B. benzethonium chloride.
   - C. dinitrophenol.
   - D. iodine.
   - E. potassium permanganate.

A = 1,2,3; B = 1,3; C = 2,4; D = 4; E = All

4. Antiseptics may be effective because they
   1. inactivate enzymes.
   2. precipitate proteins.
   3. increase membrane permeability.
   4. kill microorganisms.
5. When methenamine is given as a urinary antiseptic, its effect
   1. is increased by administering mandelic acid.
   2. depends on the release of formaldehyde.
   3. is increased by administering ammonium chloride.
   4. is increased by administering urea.

67

JERROLD A. TURNER

Drugs Used to Treat Protozoal Diseases

The treatment of protozoan infections often requires a thorough understanding of the disease and the criteria for a satisfactory clinical response. In some instances, the use of highly toxic drugs may be needed, and their potential benefit must be weighed carefully against the risk of continued infection. Most antiprotozoan drugs have not been proved safe in pregnancy, and thus their use must be individualized. Consultation with a clinical parasitologist is frequently valuable before initiating treatment with an unfamiliar drug.

Many drugs used to treat parasitic infections are not available commercially in the United States but can be obtained on an investigational basis for the treatment of specific infections from the Parasitic Disease Drug Service, Centers for Disease Control, Atlanta, Georgia (Table 67-1).

MALARIA

Malaria continues to be a major cause of morbidity and mortality. It is endemic in more than 90 countries, and although control measures have been successful in many areas a dramatic resurgence in malaria prevalence has taken place within the past few years, especially in Southern Asia and Latin America.

THE MALARIA PARASITE

Four species of the genus *Plasmodium* may cause malaria in humans: *Plasmodium vivax, P. malariae, P. falciparum,* and *P. ovale.* These parasites have complex life cycles (Fig. 67-1), and several stages of development occur in the human host. Humans are infected when forms of the parasite (sporozoites) are introduced in the saliva of the mosquito vector. The sporozoites pass to the liver, where they penetrate hepatocytes and undergo asexual multiplication. The liver stage (exoerythrocytic stage) matures and organisms rupture from hepatocytes to parasitize erythrocytes, where asexual multiplication continues. Parasitized red blood cells eventually rupture, releasing parasites to enter other erythrocytes to begin the cycle again. The duration of the cycles depends on the species of malaria. Some organisms do not divide asexually in the erythrocytes but develop into male and female

TABLE 67-1. Investigational Drugs for Protozoal Infections Available from the Parasitic Disease Drug Service*

Drug	Disease
Dehydroemetine	Amebiasis
Diloxanide furoate	Amebiasis
Nifurtimox	American trypanosomiasis
Melarsoprol	African trypanosomiasis
Pentamidine	Leishmaniasis
	Pneumocystis infection
Sodium stibogluconate	Leishmaniasis
Suramin	African trypanosomiasis

* Centers for Disease Control, Atlanta, GA 30333 (phone: 404-329-3311).

gametocytes. Gametocytes remain intact in the circulating blood and, when ingested by a mosquito, will complete the sexual cycle in the insect host.

An important difference exists between species of malaria in their capacity to maintain exoerythrocytic infection. *P. falciparum* and *P. malariae* do not persist within the liver cells after erythrocytes have become infected, whereas *P. vivax* and *P. ovale* do and thus may produce true relapses months or years later. Recurrence of symptoms (recrudescence) in infections with *P. falciparum* or *P. malariae* results from a persisting, low-grade, subclinical erythrocytic infection that abruptly increases to clinically significant levels. Recrudescence is differentiated from the true relapse of *P. vivax* and *P. ovale*.

If infection arises from the direct transfer of parasitized red blood cells in blood transfusions, by the use of contaminated needles, or transplacentally, no exoerythrocytic infection occurs.

PATHOGENIC EFFECTS OF MALARIA

Exoerythrocytic infection produces no liver dysfunction and no clinical symptoms. Asexual maturation in the erythrocytes, however, produces cyclic hemolysis that coincides with the onset of characteristic chills and fever of the malarial paroxysm. Hyperplasia of the reticuloendothelial system results in hepatosplenomegaly, and immunoglobulin levels are elevated. *P. falciparum* infections tend to be more severe because higher parasitemias occur than with other species, and parasitized red blood cells tend to occlude capillaries, causing local ischemia. This phenomenon, occurring in the brain, produces *cerebral malaria,* an often fatal condition.

TREATMENT OF MALARIA

Treatment can be divided into *chemoprophylaxis* (Table 67-2), *treatment of the clinical attack,* and *radical cure* (elimination of all parasites from the body).

Chemoprophylaxis

An ideal prophylactic agent would destroy sporozoites upon inoculation by the mosquito, but no such agent is available. Current prophylaxis is actually *suppressive prophylaxis* that prevents maturation of the erythrocytic infection but may have no effect on stages in liver cells. Although pyrimethamine and chloroguanide have been widely used in suppressive prophylaxis, resistance to these drugs is found in many parts of the world; therefore chloroquine is considered the chemosuppressive agent of choice. If suppressive prophylaxis is carried out for a sufficiently long period, after leaving an edemic area, infections with *P. malariae* and *P. falciparum* may be totally eliminated (*suppressive cure*). However, to eliminate persisting liver stages of *P. vivax* and *P. ovale* and prevent relapses of these species, primaquine must be given. A combination of chloroquine and primaquine has been used for chemoprophylaxis in military personnel, but its

FIG. 67.1. Life cycle of malaria parasites.

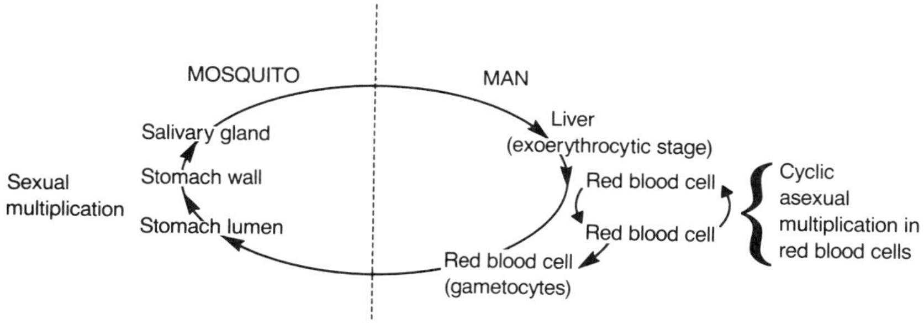

TABLE 67-2. Drugs and Doses for Malaria Chemoprophylaxis*

	Adult Dosage	Comments
4-Aminoquinolines		
Chloroquine phosphate and chloroquine sulfate	500 mg (300 mg base) weekly, continued for 6 weeks after leaving endemic area.	Effective in suppressing erythrocytic stages; when taken for 6 weeks after last exposure, suppressive cure of *P. malariae* and sensitive strains of *P. falciparum* occurs. These drugs will not prevent relapses of *P. vivax* and *P. ovale* infection.
Hydroxychloroquine sulfate	400 mg (310 mg base) weekly, continued for 6 weeks after leaving endemic area.	
Amodiaquine hydrochloride	520 mg (400 mg base) weekly, continued for 6 weeks after leaving endemic area.	
Dihydrofolate reductase inhibitors		
Pyrimethamine	25 mg weekly, continued for 6 weeks after leaving endemic area.	Resistance to these drugs is found in *P. vivax* in many areas.
Chloroquanide	100 to 200 mg daily, continued for 6 weeks after leaving endemic area.	
Pyrimethamine–sulfadoxine	25 mg of pyrimethamine and 500 mg of sulfadoxine every week, continued for 6 weeks after leaving endemic area.	Used only in chemoprophylaxis of chloroquine-resistant strains of *P. falciparum.* Should not be used longer than 6 months. Chloroquine should also be given if in an area where pyrimethamine resistance occurs in *P. vivax.*
8-Aminoquinoline		
Primaquine phosphate	26.3 mg (15 mg base) daily for 14 days or 79 mg (45 mg base) weekly for 8 weeks. To be given upon return from endemic area concurrently with, or immediately after the course of suppression with chloroquine or similar drug.	Prevents later development of clinical attacks of *P. vivax* and *P. ovale* infection. Recommended for travelers with known significant exposure to *P. vivax* or *P. ovale* infection.

* For travelers, drug therapy is begun 2 weeks before departure to assess any untoward reactions.

use for residents in endemic areas or for travelers is not recommended because of increased risk of toxicity. To prevent relapsing malaria, a course of primaquine may be added to the usual chemosuppressive regimen with chloroquine when a traveler returns from an endemic area.

Chloroquine-resistant strains of *P. falciparum* have been found in Central and South America, Southeast Asia, areas of the Philippines, Indonesia, New Guinea, Bangladesh, Eastern India, Kenya, and Tanzania. Because of the continued spread of chloroquine resistance, current information should be sought from authorities such as the Centers for Disease Control, Atlanta, Georgia, before advising travelers on malaria chemoprophylaxis. The drug combination currently used for chemoprophylaxis for resistant *P. falciparum* is pyrimethamine and sulfadoxine.

Acute Malaria

Chloroquine, U.S.P., is the drug of choice for treating acute attacks of malaria caused by all species except chloroquine-resistant *P. falciparum.* Chloroquine phosphate is administered orally in the following dosage: 1 g (600 mg base) immediately, followed in 6 hours by 500 mg (300 mg base), and 500 mg (300 mg base) again in 24 hours and 48 hours. This regimen is adequate for radical cure of *P. malariae* and chloroquine-sensitive *P. falciparum* infections. If the infection is caused by *P. vivax* or *P. ovale,* the course of chloroquine is immediately followed by primaquine phosphate, 26.3 mg (15 mg base) daily for 14 days, to eliminate any persisting exoerythrocytic organisms (radical cure).

The treatment of acute chloroquinine-resistant *P. falciparum* infection requires multiple drug therapy. Most infections will be eliminated by the concomitant use of quinine sulfate, 650 mg every 8 hours for 3 days; pyrimethamine, 25 mg every 12 hours for 3 days; and sulfadiazine, 500 mg every 6 hours for 5 days. Less effective alternative courses of therapy are quinine sulfate, 650 mg every 8 hours for 3 days, plus tetracycline, 500 mg every 6 hours for 7 days, or quinine sulfate, 650 mg every 8 hours plus co-trimoxazole (320 mg of trimethoprim, 1.6 g of sulfamethoxazole) every 12 hours for 5 days.

Effect of Drugs on Sexual Stages of Malaria Parasites

Gametocytes of *P. falciparum* may remain in the circulation for prolonged periods after the patient has been treated with chloroquine alone. These gametocytes are rapidly destroyed by a single dose of 79 mg of primaquine phosphate (45 mg base). Pyrimethamine and chloroguanide, although they do not destroy gametocytes, will prevent their development in the mosquito.

ANTIMALARIAL DRUGS

Cinchona Alkaloids: Quinine, U.S.P.

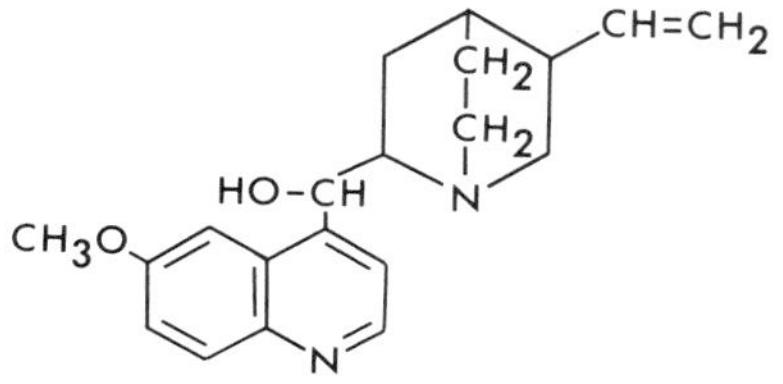

QUININE

Quinine, one of many alkaloids derived from the bark of the South American cinchona tree, and its d-isomer, quinidine, are the only cinchona alkaloids currently in use. Quinine has largely been replaced by less toxic synthetic antimalarial agents; however, it is still extremely useful in treating chloroquine-resistant *P. falciparum* infections.

Antimalarial Actions. Quinine acts only on erythrocytic asexual organisms. Its mechanism of action is not known, but it forms a complex with DNA that inhibits protein synthesis.

Nonantimalarial Actions. High doses of quinine may produce a quinidinelike effect on the heart (*see* Chap. 34) or a curarelike effect on skeletal muscle (*see* Chap. 19). Quinine has been used therapeutically in nocturnal muscle cramps, myokymia, myotonia congenita, dystrophia myotonia, and torsion spasm.

Although the gravid uterus shows little responsiveness to quinine, oxytoxic effects become more prominent as pregnancy progresses. Although the drug was used at one time to induce labor, this action is unreliable. Toxic doses of quinine may induce abortion, but whether this is due to myometrial stimulation or fetal toxicity is unclear.

Absorption, Metabolism, and Excretion. Quinine is readily and almost totally absorbed from the upper small intestine when given orally. Intramuscular and s.c. administration of quinine is contraindicated because of local tissue injury, including sloughing of the skin and production of sterile abscesses. Following a single oral dose, peak plasma concentrations are reached in 1 to 3 hours. About 75% is bound to plasma proteins, and only small amounts are found in the cerebrospinal fluid. The drug is largely metabolized in the liver, and degradation products are excreted in the urine; less than 5% is excreted unchanged. Because quinine is a base, its rate of excretion is influenced by urinary *p*H (*see* Chap. 2).

Adverse Effects. Toxic side-effects, termed *cinchonism,* usually develop when plasma levels of quinine exceed 10 μg/ml. Rarely cinchonism may follow a single oral dose (idiosyncratic reaction). Cinchonism consists of impairment of auditory and vestibular function, some visual abnormalities, nausea, vomiting, abdominal pain, and diarrhea. Idiosyncratic reactions may be accompanied by pruritus, angioedema, fever, and cutaneous flushing. Other adverse side-effects include hemolysis, leukopenia, thrombocytopenia, and agranulocytosis. Massive hemolysis and hemoglobinuria (blackwater fever) have been linked to undertreatment of *P. falciparum* infections.

Preparations and Administration. Quinine sulfate, U.S.P., is available in tablets and capsules that contain 130, 200, or 325 mg. Totaquine, a less refined, cheaper preparation of cinchona bark alkaloids that contains about 10% quinine, is used in many areas where the cost of pure quinine salts would be prohibitive. Quinine dihydrochloride is available for i.v. use (600 mg in 300-ml normal saline infused over 1 hour) in patients with chloroquine-resistant falciparum malaria who are unable to take oral medication. It may be repeated in 6 to 8 hours with a maximum dose of 1800 mg/day. Patients who receive i.v. quinine should be monitored electrocardiographically, and blood levels should be obtained periodically if there is evi-

---

Cinchona bark, also known as Jesuit's bark or quina-quina, was introduced to Europe from Peru in the 17th century for treating fevers. Quinine was purified from this in France in 1820. Linnaeus named the genus *Cinchona* in honor of the Spanish Countess of Chinchon, who was said to have introduced the bark to Europe, having been cured of malaria by it in Peru. The story is now believed to be a romantic fable.

dence of impairment of renal or hepatic function.

4-Aminoquinolines: Chloroquine, U.S.P.

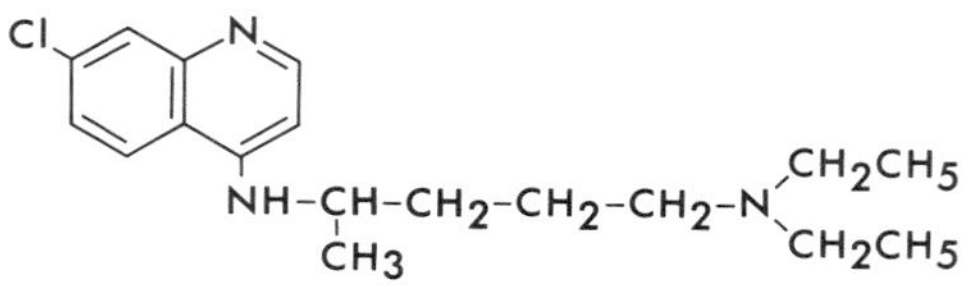

CHLOROQUINE

Hundreds of 4-aminoquinoline compounds have been tested for antimalarial activity. Of these, *chloroquine* (Aralen, Avloclor, Nivaquine B, Resochin, Roquine), *hydroxychloroquine* (Plaquenil), and *amodiaquin* (Camoquin) are commonly used. Although chloroquine was first synthesized in Germany in 1934, its use as an antimalarial was not pursued until its "rediscovery" during the search for effective synthetic antimalarials during World War II. The 4-aminoquinolines contain the alkyl side-chain present in quinacrine (*see* below). Chloroquine has also been used in hepatic amebiasis and in some collagen disorders.

Mode of Action. The exact antimalarial action of chloroquine on erythrocytic parasites is not known, but it does bind to double-stranded DNA, inhibiting DNA and RNA polymerase. Chloroquine is concentrated in parasitized red cells, possibly because of enhancement of passive diffusion by some metabolic activity of the parasite; lysosome stabilization; or the development of specific drug-binding sites. Chloroquine inhibits several enzyme systems, binds to and stabilizes lysosomes, and inhibits cell growth in many different organisms and in some mammalian cells. It also has antihistaminic and antiinflammatory properties.

Antimalarial Actions. Chloroquine is the most widely used drug for suppressive prophylaxis and for treatment of acute clinical attacks in all species of malaria except chloroquine-resistant falciparum strains. Relief from symptoms of the acute attack usually occurs within 48 hours of administration.

Absorption, Metabolism, and Excretion. Chloroquine is nearly completely absorbed from the gastrointestinal tract, and 50% is bound to plasma proteins. Chloroquine avidly binds to melanin, and therefore is concentrated in the retina. The drug is also found in high concentrations in liver, spleen, kidney, and lung. Because of this binding, loading doses must be used to treat acute malaria and hepatic amebiasis. About 30% of chloroquine is degraded in the body to several compounds, many of which have significant antimalarial activity. Chloroquine is excreted slowly in the urine. Excretion may be enhanced by urinary acidification. Patients on high-dose, chronic therapy may continue to excrete chloroquine for several years after the cessation of treatment.

Adverse Effects. Reactions to low doses of chloroquine used in malaria prophylaxis are very rare. The higher doses used for short-term treatment of acute malaria may produce anorexia, nausea, vomiting, headache, and pruritus. Chronic therapy with chloroquine in high doses such as those used in collagen disorders may cause reversible corneal opacities. Narrowing of the retinal arterioles and macular lesions, including edema and hyperpigmentation, are irreversible complications. Retinal examinations and visual tests should be done every 3 months when chloroquine is used in high doses. Other untoward side-effects associated with high-dose chloroquine therapy have been deafness, neuromyopathy, blood dyscrasias, skin eruptions, and toxic psychoses.

Preparations and Administration. Chloroquine is supplied as the diphosphate salt in tablets of 250 mg and 500 mg (500-mg salt is equivalent to 300-mg base). Chloroquine is also available for parenteral use as the dihydrochloride in 5-ml ampules that contain 50 mg of the salt (40 mg base/ml). Chloroquine dihydrochloride is given intramuscularly and should be used only in patients who are unable to take oral medication. It must be used with extreme caution in children. *Amodiaquine hydrochloride* (Camoquin) and *hydroxychloroquine sulfate* (Plaquenil) are other 4-aminoquinolines that have uses and toxicity similar to chloroquine.

8-Aminoquinolines: Primaquine, U.S.P.

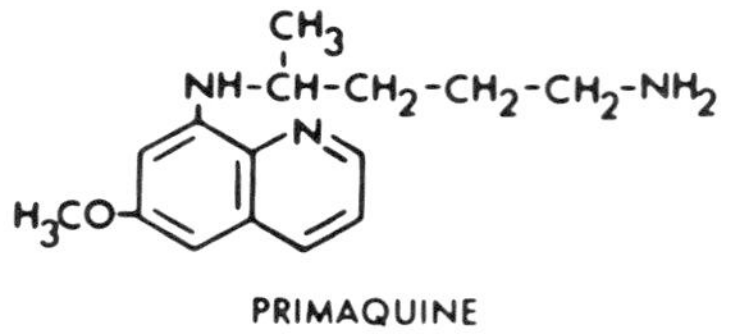

PRIMAQUINE

Although several 8-aminoquinoline compounds have been used therapeutically, primaquine, because of its relative safety and lower toxicity, is the only one in current use.

Actions. Primaquine is the only available drug that has activity against the exoerythrocytic stages of malaria. It is used to prevent relapses of *P. vivax* and *P. ovale* infection and is also effective in eliminating the gametocytes of *P. falciparum*. Although primaquine binds to DNA, there is no evidence that it interferes with DNA or RNA function. Certain geographic strains of *P. vivax* have relative resistance to primaquine.

Absorption, Metabolism, and Excretion. Primaquine is essentially completely absorbed from the gastrointestinal tract and completely metabolized, less than 1% being excreted unchanged in the urine. There is evidence that primaquine metabolites are the active agents. Some concentration of the drug occurs in the liver, lungs, brain, heart, and skeletal muscle.

Adverse Effects. Persons with glucose-6-phosphate dehydrogenase (G-6-PD) deficiency (*see* Chap. 6) develop some hemolysis when they receive therapeutic doses of primaquine. Patients who require therapy with primaquine should be screened for G-6-PD deficiency, and, if found, their course should be monitored carefully. Primaquine induces methemoglobinemia in persons genetically deficient in NADH methemoglobin reductase. Because quinacrine and biguanide compounds delay the metabolism of primaquine and increase its toxicity many times, these drugs should never be used concomitantly.

Common reactions to primaquine include nausea, cramping abdominal pain, headaches, visual disturbances, and pruritus. Leukocytosis or leukopenia are unusual manifestations, and agranulocytosis occurs rarely.

Preparation and Administration. Primaquine is supplied as the diphosphate salt in a 26.3-mg (15 mg base) tablet. There are no parenteral formulations.

Dihydrofoalate Reductase Inhibitors: Biguanides

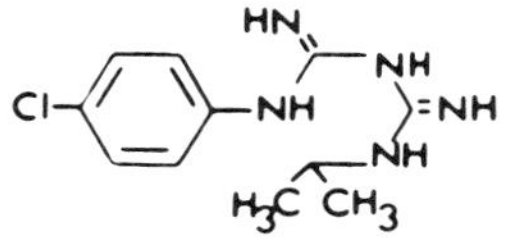

CHLOROGUANIDE

Chloroguanide was synthesized by the British during World War II in a search for effective synthetic antimalarial compounds.

Mode of Action. Chloroguanide is inactive as an antimalarial until it is metabolized into a triazine ring compound, cycloquanil. Cycloquanil inhibits dihydrofolate reductase, a necessary enzyme in folic acid metabolism. This effect prevents nuclear division in the malaria parasite.

Antimalarial Actions. Chloroguanide acts slowly and should not be used to treat acute malaria in nonimmune persons. It is an effective chemosuppressive agent against susceptible strains of *Plasmodium*. Unfortunately, resistance to chloroguanide has developed in many areas of the world. Chloroquine-resistant strains of *P. falciparum* are also resistant to chloroguanide. Cross-resistance exists between chloroguanide and pyrimethamine. The drug damages gametocytes so that they fail to develop and complete their cycle in the mosquito.

Absorption, Metabolism, and Excretion. Chloroguanide is slowly absorbed from the gastrointestinal tract. Peak plasma concentrations are reached in 2 to 4 hours. The drug is preferentially concentrated in erythrocytes. About 50% of chloroguanide is excreted in the urine and 10% in the feces. Chloroguanide is metabolized to the antimalarial compound cycloguanil (*see* above).

Adverse Effects. Untoward reactions to chloroguanide as a prophylactic agent are rare. High doses may cause vomiting, abdominal pain, diarrhea, hematuria, and proteinuria.

Preparation and Administration. Chloroguanide hydrochloride (Proguanil, Biguanide, Chloroguanil, Diguanyl, Paludrine, and Proguanide) is supplied in 100-mg tablets for oral administration.

Cycloguanil embonate, U.S.P. (cycloguanil pamoate, Camolar), is supplied in a relatively insoluble formulation that, when given intramuscularly has a duration of action of 3 months. Local reactions at the injection site and the development of drug resistance have limited its use.

Dihydrofoalate Reductase Inhibitors: Diaminopyrimidines

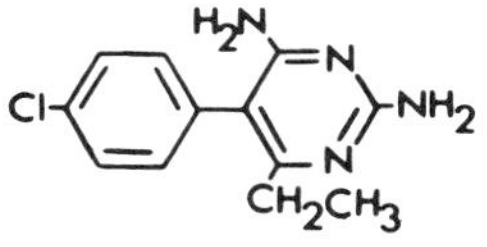

PYRIMETHAMINE

Pyrimethamine, U.S.P. (Daraprim, Malocide), is the most widely used diaminopyrimidine. It is closely related in structure to chloroguanide and has a similar inhibitory action on dihydrofolate reductase.

Mode of Action. Pyrimethamine and other diaminopyrimidines inhibit the conversion of dihydrofolate to tetrahydrofolate in the biosynthesis of purines and pyrimidines. Dihydrofolate reductase varies in its susceptibility to diaminopyrimidines depending on the source. The dihydrofolate reductase of malaria parasites, for example, may be very sensitive to inhibition by pyrimethamine, but the enzyme in bacteria may be relatively resistant.

Because mammalian cells can use exogenous folate whereas susceptible protozoa must synthesize folate from para-aminobenzoic acid (PABA), folinic acid may be used concomitantly with pyrimethamine to overcome the potential toxicity of the drug on the host without interfering with its action on the parasitic organism. Diaminopyrimidines are frequently combined with sulfonamides for synergistic effect. The sulfonamides act at a different step (*see* Chap. 57).

The antimalarial actions of the diaminopyrimidines are similar to those of chloroguanide. Cross-resistance exists between pyrimethamine and chloroguanide. Pyrimethamine is more potent than chloroguanide and has a much longer duration of action because of its slower excretion. The drug is well absorbed from the gastrointestinal tract, and a significant portion is bound to tissue. Little is known about the metabolism of pyrimethamine; however, some of the drug is slowly excreted unchanged in the urine.

Adverse Effects. The standard weekly dose of pyrimethamine used in malaria chemosuppression is free from side-effects. Higher doses and prolonged courses of pyrimethamine may produce a megaloblastic anemia. Patients on high-dose, chronic regimens, such as those used in toxoplasmosis, should have their hematologic status assessed frequently.

Preparation and Administration. Pyrimethamine is available in 25-mg tablets for oral use.

Trimethoprim, U.S.P.

Trimethoprim was developed as an antibacterial agent and is used in a fixed combination with sulfamethoxazole (*see* Chap. 64). This combination is used in malaria only as an alternative form of therapy for chloroquine-resistant *P. falciparum* infection in conjunction with quinine. The combination (co-trimoxazole is useful in treating pneumonia caused by *Pneumocystis carinii*. (For further details, *see* Chapter 64.)

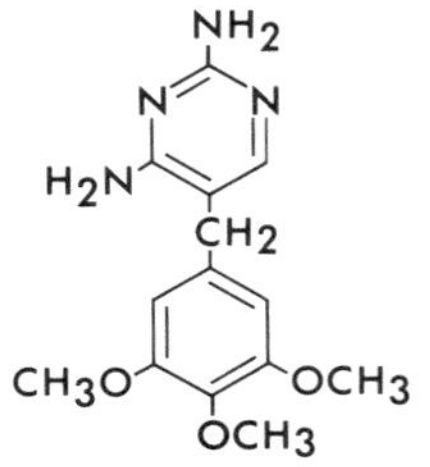

TRIMETHOPRIM

Pyrimethamine-sulfadoxine (Fansidar, Falcidar, Methipox, and Antemal), a fixed combination of pyrimethamine, 50 mg, and sulfadoxine, 1000 mg, is the only currently available chemoprophylactic for chloroquine-resistant *P. falciparum* infections. In many areas, pyrimethamine–sulfadoxine is adequate chemoprophylaxis for all strains of malaria; however, if pyrimethamine resistance is present in local strains of *P. vivax*, chloroquine should be added to the regimen.

Miscellaneous antimalarial drugs.

Dapsone (*see* Chap. 65) was used as part of the chemoprophylactic regimen for chloroquine-resistant *P. falciparum* infection among military personnel in Vietnam. *Tetracycline, minocycline, clindamycin,* and *lincomycin* have some antimalarial activity. A combination of *quinine* and *tetracycline* has been used to treat the clinical attack of chloroquine-resistant *P. falciparum* infection. *Mefloquin,* a quinoline compound, has shown great promise in chloroquine-resistant *P. falciparum* infections. It is currently undergoing extensive testing in humans.

AMEBIASIS

Infection with the protozoan parasite *Entamoeba histolytica* is termed *amebiasis*. The infection is acquired by the ingestion of amebic cysts in food or water contaminated by the feces of carriers. Amebiasis is found in all parts of the world, but areas with high prevalance rates are correlated with inadequate sanitation and poor hygienic standards. The large intestine is the primary site of parasitization. In most infections, the trophozoites (vegetative forms) appear to feed on bacteria and multiply within the colonic lumen without causing disease. Some of these motile forms transform into cysts that are passed in the feces and may remain infectious for several weeks under optimal conditions. When invasion of the colonic mucosa occurs, a variety of syndromes may develop, including acute amebic colitis (amebic dysentery), chronic colonic dysfunction, acute colonic perforation, insidious peritonitis, mass lesions in the cecum or colon (amebic granuloma or ameboma), and colonic strictures. Amebic liver abscess is the most common extraintestinal manifestation of invasive amebiasis, and this condition often develops in the absence of intestinal symptoms. Hepatic abscesses may be complicated by rupture or extension to adjacent organs or structures. Pleuropulmonary involvement is most frequent, but rupture into the pericardium, peritoneal cavity, bowel, or other areas may occur. Cerebral abscesses and cutaneous infections have been reported rarely.

Drugs used in amebiasis (Table 67-3) are classified according to their site of action; those effective against organisms in the bowel lumen are termed *luminal amebicides* and those effective in the bowel wall, liver, and other tissues, are termed *tissue amebicides*. The nitromidazoles must be followed with a course of a luminal amebicide to be certain that all parasites are eliminated.

All treatment regimens (Table 67-4) contain a highly effective luminal amebicide to ensure eradication of luminal parasites. All patients with intestinal infections should be followed with a series of three stool examinations performed 4 weeks after treatment, or sooner if symptoms persist or recur.

In addition to chemotherapy, many authorities recommend that large liver abscesses be aspirated percutaneously. This is especially important for abscesses that threaten to rupture intraperitoneally or through the diaphragm.

TABLE 67-3. Drugs Used in Amebiasis

Luminal amebicides
1. 8-hydroxyquinolines
Diiodohydroxyquin
Iodochlorhydroxyquin
Dibromohydroxyquinoline
2. Antibiotics
Paromomycin
(Tetracycline)*
(Erythromycin)*
3. Amides
Diloxanide furoate
Chlorbetamide
Chlorphenoxamide
Teclozan
4. Alkaloid
Emetine bismuth iodide
5. Arsenicals
Carbarsone
Glycobiarsol
Difetarsone
6. Quinone
Phanquone
7. Nitroimidazole*
Metronidazole
Tinidazole
Tissue amebicides
1. Nitroimidazole
Metronidazole
Tinidazole
2. Alkaloids
Emetine
Dehydroemetine
3. 4-Aminoquinoline
Chloroquine

* Not highly effective when used alone.

Ipecacuanha Alkaloids: Emetine, U.S.P.

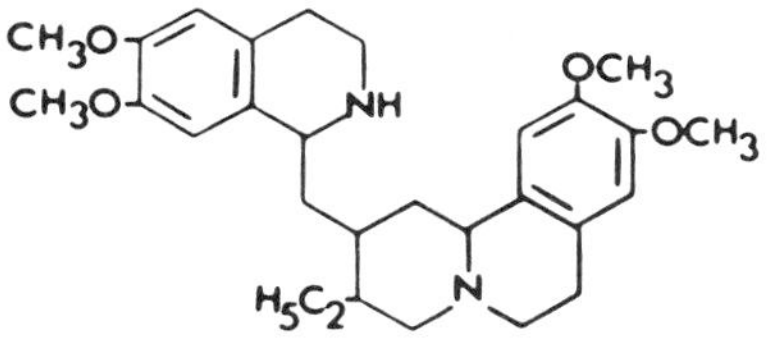

EMETINE

The root of the ipecac plant (*Cephaelis ipecacuanha* or *C. acuminata*) contains antiamebic alkaloids. Its principal and most active alkaloid is emetine. The ipecac plant is native to Brazil and Central America and was used by Brazilian natives as an antidiarrheal compound. It was introduced into Europe in the 17th century, where its use spread as a treatment for "tropical dysentery." In 1912, the specific antiamebicidal activity of the drug was demonstrated *in vitro*. Despite considerable toxicity, this drug was a mainstay tissue amebicide until the development of the nitromidazoles.

Mode of Action. Emetine interferes with protein synthesis by blocking transfer of amino acids from RNA to ribosomes. It is lethal *in vitro* to trophozoites of *E. histolytica* but is less active against cysts. Emetine is a highly effective tissue amebicide, but its use fails to eradicate organisms from the lumen of the intestine, possibly because of inadequate concentration of the drug in that area.

Emetine causes nausea and vomiting, probably of central origin, adrenergic and cholinergic blockade, and alteration of cardiac conduction.

TABLE 67-4. Treatment Regimens for Amebiasis

Clinical Status	Regimen of Choice	Alternate Regimens
Asymptomatic carrier	Diloxanide furoate, 500 mg q 8 hours X 10 days	1. Diiodohydroxyquin, 650 mg q 8 hours X 20 days 2. Paromomycin, 25 to 35 mg/kg/day in three divided doses X 5 to 10 days
Mild to moderate* intestinal disease	Metronidazole, 750 mg q 8 hours X 5 to 10 days, plus diiodohydroxyquin†, 650 mg q 8 hours X 20 days	1. Paromomycin, 25 to 35 mg/kg/day X 5 to 10 days, plus chloroquine, 250 mg q 6 hours X 2 days, then 250 mg q 12 hours X 12 days 2. Tetracycline, 500 mg q 6 hours X 10 days, plus diiodohydroxyquin†, 650 mg q 8 hours X 20 days, plus chloroquine, 250 mg q 6 hours X 2 days, then 250 mg q 6 hours X 12 days
Severe intestinal* disease	Metronidazole, 750 mg q 8 hours X 5 to 10 days, plus diiodohydroxyquin†, 650 mg q 8 hours X 20 days	1. Tetracycline, 500 mg q 6 hours X 10 days, plus diiodohydroxyquin†, 650 mg q 8 hours X 20 days, plus chloroquine, 250 mg q 6 hours X 2 days, then 250 mg q 12 hours X 14 days. 2. Emetine‡, 1 mg/kg/day (maximum, 60 mg), up to 5 days, for control of symptoms, plus diiodohydroxyquin†, 650 mg q 8 hours X 20 days, plus chloroquine, 250 mg q 6 hours X 2 days, then 250 mg q 12 hours X 12 days.
Hepatic abscess	Metronidazole, 750 mg q 8 hours X 5 to 10 days, plus diiodohydroxyquin†, 650 mg q 8 hours X 20 days	Emetine‡, 1 mg/kg/day (maximum, 60 mg) X 10 days, plus chloroquine, 250 mg every 6 hours X 2 days, then 250 mg every 12 hours X 26 days, plus diiodohydroxyquin†, 650 mg q 8 hours X 20 days.

* A tissue amebicide should be used in both mild and severe intestinal disease to prevent the development of liver abscess.

† Diiodohydroxyquin is listed because of its availability, but it is probably less effective and potentially more toxic than diloxanide furoate.

‡ Dehydroemetine may be less toxic than emetine and can be substituted for emetine at a dosage of 1 to 1.5 mg/kg/day for up to 5 days in severe intestinal disease and 1.5 mg/kg/day for 10 days (maximum total dose of 1.0 g) in hepatic abscesses.

Absorption, Metabolism, and Excretion. Emetine is concentrated in the liver, lung, kidney, and spleen after parenteral administration. The drug is excreted extremely slowly; therefore doses tend to be cumulative. Emetine may be detectable in the urine several months after cessation of treatment.

Adverse Reactions. Local reactions of the injection site are common and include pain, tenderness, and muscle weakness. Systemic effects of nausea, vomiting, and diarrhea are relatively common. Generalized muscular tenderness, weakness, stiffness, and aching may persist for several weeks following treatment. Electrocardiographic changes (T-wave flattening and lengthening of the P-R and Q-T intervals) are common. If toxic levels of emetine are reached, significant impairment of myocardial function may occur with arrhythmias, chest pain, dyspnea, congestive heart failure, and hypotension. Deaths that occur during emetine administration are related to myocardial toxicity. Although electrocardiographic abnormalities occur at therapeutic doses, these changes revert to normal within weeks after the last dose. Emetine should be avoided in persons with preexisting cardiovascular disease. Bed rest and electrocardiographic monitoring are considered appropriate for all patients undergoing emetine therapy.

Preparations and Administration. Emetine hydrochloride, U.S.P. in 1-ml ampules (65 mg/ml) is given intramuscularly or by deep s.c. injection.

Emetine bismuth iodide was developed as a luminal amebicide. The compound contains approximately 25% anhydrous emetine and 20% bismuth. It is taken orally, and emetine is slowly released in the intestinal lumen. Because of frequent adverse side-effects, the drug has been replaced by the less toxic diloxanide furoate or 8-hydroxyquinolines.

Dehydroemetine is a synthetic compound that has been used since 1962. Although its effects are similar to those of emetine, many authorities believe that the toxicity is somewhat less. In experimental animals, dehydroemethine is cleared more rapidly than is emetine. The drug disappears from the urine in about 10 days compared with 30 days for emetine. Dehydroemetine is supplied as the dihydrochloride in 2-ml ampules that contain 30 mg/ml. Dehydroemetine should not be administered until 45 days after a previous course of emetine or 14 days after a previous course of dehydroemetine.

4-Aminoquinoline: Chloroquine

Chloroquine (*see* above) is a tissue amebicide, with major activity occurring in the liver where it is concentrated. It is used in conjunction with emetine to treat amebic hepatic abscesses and is used with other amebicides in the treatment of invasive intestinal amebiasis to prevent the development of liver abscess (Table 67-3).

8-Hydroxyquinoline: Diiodohydroxyquin

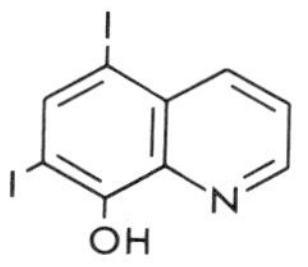

DIIODOHYDROXYQUIN

The halogenated hydroxyquinoline compounds are effective luminal amebicides. They are directly amebicidal, but their mode of action is unknown.

Absorption, Metabolism, and Excretion. After oral administration, probably less than 10% of diiodohydroxyquin is absorbed, with most being excreted unchanged in the stool. Little information is available on its metabolism and excretion.

Adverse Reactions. In recommended doses, side-effects are rare and consist of nausea, occasional vomiting, abdominal discomfort, diarrhea, pruritus ani, and headache. Persons sensitive to iodine may develop rashes, furunculosis, chills, and fever.

The most serious side-effect is neurotoxicity. An epidemic of a neurologic disorder called *subacute myelo-optic neuropathy* (SMON) occurred in Japan in the 1960s. It was associated with high-dose, long-term use of iodochlorhydroxyquin. Although the cause and effect relation has not been clearly defined, the association between SMON and iodochlorhydroxyquin has led to its withdrawal from the market in Japan and the United States. Following its withdrawal in Japan, the incidence of SMON decreased abruptly. Optic atrophy has been seen in young children receiving high-dose, chronic administration of diiodohydroxyquin. Because of its iodine content, diiodohydroxyquin may interfere with certain thyroid function tests.

Preparation and Administration. Diiodohydroxyquin (iodoquinol, Yodoxin, Embequin, Lanodoxin, Savorquin, Sebaquin) is available in tablets of 210 mg and 650 mg. Iodochlorohydroxyquin (clioquinol, Entero-vioform, Nioform, Vioform) is similar to diiodohydroxyquin except for the replacement of iodine with chlorine. A higher percentage of iodochlorohydroxyquin is absorbed than diiodohydroxyquin. In many parts of the world, iodochlorohydroxyquin has been used indiscriminately as a nonspecific treatment of diarrhea. This use is inappropriate and possibly hazardous.

Other halogenated hydroxyquinolines are dibromoquin (Intestopan), chinifon (Chinioform, Yatren), and chloroquinaldol (Sterosan).

Analines: Diloxanide Furoate (Furamide)

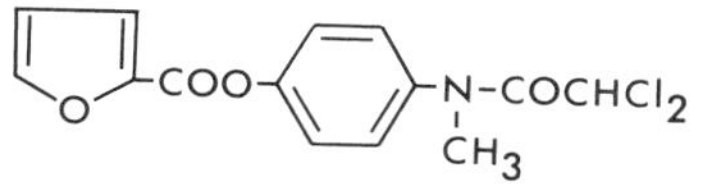

DILOXANIDE FUROATE

Diloxanide (Entamide) was developed through experimentation with substituted acetanlides. Studies of diloxanide esters show that the furoate form is less soluble and more active. It is currently the luminal amebicide of choice. It is amebicidal, but its mode of action is unknown.

Absorption, Metabolism, and Excretion. Following oral administration, most diloxanide is hydrolyzed from the furoate ester and rapidly absorbed. Up to 90% is excreted in the urine within 48 hours of administration as the glucuronide. Less than 10% is excreted in the stool.

Adverse Reactions. Significant symptoms, other than flatulence, are unusual. Rarely, nausea, abdominal cramps, esophagitis, xerostomia, diarrhea, pruritus, and urticaria occur. The drug is contraindicated in pregnancy and should not be administered to children under 2 years of age.

Preparation and Administration. Diloxanide furoate is available in 500-mg tablets for oral administration.

Nitromidazoles: Metronidazole, U.S.P. (Flagyl)

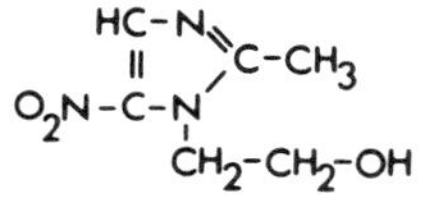

METRONIDAZOLE

Metronidazole was used for several years to treat trichomoniasis before it was found to be a highly effective tissue amebicide. It is the drug of choice for invasive amebiasis in conjunction with a luminal amebicide.

Mode of Action. After uptake by the protozoan cell, the nitrogroup is reduced, and the resultant metabolites are bound to DNA and to cytoplasmic protein. Nucleic acid synthesis is inhibited. Metronidazole has clinically significant activity against anaerobic bacteria, *Trichomonas vaginalis*, *Entamoeba histolytica*, and *Giardia lamblia*. It also has been used in dracunculiasis, balantidiasis, and some forms of leishmaniasis, but its efficacy in these conditions is uncertain.

Absorption, Metabolism, and Excretion. Metronidazole is well absorbed after oral administration, and it is distributed in total body water. Therapeutic levels are attained in many sites, including cerebrospinal fluid, bone, and bile. The drug can be recovered in the placenta, saliva, semen, and milk. About 70% is excreted unchanged in the urine; the remainder is excreted by the kidney predominantly as glucuronides. An unidentified metabolite may color the urine reddish brown. Only trace amounts of metronidazole are found in feces.

Adverse Effects. Commonly occurring are a metallic taste, nausea, and diarrhea and, less frequently, vomiting and abdominal pain. Headache, insomnia, dizziness, ataxia, vertigo, confusion, and paresthesiae are rare. Occasionally patients taking metronidiazole may experience a disulfiramlike reaction after the ingestion of alcohol (*see* Chap. 27).

Metronidazole is mutagenic in bacteria and carcinogenic in rodents; however, the precise cancer risk, if any, in humans exposed to metronidazole is unknown. Although adverse effects on the fetus have yet to be demonstrated, metronidazole is contraindicated in the first trimester of pregnancy. It should not be used in the presence of blood dyscrasias or central nervous system disorders.

Preparations and Administration. Metronidazole is supplied in 250-mg tablets for oral use and as the hydrochloride in vials containing 500 mg for i.v. use after reconstitution. Intravenous metronidazole is used in some bacterial infections and occasionally in invasive amebiasis when oral medication is not possible.

Tinidazole (Fasigyn), *nimorazole* (Naxogin), and *ornidazole* (Tiberal) are closely related to metronidazole with similar actions. They are not yet available in the United States.

Arsenicals

Several organic arsenical compounds have been used in amebiasis: The most widely known are *carbarsone*, a phenylarsonic acid derivative; *glycobiarsol* (Milibis), a bismuth salt of a phenylarsonic acid; and *diphetarsone*, closely related to carbarsone. Although the arsenicals have been reliable luminal amebicides, reports of occasional severe reactions, including fatalities, have led to substitution of drugs with less toxicity.

Antibiotics: Paromomycin, U.S.P.

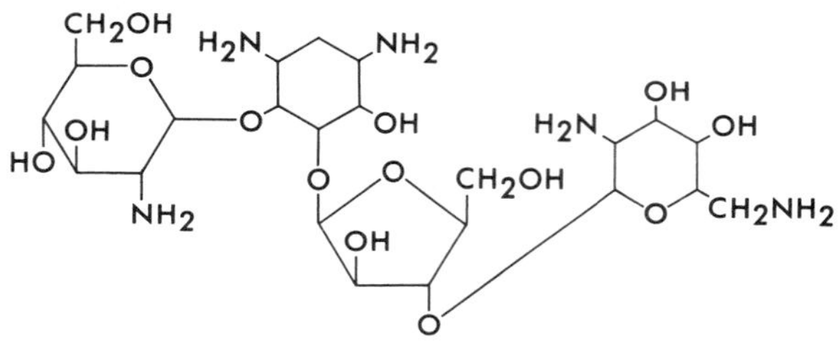

PAROMOMYCIN

Paromomycin sulfate (Humatin) is an amebicidal aminoglycoside antibiotic derived from *Streptomyces rimosus*. It also has antibacterial activity probably similar to the action of other aminoglycosides. The drug is a useful luminal amebicide effective in mild to moderate symptomatic disease. Little absorption occurs after oral administration unless significant ulceration is present. If the drug is appreciably absorbed or inappropriately administered parenterally, severe ototoxicity and nephrotoxicity may result. Therapeutic oral doses of paromomycin commonly result in diarrhea and anorexia. Less frequently, nausea, vomiting, abdominal pain, and pruritus ani result. Paromomycin sulfate is available in capsules that contain 250 mg of the base and in a syrup that contains 125 mg of the base per milliliter.

Other Amebicides

Phanquone (Entobex), A quinone derivative, and benzylamine derivatives such as *chlor-*

phenoxamine (Clefamide, Mebinol), *chlorphenoxamide ethyl ether* (Etofamide), *chlorbetamide* (Mantomide, Pontalin), and *Teclozan* (Falmonox) are synthetic amebicides used in some countries, mainly as luminal amebicides. None of these drugs offer significant advantages over those listed in the recommended therapeutic regimens (Table 67-3).

DIENTAMOEBA INFECTION

Nonspecific gastrointestinal complaints, including diarrhea, may accompany infection with the intestinal flagellate *Dientamoeba fragilis*. The organisms may be eliminated by tetracycline, 500 mg every 6 hours for 10 days, or diiodohydroxyquin, 650 mg every 8 hours for 10 days.

GIARDIASIS

Giardiasis (infection with *Giardia lamblia*) may be asymptomatic or may produce complaints of diarrhea, anorexia, bloating, and flatulence. Rarely malabsorption occurs. The infection is common throughout the world. Transmission occurs after ingestion of cysts in contaminated food or water. The drugs most commonly used are quinacrine or metronidazole; tinidazole has been highly effective in a single dose of 2.0 g.

Quinacrine (Mepacrine, Atabrine) was the first synthetic compound to be widely used for malaria chemosuppression. It is now obsolete for use in malaria because of the development of the less toxic 4-aminoquinolines such as chloroquine. Quinacrine is also obsolete in treating tapeworm infections but is still used in giardiasis.

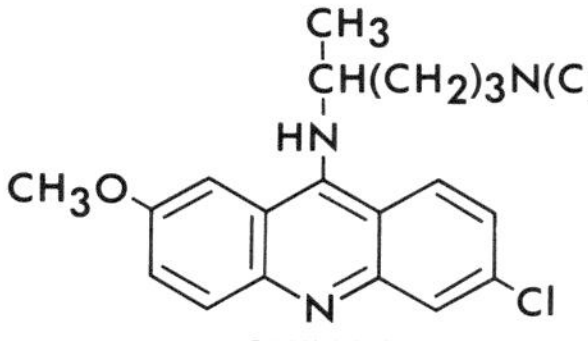

QUINACRINE

Quinacrine is rapidly and completely absorbed from the intestinal tract; the drug binds to plasma proteins and accumulates in many tissues, especially the liver, spleen, lungs, and adrenal glands. Quinacrine is also deposited in the nails and hair, where its presence may be detected by fluorescence under ultraviolet light. The metabolic degradation of quinacrine is not known. It is slowly excreted in the urine, and detectable amounts may be present as long as 2 months after cessation of therapy.

Gastrointestinal symptoms, including nausea, vomiting, and diarrhea, may occur with the dosage used to treat giardiasis but may be ameliorated by taking the drug with meals. Headaches, fever, myalgia, arthralgia, insomnia, and skin rashes have been reported, and a yellow discoloration of the skin, nails, and sclera may occur with chronic administration. Quinacrine should be used with caution in persons with central nervous system disease because it may induce a toxic psychosis. Quinacrine may exacerbate psoriasis. Quinacrine should never be used with primaquine or other 8-aminoquinolines because it inhibits their excretion and allows them to reach toxic levels readily.

Quinacrine hydrochloride is supplied as tablets containing 100 mg of the dihydrochloride.

Furazolidone, N.F. (Furoxone), a nitrofuran derivative (*see* below), has been used in giardiasis.

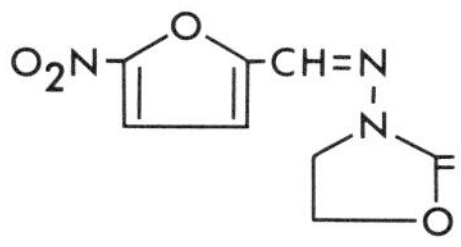

FURAZOLIDONE

Although it is somewhat less effective than the drugs mentioned above, its liquid formulation (50 mg/15 ml) makes it more easily administered to children. It also is supplied in tablets of 100 mg. The dosage for children is 1.25 mg/kg every 6 hours for 7 days. Adverse effects include nausea, vomiting, and headache. Rarely hypersensitivity reactions occur. The drug inhibits monoamine oxidase (MAO) and should not be used with other MAO inhibitors. If a course of treatment exceeds 5 days, foods with high tyramine content should be avoided (*see* Chap. 8). A disulfiramlike reaction may occur in patients who ingest alcohol during therapy or within 4 days after cessation of treatment (*see* Chap. 27). Furazolidone may cause hemolysis in G-6-PD deficient persons (*see* Chap. 6).

Paromomycin, U.S.P. (*see* above), is also active in giardiasis. It is administered in quantities of 25 to 35 mg/kg divided into three doses daily for 5 to 10 days.

TRICHOMONIASIS

Infection with *Trichomonas vaginalis* is usually acquired by sexual contact, but transmission occasionally occurs from contact with fomites such as contaminated moist towels or washcloths. Males are usually asymptomatic carriers, but females often develop severe vaginitis and cervicitis. Metronidazole and other nitromidazoles are the only effective drugs when given orally. Although *Trichomonas vaginitis* may respond to substances administered as douches, the problem of reinfection from sexual partners remains. Metronidazole is given either as 250 mg every 8 hours for 7 days or in a single dose of 2.0 g. It is important that male sexual partners be treated simultaneously.

TOXOPLASMOSIS

Ingestion of oocysts of *Toxoplasma gondii* from the feces of infected cats or ingestion of cysts from infected rare or raw meat causes human infection. Congenital toxoplasmosis may occur if the mother acquires the infection during pregnancy, particularly during the second and third trimesters.

Treatment involves the simultaneous use of pyrimethamine, U.S.P. (*see* above), 25 mg daily, and sulfadiazine or trisulfapyrimidines (*see* Chap. 64), 2 to 6 g daily, in divided doses for 3 to 4 weeks. Treatment of ocular toxoplasmosis usually includes simultaneous administration of corticosteroids. Leukovorin calcium (folinic acid) may be given in doses up to 10 mg/day intramuscularly to prevent any adverse hematologic effects of pyrimethamine. Co-trimoxazole also appears to be effective.

Spiramycin, a macrolide antibiotic closely related to erythromycin, is often used in France. It is given in doses of 2 to 4 g/day for 3 to 4 weeks and may be used as an alternative to, or in conjunction with, the pyrimethamine-sulfa regimen.

Congenital toxoplasmosis in the newborn, active ocular toxoplasmosis, and systemic acquired toxoplasmosis usually require treatment. Simple lymphadenopathy usually resolves slowly without treatment. Pyrimethamine is contraindicated in pregnancy under most circumstances; it may, however, be required to reduce the risk of disease in the fetus when toxoplasmosis is acquired in pregnancy. Toxoplasmosis in pregnancy must be evaluated carefully on an individual basis.

PNEUMOCYSTIS CARINII INFECTION

Co-trimoxazole has been effective both in treatment and prophylaxis of *Pneumocystis carinii* infection in high-risk patients. The following regimen is used for established infections: trimethoprim, 20 mg/kg/day, and sulfamethoxazole, 100 mg/kg/day, given in four divided doses daily for 14 days. An alternative treatment is pentamidine, 4 mg/kg/day intramuscularly for 14 days.

LEISHMANIASIS

Leishmania are transmitted to humans by the bite of sand flies (*Phlebotomus* and related genera). *Leishmania donovani* produces visceral leishmaniasis (kala-azar), *Leishmania tropica* causes skin ulcerations, *Leishmania mexicana* and *Leishmania braziliensis* occur in the Western Hemisphere and cause cutaneous lesions, but certain strains of *L. braziliensis* secondarily involve mucous membranes of the oral cavity and nasopharynx.

The responsiveness of different geographic strains to chemotherapy varies significantly; for example, in East Africa, visceral leishmaniasis is usually highly resistant to antimonial treatment, but the same form of disease in India responds readily. Table 67-5 outlines treatment regimens for the common forms of leishmaniasis.

Antimonials: Sodium Stibogluconate

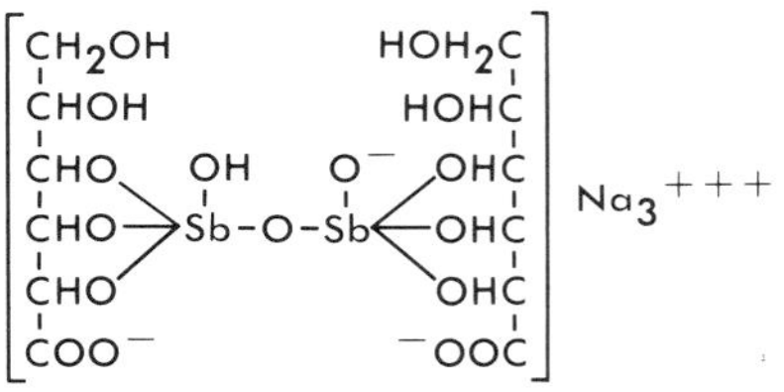

SODIUM STIBOGLUCONATE

Although trivalent antimonials such as potassium antimony tartrate (tartar emetic) and stibophen (Fuadin) have been used in leishmaniasis, they have been replaced by the pentavalent antimonials sodium stibogluconate (Pentostam, Solustibosan); N-methyl glucamine antimoniate (meglumine antimonate, Glucantime); urea stibogluconate (Stiburea); and ethyl stibamine (Neostibosan). Sodium stibogluconate is the most widely used. Although antimonial compounds inhibit several enzyme systems, the exact mode of action in protozoal infections is unknown.

CHARLES DONOVAN, 1863– . An Irish surgeon in the Indian medical service and later a distinguished entomologist. In 1903 followed Leishman in identifying the Leishman–Donovan bodies, the parasite of kala-azar, now called *Leishmania donovani*.

TABLE 67-5. Treatment of Leishmaniasis

	Treatment of Choice	Alternate Therapy
Visceral leishmaniasis (*L. donovani* infection)	Sodium stibogluconate, 600 mg i.m. or i.v. daily for 6 to 10 days. Repeat course may be needed.	Pentamidine, 2 to 4 mg/kg i.m. daily for up to 15 days.
Cutaneous leishmaniasis (*L. tropica* infection)*	Sodium stibogluconate, as in visceral leishmaniasis. (Treatment may not be indicated if spontaneous healing is occurring.)	Local treatment Heat Intralesional injections x-ray
American cutaneous leishmaniasis (*L. mexicana* infection)†	Cycloguanil embonate† in oil, 350 mg base i.m.	Sodium stibogluconate, as in visceral leishmaniasis.
American mucocutaneous leishmaniasis (*L. braziliensis* infection)	Sodium stibogluconate, as in visceral leishmaniasis.	Amphotericin B, 0.25 to 1 mg/kg by slow i.v. infusion daily or every 2 days for up to 8 weeks

* Treatment for cutaneous leishmaniasis with systemic drugs is usually not indicated; it may be necessary in lesions that are cosmetically significant or in cases where spontaneous healing does not occur.

† If the infection is acquired in a geographic area where only *L. mexicana* occurs, treatment of skin lesions with systemic drugs is not warranted unless the external ear is involved.

Absorption, Metabolism, and Excretion. Absorption of antimonials from the gastrointestinal tract is slow and accompanied by severe mucosal irritation. Therefore these drugs are administered parenterally. Sodium stibogluconate is concentrated in the liver and spleen. A small amount is metabolized to trivalent antimony. Excretion is largely through the kidney, with more than 50% of a single dose appearing in the urine with 24 hours of administration.

Adverse Reactions. Nausea, vomiting, and abdominal pain are not uncommon. Although antimonials are contraindicated in liver disease, hepatotoxicity from sodium stibogluconate is extremely rare. Fever, urticarial rash, proteinuria, and minor electrocardiographic T-wave changes have been reported. Coughing may occur immediately after i.v. administration. Anaphylactoid reactions have been seen, usually occurring after the fifth or sixth injection.

Preparation and Administration. Sodium stibogluconate is supplied in a solution containing 100 mg of the pentavent antimony per milliliter for i.m. or i.v. use.

Aromatic Diamidines: Pentamidine

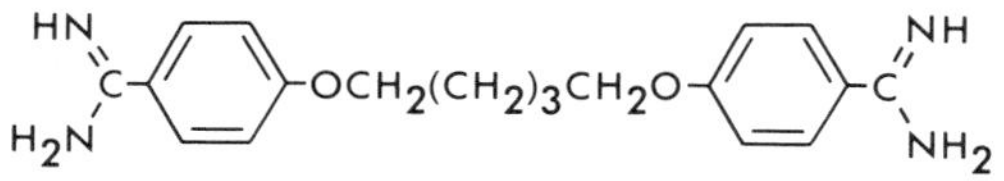

PENTAMIDINE

Pentamidine isethionate (Lomidine) is the most widely used of the amidine compounds. Its mode of action is unknown. The drug is significantly bound to tissue and is found in high concentration in the kidney. It is very slowly excreted unaltered in the urine. Pentamidine does not cross the blood–brain barrier. Adverse effects include hypotension, tachycardia, nausea, and vomiting; these effects are less common when the drug is given intramuscularly rather than intravenously. Hypoglycemia may occur, especially between the fifth and seventh days of treatment. Pentamidine also may produce hyperglycemia in both diabetic and nondiabetic persons. Nephrotoxicity has been reported in persons receiving concomitant nephrotoxic drugs or who have preexisting renal disease. Patients with normal renal function may have mild, reversible azotemia. Pentamidine isethionate is available as a dry powder to be diluted with distilled water to a 10% solution; it must be refrigerated and used within 5 to 7 days. The preferred route of administration is intramuscular.

Amphotericin B (*see* Chap. 69) has been used successfully in leishmaniasis resistant to other forms of therapy.

TRYPANOSOMIASIS

West African trypanosomiasis, caused by *Trypanosoma gambiense*, evolves slowly with the appearance of trypanosomes in the blood, lymphatics, and eventually in the cerebrospinal fluid. Progressive neurologic deficits end in somnolence, coma (sleeping sickness), and death.

East African trypanosomiasis causes *Trypanosoma rhodesiense* and is rapidly progressive, death usually being due to myocarditis or encephalitis. Both forms of African trypanosomiasis are transmitted by the bite of the tse-tse fly (*Glossina* species).

American trypanosomiasis (Chagas disease) is caused by *Trypanosoma cruzi* and transmitted by kissing bugs.

Treatment regimens for the trypanosomiases are outlined in Table 67-6. Both suramin and pentamidine have been used prophylactically in African trypanosomiasis because they maintain adequate blood levels for several months after a single injection.

Suramin

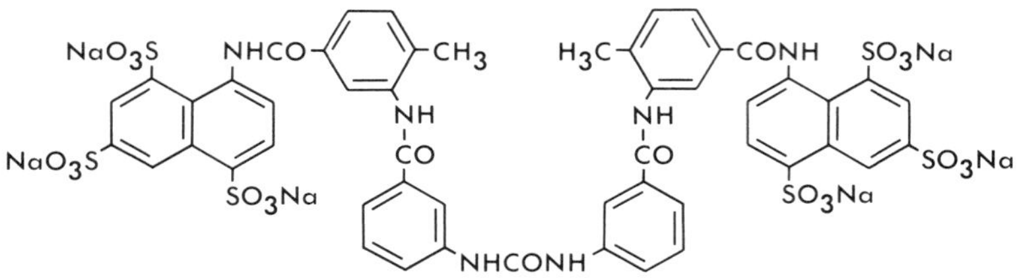

SURAMIN SODIUM

Suramin sodium (Antrypol, Bayer 205, Germanin, Naphuride, Moranyl, Belganyl) is a complex urea compound used in treating early African trypanosomiasis when there is no evidence of central nervous system involvement. Although suramin has been used in prophylaxis of African trypanosomiasis, pentamidine is generally preferred. Suramin is also used to eliminate the adult forms of *Onchocerca volvulus* (*see* Chap. 68).

Suramin competitively inhibits enzymes in the glycolytic pathway. Trypanosomes rely entirely on glycosis for an energy source. However, the exact mode of action of suramin is unknown, and antitrypanosomal activity can be demonstrated only *in vivo*. Suramin binds to plasma proteins. It is concentrated in the kidney in experimental animals. Suramin is very slowly excreted unchanged in the urine over a period of months. Nausea, vomiting, hypotension, loss of consciousness, and seizures may occur in sensitive persons. A test dose of 100 mg given intravenously will detect such persons, and this test should always be done before the start of therapy. Albuminuria is common during treatment but usually disappears within a few weeks after cessation of therapy. A burning sensation in the palms and soles is fairly common. Fever, rashes, pruritus, and edema may occur; these symptoms are common in onchocerciasis when the patient has not received diethylcarbamazine before suramin therapy. The drug must be used cautiously in patients with hepatic or renal disease.

Suramin sodium is supplied as a powder in ampules containing 1.0 g for reconstitution as a 10% solution in distilled water. It must immediately be given intravenously after the solution has been prepared. It is highly irritating to tissues if extravasated.

Arsenicals: Melarsoprol

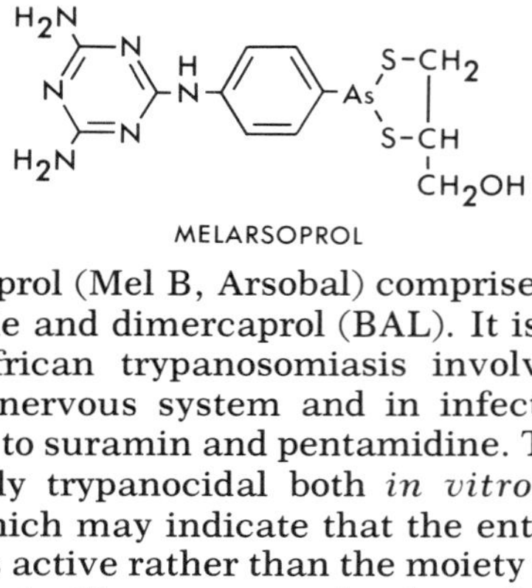

MELARSOPROL

Melarsoprol (Mel B, Arsobal) comprises melarsen oxide and dimercaprol (BAL). It is used to treat African trypanosomiasis involving the central nervous system and in infections refractory to suramin and pentamidine. The drug is rapidly trypanocidal both *in vitro* and *in vivo*, which may indicate that the entire compound is active rather than the moiety containing arsenic. The exact mechanism of action is unknown, but the drug inhibits essential sulfhydryl enzymes. The selective toxicity for protozoa over mammalian cells may be related to differing sensitivity of the enzyme systems, more rapid penetration of the drug into the protozoal cell, or a combination of these factors. Strains of protozoa with relative resistance to arsenic are less permeable to organic arsenicals than are susceptible strains.

Although melarsoprol is fairly well absorbed from the gastrointestinal tract, it is used by slow i.v. infusion clinically. A small, but therapeutically active, fraction of the drug enters the cerebrospinal fluid. Up to 7% is excreted unchanged in the urine, and 10% to 20% of the

CARLOS CHAGAS, 1879–1934. Brazilian physician. In 1909 discovered *Trypanosoma cruzi*, the causative agent of American trypanosomiasis, Chagas disease. Charles Darwin may have contracted this disease during the Beagle voyage of 1831–1836.

OSWALDO CRUZ, 1872–1917. Braziliana physician. After study in Paris at the Institut Pasteur, Cruz returned to Brazil to set up a similar institution in 1901, to found the national public hygiene service, and to clear the major cities of yellow fever, bubonic plague, and smallpox.

TABLE 67-6. Treatment of the Trypanosomiases

	Regimen of Choice	Alternate Regimen
African trypanosomiasis (*T. gambiense* and *T. rhodesiense* infection)		
Early disease without CNS involvement	Suramin*, 1 g i.v. on Days 1, 3, 7, 14, and 21.	Pentamidine, 4 mg/kg/day i.m. X 10 days
With CNS involvement	Melarsoprol†, 2 to 3.6 mg/kg i.v. daily for 3 days. After 1 week 3.6 mg/kg daily for 3 days. Repeat again after 10 to 21 days.	Tryparsamide, 30 mg/kg i.v. every 5 days for 12 doses. May repeat after 1 month. Plus Suramin*, 10 mg/kg i.v. every 5 days for 12 doses. May repeat after 1 month.
American trypanosomiasis (*T. cruzi* infection)	Nifurtimox, 5 to 7 mg/kg daily in four divided doses. Increase by 2 mg/kg/day every 2 weeks until dose reaches 15 to 17 mg/kg/day. Duration of total course, 90 to 120 days.	None.

* Suramin treatment should always be preceded by a test dose of 100 mg intravenously to determine whether sensitivity exists.

† If the patient is severely ill from systemic trypanosomiasis, many authorities recommend a short course of suramin before melarsoprol therapy.

arsenic is also excreted in the urine. Some arsenic probably accumulates in the body during a course of therapy.

Adverse effects include toxic encephalopathy, nausea, vomiting, hepatotoxicity, and nephrotoxicity. Thrombophlebitis may develop at injection sites.

The drug is supplied in ampules containing 6 ml of a 3.6% solution (36 mg melarsoprol per milliliter) in propylene glycol. It should be stored in the dark and below 25°C. Patients should be hospitalized while undergoing therapy.

Melarsonyl (Mel W, Trimelarsan), a water-soluble derivative of melarsoprol, may be administered intramuscularly. However, it has no other advantages over melarsoprol, and relapses following melarsonyl treatment are refractory to melarsoprol.

Tryparsamide, a drug that contains 25% pentavalent antimony, was widely used in West African trypanosomiasis.

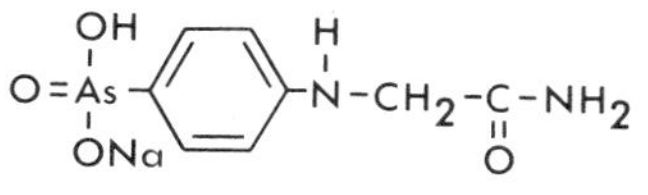

TRYPARSAMIDE

Because of frequent toxicity, often with optic nerve damage, it has been replaced by suramin and pentamidine. The drug readily enters the cerebrospinal fluid and is still valuable as an alternative to melarsoprol, when used in conjunction with suramin, for central nervous system involvement. It is supplied as a powder to be made up to a dose of 30 mg/kg in 10 ml of water intravenously.

Nitrofurans: Nifurtimox

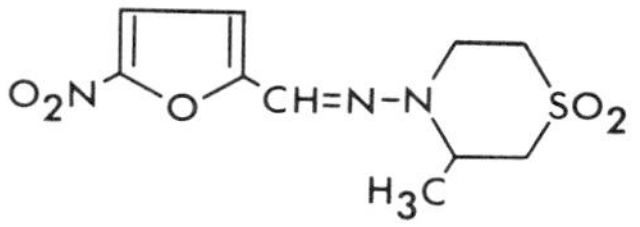

NIFURTIMOX

Nifurtimox (Bayer 2502, Lampit) is used in acute and chronic American trypanosomiasis. Its mode of action is unknown, but the drug can kill the intracellular parasites in tissue culture. Acute disease responds better to treatment than does chronic disease. Serologic tests often revert to negative in persons treated early during the illness. In chronic infections, parasitemia may be eliminated during therapy, but relapses occur in 20% or more of patients after the drug has been withdrawn.

The drug is rapidly absorbed from the gastrointestinal tract but attains only low concentrations in the blood, tissues, and urine. Peak blood levels occur 1 hour after ingestion, and nifurtimox has a T½ of about 8 hours. Little is known about its metabolism or the trypanocidal activity of its metabolites.

Common side-effects are anorexia, nausea, vomiting, and weight loss. Usually these symptoms are not severe enough to cause interruption of treatment. Less common are seizures, headache, nervousness, insomnia, drowsiness, peripheral neuropathy, and other neurologic abnormalities. The drug is supplied in 100-mg tablets for oral use.

Nitrofurazone (Furacin) is used to treat special cases of African trypanosomiasis resistant to other drugs. It is toxic.

FURTHER READING

1. Chemoprophylaxis of malaria. Morbidity and Mortality Weekly Report 27, No. 10:81–90, 1978.
2. Drugs for parasitic infections. Med Lett 21, No. 26:105–112, 1979.
3. Goldman P: Metronidazole. N Engl J Med 303, No. 21:1212–1218, 1980
4. Health information for international travel. Morbidity and Mortality Weekly Report (Suppl) Vol 29, 1980
5. Informational Material for Physicians (Dehydroemetine, Diloxanide furoate, Melarsoprol, Nifurtimox, Pentamidine, Sodium stibogluconate, Suramin). Atlanta, Parasitic Disease Drug Service, Centers for Disease Control.
6. Steck EA: The Chemotherapy of Protozoan Diseases, Vols I–IV. Washington, DC, Division of Medicinal Chemistry, Walter Reed Army Institute of Research, U.S. Government Printing Office, 1972
7. Woolfe G: The chemotherapy of amebiasis. Prog Drug Res 8:11–52, 1965

CHAPTER 67 QUESTIONS

(*See* P. 7 for Full Instructions)

Select the One Best Answer

1. In the treatment of malaria,
   - A. quinine will produce a radical cure of a *P. vivax* infestation.
   - B. primaquine cannot produce hemolytic anemias unless there is a genetic deficiency of glucose-6-phosphate dehydrogenase.
   - C. sulphomethoxine increases the effect of pyrimethamine on folic acid metabolism.
   - D. chloroquine is contraindicated in the presence of an amebic abscess.
   - E. only primaquine can produce a radical cure of *P. falciparum*.

2. Each of the following drugs is effective in intestinal amebiasis EXCEPT
   - A. tetracycline.
   - B. chloroquine.
   - C. diiodohydroxyquin.
   - D. carbarsone.
   - E. paromomycin.

3. An alkaloidal antiparasitic drug with considerable cardiac toxicity is
   - A. piperazine.
   - B. emetine.
   - C. diethylcarbamazine.
   - D. thiabendazole.
   - E. pyrvinium pamoate.

4. Which of the following agents has no place in the treatment of trypanosomiasis?
   - A. Melarsoprol
   - B. Pentamidine
   - C. Suramin
   - D. Tryptamine
   - E. Tryparsamide

A = 1,2,3; B = 1,3; C = 2,4; D = 4; E = All

5. Which of the following drug combinations are useful for the reasons stated?
   1. Pyrimethamine plus a sulfonamide to treat malaria because both inhibit folic acid metabolism
   2. Quinine plus chloroquine to treat *Plasmodium vivax* because their combined actions will destroy both the exoerythrocytic and erythrocytic parasites
   3. Primaquine plus chloroquine to reduce the incidence of resistant strains of *Plasmodia*
   4. Quinine plus quinidine to treat cardiac arrhythmias to reduce toxicity

6. Chloroquine
   1. is recommended for tourists going to a region where malaria is endemic.
   2. prevents malarial infection of the liver.
   3. is generally a curative agent for sensitive strains of *P. falciparum* malaria.
   4. causes yellow skin.

7. Metronidazole (Flagyl) is effective against
   1. invasive *E. histolytica* in gut.
   2. *E. histolytica* in liver.
   3. *T. vaginalis*.
   4. *G. lamblia*.

8. Emetine
   1. can terminate the symptoms of a severe acute attack of amebiasis.
   2. is the ingredient in Syrup of Ipecac responsible for its emetic effect.
   3. in large therapeutic doses may produce electrocardiographic changes.
   4. rapidly eliminates *E. histolytica* cysts that persist in the lumen of the intestine.

9. Diiodohydroxyquin
   1. will eradicate *E. histolytica* cysts from the lumen of the intestine.
   2. is effective in suppressing severe amebic dysentery.
   3. should not be used in patients hypersensitive to iodine-containing drugs.
   4. is effective for treating amebic abscess in brain.

JEREMY H. THOMPSON

68

Drugs Used to Treat Helminthiasis

Worm infection (helminthiasis) includes parasitization with cestodes (tapeworms), nematodes (roundworms), and trematodes (flukes) (Table 68-1). Helminthiasis is present in about half the world's population and is not limited to tropical or subtropical countries but is endemic in many areas because of poor sanitation, poor family hygiene, malnutrition, disease, and crowded living conditions. Further, with increasing travel, and especially with the recent large emigration from countries in Southeast Asia to America, physicians may expect now to see infections caused by exotic parasites. The anthelmintic drugs are toxic compounds that act directly on the parasite. Anthelmintic agents that act against intestinal helminths (vermifuges) kill or sterilize the worms, paralyze them so that they lose hold of the intestinal mucosa and are expelled, or interfere with egg production or influence chemotaxis. Host immunity seems unimportant for recovery. Treatment is frequently complicated by drug toxicity, "Jarish–Herxheimer-like" reactions to liberated helmintic protein, coincident disease, especially malnutrition, and anemia or dehydration. Improvement of the patient's general condition nutritionally and correction of anemia and electrolyte imbalance are important aspects of therapy. In every case the need for treatment must be balanced against potential toxicity. *The mere presence of a parasite does not mean that it must be treated.*

The drug package insert should be consulted for special precautions about dosage or administration, since herein only principal adverse effects are given for each agent, and no attempt is made to list all precautions and contraindications to therapy. Infection with more than one type of worm is common. Thus drug therapy must take into account a possible effect on a second parasite. When selecting a drug, cost should be considered because many patients who need these agents are financially destitute. The drugs are discussed alphabetically (Table 68-2).

(*Text continues on p. 699*)

TABLE 68-1. Cause and Treatment of Helminthic Infections in Humans

Disease	Helminth	Drugs Used in Treatment: *Primary*	Drugs Used in Treatment: *Secondary*
Cestode (tapeworm) infections			
Intestinal taeniasis	*Diphylobothrium latum*	Paramomycin	
	Hymenolepsis nana	Paramomycin	
	Taenia saginata	Paramomycin	
	Taenia solium	Paramomycin	
Somatic taeniasis (cysticercosis)	*T. solium*	None	
Nematode (roundworm) infections			
Ancylostomiasis	*Ancylostoma duodenale*	Bephenium Mebendazole Pyrantel	Hexylresorcinol
	Necator americanus	Bephenium Mebendazole Pyrantel	Hexylresorcinol
Cutaneous larva migrans	*Ancylostoma braziliene*	Thiabendazole	
	Ancylostoma caninum	Thiabendazole	
Ascariasis	*Ascaris lumbricoides*	Mebendazole Piperazine Pyrantel	Bephenium Diethylcarbamazine
Enterobiasis	*Enterobius vermicularis*	Piperazine Pyrantel Pyrvinium	
Filariasis	*Wuchereria bancrofti*	Diethylcarbamazine	
	B. malayi	Diethylcarbamazine	
	Loa loa	Diethylcarbamazine	
Onchocerciasis	*Onchocerca volvulus*	Diethylcarbamazine + suramin	
Dracunculiasis	*Dracunculus medinensis*	Niridazole	
Strongyloidiasis	*Strongyloides stercoralis*	Thiabendazole	Pyrvinium
Trichiniasis	*Trichinella spiralis*	Corticosteroids + mebendazole	
Trichuriasis	*Trichuris trichiura*	Mebendazole	
Trematode (fluke) infections			
Clonorchiasis	*Clonorchis sinensis*	Bithionol	
Fascioliasis	Fasciola hepatica	Bithionol	
	Fasciolopsis buski	Hexylresorcinol	Tetrachloroethylene
Paragonimiasis	*Paragonimus westermani*	Bithionol	Sulfonamides + emetine
	P. kellicotti	Bithionol	Sulfonamides + emetine

(continued)

TABLE 68-1. *(Continued)*

Disease	Helminth	Drugs Used in Treatment	
		Primary	***Secondary***
Schistosomiasis (bilharziasis)	*Schistosoma haematobium*	Metrifonate Praziquantel	Hycanthone Niridazole Stibocaptate Stibophen Lucanthone
	S. mansoni	Niridazole Oxamniquine Praziquantel	Hycanthone Stibocaptate Stibophen Lucanthone
	S. japonicum	Niridazole Praziquantel Tartar emetic	Stibocaptate Stibophen

PATRICK MANSON, 1844–1922. British physician and parasitologist. Often described as the "father of modern tropical medicine." In 1879 proved the mosquito to be the vector and filaria the agent of elephantiasis. First to suggest that mosquito was also the malaria vector.

TABLE 68-2. Anthelmintic Drugs

Drug	Properties	Adverse Effects	Preparations, Dosage, and Use
Antimony compounds	Potassium and sodium antimony tartrate, stibophen, and antimony-containing compounds may all be used. Properties are discussed in Chapter 67. They selectively inhibit schistosomal phosphofructokinase, which catalyses the conversion of fructose-6-phosphate to fructose-1-6-diphosphate.	Muscle pain and stiffness. Cough and vomiting with too rapid i.v. injection. Pain, sloughing, and local irritation following leakage on i.v. injection; bradycardia. Rarely produced are colic, diarrhea, various skin rashes, pruritus, liver, renal and myocardial damage, hemolytic anemia, shock, sudden death. See also Chapter 67.	Potassium and sodium antimony tartrate are given i.v. in increasing doses from 60 to 120 mg every 2nd day. Used in some cases of schistosomiasis. Stibophen is given i.m. in doses of 100 mg every 2nd day for 1 to 3 weeks.
Bephenium hydroxynaphthoate 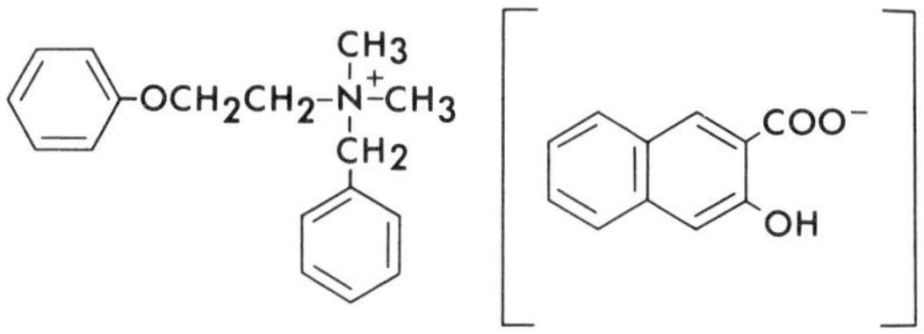 BEPHENIUM HYDROXYNAPHTHOATE	A quaternary ammonium compound, the drug of choice for treating infections with hookworms in humans because it is less toxic than tetrachloroethylene. It is more active against *Ancylostoma duodenale* than against *Necator americanus*. Several related drugs are used as anthelmintics in veterinary practice. A single oral dose is often effective, but, because the drug is relatively nontoxic, little is lost by continuing therapy for 3 to 7 days.	Bephenium has a bitter taste and may produce nausea, vomiting, diarrhea, and abdominal pain.	Bephenium (Alcopar) is given orally in 5-g doses for 3 to 7 days. Special attention to diet is not required, and no sequential catharsis is necessary. It can be used safely if concomitant ascariasis is present because it does not stimulate *A. lumbricoides*.
Bithionol	A phenolic compound developed in Japan. The drug of choice for paragonimiasis and occasionally in fascioliasis.	Vomiting, colic, diarrhea, urticaria, and photodermatitis.	The usual oral dose is 50 mg/kg every 2nd day for 10 doses.

Carbon tetrachloride	A halogenated hydrocarbon obsolete in the treatment of helminthiasis but still frequently used in the dry cleaning industry (as a cleaner) and as a solvent in rubber and paint industries. Thus accidental and occupational exposure are important toxicologically.	Highly hepatotoxic, and fatalities have resulted from occupational exposure.	None
Chloroquine	Chloroquine has been used in clonorchiasis but with limited success. It may depress ova output but does not kill the worms. *See* Chapter 67.	*See* Chapter 67.	*See* Chapter 67.
Dichlorophen 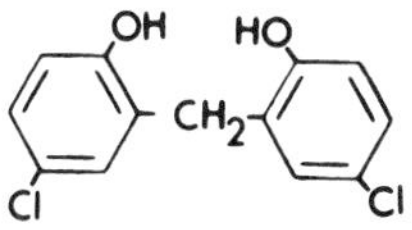 DICHLOROPHEN	A new taeniacide whose mode of action is unknown. It detaches the scolex from the bowel wall so that the worm dies and is rapidly digested. Thus fecal examination is valueless in determining success of treatment.	Gastrointestinal irritation, urticarial skin rashes, lassitude, and depression may develop. Since the worm is digested intraluminally, cysticercosis may result from autoinfection by ova liberated from *T. solium*.	Dichlorophen (Anthiphen) is available only in Europe. The usual dose is 6 g orally, repeated twice. No bowel preparation required, but a saline cathartic should be given 2 to 4 hours after the drug to minimize the danger of cysticercosis.
Diethylcarbamazine 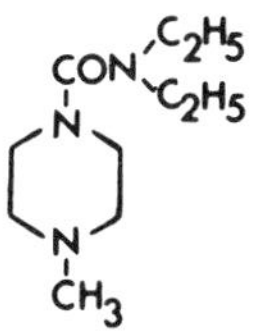 DIETHYLCARBAMAZINE	A piperazine ring-containing phenothiazine effective against several species of filarial parasite. It is inactive *in vitro* but highly active *in vivo*, probably sensitizing the microfilaria so that they become phagocytozed by fixed tissue macrophages. No phagocytosis occurs in the blood stream. The drug kills adult *Brugia malayi* and *Loa loa* and most adult *Wuchereria bancrofti*; it has minimal activity against adult *Onchocerca volvulus*.	Adverse reactions are frequent but rarely necessitate discontinuance of therapy. Commonly seen are headaches, arthralgia, lymphadenopathy, gastrointestinal upsets, a general feeling of weakness, dermatitis, and fever. Transient leukocytosis and eosinophilia may appear. An encephalopathy is rare. In initial therapy for onchocerciasis and filariasis, severe allergic or	Diethylcarbamazine citrate, U.S.P. (Banocide, Hetrazan), is highly stable under extremes of heat and humidity. The usual dose is 2 mg/kg q 8 hours for 1 to 3 weeks depending on the type of infection. *W. bancrofti* and *B. malayi* are usually cured by one course of therapy. Loaiasis may require several spaced courses for complete cure; in onchocerciasis repeated courses, usually combined with suramin, are required to keep the disease in

(*continued*)

TABLE 68-2. (*Continued*)

Drug	Properties	Adverse Effects	Preparations, Dosage, and Use
Diethylcarbamazine (*continued*)	Rapidly absorbed following oral administration with diffusion throughout most tissues and tissue compartments. It is excreted as the free drug and as a mixture of four metabolites, all of which contain a piperazine ring but are therapeutically inactive.	febrile reactions may occur owing to release of helmintic protein on worm disintegration; corticosteriods or H_1-blockers may be useful in controlling these reactions.	check. Diethylcarbamazine is also of value in ascariasis, visceral larva migrans, and tropical pulmonary eosinophilia.
Hexylresorcinol 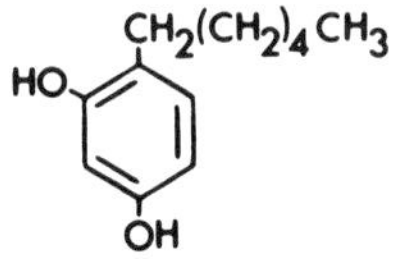 HEXYLRESORCINOL	Introduced originally as a urinary antiseptic but subsequently found to paralyze various worms, in particular *Ascaris lumbricoides, Ancylostoma duodenale, Taenia saginata, Hymenolepsis nana, Trichuris trichiura,* and *Fasciolopsis buski.* Many of the newer drugs are more effective anthelmintics, but hexylresorcinol may be used rarely in cases of mixed infection where the use of a more potent drug acting against a single parasite might be dangerous. About 30% of an oral dose is absorbed.	Glossal and buccal ulceration may develop if the tablets are chewed and not swallowed whole or are held in the mouth. Gastrointestinal irritation is common, and the drug should not be used in patients with ulcerative or obstructive conditions of the intestine. Coating of the buttocks with petroleum jelly before use of hexylresorcinol enemas may prevent perianal irritation and ulceration. Hexylresorcinol may be mutagenic and carcinogenic.	Hexylresorcinol, N.F. (Caprokol), is available as 100- and 200-mg gelatin-coated tablets. The usual dose for adults, 1 g, should be followed 2 to 4 hours later by a saline cathartic. It should be given after an overnight fast since fatty food depresses intraluminal activity. Hexylresorcinol can be administered as an enema (1:100) in water.
Hycanthone	The hydroxymetabolite of lucanthone possesses marked schistosomicidal activity. It may replace lucanthone.	Gastrointestinal upsets, headache, myalgia, dizziness, and altered liver function.	Hycanthone (Etrenol) used rarely in treating *S. mansoni* and *S. haematobium* infections.

Lucanthone 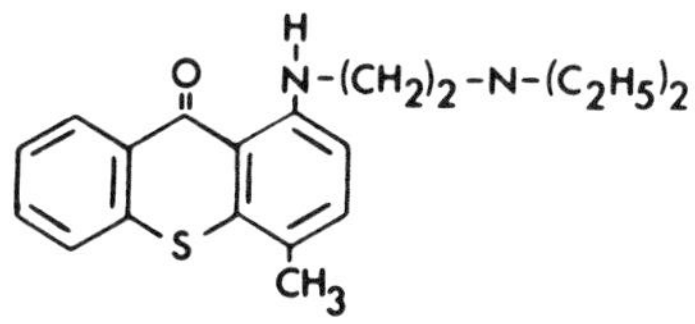 LUCANTHONE	Effective against adult *Schistosoma haematobium* and *S. mansoni* but only weakly, if at all, effective against *S. japonicum*. It prevents helmintic ova production or release and subsequently destroys the parasite. Fully absorbed following oral administration, passing into most tissue spaces. Only about 10% to 15% is excreted unchanged into the urine.	Children tolerate lucanthone better than do adults, and tolerance is poor among Egyptians and Latin Americans. Gastrointestinal irritation develops in 15% to 20% of patients. The drug has a bitter taste. Vertigo, tinnitus, convulsions, acute psychoses, and circulatory failure are rare. H_1-blockers or atropine may protect against the development of some of these adverse effects. The skin and sclerae may turn yellow or orange (drug pigment) during therapy; this usually requires 4 to 6 weeks to regress. The drug should be used with caution if severe renal disease is present.	Lucanthone hydrochloride, U.S.P. (Miricil D), is given in doses of 5 mg/kg two or three times a day for 5 to 10 days. It is of use only in schistosomiasis.
Mebendazole	A new broad-spectrum anthelmintic showing activity in ascariasis, ankylostomiasis, trichuriasis, and filariasis. Mebendazole kills helminths by inhibiting glucose uptake and by destroying microtubules. It is essentially nonabsorbed, only 10% appearing in the urine.	Nausea, colic, diarrhea, headache, and drowsiness. Dysmorphogenic in animals.	Mebendazole (Vermox) is usually given in doses of 100 mg q 12 hours for 3 days.
Metrifonate 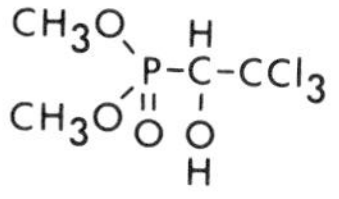 METRIFONATE	An organophosphorus cholinesterase inhibitor effective against *S. haematobium*. Available on an investigational basis from the Centers for Disease	Nausea, colic, diarrhea, vomiting, "weakness," fatigue, and bronchospasm appear within 6 hours of oral administration and disappear	Metrifonate (Bilarcil), 10 mg/kg (for adults and children), for three doses at 2-week intervals. Erythrocyte cholinesterase levels should be measured 2 days

(*continued*)

TABLE 68-2. (*Continued*)

Drug	Properties	Adverse Effects	Preparations, Dosage, and Use
Metrifonate (*continued*)	Control. Metrifonate paralyzes adult schistosomes, which become encased and die when trapped in small arterioles.	within 24 hours. Because host cholinesterase activity is depressed, skeletal muscle relaxants should be used carefully (see Chap. 19).	before the administration of each dose and 6 months after treatment.
Niclosamide 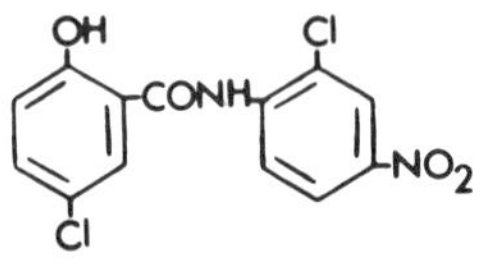 NICLOSAMIDE	Taeniacidal in humans and effective against *Echinococcus granulosus* in dogs. Poorly absorbed following oral administration. Mode of action to depress respiration and block glucose uptake, leading to detachment of the scolex from the mucosa, permitting worm expulsion. Not absorbed.	Gastrointestinal irritation. May initiate cysticerosis (*see* above, dichlorophen).	Niclosamide (Cestocide, Yomesan) is available only in Europe; it is used in the U.S. on an investigational basis, but its use is prohibited for treating *T. solium* infections. The usual dose is 2 g (four tablets) in the morning after an overnight fast. In the U.S., niclosamide is under investigation for treatment of beef and fish tapeworm infection and infection with *H. nana*.
Niridazole 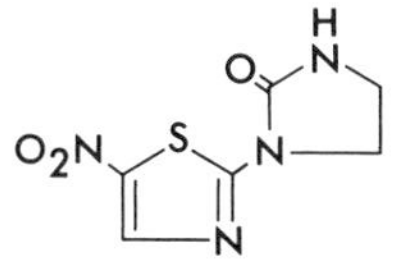 NIRIDAZOLE	A relatively new drug related to the nitrofurans and metronidazole, which has been used mainly in Africa. In schistosomes it prevents maturation of the egg and shell in females and produces degeneration of the testes in males. Niridazole is well absorbed following oral administration but largely metabolized by the liver on its first passage. The parent drug and its metabolites are avidly protein bound; excretion is by kidney and liver. Inhibits uptake of glucose by the parasite.	Gastrointestinal upsets (nausea, anorexia, vomiting, abdominal pains, diarrhea), various skin rashes, and paresthesias are common. Flattening and inversion of T waves may appear on electrocardiographic examination without any other evidence of myocardial toxicity. Rarely central effects of insomnia, aggitation, visual and auditory hallucinations, confusion, and epileptiform convulsions may develop. Hemolytic anemia	Niridazole (Ambilhar) is not available in the U.S. The usual dose is 25 mg/kg/day for 5 to 10 days. It is schistosomicidal in *S. haematobium* and *S. mansoni* infections, but a poor response other than a decreased cell count is seen in *S. japonicum* parasitization. Niridazole is of some value in guinea worm infection, cutaneous leishmaniasis, and possibly intestinal and extra-intestinal amebiasis and onchocerciasis.

		occurs in subjects with glucose 6-phosphate dehydrogenase deficiency. Patients may complain of an objectionable body odor, and the urine may be colored dark.	
Oxamniquine	An investigational synthetic derivative of lucanthone effective orally in a single dose against *S. mansoni,* where it kills the early larval stage. More active against Brazilian than African disease and more effective in adults than in children.	Dizziness, nausea, drowsiness, hallucinations, hematuria, proteinuria, elevation of serum SGOT and SGPT levels.	Oxamniquine (Vansil; Mansil), a single dose of 15 mg/kg (Brazilian disease) or 60 mg/kg in divided doses over 2 days (African disease).
Paromomycin	*See* Chapter 67	*See* Chapter 67	*See* Chapter 67
Piperazine 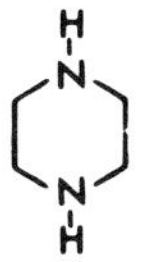 PIPERAZINE	Highly effective against *Ascaris lumbricoides* and *Enterobius vermicularis.* In *A. lumbricoides,* it blocks the effect of acetylcholine at the myoneural junction, causing relaxation of the worm's hold on the mucosa with subsequent expulsion by normal peristaltic activity or cathartics. Its mode of action in enterobiasis is not known. Readily absorbed following oral administration but still highly effective against *A. lumbricoides* in the small bowel and *E. vermicularis* in the colon. Most of the drug is excreted unchanged.	Gastrointestinal irritation and headaches are common. Urticaria, skin rashes, amblyopia, and transient muscle weakness may develop but are rare. Cerebellar ataxia ("worm wobble") is a rare but serious adverse effect and is more likely to develop if other phenothiazine compounds are administered concomitantly.	Piperazine citrate, U.S.P. (Antepar), and piperazine adipate (Entacyl) are popular among the many available preparations. In enterobiasis the usual dose is 65 mg/kg. Two short courses of therapy lasting 7 days, with a week's rest in between, are probably sufficient. Simultaneous treatment of the whole family is probably not necessary. In ascariasis, 3 to 5 mg daily for 1 to 3 days for adults usually results in complete cure. The usual dose for children is 50 to 75 mg/kg daily for 1 to 3 days.

(*continued*)

TABLE 68-2. *(Continued)*

Drug	Properties	Adverse Effects	Preparations, Dosage, and Use
Praziquantel	An investigational acetylated isoquinoline-pyrazine effective in various cestode infections in humans, and in animals against all three types of schistosomiasis.	Not fully known.	Praziquantel (Droncit), 15 to 25 mg/kg.
Pyrvinium 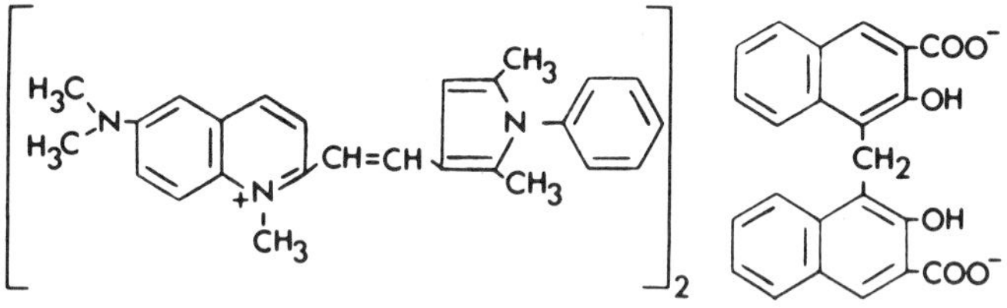 PYRVINIUM PAMOATE	A poorly absorbed red cyanine dye that selectively depresses essential anaerobic metabolic reactions in *Trichuris trichiura*, *Strongyloides stercoralis*, *Ascaris lumbricoides*, and *Enterobius vermicularis*. The pamoate is more effective and less irritating than the chloride. One dose cures 80% to 95% of cases of enterobiasis for a 2- to 3-week period.	Gastrointestinal irritation and photodermatitis may occur. Feces are colored red. Underclothes may also become heavily stained.	Pyrvinium Pamoate, U.S.P. (Povan), is available as a 50-mg tablet and as a suspension of 10 mg/ml. For enterobiasis the drug is given orally in doses of 5 mg/kg (maximum 300 mg) every 2 weeks. Attempts to prevent reinfection with pinworms by simultaneous treatment of the whole family is often undertaken but is rarely successful. It is also occasionally used in stronglyoidiasis.
Pyrantel	A new drug for the treatment of enterobiasis and ascariasis probably acts by producing neuromuscular blockade (cholinesterase inhibition) in the worms, permitting their expulsion. It is also effective in the treatment of hookworm, although not approved for this disease. It is poorly absorbed following oral administration, only about 10% of any given dose being excreted in the urine as free drug or metabolites.	Gastrointestinal upsets; fever, headache, lassitude, elevation of liver function tests, and various skin rashes may develop.	Pyrantel pamoate (Antiminth) is given in a single dose of 11 mg/kg, with a maximum dose of 1.0 g. Many physicians consider it to be the drug of choice for enterobiasis and ascariasis.

Sulfonamides	*See* Chapter 64.	*See* Chapter 64.	The sulfonamides (*see* Chap. 64) are occasionally combined with emetine in the treatment of paragonimiasis.
Suramin	*See* Chapter 58.	*See* Chapter 58.	Suramin (*see* Chap. 58) can be combined with diethylcarbamazine in the treatment of onchocerciasis. The recommended dose is 1.0 g/week for 5 to 10 weeks after a 200-mg test dose.
Tetrachloroethylene 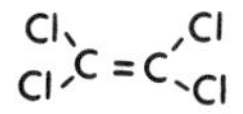 TETRACHLOROETHYLENE	An unsaturated chlorinated hydrocarbon chemically related to carbon tetrachloride and chloroform but of no value as an anesthetic because of its low vaporization and high boiling point. Essentially of historical interest only except for fluke infections in humans, and in veterinary practice. Intestinal absorption is minimal in the absence of fat or alcohol.	Gastrointestinal irritation (burning pain, nausea, vomiting, and diarrhea) is common. Rarely excessive absorption occurs, producing chloroform-like central nervous system effects (giddiness, drowsiness, vertigo, progressive coma).	Tetrachloroethylene, U.S.P., is available in gelatin capsules, which are heat and light labile. The usual dose is 0.12 ml/kg (maximum 5 ml) orally. The capsules should be emulsified and given orally or by duodenal tube since, if swallowed whole, they may dissolve caudal to the worm; subsequent catharsis is probably not necessary. The patient should be on an alcohol- and fat-free diet at least 36 hours before and after therapy.
Thiabendazole 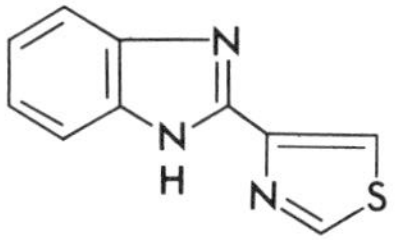 THIABENDAZOLE	A potent anthelmintic *in vitro*, possessing marked activity against *Strongyloides stercoralis* and *Trichinella spiralis;* in animal muscle *in vivo*, it kills *Trichinella spiralis* larvae. Thiabendazole is rapidly absorbed following oral administration, with peak serum levels developing within 1 hour.	Adverse effects are frequent and often severe. Gastrointestinal upsets (nausea, anorexia, vomiting, crampy abdominal pain, diarrhea), lassitude, headache, dizziness, tinnitus, paresthesias and hallucinations, olfactory disturbances, and sleepi-	Thiabendazole, U.S.P. (Mintezol), is available as a suspension of 100 mg/ml. The usual dose is 25 mg/kg/day with 3.0 g maximum daily dose. It is of value in the treatment of multiple parasitic infections, particularly strongyloidiasis, ancylostomiasis, trinchinosis, and trichuri-

(*continued*)

TABLE 68-2. *(Continued)*

Drug	Properties	Adverse Effects	Preparations, Dosage, and Use
Thiabendazole (*continued*)	About 90% of the drug is excreted in the urine in the free form or as glucuronide and sulfate conjugates. Produces only a temporary effect on the worm, and the egg count reverts to normal upon stopping therapy. *Trichiuris trichiura* eggs become deformed and irregular in shape during treatment. Mebendazole is preferred because it usually produces a complete cure.	ness may develop. A variety of hypersensitivity phenomena may appear owing to allergy to the drug or to a parasitic protein. Skin lesions (urticaria, maculopapular rashes); leukopenia, fever, and lymphadenopathy may develop. Rarely hypotension, altered liver function tests, Stevens–Johnson syndrome, hyperglycemia, and xanthopsia may appear.	asis. Also used in visceral and cutaneous larva migrans.

ALBERT MASON STEVENS, 1884–1945. New York pediatrician. In 1922 described, with Frank Chambliss Johnson (1894–1934), the Stevens–Johnson syndrome, a severe form of erythema multiforme, probably drug-induced.

FURTHER READING

1. Botero D: Chemotherapy of human intestinal parasitic diseases. Am Rev Pharmacol Toxicol 18:1–15, 1978
2. Katz M: Anthelmintics. Drugs 13:124–136, 1977
3. Keystone JS, Murdoch JK: Mebendazole. Ann Intern Med 91:582–586, 1979
4. Mansour TE: Chemotherapy of parasitic worms: New biochemical strategies. Science 205:462–469, 1979
5. The Medical Letter 21:105–112, 1979

CHAPTER 68 QUESTIONS

(See P. 7 for Full Instructions)

Select the One Best Answer

1. The effectiveness of piperazine citrate against *Ascaris lumbricoides* infestation is due to its
   A. cuticular blistering effect.
   B. neuromuscular blocking effect.
   C. blockade of glycolysis.
   D. cathartic effect.
   E. inhibition of respiration.

2. The drug recommended for treating a mixed infestation of *Ascaris* and *Trichuris* is
   A. piperazine.
   B. bephenium.
   C. thiabendazole.
   D. hexylresorcinol.
   E. tetrachloroethylene.

3. Niridazole is
   A. very effective against an infestation with *Schistosoma haematobium.*
   B. administered only intravenously.
   C. curative for schistosomiasis in a single dose.
   D. the drug of choice for tapeworms.
   E. rapidly eliminated by the parasite.

4. A broad-spectrum anthelmintic having larvicidal activity is
   A. pyrvinium.
   B. emetine.
   C. thiabendazole.
   D. piperazine.
   E. diethylcarbamazine.

A = 1,2,3; B = 1,3; C = 2,4; D = 4; E = All

5. Piperazine is an effective drug for treating
   1. ascariasis.
   2. trichuriasis.
   3. enterobiasis.
   4. strongyloidiasis.

6. *Enterobius vermicularis* (pinworm) infections are effectively treated with
   1. pyrvinium pamoate.
   2. piperazine citrate.
   3. mebendazole.
   4. diethylcarbamazine.

7. Actions of piperazine on *A. lumbricoides* include that it causes
   1. flaccid paralysis.
   2. malformation of eggs.
   3. inhibition of muscle response to acetylcholine.
   4. injury to male reproductive tract.

8. Drugs of some therapeutic benefit in schistosomal infections include
   1. niridazole.
   2. antimony compounds.
   3. hycanthone.
   4. carbon tetrachloride.

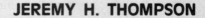

JEREMY H. THOMPSON

69 Drugs Used to Treat Mycotic Disease

Various fungi can infect humans. Broadly, they can be classified into those that produce *superficial infections* of the keratinized tissues (stratum corneum, hair, nails); *systemic infections* that involve the lungs, bones, viscera, and meninges; and *local infections*.

Superficial infections are produced by fungi that penetrate keratinized tissue and grow within it. In hair and nails, where keratin is more compact, infection tends to occur at the zone where new keratin is being formed in the hair follicle and in the nail bed, respectively; some involvement may occur only at the distal portion of the nail. Superficial disease is caused by various fungi; ringworm (*e.g.*, tinea capitis, tinea corporis, tinea cruris, tinea unguium) is caused by various strains of *Microsporum, Trichophyton,* and *Epidermophyton;* tinea versicolor, by *Malassezia furfur;* candidiasis, by *Candida albicans;* and tinea nigra, by *Cladosporium wernickii.*

Systemic infections are produced by various fungi (*see* Table 69-3). *Local infections,* usually caused by *Candida albicans,* typically develop in the mouth, bowel, or vagina.

Fungal infections are commonly precipitated by an easily recognizable cause, *and their control or elimination is often of more importance than antifungal therapy itself* (Fig. 69-1). Predisposing factors for superficial dermatitic infections include skin maseration, poor hygiene, diabetes mellitus, corticosteroid therapy, chafing, and occlusive shoes. Predisposing factors for systemic fungal disease include malignancy, uremia, tuberculosis, sarcoidosis, diabetes mellitus, hypoparathyroidism, therapy with broad-spectrum antibiotics, glucocorticosteroids or antineoplastic drugs, malnutrition, burns, debilitation, or radiation exposure.

Candida spp. are part of the normal body flora. Local infection, however, may be precipitated by many of the factors listed above for systemic fungal infections and by several local factors; with oral infection (reduced salivary flow, poor fitting dentures, the use of inhaled corticosteroids, and latent iron or vitamin deficiency); with gastrointestinal infection (broad-spectrum antibiotic therapy); with vaginal infection (therapy with oral contraceptives or

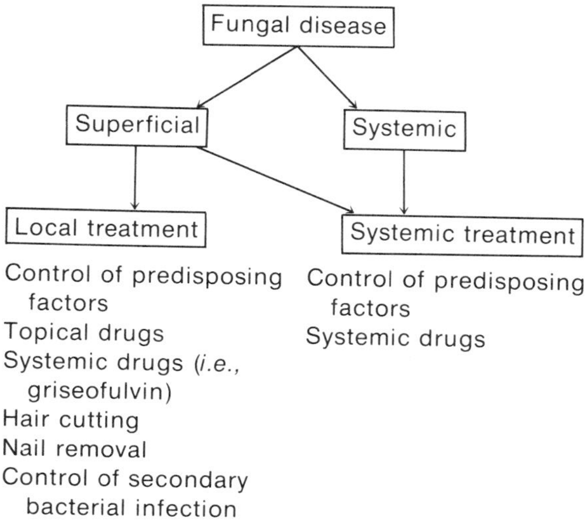

FIG. 69-1. Summary of the treatment of superficial and systemic fungal disease.

broad-spectrum antibiotics); and with skin infection (intertrigo).

CHEMOTHERAPY OF SUPERFICIAL MYCOSES

INTRODUCTION AND GENERAL PRINCIPLES

Many preparations are available for treating superficial fungal disease. Use of *topical agents* (Table 69-1) is usually sufficient for infections of glabrous skin. Deeper infections, particularly of the toe webs, hair, and nails, require systemic treatment often accompanied by topical agents. Griseofulvin is the only systemic agent currently available. Cure of superficial mycoses, particularly those of the toe webs, nails and hair, is difficult because the drug may not be able to reach the site of infection deep within hyperkeratotic epidermis, nail, or hair follicle and because of continuing reinfection. Additionally, *in vitro* susceptibility testing is relatively valueless since such results and *in vivo* response correlate poorly. Despite this, some classify antimycotic agents into *fungistatic* and *fungicidal* categories (*see* Chap. 56).

Keratolytic agents, for example, salicylic acid, are often used concomitantly with topical drugs to increase their penetration and to hasten the shedding of heavily infected stratum corneum. Similarly, drugs that reduce hyperhidrosis may be valuable adjunctive agents. Bacterial suprainfection is common and demands prompt treatment. It can often be controlled by soaks or compresses of Burow's or warm potassium permanganate solutions (1 : 10,000), or by adequate débridement of heavily infected stratum corneum. Some authorities have recommended a short course of antibiotic therapy, but antibiotics may initiate further suprainfection and may cross-react with fungal products, producing "id" reactions. Preliminary corticosteroid therapy has been suggested for progressive eczematous lesions and to control dermatophytids and allergic phenomena. Systemic corticosteroids (plus antifungal therapy) may be of special value in human cases of animal ringworm, since by their antiinflammatory activity steroids minimize the degree of final scarring.

SYSTEMIC DRUGS FOR TINEA INFECTIONS

GRISEOFULVIN

Griseofulvin, obtained from *Penicillium griseofulvum dierckx* and *P. janczewski*, is the only available systemic agent for treating superficial mycoses due to most strains of *Microsporum*, *Trichophyton*, and *Epidermophyton*. It is ineffective against *Candida* spp. and fungi that cause systemic disease. Griseofulvin is fungicidal for growing cells and fungistatic for resting cells.

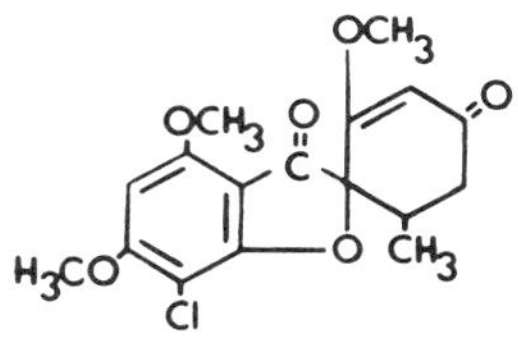

GRISEOFULVIN

Mode of Action

Griseofulvin may act by depressing nucleic acid synthesis and by interfering with microtubular function. *In vivo* it selectively accumulates within the stratum corneum, binding to keratin precursor cells and making them resistant to fungal infection. Greater accumulation occurs during summer than winter months. Thus new skin, hair, and nails are the first to become free of fungal elements, and

(*Text continues on p. 708*)

KARL AUGUST VON BUROW, 1809–1874. Königsberg surgeon. In 1857 described his solution of mild aluminum acetate for treating scalp wounds.

TABLE 69-1. Topical Drugs for Tinea Infections

Drug	Properties	Adverse Effects	Preparations
Heavy metals	Penetrate fungal cytoplasm and oxidize enzyme sulfhydryl groups (*see* Chap. 66)		Ionic copper, thiomerosal, bismuth
Iodine	Used on tinea corporis. Not used on toes or in groin because severe blistering may develop	Iodine should never be mixed with a mercuric salt because the highly irritating red iodide of mercury is formed	Alcoholic iodine 2%
Detergents (surface active agents)	Polar compounds that possess hydrophobic and hydrophilic groups that disturb osmotic functions of cell membrane (see Chap. 57)		Benzalkonium chloride and cetyltrimethylammonium bromide (*see* Chap. 66)
Selenium	Used to control dandruff and nonspecific dermatoses. Selenium sulfide lotion 2.5% for tinea versicolor	Poisonous if ingested	Selenium sulfide, U.S.P.
Castellani's paint	Mixture of 0.3% basic fuchsin, 1.0% boric acid, 10% resorcinol, and 4.5% phenol. Of some use in tinea pedis, cruris, and axilaris and in nonspecific dermatoses	Stains clothes deeply	Carbol-fuchsin Solution, N.F.
Fatty acids	Fungistatic activity increases with an increase in the number of carbon atoms up to 11. Straight chains are more active than branched chains. The antifungal activity of sebum is due to propionic and caprylic acids. Used in tinea pedis and corporis (undecylenic and caprylic acids) or in bakery products (propionates)	Possesses unpleasant, rancid, sweatlike oder. Rarely produces sensitization	Undecylenic acid, N.F.; zinc undecylenate, N.F.; caprylic acid; caprylic compounds (10% sodium caprylate plus 5% zinc caprylate). Sodium and calcium propionates

Whitfield's ointment	Fungistatic (benzoic acid 6%) and keratolytic (salicylic acid 3%) agent used in tinea versicolor and ringworm		
Salicylanilide 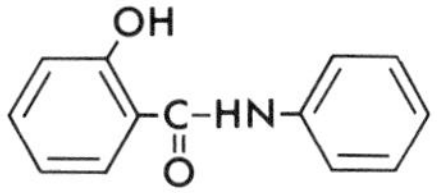	Salicylic acid derivative of aniline. Weak fungistatic agent often combined with undecylenic acid	Photosensitivity reactions	Salicylanilide, N.F., 5% ointment. Present in many soaps.
Glyceryl triacetate	Releases acetic acid locally under influence of host and mycotic esterases. Weakly active against ringworm fungi but not *C. albicans*		Triacetin ointment 25%. Triacetin powder 33%
Tolnaftate 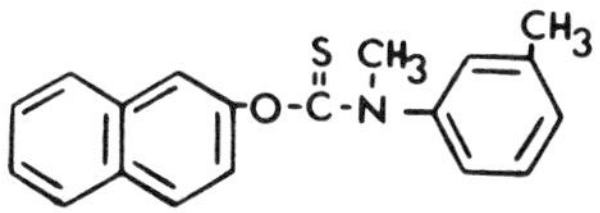	Effective against most dermatophytoses, and erythrasma. No effect on tinea of the hair or nails or on *C. albicans*. Should be combined with keratolytics to treat tinea of palms and soles		Tolnaftate, U.S.P., 1% solution
Haloprogin	A synthetic iodinated trichlorophenol compound. Effective in dermatophyte, candida, and tinea versicolor infections of the skin		Haloprogin, 1% cream or solution
Acrisorcin	Used in tinea versicolor. Antifungal activity reduced by soaps. Should be applied twice daily for at least 1 month after the infection has cleared	Sensitivity reactions	Acrisocin 2% cream
Thymol	Used in many dermatophytoses. Often added to Whitfield's ointment		Thymol, U.S.P., 1% alcoholic solution or 2% powder
Miconazole nitrate	Used in tinea infections (*see* imidazoles in text)		Miconazole nitrate 2% cream
Zinc pyrithione	Effective for Tinea versicolor and *Pityrosporum ovale*	Irritation	1% solution

ALDO CASTELLANI, 1875–1971. Italian-born physician. In 1903 demonstrated the cause and transmission of sleeping sickness, discovered the yaws spirochete in 1905, and investigated parasitic skin diseases. In 1912 described bronchospirochetosis, Castellani's bronchitis.

therapy must be continued until the infected keratin has been replaced by keratin containing griseofulvin, which usually takes 3 to 10 weeks for skin and hair infections and up to 18 months for nail disease. Infection of the soles of the feet is rarely cured by griseofulvin alone. The clinical effectiveness of griseofulvin depends on the occurrence of normal epithelial cell turnover and intact host defense mechanisms. Mycotic resistance is rare.

Absorption, Metabolism, and Excretion

The *rate,* but not the *degree,* of griseofulvin absorption depends on the particle size of the formulation. Small-sized particles (<3.0 μm in diameter; microcrystalline form) are absorbed two to three times as rapidly as large particles (<10 μm). A recently introduced ultramicrocrystalline formulation is absorbed most rapidly of all. Fatty meals increase absorption since the agent is lipophilic. After standard doses, blood levels of 1 to 2 μg/ml are reached within 2 to 4 hours. The drug has a V_d of 1.5 liters/kg and a T½ of between 10 and 30 hours. Griseofulvin is metabolized in the liver to the inactive product 6-demethylgriseofulvin and excreted in the urine. Loss also occurs in the feces. Barbiturates and primidone may accelerate the hepatic microsomal catabolism of griseofulvin through enzyme induction, and phenobarbital reduces the gastrointestinal absorption of griseofulvin.

Adverse Effects

Gastrointestinal upsets, headache, low-grade fever, and malaise may develop in up to 5% of patients. Headaches tend to be severe during early therapy but usually diminish in frequency and severity with continued exposure. Thirst (xerostomia), frequency of micturition, chest pain, dyspnea, skin lesions (lupus erythematosus-like eruptions, urticaria, lichen planus, erythema multiforme, and photodermatitis), and serum sickness are not uncommon. Griseofulvin has a structural similarity to colchicine, but, although it depresses spermatogenesis in mice, it has not been shown to do so in humans. Cross-sensitivity has not been described in patients sensitive to penicillin. Forgetfulness, apathy, amblyopia, vertigo, and disorientation develop rarely but are potentiated by concomitant alcohol ingestion. Leukopenia and granulocytopenia are rare, but periodic blood counts during long-term therapy are advisable. Griseofulvin may also produce polyarteritis, peripheral neuritis, gynecomastia, and hyperpigmentation of the nipples, areolae, and external genitalia from "estrogen-like" effects. Suprainfection with *Candida albicans* is seen occasionally.

Griseofulvin is a potent enzyme-inducing agent (*see* Chap. 11) and may precipitate symptoms of porphyria in patients with this disease or with advanced liver disease because it induces hepatic δ-aminolevulinic acid (ALA) synthetase. Griseofulvin may also reduce the gastrointestinal absorption of warfarin and reduce the cutaneous response to the tuberculin test.

Preparations and Dosage

Griseofulvin, U.S.P., is the official form; there are many proprietary preparations. Because of irregular gastrointestinal absorption, the total daily dose should be divided into three or four portions and administered after meals. Duration of therapy depends on the location of the fungus. The usual daily doses for adults and children are 0.5 to 1.0 g and 10 mg/kg, respectively.

Uses

Griseofulvin is highly effective in treating fungal infections of the skin, hair, and nails caused by *Microsporum, Tricophyton,* and *Epidermophyton* species. Pruritus and burning are usually relieved within 1 to 3 days, which coincides with the time griseofulvin appears within the basal layers of the stratum corneum.

Treatment should be continued for about 3 to 4 weeks if the nails, palms, and soles are not involved. Infection of the highly keratotic palms and soles, and of the nails, requires therapy for 4 to 12 weeks and 4 to 12 months, respectively. Griseofulvin should not be used if the tinea will respond to topical agents (Table 69-1) because a potentially toxic drug cannot be justified when less dangerous chemicals will suffice. A definite mycologic diagnosis should always be required before the start of therapy, since treatment is often prolonged and costly.

Experimentally, griseofulvin has been reported to be of some symptomatic benefit in Raynaud's disease and *herpes zoster* infection.

Basic Principles of Treatment of Tinea

Griseofulvin is the drug of choice for uncomplicated tinea capitis, for favus, and for kerions.

A. G. Maurice Raynaud, 1834–1881. French physician. Described the disease named for him, a bilateral ischemia of the toes or fingers caused by a vascular disorder, in his doctoral thesis in 1862. Also wrote on the history of medicine.

Some authorities recommend an initial trial of topical drug therapy in tinea barbae, corporis, cruris, and manuum, with the addition of griseofulvin if local therapy fails, but for severe tinea both topical and systemic drugs can be used concomitantly. Other adjunctive procedures are hair clipping or shaving plus warm compresses and débridement in tinea barbae and application of mild keratolytic agents in tinea corporis. Tinea pedis is a chronic therapeutic problem, the infection persisting because of the thick stratum corneum and constant reinfection. Apart from griseofulvin and tolnaftate, haloprogin, clotrimazole, miconazole, and Whitfield's ointment are most valuable; undecylenic acid and zinc undecylenate are not as effective. Foot hygiene, avoidance of reinfection from communal shower rooms, and avoidance of wool and synthetic fiber socks is of greater importance. Dusting powders can also be valuable. Tinea unguium is difficult to cure. Griseofulvin is the drug of choice, combined in selected cases with nail avulsion. Tinea versicolor tends to recur, but Whitfield's ointment, haloprogin, acrisorcin, 2.5% selenium sulfide lotion, and 10% sodium thiosulfate are of some value. Tinea nigra may respond to Whitfield's ointment.

TOPICAL DRUGS FOR SUPERFICIAL CANDIDIASIS

Candida albicans may cause superficial, local, or systemic infection. Several drugs are available for topical therapy, some of which may also be given systemically. Nystatin is the most important; other agents are indicated in Table 69-2.

NYSTATIN

Origin and Mode of Action

Nystatin, so named because it was located in the New York State Department of Health (1951), is a polyene antibiotic obtained from *Streptomyces noursei*. Polyenes are complex molecules with a large conjugated lipophilic double-bond system (—CH=CH—) in a lactone ring linked to an amino sugar. Nystatin is a conjugated tetraene linked to the amino sugar mycosamine. Nystatin exhibits both fungistatic and fungicidal activity, depending on the drug concentration, the presence of blood, pus, or tissue fluid that reduces activity, and the susceptibility of the fungus. It is measured in milligrams or units (1 mg = >2000 units). Fungi generally sensitive *in vitro* include *Candida albicans*, fungi causing ringworm, *Histoplasma capsulatum*, and *Cryptococcus neoformans*.

Nystatin may act by altering fungal cell membrane permeability, probably by complexing with membrane ergosterol (*see* Chap. 57). Its lack of antibacterial activity may be related to the relative absence of sterols in bacterial cell membranes. Fungal resistance develops rarely. Cross-resistance occurs with amphotericin B (*see* below).

Nystatin is usually given orally for a local effect in the mouth, esophagus, or bowel lumen or applied topically in various formulations onto the skin or into the vagina. Parenteral administration is undertaken very rarely because the drug is highly toxic by this route.

Adverse Effects

Even in large doses, nystatin is relatively innocuous when applied topically, but cutaneous irritation may develop after repeated exposure. Contact sensitivity is very rare. Minor symptoms of nausea and diarrhea may follow oral administration. Suprainfection is never a problem. Intramuscular nystatin is painful and produces hemolytic anemia, probably through complexing with red blood cell membrane sterols.

Preparation and Dosage

Nystatin, U.S.P. (Mycostatin), is present in various topical formulations often combined with gentian violet, procaine hydrochloride, antibiotics, or hydrocortisone. The oral dose is 0.5 to 1 million units every 8 hours. Topical powders, ointments, creams, and suppositories are applied every 8 hours. In esophageal infection, the drug should be given hourly, at least for the first several days.

Uses

The main use of nystatin is in treating candidiasis of the skin, mouth, intestine, conjunctival sac, and vagina. In treating vaginal infections, the use of specific formulations should be accompanied by the use of vulval creams and oral therapy to minimize reinfection from the bowel. In sexually active women, male partners should also be treated with topical genital creams. Several preparations of broad-spectrum antibiotics (tetracyclines, neomycin) are

---

ARTHUR WHITFIELD, 1868–1947. English dermatologist. His ointment, described in 1907, was composed of benzoic and salicylic acids in lanolin.

TABLE 69-2. Drugs Used to Treat Candidiasis

Drug	Properties	Adverse Effects	Preparations
Nystatin	*See* text		Ointment or cream 3% to 5%
Chloroquinaldol	Has mild gram-positive antibacterial, anticandidal, and keratoplastic activity		
Hexetidine (Sterisil)	Used to treat vulvovaginal candidiasis and trichomoniasis (*see* Chap. 67). Detergents reduce its antifungal activity	Vulval or vaginal irritation	Hexetidine gel 0.1% for vaginal use only. The usual dose is 7 ml of the gel inserted high in the vaginal vault daily for 1 week
Gentian Violet, U.S.P.	Effective in some cases of aural, oral, vaginal, or cutaneous candidiasis	Stains deeply. Rarely sensitizing	Available as a 2% solution, and for vaginal infections as a 1% solution in glycerine
Chlordantoin	A derivative of an agricultural fungicide. Used in cutaneous, paronychial, and vaginal candidiasis	Cutaneous irritation	Combined with benzalkonium chloride (Sporostacin)
Candicidin (Candeptin)	A heptaene fungistatic and fungicidal antibiotic obtained from *Streptomyces griseus* with an antifungal spectrum similar to that of amphotericin B and nystatin. It is 15 to 30 times more active, however, then either of those agents against *C. albicans in vitro.* Probably acts by complexing with cell membrane sterols (*see* Chap. 57). Not absorbed after topical, vaginal, or oral administration	Cutaneous sensitivity rare. Vulvovaginitis following local therapy. Cross-sensitivity not reported	Available as an ointment (0.06%) and as tablets (0.30 mg)
Miconazole nitrate (Monistat)	Used in vulvovaginal candidiasis; *see* text (imidazoles)	Vulvovaginal irritation	Cream 2%
Amphotericin B	*See* text		
Clotrimazole	*See* text (imidazoles)		
Natamycin	*See* text		
Iodochlorhydroxyquin	Weak, anticandidal activity. *See* Chap. 67		

available in combination with nystatin (*see* Chap. 60) to reduce the *candida* suprainfections that occasionally develop. The effectiveness of these combinations is doubtful. Nystatin can be given parenterally for the very rare systemic case of candida infection resistant to other drugs.

NATAMYCIN

Natamycin is a tetraene antifungal antibiotic obtained from *Streptomyces natalensis*, which acts like nystatin. Natamycin possesses a wide antifungal spectrum against common dermatophytes. It is also active against *Trichomonas vaginalis* but possesses no antibacterial activity. Natamycin can be used orally, topically on the skin and in the eye, and vaginally; it is not absorbed after oral administration but is occasionally given by this route to treat intestinal candidiasis. Adverse reactions have not been described after topical or vaginal applications, but minor symptoms of gastrointestinal irritation may follow oral administration.

Natamycin is available in various preparations in a strength of 2% (pimafucin, pimaricin). It is effective in treating chronic candidal paronychia and vulvovaginitis. It may also be used to treat tinea versicolor.

Natamycin (Natacyn) ophthalmic suspension 5% is an approved drug for treating keratitis, conjunctivitis, and blepharitis due to various fungi, including *Fusarium, Cephalosporium, Candida,* and *Aspergillus* spp. The dose is one drop of the suspension every 1 to 2 hours for 3 days, and then one drop every 3 to 4 hours for up to 4 weeks. Mild irritation and chemosis may develop.

CHEMOTHERAPY OF SYSTEMIC MYCOSES

Systemic mycotic diseases are becoming more common. They can be divided into two types: infection with opportunistic pathogens (*Aspergillus, Mucor,* and *Candida* spp. and *Cryptococcus neoformans;* and infections with primary pathogens (*e.g., Coccidioidis immitis, Histoplasma capsulatum,* and *Sporothrix schenckii*).

Chemotherapy of systemic fungus disease is unsatisfactory: Only a limited number of drugs is available (Table 69-3), and their use is associated with severe toxicity. The control of predisposing factors (Fig. 69-1) and continuance of drug therapy long enough to reduce the likelihood of relapse are of prime importance.

POTASSIUM IODIDE

Potassium iodide, U.S.P., resolves chronic granulomas, a property that is obsolete in treating syphilis but still of value in some systemic fungal diseases. It is available as a saturated solution of 1 g/ml. The starting dose is 1 g every 8 hours, which is gradually increased to 3 to 4 g every 8 hours in severe cases. Therapy should be continued for 4 to 6 weeks after all lesions appear to have healed; this may take several months. Potassium iodide is particularly valuable in cutaneous and lymphatic sporotrichosis but should be used cautiously in pulmonary or disseminated disease. If iodism (a metallic taste in the mouth, parotitis, gastrointestinal upsets, acneiform skin rash, and coryza) develops, therapy should be discontinued for several days and resumed at a lower dosage.

BENJAMIN ROBINSON SCHENCK, 1872–1920. American gynecologist. Described Schenck's disease, a form of sporotrichosis, in 1898 and discovered the causative agent, *Sporotrichum schenckii.*

AMPHOTERICIN B

Of the two amphotericins, A and B, isolated in 1958 from *Streptomyces nodosus,* only the conjugated heptaene amphotericin B is used in therapeutics. It is a *heat-labile* and *light-sensitive* fungistatic antibiotic with a wide spectrum of activity (Table 69-3). The antifungal effects are maximal between *p*H 6.0 and 7.5. Resistance *in vivo* is rare. Cross-resistance occurs with nystatin but is uncommon. Rifampin, which has no direct antifungal effects, reduces the concentration of amphotericin B needed to produce fungistasis *in vitro* in various *Candida, Histoplasma,* and *Aspergillus* spp.

Mode of Action

Amphotericin B exhibits two types of binding to sensitive fungi *in vitro:* nonreversible, energy-dependent binding occurs at high drug concentrations and leads promptly to cell death; and reversible and non-energy-dependent binding is seen at low drug concentrations. Here amphotericin B binds to sterols, predominantly ergosterol, in the cell membrane, producing physical changes that in turn, lead to a gradual loss of essential intracellular nutrients, cell lysis, and death. It is not clear which of these actions, if either, is responsible for its *in vivo* antifungal effect. Miconazole (*see* below) may antagonize the actions of amphotericin B *in vivo* by depressing ergosterol synthesis. *In vivo* amphotericin B augments delayed hypersensitivity reactions and increases cell-mediated immunity, but the clinical significance of these effects is not clear.

Absorption, Metabolism, and Excretion

When used topically, orally, or locally, amphotericin B has no significant absorption. Thus, when systemic disease is being treated, amphotericin B must be given by i.v. infusion or intrathecally, when the central nervous system is involved. After i.v. injection, the drug passes poorly into the cerebrospinal fluid, levels typically reaching one-thirtieth or one-fiftieth simultaneous plasma levels, and it does not cross the placental barrier. Amphotericin B is bound 90% to plasma proteins, especially lipoproteins, and has a T½ of 24 to 48 hours. It is partially metabolized in the liver and ex-

TABLE 69-3. Cause and Treatment of Systemic Mycoses

Disease	Fungus	Drugs of Choice[1]	Alternative Agents[2]
Actinomycosis	*Actinomyces israelii* (not a true fungus)	Penicillin G[3]	A cephalosporin,[4] chloramphenicol, a tetracycline[5]
Aspergillosis	*Aspergillus fumigatus, A. niger*	Amphotericin B ± rifampin	None
Blastomycosis (North American)	*Blastomyces dermatitidis*	Amphotericin B ± rifampin	Hydroxystilbamidine[6]
Blastomycosis (South American)	*Blastomyces brasiliensis*	Amphotericin B	Miconazole
Candidiasis (moniliasis)	*Candida albicans*	Amphotericin B ± flucytosine[7]	Amphotericin B + rifampin
Chromoblastomycosis	*Fonsecaea, Phialophora, Cladosporium*	Flucytosine	Amphotericin B + potassium iodide
Coccidioidomycosis	*Coccidioides immitis*	Amphotericin B	hydroxystilbamidine, miconazole[8]
Cryptococcosis (torulosis)	*Cryptococcus neoformans*	Amphotericin B + flucytosine[7]	Amphotericin B + rifampin
Geotrichosis	*Geotrichum candidum* and other *Geotrichum* spp.	Amphotericin B	Potassium iodide
Histoplasmosis	*Histoplasma capsulatum*	Amphotericin B	Amphotericin B + rifampin, hydroxystilbamidine, a sulfonamide
Maduromycosis	*Madurella mycetomi, Madurella grisea, Petriellidium boydii*	Amphotericin B	A sulfonamide, a tetracycline[5]
Phycomycosis	*Mucor* spp.	Amphotericin B	Hydroxystilbamidine
Nocardiosis	*Nocardia asteroides* (not a true fungus)	A sulfonamide + amoxicillin or erythromycin	Co-trimoxazole, a sulfonamide + minocycline, a tetracycline[5] ± cycloserine, rarely capreomycin
Penicilliosis	*Penicillium* spp.	Amphotericin B	None
Rhinosporidiosis	*Rhinosporidium seeberi*	Amphotericin B	None
Sporotricosis	*Sporothrix schenckii*	Amphotericin B, potassium iodine[9]	None

James Israel, 1848–1926. German surgeon. In 1878 proved for the first time the presence of actinomycosis in humans. Most of his work after this period was in urology.

[1] All drugs listed alphabetically.
[2] All drugs listed alphabetically.
[3] Oral therapy must not be relied on for serious disease. Usual doses are 10 to 20 mega units/day intravenously. In patients allergic to penicillin, erythromycin, minocycline, a cephalosporin, clindamycin, or streptomycin may be used.
[4] Cephalosporins (other than moxalactam) do not pass into the cerebrospinal fluid in therapeutic amounts.
[5] Tetracycline hydrochloride is usually the best agent.
[6] For cutaneous disease only.
[7] Some strains may be resistant, or resistance may appear during therapy.
[8] Preferred over hydroxystilbamidine.
[9] For lymphocutaneous disease only.

creted in the bile and feces. About 3% of the drug is excreted in the urine unchanged. It is not removed by hemodialysis.

Adverse Effects

With systemic therapy, adverse reactions develop in almost all patients. Generally, crystalline preparations are less toxic than solubilized preparations. Adverse effects commonly seen during or shortly after infusions have stopped include fever, general malaise, chills, myalgia, arthralgia, nausea, diarrhea, headaches, vertigo, hypotension, flushing, and sweating. Thrombophlebitis is usual and may be reduced by adequate drug dilution, a slow infusion rate, and heparin use. Ventricular fibrillation and cardiac arrest rarely may follow too rapid infusion. Hypersensitivity and maculopapular skin rashes, anaphylactic shock, leukopenia, thrombocytopenia, hemolytic and hypochromic anemias, peripheral neuritis, amblyopia, convulsions, and acute hepatic failure are rare.

More than 80% of patients develop some impairment of renal function, as indicated by proteinuria, hematuria, hypokalemia, hypomagnesemia, and elevated blood urea nitrogen or creatinine levels, owing to a direct toxic effect of the antibiotic on the renal tubules and to renal vasoconstriction. Renal lesions are usually reversible but may progress to tubular acidosis and nephrocalcinosis. Intrathecal amphotericin B may be followed by lumbar pain, amblyopia, diplopia, chemical meningitis, paresthesias, nerve palsies, urinary retention, and severe headaches. Death has occurred. Concomitant therapy with cortisone, antipyretics, H_1-antagonists, and antiemetics may counteract some of these adverse reactions. Amphotericin B potentiates bone marrow toxicity of flucytocine (*see* below).

Preparations and Dosage

Amphotericin B is available as a microcrystalline suspension and an aqueous colloid suspension. The microcrystalline preparation is available either as a 3% amphotericin preparation for topical application in candidiasis (*see* above) or as an oral preparation combined with neomycin or a tetracycline. The colloidal preparation amphotericin B, *U.S.P.* (Fungizone), contains about 0.8% sodium desoxycholate per milligram (to allow dispersion of the highly insoluble antifungal agent) plus a phosphate buffer and sodium chloride. It is the only preparation available for i.v. or intrathecal therapy.

Colloidal amphotericin B should be freshly prepared in sterile water or 5% dextrose, where it is stable for several hours in the cold. Normal saline or solutions with electrolytes or an acid *p*H or that contain other drugs or preservatives should not be used because amphotericin B may precipitate. A trial dose of 1 to 5 mg should always be given, but there is no consensus as to the subsequent dose or dosing schedule.

The objective is to establish an effective dose as rapidly as possible while minimizing renal toxicity. Several disparate techniques have been recommended, including alternate-day therapy, rapid i.v. infusions ("pulse" therapy), and slow step-wise increments in dosage. Generally, the dose and dosing schedule depend on several factors, particularly the type of fungus, the locus and severity of the infection, and the degree of toxicity, especially renal dysfunction that develops. Various maneuvers have effectively minimized renal damage—keeping the patient hydrated, prolonging the infusion time, giving the drug on alternate days, alkalinizing the urine, and concomitantly using manitol. In practice, drug dosage is usually modulated by monitoring the creatinine clearance.

For intrathecal use, 0.5 mg of amphotericin B should be diluted in distilled water or cerebrospinal fluid (0.1–0.25 mg/ml) and slowly injected with hydrocortisone two or three times weekly for several months. It may be advisable to alternate between lumbar and cisternal injection sites. Intralesional amphotericin B is the treatment of choice for local chromomycoses.

Uses

Amphotericin B is an important drug because it is the only currently available agent for treating progressive systemic mycoses. Parenteral amphotericin B should be reserved for severe infections, but duration of treatment varies with disease severity and with the occurrence of adverse effects that may necessitate interruption of therapy. The minimal duration of treatment is 4 to 6 weeks, but severe fungal disease may require 5 to 6 months of therapy. Patients must be hospitalized and their renal function and serum electrolytes carefully monitored.

Amphotericin B is often given with flucytosine. Potassium, magnesium, and calcium supplements will minimize muscle and neurologic toxicity. Amphotericin B antagonizes the action of miconazole (*see* below).

Amphotericin B is used topically and locally to treat superficial infections with *Candida* and other fungi, in some cases of visceral leishmaniasis, and infection with the ameba *Naegleria*.

5-FLUOROCYTOSINE (FLUCYTOSINE)

Flucytosine is a synthetic drug unlike other fluorinated compounds such as 5-fluorouracil and the riboside and deoxyriboside of fluorocytosine in that it lacks significant cytotoxic properties in humans. It is fungistatic or fungicidal

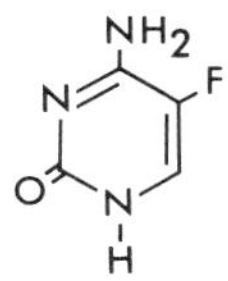

FLUCYTOSINE

depending on its concentration, duration of exposure, and sensitivity of the fungus.

Mode of Action

Flucytosine is readily taken up into sensitive fungal cells and converted into intermediaries that block thymidylate synthetase and disrupt protein synthesis (Fig. 69-2). Synergism may be observed when flucytosine is combined with amphotericin B since amphotericin B, by disrupting the fungal cell membrane (*see* Chap. 57), allows greater uptake of the more potent agent.

Resistance

Cytosine deaminase activity (Fig. 69-2) is low or absent in mammalian cells, thus explaining why the drug has minimal toxicity in humans. Some resistant fungi lack cytosine deaminase, cytosine permease, or uridine monophosphate pyrophosphorylase. Fungal resistance develops rapidly and can be minimized by the concomitant use of amphotericin B.

Antifungal Spectrum

Flucytosine is effective against various fungi, particularly yeasts (*Candida albicans*, *Cryptococcus neoformans*, and *Sporothrix schenckii*) and some species of *Aspergillus* and *Chromomyces*. It is inactive against *Blastomyces dermatitidis*, *Coccidiodioides immitis*, and *Histoplasma capsulatum*. *In vitro* culture media that contain beef and yeast extracts and peptones that contain pyrimidines such as cytosine effectively compete with flucytosine and thus will alter sensitivity results.

Absorption, Metabolism, and Excretion

Flucytosine is well absorbed after oral administration, with peak levels developing within 4 to 6 hours. Doses should be adjusted to keep blood levels between 50 and 75 μg/ml (*see* hematologic toxicity below). Flucytosine has a V_d of about 0.6 liters/kg and is protein bound about 5%; thus it is widely distributed even in the cerebrospinal fluid. Flucytosine has a T½ of 4 to 6 hours and is minimally metabolized, 80% to 90% being excreted unchanged by glomerular filtration, yielding urinary concentrations of 200 to 400 μg/ml. Doses of flucytosine must be drastically reduced in renal impairment since in anuria the drug has a T½ of 3 to 4 days. Flucytosine is removed by hemodialysis and peritoneal dialysis.

FIG. 69-2. Proposed mechanisms of action of flucytosine.

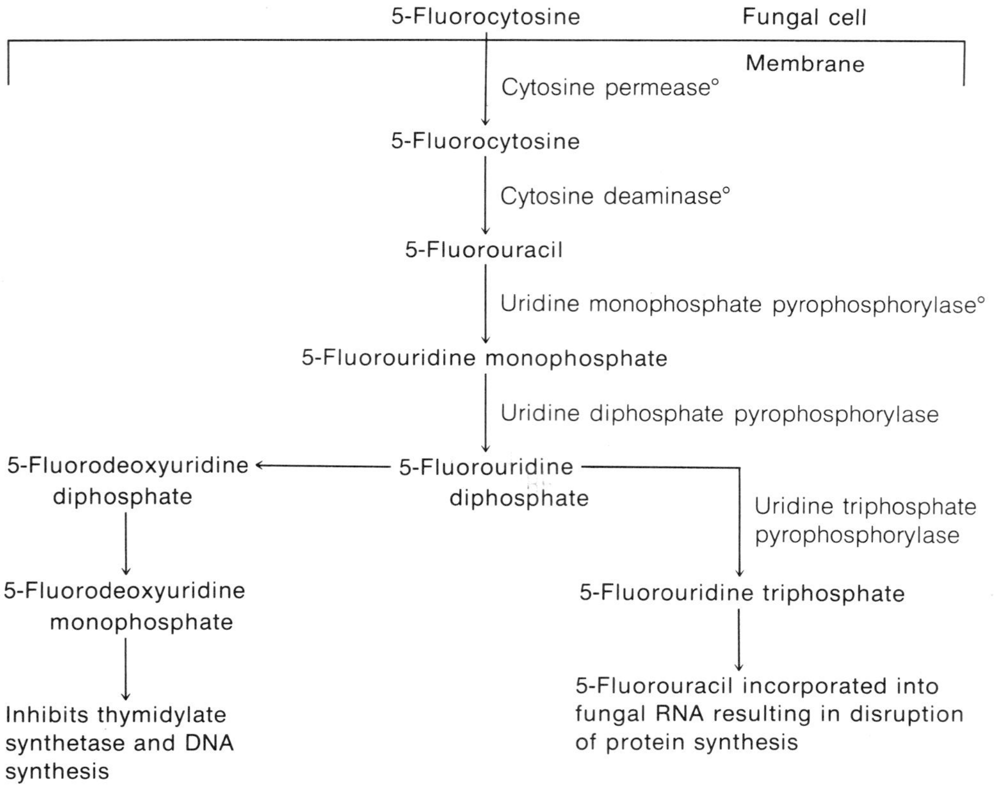

° Enzymes that may be deficient in flucytosine-resistant fungi.

Adverse Effects

Flucytosine commonly produces nausea, anorexia, crampy abdominal pains, and vomiting; occasionally it produces generalized malabsorption and rarely intestinal perforation. Reversible liver dysfunction with elevation of serum glutamic oxalacetic transaminase and alkaline phosphatase activity occurs in 10% of patients. Flucytosine has been associated with progressive leukopenia, thrombocytopenia, confusional states, hallucinations, severe headaches, and vertigo. Hematologic damage is more likely in those patients who concomitantly receive cytotoxic drugs or irradiation, in those who have some hematologic disease, or in those in whom blood levels of flucytosine exceed 100 μg/ml. Blood counts should be performed twice weekly during therapy.

In rodents, which metabolize flucytosine to 5-fluorouracil, the drug is teratogenic; the human organism does not metabolize flucytosine to 5-fluorouracil.

Preparations, Dosage, and Uses

Flucytosine (Ancobon) is available in capsules of 250 and 500 mg. An average dose is 25 to 35 mg/kg every 6 hours. Flucytosine has been particularly valuble in treating *Candida albicans* endocarditis, cryptococcal meningitis, pulmonary disease, and various infections caused by *Aspergillus*. Flucytosine probably should not be given alone because resistance develops rapidly. By combining flucytosine and amphotericin B, lower doses of amphotericin B can be used (producing fewer side-effects), an additive or possibly a synergistic antifungal effect is obtained, and mycotic resistance to flucytosine is less likely to develop.

The main advantages of flucytosine are its rapid absorption after oral administration, its wide tissue distribution, and its relative lack of serious adverse effects. Clinical effectiveness is limited by the development of resistance and by the high incidence (10%) of resistance in initial isolates of *Candida albicans*.

IMIDAZOLES

Three imidazoles are of therapeutic importance: *clotrimazole*, *miconazole*, and *ketoconazole*.

Clotrimazole

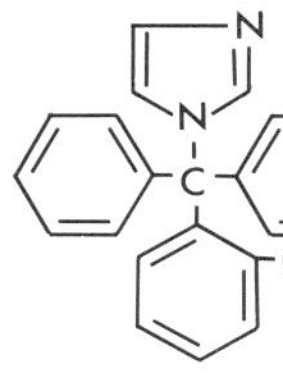

CLOTRIMAZOLE

Clotrimazole is fungistatic, inhibiting *in vitro Histoplasma capsulatum*, *Cryptococcus neoformans*, *Coccidioidis immitis*, *Aspergillus fumigatus*, *Blastomyces dermatitidis*, *Candida albicans*, *Microsporum* spp., *Epidermophyton floccosum*, and *Trichophyton*. *In vivo*, however, severe toxicity (hallucinations, disorientation) and rapid hepatic metabolism limit its usefulness to topical and local application.

Topical clotrimazole penetrates deeply into the dermis and is nonsensitizing but may produce some burning pain or local irritation for the first few days; it is of some value (1% cream or solution, Lotrimin; Mycelex) in treating various dermatophytes and in vaginal candidiasis (Gyne-Lotrimin; Mycelex G), where a 7-day course is usually satisfactory.

Miconazole

Miconazole has a broad spectrum. It is used topically in cutaneous candidiasis, infections by *Tricophyton mentagrophytes* and *Epidermophyton floccosum*, systemic coccidioidomycosis, candidiasis, histoplasmosis, cryptococosis, South American blastomycosis, and

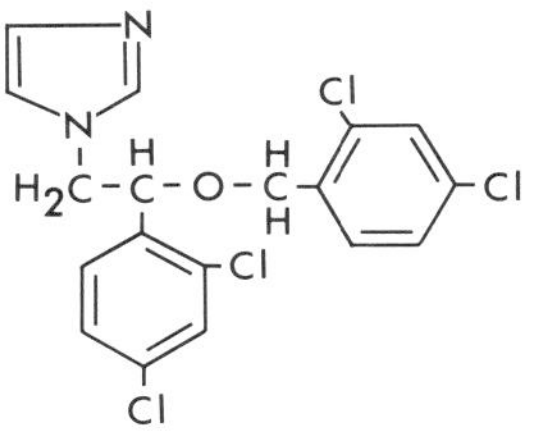

MICONAZOLE

nocardiosis. Intrathecal administration may be needed for meningeal infection.

Miconazole damages fungal cell membranes (possibly by inhibiting ergosterol biosynthesis), resulting in a loss of essential cell nutrients. Additionally it interferes with mitochondrial enzymes, leading to an accumulation of toxic peroxide compounds.

Miconazole is only partially absorbed (25–35%) after oral administration; thus i.v. therapy is mandatory for severe systemic disease. The drug passes to most tissue compartments but poorly into saliva, sputum, and cerebrospinal fluid. Miconazole is rapidly metabolized by microsomal enzymes, the major metabolite being α-(2,4-dichlorophenyl)-1H-imidazole ethanol. Miconazole is about 90% protein bound and thus is not significantly cleared by hemodialysis.

Because of the potential risk of anaphylaxis, all patients should receive an initial test dose of not more than 200 mg.

Toxicity from topical application is low. Burning pain and irritation may appear, but the drug is probably nonsensitizing. After i.v. administration, severe thrombophlebitis develops in 30% to 40% of patients, necessitating the subsequent use of deep veins for continued therapy. Rotation of the i.v. sites, use of large veins, concomitant use of heparin or hydrocortisone in the infusate, dilution of miconazole in large volumes of normal saline or 5% dextrose, and an infusion time of 30 to 60 minutes will minimize the severity of phlebitis. Postinfusion nausea (20% of patients) can be minimized by slowing the rate of infusion, by infusing miconazole between meals, or by using antiemetics prophylactically. Pruritus (25% of patients) is occasionally severe and persistent despite both systemic and local therapy. Erythematous, maculopapular, and urticarial skin rashes (10% of patients) may disappear during therapy or require termination of drug exposure. Anemia, thrombocytosis, and erythrocyte aggregation develop in 10% to 30% of patients, and on direct examination plasma has a bluish appearance. Hyponatremia may appear because of inappropriate ADH secretion. Rarely observed adverse effects are drug fever, gastrointestinal upsets, flushing, mental changes (euphoria, anxiety, increased libido, acute psychoses), headaches, hyperesthesia, increased bruisability and bleeding gums, eosinophilia, jaundice, elevation of serum SGOT and SGPT, cardiorespiratory depression, arrhythmias, and anaphylactic shock.

An excipient, the vehicle *cremophor-EL*[R] (a polyoxyethylated castor oil mixture), may cause most of the adverse effects of miconazole, including hyperlipidemia (hypercholesterolemia and hypertriglyceridemia).

Miconazole is available as a cream or lotion for topical use in ringworm and candidiasis (Mica Tin) and for local treatment of vaginal candidiasis (Monistat). For systemic fungal infections, the usual i.v. dose is 0.2 to 0.4 g every 8 hours diluted in at least 200 ml of dextrose or normal saline, and infused over 30 to 60 minutes.

Miconazole antagonizes the activity of amphotericin B possibly by inhibiting fungal synthesis of ergosterol, thus decreasing the binding sites for the polyene.

Ketoconazole

Ketoconazole (Nizoral) is a promising water-soluble imidazole for treating systemic fungal infections and chronic mucocutaneous candidiasis. It is well absorbed after oral administration, its bioavailability being increased by food. After a dose of 200 mg orally, peak plasma levels of about 3.5 μg/ml develop within 60 to 120 minutes. Ketoconazole has a T½ of about 8

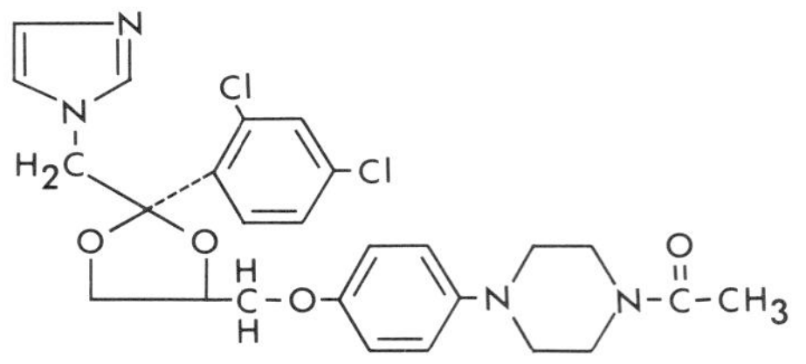

KETOCONAZOLE

hours, penetrates poorly into the cerebrospinal fluid, and is extensively degraded in the liver, with metabolites being excreted in bile and feces. Only about 3% of a single dose is cleared unchanged by the kidney.

Side-effects appear to be minimal. Nausea, vomiting, and dyspepsia are reduced if the drug is taken with food. Rarely reported have been abdominal pain, pruritus, photophobia, headaches, dizziness, drug fever, insomnia, transient hypocholesterolemia, and skin rashes. It may very rarely produce hepatocellular necrosis.

Ketoconazole has a similar antifungal spectrum to miconazole and *in vitro* possesses three to five times more activity against *Coccidioides immitis* than does that agent. It is supplied in 200-mg tablets, the usual dose being 200 to 400 mg/day.

EXPERIMENTAL AGENTS

Hamycin

Hamycin, an experimental polyene antibiotic related to amphotericin B, is obtained from *Streptomyces pimprima*. It is well absorbed after oral administration and possesses activity against various fungi, particularly *Blastomyces dermatitidis*, *Histoplasma capsulatum*, *Aspergillus fumigatus*, *Cryptococcus neoformans*, and *Candida albicans*. Adverse reactions reported to date have been limited to the gastrointestinal tract.

Hamycin (Primamycin) is available experimentally for oral and topical use. Relapses are common, particularly in the treatment of deep fungal infections. Hamycin may be applied topically in treating vaginal candidiasis.

X-5079C

X-5079C (RO-2-7758: Saramycetin) is a sulfur (13%)-containing fungistatic polypeptide antibiotic derived from a strain of streptomyces. It has been found effective in treating some deep mycoses, particularly *Blastomyces dermatitidis*, *Histoplasma capsulatum*, and *Sporothrix schenckii*. It has no activity against *Cryptococcus neoformans*. The potential of this agent has not yet been fully explored because of its relative unavailability. Side-effects reported with X-5079C have included skin rashes, particularly urticaria, and liver damage. It is usually given in doses of 3 to 5 mg/kg for 4 to 6 weeks.

FURTHER READING

1. Atkinson AJ, Bennett JE: Amphotericin B pharmacokinetics in humans. Antimicrob Agents Chemother 13:271–276, 1978
2. Hamilton–Miller JMT: Chemistry and biology of the polyene macrolide antibiotics. Bacteriol Rev 37:166–196, 1973
3. Medoff G, Kobayashi GS: Strategies in the treatment of systemic fungal infections. N Engl J Med 302:145–155, 1980

CHAPTER 69 QUESTIONS

(See P. 7 for Full Instructions)

Select the One Best Answer

1. The drug effective for systemic mycotic infections is
   A. griseofulvin.
   B. polymyxin B.
   C. tolnaftate.
   D. sulfacetamide.
   E. amphotericin B.
2. The drug administered orally for systemic therapy for dermatomycotic infections is
   A. amphotericin.
   B. griseofulvin.
   C. demeclocycline.
   D. nystatin.
   E. tolnaftate.
3. For an uncomplicated infection with *Histoplasma capsulatum*, therapy should begin with
   A. penicillin.
   B. griseofulvin.
   C. amphotericin B.
   D. ampicillin or amoxicillin.
   E. a sulfonamide.
4. Each of the following statements about griseofulvin is true EXCEPT that it
   A. is absorbed best after a fat meal.
   B. is useful against systemic histoplasmosis.
   C. is effective orally against ringworm infection of the scalp.
   D. is deposited in keratin precursor cells.
   E. can produce photosensitivity to ultraviolet light.

A = 1,2,3; B = 1,3; C = 2,4; D = 4; E = All

5. Which of the following antifungal agents can be useful in treating nonsystemic candidiasis?
   1. Miconazole
   2. Haloprogin
   3. Nystatin
   4. Tolnaftate
6. Agents effective in treating cryptococcal meningitis include
   1. amphotericin B.
   2. griseofulvin.
   3. flucytosine.
   4. nystatin.
7. Drugs used topically only for fungal infections include
   1. amphotericin B.
   2. tolnaftate.
   3. griseofulvin.
   4. undecylenic acid.
8. Gastrointestinal candidiasis occurring in a patient under prolonged therapy with tetracycline may be effectively treated orally with
   1. neomycin.
   2. nystatin.
   3. griseofulvin.
   4. amphotericin B.

A. Griseofulvin
B. Penicillin G
C. Both
D. Neither

9. Is (are) the treatment of choice for *actinomycosis israeli* infections.
10. May cause severe headaches.

11. CNS side-effects are potentiated by alcohol.

12. May precipitate porphyria.

A. Nystatin
B. Amphotericin B
C. Both
D. Neither

13. Block(s) reduplication of fungal cell wall.

14. Is (are) highly toxic when given systemically.

15. Is (are) the drug of choice for deep tinea infections of keratinized tissues.

16. Is (are) a polyene antibiotic.

A. Amphotericin B
B. Sulfonamides
C. Both
D. Neither

17. Cross-resistance with nystatin is unlikely.

18. Is (are) light sensitive.

19. Activity is potentiated by miconazole.

20. Renal toxicity is reduced by alkalinizing the urine.

A. Flucytosine
B. Miconazole
C. Both
D. Neither

21. Is (are) synergistic with amphotericin B.

22. Require(s) metabolism to an active intermediary.

23. Block(s) fungal thymidylate synthetase.

24. Fungal resistance develops rapidly.

JEREMY H. THOMPSON

70

Drugs Used to Treat Viral Diseases

The true viruses, of which more than 200 have been associated with various infectious diseases in humans, contain a core (single- or double-stranded) of either DNA (smallpox, chickenpox, herpes simplex, herpes zoster) or RNA (poliomyelitis, mumps, measles, rabies), but not both, and can replicate only inside host cells predominantly through the use of host enzyme systems (*see* below).

Several obstacles have hampered the development of effective antiviral therapy.

1. Since viral replication is intracellular, antiviral drugs must be highly selective and not seriously interfere with normal cellular functions of the host.
2. Antiviral drugs must be able to readily enter host cells intact.
3. Most viral diseases are of short duration and, because rapid effective techniques of diagnosis are not available, treatment begun at the height of symptoms is already late in the course of disease.
4. As the prodromal phase of many virus infections is relatively asymptomatic and corresponds with the period of maximum virus growth, spread of disease is difficult to control.
5. There is a relative lack of knowledge on specific virus enzyme systems that may serve as targets for drugs.
6. There is great difficulty in demonstrating efficacy of treatment in viral diseases that are commonly self-limiting.
7. There is often poor correlation between *in vitro* antiviral activity and *in vivo* response.
8. There is limited knowledge on the pathogenesis of many virus infections and virus:host cell relationships and on the natural history of many virus infections.
9. Development of predictive *in vitro* or *in vivo* laboratory tests of antiviral drug efficacy has been slow.

For these reasons, most of the major advances in the treatment of viral diseases have been in the area of *prevention,* for example, vector control. Some success has been achieved by *active immunization* (*see* Chap. 76) and by *passive immunization*. Passive immunization involves the use of antibodies. Antibodies can be prepared in animals (high titer hyperimmune gamma globulin or in humans, but the former are rarely used to treat human viral diseases since they may induce allergic reactions. Human gamma globulin is prepared from pooled blood of healthy donors or from convalescent patients. Antibodies are most effective when used prophylactically in persons who have been exposed to such viral diseases as measles, rubella (particularly pregnant women), rabies, infectious hepatitis, mumps, and occasionally varicella.

Neither active nor passive immunization is of value once disease has appeared, and, with few exceptions, the treatment of viral disease consists of alleviating symptoms rather than attacking the causative organism. Little is known about the effects of antiviral drugs on virus persistence, latency, or oncogenicity.

BIOLOGY OF VIRUSES

A knowledge of the biology and reproduction of the true viruses facilitates understanding of antiviral drug action.

VIRAL STRUCTURE

Viruses contain a core (genome) of nucleic acid (either RNA or DNA, but not both) surrounded by a coating of protein subunits or capsomers (capsoids), the viral antigens. The capsomeres protect the nucleic acid and may be responsible for viruses attaching (adsorption) onto host cells.

VIRAL SPECIFICITY

Like the more complicated bacteria, viruses have a wide range of host and tissue specificity. Thus mumps virus is pathogenic for humans only, and polio virus has a marked affinity for anterior horn cells. This implies that capsomeres are not merely a protective envelope but have configurations that lead to discriminatory cell attachment, and possibly enzymes important in the process of penetration (*see* below).

VIRAL REPRODUCTION

Since viruses contain few intracytoplasmic enzymes capable of reproducing viral nucleoprotein, the virus must invade a host cell and direct its synthesizing mechanisms to produce viral rather than host components. The cycle of viral reproduction (Fig. 70-1) is readily divided into the phases described below.

Free Viral Particle

At present no major drugs are active against the free virus particle, but it can be destroyed *in vitro* by heat, ultraviolet light, x-irradiation, and β propiolactone.

Viremia

After the free virus particles have entered the host, a viremia occurs, and the particles localize in their preferred tissue. While the particles are in this extracellular environment, they may be inactivated by endogenous or exogenous (gamma globulin) antibodies, for example, poliomyelitis antibody attacks viral intercapsomeric junctions. No drugs other than antibody are known to act at this stage.

Attachment

Typically, before a virus can penetrate a cell, it must become attached onto the cell's surface, presumably at specialized receptor areas. Immunoglobulins and heparin are effective in removing some viruses that have attached to host cell membranes, but the clinical significance of this effect is not clear.

Penetration and Uncoating

Viral penetration may depend on a process analogous to phagocytosis (pinocytosis), and a single virus may use different mechanisms of penetration in the same cell type. Viruses may penetrate *in toto* or leave behind some of their outer coat proteins. After penetration, the virus particle "uncoats" with separation of the genome and capsomere, releasing viral nucleic acid. Uncoating may be a complex two-step process, as seen with vaccinia virus, or a simpler one-step event, as shown with polio virus.

Transcription and Replication

Specific mRNA is synthesized, coding for enzymes and proteins necessary for the formation of viral components. The length of these phases may be as short as 10 minutes for some bacteriophages or as long as 9 hours for herpesviruses.

Generally DNA viruses first code for mRNA (transcription), which then attaches to host cell ribosomes, initiating protein synthesis (translation). The nucleic acid of RNA viruses may serve indirectly as mRNA, or the RNA can be transcribed to a complementary messenger.

Because of their complexity, the transcription and replication phases offer the most likely

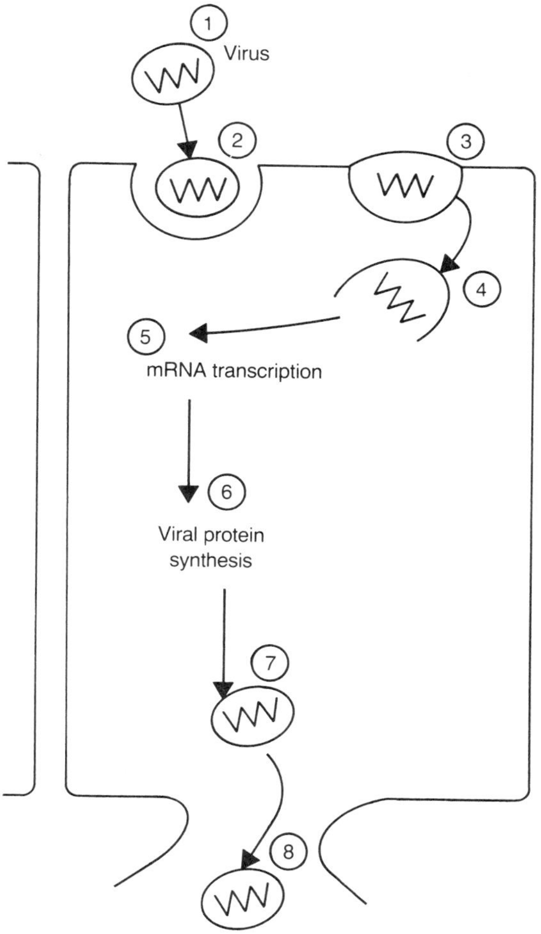

Step	Antiviral drugs
1. Free virus	Immune serum
	Immune serum
2. Attachment	Heparin
3. Penetration	Amantadine Rimantadine
4. Uncoating of viral nucleic acid	Amantadine Rimantadine
5. Viral mRNA transcription	Interferon
6. Viral protein synthesis	Acyclovir Ara-A (vidarabine) Ara-C (cytarabine) IDUR (idoxuridine) Trifluridine Interferon
7. Virus assembly	Methisazone
8. Release	Interferon

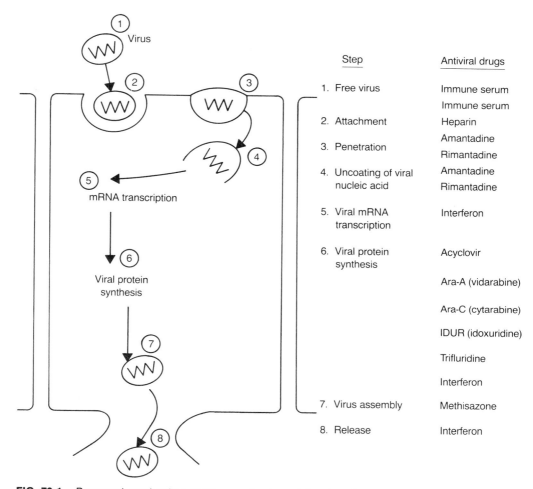

FIG. 70-1. Proposed mechanism of virus synthesis and the site of action of antiviral drugs.

target sites for the development of antiviral drugs that possess selective toxicity. Replication of DNA viruses may be catalyzed by specific viral DNA polymerases that are different from host cell DNA polymerases. Adenine arabinoside, for example, is a more effective inhibitor of this enzyme from viral than from human cells.

Assembly and Maturation

An aggregation of newly synthesized viral components, and their assembly into a precisely defined structure, the viral nucleocapsoid occur in the nucleus (*e.g.*, adenoviruses), in the cytoplasm (*e.g.*, poxviruses), or at the cell surface (*e.g.*, influenza virus).

Release

Virus infections may propagate with or without host cell death. If release of progeny virions occurs, the host cell usually dies. On release the virions may spread both locally or hematogenously. Some virions spread through cell-to-cell contact, and with some animal viruses the formation of a syncytium of host cells may facilitate virus spread without full virus maturation—that is, subvirus units may propagate an infection.

VIRAL INTERFERENCE

The ability of one virus to interfere with the development of a second virus in the same tissue or host is called *viral interference*. It was first observed by Jenner, who showed that vac-

---

EDWARD JENNER, 1749–1823. English physician. Performed the first vaccination for smallpox (using a cowpox vaccine) in May 1796. In 1771 Jenner had prepared and cataloged the specimens from Cook's first Pacific voyage.

cinia reacted weakly on skin involved in a herpetic eruption. *Interferons* were discovered in 1957 by Isaacs and Lindeman, who demonstrated that cells exposed to infectious or inactivated influenza virus produced and secreted a soluble substance that could inhibit virus multiplication. Interferon production *in vivo* may play an important role in the recovery from some viral infections and in the regulation of various immune functions (*see* below).

ANTIVIRAL DRUGS

1-ADAMANTANAMINE HYDROCHLORIDE (AMANTADINE HYDROCHLORIDE)

Amantadine, marketed in 1966, is a symmetrical, heterocyclic, water-soluble, primary amine with a novel "cagelike" structure. In tissue culture, amantadine inhibits the growth of several unrelated viruses (*e.g.*, influenza A and C, parainfluenza, pseudorabies, rubella, arenaviruses, and oncornaviruses). *In vivo,* however, amantadine is effective only against in-

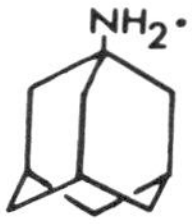

AMANTADINE HYDROCHLORIDE

fluenza A, particularly A_2 (Asian H2N2) and its antigenic variants such as swine virus (HSW1N1) and Russian virus (H1N1). It has no activity against influenza B. *Rimantadine*

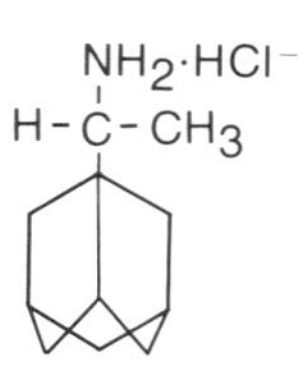

RIMANTADINE HYDROCHLORIDE

is an experimental congener similar to amantadine.

Mode of Action

Amantadine prevents penetration of viral particles into host cells. In addition, it may prevent virus uncoating and virus release under certain circumstances. Amantadine has no curative properties and acts only as a partial prophylactic in some persons. It is effective only when given within 24 to 48 hours of infection; the earlier it is given, the better. It has no effect on the production or action of antibody. Among sensitive viruses *in vitro,* complete prophylaxis is rare even at the maximum nontoxic concentration of about 50 mg/ml. Its action in Parkinson's disease is discussed below.

Absorption, Metabolism, and Excretion

Amantadine is completely absorbed from the gastrointestinal tract. Following a dose of 100 mg, peak blood levels are reached after 2 to 4 hours. Amantadine has a large volume of distribution, readily passing to most tissues and fluids, including the cerebrospinal fluid, saliva, and nasal secretions. Thus far no patterns of drug metabolism have been identified, and 90% of any dose appears in the urine unchanged. Renal tubular secretion accounts for 80% of the renal clearance, and, since the drug is a base, its excretion is *p*H dependent (*see* Chap. 3). Amantadine is also cleared into the milk. The biologic half-life of amantadine is about 20 hours. Because of its dependence on renal excretion, amantadine accumulates in the presence of diminished renal function. The drug is cleared slowly by hemodialysis, since little is available immediately because of its large volume of distribution.

Adverse Effects

Adverse reactions to amantadine are usually dose-related, mild, appear within 48 hours of the start of therapy, and reversible. With standard doses, reactions are seen in 4% to 8% of patients, namely, skin rashes, urinary frequency, xerostomia, and gastrointestinal upsets. Serious adverse effects are seen in the central nervous and cardiovascular systems, especially with doses greater than 400 mg/day; slurred speech, somnolence, confusion, headaches, inability to concentrate, jitteriness, aggressiveness, ataxia, a drunken feeling, insomnia, epileptiform seizures, blurred vision, vertigo, nervousness, tremor, oculogyric crises, and some psychic reactions (depression, feeling of detachment, lilliputian hallucinations, and paranoia) may occur. However, such symptoms may develop in patients on conventional dosage schedules, particularly when alcohol or other centrally acting agents are used concomitantly. With chronic therapy, peripheral edema and livedo reticularis may be seen; only rarely will congestive cardiac failure, orthostatic hypotension, cardiac arrhythmias, and leukopenia occur.

Generally, toxic doses of amantadine are

ALICK ISAACS, 1921–1967. London virologist. With Jean Lindenmann, a Swiss microbiologist, published the discovery of interferon in 1957.

very near therapeutic doses, and geriatric patients or those with a history of psychic upsets or seizures should not be given the drug. Amantadine should be used cautiously in patients with diminished renal function. Rimantadine may be less toxic than amantadine.

Preparations, Dosage, and Uses

Amantadine hydrochloride (Symmetrel) is of some use (50–70%) in the prophylaxis and treatment of influenza infection in humans. However, influenza is usually a self-limiting mild disease, and amantadine does produce side-effects. Amantadine is indicated for prophylaxis in a proven epidemic of influenza type A, where it should be given to unvaccinated children and adults at high risk (with cardiac, pulmonary, and immunodeficiency states), all adults whose activities are vital to the community (policemen, firemen, soldiers, doctors, nurses), and susceptible persons confined in a semiclosed institutionalized environment. It must be given no later than 48 hours after the onset of symptoms. The chemoprophylaxis of influenza has one theoretical advantage over active immunization: For vaccination to be successful, it must be administered 4 to 8 weeks before the expected time of infection, whereas chemoprophylaxis can be initiated immediately. Since amantadine is not 100% effective, however, it seems prudent in prophylaxis to use a vaccine that contains a current strain of influenza virus, rather than amantadine. Other important factors against amantadine use prophylactically are its cost, inconvenience, side-effects, and concern about increasing viral resistance. The usual adult dose of amantadine is 200 mg/day for 10 days or for as long as the local epidemic persists. In children 1 to 9 years old, the daily dose is 4 to 8 mg/kg/day, with a maximum of 150 mg/day. In the case of 9 to 12 year olds, the dose of amantadine is 100 mg every 12 hours.

Amantadine may offer some benefit in combating akinesia in Parkinson's disease, but it may exacerbate tremor. Amantadine may act by increasing the release of dopamine and by reducing its reuptake. Thus patients who respond to amantadine (indicating that they have functionally responsive dopamine receptors) will also respond to levodopa; amantadine is less potent than levodopa (*see* Chap. 30), and its effectiveness may wear off within a couple of months. Sensitivity is usually restored by a brief interruption of therapy. Rimantadine has no activity in Parkinson's disease.

Amantadine has also been used with limited success to treat subacute sclerosing panencephalitis and Creutzfeldt–Jakob disease. It has had some abuse as a psychedelic agent.

VIDARABINE

Vidarabine (9-β-D-arabinofuranosyladenine: adenine arabinoside: Ara-A: Vira-A), a purine nucleoside related to idoxuridine and Ara-C,

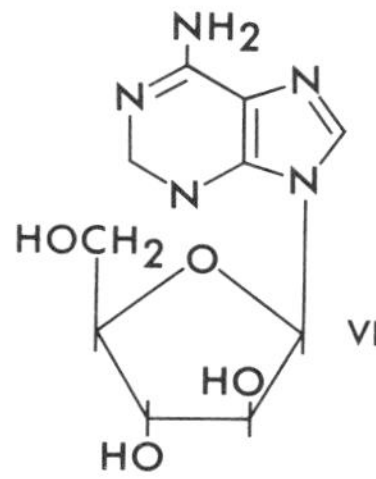

VIDARABINE

can be produced by fermentation of *Streptomyces antibioticus*. It was developed originally as an anticancer drug.

Antiviral Spectrum

Vidarabine has a wide spectrum of activity against DNA viruses in tissue culture (*H. simplex* 1 and 2, varicella/zoster, Epstein-Barr virus, B virus, cytomegalovirus, vaccinia, and pseudorabies), but RNA-containing viruses, with a few exceptions (*i.e.*, vesicular stomatitis virus), are not affected. Viral resistance has not been described.

Mode of Action

The precise mode of action of vidarabine is not known, and its measurement and study are complicated by the fact that a major metabolite, arabinosyl hypoxanthine (araHx), has a similar spectrum of activity but is less potent. Both vidarabine and araHx can be taken up into cells and phosphorylated into monophos-

---

ALFONS JAKOB, 1884–1931. German psychiatrist. Worked on the identification of physical causes for mental disease, on functional localization in the brain, histopathology, and neurophysiology. Known for his work on the scleroses and the degenerative viral encephalopathy, Jakob–Creutzfeldt's disease.

HANS-GERHARD CREUTZFELDT, 1885–1964. German psychiatrist and neurologist. Worked on encephalitis, neurologic changes in morphinism, and in 1920 described Jakob–Creutzfeldt's (or Creutzfeldt–Jakob's) disease, which usually affects middle aged or elderly persons.

MICHAEL ANTHONY EPSTEIN, 1921– English physician, pathologist. With Y. M. Barr, reported discovery of the Epstein–Barr virus in cultured Burkitt's lymphoma cells.

phate, diphosphate, and triphosphate forms. Each form may act differently. Vidarabine inhibits viral DNA synthesis possibly by suppressing DNA polymerase or viral-induced ribonucleotide reductase. Viral DNA is inhibited at concentrations of vidarabine that have virtually no effect on host cell DNA, RNA, or protein synthesis. Vidarabine may also act as a chain terminator, particularly in herpes simplex DNA strands.

Absorption, Metabolism, and Excretion

Vidarabine is not effective when given orally. The drug is poorly soluble and must be infused at a concentration not greater than 0.5 to 0.7 mg/ml. Vidarabine is widely distributed and accumulates in several cell types, such as the erythrocyte, and in tissue fluids, such as aqueous humor. Cerebrospinal fluid levels are 50% those achieved in blood. Vidarabine is rapidly deaminated by adenosine deaminase to arabinosyl hypoxanthine in serum and red blood cells; it is also phosphorylated and oxidized. Vidarabine has a biologic half-life of about 2 to 4 hours. About 50% of any dose is excreted by the kidney unchanged or as araHx.

Adverse Effects

Minimal toxicity has been observed with 12-hour infusions of vidarabine in doses of 5 to 15 mg/kg. Nausea, vomiting, diarrhea, weight loss, skin rashes, and thrombophlebitis may be seen (14% of patients). With higher doses, ataxia, dizziness, painful paresthesias, encephalopathy (tremors, hallucinations, confusion, psychoses, EEG changes), leukopenia, thrombocytopenia, and a megaloblastic bone marrow may develop. Dysmorphogenesis has been shown in rats and rabbits but not in humans or rhesus monkeys, which have the same metabolic pathways for vidarabine. Because of the drug's poor solubility, problems of fluid overload may occur.

Preparations and Uses

The full therapeutic potential of vidarabine has not yet been determined. Application of vidarabine ointment 3% every 3 hours until healing occurs, and then every 8 hours daily for 7 days, is of value in superficial herpes simplex keratitis (dendritic or geographic types); it is of little value in stromal disease unless given parenterally. Vidarabine may be more effective than idoxuridine, may be effective in idoxuridine failures, and may cause less inhibition of corneal healing than idoxuridine.

Vidarabine is often lifesaving in proven (brain biopsy positive) herpetic encephalitis, and the earlier the drug is given the better. Prognosis is poor if the patient is already comatose, since brain damage usually has already occurred. Doses of 15 to 20 mg/kg are given over a 12- to 24-hour period for 10 days. The volume of fluid necessary for this dose is about 1.5 liters (2.22 ml of fluid/mg), which may cause some problems in itself.

Neonatal herpes simplex infections of several types have also responded to vidarabine, but it should not be used to treat similar infections in the immunocompetent host with uncomplicated disease. Vidarabine is of no benefit prophylactically (5 mg/kg/day) in cytomegalovirus pneumonia or in recurrent or primary herpes genitalis infection but decreases the pain and accelerates the healing of cutaneous lesions of varicella zoster infection in immunocompromised patients. *Ara AMP*, an experimental derivative of vidarabine, is more soluble than the parent compound and also has greater bioavailability.

ACYCLOVIR

Acyclovir (9-(2-hydroxyethoxymethyl) guanine; acycloguanosine; ACV) is a recently introduced experimental agent with *in vitro* and

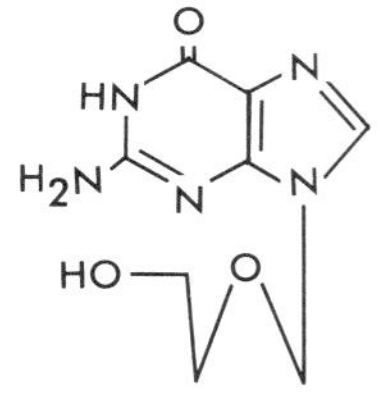

ACYCLOVIR

in vivo activity against herpesviruses. Acyclovir offers promise because it is minimally toxic and is not rapidly metabolized *in vivo*.

Antiviral Spectrum

Acyclovir inhibits the multiplication of herpes simplex types 1 and 2, cytomegalovirus, varicella/zoster virus, Epstein–Barr virus, and B virus. Sensitive viruses have a specific thymidine kinase (*see* below), and herpes simplex acyclovir-resistant mutants lack this enzyme. Host cells are 3000-fold less sensitive to acyclovir than susceptible herpes simplex cells.

Mode of Action

Sensitive viruses encode for a specific thymidine kinase that converts acyclovir to acycloguanosine monophosphate, which in turn is further phosphorylated by other kinases to acycloguanosine triphosphate (acyclo GTP). Acyclo GTP is an inhibitor of herpesvirus-encoded DNA polymerase, inhibiting this enzyme 10 to 30 times more effectively than it inhibits host DNA polymerase. Acyclo GTP may also serve as a false substrate for viral DNA polymerase, leading to chain termination.

Preparations and Use

Acyclovir is undergoing clinical trials in humans for treatment of herpes simplex cutaneous and systemic disease, where it offers early promise. A 3% ointment in a petrolatum base has been reported to give better results in herpetic keratitis than either idoxuridine or vidarabine.

N-METHYLISATIN β-THIOSEMICARBAZONE (METHISAZONE)

Methisazone has a wide *in vitro* antiviral spectrum, but activity *in vivo* is confined to treatment of infections caused by the pox viruses. Methisazone protects against smallpox and alastrim (variola minor) and may be useful in complications of primary vaccination. In one

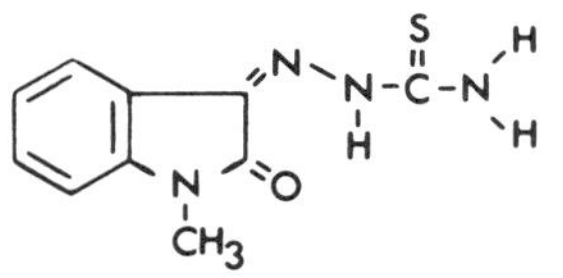

N-METHYLISATIN β-THIOSEMICARBAZONE

early series reported from Madras, India, 6 mild cases of smallpox with 2 deaths developed in 2297 patients treated with methisazone, in contrast to 114 cases of smallpox with 20 deaths in 2842 nontreated control subjects. With the eradication of smallpox and the limited use of vaccination (*see* Chap. 76), the need for this drug is small.

Mode of Action

Methisazone may prevent the synthesis of a protein required for normal virus assembly, morphogenesis, or maturation. It may act as a ligand for metallic ions.

Pharmacology and Adverse Effects

Methisazone is absorbed after oral administration, with peak plasma levels developing within 4 to 7 hours. Little is known about its metabolism; one metabolite, isatin-3-thiosemicarbazone, has about half the antiviral activity of methisazone. In limited clinical use, the only adverse effects have been nausea and vomiting, some impairment of mentation, dermatitis, and jaundice (methisazone prevents the conjugation of bilirubin with glucuronic acid).

Uses

Methisazone (Marboran) in doses of 1.5 to 3.0 g daily is effective in smallpox prophylaxis when given before the 8th or 9th day of the incubation period. It also effectively prevents the development of variola minor in contacts of the disease. Combined with antivaccinal gamma globulin, methisazone may be of value in patients with complications of vaccination (vaccinia gangrenosa and eczema vaccinatum) and in the modification of primary vaccination in a patient who *must* be vaccinated in the presence of some contraindication (eczema and myeloproliferative disease, among others). Since routine primary vaccination is no longer recommended (*see* Chap. 76), the need for methisazone will be small.

5-IODO-2′-DEOXYURIDINE

Of the four halogenated pyrimidine deoxyribosides—iododeoxyuridine, fluorodeoxyuridine, bromodeoxyuridine, and chlorodeoxyuridine—iododeoxyuridine is the most important and effective (Fig. 70-2).

5-Iodo-2′-deoxyuridine (2′-deoxy-5-iodouridine, IDU, IDUR, idoxuridine) inhibits the replication of DNA viruses *in vitro* (particularly herpes simplex and *Vaccinia*). Generally, RNA viruses, with one or two possible exceptions (*e.g.*, Rous sarcoma virus), are not affected.

Mode of Action and Viral Resistance

Idoxuridine inhibits various enzymes involved in DNA synthesis, including thymidylic synthetase, thymidine kinase, thymidylic phosphorylase, nucleoside diphosphate reductase, and DNA polymerase. Its most important action, however, is almost certainly that of competing with thymidine-5′-phosphate.

In vivo, idoxuridine is sequentially converted by kinases into monophosphate, diphos-

---

FRANCIS PEYTON ROUS, 1879–1970, New York physician and virologist. Best known for his discovery of the first known tumor-inducing virus, the Rous fowl sarcoma virus, in 1910. With others, Rous developed techniques for blood preservation that enabled him to set up the world's first blood banks, behind the lines in France and Belgium during World War I. Received the Nobel Prize in 1966.

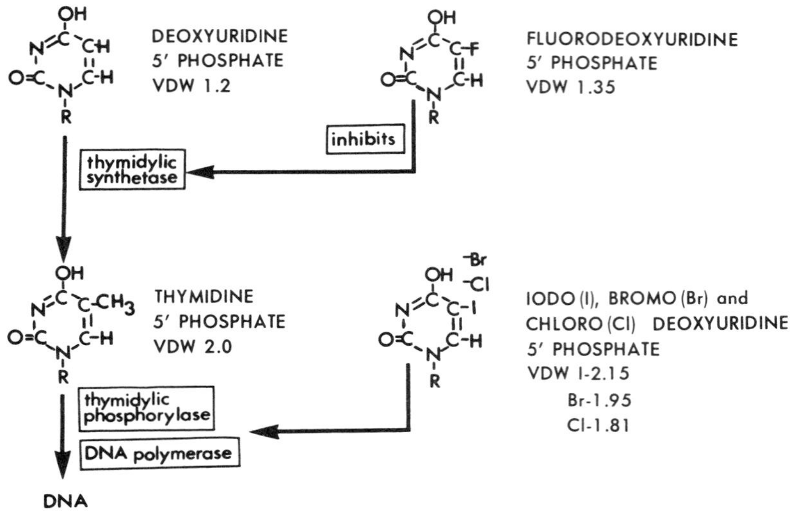

FIG. 70-2. Mode of action of the deoxyuridines. *VDW* = van der Waals radius (*see* footnote on this page)

phate, and triphosphate forms. The triphosphate competes with thymidine-5′-phosphate (Fig. 70-2) in the formation of DNA by DNA polymerase. DNA polymerase is unable to distinguish between idoxuridine and thymidine because the van der Waals radius of iodine (2.15) is essentially similar to that of the methyl group of thymidine (2.0). It is generally understood that idoxuridine DNA does not function properly but leads to the production of defective nucleic acid (lethal viral synthesis). Resistance to idoxuridine has been described for some isolates of herpes simplex.

Pharmacology

Because idoxuridine is rapidly incorporated into host DNA following systemic administration, current use of this drug is confined to topical therapy in the conjunctival sac or on the skin. Small quantities of the drug may be absorbed but are rapidly excreted in the urine as iodine, ribose, and uracil.

Adverse Effects

Adverse effects that result from topical conjunctival therapy are usually minimal. Periorbital burning, tingling pain or discomfort, lacrimation, edema, and erythema, accompanied by photophobia, are common and may reflect irritation from the drug base and not the idoxuridine itself. There may be an increased occurrence of subepithelial opacities following its use, but this has not been proved. The insoluble petrolatum base must not be incorporated into deep corneal lesions.

Preparations and Uses

Iodoxuridine, U.S.P., is available in a 0.1% solution (Dendrid, Herplex, Stoxil); in a 0.1% solution in polyvinyl alcohol (Herplex);

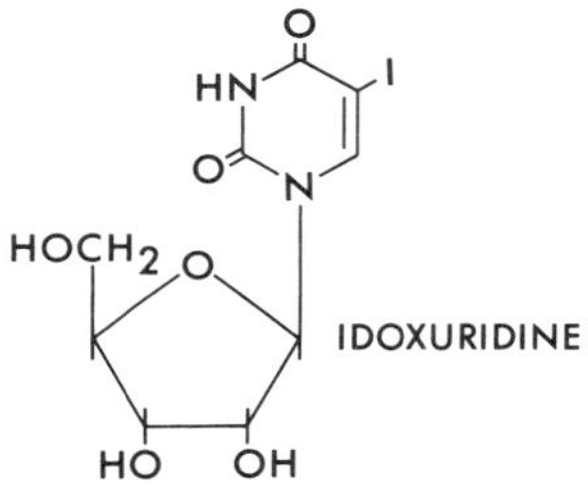

and as a 0.5% ointment in a petrolatum base (Stoxil). The solution is heat- and light-sensitive and should be kept refrigerated. The ointment is heat-stable.

Idoxuridine is effective in some cases of primary and recurrent herpes simplex and vaccinia keratitis, but when the disease is chronic or accompanied by deep stromal lesions the drug is of doubtful value. The 0.1% solution is probably more effective than the ointment; the usual dose in herpetic keratitis is 1 drop hourly during the day and every 2 hours at night. Dosage is gradually reduced to 1 drop every 2 to 4 hours. If no obvious effect is seen after 1 week, therapy should be discontinued. If there is deep stromal involvement, combination with corticosteroids, cycloplegics, or antibacterial drugs (if secondary infection is present) may be desir-

---

Johannes Diderik van der Waals, 1837–1923. Dutch physicist. Won Nobel Prize in 1910 for his work on the behavior of gases. Also studied surface tension, capillarity, and the theory of mixtures.

able. Even if a satisfactory response is being obtained, idoxuridine therapy should probably not be continued for longer than 3 weeks.

Topically administered, idoxuridine sensitizes herpesviruses to the lethal effects of irradiation, an effect that can be seen in herpes keratitis. The clinical efficacy of a combination of idoxuridine plus irradiation is unclear.

Idoxuridine has been used to treat other herpetic infections (mucocutaneous herpes, including genital herpes) and infections due to cytomegalovirus, but the results have not been impressive. Idoxuridine in 40% dimethylsulfoxide (DMSO) was shown in England to be of some benefit in herpes zoster, reducing the duration of pain and accelerating healing, in primary herpetic whitlow, and in Kaposis varicelliform eruption. Idoxuridine in 5% DMSO shortens the course of some cutaneous herpetic lesions in humans. It has no effect in genital herpes.

DMSO, a primary irritant, produces skin maceration with prolonged treatment and whealing due to histamine release (Table 51-2). DMSO (RIMSO-50) is approved for the symptomatic treatment of interstitial cystitis; otherwise it is an experimental agent. After topical or intravesical administration most patients complain of a garlic-like odor to their breath due to exhaled dimethylsulfide. *DMSO must not be applied to the eye or within the mouth and should not come into contact with rubber, nylon, plastics, or other synthetic fibers.*

TRIFLURIDINE

Trifluridine (Trifluorothymidine; Viroptic R; F_3TdR) is a new pyrimidine nucleoside originally introduced as an anticancer drug. Trifluridine inhibits DNA synthesis similarly to IDUR but is incorporated more efficiently into virus DNA than into host DNA. It demonstrates activity *in vitro* against *Herpes simplex* types 1 and 2.

Topically in the eye, trifluridine causes stinging or burning pain and palpebral edema. Rarely hypersensitivity reactions and an epithelial keratopathy have been observed.

Trifluridine has been used for topical treatment of primary and recurrent herpes simplex keratitis and keratoconjunctivitis; it has not been tested against other herpetic infections. Trifluridine appears to heal corneal ulcers more effectively than does idoxuridine or vidarabine and appears to be effective in some cases of IDUR resistance.

CYTARABINE

Cytarabine (1-β-D-arabinofuranoxylcytosine: Ara-C; Cytarabine, Cytosar) was originally developed as an antileukemic drug. It is now available experimentally for topical administration in some virus diseases. Cytarabine has an antiviral spectrum similar to that of idoxuridine, but antiviral resistance has been reported only rarely. The drug inhibits nucleoside di-

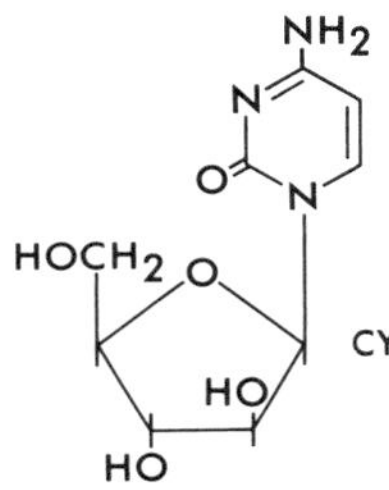

CYTARABINE

phosphate reductase and DNA polymerase and depresses the reduction of cytidilic acid to deoxycytidilic acid, thus depleting the pool of deoxycytidine triphosphate available for DNA synthesis. Its primary site of action is, however, not clear. Following i.v. administration, Ara C is rapidly deaminated to the antivirally inactive uracil arabinoside.

Adverse Effects

Adverse effects following topical administration have been minimal and parallel those seen with idoxuridine.

Uses

Cytarabine has been used in the conjunctival sac to treat herpetic keratitis. It has also been used to treat topically other localized and generalized infections caused by herpes simplex and herpes zoster/varicella viruses, but convincing proof of clinical efficacy is lacking. Results in the treatment of cytomegalovirus infections have not been encouraging, but cytarabine has been used successfully to treat smallpox. It has no value systemically.

Cytarabine has two advantages over idoxuridine. First, herpesviruses, particularly type 2, are generally more sensitive to cytarabine than to idoxuridine. Second, resistance develops

---

MORITZ KAPOSI–KOHN, 1837–1902. Austrian dermatologist. Described Kaposi's sarcoma of the skin in 1872; xeroderma pigmentosum (Kaposi's dermatosis) in 1882; and many other specific diseases.

rapidly to idoxuridine but has not been a problem with cytarabine.

INTERFERONS

The interferons are a group of cellular glycoproteins, one of a class of cytokines similar to other hormone-like agents such as erythropoietin, osteoclast activation factor, and epithelial growth factor. Interferons are produced by vertebrate cells in response to virus infection or after stimulation by various nonvirus inducers. All interferons have antiviral effects but differ physiochemically and antigenically depending on the cell of origin and the inducer used. Although "interferons" were discovered in 1957, only recently has the spectrum of their activity in response to viral disease, in immunoregulation, in growth inhibition, and in the inhibition of embryogenesis been recognized. Cost factors and problems in production and purification have retarded the availability of interferons and the widespread study of their properties and full therapeutic potential.

Source

There appear to be two main types of interferon: *Type I interferon* is produced by cell cultures or in animals, including humans, that have not been sensitized to the inducer. *Type II interferon* is produced by T and B lymphocytes or macrophages previously sensitized to a specific antigen; type II interferon may be related to migration inhibitory factor. The interferon gene is normally repressed, but interferon production may be initiated by various inducers, including virus infections, exposure to antigens, or mitogens, and various artificial inducers such as poly (I): poly (C) and tilorone (*see* below).

There are several differences between type I and type II interferon, such as in heat stability, host range, and *p*H properties; whereas both types inhibit a variety of viruses, type II interferon possesses more potent immunoregulatory properties. Type I interferon has been isolated from human leukocytes (HLI) and from human diploid fibroblasts in cell culture (HFI). HLI and HFI differ somewhat biologically and immunologically. HLI has a molecular weight of about 20,000 daltons and has been the interferon used predominantly in clinical trials because of its absorption from i.m. sites. Type I interferon has been prepared from fresh buffy-coat leukocytes, induced with Sendai virus.

JOHN DALTON, 1766–1844. English chemist. Best known for his work in physics and chemistry: the law of partial pressures, atomic theory, and composition of ether. Was color blind and in 1794 wrote the first detailed report on this problem, sometimes known as daltonism.

Mode of Action

As antiviral agents, interferons bind to specific host-cell plasma membrane receptors and induce *functional* and *structural* changes therein, possibly through derepressing a gene on chromosome 21. *Functionally* several enzymes are produced that block virus replication, assembly, and release; alterations in membrane charge, density, substrate binding, nucleoside transport, and histocompatibility antigen expression are also seen. Virus attachment, penetration, and uncoating, however, proceed unimpeded. *Structurally,* alterations are observed in cytoplasmic fibers.

Properties

Interferons possess at least three properties: antiviral effects; immunoregulatory properties; and inhibition of cell growth.

Antiviral Effects. Interferons are relatively species specific but not virus specific in interfering with various RNA and DNA viruses. Several clinical studies have demonstrated some benefit when interferon is used either therapeutically or prophylactically (*see* below). Myxoviruses are very sensitive to interferon, whereas adenoviruses are relatively resistant.

Immune Regulation and Growth Inhibition. Both antigen- and virus-induced interferon suppress precursor T- and B-cell lymphocytes, sensitized T and B cells, and macrophages. In particular, interferons may be important immunoregulatory signals for natural killer (NK) cell activity. In animals, interferons inhibit graft-versus-host disease, but this is of limited benefit in humans because marrow cell growth inhibition is also seen.

Interferons are growth inhibitors. In osteosarcoma cell lines, for example, HFI possesses greater inhibitory effects than does HLI.

Pharmacology

Interferons are not absorbed after oral administration or when applied topically to intact skin or mucosae. After i.m. or s.c. injection of 2×10^4 units/kg, peak blood levels develop within 5 to 8 hours, and levels of 100 units/ml are still present 12 hours later. After constant i.v. infusion, the drug has a biologic half-life of 2 to 4 hours. No major metabolites have been identified. Interferons have poor tissue penetration in animals and humans. Cerebrospinal fluid levels are about 1/30th of simultaneous blood levels. Measurement of serum interferon levels correlates poorly with response, since antiviral effects persist after interferon becomes unmeasurable.

Adverse Effects

Nonspecific toxicity (fever, malaise, fatigue, lassitude, nausea, and vomiting), is frequently seen after parenteral therapy but is becoming less common as interferon preparations become more pure. Pain, myalgia, induration, and local erythema may be seen at the injection site, and rapid i.v. injection may result in hypotension. Transient elevation of serum transaminases has been reported in children. Growth inhibition is dose related. Doses of 8.5 units/kg/day or more result in some bone marrow suppression, with the development of leukopenia after 3 to 5 days, and subsequently thrombocytopenia and a fall in the reticulocyte count; these all revert to normal within 1 week of stopping therapy. Marrow toxicity is more common in those patients who receive other marrow suppressants—that is, in the treatment of renal transplant recipients.

Preparations and Uses

The interferons are experimental agents. HLI has been used prophylactically and therapeutically following topical, i.v., s.c., and i.m. administration. HFI must be given intravenously or topically because it is destroyed after i.m. administration. Interferon has been beneficial in some viral infections, including varicella/zoster disease in immunocompromised patients, chronic active hepatitis, and herpes simplex keratitis. Prophylactically interferon has been shown to be of some benefit against cytomegalovirus, rubella, Epstein–Barr virus, herpesvirus infections, and rhinovirus type-4 infection. Topically interferon is effective in treating herpetic keratitis, particularly when combined with adequate débridement.

In the treatment of cancer, some response has been observed against osteosarcoma, non-Hodgkin's lymphoma, melanoma, multiple myeloma, juvenile laryngeal papilloma, and breast carcinoma. Various multicenter trials are currently in progress.

INTERFERON INDUCERS/INHIBITORS

Because the supply of interferon is limited, various attempts have been made to develop synthetic inducers to stimulate the production of endogenous interferon. Numerous inducers have been described, but only a few have been tried in humans: Tilorone (bis-diethyl-aminoethylfuorenone); poly [1]: poly [C] (poly riboinosinicpolyribocytidylic acid); a complex of poly [1]: poly [C] with poly-L-lysine and carboxymethyl cellulose; and a substituted propanedinane. Drawbacks to the use of interferon inducers *in vivo* are their toxicity (primarily pyrogenicity) and the inconsistent interferon response. *Enhancer agents* and *stimulon* have been found in virus-infected cells, and these substances counteract the effectiveness of interferon.

ANTIVIRAL DRUGS UNDER INVESTIGATION

Ribavirin

Ribavirin (1-β-D-ribofuranosyl-1, 2, 4, triazole-3-carboxamide, Virazole) is a synthetic nucleoside with *in vitro* antiviral properties against various RNA and DNA viruses. After phosphorylation, ribavirin competitively inhibits inosine-5-phosphate dehydrogenase, thus depleting the intracellular pools of dGTP and GTP, thereby depressing guanosine synthesis. Clinical results have been somewhat disappointing.

Isoprinosine

Isoprinosine (Inosiplex), a compound formed from the p-acetamidobenzoate salt of N,-N diethylamino-2-propanol and inosine in a 3:1 ratio, may be beneficial prophylactically against rhinoviruses, herpes simplex, and influenza type A infections. It also has some immunostimulatory properties.

6-Azaruridine

6-Azaruridine inhibits orotidylic acid decarboxylase and has been shown to inhibit several DNA and RNA viruses *in vitro*. It is undergoing trials for the treatment of measles and subacute sclerosing panencephalitis. *5-Trifluoromethyl-2-deoxyuridine* and *5-ethyl-2′-deoxyuridine* are congeners of idoxyuridine and show promise in DNA virus infections.

Rifampin

Rifampin (*see* Chap. 65) inhibits the replication of poxviruses and adenoviruses *in vitro*, but clinical trials have been disappointing. It probably interferes with the assembly of virus DNA and protein when the virus envelope is formed. *Quinacrine* (*see* Chap. 67) has been used experimentally against arborviruses. *Flumidin* (*N′N′-anhydrobis*[*β-hydroxyethyl*] *biguanide hydrochloride, ABOB*) has been reported in early studies to have some prophylactic activity against influenza. *Xenalamine* may have some prophylactic and therapeutic activity in influenza and chickenpox. *Phagicin*, a polypeptide produced by bacteriophage-infected *Escherichia coli*, may be useful in systemic viral disease.

Other agents under investigation are *phosphonoacetic acid* and *2-deoxy-D-glucose*. Megadoses of *ascorbic acid* (*see* Chap. 73) do not reduce infection with the common cold viruses. *Photodynamic inactivation* of viruses is obsolete because it encourages oncogenicity.

FURTHER READING

1. Bryson YJ: Antiviral agents. In Feigin RD, Cherry JD (eds): Textbook of Pediatric Infectious Disease, pp 1713–1735. Philadelphia, WB Saunders, 1981
2. Chang T-W, Snydman DR: Antiviral agents: Action and clinical use. Drugs 18:354–376, 1979
3. Hirsch MS, Swartz MN: Antiviral agents. N Engl J Med 302:903–907, 949–953, 1980
4. Issacs A, Lindenmann J: Virus interference: 1. The interferons. Proc R Soc Lond [Biol] 147:258–267, 1957
5. Pollard RB, Merigan TC: Experience with clinical applications of interferon and interferon inducers. Pharmacol Ther 2:783–811, 1978
6. Smith RA, Sidwell RW, Robins RK: Antiviral mechanisms of action. Annu Rev Pharmacol Toxicol 20:259–284, 1980

CHAPTER 70 QUESTIONS

(*See* P. 7 for Full Instructions)

Select the One Best Answer

1. Each of the following associates a mechanism for inhibiting a viral disease with an agent that acts by the stated mechanism EXCEPT
   A. prevents attachment of virus to cell—antibody.
   B. prevents assembly of mature virus particle—methisazone.
   C. prevents viral infection only indirectly through the immune system—interferon.
   D. prevents viral transcription—idoxuridine.
   E. prevents viral penetration into cells—amantadine.
2. Drugs effective in treating herpes simplex infections include each of the following EXCEPT
   A. idoxuridine.
   B. acyclovir.
   C. cytarabine.
   D. amantadine.
   E. trifluridine.
3. A drug that inhibits penetration of host cells by influenza A_2 virus is
   A. methisazone.
   B. idoxuridine.
   C. amantadine.
   D. vitamin C.
   E. vidarabine.
4. Each of the following statements is true for amantadine EXCEPT that
   A. high doses may lead to the development of lilliputian hallucinations.
   B. it may be of some benefit in reducing akinesia in Parkinson's disease.
   C. it may reduce tremor in Parkinson's disease.
   D. it has been "abused" as a psychedelic agent.
   E. its central nervous system side effects are potentiated by alcohol.

A = 1,2,3; B = 1,3; C = 2,4; D = 4; E = All

5. Amantadine is
   1. useful in prophylaxis against A_2 influenza.
   2. ineffective in type B influenza strains, rubella, and measles.
   3. effective in the therapy of parkinsonian akinesia.
   4. neurotoxic when given in high doses.
6. Cytarabine
   1. is inactivated very rapidly after i.v. administration.
   2. is active against *Herpes zoster*.
   3. is the agent of choice in *Herpes simplex* encephalitis.
   4. rapidly induces emergence of resistant viruses.
7. Which of the following has clinical antiviral activity against smallpox?
   1. Idoxuridine
   2. Amantadine
   3. Cytarabine
   4. Methisazone
8. Passive immunization is of some therapeutic value in
   1. measles.
   2. mumps.
   3. rabies.
   4. rubella.

9. Amantadine is useful in the prophylaxis of
   1. swine flu.
   2. Russian flu.
   3. Asian flu.
   4. parainfluenza.

10. Actions of amantadine include
    1. preventing penetration of virus particles into cells.
    2. preventing virus uncoating.
    3. preventing virus release.
    4. preventing virus reassembly.

A. Vidarabine
B. Acyclovir
C. Both
D. Neither

11. Interfere(s) with viral DNA polymerase.
12. One of its metabolites is antivirally active.
13. Is effective against herpes viruses.
14. Antiviral activity depends on a specific thymidine kinase.

71

CHARLES M. HASKELL

Anticancer Drugs

The modern era of cancer chemotherapy dates from 1941 with the demonstration by Huggins and Hodges that estrogen could modify the course of prostatic cancer. Subsequently, the polyfunctional alkylating agents were developed as a result of experimental work during World War II (Gilman and Goodman), and shortly thereafter the antimetabolites were discovered through observations by Dr. Sidney Farber in patients with acute leukemia.

Now more than two dozen drugs have value in the treatment of cancer. This chapter summarizes the biochemical and clinical pharmacology of anticancer agents.

SELECTIVE TOXICITY

The clinically useful anticancer agents have a greater cytotoxicity for malignant tissues than for normal cells of the tumor-bearing host. They are therefore said to exhibit *selective toxicity,* made possible by metabolic differences between malignant and normal cells. Unfortunately, these differences are *quantitative* rather than *qualitative,* leading to at least some degree of drug-induced toxicity to normal tissues. Most of the quantitative differences between normal and cancer cells relate to *biochemical pathways, transport processes,* and *DNA-repair mechanisms.* For example, the synthesis of major macromolecules, including DNA and RNA, is more easily damaged by some anticancer drugs in certain cancer cells than in normal cells. In addition, there may be

---

CHARLES BRENTON HUGGINS, 1901– . Canadian-born Chicago surgeon. In 1941 introduced the concept of the hormonal dependence of cancers with his treatment of prostatic cancer with estrogens and castration.

CLARENCE VERNARD HODGES, 1914– . American surgeon. Worked with C. B. Huggins on the use of stilbestrol to treat metastatic carcinoma of the prostate.

ALFRED GILMAN, 1908– . American pharmacologist. In 1946 introduced, with F. S. Philips, the use of nitrogen mustards in Hodgkin's disease therapy. Was the author, with L. S. Goodman, of *The Pharmacological Basis of Therapeutics,* first edition, 1941.

SIDNEY FARBER, 1903–1973. Pathologist at Children's Hospital, Boston. In 1948 introduced the antifolate aminopterin, an antimetabolite, which led to the development of similar but more effective agents such as methotrexate. Is also remembered for a ceramide lipidosis, Farber's disease.

differences in the ability of normal cells and cancer cells to repair damage to these critical molecules.

The selective toxicity of tumor drugs depends on *patient factors*, (*biologic*) *factors*, and *pharmacologic factors*.

PATIENT FACTORS

The clinician's first responsibility in deciding about the use of anticancer drugs is to assess the individual patient, since drug toxicity, or safety, may be modified by factors such as nutrition, the use of concomitant drugs, and the presence of hepatic, renal, or pulmonary disease. Dosage may have to be adjusted according to age because younger patients generally tolerate chemotherapy better than older ones. The tolerance for certain forms of chemotherapy may differ between women and men, particularly as it relates to the psychological acceptance of certain toxic reactions. Psychological and social factors may be very important for the acceptance of certain regimens of chemotherapy.

TUMOR (BIOLOGIC) FACTORS

The cancer cell is a variable and fluctuating target, and its sensitivity to various drugs differs from one form of cancer to another.

One of the major factors influencing the response of a cancer to drug therapy is the fraction of the tumor cells in the replicative cycle. Thus the cell cycle (Fig. 71-1) of an individual tumor cell and the kinetics of growth of a tumor cell population must be considered in evaluating selective toxicity. Specifically, the activity of drugs during different phases of the cycle (phase specific) must be differentiated from drugs that kill cells during all or most phases of the cell cycle (phase nonspecific).

FIG. 71-1. Schematic diagram of the cell life cycle. G_1 is the first "gap" period and G_2, the second "gap" period. (Morton DL: Ann Intern Med 77:443, 1972)

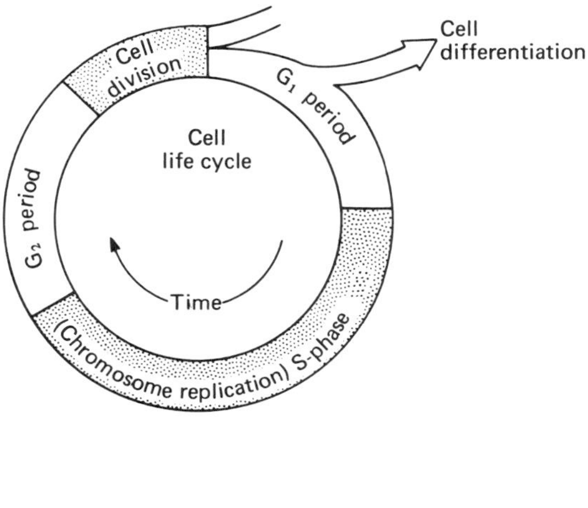

Although dividing normal cells and cancer cells go through the same phases, they differ in the number and distribution of cells in cycle. Normal and neoplastic cells may be influenced by certain growth factors; both appear to divide more rapidly when the population size is small and more slowly when it is large. The quantitative rates of growth of both experimental and human tumors have been measured: When the tumor size is small and growing rapidly, a relatively high proportion of cells is synthesizing DNA (in S phase) at any given time. At this stage in the life history of a cancer, the use of phase-specific drugs effective against rapidly dividing cells is logical. In contrast, an advanced tumor with very low growth fraction and a slow increase in size may respond better to a phase nonspecific drug.

Cancer is generally considered a clonal expansion of a single cell that has become neoplastic. The ultimate clone that causes clinical problems, however, may be the result of additional somatic mutations, and the clinical mass of tumor may contain a heterogeneous cell population. Some cells within that population may be sensitive to chemotherapy, whereas others may not. Thus an additional biologic factor of importance is the possible heterogeneous response of tumors to chemotherapy.

The differences between normal tissues and the malignant tissue may be slight. Many normal tissues have a high proliferative capacity rivaling, and in some instances exceeding, that of malignant tissues. Such normal tissues, including bone marrow elements, gastrointestinal epithelium, and hair follicles, bear the brunt of the toxic effects of certain anticancer drugs. Fortunately, the rapidly proliferating normal and cancer cells are not always equally vulnerable, and the principle of selective toxicity can still be used. Apparently, however, the margin of safety is a narrow one.

PHARMACOLOGIC FACTORS

Drug action depends on a direct interaction of the anticancer drug or a metabolite with a specific receptor, which, in nearly all cases, is found within the cancer cell. The ability of a given drug or drug combination to reach cellular receptors is affected by variations in drug absorption, distribution, metabolism, and excretion (Fig. 71-2).

Ultimately it is the concentration of the drug or a metabolite for a given time of exposure at the receptor site that is critical in determining the effectiveness of drug action. This relation is sometimes expressed as the product of drug concentration multiplied by drug exposure time, or the C × T function. For any given antineoplastic drug, the net effect in the host is the drug's therapeutic index.

Factors That Affect the Therapeutic Index

Route of Administration and Absorption. Various routes (p.o., i.v., i.m., or i.a.) of administration may be chosen to optimize availability; drugs also may be instilled into a local site (*e.g.*, a malignant effusion in the pleural space or into the spinal fluid). Antitumor activity may be improved by carefully selecting the route of administration, thereby allowing a drug to reach higher concentrations in the tumor area. One very specialized example of this approach is isolation–perfusion of an extremity with high doses of alkylating agents for regional malignant melanoma.

Distribution and Transport. After a drug is absorbed, it may enter or pass through various compartments, including vascular spaces, extracellular spaces, and cells. Drugs may either accumulate in certain areas or be excluded as a result of binding, active transport, or fat solubility.

Because most anticancer drugs exert their effect directly on an intracellular target molecule, their ability to get to the cancer cell is vital. If tumor cells are in an area of the body inaccessible to anticancer drugs, then the product of the concentration multiplied by the time factor for these drugs will be negligible and the cancer cells will survive ("sanctuary" effect). An example of such a sanctuary is the cerebrospinal fluid, in which tumor cells appear to be inaccessible to many anticancer drugs because of the blood–brain barrier. Most commonly used anticancer drugs are relatively lipid insoluble (*see* Chap. 2). Access to the brain is largely restricted to molecules that are highly fat soluble.

FIG. 71-2. Factors that contribute to selective toxicity. (Modified from Haskell CM: In *Cancer Treatment.* Philadelphia, W B Saunders, 1980)

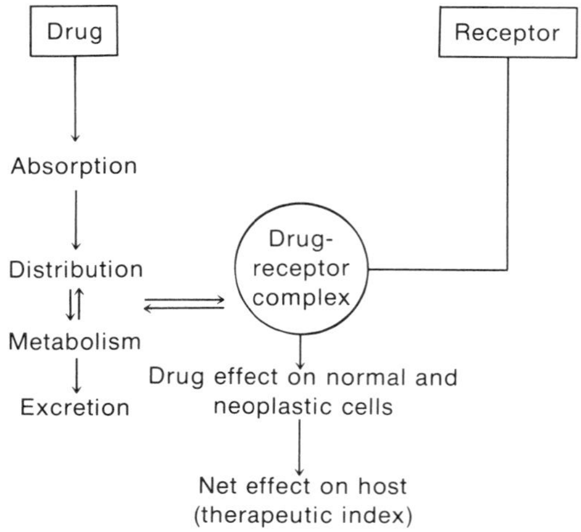

Biotransformation. Some drugs are inactive and require biotransformation—for example, cyclophosphamide, which is metabolized in the liver. Other drugs can modify the activation process, including barbiturates and corticosteroids (*see* Chap. 8).

Excretion. Methotrexate is primarily excreted by the kidneys. Thus even a moderate elevation of blood urea nitrogen may be associated with major hematologic toxicity from the use of relatively low doses of methotrexate. Similarly, vincristine or doxorubicin, excreted primarily in bile, may lead to severe toxicity when administered in full doses to patients with biliary disease.

Drug Interactions. Most patients with cancer receive potent drugs for the control of symptoms that result from treatment. These drugs may be responsible for the following significant drug interactions.

1. Direct chemical or physical interaction (*e.g.*, nitrogen mustard destroyed in aqueous solutions)
2. Interaction during intestinal absorption (*e.g.*, methotrexate and antibiotics)
3. Interaction at plasma protein transport site (*e.g.*, methotrexate and aspirin displace each other)
4. Interaction at the cellular receptor site (*e.g.*, folic acid and methotrexate)
5. Interaction by accelerated or inhibited metabolism (*e.g.*, allopurional retards the degradation of 6-mercaptopurine)
6. Alterations in acid–base balance leading to changes in drug distribution and renal clearance (*e.g.*, theoretical not established for anticancer drugs)
7. Alterations of renal function that influence rates of renal excretion (*e.g.*, methotrexate excretion)

8. Alterations in cellular transport mechanisms (*e.g.*, L-asparaginase inhibits methotrexate uptake)
9. Alterations in cellular biochemical pathways and drug resistance (*e.g.*, 6-mercaptopurine and allopurinol, *see* 5 above).

Drug Resistance. Often the first trial of a given drug is successful, but subsequent doses are progressively less successful until there is no apparent beneficial effect.

A number of cellular mechanisms are probably involved in drug resistance: *altered drug metabolism* (increase in deactivation, decrease or loss of the essential activation process), *cell impermeability* to the active compound, *altered specificity* of an inhibited enzyme, *increased production of a target molecule*, *repair of cytotoxic lesions*, and in some cases *alternative biochemical pathways* that bypass an inhibited reaction. Obviously the development of anticancer drug resistance and the appearance of bacterial resistance are analogous (*see* Chap. 56). Treatment strategy is often similar: change the drug or, less often, use larger doses of the same drug.

Drug Toxicity. The usefulness of cancer chemotherapy is often limited by toxic reactions in normal cells. Although it would be preferable to use drugs with a high therapeutic index (maximum therapeutic benefit with virtually no toxicity), this ideal is rarely achieved clinically. Thus one must be familiar with the spectrum of toxicity seen with anticancer drugs.

Bone Marrow Toxicity. Leukopenia with an attendant high risk of infection and thrombocytopenia and bleeding may occur and be life-threatening. Because of the *critical importance* of bone marrow toxicity in cancer chemotherapy, a classification of drugs according to their myelosuppressive potential and the time-course of recovery from granulocytopenia are given in Table 71-1.

Some drugs (particularly the alkylating agents, including the nitrosoureas and mitomycin-C), cause cumulative, delayed myelosuppression, which rarely may lead to prolonged, severe pancytopenia.

Gastrointestinal Toxicity. Anorexia, nausea, and vomiting occur commonly with some anti-

TABLE 71-1. Drug-Induced Myelosuppression*

Category*	Drug	Nadir of Granulocytes	Recovery
		days	
I	Mechlorethamine	7–15	28
	Melphalan	10–12	—
	Busulfan	11–30	24–54
	Carmustine	26–30	35–49
	Lomustine	40–50	60
	Semustine†	28–63	82–89
	Cytarabine	12–14	22–24
	Vinblastine	5–9	14–21
II	Cyclophosphamide	8–14	18–25
	5-Fluorouracil	7–14	20–30
	6-Mercaptopurine	7	14–21
	Methotrexate	7–14	14–21
	Dactinomycin	15	22–25
	Procarbazine	25–36+	35–50+
III	Vincristine	4–5	7
	Bleomycin	—	—
	L-Asparaginase	—	—
	cis-Dichlorodiammine-platinum II	—	—
	Hormones	—	—

* Modified from Henderson ES: In Dimitrov NV and Nodine JH (eds): *Drugs and Hematologic Reactions.* New York, Grune & Stratton, 1974 and Creaven PJ, Mihich E: *Semin Oncol* 4:147, 1977.

* Categories: I, primarily myelosuppressive toxicity; II, myelosuppressive but other toxicities equally important; III, rarely cause granulocytopenia.

† Experimental drug.

neoplastic agents, and suppression with antiemetics is only variably effective. Stomatitis, esophagitis, peptic ulcer disease, and diarrhea may also occur.

Immunosuppression. In view of evidence implicating host immunologic factors in the control of small numbers of tumor cells, the potential immunosuppressing effect of cancer chemotherapeutic drugs on cellular and humoral immunity becomes increasingly important. Experimentally the preservation, and in some cases the augmentation, of immunity is important to therapy. Immunosuppression may also place the patient at risk from various infections.

Immunosuppression may vary depending on the dose and schedule of the administered drug, either by itself or in combination with other drugs. Intermittent, intensive courses of chemotherapy appear to suppress cellular immunity much less than do continuous low doses of chemotherapy. Generally the immunosuppressive effects of most of the common anticancer drugs do not extend beyond the period of active drug administration, although some patients demonstrate an "immunologic overshoot" afterward. Thus when short courses of combination chemotherapy are given every 2 to 4 weeks, the patient's immunologic function may predominantly be normal.

Skin Reactions. Local tissue necrosis from extravasation, hyperpigmentation, hyperkeratosis, dermatitis, urticaria, vasculitis, flushing, and nail changes, including transverse banding and, rarely, nail loss, may occur.

Alopecia. Doxorubicin, cyclophosphamide, and other agents frequently produce alopecia. It is nearly always reversible.

Liver Toxicity. Liver toxicity is uncommon but may be serious, ranging from minimal elevations of transaminases (cytarabine) to cirrhotic changes (methotrexate) and even necrosis (6-mercaptopurine).

Lung Toxicity. Methotrexate and alkylating agents occasionally lead to lung toxicity, but bleomycin results in this problem most often. In some patients lung toxicity occurs as severe pulmonary fibrosis.

Heart Toxicity. Doxorubicin, daunomycin, and very high doses of cyclophosphamide may cause serious cardiac damage.

Genitourinary Toxicity. Hemorrhagic cystitis is rare except in about 10% of patients treated with cyclophosphamide. Nephrotoxicity occurs with standard doses of mithramycin, streptozocin, L-asparaginase, and cisplatin, and with high doses of methotrexate or 6-mercaptopurine. Uric acid nephropathy may develop but can generally be prevented by allopurinol and hydration.

CNS Toxicity. Mild to moderate neurologic problems may occur with some drugs, but these are generally reversible. Severe neurotoxicity is most commonly seen with excessive doses of vincristine.

Second Malignancies. Many of the antineoplastic drugs are mutagenic as well as teratogenic, and some, (*e.g.*, procarbazine and alkylating agents) are carcinogenic in animals. Because patients are living longer after treatment, the potential carcinogenicity of anticancer agents is increasingly of concern. For example, delayed acute leukemia has been found to occur in patients treated with alkylating agents for Hodgkin's disease or multiple myeloma.

Miscellaneous Complications. Various other complications may occur, including coagulation problems, the syndrome of inappropriate antidiuretic hormone secretion, electrolyte problems, pancreatitis, diabetes mellitus, pituitary insufficiency, adrenal insufficiency, fever, anaphylaxis, aseptic necrosis of the femoral heads, pathologic fractures, hemolytic anemia, cataracts, and suppression of growth. Indeed, the prudent physician should be alert to both the known complications of cancer chemotherapy and those that are currently unrecognized as part of this emerging discipline.

LOG-CELL KILL HYPOTHESIS

Anticancer drugs are thought to be incapable of killing all cancer cells at any given exposure. Rather, they kill a variable fraction of cells, anywhere from a small percentage up to a maximum of 99.999%. The observed fractional tumor cell kill can frequently be graphed as a line with a negative exponential slope; therefore, experimental chemotherapeutic data are often expressed in logarithmic terms. Because the body burden of tumor cells in humans with an advanced malignancy may be greater than 10^{12} cells (1 kg) and a single maximal exposure of tumor cells to a drug achieves at best somewhere between 2 and 5 logs of cell kill, treatment must be repeated multiple times to achieve even partial control.

DRUG SCHEDULES AND COMBINATION CHEMOTHERAPY

Studies with experimental animal tumors have conclusively demonstrated the importance of drug scheduling in therapy. Cytarabine, an antimetabolite that kills cells only in the S phase (phase specific), must be given frequently to assure contact with cancer cells during this critical period. When this drug is so used, some forms of murine leukemia can be cured, whereas maximally tolerated doses of the drug given at less frequent intervals fail to prolong survival. On the other hand, cyclophosphamide (phase nonspecific) achieves optimal suppression of most experimental animal neoplasms when given on a high-dose intermittent schedule.

A second factor related to drug scheduling is the growth status of any given tumor. In general, solid tumors with a large tumor mass grow slowly and have a small growth fraction (less than 10%). Because relatively few of these cells are actually dividing, the tumors are generally insensitive to phase-specific drugs. Thus the usual treatment for advanced nonhematologic tumors has been with phase-nonspecific drugs such as alkylating agents. Successful treatment with such phase nonspecific drugs may, however, render the tumor more susceptible to phase-specific drugs by reducing the size of the tumor so that it has a high growth fraction with many cells in S phase.

The optimal treatment for many kinds of tumors is the use of drug combinations. Several theoretical and practical advantages to combination chemotherapy have emerged after active study of various drug combinations for the primary therapy of advanced neoplasms and as early therapy in combination with surgery and radiation therapy. At the risk of oversimplification, it may be useful to amplify this principle by thinking of a population of malignant cells as resembling a culture of bacteria. In both, combinations of agents can delay or suppress the emergence of drug-resistant cells and can prolong the time necessary for the population of dividing cells to reach a density that produces clinically apparent disease. Addition of an anticancer drug to malignant cells results in the killing of the drug-sensitive cells, just as the addition of an antibiotic to bacteria results in the killing of the susceptible bacteria (*see* Chap. 55). If the drug is not completely effective, a portion of the cancer survives. The surviving population contains drug-resistant cells that, if capable of replication, give rise to a drug-resistant tumor. The administered drug thus has a selective mode of action leading to the emergence of a resistant cell line.

It is not easy to determine the frequency of drug resistance in cancer cells. However, the chances for the development of a drug-resistant line are not as good if two or more drugs of dissimilar modes of action are used in treatment combination. For example, a patient with acute lymphocytic leukemia may have 10^{12} tumor cells in his body. If a single drug, for example, prednisone, is 99.999% effective (*i.e.*, if it kills 99,999 of every 100,000 tumor cells), then 10^7 malignant cells remain after prednisone therapy. If, in addition, a second agent with a different mode of action, such as vincristine, is 99.9% effective, the population of malignant cells can be further reduced to 10^4 cells. If still more agents are used, it is theoretically possible to reduce the cell population to nearly zero. At present, this goal is not attainable because of limitations imposed by toxicity; malignant cells are often concentrated in sites not reached by the drug (*i.e.*, the CNS); and unsusceptible cells may be in a prolonged G_1 and G_0 phase.

PRINCIPLES OF COMBINATION CHEMOTHERAPY

Successful programs must be designed with care to minimize dangerous effects. Thus only drugs active against the tumor in question are included, drugs must have different mechanisms of action to minimize drug resistance; and drugs should have different spectra of clinical toxicity, allowing the administration of full or nearly full doses of each agent. Additionally, most oncologists prefer to use intermittent rather than continuous programs of drug administration. This approach tends to maximize tumor cell killing and appears to be tolerated better by patients and cause less immunosuppression.

CLASSES OF DRUGS AND MECHANISMS OF ACTION

Antineoplastic drugs act predominantly on *enzymes* and *substrates* (Fig. 71-3). Thus drugs

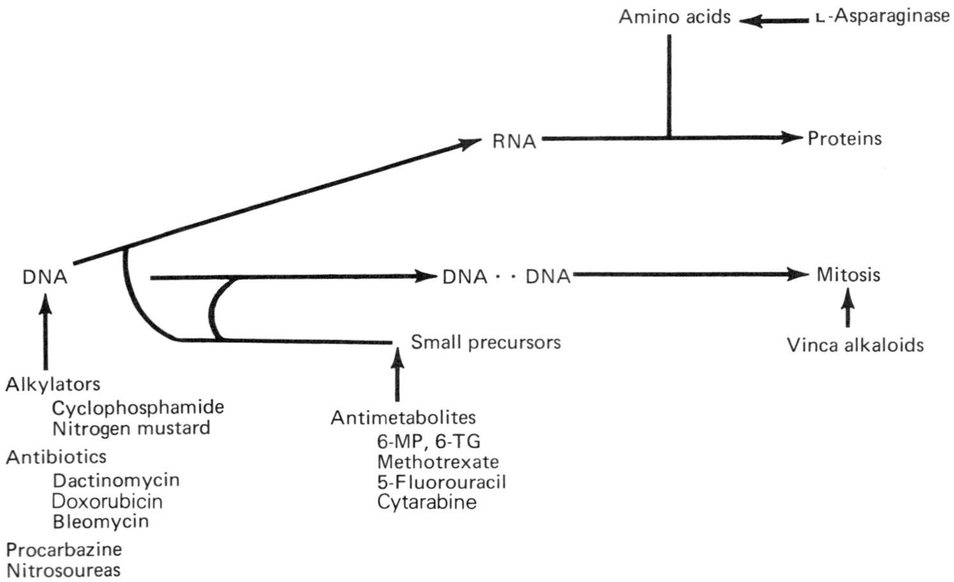

FIG. 71-3. Site of action of chemotherapeutic agents. Red arrow indicates drugs acting primarily as inhibitors of enzymes, black arrows indicate specific substrates acted upon by drugs of that class. (Modified from Cline MJ, Haskell CM: *Cancer Chemotherapy,* (3rd ed). Philadelphia, W B Saunders, 1980).

may act as *false precursors* for an enzyme or as *inhibitors* of the active site of an enzyme or of its controlling (allosteric) site; these drugs are usually structural analogues of normal metabolites and are commonly referred to as antimetabolites. Additionally, at least five major chemical classes of drugs, including alkylating agents, antitumor antibiotics, vinca alkaloids, and antitumor enzymes, appear to act by binding to specific substrates, usually DNA or proteins.

The chemical structures of selected anticancer agents, their pharmacologic characteristics, and some details of their clinical use in terms of dosage, acute and delayed toxicity, and major indications are provided in Figure 71-4 and Tables 71-2 and 71-3, respectively. Further details on the more important anticancer drugs follows.

ALKYLATING AGENTS

The alkylating agents are highly reactive compounds with the ability to substitute alkyl groups (*e.g.*, $R-CH_2-CH_2+$) for the hydrogen atoms of certain organic compounds. Although many cellular substances can undergo this type of reaction, alkylation of DNA is the crucial cytotoxic mechanism. Alkylation produces breaks in the DNA molecule and creates cross-linkage of its twin strands, thus interfering with its replication and transcription. Similar effects are produced by certain kinds of ionizing radiations so that the alkylators are said to be *radiomimetic*.

There are six chemical subclasses of alkylating agents: nitrogen mustard derivatives (mechlorethamine, cyclophosphamide, chlorambucil, melphalan); ethylenimine derivatives (thio-TEPA); alkyl sulfonates (busulfan); triazene derivatives (dacarbazine); nitrosoureas (BCNU, CCNU, methyl-CCNU); and derivatives of *cis*-diamminedichloroplatinum. Most of these drugs are considered polyfunctional alkylating agents because they contain more than one alkylating group. Moreover, the nitrosoureas and dacarbazine appear to have additional mechanisms of cytotoxicity separate from their ability to alkylate nucleic acids.

As a class, the alkylating agents are considered to be cell cycle phase nonspecific. Their pharmacologies and clinical uses differ markedly; nevertheless, nitrogen mustard derivatives administered to the same level of toxicity produce similar antitumor effects. With rare exceptions, tumor cell resistance to one nitrogen mustard derivative indicates resistance to others, but not dacarbazine and the nitrosoureas. The known mechanisms responsible for resistance involve the development of DNA repair enzymes and modification of drug transport.

ALKYLATING AGENTS

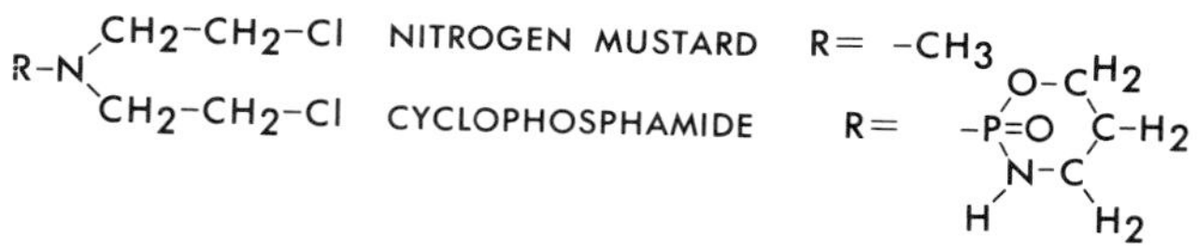

ANTIMETABOLITES

NORMAL METABOLITE

STRUCTURAL ANALOG

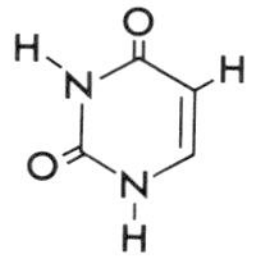

URACIL

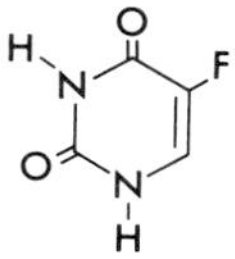

5-FLUOROURACIL

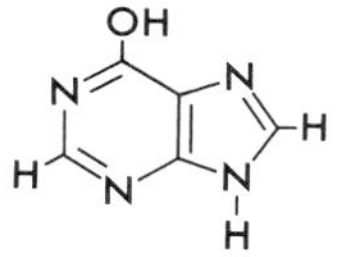

HYPOXANTHINE

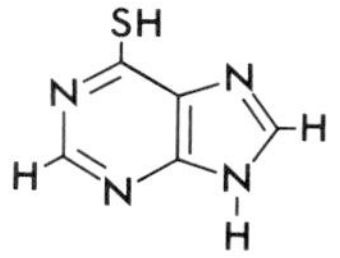

6-MERCAPTOPURINE

VINCA ALKALOIDS

VINCRISTINE
VINBLASTINE

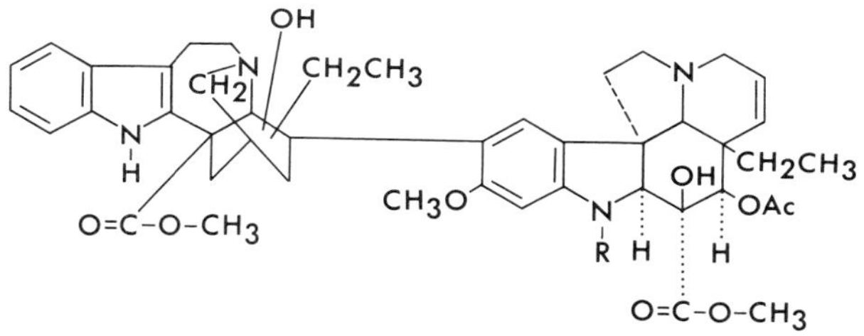

VINCRISTINE
R is O=C–H

VINBLASTINE
R is CH_3

ANTIBIOTICS

ACTINOMYCIN-D

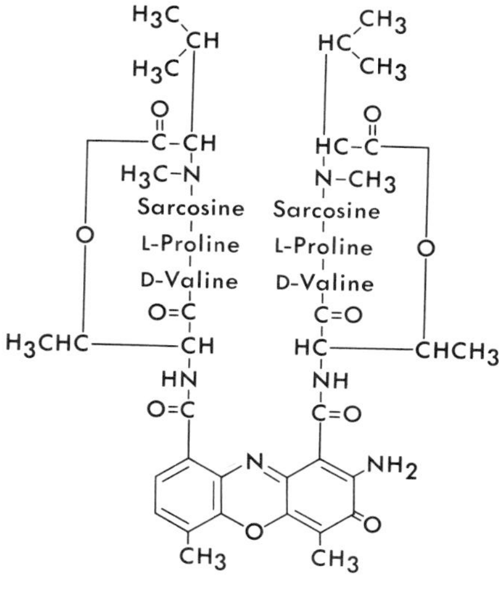

FIG. 71-4. Chemical structures of selected anticancer drugs.

TABLE 71-2. Pharmacologic Characteristics of Selected Anticancer Drugs

Drug	Cell-Cycle Phase Specificity	Plasma T½	Plasma Protein Binding %	Entry into CNS†	Biotransformation		Main Route of Excretion	Major Toxicities
					Activation	*Degradation*		
Alkylating agent								
Cyclophosphamide	NS	6.5 hr	10	Moderate	Oxidized by hepatic microsomal enzymes to biologically active and inactive products		Renal	Myelosuppression; cystitis; alopecia
Antimetabolites								
Methotrexate	S	12 hr	50	Minimal	None	None	Renal	Myelosuppression; stomatitis; hepatic dysfunction
6-Mercaptopurine	S	90 min	10–20	Moderate	To nucleotide	Oxidation to 6-thiouric acid via xanthine oxidase	Renal	Myelosuppression; stomatitis; hepatic dysfunction
Cytarabine	S	2 hr	Negligible	Moderate	To nucleotide	Deamination to uracil arabinoside	Renal	Myelosuppression
5-Fluorouracil	NS	20 min	? negligible	Extensive	To nucleotide	Extensive	Lung and renal	Myelosuppression; gastrointestinal; integument
Vinca alkaloids								
Vincristine	S	A few min	? negligible	? negligible	? extensive		Bile	Neuropathy; alopecia
Antibiotics								
Dactinomycin	NS	A few min	? negligible	Low	None	None	Bile	Myelosuppression; gastrointestinal; integument
Doxorubicin	NS	27 hr	Extensive	? negligible	Extensive biotransformation to active and inactive metabolites		Bile	Myelosuppression; stomatitis; alopecia; cardiac damage
Hormones								
Prednisone	NS	24 hr	90	Low	—	Conjugation and reduction in liver	Renal	Peptic ulcer; psychosis; diabetes mellitus; electrolyte problem; myopathy

Cline MJ, Haskell CM: Cancer Chemotherapy, 3rd ed. Philadelphia, W B Saunders, 1980.

* S = phase specific; NS = phase nonspecific; † CNS = central nervous system; ? = undetermined or estimated from known properties of the drug or a closely related drug.

ANTIBIOTICS

The clinically useful antibiotics come from various strains of *Streptomyces*. They are tumoricidal by directly binding to DNA through a process called intercalation, inhibiting DNA and RNA synthesis. As a class, the antibiotics have a number of effects on different phases of the cell cycle, but they behave as cell cycle phase-nonspecific agents. Their clinical usefulness and major toxic reactions are diverse, as shown in Table 71-3.

VINCA ALKALOIDS

Plants have provided some of the most useful antineoplastic agents. For example, vincristine (Oncovin) and vinblastine (Velban) are alkaloids extracted from the common periwinkel plant (Fig. 71-4).

Vinca alkaloids appear to act by binding to cellular microtubular proteins. Because these are essential components of the mitotic spindle in dividing cells, drug binding leads to mitotic arrest. Similar proteins are an important part of nervous tissue. Although the kinetic effects of vinca alkaloids are difficult to classify, most clinicians consider them to be cell cycle phase specific.

Despite the many similarities in chemical structure and action shared by vincristine and vinblastine, their antitumor spectra are different and they are not cross-resistant. Vincristine use is usually limited by neurotoxicity, whereas the dose-limiting toxicity of vinblastine is usually bone marrow suppression.

Antitumor Enzymes (L-Asparaginase)

In 1953 Kidd discovered that guinea-pig serum inhibited several rodent neoplasms. The antitumor component of guinea-pig serum was later shown to be the enzyme L-asparaginase. Related enzymes with antitumor activity have since been extracted from various bacteria. L-Asparaginase is effective in humans through its ability to destroy extracellular supplies of L-asparagine resulting in the death of cancer cells that lack the enzymatic ability to make this amino acid. L-Asparaginase is usually considered to be cell cycle phase nonspecific, although it may block some cells in the G_1 or S phase.

The current use of L-asparaginase is limited to the treatment of acute lymphoblastic leukemia, either in relapse or in initial diagnosis. Toxic effects include anaphylaxis and suppressed protein synthesis.

MISCELLANEOUS AGENTS

Procarbazine

Procarbazine is a unique antineoplastic agent initially synthesized as a potential monoamine oxidase inhibitor. It must be metabolically activated, and it may interfere with a wide variety of biochemical processes. The mechanism of procarbazine action is uncertain, although metabolites can depolymerize DNA. It is a potent carcinogen in experimental animals. Procarbazine is not cross-resistant with the alkylators or to other commonly used antineoplastic drugs. It is cell cycle phase nonspecific.

Procarbazine is an extremely useful drug in treating advanced Hodgkin's disease but may cause CNS and bone marrow toxic reactions. Neurotoxicity may depend on its weak monoamine oxidase inhibitory activity and the decreased pyridoxal phosphate levels that follow its use.

Mitotane (o,p'DDD, Lysodren)

Mitotane, a derivative of DDT, causes necrosis and atrophy of the adrenal cortex and is primarily used to treat adrenal carcinomas. It is tightly and rapidly bound to mitochondria of the adrenal cortex, inhibiting the conversion of cholesterol to ACTH-induced steroids. Mitotane stimulates peripheral extraadrenal cortisone metabolism and may also modify peripheral androgen metabolism.

Antineoplastic hormonal agents

Androgens, estrogens, antiestrogens, and glucocorticosteroids have been used as therapeutic agents in various neoplastic diseases. To be effective, they all seem to need the presence of specific steroid hormone receptors, and they are therefore best considered in the category of substrate active agents.

Antimetabolites

The antimetabolites are structural analogues of normal metabolites required for cell function and replication. Antimetabolites may interact with enzymes and thereby damage cells in three ways: by substrating for a metabolite normally incorporated into a key molecule, making the molecule function abnormally; by competing successfully with a normal metabolite for a key enzyme; and by competing with a normal metabolite that acts at an enzyme regu-

(*Text continues on p. 740*)

TABLE 71-3. Clinical Characteristics of Selected Anticancer Drugs

Drug	Usual Dosage	Toxicity: *Acute*	Toxicity: *Delayed*	Major Indication for Use
Alkylating agents				
Cyclophosphamide (Cytoxan)	30–40 mg/kg i.v. every 3–4 weeks. 2–4 mg/kg/day p.o.	Nausea and vomiting	Myelosuppression; alopecia; cystitis	Hodgkin's and non-Hodgkin's lymphomas; multiple myeloma; lymphocytic leukemia; many solid tumors
Melphalan (Alkeran)	0.25 mg/kg/day X 4 p.o. every 4–6 weeks	None	Myelosuppression	Multiple myeloma; breast and ovarian cancer
Mechlorethamine (nitrogen mustard; Mustargen)	0.4 mg/kg i.v. or i.p. in single or divided doses	Nausea and vomiting; local irritant	Myelosuppression	Hodgkin's disease; locally for malignant effusions
Antimetabolites				
Methotrexate (MTX)	0.4 mg/kg/day i.v. push X 4–5 or 0.4 mg/kg i.v. push 1 or 2 times/week	Occasional diarrhea	Oral and gastrointestinal ulcers; myelosuppression; hepatotoxicity	Choriocarcinoma; acute lymphocytic leukemia; carcinoma of cervix and head and neck
Fluorouracil (5-FU)	12.5 mg/kg/day i.v. X 3–5 days or 15 mg/kg/wk i.v.	Nausea	Myelosuppression; stomatitis; diarrhea	Carcinomas of breast, ovary, and large bowel
Cytarabine (Cytarabine HCl; arabinosyl cytosine; ara-C; Cytosar)	2–3 mg/kg/day i.v. until response or toxicity	Nausea and vomiting	Bone marrow depression	Acute leukemia
6-Thioguanine (6-TG)	2 mg/kg/day p.o.	Occasional nausea and vomiting	Myelosuppression	Acute leukemia

Vinca alkaloids				
Vincristine sulfate (Oncovin)	0.01–0.03 mg/kg/week i.v.	Local irritant	Mild myelosuppression; neuropathy; constipation; alopecia	Acute leukemia; Hodgkin's disease; other lymphomas and solid tumors
Vinblastine sulfate (Velban)	0.1–0.2 mg/kg/week i.v.	Nausea; local irritant	Alopecia; neuropathy; myelosuppression	Hodgkin's disease; miscellaneous solid tumors
Antibiotics				
Dactinomycin (actinomycin D; Cosmegen)	0.015–0.05 mg/kg/week i.v.	Nausea; vomiting;	Myelosuppression; alopecia; gastrointestinal ulcers	Wilms' tumor; sarcomas; testicular carcinomas
Mithramycin (Mithracin)	0.025–0.050 mg/kg i.v. every other day for up to 8 doses	Nausea and vomiting; hepatotoxicity	Myelosuppression; hypocalcemia	Embryonal carcinoma of testis
Doxorubicin	60 mg/m^2 body surface area i.v. every 3–4 weeks	Nausea and vomiting; local irritant	Myelosuppression; alopecia; cardiac damage; stomatitis	Sarcomas; lymphomas; breast cancer; thyroid cancer
Bleomycin	10–15 units/m^2 1 or 2 times/week	Nausea, vomiting; fever, anaphylaxis	Pulmonary fibrosis; alopecia; stomatitis; edema	Hodgkin's and non-Hodgkin's lymphomas; cancer of head and neck
Hormones				
Prednisone	10–100 mg/day p.o.	None	Hyperadrenocorticism	Leukemia; lymphoma; multiple myeloma; breast cancer
Diethylstilbestrol (DES)	1, 5, or 15 mg/day p.o. (1 mg in prostate)	None	Hypercalcemia; fluid retention; feminization; uterine bleeding; may cause vaginal carcinoma of offspring when given during pregnancy	Breast and prostatic carcinoma
Medroxy progesterone acetate (Provera)	100–200 mg/day p.o.; 200–600 mg 2 times/week	None	None	Endometrial carcinoma; renal cell carcinoma

latory site to alter the catalytic rate of the enzyme.

Of the many antimetabolites developed and tested in the last 30 years, only 5 are commercially available and widely used in the treatment of cancer: methotrexate (MTX, Methotrexate); 5-fluorouracil (5-FU, Fluorouracil); cytarabine (ara-C, Cytosar); 6-mercaptopurine (6-MP, Purinethol); and 6-thioguanine (6-TG, Thioguanine).

With the exception of 5-fluorouracil, the clinically useful antimetabolites are cell cycle phase specific.

Methotrexate

Methotrexate is a structural analogue of folic acid and competes avidly for the folate binding site of dihydrofolate reductase (DHFR). Tight but reversible binding by methotrexate blocks the synthesis of tetrahydrofolate and depletes folate cofactors, resulting primarily in the decreased synthesis of thymidine and purine nucleotides.

The cytotoxicity of methotrexate can be reversed by leukovorin (citrovorum factor, 5-formyl tetrahydrofolate). Leukovorin is readily converted to other forms of reduced folate within the cell, which can then act as methyl donors for various biochemical reactions. Methotrexate may be given in massive doses followed by citrovorum factor as a "rescue" therapy. This procedure is currently experimental, although the use of leukovorin after intrathecal methotrexate administration for patients with central nervous system leukemia is a well-accepted regimen.

5-Fluorouracil

5-Fluorouracil is a structural analogue of the DNA precursor uracil. Other analogues are available, including FUdR (floxuridine) and the experimental agent ftorafur.

5-Fluorouracil works primarily as an irreversible inhibitor of thymidylate synthetase, but only after intracellular conversion to the active metabolite 5-fluorodeoxyuridylate. A lesser and probably undesirable action is the formation of 5-fluorouridylate, which can inhibit RNA synthesis. 5-Fluorouracil is degraded in the liver and some other tissues. The degradative enzymes are found in high concentrations in the gut but not in colonic carcinomas; this finding may partly explain the susceptibility of colonic carcinomas to 5-FU. The balance between the degradative and activating pathways of 5-FU may have clinical relevance.

Cytarabine

Cytarabine is a nucleoside analogue of cytosine that requires activation by intracellular kinases to ara-CTP triphosphate. The activated triphosphate, which competitively inhibits DNA polymerase, is highly phase specific for the S phase of the cell cycle. Thus cytarabine is most effective when given as a continuous infusion or as multiple small doses rather than as a single, large intermittent dose.

Purine Analogues

Mammalian cells require preformed purines or those made *de novo* within the cells as essential components of RNA, DNA, and coenzymes. Two purine antagonists, *6-mercaptopurine* (6-MP; Purinethol) and *6-thioguanine* (6-TG; Thioguanine) developed by Hitchings in 1952 remain useful today. Closely related compounds of clinical importance are *azathioprine* (Imuran) and *allopurinol* (Zyloprim). Azathioprine is a structural analogue of 6-MP with important immunosuppressive properties. Allopurinol is a potent xanthine oxidase inhibitor useful in oncology.

Both 6-MP and 6-TG undergo extensive metabolic changes *in vivo*. Both require activation to their respective ribonucleotides for cytotoxicity. 6-Thioguanine undergoes subsequent metabolism leading to incorporation into DNA as a false purine base. This appears to be its major mechanism of action, although an additional cytotoxic effect relates to its incorporation into RNA. After phosphorylation to the ribotide, 6-MP may be converted to 6-TG ribotide or one of its products, and thus be incorporated into DNA. However, it may also directly inhibit the conversion of aminoimidazolecarboxamide ribotide (AICR) to inosine or may indirectly inhibit AICR synthesis after conversion to a methylated form, 6-methyl-mercaptopurine-ribotide (6MMPR).

Xanthine oxidase is necessary to degrade 6-MP and 6-MMPR. Thus the dose of 6-MP must be reduced by 60% or 70% in the patient who receives allopurinol. Such a dose reduction is not necessary with 6-TG because its catabolism is not mediated by xanthine oxidase.

Both 6-MP and 6-TG are used almost exclusively to treat acute leukemia and are considered to be cell cycle phase specific. The

---

GEORGE HERBERT HITCHINGS, 1905– . American biochemist. Inventor of many chemotherapeutic drugs, including mercaptopurine. Also developed antimalarials, allopurinol for gout therapy, and azathioprine for autoimmune disease and transplantation.

6-thiopurines are not cross-resistant to other chemotherapeutic drugs but are cross-resistant to each other. Both are immunosuppressive and mutagenic.

CLINICAL USE OF ANTICANCER DRUGS

Before initiating therapy for any patient with cancer, it is essential to define clearly the goals of therapy. Both the *quality* and *quantity* of life are important considerations. In general, the effect of treatment on the quantity of life has traditionally been assessed by the duration of expected survival for finite periods of time, and frequently the word "cure" is evoked for patients who are expected to live for 5 or more years. Increasingly, however, the word cure is being limited to the situation where a population of patients with a given kind of cancer may be expected to have a survival curve parallel to that of the normal age- and sex-matched population at some subsequent point after therapy. Death may come early, but at some point in the future course of the group of patients the survival curves should parallel each other.

In this sense cure is not a common accompaniment of cancer chemotherapy but nevertheless does occur in some selected neoplasms, including some forms of acute leukemia and malignant lymphomas, choriocarcinoma, testicular cancer, and some tumors of childhood. Nevertheless, substantial prolongation of life may be possible with chemotherapy so that cure is not the only consideration in deciding whether to use an aggressive and potentially dangerous form of chemotherapy. On the other hand, when one considers primarily the quality of life without any great expectation of prolonged survival, the goal of therapy is palliation. In this setting, treatment is primarily directed at reducing symptoms and improving the quality of life.

Although a detailed statement of the principles of clinical treatment are beyond the scope of this book, certain basic tenets for the use of cancer chemotherapeutic agents in the clinical setting should be clear. Generally the following guidelines have proved useful.

1. Use chemotherapeutic agents only when a diagnosis of malignancy has been established histologically.
2. Determine whether the particular malignancy is known to respond to treatment in a reasonable percentage of cases with a beneficial outcome for the patient or whether the treatment is a useful adjunct to surgery or radiation therapy in the management or cure of malignancy.
3. Do not use chemotherapeutic agents unless there are adequate facilities to monitor the potential toxicity of the agents to the patient's normal tissues.
4. Follow objective markers of the tumor, if possible, to determine tumor response to chemotherapy.

Table 71-4 summarizes the current role of antineoplastic drugs in the treatment of can-

TABLE 71-4. Role of Antineoplastic Agents in the Treatment of Cancer

*Chemotherapy Very Useful (Patient Benefit > 50%)**
Trophoblastic tumors
Burkitt's lymphoma
Acute lymphoblastic leukemia
Hodgkin's disease
Histiocytic lymphoma
Lymphocytic lymphoma
Testicular tumors
Wilms' tumor
Ewing's sarcoma
Osteosarcoma (adjuvant chemotherapy only)
Embryonal rhabdomyosarcoma of childhood
Carcinoma of breast
Chemotherapy Moderately Useful (Patient Benefit 20–50%)
Acute nonlymphocytic leukemia
Carcinoma of ovary
Chronic myelogenous and lymphocytic leukemia
Multiple myeloma
Carcinoma of prostate
Carcinoma of endometrium
Adrenal carcinoma
Adult sarcomas
Oat-cell carcinoma of lung
Islet-cell carcinomas
Chemotherapy Rarely Useful (Patient Benefit < 20%)
Carcinoma of bowel and stomach
Bronchogenic carcinoma other than oat cell
Head and neck carcinoma
Carcinoma of cervix
Melanoma
Neuroblastoma
Brain tumors
Bladder carcinomas
Renal carcinomas
Pancreatic, liver, and bile duct carcinomas
Carcinoid tumors

(Haskell CM: Cancer Treatment. Philadelphia, W B Saunders, 1980)

* An objective partial or complete response with subjective benefit lasting 6 months or longer is required for "patient benefit." The approximate percentage of patients who benefit is given for each group.

cer. Those readers interested in a more thorough discussion of the principles and implementation of cancer chemotherapy in clinical medicine are referred to standard works on this subject (*see* Further Reading).

FURTHER READING

1. Cline MJ, Haskell CM: Cancer Chemotherapy, 3rd ed. Philadelphia, W B Saunders, 1980
2. Haskell CM (ed): Cancer treatment, 2nd ed. Philadelphia, W B Saunders, 1984.
3. Livingston RB, Carter SK: Single Agents in Cancer Chemotherapy. New York, Plenum Publishing Corporation, 1970
4. Pratt WB, Ruddon RW: The Anticancer Drugs. New York, Oxford University Press, 1979

CHAPTER 71 QUESTIONS

(*See* P. 7 for Full Instructions)

Select the One Best Answer

1. Drugs effective in the treatment of acute leukemias include all of the following EXCEPT
   - *A.* 6-mercaptopurine.
   - *B.* methotrexate.
   - *C.* 5-fluorouracil.
   - *D.* prednisone.
   - *E.* vincristine.
2. An agent characterized by its usefulness in treating leukemia and by its increased toxicity in the presence of allopurinol is
   - *A.* azothioprine.
   - *B.* thioguanine.
   - *C.* arabinosylcytosine.
   - *D.* methotrexate.
   - *E.* 6-mercaptopurine.
3. Treatment of choriocarcinoma was revolutionized by the introduction of
   - *A.* 5-fluorouracil.
   - *B.* vincristine.
   - *C.* nitrogen mustard.
   - *D.* cytarabine.
   - *E.* methotrexate.
4. Cancer chemotherapeutic agents considered antimetabolites include all of the following EXCEPT
   - *A.* busulfan.
   - *B.* 6-mercaptopurine.
   - *C.* methotrexate.
   - *D.* thioguanine.
   - *E.* arabinosylcytosine.
5. The toxic effects of methotrexate can be counteracted by
   - *A.* adenine.
   - *B.* folinic acid (citrovorum factor).
   - *C.* cyanocobalamin.
   - *D.* para-aminobenzoic acid.
   - *E.* glutamic acid.

A = 1,2,3, B = 1,3, C = 2,4, D = 4, E = All

6. 6-Thioguanine
   1. must be converted to a ribotide for antitumor activity.
   2. has antitumor action that is antagonized by allopurinol.
   3. is incorporated into DNA as a "false" precursor base.
   4. must be given parenterally for therapeutic effect.
7. Cancer cells are killed in only one portion of the cell cycle if the chemotherapeutic agent is
   1. nitrogen mustard.
   2. methotrexate.
   3. doxorubicin.
   4. arabinosylcytosine.
8. Anticancer agents that are antimetabolites include
   1. vincristine.
   2. 5-fluorouracil.
   3. dactinomycin.
   4. 6-mercaptopurine.
9. Resistance to methotrexate may develop in tumor cells by a mechanism involving
   1. impaired influx of methotrexate into the cell.
   2. altered affinity of dihydrofolate reductase for methotrexate.
   3. increased levels of dihydrofolate reductase.
   4. the emergence of repair enzymes.
10. Which of the following drugs must be transformed in the body before it becomes a biologically active antiproliferative agent?
    1. Azathioprine
    2. L-arparaginase
    3. Cyclophosphamide
    4. Methotrexate

THREE

Special Topics and Reference Material

72

JAY M. ARENA

General Principles of Treatment of Poisons and Their Available Antidotes

The causes of poisoning are many: accidental and deliberate, civilian and industrial. In pediatric patients, the chief etiologic factors are poor or faulty child supervision and parental unawareness of the problem. Each year more than 1 million incidents of poisoning occur in the United States, with over 3000 deaths, including those from gases and vapors. About one half of those deaths are accidental, and one third occur in children younger than 5 years of age. In fact, poisoning is the most common *medical* emergency among young children. These are somber statistics for a mechanism of injury and death that is largely preventable.

The above figures are undoubtedly much too low. Many more children die each year from the accidental ingestion of, or exposure to, toxic chemicals in household agents or drugs, but the correct diagnosis is never made because incriminating evidence is not detected or recognized. The natural curiosity of children to learn by exploration, questioning, sampling, and trial and error leads them to investigate more than a quarter of a million household products and a myriad of drugs that are now available. With the increasing number of potentially toxic household agents and family drugs in our homes, this problem, enormous now, promises to be even more serious in the next decade.

When an acutely ill person (particularly a child) with a bizarre chain of signs and symptoms is seen and presents an obscure and uncertain diagnosis, ingestion of a drug or exposure to a toxic chemical compound should always be considered. In patients who have not been observed to ingest or to have contact with a poison, the problem of an accurate diagnosis can be a most difficult one. Many symptoms and signs are tabulated as a quick aid in diagnosis (Table 72-1).

Treatment for acute poisoning, whether drug or chemical, is mainly symptomatic and supportive. Overtreatment of the poisoned patient with large doses of stimulants, sedatives, and other therapeutic agents (nonspecific antidotes) often does much more damage than the

(Text continues on p. 748)

OREY H. COSTILL. Wrote his inaugural dissertation on chlorosis in 1821. The first edition of his *A Practical Treatise on Poisons* appeared in 1848, a book that, for the first time, set out the symptoms and treatment for various types of poisoning as a ready reference for physicians.

TABLE 72-1. Signs and Symptoms of Poisoning*

Sign or Symptom	Poison
Eye	
Dilatation of pupil (mydriasis)	Belladonna group, meperidine, alcohols, ether, chloroform, papaverine, sympathomimetics, parasympatholytics, antihistamines, gelsemium, cocaine, camphor, aconitine, benzene, barium, thallium, botulinus toxin, cyanide, carbon monoxide, carbon dioxide
Constriction of pupil (miosis)	Opium, morphine group, sympatholytics (ergot), parasympathomimetics, dibenamine, barbiturates, cholinesterase inhibitors, chloral hydrate, picrotoxin, nicotine, caffeine
Purple-yellow vision	Marihuana, digitalis, carbon monoxide, santonin
Blurred vision	Belladonna group (atropine), methyl alcohol, ethyl alcohol, ergot, carbon tetrachloride, irreversible cholinesterase inhibitors (DFP, TEPP, HETP), vesicant war gases (mustard gas), camphor
Partial or total blindness	Methyl alcohol
Photophobia, lacrimation, pain	Vesicant war gases (mustard gas), Mace, tear gases (bromacetone, others)
Face and scalp	
Dull and masklike expression	Barbiturates, bromides, gelsemine, manganese, thallium
Facial twitchings	Lead, mercury
Alopecia	Thallium, arsenic, ergot, hypervitaminosis A, gold, lead, boric acid, thiocyanates
Skin and mucous membranes	
Pale	Aniline derivatives, colchicine, sympathomimetics (epinephrine), insulin, pilocarpine
Livid, ashy pale	Dinitrocresol, dinitrophenol, ergot, lead, phenacetin
Cyanotic, brown-bluish (in absence of respiratory depression and shock)	Nitrobenzene, chlorates, acetanilids, carbon dioxide, methane, nitrous oxide, aniline derivatives, nitrites, morphine, sulfides, ergot, amyl nitrite, and well over 100 other drugs and chemicals
Pink	Carbon monoxide, cyanides
Yellow	Atabrine; jaundice from hepatic injury (chlorinated compounds, arsenic and other heavy metals, chromates, mushrooms, and many drugs); jaundice from hemolytic anemias (aniline, nitrobenzene, quinine derivatives, arsine, fava beans, and many drugs)
Sweating	Pilocarpine, nicotine, physostigmine, picrotoxin
Dry, hot skin	Belladonna group (atropine), botulinus toxin
Blue-gray	Silver salts
Local coloring of the skin	
Brown, black	Iodine, silver nitrate
Deep brown	Bromine
Yellow	Nitric acid, picric acid
White	Phenol derivatives
Gray	Mercuric chloride
Nervous system	
Coma	Morphine derivatives and analogues, all hypnotics, sedatives and general anesthetics, barbiturates, chloral hydrate, sulfonal, trional, paraldehyde, chloroform, ethers, bromides, alcohols, lead, cyanide, carbon monoxide, carbon dioxide, nicotine, benzene, atropine, phenols, scopolamine, xylene, irreversible cholinesterase inhibitors, (DFP, TEPP, HETP, parathion), insulin, aniline derivatives, mushrooms, salicylates, copper salts
Delirium, mental disturbances	Belladeonna group (atropine, hyoscine), cocaine, alcohol, lead, marihuana, arsenic, ergot, amphetamine and derivatives, antihistamines, camphor, benzene, barbiturates, DDT, aniline derivatives, physostigmine, veratrine, nerve gases (DFP, TEPP)
Convulsions	Strychnine, picrotoxin, camphor, santonin, cocaine, belladonna group (atropine), veratrine, aconite, irreversible cholinesterase inhibitors (DFP, TEPP, HETP, parathion), pentylenetetrazol, amphetamine and derivatives, ergot, nicotine, lead, antipyrine, barium, sodium fluoroacetate, mushrooms, caffeine, carbon monoxide, cyanides, salicylates, copper salts

(continued)

TABLE 72-1. (*Continued*)

Sign or Symptom	Poison
Headache	Carbon monoxide, phenol, benzene, nitrobenzene, nitrates, nitrites, aniline, lead, indomethacin (Indocin)
Muscle spasms	Atropine, cadmium, strychnine, copper salts, bites of black widow spider, scorpion, and sting ray
General or partial paralysis	Carbon monoxide, carbon dioxide, botulinus toxin, alcohols, physostigmine, curare group, DDT, aconite, nicotine, barium, cyanide, mercury, arsenic, lead
Gastrointestinal tract	
Nausea, vomiting, diarrhea, dehydration, abdominal pain	Heavy metal salts, corrosive acids and alkalies, halogens, cathartics (croton oil, castor oil), ergot, nicotine, aconitine, cantharides, solanine, acetanilid and derivatives, phosphorus, phenols, cresol, methyl alcohol muscarine, cardioactive glycosides (digitalis), fluorides, morphine and analogues, DDT, irreversible cholinesterase inhibitors (DFP, TEPP, HETP, OMPA, parathion), pilocarpine, veratrine, colchicine botulinus toxin, mushrooms, boric acid and sodium borate, cocaine, procaine and local anesthetics, salicylates
"Burning" throat and stomach	Camphor, picrotoxin, iodine, arsenicals, antimony compounds
Abnormal color of feces	
Pink to red to black (resulting from internal bleeding)	Salicylates, anticoagulants
Orange-red	Phenazopyridine (Pyridium)
Whitish	Antacids, such as aluminum hydroxide preparations
Blue	Dithiazinine (Delvex)
Red	Pyrvinium pamoate (Povan)
Black	Bismuth sodium triglycollamate (Bristrimate), bismuth glycolylarsanilate (Milibis), bismuth subsalicylate (Pepto-Bismol), iron preparations
Brownish staining of rectal mucosa	1,8-Dihydroxyanthraquinone (Dorbane, Doxan)
Odor of vomitus, breath, or body fluids	
Phenolic	Phenols, cresol
Etheric, ethereal sweet	Ether
Sweet	Chloroform, acetone
Bitter almondlike	Cyanides, Laetrile
Stale tobaccolike	Nicotine
Pearlike	Chloral hydrate
Alcoholic	Alcohols
Garliclike	Phosphorus, tellurium, arsenic, malathion
Shoe polishlike	Nitrobenzene
Violets	Turpentine
Colored material in gastric lavage or vomitus	
Pink or purple	Potassium permanganate
Blue, green	Copper salts, chemical dyes added to fluorides or mercury bichloride
Green	Nickel salts
Pink	Cobalt salts
Yellow	Picric acid, nitric acid
Bright red	Mercurochrome, nitric acid
Black, coffeelike grounds	Sulfuric acid, oxalic acid, nitric acid
Brown	Hydrochloric acid
Luminescent in dark	Yellow phosphorus
Discolored, bloody	Alkalis
Mouth	
Excess salivation	Ammonia, cantharides, pilocarpine, arecoline, physostigmine, muscarine, nicotine, mercury, irreversible cholinesterase inhibitors (DFP, HETP, TEPP), salicylates
Dry mouth	Belladonna group (atropine), botulinus toxin, barium, diphenhydramine, ephedrine

(*continued*)

TABLE 72-1. *(Continued)*

Sign or Symptom	Poison
Ears	
Impaired hearing ("roaring")	Salicylates, quinine, streptomycin, and other aminoglycoside antibiotics
"Buzzing"	Camphor, tobacco, ergot, methyl alcohol, quinidine
Genitourinary system	
Uterine cramps, uterine bleeding, abortion	Phosphorus, lead, pilocarpine, physostigmine, nicotine, ergot, quinine, mustard, cantharides, apiol, cathartics (croton oil, castor oil)
Abnormal color of urine:	
Blue	Methylene blue
Brown to black	Aniline dyes, cascara, chlorinated hydrocarbons, hydroxyquinone, melanin, methocarbamol (Robaxin), naphthalene, naphthol, nitrites, nitrofurans—furazolidone (Furoxone), nitrofurazone (Furacin)—phenol, phenyl salicylate (salol), pyrogallol, quinine, resorcinol (resorcin), rhubarb, santonin, senna, thymol
Green (blue plus yellow)	Anthraquinone, arbutin, bile pigments, eosins, methocarbamol (Robaxin), methylene blue, resorcinol (resorcin), tetrahydronaphthalene, thymol
Magenta to purple	Fuchsin, phenolphthalein
Orange	Indandione derivatives in alkaline urine: anisindione (Miradon), diphenadione (Dipaxin), phenindione (Danilone, Eridione, Hedulin)
Orange to orange-red	Phenylazopyridine (Pyridium)
Orange to red-brown	Combinations of phenylazopyridine (Pyridium) and other drugs used as urinary antiseptics; many of the trade names begin with Azo-; also santonin
Pink and red to red-brown	Aminopyrine, dipyrone, anthraquinone and its dyes, antipyrine (Pyrazoline), beets, chrysarobin (alkaline urine), cinchophen, danthron (Dorbane) (pink to violet in alkaline urine), deferoxamine (Desferal) (with elevated serum iron), phenytoin (Dilantin), emodin (alkaline urine), eosins (red with green fluorescence), hematuria producers (mercuric salts, irritants, others), hemolysis producers, phenindione (Danilone, Hedulin), phenolic metabolites (glucuronides), phenolphthalein (alkaline urine), phensuximide (Milontin), porphyrins, prochlorperazine (Compazine), rhodamine B (a food dye), santonin (alkaline urine), thiazolsulfone (Promizole), urates (especially in newborn infants and during tumor lysis)
Rust	Chlorzoxazone (Paraflex)
Yellowish or brownish	Danthron (Dionone, Dorbane, Istizin) (acid urine), heavy metals (bismuth, mercury), liver poisons (jaundice)—alcohol, arsenicals, carbon tetrachloride, chloral hydrate, chlorinated hydrocarbons, chlorobutanol (chlorbutol, Chloretone), chloroform, cinchophen—naphthalene, neocinchophen, nitrofurantoins, pamaquine (Aminoquin), Beprochine, Gamefar, Plasmoquine, Praequine, Quipenyl, sulfonamides, tribromomethanol with amylene hydrate (Avertin)
Yellow or green	Carotene-containing foods, methylene blue, riboflavin, vitamin B complex, yeast concentrate
Respiratory system	
Slow respiration	Opium, morphine derivatives and analogs, chloral hydrate, alcohols, picrotoxin, fluorides, cyanides
Rapid or deep respiration, or both	Belladonna group (atropine), cocaine, amphetamine and derivatives, strychnine, carbon dioxide, lobeline, salicylates, nikethamide, camphor
Dyspnea	Cyanides, carbon monoxide, volatile organic solvents (benzene), snake venoms, suffocating war gases (phosgene), carbon dioxide
Respiratory paralysis	Morphine derivatives and analogues, general anesthesia, hypnotics and sedatives (barbiturates), alcohols, snake venoms, carbon monoxide
Edema (pulmonary)	Chlorine, bromine, phosgene, methyl perchloroformate
Burning pain in chest and throat	Tear gases
Sneezing	Adamsite, Clarc I, Clarc II
Restlessness	Caffeine, amphetamines
Laryngitis, coughing	Vesicant war gases (mustard gas, Lewisite, others), nerve gases (DFP, TEPP)
Difficult breathing	Alkalis

(continued)

TABLE 72-1. (*Continued*)

Sign or Symptom	Poison
Cardiovascular system	
Slow pulse (bradycardia)	Barium, aconite, cardioactive glycosides (digitalis), muscarine, physostigmine, pilocarpine, quinine, quinidine, veratrine, picrotoxin, lead
Fast pulse (tachycardia)	Amphetamine and derivatives, atropine, cocaine, sympathomimetics (ephedrine), epinephrine, phenylephrine, caffeine, alkalis
Angina pectoris-type pain	Nicotine
Pain in heart area	Sternutators (Adamsite, Clarc I, Clarc II)
Hypotension	Chloral hydrate, alkalies, nitrites, nitrates, quinine, volatile oils, iron salts, chlorpromazine (Thorazine)
Hypertension	Epinephrine or substitute, veratrum (large doses), ergot, cortisone, vanadium, lead, nicotine, amphetamines
Vascular collapse	Leads, acids, alkalis

* Material taken largely from Arena JM: Poisoning: Toxicology, Symptoms, Treatment, 4th ed. Springfield, Illinois, Charles C Thomas, 1979.

poison itself. A calm attitude with the judicious use of drugs, electrolytes, and the maintenance of an adequate airway is far more effective than heroic measures, which usually are unnecessary. As a matter of fact, it is impossible at times to determine whether recovery occurred because of, or despite, the treatment used.

SPECIFIC THERAPEUTIC MEASURES

VOMITING

When poisons have been taken orally, the stomach should be emptied quickly. This is the most important treatment that one can use, and there should be no procrastination. Most poisons are in themselves emetics, but if vomiting does not occur spontaneously it should be induced where possible, if not contraindicated. (Contraindications include ingestion of corrosives, strychnine, or petroleum distillates (unless containing toxic chemicals or pesticides or an unusually large amount has been ingested); and coma.) In children, when syrup of ipecac is not available in the home, vomiting is best induced by having them drink a glass of water or milk, then gagging them with a finger (with precautions to prevent biting) or by stroking the posterior pharynx with a blunt object. To prevent aspiration in small children, the body should be inverted with the head down, but supported, and the feet elevated. Syrup of ipecac (not the fluid extract), if available, may be given in doses of 10 to 15 ml and repeated once in 15 to 30 minutes if emesis does not occur. Fluids (1–2 glasses) should be given several minutes before the ipecac is swallowed, since emesis may not occur if the stomach is empty. For adults, the ipecac may be given in one dose (30 ml) and before the fluids, but children are stubborn about taking anything after they have been forced to swallow ipecac. Use of larger doses of ipecac, if ineffective, makes gastric lavage doubly imperative because, when left in the stomach, it is an irritant and, when absorbed, it is a specific cardiotoxin that can produce disturbances of conduction, atrial fibrillation, or fatal myocarditis. The contraindications for using ipecac are the same as those for gastric lavage. If more than 1 hour has elapsed since an antiemetic drug has been ingested, ipecac should not be used. Salt water as an emetic may be dangerous (hypernatremia) and should not be used in children, and mustard is impractical.

The injection of apomorphine, 0.066 mg/kg subcutaneously, for prompt emesis followed by naloxone HCl, 0.01 mg/kg intravenously, intramuscularly, or subcutaneously to terminate both the emetic and narcotic effects of apomorphine (the use of this narcotic antagonist can be omitted in most instances) is gaining widespread acceptance and is being used at many poison control centers. For best results, water (1–2 glasses) should be given beforehand (also true for the use of syrup of ipecac), since emesis does not occur readily if the stomach is empty. This therapy has three very distinct advantages: rapid vomiting (within 3–5 minutes) with emptying of all gastric contents; no obstruction of lavage tubes that may produce delays and incomplete emptying; and reflux of contents (*e.g.*, enteric coated tablets) from the upper intestinal tract into the stomach. This treatment, however, should not be used if the patient is greatly depressed or comatose or if the apormorphine solution is green, which indicates decomposition of the tablet.

GASTRIC LAVAGE

If vomiting cannot be induced or is contraindicated, gastric lavage should be instituted at once. Gastric lavage is clearly indicated within 3 hours after ingestion of a poison and even later (up to 8 hours) if enteric coated drugs or large amounts of milk or cream have been recently taken. There are, however, certain contraindications, including [1] ingestion of strong corrosive agents, such as alkali (concentrated ammonia, lye) or mineral acids (lavage probably can safely be carried out within 1 hour of ingestion); [2] ingestion of strychnine (a convulsion may be induced if much time has elapsed); [3] ingestion of clear petroleum distillates (kerosene, mineral seal oil); and [4] coma with depression of cough reflex (aspiration pneumonia may occur).

In children, the only equipment needed is a common urethral catheter (8–12 French) and a syringe (20 or 50 ml). Davol plastic duodenal tubes are preferable because of their durability, flexibility, and ease of passage with lubrication. For adults, a tube with a diameter between $^{5}/_{16}$ and $^{1}/_{2}$ (about 1 cm), 24F or greater, is usually satisfactory. The larger the tube that can be passed, the more rapidly the lavage can be completed.

In older children and adults the nasal route is preferred. However, oral passage is easier and less traumatic for infants and young children. The distance from the bridge of the nose to the tip of the xiphoid process should be marked on the lavage tube with adhesive tape before passage. Passage will be facilitated by immersing the tube in cold water or a water miscible jelly (avoid oils). Dentures and other foreign objects should be removed from the mouth. Restraints will be needed for most children. In centers where anesthesiologists are readily available, patients can be lightly anesthetized, given succinylcholine, and lavaged after inserting into the trachea an endotracheal tube with an inflatable cuff; or a fiberoptic endoscope can be used. (In most community hospitals and in physicians' offices, this method, although ideal, is impractical.)

The patient should be placed on his left side with his head hanging over the edge of the examining table and with his face down. If possible, the foot of the bed or table should be elevated. This position is particularly important if the patient is drowsy, since the chances of aspiration are thus minimized. The tube should be passed gently since no great force is necessary. If the patient will cooperate, have him swallow frequently; this allows the tube to move easily and rapidly. If the catheter enters the larynx instead of the esophagus, dyspnea and severe coughing are produced, but not if the patient is deeply narcotized. If the tube enters the larynx, it should be partially withdrawn before proceeding. If in doubt as to the placement of the tube, one should dip the free end in a glass of water; continuous bubbling on expiration implies placement in the trachea, whereas gas from the stomach is usually expelled in two or three bursts. In every instance, aspiration should be performed before instilling the lavage solution or antidote. When the tube has reached the stomach, the glass syringe is then attached and the stomach contents aspirated.

The fluid ordinarily used for lavage is tap water that contains an antidote, if one is available. However, the substitution of isotonic or one-half isotonic saline solution is far safer, particularly for children who have a limited tolerance for electrolyte depletion. A 5% increase in body fluid volume with electrolyte free water is sufficient to initiate the cardinal symptoms of water intoxication, which are tonic and clonic seizures with coma. These may start without prodromes.

Only small amounts of fluids should be instilled at once so that the passage of the poison into the upper intestinal tract will not be promoted. Lavage should be repeated 10 to 12 times or until the returns are clear. All washings should be saved, with the first separated from the others, for any analyses that might be indicated. As soon as the lavage is completed, an antidote, if indicated, should be instilled through the tube and allowed to remain in the stomach. Before the catheter is withdrawn, it should be pinched off or suction should be maintained to prevent aspiration.

Recently, a device consisting of a double lumen tube designed to deliver and aspirate simultaneously (or separately) has allowed the entire procedure of gastric lavage to be done in as little as 5 minutes.

Lavaging Fluids

The following substances are useful but seldom needed in gastric lavage.

1. *Tannic acid* is mildly acidic (for neutralizing strong alkalis, diluted acetic acid is more effective) and precipitates a large number of organic and inorganic compounds, including alkaloids, metals, and

some glucosides. The tannates formed often redissolve and hydrolyze later, and therefore should not be allowed to remain in the stomach. About 30 to 50 g of tannic acid in 1000 ml of water is an effective concentration. Among the compounds rapidly precipitated by tannic acid are apomorphine, hydrastine, strychnine, veratrine, cinchona alkaloids, and salts of aluminum, lead, and silver. Because of its hepatotoxic properties, tannic acid should be used carefully and only in the recommended dilutions.

2. *Potassium permanganate* is an oxidizing agent that reacts well with organic substances. It effectively neutralizes such compounds as strychnine, nicotine, physostigmine, and quinine. Because potassium permanganate is itself a strong irritant, it must be well diluted (about 1:10,000, and not stronger than 1:5000) and no undissolved particles should come in contact with the stomach or other tissues. A thoroughly dissolved 5% solution should be kept on hand to be diluted to the needed strength. A 1:10,000 solution may be prepared by dissolving 0.1 g in 1 liter of water or 1 g may be dissolved in 100 ml of water and 10 ml of this solution added to 1000 ml of water to make a 1:10,000 solution.
3. *Dairy or evaporated milk* may be used. Evaporated milk may be diluted with equal parts of water or used without dilution, particularly when the demulcent action is desired—for example, with copper sulfate, croton oil, chlorates, and thioglycollic acid.
4. *Sodium bicarbonate* in a 5% solution is advised for gastric lavage in cases of ferrous sulfate poisoning since it forms the less corrosive and more insoluble ferrous carbonate. The bicarbonate, although an effective alkaline solution, is usually not recommended for neutralizing acids because the liberated CO_2 might cause increased gastric distension and thus predispose the patient to perforation if the stomach wall has been partly corroded by the acid.
5. *Calcium salts* are helpful in fluoride and oxalate poisoning and in preventing tetany from hypocalcemia in certain types of poisoning. Lavage with a dilute solution of calcium lactate is recommended for many of these toxic substances. About 15 to 30 g of calcium lactate (or gluconate) in 1000 ml of water may be used. Calcium chloride, 4 g in 1000 ml of water, is an alternate treatment.
6. *Magnesium oxide* (or hydroxide) is used primarily as a neutralizing agent for acidic substances, including aspirin, sulfuric and other mineral acids, and oxalic acid. It does not release CO_2 to distend the stomach, and if too much is not allowed to remain in the stomach the depressant effect of magnesium on the central nervous system is negligible. About 25 g of magnesium oxide in 1000 ml of water is the recommended concentration.
7. *A starch solution* is considered particularly effective in neutralizing iodine. About 75 to 80 g of starch in 1000 ml of water is used and the lavage continued until the return fluid is no longer blue.
8. *Ammonium acetate* or dilute ammonia water, about 4 ml in 500 ml of water, combines with formaldehyde to form relatively harmless methenamine.
9. *Normal saline solution* (0.8% or about 1 teaspoon of salt in 1 pint of water) is an effective gastric lavage solution for silver nitrate because it reacts with it to form a relatively insoluble and noncorrosive silver chloride.
10. *Activated charcoal* is the residue from destructive distillation of various organic materials, treated to increase its absorptive powers; vegetable charcoals made from wood pulp, which has a low ash content, are particularly useful. This is a potent absorbent that rapidly inactivates many poisons, if given early before much of the poison has been absorbed (Table 72-2). It is effective for virtually all chemicals (except cyanide, ferrous sulfate, alcohols, boric acid, and corrosives), whether they be organic, inorganic, large or small molecule compounds (Table 72-3). The potency of absorption is not reduced by the acidity or alkalinity of the poison or by a wide range of *p*H in the gastrointestinal tract. Absorbed material is retained tenaciously throughout passage in the gut.

Activated charcoal is one of the best, least expensive, and most practical emergency antidotes available. One to two tablespoonsful in an 8-ounce glass of water or a mixture of soupy consistency would be a suitable concentration for oral use or lavaging. Bone chars are not effective because of their high mineral content, and mineral charcoals are little used.

We have had favorable experience with five commercial activated charcoals on the American market: Activated Charcoal (Merck Sharp

TABLE 72-2. Approximate Amount of Substance Adsorbed by 1 g of Charcoal

Adsorbendum	Maximum Adsorption
	mg
Mercuric chloride	1800
Sulfanilamide	1000
Strychnine nitrate	950
Morphine hydrochloride	800
Atropine sulfate	700
Nicotine	700
Barbital (Veronal)	700
Barbital sodium (Medinal)	150
Phenobarbital sodium (Luminal)	
Alurate sodium	
Dial sodium (Dial)	300–350
Evipal sodium	
Phanodorn calcium	
Salicylic acid	550
Phenol	400
Alcohol	300
Potassium cyanide	35

& Dohme, West Point, PA; most effective in *in vivo* tests); Norit A (American Norit Co., Jacksonville, FL); Darco G 60 (Atlas Powder Co., Wilmington, DE); Nuchar C (West Virginia Pulp and Paper Co., New York, NY); and Requa's (Requa Manufacturing Co., Brooklyn, NY). Undoubtedly other good ones are available as well.

A minor drawback to activated charcoal is that it is black; thus many children will refuse to drink it, and, if spewed, it spots uniforms, clothes, walls, and personnel. It is hoped that an effective palatable, easier to administer suspension preparation will soon be on the market.

Activated charcoal should not be used simultaneously with syrup of ipecac because it can adsorb the emetic principle and inactivate it. It should be administered only after emesis has been induced successfully.

TABLE 72-3. Some Substances Effectively Adsorbed by Activated Charcoal

Organic Compounds		Inorganic Compounds
Aconite	Muscarine	Antimony
Alcohol	Nicotine	Arsenic
Antipyrine	Opium	Iodine
Atropine	Oxalates	Lead (to limited extent)
Barbiturates	Parathion	
Camphor	Penicillin	Mercuric chloride
Cantharides	Phenol	Phosphorus
Cocaine	Phenolphthalein	Potassium permanganate
Delphinium	Quinine	
Digitalis	Salicylates	Silver
Elaterin	Stramonium	Tin
Hemlock	Strychnine	Titanium
Ipecac	Sulfonamides	
Methylene blue	Veratrum	
Morphine		

ANTIDOTES

Effective and useful specific antidotes for poisoning (Table 72-4) are limited in number, and often their overuse may complicate the initial injury by producing other forms of poisoning. The sensible selection and use of drugs and therapeutic measures for the general and supportive treatment of poisoning are more likely to save lives than the ill-considered and heroically applied specific antidotes. The most useful and practical antidotes now available to the physician for emergency use are outlined in Table 72-5. Because of the frequency of occurrence of barbiturate intoxication its treatments are summarized in Table 72-6, and these treatments, combined with the symptomatic and supportive drugs and measures on hand, are generally all that are needed.

ANTIBIOTICS

Antibiotics are often of considerable value in such inflammatory conditions as pneumonitis, mediastinitis, and peritonitis, which often follow the ingestion of certain toxic substances—petroleum distillates, turpentine, cedar oil, lye, acids, and other corrosives.

An antibiotic should be selected on an individual basis, depending on the severity and nature of the poison. In the hope of forestalling infection, some physicians advise that these antibiotics be administered before the onset of signs and symptoms of infection when it is certain that substantial amounts of the particularly dangerous substances have been swallowed or aspirated into the lungs. Others believe that skilled and discriminating use of antibiotics would exclude their prophylactic use, except in already infected persons, if aspiration occurs or if any indwelling catheter is needed.

(*Text continues on p. 756*)

TABLE 72-4. Antidotes

Antidote	Dose	Poison	Reaction (Antidote) and Comments
Acids, weak	100–200 ml	Alkali, caustic	
Acetic acid, 1%			
Vinegar, 5% acetic acid (diluted 1:4 with water)			
Hydrochloric acid, 0.5%			
Activated charcoal Darco G (Atlas Chem) Nuchar C (W Va Pulp & Paper) Norit A (Am Norit Co)	1–2 tbs to glass water or a mixture of soupy consistency	Effective for virtually all poisons, organic and inorganic compounds of large and small molecules	Broad spectrum of activity No reaction except staining. Not effective for cyanide, corrosives, iron, and boric acid
Alcohol, ethyl	i.v. as 5% solution in bicarbonate or saline solution p.o. as 3–4 oz of whiskey (45%) every 4 hr for 1–3 days	Methyl alcohol Ethylene and other glycols	Competes with methyl alcohol for the hepatic enzyme alcohol dehydrogenase and prevents formation of toxic formic acid and formates; glycols into oxalates
Alkali, weak			
Magnesium oxide (preferred)*	2.5% solution (25 g/liter)	Acid, corrosive	Gastric distension from liberated CO_2 (from use of $NaHCO_3$)
Sodium bicarbonate	5% solution (50 g/liter)		
Ammonium acetate	5 ml in 500 ml water	Formaldehyde (formalin)	Forms relatively harmless methenamine
Ammonium hydroxide	0.2% solution Both are for gastric lavage		
Atropine sulfate	1–2 mg i.m. and repeat in 30 min	Organic phosphate esters and other cholinesterase inhibitors	Atropinization
Barbiturate antidotes			See Table 72-6
Bromobenzene	Adult: 1 g Child: 0.25 g (in lavage solution)	Selenium	
Calcium EDTA	25 to 50 mg/kg, 2% solution 2 times a day	Cadmium	Nephrotoxic
or	for 5 days	Cobalt	Increases urinary potassium excretion
Versene (ethylenediamine tetra-acetate)	50 mg/kg, 20% solution (0.5% procaine) i.m. daily for 5–7 days	Copper Nickel, and other metals Iron	Oral EDTA should not be used until all lead has been removed or absorbed from the gastrointestinal tract
[DTPA: (diethylenetriamine penta-acetic acid), more promising analogue]	Repeat these courses after 2-day rest period	Lead (combined therapy with BAL for encephalitis)	
Calcium lactate	10% solution (in lavage solution	Chlorinated hydrocarbons Fluoride Oxalates	
Calcium gluconate	10% solution, 5–10 ml i.m. or i.v., may be repeated in 8–12 hr	Black widow spider and other insect bites	Muscle relaxant Bradycardia Flushing Local necrosis from perivenous infiltration (methocarbamol, and others also effective)

(continued)

TABLE 72-4. *(Continued)*

Antidote	Dose	Poison	Reaction (Antidote) and Comments
Chlorpromazine†	1–2 mg/kg i.m.	Amphetamine	Drowsiness Hypotension Neuromuscular (parkinsonian)
Copper sulfate	0.25–3.0 g in glass of water	Phosphorus	Forms insoluble copper phosphide
Cyanide poison kit (Eli Lilly stock M76)		Cyanide, Laetrile	Hypotension
Amyl nitrite pearls Sodium nitrite	0.2 ml (inhalation) follow with 3.0% solution (10 ml) in 2–4 min and		
Sodium thiosulfate	25% solution (50 ml) in 10 min through same needle and vein. (repeat with ½ doses if necessary)	Iodine	Sodium thiosulfate used alone for iodine; forms harmless sodium iodide
Deferoxamine B Desferal isolated from *Streptomyces pilosus*	1–2 g i.m. or i.v. (adults), repeat if necessary every 4–12 hr; also 5–10 g via nasogastric tube after gastric lavage	Iron Hemochromatosis	Diarrhea Hypotension
Dimercaprol (BAL)	Severe intoxication Day 1: 3.0 mg/kg every 4 hr (6 inj) Day 2: same Day 3: 3.0 mg/kg every 6 hr (4 inj) Days 4–13 (or until recovery): 3.0 mg/kg every 12 hr (2 inj) Mild intoxication Day 1: 2.5 mg/kg every 4 hr (6 inj) Day 2: same Day 3: 2.5 mg/kg every 12 hr Days 4–13 (or until recovery): 2.5 mg/kg daily (1 inj.)	Antimony Arsenic Bismuth Gold Mercury (acrodynia) Nickel Lead (combined therapy with EDTA for encephalitis) Contraindicated for iron	Flushing Myalgia Nausea and vomiting Nephrotoxicity Hypotension Pulmonary edema Salivation and lacrimation Fever (children)
Diphenhydramine hydrochloride	10–50 mg i.v. or i.m.	Phenothiazine tranquilizers (for extrapyramidal neuromuscular manifestations)	Atropine-like effect Drowsiness
Dithizon	10 mg/kg twice a day orally with 100 ml 10% glucose solution for 5 days	Thallium	Diabetogenic Not available for therapeutic use; may be obtained through a chemical supply company

(continued)

TABLE 72-4. (*Continued*)

Antidote	Dose	Poison	Reaction (Antidote) and Comments
Household antidotes Milk Raw eggs Flour Starches		Arsenic Mercury and other heavy metals Iodine	These are useful and readily available antidotes that can be used in an emergency; all have demulcent properties
Hydrogen peroxide	3% solution (10 ml in 100 ml water as lavage solution)	Potassium permanganate Oxidizing agent for many other compounds	Irritation of mucous membranes Distension of abdomen from release of gas
Iodine, tincture	15 drops in 120 ml water	Precipitant for: Lead Mercury Quinine Silver Strychnine	Precipitants must be thoroughly removed by gastric lavage
Magnesium sulfate	2–5% solution for lavage	Precipitant for: Barium Lead	
Sodium sulfate	10% solution i.m. and repeat in 30 min; also as catharsis for rapid elimination of toxic agent from gastrointestinal tract	Hypervitaminosis D Hypercalcemia (glucocorticoid therapy preferable)	
Methylene blue	i.v.: 1% solution given slowly (2 mg/kg) and repeat in 1 hr if necessary Orally: 3–5 mg/kg (action much slower)	Methemoglobinemia produced by: Acetanilid Aniline derivatives Chlorates Dinitrophenol Nitrites Pyridium Over 100 other chemicals and drugs	Perivenous infiltration can produce severe necrosis Hypertension Hemolysis
Monoacetin (glyceryl monoacetate)	0.5 ml/kg i.m. or in saline solution i.v.; repeat as necessary	Sodium fluoroacetate "1080"	Not available commercially; if parenteral therapy not feasible, can give 100 ml of monoacetin in water
Nalorphine	Adult: 5–10 mg i.m. or i.v. and repeat in ½ hr Child: 0.1–0.2 mg/kg i.m. or i.v. and repeat in ½ hr	Codeine Demerol Dionin Heroin	Withdrawal symptoms Depressant effects in other than narcotic compounds
Levallorphan and	Adult: 0.5–1.0 mg i.m. or i.v. Child: 0.01–0.02 mg/kg i.m. or i.v.	Methadone Morphine Pantopon	
Naloxone	0.01 mg/kg i.v., i.m., or s.c.	(For respiratory and cardiovascular depression)	Naloxone produces no respiratory depression, psychotomimetic effects, circulatory changes or miosis and is preferable

(*continued*)

TABLE 72-4. (*Continued*)

Antidote	Dose	Poison	Reaction (Antidote) and Comments
Petrolatum, liquid (mineral oil)		Stomach concretion (castor oil preferred)	Solvent Demulcent
Pralidoxime iodine (2-PAM iodine)	Adult: 1–2 g	Organic phosphate esters	Diplopia
Pralidoxime chloride (2-PAM chloride)	Child: 25–50 mg/kg i.m. or i.v. as 5% solution	Cholinesterase inhibition by any agent: chemical, drug, etc	Dizziness Headache
Penicillamine and its derivatives	1–5 g orally	Mercury and other heavy metals Lead (investigational drug permit necessary)	Fever Stupor Nausea and vomiting Myalgia Leukopenia, thrombocytopenia Nephrosis, reversible Optic axial neuritis, reversible Ineffective when severe vomiting is prominent
Physostigmine	1–2 mg i.v.	Anticholinergic compounds (peripheral and central effects)	Only cholinergic drug that crosses the blood-brain barrier
Pilocarpine (available only as a powder—Wyeth Lab)	Orally: 2–4 mg	Atropine and related alkaloids	Antagonizes the parasympathetic (mydriasis and dry mouth), not central, effects of atropine
Potassium permanganate	1:5,000 and 1:10,000 solution for gastric lavage	Nicotine Physostigmine Quinine Strychnine Oxidizing agent for many alkaloids and organic poisons	Severe irritant and should not be used in stronger dilutions or with any residual particles
Protamine sulfate	1% solution i.v. slowly (mg/mg) to that of heparin	Heparin	Sensitivity effects
Sodium chloride	1 tsp salt to 1 pt water (approximately normal saline solution) 6–12 g orally in divided doses or in isotonic saline i.v.	Silver nitrate Bromides	Forms noncorrosive silver chloride Hypernatremia
Sodium formaldehyde sulfoxalate	5% in lavage solution (preferably combined with 5% sodium bicarbonate)	Mercury salts	BAL therapy should follow gastric lavage
Sodium thiosulfate	Orally: 2–3 g or i.m.: 10 or 25% solution Repeat in 3–4 hr	Iodine Cyanide	
Starch	80 g/1000 ml water	Iodine	
Tannic acid	4% in lavage solution; never use in greater concentrations	Precipitates alkaloids, certain glucosides, and many metals	Hepatotoxic Tannates formed should not be allowed to remain in the stomach Because of its hepatotoxicity, should be used cautiously and in no greater than 4% solution

(continued)

TABLE 72-4. *(Continued)*

Antidote	Dose	Poison	Reaction (Antidote) and Comments
Universal antidote (activated charcoal alone preferable)	Two parts pulverized charcoal (burned toast); One part magnesium oxide (milk of magnesia); One part tannic acid (strong tea solution)		Overrated and ineffective; may actually be harmful in that it can give false sense of security to those who use it; mentioned here only to negate its popularity in lay journals and books
Vitamin K_1	25–150 mg i.v. Rate not to exceed 10 mg/min	Coumarin derivatives: Coumarin, Marcoumar, Warfarin, others	Bleeding; Focal hemorrhages

* Although seemingly paradoxical, magnesium oxide should be used for (alkali) hypochlorite (bleaches) ingestion to prevent the formation of irritating hypochlorous acid.

† Recent reports have indicated that haloperidol is more effective in much smaller doses than chloropromazine for treating amphetamine intoxication.

INCREASING THE EXCRETION OF POISONS

DIALYSIS

Hemodialysis (Artificial Kidney)

Dialysis can be used in cases of severe poisoning from dialyzable substances as well as for nondialyzable nephrotoxic compounds that produce acute tubular damage and renal failure. Generally, poisons that circulate in the blood or that are reversibly bound to tissue or colloids in equilibrium with the unbound poison can be removed by dialysis, whereas those irreversibly bound cannot. Dialyzable poisons include barbiturates, borates, bromates, bromides, ethylene glycol, glutethimide, methanol, salicylates, salt, thiocyanates, and many others. Nephrotoxic compounds are not dialyzable.

Contraindications to this procedure are an inexperienced operator and inadequate knowledge of the problem to which the apparatus is to be applied; bleeding, particularly from the gastrointestinal tract; and destruction of platelets and white blood cells by the cellophane membrane during hemodialysis.

Lipid Dialysis

Lipid dialysis is a technique used to treat poisonings by glutethimide, pentobarbital, secobarbital, phenothiazines, camphor, and other lipid soluble substances that cannot be removed effectively by hemodialysis using an aqueous dialysate. Lipid dialysis is similar to aqueous hemodialysis except that oil is circulated on the dialysate side of the membrane. An inexpensive and readily available effective, safe, nontoxic, and nonpyrogenic dialysate is soybean oil. The oil does not cross the celephone membrane and will absorb large quantities of lipid soluble substances.

A Klung or Kiil membrane can be used easily for lipid dialysis with only a few modifications. Two gallons of soybean oil will absorb a large quantity of the drug and compounds, and only a slow flow of the oil past the membrane is necessary for complete removal of lipid soluble substance in each circulation of the blood through the membrane. Glutethimide is highly soluble in alcohols and lipids but is very poorly soluble in water.

Peritoneal Dialysis

Peritoneal dialysis is much more efficient than the natural kidney (but less efficient than the artificial kidney) for ridding the body of overdoses of many exogenous poisons. The artificial kidney is always preferable for dialysis but is not always available. Peritoneal dialysis, therefore, because of its availability and simplicity, is used much more frequently for dialysis. The development and use of simple disposable equipment with accompanying solutions for patients with or without edema have brought this type of therapy within the reach of every physician and hospital. An automatic peritoneal dialysis system (Drake–Willock, Portland, OR) is now available for acute as well as chronic conditions. Contraindications are

TABLE 72-5. Treatment of Convulsions Due to Poisoning*

Drug	Method of Administration and Dosage	Advantages	Disadvantages
Ether	Open drop	Dosage easily determined; good minute-to-minute control; no sterile precautions	Difficult to give in presence of convulsion; requires constant supervision by physician
Thiopental sodium (Pentothal sodium)	Give 2.5% sterile solution i.v. until convulsions are controlled; maximum dose: 0.5 ml/kg	Good minute-to-minute control; can be given easily during convulsion	Doses larger than recommended may cause persistent respiratory depression; requires sterile equipment and administration
Pentobarbital sodium (Nembutal sodium)	Give 5 mg/kg gastric tube, rectally, or i.v. as sterile 2.5% solution at a rate not to exceed 1 ml/min until convulsions are controlled	Good control of initial dose	No control of effects after drug has been given; requires sterile precautions; may produce severe respiratory depression
Phenobarbital sodium	Give 1–2 mg/kg i.m. or gastric tube and repeat as necessary at 30 min intervals up to a maximum of 5 mg/kg	Effect lasts 12–14 hr	Causes severe persistent respiratory depression in overdoses
Succinylcholine chloride	Give 10–50 mg i.v. slowly and give artificial respiration during period of apnea; repeat as necessary	Will control convulsions of any type; effect lasts only 1–5 min; circulation not ordinarily affected	Artificial respiration must be maintained during use; no antidote is available; apnea may persist for several hours in some cases
Trimethadione (Tridione)	Give 1 g i.v. slowly; maximum dose: 5 g	Little depression of respiration	Not effective in all types of convulsions
Tribromoethanol (Avertin)	Only by rectal instillation; 50–60 mg/kg causes drowsiness, amnesia; 70–80 mg/kg produces light unconsciousness and analgesia	Ease of administration and pleasant induction with out mental distress and respiratory irritation	A nonvolatile anesthetic given by a route which prevents adequate control once it is administered; contraindicated when renal or hepatic injury exists
Amobarbital sodium (Amytal)	Give 2% sterile solution; dose range 0.4–0.8 g	Immediate action and lasts 3–6 hr	Inhibits cardiac action of vagus; may produce severe respiratory depression
Phenytoin sodium (Dilantin)	Give i.v. slowly 150–250 mg from steri-vial and repeat 30 min later with 100–150 mg if necessary	Lack of marked hypnotic and narcotic activity	Solution is highly alkaline and perivenous infiltration may cause sloughing; not always effective and other anticonvulsants frequently must be used; cardiac arrest has been reported after i.v. therapy
Paraldehyde	Give 5–15 ml gastric tube, rectally or i.m.	Little depression of respiration, effects last 12 hr	Harmful in presence of hepatic disease; old and loosely stoppered solutions can break down to acetic acid and produce serious intoxication
Diazepam (Valium)	Give 2–5 mg i.v. or i.m.; repeat 2 hr later if necessary	Good muscle relaxant for skeletal muscle spasm	Hypotension; respiratory depression or muscular weakness may occur if used with barbiturates

* Convulsions may occur with almost any compound in a toxic dose.

TABLE 72-6. Management of Barbiturate Poisoning

Condition	Treatment	Guides
Respiratory insufficiency	Airway, suction; endotracheal intubation, cuffed tube, lavage; humidified oxygen; mechanical ventilation, pressure or volume controlled ventilator	Arterial Po_2, O_2 saturation, Pco_2, *p*H, minute ventilation; x-ray film of chest; airway pressure
Hypovolemia	Albumin, 5% solution, 1 liter, then dextrose, 10% in sodium chloride 0.9% solution; potassium chloride supplement, 40–120 mEq	Central venous pressure, arterial pressure, urine output and osmolality
Low urinary output	Fluid infusion; furosemide, 40 mg i.v. or ethacrynic acid, 25 mg i.v.	Urinary output and osmolality
Heart failure	Digoxin, 0.5 mg i.v., followed by 1–4 doses of 0.25 mg digoxin at 1–2 hr intervals	Central venous pressure, ECG
Pneumonia	Ampicillin sodium, 1 g every 4 hr i.v.; methicillin sodium, 1 g every 6 hr i.v.; chloramphenicol sodium succinate, 500 mg every 6 hr i.v.; gentamicin sulfate, 0.75 mg/kg every 6 hr i.m.	Sputum and blood culture, with antibiotic sensitivity; chloramphenicol after aspiration of gastric contents, gentamicin for gram-negative bacteria resistant to other antibiotics
Dialysis	Peritoneal Lipid Hemodialysis (preferred)	Barbiturate levels of 3.5 mg/dl for short acting drugs and 8–10 mg/dl for long acting agents; impaired hepatic and renal function

absolute—infection of the peritoneal cavity—and *relative*—recent or extensive abdominal surgery.

EXCHANGE TRANSFUSION

Blood transfusion is effective particularly when the toxic products of the poison tend to remain in the circulating bloodstream rather than become fixed or deposited in the viscera, bones, or other tissues: specifically, the various types of drugs that cause methemoglobinemia, for example, the aniline dyes and their derivatives, such as acetanilid and phenacetin, nitrites, nitrates, bromates, chlorates, sulfanilamide, Pyridium (phenazopyridine), and nitrobenzene and related nitro compounds. The object is to supply normal hemoglobin that can transport oxygen. In more severe instances, exchange or exsanguination transfusions may be lifesaving if facilities and blood are available. This procedure offers certain advantages over other methods, such as hemodialysis, in that it is familiar to most physicians, requires little specialized equipment, and does not require exceptional experience as does the safe use of hemodialysis. Except in very small children, it has obvious limitations, is technically difficult, and presents the hazard of blood transfusion reaction, since it may be necessary to use blood from several sources. It is used with best results in infants younger than 1 year of age poisoned from salicylates, barbiturates, or other dialyzable drugs.

FORCED DIURESIS

Forced osmotic diuresis and alkalinization of the urine with large quantities of parenteral fluids are now being used effectively to treat barbiturate and other intoxications.

GENERAL THERAPEUTIC MEASURES

1. An adequate airway should be established by inserting an oropharyngeal or endotracheal tube. Often, however, extension of the head and forward displacement of the mandible are sufficient. Mouth-to-mouth breathing or mechanical respiratory equipment may be needed. Physiologic improvement of the patient's condition is often notable when tissues receive adequate oxygen.
2. Generally, legs and head are elevated to the level of the right atrium to allow venous drainage of the lower extremities and to promote circulatory pooling in the head and thorax. Cardiac failure may necessitate alterations in position.
3. Elastic bandaging of the legs prevents venous stasis. Passive leg exercises are advis-

able if depression is extreme. The patient is turned from side to side every 2 hours to promote pulmonary drainage and to reduce atelectasis.

4. Homeostasis is maintained by parenteral fluid according to blood electrolyte concentrations and urine output. An indwelling urethral catheter is placed in the bladder to allow accurate hourly measurement of output. When the kidney is not damaged, fluid therapy is aided by hourly measurement of urine specific gravity.
5. If oliguria is associated, electrocardiographic examination and frequent measurement of serum potassium are required.
6. Vital signs are recorded every 15 minutes, or more frequently, if values are labile or vasopressors are administered.
7. CNS stimulants should not be used to improve respiration. These drugs impart a false sense of security, and harmful reactions, such as rebound depression or convulsions, may occur. If the myocardium is hypoxic, epinephrine may induce fatal ventricular fibrillation.
8. Intravenous vasopressors such as phenylephrine, methoxamine, or other adrenergic drugs may be needed if the patient has tachycardia above 110 pulse beats per minute, prolonged capillary filling time, pallor, or diaphoresis. Moderate hypotension as low as 80 mm Hg does not necessitate vigorous therapy with vasopressors unless urinary output is depressed. Extremely potent agents, such as levarterenol bitartrate, are used for severe shock, but vasoconstrictors may significantly depress urinary output.
9. Convulsions can occur with almost any compound in a toxic dose. Table 72-5 gives the various types of treatment available for convulsions.

TREATMENT OF NONORAL POISONING

ABSORBED DERMAL POISONS

A number of poisonous compounds can produce intoxication through transcutaneous absorption as well as local dermatitis. These compounds include chlorinated and organic phosphate insecticides, halogenated hydrocarbons, caustics, and corrosives. Contaminated skin should be thoroughly washed with water from a hose or shower or even poured from a bucket. Clothing should be removed while a continuous stream of water is played on the skin. A 24-hour continuous shower has not been found effective for chemical burns. Chemical antidotes could increase the extent of injury. Corroded and burned areas should be treated as any burn.

INHALED POISONS

In cases of gas poisoning, one should first move the victim from the presence of the gas and then apply artificial respiration, if needed.

INJECTED POISONS

If a poison has been injected, application of tourniquets central to the point of injection may slow absorption. Quantities of unabsorbed poison may be removed by surgery and suction similar to that commonly advised for the treatment of snake bite. Cryotherapy is also beneficial in delaying absorption.

CHEMICAL EYE BURNS

A chemical burn of the eye results from local contact with a chemical—solid, liquid, dust, mist, or vapor—of such a degree as to alter the structure of the cornea and conjunctiva. Some alterations not visualized readily may be seen by staining with a 2% solution of fluorescein after a local anesthetic. The basic treatment of all types of chemical eye injuries is the quick, thorough irrigation of the eye with water at the nearest source of supply for 15 minutes. Neutralizing agents should not be used. An ophthalmologist should be consulted for degree of damage and specific therapy.

COMMON POISONS AND THERAPY*

ACETAMINOPHEN

An overdose of acetaminophen is hepatotoxic. Treatment is symptomatic and supportive and includes early use of acetylcysteine.

Oral methionine (Pedameth), 2.5 every 6 hours up to 10 g, has been found to be effective in reducing the frequency and severity of acetaminophen-induced liver damage. (This use of methionine is not listed in the manufacturer's

* Modified from Arena JM: Poisoning: Toxicology, Symptoms, Treatment, 4th ed. Springfield, Illinois, Charles C Thomas, 1979

official directive.) Although this compound has few side-effects and is of low toxicity, it may aggravate a preexisting hepatic disease, and therefore should be given early (before 12 hours) after ingestion, before the likely acetaminophen hepatic effects occur.

N-Acetylcysteine (Mucomyst) appears to act as a glutathione substitute and to combine directly with the toxic acetaminophen epoxide. It is currently recommended as the oral drug of choice (loading dose of 140 mg/kg, followed by 70 mg/kg every 6 hours for a total of 18 doses) if given within 12 hours after ingestion. (This use of N-acetylcysteine is not listed in the manufacturer's official directive.)

ACETYLSALICYLIC ACID (ASPIRIN)

1. Immediate (emesis or gastric lavage)
   - Evaluate severity of intoxication (extrapolation method of Done)
   - Appraise status of dehydration
   - Determine acid–base imbalance. Test urine with Phenistix paper and Nitrazene paper
   - Measure blood electrolytes
   - Draw blood for salicylate level and blood gases; P_{CO_2}; P_{O_2}; pH
2. Pending laboratory report
   - Start i.v. fluids (5% glucose in 1/3 isotonic saline solution)
   - If dehydration is severe, give hydrating solution at the rate of 8 ml/m² body surface/min, for 30 to 45 minutes. Slow hydrating solution to 2 ml/m²/min.
   - Correct bicarbonate and potassium deficits as indicated (average requirement, 5 mEq $NaHCO_3$/kg and 2 mEq K/kg/12 hr)
   - In presence of clinical acidosis and acid urine, give $NaHCO_3$ in initial hydrating solution
   - Sponge body with cool water for hyperpyrexia
3. In life-threatening intoxication
   - Consider exchange transfusion in young children, peritoneal dialysis with 5% albumin solution (Albumisol), or hemodialysis
4. Vitamin K and vitamin B complex
5. Maintenance management

AMPHETAMINE

1. Gastric lavage or emesis.
2. Activated charcoal.
3. Sedation or short-acting barbiturates with caution.
4. Chlorpromazine (Thorazine), 1 to 2 mg/kg intramuscularly (repeat if necessary) or, preferably, haloperidol (Haldol), 0.5 to 2.0 mg every 8 hours.

ANTIHISTAMINICS (H_1 BLOCKERS)

1. Gastric lavage or emesis.
2. Activated charcoal.
3. Saline cathartic.
4. Do not use stimulants.
5. Levarterenol for hypotension.
6. Short-acting barbiturates with caution.

ATROPINE

1. Gastric lavage with 4% tannic acid solution or emesis.
2. Pilocarpine or physostigmine (preferable) for parasympathomimetic effects.
3. Miotic for eyes.
4. Oxygen.
5. Small doses of barbiturates, chloral hydrate, or paraldehyde for delirium or convulsions.
6. Cold packs or alcohol sponging for hyperpyrexia.
7. Indwelling urethral catheter.

BARBITURATES AND NONBARBITURATE HYPNOTICS

There is no specific antidote for barbiturates and nonbarbiturate hypnotics. In acute poisoning, the immediate establishment of adequate pulmonary ventilation and the control of shock are of prime importance; analeptics are considered subsidiary, if not actually contraindicated. The most favorable results are obtained by careful attention to respiratory and circulatory functions.

Forced diuresis (i.v. fluids) with alkalinization of the urine and diuretics (acetazolamide [Diamox] or mercurials) reduces the need for vasopressor drugs, prevents renal complications and hyperthermia, and lessens crust formation in the respiratory tract. Contraindications are cardiac and renal disease. Pulmonary edema does not seem to be a serious hazard. Hemodialysis should be resorted to when indicated. Dialysis need be considered only in the presence of compromised renal function.

With nonbarbiturate hypnotics (including glutethimide and methyprylon), a history is of paramount diagnostic importance. Intoxication with these drugs should be considered if lethargy, mydriasis, hypotension, flaccid paralysis, and respiratory depression are present. Glutethimide also produces alternating periods of coma and relative alertness owing to an enterohepatic circulation. Lethal plasma levels of glutethimide and methyprylon are not known. The approximate fatal dose of glutethimide is 10 to 12 g and that of methyprylon, more than 6 g. Supportive measures, forced diuresis, and dialysis are the most effective means of treatment.

1. Gastric lavage with a solution of saline and activated charcoal.
2. Continue lavage with isotonic saline until the return is clear.
3. Use castor oil for instillation and withdrawal to increase solubility of sedatives and to dissolve concretions.
4. Ensure clear airway.
5. Respiratory stimulants such as picrotoxin or pentylenetetrazol (Metrazol), administered in subconvulsive doses, are not often used in present-day therapy.
6. Artificial respiration.
7. Administer 100% oxygen.
8. For circulatory depression and shock caused by depression of vasomotor center, as well as indirect action on smooth muscle in blood vessel wall, give pressor amines, such as levarterenol.
8. Intravenous hydrocortisone.
9. Blood transfusion.
10. Trendelenburg position.
11. For water loss from skin and lungs, decreased urine output, variable electrolytes, be sure that hydration is adequate, with 5% to 10% glucose in water to facilitate renal elimination of barbiturates.
12. Base the use of electrolytes on analysis of plasma.
13. For depression of kidney function resulting from hypotension and central antidiuretic action of barbiturates, exchange transfusion (children).
14. Intermittent peritoneal dialysis.
15. Artificial kidney (lipid dialysis).
16. For cerebral edema, use mannitol or urea.

CANTHARIDIN (SPANISH FLY, RUSSIAN FLY)

1. Gastric lavage (cautiously because of corrosive effects) or emesis.
2. Demulcents.
3. Therapy for shock.
4. Short-acting barbiturates.
5. Adequate fluids for diuresis.
6. Avoid morphine because of respiratory depression.

CARBON MONOXIDE

1. Move patient from exposure immediately.
2. Artificial respiration and oxygen.
3. Administer 100% oxygen in a pressure chamber, if available.
4. Hypothermia.
5. Give blood transfusion or washed red blood cells early.
6. Chronic carbon monoxide poisoning and therapy are questionable.

CHLORDANE

1. Gastric lavage or emesis.
2. Short-acting barbiturates.
3. For skin contamination, wash skin thoroughly and remove contaminated clothing.
4. Avoid fats, oils, demulcents, and epinephrine, which should never be used in any halogenated insecticide poisoning.

CHLORINATED ALKALIS (HYPOCHLORITES, CHLORINE)

1. Careful gastric lavage or emesis for large amounts only.
2. Diluted vinegar and fruit juice.
3. Demulcents.
4. Move from exposure and wash skin thoroughly.
5. Antibiotics and corticosteroids for pulmonary edema and pneumonitis from chlorine inhalation.
6. Oral magnesium oxide (paradoxical as it may sound) to prevent formation of irritating hypochlorous acid in the stomach.

COCAINE

1. Gastric lavage or emesis.
2. Remove drug from skin or mucous membranes.
3. Short-acting barbiturates.
4. Artificial respiration and oxygen.

CODEINE

1. Gastric lavage or emesis.
2. Saline cathartic.
3. Antagonist naloxone (Narcan).
4. Artificial respiration and oxygen.
5. Maintain body heat and fluid balance.

COSMETICS

1. For deodorants (aluminum salts, titanium dioxide, antibacterial agents) and depilatories (soluble sulfides or calcium thioglycolate), gastric lavage or emesis, if large amount ingested.

CYANIDES (HYDROGEN, POTASSIUM, SODIUM)

1. Gastric lavage or emesis, if ingested. (*See* Table 72-4 for cyanide poison kit.)
2. Kelocyanor (dicobalt tetracemate) is being used effectively in Europe but has not been approved for use in the United States at present.
3. Artificial respiration and oxygen.
4. Remove contaminated clothing and wash skin thoroughly.

DDT (CHLOROBENZENE INSECTICIDE, TDE, DFDT, DMC, METHOXYCHLOR, NEOTRANE, OVOTRAN, DILAN, DIMITE)

1. Gastric lavage or emesis.
2. Saline cathartic.
3. Short-acting barbiturates.
4. Artificial respiration and oxygen.
5. Remove contaminated clothing and wash skin thoroughly.
6. Avoid fats, oils, demulcents, epinephrine, and related compounds.

DETERGENTS (ANIONIC AND NONIONIC SUFFACTANTS, PHOSPHATE SALTS, SODIUM SULFATE AND CARBONATE, FATTY ACID AMIDES)

1. Unless taken in large quantities, no serious toxicity other than gastrointestinal symptoms.
2. At present causing havoc with public water supplies.
3. Milk, egg whites, mild soap solution by mouth.

DIGITALIS (PURPLE FOXGLOVE)

1. Gastric lavage or emesis for accidental or suicidal ingestion.
2. Artificial pacemaker.
3. Potassium chloride, orally or intravenously, under electrocardiographic observation.
4. Procainamide, quinidine, phenytoin, propranolol, lidocaine, or atropine.

ETHYL ALCOHOL (PURE) (WHISKEY = 40% to 50% ALCOHOL; WINES = 10% TO 20% ALCOHOL; BEERS = 2% TO 6% ALCOHOL

1. Gastric lavage or emesis.
2. Sodium bicarbonate, 1 teaspoonful to 1 pint of water, every 1 to 2 hours to prevent acidosis.
3. Intravenous bicarbonate for acidosis.
4. Caffeine and sodium benzoate or strong coffee.
5. Hypertonic glucose or urea for cerebral edema.
6. Intravenous glucose for hypoglycemia.
7. Avoid depressant drugs and potent respiratory stimulants.

FERROUS SULFATE (COPPERAS, GREEN VITRIOL; ABOUT 20% ELEMENTAL IRON)

1. Maintenance of open airway.
2. Control of shock with i.v. fluids, blood or plasma, and oxygen.
3. Gastric lavage with concentrated solution of sodium bicarbonate, 5% disodium phosphate, or milk until returning fluid is clear.
4. Critically ill patients should receive calcium disodium edetate (edathamil), 70 to 80 mg/kg/24 hours in dextrose or isotonic saline solution in a 0.5% to 2% concentration intravenously; if used orally (and rate of its absorption through a gut wall damaged by iron is not known), only one half the aforementioned dose should be used.
5. Duration of treatment with calcium disodium edetate should not be longer than 5 days.
6. Deferoxamine (Desferal), a chelating agent, is effective in acute iron poisoning in doses of 1 to 2 g intravenously (slowly to avoid hypotensive effects) or intramuscularly.
7. Repeat parenteral therapy if serum iron levels remain high.

FLUORIDES (FLUORINE, HYDROGEN FLUORIDE, FLUOROSILICATES [INSOLUBLE])

1. Gastric lavage or emesis with lime water (0.15% calcium hydroxide), calcium chloride solution (1 teaspoonful per liter of water), or milk.

2. 10% calcium gluconate intravenously or intramuscularly.
3. Demulcents.
4. For inhalation, move to fresh air.
5. Artificial respiration and oxygen.
6. Prophylactic antibiotics and corticosteroids for pulmonary irritation and edema.
7. Wash skin immediately and thoroughly with water and apply magnesium oxide paste with 20% glycerin.

METHYL ALCOHOL

1. Ethyl alcohol, 10 ml/hr, can suppress the metabolism of methyl alcohol to formic acid and formates.
2. In severe poisoning, give ethyl alcohol intravenously in a 5% concentration in bicarbonate or saline solution plus 90 to 120 ml (3–4 oz) of whiskey (45% alcohol) orally every 4 to 6 hours for 1 to 3 days.
3. Combat acidosis.
4. Hemodialysis is paramount in serious poisoning.

MORPHINE (CODEINE, HEROIN, PROPOXYPHENE [DARVON], MEPERIDINE [DEMEROL], DIHYDROMORPHINONE [DILAUDID], OPIUM ALKALOIDS [PANTOPON])

1. Gastric lavage (before loss of consciousness).
2. Do not use syrup of ipecac or apomorphine.
3. Activated charcoal.
4. Saline cathartic.
5. Delay absorption of i.m. drug with tourniquet and cryotherapy.
6. Maintain adequate airway, body temperature, fluids, and electrolytes.
7. Give antagonist naloxone hydrochloride (Narcan).
8. Give ephedrine for hypotension and bradycardia; methoxamine or phenylephrine if pulse is rapid.
9. Doxapram hydrochloride (Dopram), 3 to 5 ml intravenously, is the respiratory stimulant of choice but has short-lasting effects (3–5 minutes).

PARAQUAT AND DIQUAT

1. Induce vomiting with syrup of ipecac or perform gastric lavage if vomiting has not occurred.
2. If lavage is performed, care must be taken, because paraquat may be corrosive to the esophagus.
3. Immediately following vomiting or lavage, give about 200 to 500 ml of a 30% aqueous suspension of an adsorbent clay (such as Robinson's bentonite, U.S.P., or Robinson's fuller's earth, U.S.P.) plus an effective dose of cathartic—for example, magnesium sulfate to remove paraquat from the entire gastrointestinal tract.
4. Repeat as often as is practical (every 2–4 hours for several days until paraquat can no longer be detected in blood, urine, or dialysate).
5. If bentonite or fuller's earth is not immediately available, an adsorbent such as powdered activated charcoal should be used until better clays are obtained.
6. Use oxygen sparingly and cautiously for dyspnea or cyanosis because it may aggravate lung lesions.
7. Start forced diuresis as soon as possible to remove paraquat from the blood.
8. If renal function is impaired, hemodialysis or peritoneal dialysis may be of value.
9. For skin contamination, remove clothing and wash skin thoroughly with soap and water for several minutes.
10. If the eyes are involved, irrigate them immediately for 10 to 15 minutes and then have an ophthalmologist examine them.

PARATHION (PHOSPHATE ESTER INSECTICIDES) (MALATHION, SYSTOX, EPN, DIAZINON, GUTHION, TRITHION, TEPP, OMPA, CO-RAL, PHOSDRIN)

1. Promptly induce emesis or gastric lavage with 5% $NaHCO_3$ for ingestion only.
2. Decontaminate by removing all soiled clothes and thoroughly washing the skin.
3. Maintain clear airway and respiration with laryngeal intubation and artificial respiration and oxygen.
4. Give atropine, 1 to 2 mg intramuscularly or intravenously, and repeat at 20- to 30-minute intervals as soon as cyanosis has cleared (chance of ventricular fibrillation).
5. Continue atropine until definite improvement occurs and is maintained (sometimes 2 days or more).
6. Total dosage required may be phenomenal (over 1000 mg).
7. Use pralidoxime chloride (Protopam chloride), a cholinesterase reactivator, as 5% solution intravenously.
8. Avoid narcotics, barbiturates, epinephrine,

aminophyline, ether, and phenothiazine derivates because they further reduce cholinesterase activity and some are respiratory depressants.

TEAR GASES

The most commonly used preparations are chloracetophenone, ethylbromoacetate, bromoacetone, bromobenzyl cyanide, and bromomethylethylketone. *Alpha-chloroacetophenone*, even though called a "gas," is actually a fine powder. In commercial blast-dispersion cartridges, it is mixed half and half with silica anhydride, and a standard shotgun prime is used as a propellant. The mixture is an effective lacrimator in concentrations as low as 2 parts per million (ppm) of air. It causes extreme irritation and edema of the mucous membranes of the nose and eyes if discharged into the face, and temporary blindness may result. *Mace* contains recrystallized 2-chloroacetophenone (0.9% 1,1,1-trichloroethane), solvents, and propellants—Freon, kerosene, methylchloroform 4.0%.

The eyes should be irrigated for 15 minutes with isotonic saline solution or water, followed by an antiinflammatory eye ointment. For clothing and skin contamination, the clothes should be removed and a thorough shower taken.

TRICYCLIC (DIBENZAZEPINE) COMPOUNDS

Symptoms of convulsions, coma, signs of atropinism, and cardiac arrhythmias should suggest tricyclic antidepressant poisoning specifically and intoxication by other anticholinergic drugs and chemicals generally.

Treatment is supportive and symptomatic, with particular attention given to the correction of cardiac arrhythmias and maintenance of blood pressure and respiration.

Cardiac arrhythmias may progress to cardiac arrest because of ventricular fibrillation or asystole. Although documentation is limited, some arrhythmias are controlled by use of parasympathomimetic drugs: physostigmine (drug of choice; 1 mg intravenously); pyridostigmine (Mestinon); neostigmine (Prostigmin); and the beta-adrenergic blocking agent propranolol (Inderal) are also effective. Because it is not possible to predict which patient will respond, more than one antiarrhythmic drug may have to be tried. Intravenous phenytoin has had dramatic antiarrhythmic properties and may also be useful in preventing convulsions, which occur frequently. Congestive heart failure is treated by digitalization. However, rapid digitalization should be avoided when multiple ventricular ectopic beats are likely to occur. The administration of sodium bicarbonate and potassium may aid in treating the cardiovascular effects. Convulsions may cause a dangerous increase in the cardiac workload. Agitation, tremors, and convulsions have been successfully treated with parenteral barbiturates. However, use of barbiturates is questionable if drugs that inhibit monoamine oxidase have been taken recently. Diazepam has been used as an alternative to barbiturates for controlling convulsions and is considered the drug of choice by some. Hypotension and shock may be treated by i.v. glucose, saline, or plasma and by cautious administration of vasopressor agents such as levarterenol (l-norepinephrine; Levophed), phenylephrine, or metaraminol, which will increase blood pressure without increasing heart rate. Any of these sympathomimetic drugs may induce cardiac arrhythmias. Other sympathomimetic drugs such as epinephrine and isoproterenol, which stimulate the cardiac beta-receptor, should be avoided because they further increase the heart rate and may lead to fatal ventricular fibrillation. Respiration must be maintained. Intratracheal artificial respiration is effective. Patients should be observed for possible recurrence of respiratory distress after resumption of spontaneous breathing. Various methods have been attempted to hasten excretion of these drugs, such as exchange transfusion, repeated gastric lavage, and osmotic diuresis with mannitol. Catheterization should be considered if diuresis is attempted. Hemodialysis and peritoneal dialysis are not effective in removing significant amounts of these drugs.

In children, tricyclic drugs are especially treacherous. When a verified ingestion occurs, the child should be hospitalized for monitoring for at least 48 hours, even though the patient may be asymptomatic at admission.

FURTHER READING

1. Arena JM: Poisoning: Toxicology, Symptoms, Treatment, 4th ed. Springfield, Illinois, Charles C Thomas, 1979
2. Berry FA, Labdin MA: Apomorphine and levallorphan tartrate in acute poisonings. Am J Dis Child 105:160, 1963
3. Lasagna L: (*N*-allylnormorphine): Practical and theoretical considerations. Arch Intern Med 94:532, 1954
4. Robertson WO: Syrup of ipecac—slow or fast emetic? Am J Dis Child 103:136, 1962

CHAPTER 72 QUESTIONS

(See P. 7 for Full Instructions)

Select the One Best Answer

1. The most appropriate agent for inducing emesis in children in the home is
   A. warm salt water.
   B. apomorphine.
   C. digitalis.
   D. syrup of ipecac.
   E. copper sulfate.

2. For overdosage by the oral route, the agent that can be used to absorb the largest variety of drugs is
   A. activated charcoal.
   B. mineral oil.
   C. cholestyramine.
   D. kaolin with pectin.
   E. aluminum hydroxide.

3. The principal toxic effect observed in humans exposed to chlorophenothane (DDT) is
   A. central nervous system stimulation.
   B. voluntary muscle paralysis.
   C. bronchial constriction.
   D. hepatocellular damage.
   E. lowering of blood cholinesterase.

4. Dimercaprol (BAL) is indicated for the treatment of poisoning by each of the following EXCEPT
   A. arsenic.
   B. antimony.
   C. lead.
   D. cadmium.
   E. gold.

5. Edetate (EDTA) is an effective agent for increasing the urinary elimination of
   A. mercury.
   B. arsenic.
   C. lead.
   D. antimony.
   E. gold.

A = 1,2,3; B = 1,3; C = 2,4; D = 4; E = All

6. With reference to poisonings with cyanide or carbon monoxide,
   1. 50% methemoglobin is more detrimental than 50% carboxyhemoglobin.
   2. artificial respiration with hyperbaric oxygen is very effective for both poisonings.
   3. sodium nitrite intravenously is indicated in the treatment of both poisonings.
   4. fatalities occur more rapidly with cyanide than with carbon monoxide.

7. Both the organophosphate and chlorinated hydrocarbon insecticides
   1. can produce convulsions.
   2. produce effects anatagonized by atropine.
   3. are absorbed through mucous membranes.
   4. are water soluble.

8. Deferoxamine
   1. is effective intramuscularly against systemic iron toxicity.
   2. is administered parenterally for treating arsenic poisoning.
   3. is given orally to decrease absorption of iron in the intestine.
   4. inhibits cytochrome oxidase activity.

9. Penicillamine (Cuprimine; dimethylcysteine)
   1. is allergenic in many patients.
   2. reduces lead accumulation in plumbism.
   3. prevents copper accumulation in Wilson's disease.
   4. is effective orally.

10. Pentavalent arsenicals
    1. are least toxic of the arsenicals.
    2. may cause liver damage.
    3. may cause kidney damage.
    4. are used to treat schistosomiasis.

73

CARL E. ANDERSON

The Vitamins

Until the early 1900s it was believed that only carbohydrates, protein, some minerals, water, and fat were needed to maintain health. It is now known that such a diet will not sustain life and that additional "accessory food factors" (vitamins) are essential.

Vitamins are organic substances needed in small amounts for metabolism that cannot be synthesized by the body in sufficient quantity. Mostly they are not related chemically and differ in their physiological role.

Casimir Funk, a Polish biochemist working in the Lister Institute in London, prepared the first successful essential "accessory food factor." He obtained a potent antiberiberi substance from rice polishings. Since it was an amine and necessary for life, he called it a "vitamine." As other "vitamines" were discovered, only a few were found to be "amine" in nature, and thus the final *e* was dropped, leaving the now general term *vitamin*.

During 1913–1914, McCollum and Davis extracted a fraction from butter fat that they called "fat-soluble A" to distinguish it from the water-soluble unidentified dietary essential called the antiberiberi substance. These two dietary essentials became vitamins A and B. As the vitamins were discovered one by one, each was assigned a letter. The antiscorbutic factor became vitamin C, the antirachitic factor vitamin D, the antihemorrhagic factor vitamin K, and so on. When through isolation and synthesis the chemical structure of the vitamin became known, it was given a specific chemical name. Vitamin B_1 became thiamine and the antiscorbutic vitamin C became L-ascorbic acid. It was assumed that the chemical name assigned to the vitamin applied to a single chemical substance of definite activity. It is now clear that some vitamins comprise several closely related compounds. The term vitamin A is now used to refer collectively to all active and synthesized forms of the vitamin. Vitamin A alcohol is now retinol, vitamin A aldehyde is retinal, and vitamin A acid is retinoic acid.

CASIMIR FUNK, 1884– . Polish-born biochemist who did much of his work in the United States. Specialized in nutrition, anemia, and the physiology of gonadotropic hormones.

CLASSIFICATION

Thirteen vitamins (or vitaminlike substances) are essential for humans, and several other

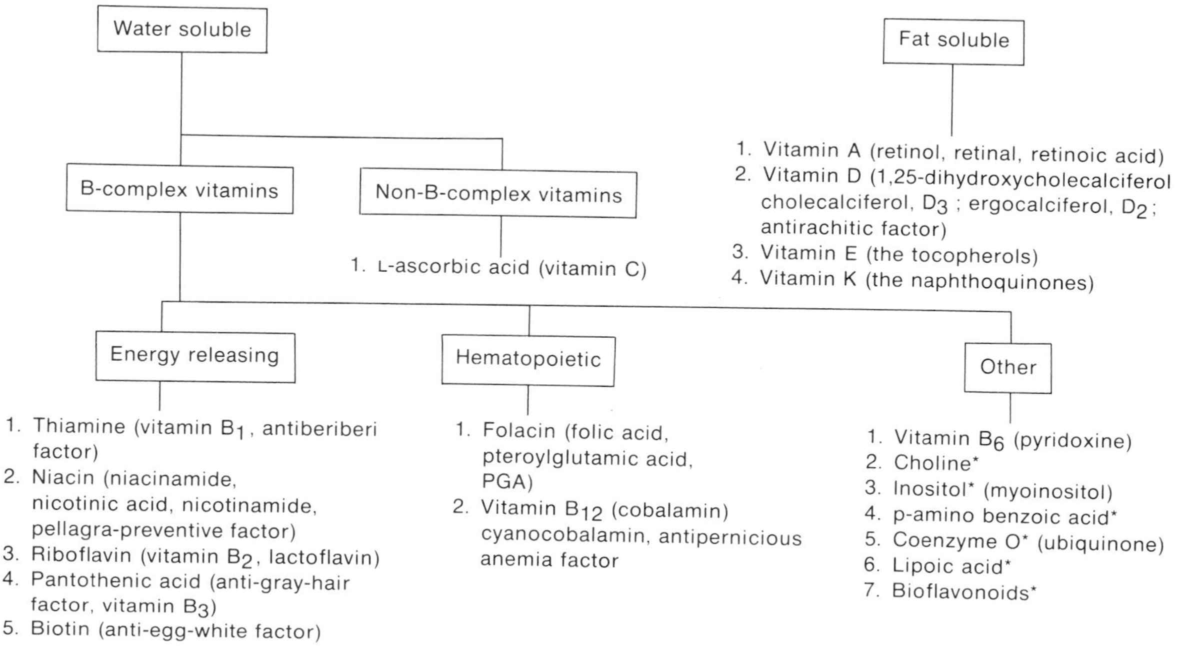

FIG. 73-1. The vitamins. *Dietary substance sometimes given vitamin status but not established as vitamins. (Schneider HA, Anderson CE, Coursin DB (eds): Nutritional Support of Medical Practice, p 25. Hagerstown, Harper & Row, 1977)

factors are important metabolically but are not yet accepted as vitamins (Fig. 73-1).

Vitamins are categorized as being fat soluble or water soluble, a classification useful because the fat-soluble vitamins have some properties in common, although physiologically and structurally they are quite different. For example, the lipid-soluble vitamins are absorbed from the intestine with dietary lipids. In malabsorption syndromes all the fat-soluble vitamins are absorbed poorly, or not at all, whereas the water-soluble vitamins may not be affected. Also, as a consequence of their lipid solubility, significant quantities of the lipid-soluble vitamins are stored in the liver, but the storage of water-soluble vitamins is not usually significant. Therefore, although a several weeks' supply of the lipid-soluble vitamins may be administred in a single dose, the water-soluble vitamins must be supplied frequently.

Although at present there is a vast body of information on the vitamins, only the most meager clues exist as to the mechanism that connects the vitamin deficiency, the tissue lesion with the biochemical defect. Much research remains to be done.

WATER-SOLUBLE VITAMINS

Energy-Releasing Vitamins

Thiamine (Vitamin B_1). *Function.* Thiamine acts principally as part of the coenzyme thiamine pyrophosphate in the oxidative decarboxylation of alpha-keto acids. In animal cells this coenzyme plays a critical role in the attainment of energy. The decarboxylation of pyruvate to "active acetate," or acetyl coenzyme A, connects the glycolytic cycle of carbohydrate metabolism with the high energy-producing Krebs (citric acid) cycle. Similarly, the decarboxylation of α-ketoglutaric acid to succinyl coenzyme A is a key step in the energy-producing Krebs cycle itself. In these steps, other energy-connected vitamins and vitaminlike substances, that is, lipoic acid, pantothenic acid, nicotonic acid, and riboflavin, are involved. Thiamine also has a role in converting tryptophan to nicotinic acid and nicotinamide; tryptophan normally contributes to the body's niacin supply.

Deficiency. Thiamine deficiency in humans is called beriberi (Singhalese *beri*, meaning "weakness" or "I can't"). It is characterized biochemically by an accumulation of pyruvic and lactic acids, particularly in the blood and brain, and impairment of the cardiovascular, nervous, and gastrointestinal systems occurs.

Beriberi has been known since earliest time. In rice-eating people, it is endemic because of the still widespread consumption of decorticated or polished rice. In the Western world, the disease is rarely seen except in alcoholism, food faddism, and sometimes in malabsorption syndromes. In alcoholic persons, the deficiency may lead to Wernicke's disease and Korsakoff's syndrome. Irreversible brain damage may occur unless the disorder is recognized early and treated promptly.

Chemical Properties. The methylene bond between the two rings of thiamine is weak and easily destroyed in an alkaline medium. The active coenzyme form is thiamine pyrophosphate.

THIAMINE: VITAMIN B_1

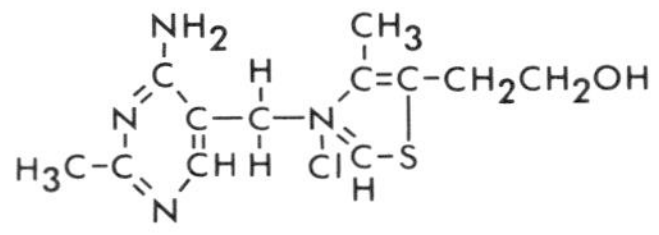

Thiamine is highly soluble in water and resists destruction at temperatures up to 100° C. It can, however, be destroyed if heated above 100° C, for example, in frying or being cooked too long under pressure. Thiamine is easily leached out of food being washed or boiled.

Absorption and Metabolism. Thiamine and its salts are easily absorbed from the small intestine. As with most of the water-soluble vitamins, the body is unable to store thiamine in any great quantity.

Liver, heart, and brain have higher concentrations of the active vitamin than does muscle tissue or other organs. A person on a high-thiamine intake regimen becomes saturated and begins to excrete increased quantities in urine.

Sources. The richest sources of thiamine are pork, whole grains, enriched cereal grains, and legumes. Green vegetables, fish, meat, fruits, and milk all contain useful quantities. In cereals the vitamin is present mainly in the germ and in the outer coat of the seed. Much of the vitamin is lost if cereals are milled or refined.

Requirement. The activity of thiamine hydrochloride is expressed in milligrams of the chemically pure and synthesized substance. From 1.2 to 1.5 mg daily is recommended for men and similar amounts for women. The following are recommended daily allowances: for infants 0.6 mg; children under 12, 0.8 to 1.4 mg; pregnant women, 1.6 mg; and lactating women 1.0 mg.

In addition the following are minimum daily requirements: infants 0.25 mg; children under 12, 0.5 to 0.75 mg; and adults 1.0 mg.

Toxicity. Taken in excessive amounts, thiamine is excreted in the urine and hence has no known toxicity. The kidney has no known threshold. Intolerance is rare, and daily doses of 500 mg have been administered for as long as 1 month without ill effects. Rarely, sensitization occurs after repeated parenteral administration.

Niacin. The discovery of niacin (nicotinic acid, nicotinamide, pellagra-preventive factor) and its association with the disease pellagra are closely linked. Pellagra was first described by Casals, a physician in Spain in 1730, soon after the introduction of corn (maize) into Europe. It was given its name (Italian *pelle,* skin ; *agra,* rough) in 1771 by the Italian physician Frapolli. The disease seems to have spread with the cultivation of corn, but not until 1917 did Goldberger, studying the disease among the poor and those in prisons in the southern United States, confirm his theory that the incidence of the disease is closely related to the quality of the diet and that certain foods (*e.g.,* yeast, milk, and meat) are pellagra preventive and can be used to treat the disease.

In 1916 T. N. Spencer, a veterinarian from Concord, North Carolina, first noted the similarity between the symptoms of a spontaneous canine disease known to veterinarians as "blacktongue" and those of human pellagra. He diagnosed blacktongue as pellagra in dogs, and from his successes in curing the animals by giving them milk, eggs, and meat he concluded that it was caused by a diet low in nitrogen.

In 1937 Elvehjem and colleagues, working at the University of Wisconsin, found that nicotinic acid was effective in curing blacktongue in dogs and pellagra in humans. Shortly there-

Carl Wernicke, 1848–1905. German neurologist. Remembered by his discovery of the speech center of the brain and Wernicke's sensory aphasia (1874), Wernicke's disease (1881), and Wernicke's paralysis (1889), a type of spastic hemiplegia.

after the use of nicotinic acid in treating human pellagra brought dramatic curative results.

Function. Niacin (nicotinic acid) is an essential part of the enzyme system concerned with hydrogen transport (oxidation) in living cells. It is the functional group of two coenzymes: *nicotinamide adenine dinucleotide* (NAD) and *nicotinamide adenine dinucleotide phosphate* (NADP). As coenzyme components of dehydrogenase enzyme systems, they assist in removing hydrogen from (oxidation of) the food substrate and then passing the hydrogens on to other components of the respiratory chain. At the end of the chain, hydrogen is united to oxygen to form water. The energy released is captured as high-energy adenine triphosphate and can then be released and transformed into other forms of energy (*e.g.*, mechanical, heat, the energy required for synthesis, and nervous energy) and can be used in other energy-requiring cellular functions.

NIACIN GROUP

NICOTINIC ACID

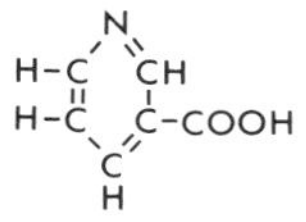

NICOTINAMIDE

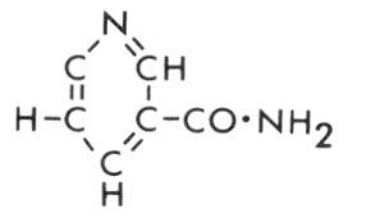

Deficiency. Niacin deficiency causes pellagra, characterized by dermatitis, diarrhea, depression, and, unless treated, death. Typical features of the disease are increasing weakness and a characteristic rash found only on the surfaces of the body exposed to the sun or heat. Early symptoms include glossitis, stomatitis, insomnia, anorexia, weakness, irritability, abdominal pain, burning sensations in various parts of the body, numbness, forgetfulness, marked fears, and vertigo. Ill-defined disturbances of the alimentary tract occur with changes of bowel function. Patients debilitated and weakened by diarrhea often die from infection or become subjected to mental disorder.

Chemical Properties. Niacin is a very stable, white compound moderately resistant to heat and to both acid and alkali.

The human body can convert tryptophan to niacin, and about 60 mg of dietary tryptophan is equivalent to 1 mg of niacin. Diets in the United States often contain 600 mg or more of tryptophan, providing a substantial contribution to the niacin pool.

Sources. Niacin is widely distributed but mostly in small amounts.

Corn is poor in niacin, and its principal protein, zein, is also very low in tryptophan. Some niacin in corn is present in a bound form that may not be bioavailable.

Requirement. Estimations of niacin requirements are complicated by the fact that tryptophan is converted to niacin in humans and by the paucity of studies of diets and of people at different ages. The allowance recommended for adults, expressed as niacin, is 6.6 mg/1000 Cal, and not less than 13 mg at caloric intakes of less than 2000 Cal. There are no data on the niacin requirements of children from infancy through adolescence. However, the following daily allowance is recommended: infants, 6 mg; children under 12, 9 to 16 mg; adults 13 to 22 mg; pregnant women, 17 mg; and lactating women, 21 mg.

The minimum daily requirement is, for children under 6, 5.0 mg; children over 6, 7.5 mg; and adults 10.0 mg.

Toxicity. Niacin is related chemically to nicotine but has quite different physiological properties. It is essentially nontoxic. Niacin (but not niacinamide) acts as a vasodilator and therefore may cause temporary cutaneous flushing, dizziness, and nausea.

Riboflavin. Riboflavin functions as a coenzyme or active prosthetic group in a group of flavoproteins concerned with tissue oxidation and respiration. Despite its fundamental role in the respiratory cycle as a hydrogen acceptor in energy and protein metabolism, no recognized disease is associated with an exclusive deficiency of riboflavin.

Riboflavin was discovered during the search for a hypothetical heat-stable vitamin B_2. Using its growth-promoting properties in the rat, Kuhn and his colleagues in 1933 finally isolated from 5400 liters of milk 1 g of active crystalline riboflavin. Unfortunately, it did not have the properties previously ascribed to vitamin B_2, for example, curing blacktongue in dogs. Clearly, riboflavin was just another of several factors present in the heat-stable fraction of the vitamin B complex.

An important clue to the nature of Kuhn's crystals was that they had a yellow color. A year earlier Warburg and Christian had described a "yellow enzyme," a respiratory catalyst that could act as a hydrogen acceptor and donor. Riboflavin and Warburg's yellow enzyme were found to be identical. The yellow enzyme proved to be a flavoprotein comprising a flavin pigment linked to a protein carrier. In 1935 riboflavin was synthesized by two independent groups: Kuhn and his colleagues in Heidelberg and Karrers' group in Basel.

Function. Riboflavin and various proteins form important enzymes that function in tissue respiration as components of the electron-transport system. These include L-amino and D-amino oxidases, xanthine oxidase, cytochrome-c reductase, and a number of dehydrogenases. The flavin coenzyme (prosthetic group) is usually flavin adenine dinucleotide (FAD) or, in some instances, flavin mononucleotide (FMN).

Deficiency. Characteristically, angular stomatitis, cheilosis, localized facial seborrheic dermatitis, glossitis (Magenta tongue), and certain functional and organic disorders of the eyes may appear. Many of these symptoms are not due to riboflavin deficiency alone but result from other deficiencies of the B complex group.

Chemical Properties and Structure. Riboflavin is an orange-yellow crystalline compound. It is water soluble and heat stable, especially in acid solution, but is easily decomposed by light. Riboflavin exhibits a yellow-green fluorescence in water solution.

RIBOFLAVIN: VITAMIN B_2

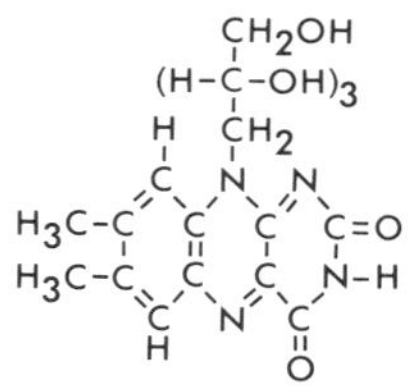

Absorption and Metabolism. Riboflavin is readily absorbed from the small intestine. It is phosphorylated in the intestine, liver, and other tissues, and some storage occurs in the liver, heart, and kidney. In humans, riboflavin is excreted predominantly in the feces where it arises both from mucosal and bacterial synthesis. It is also excreted in the urine as riboflavin or riboflavin phosphate.

Sources. Riboflavin is widely distributed in plant and animal tissues. The best food sources include milk, eggs, liver, kidney, heart, and green leafy vegetables.

Riboflavin is lost in appreciable quantities in food preparation if the food is cooked while exposed to light. Similarly it is destroyed when milk is bottled and exposed to sun or bright daylight. Losses also occur in dehydrated vegetables.

Requirements. Recommended allowances are 0.4 to 0.6 mg for infants; 0.8 to 1.2 mg for children; 1.3 to 1.8 mg for males, depending on age; and 1.1 to 1.3 mg for females. For pregnant women, 1.6 mg is recommended and for lactating women, 1.0 mg.

Minimum daily requirements are, for infants 0.6 mg; children under 12, 0.9 mg; and adults 1.2 mg.

Toxicity. There is no evidence of toxicity in humans when large amounts are consumed.

Pantothenic Acid. Pantothenic acid is an essential vitamin in humans. It is ubiquitous, hence its name from the Greek word *pantos* (meaning "everywhere"). Pantothenic acid occupies a central and basic role in carbohydrate, fat, and protein metabolism because of its position as part of the structure of coenzyme A (Fig. 73-2).

Function. As a constituent of coenzyme A, pantothenic acid is essential to a number of fundamental reactions in metabolism. It participates in this way in the release of energy from the catabolism of all three energy-yielding nutrients: carbohydrate, fat, and protein. The acetyl coenzyme A formed from the three major nutrients combines with oxalacetic acid to form citric acid, which initiates the citric acid or Krebs oxidative cycle, with the liberation and capture of the bond energies involved as high-energy adenosine triphosphate.

Pantothenic acid as a component of coenzyme A also participates in the biosynthesis of cholesterol and other sterols and of porphyrin, a component of hemoglobin. Pantothenic acid is involved in providing acetyl groups in the formation of acetyl choline and with the sulfonamides. Finally pantothenic acid is protein contained in a compound known as acyl carrier protein, required in the biosynthesis of fatty acids.

Deficiency. Pantothenic acid deficiency has been produced in human volunteers by the use of a purified diet and a specific metabolic an-

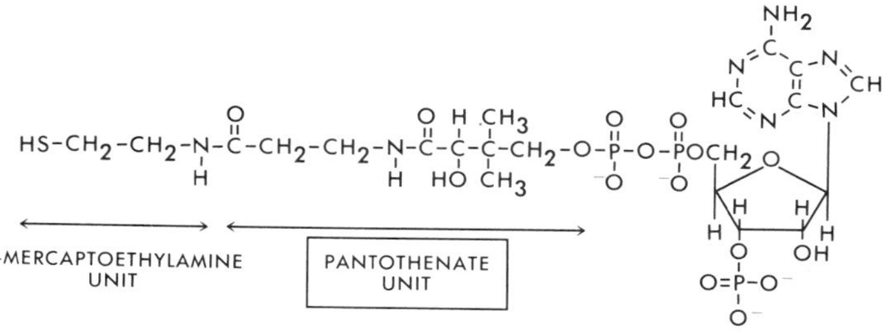

FIG. 73-2. Coenzyme A (CoA).

tagonist omega-methyl-pantothenic acid. Evidence of dietary deficiency has not been clinically recognized in humans, and the administration of a metabolic antagonist appears to be necessary to produce clinical symptoms. Symptoms and signs include fatigue, sleep disturbances, personality changes, nausea, abdominal stress, numbness and tingling of hands and feet, muscle cramps, impaired coordination, and diminished antibody production. All effects are reversed by the administration of the vitamin.

Calcium pantothenate has been used successfully to treat paralysis of the gastrointestinal tract after surgery, which causes gas to accumulate and severe abdominal pain. It may act by stimulating gastrointestinal motility. High levels of the acid (10–20 g) cause diarrhea. Intestinal bacteria synthesize considerable amounts of pantothenic acid. This, along with its widespread natural occurrence, makes a deficiency unlikely.

Chemical Properties and Structure. Pantothenic acid is a pale yellow oily liquid that has never been crystallized, although its calcium salt crystallizes readily. It is generally available in this latter form. Although stable in neutral solution, pantothenic acid is easily destroyed both on the acid and alkaline side of neutrality. It is readily soluble in water.

PANTOTHENIC ACID

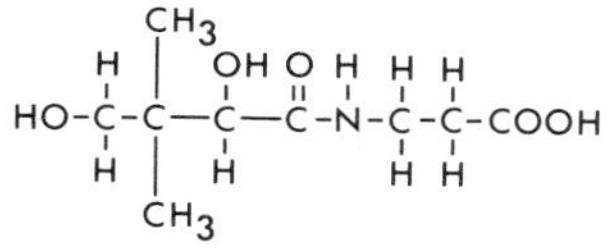

As a component of coenzyme A, pantothenic acid is involved in the intermediary metabolism of carbohydrate, fat, and protein, leading to energy release, synthesis of fatty acids and sterols, gluconeogenesis, and many other essential reactions.

Sources. Pantothenic acid is widely distributed in food, especially in foods from animal sources. The best sources are liver, kidney, egg yolk, yeast, wheat bran, and fresh vegetables (100–200 μg/g dry material); broccoli, lean beef, skimmed milk, sweet potatoes, and molasses are fair sources (35–100 μg/g dry material). It is probably synthesized by intestinal bacteria.

In most cooking and baking procedures, the vitamin loss is minimal, but temperature above the boiling point may cause considerable loss. Frozen meat may lose much of its original content in the drip that occurs with thawing.

Requirement. Pantothenic acid is readily available in most foods, and isolated dietary deficiencies are unlikely. Some subclinical deficiencies may be found in persons who are greatly malnourished.

There is no adequate evidence on which to base recommended allowance for pantothenic acid. Dietary intake in the adult population is 5 to 20 mg/day. Diets that meet nutritional needs of children contain 4 to 5 mg/day of the vitamin. A daily intake of 5 to 10 mg is thought to be adequate for adults, with the upper level suggested for pregnant and lactating women.

Toxicity. Toxicity from large intakes of pantothenic acid is not known to occur in humans.

Biotin. Biotin is a water-soluble vitamin widely distributed in nature and essential for many animal species, including man. The addition of 15% to 30% raw, dried egg-white as a source of protein to a diet low in biotin will induce symptoms of biotin deficiency. Raw egg-white contains a glycoprotein, avidin, that chelates biotin into a nonabsorbable complex.

Biotin was crystallized in 1936. It was given the name biotin because it is part of the "bios" factor needed for yeast growth, but early in the research of biotin deficiency it was also called the "anti-egg-white injury factor." Cooking denatures avidin so that it loses its ability to bind biotin.

Biotin deficiency does not occur in humans except when induced experimentally. To induce biotin deficiency with eggs, a diet must provide 30% of its calories from egg-white, which represents the egg-whites from more than two dozen eggs.

Function. Biotin is one of the most active biologic substances known. As little as 0.005 μg stimulates the growth of yeast and certain bacteria. In foods and tissues, biotin occurs bound to protein as part of several enzyme systems.

Biotin functions primarily as a coenzyme for reactions involving the addition of carbon dioxide to other units (carbon dioxide fixation) such as the carboxylation of pyruvic acid to oxalacetate in mitochondria. This bypass of the pyruvate dehydrogenase system serves to replenish oxalacetate under metabolic conditions when there is a strain on the supply of α-keto acids, as in gluconeogenesis. Biotin is also involved in the carboxylation of acetyl coenzyme A to malonyl coenzyme A in the biosynthesis of fatty acids, and in the conversion of propionyl coenzyme A to methylmalonyl coenzyme A in reactions involving the oxidation of odd-numbered carbon chains.

Biotin may be involved in carbohydrate and protein metabolism.

Deficiency. The effects of a biotin-deficient diet in animals are varied but seem to be characterized by early changes in the skin. Rats fed large amounts of egg-white develop an eczemalike dermatitis characterized by scaliness or hardening of the affected area and often starting as a characteristic alopecia around the eye. This is sometimes called "spectacle eye." Loss of hair and muscular atrophy follow these signs.

Although no evidence exists of a natural biotin deficiency in human adults, two types of dermatitis—Leiner's disease and seborrheic dermatitis (which occurs in infants)—may be caused by a lack of the vitamin. Both of these conditions respond rather dramatically to biotin therapy, although a similar condition in adults is not responsive.

Chemical Properties and Structure. Biotin is

BIOTIN

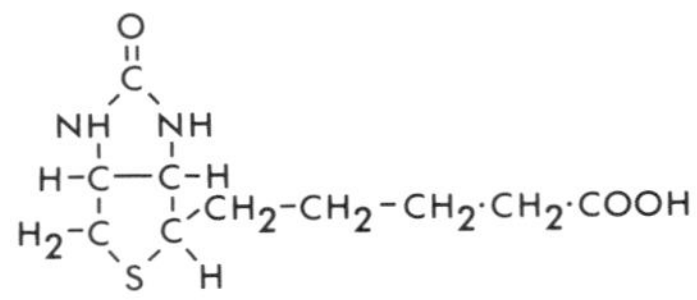

a white compound stable to heat in cooking, processing, and storage. However, being a somewhat water-soluble vitamin, losses will occur during cooking.

Biotin has been isolated in at least five active forms. One of these, biocytin, is a combination of biotin with the amino acid lysine, which may represent a fragment of the protein–coenzyme complex. Other important forms are biotin sulfone, a potent antagonist, and biotinal, which can be oxidized to an active form.

Protein-bound biotin in animal tissues is fat soluble, and the active substance in plants is water soluble. The bound form is liberated by the action of proteolytic enzymes, and therefore the linkage is believed to be peptide in nature.

Sources. Biotin is present in almost all foods, particularly those known to be good sources of the B-complex vitamins. Human milk contains an average of 0.16 μg/dl and seems little affected by variations in diet. Human milk has only one tenth as much biotin as cow's milk. Liver, kidney, milk, egg yolk, and yeast have been shown by biologic assay to be the richest sources. Pulses (peas, beans, lentils), nuts, chocolate, and some vegetables (*e.g.*, cauliflower) are fair sources. Animal meats (except for those listed above), dairy products, and cereals (unless fortified) are relatively poor sources. Except for cauliflower, nuts, and legumes, most vegetables are poorer in content than are meats. Most diets contain 150 to 300 μg of biotin, which is supplemented by bacterial intestinal synthesis that is stimulated by sucrose in the diet.

Requirement. It is believed that the body uses about 150 μg/day, an amount that appears to be adequately provided for in most diets, even without the amount of biotin provided by intestinal microorganism synthesis. Dietary intake of biotin is believed to be 100 to 300 μg/day.

Three to six times more biotin is excreted in the urine than is ingested, reflecting a major contribution of the active substance by the intestinal microflora. Humans can probably obtain all the biotin they need from the numerous microorganism present in the intestines.

Although biotin is recognized as being essential for humans, the uncertainty as to the amount contributed by intestinal microorganisms precludes a recommended daily allowance at this time.

Toxicity. Biotin has little or no toxicity. It is well tolerated by animals given large doses over prolonged periods.

Hematopoietic Vitamins

Folacin and Folic Acid. *Function and Deficiency.* Tetrahydrofolic acid plays an essential role in one-carbon transfers in metabolism. In this role it receives one-carbon radicals from such amino acids as serine, glycine, histidine, and tryptophan and transfers them at two steps in purine synthesis. In pyrimidine synthesis tetrahydrofolic acid is essential in the insertion of the methyl group in deoxyuridylic acid to form thymidylic acid, the characteristic nucleotide of DNA. Failure in this synthetic step is responsible for the megaloblastosis seen in folate and vitamin B_{12} deficiency.

Folic acid is needed for thymidylate synthesis as 5,10-methylene-tetrahydrofolate. 5,10-Methylene-tetrahydrofolate is in turn converted to 5′-methyl tetrahydrofolate, which is the methyl donor in the vitamin B_{12} dependent conversion of homocysteine to methionine. The distinction between folic acid deficiency and vitamin B_{12} deficiency is that when vitamin B_{12} is deficient, most of the folate is trapped in the methyl-tetrahydrofolate, which cannot then be used in the subsequent necessary reactions in DNA synthesis.

Chemical Properties and Structure. Folacin is a yellow crystalline substance sparingly soluble in water and stable in acid solution. When heated in neutral or alkaline solution, folacin is rapidly destroyed. Consequently it may be destroyed by some methods of cooking.

Up to seven additional molecules of glutamic acid may be attached through the α-carboxyl moiety to pteroylmonoglutamic acid.

FOLACIN
(represented by monopteroylglutamic acid)

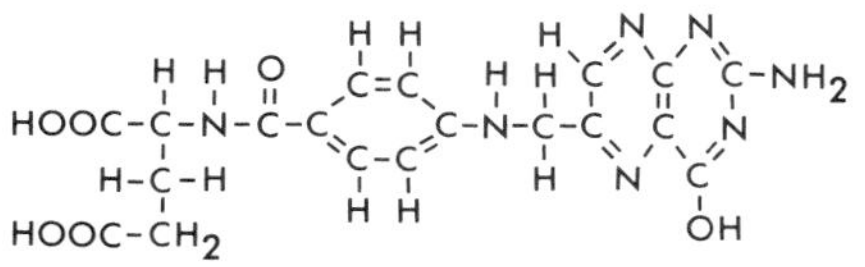

Absorption. A small intestinal mucosal conjugase (γ-L-glutamyl carboxypeptidase) hydrolyzes polyglutamyl forms of folic acid to free folic acid. Free folic acid is then absorbed from the upper part of the small intestine. During absorption it is believed that folic acid is reduced and methylated to methyl-tetrahydrofolic acid, the principal form of folate present in liver and plasma.

Sources. Good sources of folic acid are green leafy vegetables, liver, kidney, lima beans, asparagus, whole grain cereals, nuts, legumes, and yeast. The folacin content of many foods has not yet been established.

Requirement. The minimum need for adults is believed to be about 50 μg, or 0.05 mg. This allows a wide degree of difference that may be due to differences in the availability in various foods.

Toxicity. No toxic reactions to folacin have been seen when doses up to 15 mg have been taken daily for 1 month. Certain synthetic analogues are toxic, such as methotrexate.

Vitamin B_{12} (Cobalamin, Cyanocobalamin). *Function and Deficiency.* Vitamin B_{12} is essential to the proper functioning of all mammalian cells. Deficiency is most severely felt in rapidly dividing cells such as in hematopoietic tissue and in the gastrointestinal tract. A deficiency in the nervous system may lead to degeneration of nerve fibers in the spinal cord and peripheral nerves. In the bone marrow, abnormal cells—megaloblasts—can be seen. When these are present, the circulating red cells derived from them are bigger than normal (macrocytes) but usually carry a normal hemoglobin concentration (normochromic).

The formation of megaloblasts, or megaloblastosis, occurs because the formation of DNA is inhibited. Synthesis of RNA does not appear to be affected. Vitamin B_{12} deficiency depletes the cell of 5,10-methylene-tetrahydrofolate, which is necessary as a coenzyme in the synthesis of thymidylate, the nucleotide of thymidine that is the characteristic base of DNA.

The way in which vitamin B_{12} affects the nervous system is not clear. However, vitamin B_{12} also appears to be necessary for myelin formation, since a deficiency gives rise to myelin damage.

Chemical Properties and Structure. Vitamin B_{12} is present in the body in several forms. The coenzyme forms are 5-deoxyadenosyl cobalamin and methyl cobalamin. The originally isolated vitamin B_{12} was a cyanocobalamin, a form that has not been found in natural materials. In the isolation of the vitamin, cyanide was added to promote its crystallization. The natural isolated form appears to be hydroxycobalamin.

Crystalline vitamin B_{12} is freely soluble in water and is resistant to boiling in neutral solutions. It is unstable in solutions in the presence of alkali.

VITAMIN B_{12}

(represented by cyanocobalamin)

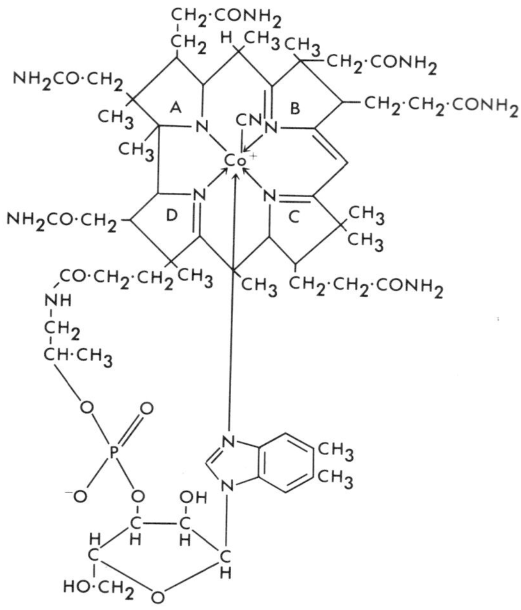

Absorption. Vitamin B_{12} requires a heat-labile glycoprotein called the intrinsic factor by Castle for intestinal absorption. This substance is secreted from the parietal cells of the stomach during the normal secretion of gastric juice. Food vitamin B_{12} released from a protein complex binds to the intrinsic factor, which it is believed helps attach the vitamin to a receptor in the intestinal mucosa of the terminal ileum. Calcium seems to be needed in this process. In the intestinal cell membrane, vitamin B_{12} is released from the intrinsic factor and absorbed into the blood.

If the gastric juice secreted by the stomach lacks intrinsic factor, absorption does not take place. Under these conditions, massive intakes of vitamin B_{12} may be given on the assumption that some diffusion into the blood will take place.

The plasma concentration of vitamin B_{12} in healthy persons normally is between 200 and 960 pg/ml. The capacity of the intestine to absorb cyanocobalamin is a valuable test (Shilling test) of absorptive capacity. Normal subjects usually absorb 30% of a test dose and excrete most of it in the urine. Persons with pernicious anemia absorb and excrete about 2% of a test dose.

Sources. Since plants cannot synthesize vitamin B_{12}, it is found only in food of animal origin. Microorganisms in the human gastrointestinal tract may synthesize the vitamin, but the site of synthesis in the colon does not allow absorption. In ruminants, microorganisms synthesize vitamin B_{12} from the plants eaten, and this can then be absorbed from the gastrointestinal tract. Therefore, domestic animals are a good food source.

The best sources of vitamin B_{12} are beef liver, kidney, whole milk, eggs, oysters, fresh shrimp, pork, and chicken.

Requirement. Humans need very small amounts of B_{12}. The recommended amount in the diet is 3 μg/day, of which 1 to 1.5 μg is absorbed. A range of 0.5 to 2.5 μg appears desirable. The average American diet contains 7 to 30 μg of the vitamin. The requirement is increased if the body metabolic rate is raised, as in fever or hyperthyroidism.

Other Water-Soluble Vitamins

Pyridoxine (Vitamin B_6). Pyridoxine owes its name to the structural resemblance to the pyridine ring. Originally, pyridoxine was used synonymously with vitamin B_6. The work of Snell and colleagues shows clearly that pyridoxine (or pyridoxol, an alcohol) is biologically converted into two other compounds: pyridoxal (an aldehyde) and pyridoxamine (an amine). All three of these compounds are active biologically as the vitamin, and pyridoxine is often used as the collective term for all three. The active coenzyme forms of pyridoxine are pyridoxal phosphate and pyridoxamine phosphate.

VITAMIN B_6 GROUP

PYRIDOXINE

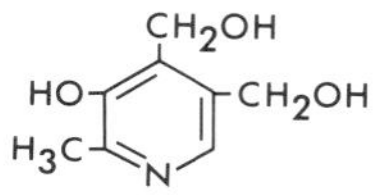

PYRIDOXAL

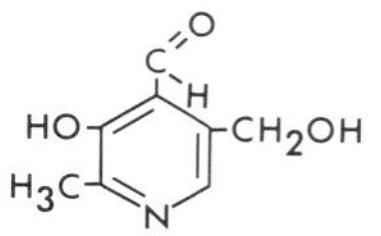

PYRIDOXAMINE

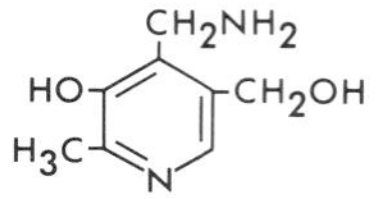

Function. Vitamin B_6 is involved primarily with reactions that include the synthesis and catabolism of amino acids and is therefore critical to protein synthesis.

Pyridoxal phosphate and pyridoxamine phosphate are very versatile coenzymes that function in a large number of different enzymatic reactions in which amino acids or amino groups are transformed or transferred. For example, pyridoxal phosphate is required as a coenzyme in transamination reactions in which the α-amino acid group of an amino acid is transferred to the α-carbon of an α-keto acid. In this manner the amino group of L-alanine in the presence of alanine transaminase transfers its amino group to α-ketoglutaric acid to form L-glutamate and pyruvate.

During the metabolic conversion of tryptophan to acetyl coenzyme A, kynureninase catalyzes the conversion of 3-hydroxykynurenine to 3-hydroxyanthranilic acid. This step requires pyridoxal phosphate and is critical in the biosynthesis of nicotinic acid, which will not be synthesized in a deficiency of pyridoxal phosphate. In deficiency states, large amounts of L-kynurenine are excreted in the urine.

Pyridoxal phosphate is a cofactor in the formation of a porphyrin precursor, an essential component of hemoglobin.

Pyridoxine appears to be involved in the metabolism of the central nervous system. Changes in electroencephalograms occur in pyridoxine deficiency. In a severe deficiency, convulsive seizures take place. Vitamin B_6 seems to be needed to prevent uncontrolled excitation of the central nervous system and eventual uncontrolled muscle seizures.

Deficiency. In adults the only symptom that can be ascribed to a lack of pyridoxine is a microcytic hypochromic anemia, which occurs with a high serum iron level. Other symptoms are weakness, nervousness, irritability, insomnia, and difficulty in walking.

Absorption and Metabolism. Pyridoxine is water soluble and heat stable but sensitive to light and alkali. As with the other B vitamins, it is absorbed in the upper part of the small intestine, where a lower *p*H facilitates passage. Once absorbed, all three forms are converted to pyridoxal phosphate, the coenzyme form. After absorption the vitamin phosphate is widely distributed.

Pyridoxine is excreted in the urine chiefly as 4-pyridoxic acid along with small amounts of pyridoxal and pyridoxamine.

Sources. Pyridoxine is widespread in nature but frequently occurs in very small amounts. Good sources of the vitamin are yeast, wheat and corn, egg yolk, liver, kidney, and muscle meats. Limited amounts are present in milk and vegetables. Vegetables that are frozen may lose as much as 20% of their original activity. Milling of cereals may lead to losses as high as 90%.

Requirement. Since there is no area in the world where pyridoxine deficiency has been defined as a problem resulting in poor nutrition, establishing a firm requirement is difficult. The Food and Nutrition Board has recommended 2 mg/day for adults. Data are not sufficient for evaluating the requirement for pyridoxine or vitamin B_6 for children and adolescents. The allowances recommended range up to 2.0 mg/day.

Toxicity. Toxicity has been described in men who received 300 mg/day. This dose far exceeds that recommended for treatment and is impossible to obtain from the diet. When pyridoxine is given intramuscularly to humans, it causes some pain, probably owing to the acidity of the solution.

Ascorbic Acid (Vitamin C). *Function.* Although it was once assumed that the metabolic role of ascorbic acid is related to its reversible oxidation and reduction properties, no role in biologic oxidation systems has been described in which ascorbic acid serves as a specific coenzyme. Ascorbic acid is, however, essential in the daily human diet. Many species of animals can synthesize ascorbic acid in their tissues and thus do not need it in their diet. However, man, other primates, and the guinea pig, by consuming food deficient in ascorbic acid, will soon develop scurvy, a potentially fatal disease characterized by deterioration of collagenous connective tissues and structures.

Connective tissue consists of system of insoluble protein fibers embedded in a continuous matrix called ground substance. Its chief function is supportive, mainly by fibrils of insoluble protein, such as collagen and elastin. Collagen is the most abundant protein in mammals, constituting one fourth of the protein of tissues and providing the major fibrous structure of skin, cartilage, tendons, ligaments, blood vessels, bone, and teeth. The intercellular cement—collagen—functions to hold the tissue cells together in discrete organized systems.

In scurvy, the hydroxylation of collagen is impaired and it cannot properly form fibers, thereby resulting in the classic skin lesions and blood vessel fragility. Similar clinical conditions include easy bruising, pinpoint peripheral hemorrhages, easy bone fracture and joint hemorrhage, poor wound healing, and friable bleeding gums with loosened teeth.

Ascorbic acid can function as a reducing agent for iron in the gastrointestinal tract and thereby enhance its absorption.

Deficiency. Scurvy is not a common disease today because of our knowledge of preventive measures. It may be seen in infants, food faddists or cranks, alcoholics, and older people. People with frank scurvy can be recognized readily, but borderline cases require experience in diagnosis. Gums are swollen, particularly between the teeth, and bleed easily. Bleeding may occur in all parts of the body, and numerous small hemorrhages or petechiae may be seen under the skin. Trivial injuries may give rise to large bruises. Large joints, such as in the knee or hip, may appear swollen because of bleeding into the joint cavity. Severe internal hemorrhages may lead to sudden death and heart failure. Adequate intake of ascorbic acid rapidly reverses these signs or symptoms.

The increased use of artificial milk products as a sole source of food for infants soon after birth has produced an increased number of cases of infantile scurvy. In older persons, declining appetite, immobility, and reduced income tend to reduce the intake of ascorbic acid and produce borderline cases of ascorbic acid deficiency. In both of the above deficiencies, the symptoms can be reversed and prevented by fruit juice or supplements of ascorbic acid.

Chemical Properties and Structure. L-Ascorbic acid is closely related to glucose. D-Ascorbic acid and many closely related compounds show very little antiscorbutic activity. It has been proposed, to avoid confusion, that D-ascorbic acid (biologically inactive) be called erythrobic acid.

ASCORBIC ACID: VITAMIN C

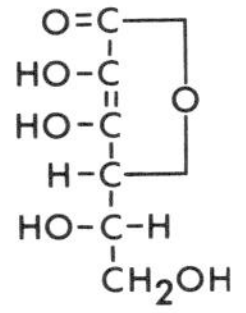

The most prominent chemical properties of L-ascorbic acid are its acidity, owing to the dissociation of the enolic hydroxyl groups, and its ready oxidation to dehydroascorbic acid. This oxidation product has about 80% of the activity of the vitamin itself. Further oxidation produces diketogulonic acid, which is inactive. This reaction is irreversible. In mammalian tissues the reversible reduction of dehydroascorbic acid to ascorbic acid appears to be aided by reducing agents, such as the sulfhydryl group of glutathione, which may be involved physiologically in maintaining the vitamin in the reduced form. Ascorbic acid is the most active reducing agent known to occur naturally in living tissues.

Most animals can synthesize ascorbic acid and thus need no dietary supply. A few species, however (man, monkeys, and the guinea pig), lack the necessary enzyme to complete the conversion of glucose or galactose to L-ascorbic acid. A dietary supply of the vitamin is therefore essential to prevent scurvy.

Absorption. Ascorbic acid is easily absorbed from the upper small intestine, probably by simple diffusion or by an active sodium-dependent transport. Apart from the adrenal cortex, tissue storage is low.

Sources. Fruits, especially citrus fruits, and tomatoes are rich sources of vitamin C. Green vegetables are also good sources, but much of the vitamin C activity may be lost in preparation and cooking.

Although rather low in ascorbic acid, potatoes and the root vegetables, if consumed in large quantities, become good sources. Storage lowers the content of ascorbic acid in potatoes, and excessive cooking completely destroys the vitamin. Animal products, such as meat, fish, eggs, and milk, are not a good source. The vitamin C contained in meat is easily destroyed by heating.

The loss of ascorbic acid by oxidation in foods is hastened by the action of ascorbic acid oxidase, which is present in raw fruits and vegetables. This enzyme becomes active when leaves or fruits are damaged by drying, bruising, or cutting.

Requirement. An intake of 30 mg/day is sufficient to replenish the quantity of ascorbic acid metabolized daily. An intake of 45 mg/day will maintain an adequate body pool. Although not known precisely, the infant's need for ascorbic acid seems to be met satisfactorily by the amount provided by the milk of the adequately fed mother, 40 to 55 mg/liter. For children up to 11 years of age, 40 mg/day is recommended. For adult males and females, 45 mg/day is recommended. Pregnant women should receive

60 mg/day, with an increase to 80 mg/day for lactating women.

Large doses of ascorbic acid (0.5–5 g/day) have reportedly reduced the frequency of the common cold, but these claims have not been sufficiently substantiated.

Toxicity. Ingestion by mouth of massive amounts of ascorbic acid has not produced direct toxicity. Because of its rapid excretion in the urine and its alteration of urinary *p*H, significant drug interactions may develop (*see* Chap. 8).

FAT-SOLUBLE VITAMINS

Vitamin A. During the early part of this century, Osborne and Mendel in New Haven and McCollum and Davis in Wisconsin and Baltimore noted that some of their rats fed purified diets grew poorly and developed inflamed eyes. When certain fats such as cod liver oil, butter, or ether extracts of egg yolk were added to their diets, the animals grew normally. This led eventually to the concept of fat-soluble vitamins as distinguished from water soluble vitamins. There are four known fat-soluble vitamins: A, D, E, and K.

Although vitamin A was one of the first vitamins to be discovered and has been known chemically since Karrer determined its structure in 1931, the chief metabolic role or function of the vitamin is still puzzling and unclear. Active preformed vitamin A is found only in foods of animal origin. However, the carotinoid pigments of plants contain inactive precursor substances, or provitamins A, that can be converted to the active vitamin when eaten and digested by animals. There are thus two sources of the vitamin: the vitamin present in animal foods; and the inactive provitamins present in foods of plant origin.

Vitamin A is a collective term now used to refer to all forms of the vitamin that are biologically active. Vitamin A alcohol is called *retinol,* vitamin A aldehyde *retinal,* and vitamin A acid *retinoic acid.*

Function. Even though at present it is not possible to relate the symptoms of vitamin A deficiency to a specific biochemical defect, except perhaps for pigments of the eye, it is possible to identify five distinct metabolic roles for the vitamin: visual purple and vision in dim light; growth; reproduction; health of epithelial cells; and a role involving the stability of membranes.

Maintenance of Visual Purple. The specific role of vitamin A in biochemical and physiological mechanisms of vision has been worked out largely by Wald and Morton. During the light reaction, rhodopsin, a photoreceptor pigment or visual purple that occurs in the rod cells of the retina, is split into a protein component, opsin, and vitamin A aldehyde (retinal). This reaction occurs during the light-bleaching reaction. As light strikes the retina, visual purple is bleached to visual yellow and retinal is separated from opsin. This light reaction excites the optic nerve, which in turn transfers the stimulus to the brain. During this process some retinal is reduced to retinol. Most of this retinol, in the presence of a dehydrogenase, is oxidized to retinal, which then can recombine with opsin to regenerate visual purple. Small losses occur through excretion, probably as retinoic acid, which must be replaced from the blood. The amount of retinal in the blood determines the rate at which rhodopsin is regenerated and made available to act as a receptor substance in the retina.

In vitamin A deficiency, a long lag in the ability of the visual mechanism to regenerate rhodopsin results in night blindness or nyctalopia. Examples of this phenomenon can be seen in the lag in adaptation of a person entering a dimly lit theater from a brightly lit street, or in the temporary blindness experienced by a driver at night meeting the headlights of an oncoming car.

The biochemical mechanism underlying color vision in the cones of the retina is analogous to that of rod vision. Again, retinal combines with a specific protein but one that differs from opsin.

Growth. An animal deprived of vitamin A will cease to grow and will die when its tissue reserves of vitamin A are depleted. A possible initial reason may be loss of appetite, which can be attributed to loss of the sense of taste resulting from keratinization of taste bud spores.

In young animals, experimentally produced vitamin A deficiency is accompanied by a cessation of bone growth. Bones fail to grow in length, and although intramembranous bone formation appears to be normal, the remodeling sequences become abnormal and stop. The defect in bone growth is thought to result from a failure in the normal conversion of osteoblasts (cells responsible for an increased number of bone cells) to osteoclasts, which causes a breakdown of bone during the process of remodeling. The bones of young vitamin A-deficient animals may be short and thick.

Bone disorders have not been observed in adults during induced vitamin A deficiency.

Nerve lesions observed in experimental vitamin A deficiency result from disproportionate growth between nerve tissues and bone. Under conditions of bone growth failure, undue pressure may occur in the brain and other nervous tissues because the protective bony framework fails to grow fast enough to accommodate these tissues. Bone growth is stimulated when vitamin A is again made available.

Reproduction. Vitamin A, either as retinol or retinal, is essential for normal reproduction. Retinoic acid does not appear to be involved in reproduction. Without vitamin A, spermatogenesis failure occurs in males and fetal resorption in females. The biochemical defect is unknown. Decreased estrogen synthesis when cholesterol is not converted to the hormone may be related to the reproductive abnormality in females. In males, vitamin A acts directly on the testes in some unknown manner, which is diminished in the deficiency.

Maintenance of Epithelial Cells. A major function of vitamin A is to maintain the health of the epithelial tissues. Epithelial cells are found in the linings of all openings into the interior of the body, for example, the alimentary tract, respiratory tract, and the genitourinary tract, as well as the glands and their ducts. They form the outer protective layer of the skin. These cells thus form an important "first line of defense" against invading bacteria and other microorganisms. The presence of degenerative changes when vitamin A is lacking is evidence that vitamin A is essential to the normal biochemical reactions that underlie the health of these cells. Epithelial cells are characterized by continuous replacement and differentiation; they produce protective mucopolysaccharides as secretory products.

When deprived of an adequate supply of vitamin A, epithelial tissues undergo changes that lead to a horny degeneration called *keratinization*. Drying of the cells of the cornea and skin occurs. The mucous membranes that line the mouth, throat, nose, and respiratory passages are damaged. This is one of the earlier signs of vitamin A deficiency. In addition to general deterioration of the epithelial cells and membranes, the cells lack normal secretions and cilia loss occurs. (By constant movement, the cilia aid in keeping the membrane surface clean.) Susceptibility to infections, such as sinus trouble, sore throat, and abscesses in ears, mouth, or salivary glands, is a common finding when vitamin A is lacking in the diet.

Stability of Cell Membranes. Vitamin A participates in an unknown way in reactions that involve the stability of the subcellular particle membranes of the lysosomes and mitochondria as well as of the cell membranes. The association between many of the changes just described and vitamin A cannot be explained with certainty. Vitamin A may have a role in cell differentiation through an influence on RNA and DNA.

Deficiency. The liver reserves of vitamin A must be depleted before symptoms of a deficiency appear. Growth ceases when the reserves are depleted. Most deficiency symptoms seen are directly or indirectly a reflection of the health of epithelial cells. A deficiency may result from [1] a low dietary intake of vitamin A for various causes; [2] interference with absorption from the small intestine owing to diseases of the pancreas, liver, gallbladder, or mucosal cells, as in malabsorption; [3] interference with the conversion of carotene to vitamin A; and [4] rapid loss of vitamin A.

In a vitamin deficiency the vitamin A concentration in plasma is usually below 20 μg/dl but may be so low as to be undetectable. It must remain low for a prolonged period to produce clinical signs of vitamin A deficiency. Normal levels are 30 to 50 μg/dl.

Night Blindness. An early symptom of vitamin A deficiency is night blindness, or nyctalopia. The visual purple pigment rhodopsin in the receptor cells or cones of the retina is necessary for vision in dim light. These receptor cells require a constant replenishment of the small amounts of vitamin A lost in the visual cycle during which a nerve impulse is transmitted to the optic nerve and rhodopsin is regenerated. A low or depleted liver reserve of vitamin A is reflected in the blood level and slower rate of regeneration of vitamin A. If continued, this will show up as slow dark-adaptation time and, eventually, night blindness.

Xerophthalmia. Xerophthalmia usually begins with a drying of the conjunctiva, which loses its shining luster. The condition may then spread to the cornea, which also becomes dull and loses its power to reflect. The lacrimal gland fails to secrete tears because of a blocked duct or a reduced ability to synthesize mucopolysaccharide. This pathologic dryness of the eye, which robs it of its normal epithelial protection, is called xerophthalmia and is a precursor of keratomalacia. If the condition remains untreated, ulceration leading to perforation, loss of intraocular fluid, and severe secondary infection may occur. Pus is exudated, and the eye will hemorrhage. This condition is known as Bitot's spots in its mildest form, as xerosis conjunctivae in moderately severe form, and as xerophthalmia in advanced stages. At this last stage, the patient is seriously ill with pyrexia and a grossly inflamed eye. Blindness in the infected eye is the inevitable result. Severe cases of xerophthalmia should be treated at once because the sight and life of the individual, usually a child, are at stake. Many children probably die of other forms of vitamin deficiency or an infection before xerophthalmia develops. Xerophthalmia occurs frequently in children in developing tropical countries where a low protein intake may be a contributive factor.

Chemical Properties and Structure. Only foods of animal origin contain preformed vitamin A. The active vitamin is a complex primary alcohol that contains a β-ionone ring with an unsaturated side-chain terminating in an alcohol group. The β-ionone ring is essential for vitamin activity, and when it is absent or altered structurally the compound may become inactive. The compound is pale yellow, almost colorless, is soluble in fat or fat solvents, and is insoluble in water. It can be destroyed by oxidation when exposed to air at high temperatures or to ultraviolet light. The vitamin A content of fats and oils can be destroyed by oxidation, since they become rancid unless protected by antioxidants or stored in a cool, dark place.

VITAMIN A (represented by retinol)

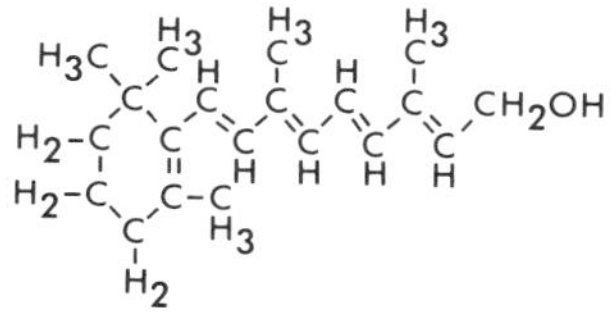

The ultimate source of vitamin A is plants. Here the provitamin form occurs as highly colored yellow or orange carotenoid pigments or carotenes. These give color to carrots, sweet potatoes, peaches, and other colored vegetables and fruits. The green color of vegetables often masks the yellow–orange color of the carotenes because of the green pigment chlorophyll, which does not have vitamin A activity. There are a number of carotenoid pigments in plants, but the three known as alpha (α), beta (β), and gamma (γ) carotene and a fourth, cryptoxanthine, the yellow pigment of corn, are important in human nutrition. Their ability to replace vitamin A in the diet depends on the integrity of the β-ionone ring. Of these forms, β-carotene is the provitamin member that when eaten and digested is theoretically cleaved in the intestinal mucosal cell into two molecules of vitamin A. Unfortunately, the ability of the human mucosal cell to split β-carotene into the two active forms of vitamin A does not approach this degree of efficiency.

Absorption and Metabolism. Both vitamin A and the carotenes are fat soluble. Their absorption from the intestine and use in tissues may therefore be decreased in the malabsorptive state. Such diseases as celiac disease, sprue, and liver disease, which interferes with bile production or flow, may induce vitamin A deficiency. Diarrhea and excessive intakes of mineral oil may also interfere with the absorption of vitamin A and the carotenes.

Preformed vitamin A in food, usually esterified with palmitic acid as retinyl palmitate, must be hydrolyzed by pancreatic enzymes before being absorbed by the muscosal cell as retinol. The carotenes and cryptoxanthine are absorbed intact in the presence of bile salts and are converted to retinol by a cleavage enzyme in the intestinal mucosal cell.

Retinol, either from dietary sources or the result of hydrolysis, is esterified inside the mucosal cell, preferentially with palmitic acid. Retinyl palmitate incorporated in chylomicrons is introduced to the bloodstream by means of the lymphatic system and thoracic duct; it is stored in the liver.

Sources. Preformed vitamin A is available only in animal products in which the animal has converted the carotene of food into active vitamin A. Food sources of preformed vitamin include liver, kidney, cream, butter, and egg yolk. The major dietary source of active vitamin A are the provitamins in yellow and green vegetables and fruits—for example, carrots, sweet potatoes, squash, apricots, spinach, collards, broccoli, cabbage, and dark leafy greens. In some defects of the intestinal tract—such as the malabsorption syndrome, lack of bile salts, defects in the epithelial cells of the intestinal mucosa, or conditions leading to diarrhea—the provitamins are not absorbed or converted to the active enzyme and are often excreted in stool.

Requirements. In the current National Academy of Sciences Table of Allowances, requirements are given in retinol equivalents. By definition, 1 retinol equivalent is equal to 1 μg of retinol or 6 μg of β-carotene or 12 μg of other provitamin A carotenoids. In terms of international units (IU), 1 retinol equivalent is equal to 3.33 IU retinol or 10 IU β-carotene. The vitamin A values of diets, expressed as retinol equivalents, can be calculated by following the example presented in the RDA. The recommended allowances are, for infants, 1500 IU; children under 12, 2000 to 4500 IU; adults, 5000 IU; pregnant women, 6000 IU; and lactating women, 8000 IU.

The minimum daily requirements (U.S.P.U.) are, for infants, 1500 IU; children under 12, 3000 IU; and adults, 4000 IU.

Toxicity. High intakes of vitamin A are toxic. Smith and Goodman have reported three cases of human vitamin A toxicity. A 4-year-old girl had been given daily doses of 25,000 units of vitamin A by her anxious, compulsive mother for 2 years before admission to a hospital. Three weeks before admission she developed increasingly severe pain in the ankles and feet, followed by transient loss of vision. On the day of admission she was found to have papilledema by her pediatrician. In addition, she had a faint yellow tint to the skin over her palms; a faint, erythematous eruption over her wrists, hands, and buttocks; and widespread excoriated areas over her entire body. Vitamin A supplement was withdrawn, and she was given a diet low in vitamin A and carotene. By the time of her discharge 9 days after admission, she no longer had visual difficulties, the dermatitis was improved, and the papilledema had disappeared. One month later she was asymptomatic except for continued scalp-hair loss.

The symptoms of vitamin A toxicity include headache, drowsiness, nausea, dry skin and loss of hair, diarrhea in adults, scaly dermatitis, weight-loss, anorexia, and, in infants, skeletal pain. Carotenoid deposits may cause a yellow dyspigmentation of the soles of the feet, palms of the hands, and nasolabial folds. Increased intracranial pressure and edema may develop. After periods of excessive intake of vitamin A in young women, hemoglobin and potassium loss from the red blood cells and cessation of menstruation occur.

Wide individual differences in sensitivity to high levels of vitamin A appear to exist. Infants have shown bulging on the head, hydrocephalus, hyperirritability, and increased intracranial pressure after doses of 25,000 IU/day for 30 days. At least one death has occurred in a food faddist.

Because of the toxicity that can be induced by high concentrations of vitamin A, the FDA has imposed a ceiling of 10,000 IU on the amount of vitamin A that can be induced in a multivitamin preparation without prescription.

Vitamin D. In 1918, Mellanby in England first clearly showed by his classic studies in puppies that rickets, a crippling bone deformity in children, is a nutritional disease that responds to a fat-soluble vitamin—vitamin D—present in cod-liver oil. If an infant lacks the vitamin, the growing portion of his bones do not harden. If the deficiency persists as the child grows, the bones cannot support the weight of the body, resulting in bowlegs, knock-knees, and enlarged joints. Other deformities of the chest, spine, and pelvis develop.

VITAMIN D (represented by cholecalciferol, vitamin D_3)†

CHOLECALCIFEROL

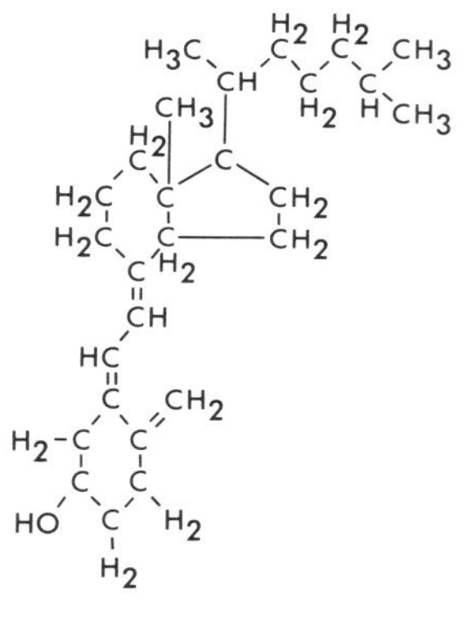

Vitamin D is actually a group of closely related steroid alcohols with vitamin D activity that promote the absorption of calcium from the small intestine and are involved in an essential way in the mineralization of bone. From the point of nutritional importance, vitamin D exists in two forms: vitamin D_2 (ergocalciferol) and vitamin D_3 (cholecalciferol). Vitamin D_1 is now known as an impure mixture of sterols.

Function. Vitamin E has been aptly described as "the vitamin in search of a disease." In a like spirit, vitamin D can be described as a vitamin with a split personality. It is present in foods and thus functions as a vitamin in the human diet. Since, in humans, cholecalciferol is formed in one organ of the body (the skin) and acts on distant target organs (the intestine and bone), it can be considered to function as a hormone.

Vitamin D is necessary for the formation of normal bone. In this role it acts on the small intestine, where it promotes the absorption of calcium and phosphorus from the intestinal lumen. It is not certain, but it may also act directly on the bone, kidneys, and other tissues. These functions of vitamin D depend on the conversion of cholecalciferol in the body into two more active substances. Dietary vitamin D is absorbed from the intestinal lumen and carried from the intestinal cell in chylomicrons. In the blood, vitamin D of both dietary and cutaneous origin is carried on an α-globulin to the liver. In the liver it is converted into 25-hydroxycholecalciferol (25-HCC). A summary of the metabolism of vitamin D is shown in Figure 73-3.

Carried in the blood from the liver to the kidney, 25-HCC is further hydroxylated to 1,25-dihydroxycholecalciferol (1,25-DCC), which is secreted by the kidney into the blood and carried to the target tissues. In the small intestine, 1,25-DCC enters the intestinal epithelial cell, where it functions apparently through DNA in the nucleus of the intestinal cell to initiate the synthesis in the cytoplasm of a specific calcium-binding protein. This calcium-binding

1,25-DIHYDROXYCHOLECALCIFEROL

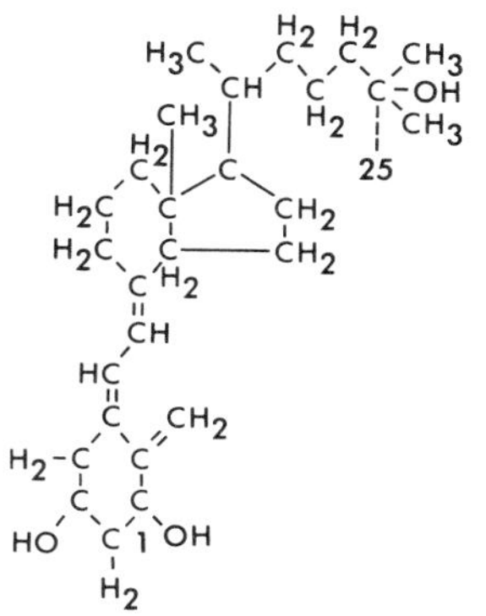

FIG. 73-3. Vitamin-D metabolism. (Schneider HA, Anderson CE, Coursin DB (eds): Nutritional Support of Medical Practice, p 44. Hagerstown, Harper & Row, 1977)

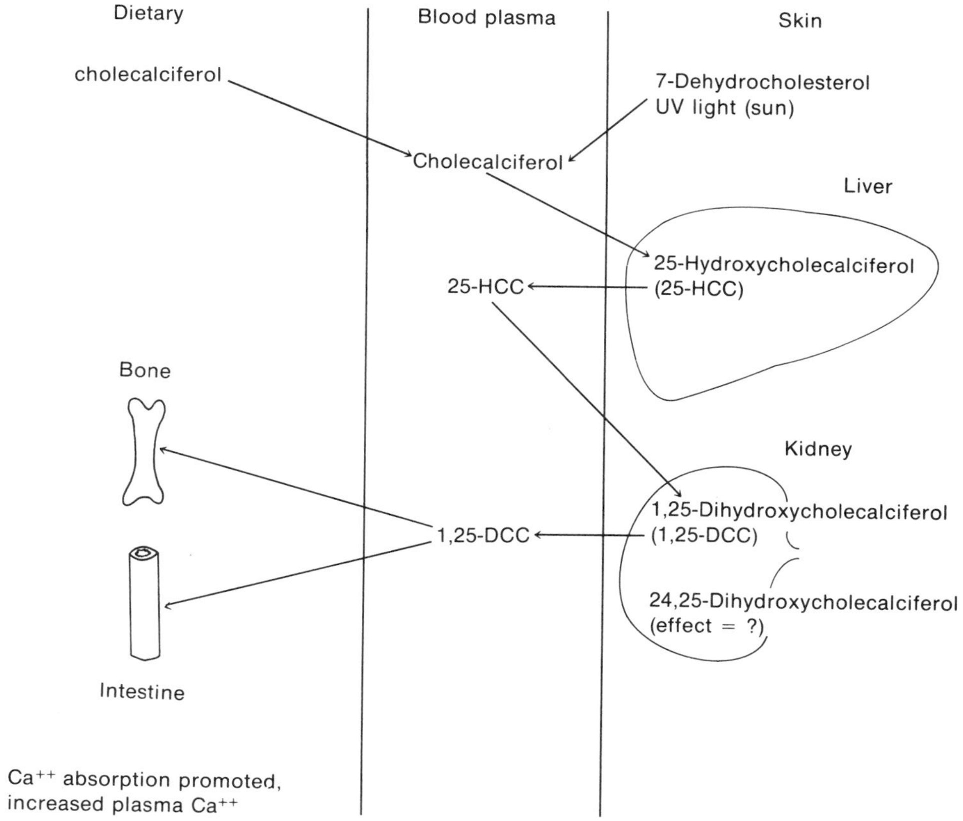

protein actively serves to transport calcium from the brush border into the blood. The increased concentration of calcium in the blood promotes bone deposits, which may be regulated by calcitonin and parathyroid hormone. The vitamin may, however, have a direct action on bone by initiating a cellular transport system for calcium.

Vitamin D also promotes tubular absorption of phosphate by the kidney. An increased urinary excretion of phosphate and a fall in plasma phosphate level may interfere with the mineralization of bone.

Deficiency. Vitamin D deficiency in children is called rickets. In adults, vitamin D deficiency is known as osteomalacia.

Rickets is essentially a disease of defective bone formation caused by inadequate deposits of calcium and phosphorus in bone. The bones are normally incompletely calcified at birth and in the deficiency remain soft and pliable. When these poorly calcified bones are needed to perform weight-bearing functions, they yield, and bowing of legs occurs when the child starts to walk or to support a weight of any kind on the incompletely mineralized bone. The ends of the large bones become enlarged, making movement difficult. At this stage, knock-knees can be seen. Deformities of the ribs result in a concave breast that causes crowding in the breast cavity. The ribs also develop irregularly spaced areas of swelling that take on the appearance of beading. The term rachitic rosary is applied to this condition. The failure of the fontanel of the skull to close, allowing rapid enlargement of the head, is also a condition of the developing deficiency. The eruption of teeth is delayed; they are poorly formed and subject to earlier decay. Growth is frequently retarded.

Rickets is primarily a deficiency of children. Unless effective measures are used early in the disease, malformation of bone may be permanent.

Osteomalacia, sometimes called adult rickets, is characterized by an accumulation of uncalcified osteoid tissue in the costochondral joints. It is prevalent in women, especially Oriental women, whose bodies have been depleted of calcium by numerous pregnancies, prolonged nursing, and long periods of protection from the sun and who receive diets low in calcium and vitamin D.

Chemical Properties and Structure. Because vitamins D_2 and D_3 and some of their related metabolites produce similar effects in the body, vitamin D is used collectively to describe the effect of this group of antirachitic vitamins. Vitamin D_3, or cholecalciferol, is the natural form of vitamin D. Humans can synthesize the vitamin by the ultraviolet irradiation of 7-dehydrocholesterol in the skin. Vitamin D_2, or ergocalciferol, is produced by exposing ergosterol, a sterol found in ergot, or black fungus, and yeast to the action of ultraviolet light. Irradiation of ergosterol gives rise to a number of related substances, some toxic, of which only ergocalciferol has marked antirachitic properties. Ergocalciferol (D_2) has the same chemical structure as cholecalciferol (D_3) except for the side-chain, which has an unsaturated double bond and an extra methyl group. Ergosterol, from which it is derived, occurs only in plants. Although ergocalciferol is used as a therapeutic agent, it rarely occurs in nature.

Sources. Vitamin D occurs naturally in such animal foods as fatty fish, eggs, liver, and butter. Milk is a poor source of vitamin D unless fortified. Much of the milk now available has vitamin D added to provide a concentration of 400 IU (10 μg of vitamin D_3) per quart. Cod-liver oil and other fish-liver oils are excellent natural sources of the vitamin. Vitamin D is present in very small quantities in green plants and mushrooms.

Although the vitamin is not widely distributed in nature, consumption of the vitamin in food or by enriched foods, the irradiation of foods that contain precursors of the vitamin, and irradiation of the skin with ultraviolet light or sunlight all ensure an adequate daily human supply.

Vitamin D is stable in foods; storage, processing, and cooking do not affect its activity.

Requirement. Because there are two sources of vitamin D—the naturally occurring form (D_3) and the synthetic (D_2)—the evaluation of minimum requirement is difficult. Only when exposure to sunlight is inadequate and dietary intake restricted do deficiency symptoms develop. The amount of vitamin D needed is thus determined by the degree of exposure to sunlight. A person primarily living and working indoors would need more vitamin D than a person working outdoors all day.

The precise requirement for vitamin D in older children and adults is not known. Normally the requirement can be met by exposure to sunlight, but if exposure to sunlight is insufficient a dietary source must be provided. An intake of 400 IU vitamin D/day is advisable for pregnant and lactating women, infants, children, and adolescents. Since the requirement for normal healthy adults seems to be satisfied by nondietary means, no recommendation is necessary. However, a dietary intake of 400 IU for normal persons of all ages incurs no risk of toxicity.

The following normal requirements and therapeutic dosage are recommended: normal requirements, 400 IU for all ages; therapeutic dosage, 400 to 4000 IU/day orally.

Toxicity. The ingestion of vitamin D in excess of the recommended amounts (hypervitaminosis) provides no benefit, and large doses can be harmful. Fat-soluble vitamins such as vitamin D can be stored in the body for a considerable time and, because they metabolize slowly, may produce toxic symptoms. The reason for this toxicity involves the difficulty of excretion rather than its storage. Excretion is gradual and by way of the bile. In contrast, the water-soluble vitamins are not stored to any great extent but when consumed in excess of needs are rapidly excreted in the urine.

There is evidence that infants are especially sensitive to the toxic effect of vitamin D. Infants need only 400 IU daily, whereas intakes such as 3000 to 4000 IU daily may produce toxic symptoms, as shown by abnormally high calcium levels in the blood, loss of appetite, and retarded growth. With daily doses of 20,000 to 40,000 IU in infants, or 75,000 to 100,000 IU for adults, toxic symptoms usually develop, including sudden loss of appetite, nausea, vomiting, intense thirst, and resulting polyuria. Diarrhea may occur, and the child may become thin, irritable, depressed, and stuporous. Fatal cases have been reported in which the arteries, renal tubules, heart, and lungs have shown evidence of considerable calcification.

Vitamin D is probably the most toxic of all vitamins. Very high doses, for example, 100,000 IU, for weeks or months may, in addition to causing deposits of calcium in many of the organs such as the arteries and kidneys, induce characteristic dense calcification of the bone along the metaphysis. Such toxic symptoms may arise when the vitamin is given in massive amounts to treat bone disease due to malabsorption caused by chronic renal disease.

The quantities of vitamin D needed to induce toxic symptoms cannot be obtained from natural sources.

Vitamin E (The Tocopherols). Current popular interest in vitamin E probably results from the hoped for, but unwarranted, expectation that results obtained and reproducible in experimental animals are directly applicable to humans. Among conditions for which vitamin E supposedly is effective are sexual impotence, sterility, habitual abortion, muscular dystrophy, arthritis, aging, and acne. Fortunately, much confirmed biochemical and metabolic information rigorously obtained by experimentation in animals can be, with reason, applied to humans, but not always. At present, there is no satisfactory evidence that any of the human ailments noted above are correctable by eating, injecting, or any other means of taking vitamin E into the human body.

Vitamin E has been known as the antisterility vitamin since its discovery in 1922. In that year, Evans and Bishop found a third unknown fat-soluble factor in lettuce, wheat germ, and dried alfalfa essential for successful reproduction in rats. A deficiency of their unknown "factor X" caused resorption of the fetus in females and atrophy of spermatogenic tissue and permanent sterility in males. Evans in 1936 isolated crystalline vitamin E from the unsaponifiable fraction of wheat germ oil and named it tocopherol, an alcohol that helps in the bearing of young (Greek *tokos,* childbirth, plus *phero,* to bear, plus *ol,* an alcohol).

In animals such as the rat, guinea pig, rabbit, and dog, the lack of vitamin E produces a condition resembling muscular dystrophy. The dystrophic muscles exhibit increased oxygen uptake, perhaps owing to increased oxidation of polyunsaturated fats, which appears to occur chiefly in the muscles. The degeneration is reported to resemble the Zenker's necrosis observed in severe infections such as typhoid fever and epidemic influenzal pneumonia. Muscle fibers may be replaced by fat and connective tissue. Increased urinary excretion of creatine may reflect the inability of skeletal muscle to use creatine. A brown discoloration occurs in the voluntary muscles of these vitamin E-deficient animals, and similar pigmentation may be seen in the uterus, ovaries, and seminal vesicles. The increased oxygen consumption of the dystrophic muscles and other abnormal findings can be lessened, sometimes dramatically, as in the rabbit, by adding the vitamin to the diet. The use of vitamin E as a curative agent to treat muscular dystrophy in humans has, without exception, met with failure.

FRIEDRICH ALBERT ZENKER, 1825–1898. German pathologist. Precisely described the muscular and intestinal forms of trichiniasis (1860) and delineated pulmonary fat embolism in 1862. Earlier, in 1851, recorded the presence of phosphate crystals in the lungs of pulmonary disease patients, the Charcot–Leyden–Zenker crystals.

Function. Vitamin E may function in tissues as an antioxidant. In tissues vitamin E may prevent the destructive nonenzymatic oxidation of polyunsaturated fatty acids by molecular oxygen. Some products that result from oxidation of fat may appear in tissues as pigments and may be associated with cell damage. They are found in tissues of older animals as well as in animals on diets lacking in vitamin E. A role for vitamin E in tissues as an agent to prevent degenerative disorders therefore cannot be discounted. Vitamin E may also function as a coenzyme or in some other manner in enzymatic reactions. Determining the functional role of vitamin E offers great opportunities for investigation.

Deficiency. At present, investigations conducted in laboratory animals have contributed to our knowledge of vitamin E. Data obtained from such animal experiments vary substantially when examined in such species as the rat, guinea pig, rabbit, dog, and chicken. Equally puzzling and seemingly unrelated are the various symptoms that involve the reproductive, muscular, vascular, nervous, and glandular systems. Only recently have vitamin E deficiencies been observed in humans, and the results are too incomplete to support firm conclusions or to verify the applicability of results obtained in animal experimentation to humans.

Deficiency in Humans. A vitamin E deficiency is rarely seen except in persons suffering from some form of malabsorption. It may be that in normal persons on a Western-style diet, vitamin E deficiency is not an important problem nutritionally.

Studies conducted in newborn infants and in children with steatorrhea have shown increased red blood cell hemolysis related to low serum tocopherol levels. Creatinuria, ceroid pigment deposits, increased hemolysis rates, and muscle lesions have been reported in persons with cystic fibrosis of the pancreas, which reduces vitamin E absorption.

Chemical Properties and Structure. Like vitamins A and D, vitamin E exists in more than one form. Of these forms, eight substances of plant origin (four tocopherols and four tocotrienols) are of interest (*see* Fig. 73-4). All are derivatives of 6-hydroxychroman and contain a 16-carbon isoprenoid side-chain. They differ structurally in the number and position of methyl groups in the ring structure, and with the tocotrienols the side-chain is unsaturated.

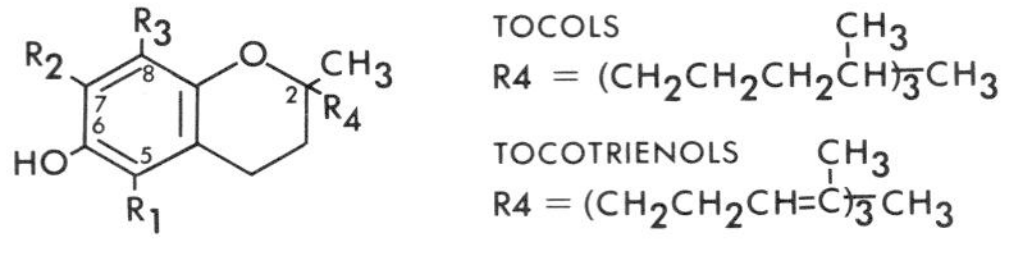

Tocol	Tocotrienol	Methyl positions
α-(alpha)	ζ-(zeta)	5, 7, 8
β-(beta)	ε-(epsilon)	5, 8
γ-(gamma)	η-(eta)	7, 8
δ-(delta)	8-methyl-tocotrienol	8

FIG. 73-4. The tocopherols. (From Schneider HA, Anderson CE, Coursin DB (eds): Nutritional Support of Medical Practice, p 48. Hagerstown, Harper & Row, 1977)

All have the same physiologic properties, but α-tocopherol is the most active of the group as a vitamin. The remaining compounds have

VITAMIN E (represented by alpha tocopherol)

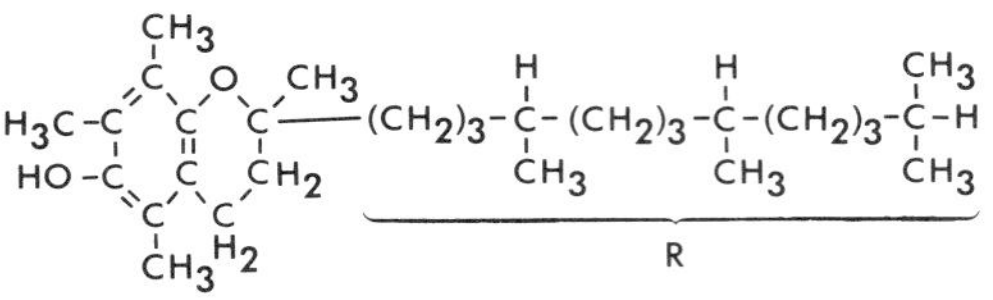

lower biologic activities estimated to be 1% to 50% of the activity of α-tocopherol. Synthesized in 1938 by Karrer in Switzerland and Smith in the United States, this is the form in which the vitamin is produced commercially. In accordance with a recommendation by the IUNS Committee on Nomenclature, the term vitamin E should be used generally for all tocol and tocotrienol derivates that exhibit qualitatively the biologic activity of α-tocopherol.

Vitamin E compounds are light yellow, viscous oils insoluble in water but freely soluble in fat solvents. They are stable to heat but readily destroyed by oxidation and ultraviolet light. They are not destroyed to any extent by temperatures used in cooking, although some loss occurs in frozen foods and processing.

Because vitamin E can take up oxygen and oxidize slowly, it can function in the body as a potent antioxidant to protect other vital metabolites such as vitamin A, the carotenes, and unsaturated fatty acids from destructive oxidation. The tocopherols are the chief antioxidants in natural fats and act to prevent fats from becoming rancid. The tocopherols are themselves easily oxidized, a property that presents difficulties in analytic procedures devised to estimate this vitamin.

Absorption and Metabolism. As a fat-soluble substance, vitamin E requires the presence of bile for absorption from the small intestine. It is absorbed best in the presence of fat. Any disease state that interferes with the absorption of fat, such as pancreatic, liver, and biliary disease or diseases of the intestinal mucosal cell and transport, will interfere with the absorption of vitamin E. Although some vitamin E may be absorbed into the portal blood, the bulk of the vitamin enters unchanged into the lymph system and is transported to the bloodstream as tocopherol attached to lipoproteins. It is stored largely in adipose tissue, muscle, liver, and in somewhat smaller amounts in heart, uterus, testes, and adrenals.

Sources. The richest sources of vitamin E are the vegetable oils. Wheat germ oil, from which α-tocopherol was first isolated, is a good source, as are salad oils and mayonnaise, beef liver, milk, eggs, butter, leafy vegetables, and cereals (particularly if fortified). Many of these foods are also excellent sources of polyunsaturated fatty acids.

Fish-liver oils are rich in vitamins A and D but low or devoid of vitamin E.

Requirement. As mentioned previously, the exact mechanism by which vitamin E functions in the body is unknown. Foods contain significant amounts of nearly all of the eight tocopherols. For this reason the milligram of α-tocopherol equivalent has been recommended as a summation term for all vitamin E activity. Vitamin E is an essential nutrient. The National Research Council's revised statement of 1974 recommends about 5 IU of vitamin E for infants, increasing to 15 IU for males and 12 IU for females.

Toxicity. Vitamin E appears to be relatively nontoxic. Human adults have been reported to consume as much as 1 g/day for months without developing signs of toxicity.

Vitamin K (the Naphthoquinones). In 1935 Henrick Dam at the University of Copenhagen, studying hemorrhagic disease in chicks fed a fat-free diet, reported that bleeding could be prevented by giving a variety of foodstuffs, especially alfalfa and decayed fish. The active material could be extracted by ether. The bleeding was not due to a lack of vitamin C (ascorbic acid). He succeeded in isolating the substance from alfalfa and showed that the antihemorrhagic substance was fat soluble but not identified with vitamins A, D, or E. He called the active substance koagulationsvitamin (after the Danish word for coagulation), which then became vitamin K.

VITAMIN K (represented by phytylmenaquinone, vitamin K_1)

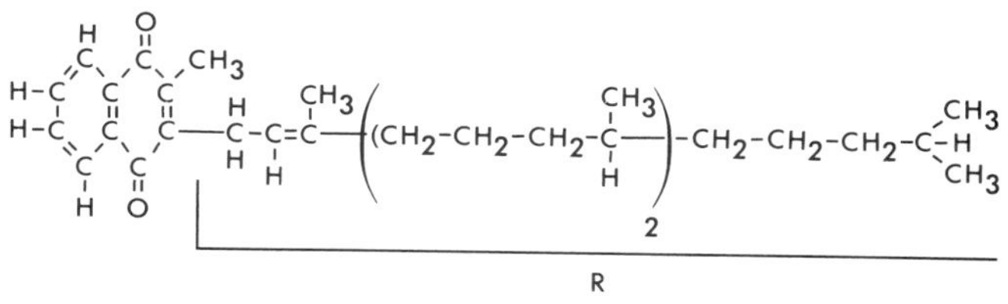

Function. The primary function of vitamin K is to catalyze the synthesis of prothrombin by the liver. Without this step, the normal process of blood clotting could not take place. In addition, the synthesis of other factors necessary in the clotting process, such as factors VII (proconvertin), IX (Christmas factor), and X (Stuart factor), depends on vitamin K. Without vitamin K, hypoprothrombinemia develops and blood clotting is greatly prolonged. In fact, defective blood coagulation is the only well-established sign of vitamin K deficiency in animals. The ability of vitamin K to alleviate hypoprothrombinemia depends on the capacity of liver cells to produce prothrombin. Advanced liver damage, as in cirrhosis or carcinoma, may be accompanied by a prothrombin deficiency that cannot be reversed by vitamin K—a normal liver is required.

The major defense of the human body against blood loss is the formation of a blood clot. Normal human blood when shed will clot in 5 to 8 minutes at 37°C. The process of forming a clot is a complex cascade of enzyme activations in which a very small amount of the first factor initiates a series of catalytic reactions until the amplified response to the injury results in formation of the clot. Prothrombin, a precursor enzyme, is in some not-yet-clear way formed as the result of the presence of vitamin K, which with thromboplastin and calcium ions is converted to the enzyme thrombin. This, in turn, catalyzes the conversion of the soluble protein dimer fibrinogen into the insoluble monomer fibrin, the basis of the clot.

The only generally accepted function of vitamin K in higher animals is that of regulating

CHRISTMAS DISEASE, a hemophilia caused by a congenital lack of coagulation factor IX, was named by Rosemary Biggs and colleagues in the 1952 paper that distinguished this condition from other hemophilias. Their first patient was a 5-year-old boy named Christmas.

the synthesis of prothrombin and other plasma-clotting factors. The vitamin regulates the rate of synthesis of prothrombin after transcription, but the nature of the control site is still undetermined. Some investigators believe that protein synthesis is not needed for the step sensitive to vitamin K in the production of prothrombin. Suttie has found data consistent with the formation of a precursor protein in the liver which is converted to prothrombin in a step requiring vitamin K.

Certain snake venoms and strains of staphylococci contain vitamin-K-like proteolytic enzymes that can cause clotting.

Deficiency. A dietary deficiency of vitamin K is unlikely because of the intestinal synthesis of the vitamin by microorganisms and because it is quite widely distributed in foods. As pointed out previously, a vitamin K deficiency may occur in biliary obstruction and in any defect in the intestinal absorption of fat, such as may occur in malabsorption syndromes (*e.g.*, sprue and celiac disease) and in conditions that give rise to steatorrhea.

Dicoumarol, which is used as an anticoagulant, resembles vitamin K in structure and can act as an antagonist to vitamin K, thereby giving rise to a hemorrhagic condition. An important therapeutic use of vitamin K is as an antidote to the anticoagulant drug. The prothrombin time, lengthened by dicoumarol use, will usually return to normal within 12 to 36 hours after the administration of the vitamin provided liver function is adequate to synthesize prothrombin.

Chemical Properties and Structure. The term vitamin K includes a group of antihemorrhagic substances with similar biologic activity. Two naturally occurring vitamins in the group, vitamin K_1 and vitamin K_2, are required for the biosynthesis of prothrombin essential in the blood-clotting process. Vitamin K_1 is present in green leaves and other plant tissues eaten in the diet. Vitamin K_2 is present in putrefying fish meal and is synthesized by intestinal bacteria. Chemically, they are quinones and related to the parent compound α-methyl-1,4-naphthoquinone (*see* Fig. 73-5).

Following the IUNS Committee on Nomenclature, vitamin K_1 is phytylmenaquinone (formerly phylloquinone or phylonadione) and vitamin K_2 multiprenylmenaquinone (formerly farnoquinone), of which there are several active forms in bacteria and in the animal body. Vitamin K_3 is menaquinone (formerly menadione), which is produced synthetically, is fat soluble, and has about twice the biologic activity of the natural forms of the vitamin. Vitamin K_2 has about 75% of the activity of vitamin K_1. It is believed that phytylmenaquinone is the biologically active form of the vitamin and that animal cells are able to convert the other forms into this active form.

When fat absorption is impaired, as in the malabsorption syndrome, several water-soluble and water-miscible preparations are available for the treatment of vitamin K deficiency. Menadione sodium bisulfite (Hykinone) and sodium menadiol diphosphate (Synkayvite) are water soluble; Mephyton, Konakin, and Monokay are water miscible.

All forms of the natural vitamin K are yellow oils quite stable to heat, air, and moisture but not to light. They are unstable in ultraviolet light and destroyed by oxidation. Cooking destroys very little of the activity because the natural forms are insoluble in water.

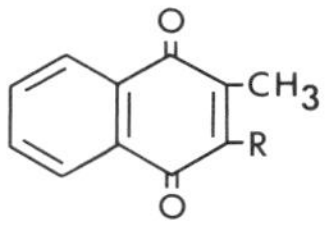

2-METHYL-1,4-NAPHTHOQUINONE

K_3 or menaquinone ———— R = H

K_1 or phytylmenaquinone ———— R = 3-phytyl-1,4-naphthoquinone

$$-CH_2-CH{=}\underset{}{\overset{CH_3}{\overset{|}{C}}}-[CH_2CH_2CH_2\overset{CH_3}{\overset{|}{C}H}]_3-CH_3$$

K_2 or multiprenylmenaquinone ———— R = 3-polyprenyl-1,4-naphthoquinone

$$-(CH_2-CH{=}\overset{CH_3}{\overset{|}{C}}-CH_2)_n-H \quad (n = 7, 8, \text{ or } 9)$$

FIG. 73-5. Chemical structure of some vitamin K compounds. (Schneider HA, Anderson CE, Coursin DB (eds): Nutritional Support of Medical Practice, p 51. Hagerstown, Harper & Row, 1977)

Cattle develop a tendency to bleed if fed on spoiled sweet clover. The substance responsible for this bleeding tendency—dicoumarol—was isolated and synthesized by Link and his students. Dicoumarol prolongs the prothrombin time of blood and so aids as an anticoagulant in the treatment of arterial and venous thromboses. Other synthetic analogues, such as warfarin (a rat poison that prevents the rat's blood from clotting) and phenindione, are antagonistic to the action of vitamin K and inhibit synthesis of prothrombin and blood-clotting factors (VII, IX, and X) in the liver.

Vitamin K_1 is thought to be an essential component of the phosphorylation processes concerned with photosynthesis in green plants, and it may have a similar role as a cofactor necessary in oxidative phosphorylation in animal tissues. It is similar in structure to coenzyme Q.

Absorption. Like vitamins A, D, and E, vitamin K is fat soluble and requires a normal supply of bile for intestinal absorption. It is absorbed in the duodenum and jejunum of the small intestine. A deficiency of vitamin K may be the result of the malabsorption syndrome, as, for example, in biliary tract obstruction or if there is a defect in fat absorption, such as in sprue and celiac disease.

Normally, vitamin K is absorbed and enters the metabolic system by way of the lacteals, lymph, and blood. It is transported from the intestine in chylomicrons and subsequently transported by the blood in β-lipoproteins.

Sources. The synthesis of vitamin K by intestinal bacteria and the levels obtained in a diet from vegetables, especially green leafy vegetables, normally supply sufficient vitamin K. In neonates, however, before the establishment of intestinal bacteria; in malabsorption syndromes such as cystic fibrosis, diarrhea, and failure of bile secretion; and in patients who require antibiotics, the amount of vitamin K in the body is reduced, and supplements of the vitamin are recommended.

Lettuce, spinach, kale, cauliflower, and cabbage are excellent sources of vitamin K. Very little vitamin K is present in most cereals, fruits, carrots, peas, meats, and highly refined foods. Breast milk particularly and cow's milk are very poor sources of the vitamin.

A primary deficiency of vitamin K in adults has never been clearly demonstrated. It must be assumed, therefore, that even a poor diet contains enough vitamin K to sustain normal human needs.

Requirement. Vitamin K is synthesized by intestinal bacteria. Although the role of the intestinal flora in synthesizing the vitamins is not fully known, absorption of synthesized vitamin K from the small intestine and of that supplied in the diet appears to be efficient in normal persons. Therefore, because of the above observations and the abundance of vitamin K in the diet, no daily recommendation of intake is made. The American Academy of Pediatrics estimates that neonates require 0.15 to 0.25 μg/kg/day. If about 10% of orally administered vitamin K is assimilated, a daily intake of 0.2 mg (200 μg) appears adequate for newborn infants. Adults are believed to require 0.3 to 15.0 μg/kg/day.

Toxicity. The natural vitamins K_1 and K_2 are nontoxic in large doses. Excessive doses (more than 5 mg) of menaquinone (formerly menadione) and its derivatives have led to hemolytic anemia in rats and kernicterus in low-birth-weight infants, probably owing to an increased breakdown of red blood cells. Vitamin K_1 seems to be free from these side-effects.

VITAMIN-LIKE COMPOUNDS

Currently, several vitaminlike substances (choline, myoinositol, coenzyme Q, α-lipoic acid, p-aminobenzoic acid, and the bioflavonoids) do not meet all the criteria necessary to be classified as vitamins (*see* above): They do not, based on present knowledge, have any essential biologic role; the animal body can synthesize sufficient amounts to meet metabolic needs; and they are present in the diet and tissues in larger amounts than the catalytically involved and established vitamins.

As knowledge increases, some of these compounds may become established as true vitamins.

Choline. Choline is synthesized in the body from glycine, provided there is another source of methyl groups, such as in methionine. The amount used is much larger than the catalytic amounts expected in metabolic reactions. Choline probably cannot be considered a vitamin because humans do not depend on a dietary source of either choline or a choline precursor. In addition, there is little evidence to suggest that in humans the administration of choline alleviates fatty liver, cirrhosis, chronic liver disease, or other defects that resemble those associated with a choline deficiency. Among alcoholic persons, however, choline may exert a protective effect in cirrhosis of the liver.

CHOLINE

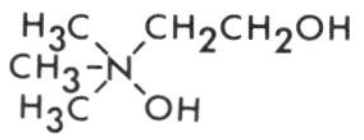

Choline is water soluble and takes up water (*i.e.*, it is hygroscopic) on exposure to air. Choline is more stable in the form of the chloride. It serves as a source of labile methyl groups. In many organic compounds the methyl group is fixed and not detachable. However, in choline the labile methyl groups may be transferred from one compound to another in a process called transmethylation. In this way, choline provides methyl groups, for example, for the synthesis of creatine and epinephrine and for methylating certain substances for excretion in the urine.

Choline is essential in the synthesis of phosphatidyl choline, a component of cell membranes and lipoproteins involved in the transport of fat-soluble substances. It is a constituent of sphinogomyelin and acetyl choline.

Choline is present in foods in which phospholipids occur, for example, egg yolk (a very rich source), whole grains, legumes such as soybeans, peas, and beans, meats of all types, and wheat germ. Vegetables and milk have small amounts. Fruits have low or no choline content.

The Food and Nutrition Board of the National Academy of Sciences does not suggest a human allowance of choline because of lack of evidence for a recommendation.

Myoinositol. The inositols are cyclic alcohols (cyclohexanols). Chemically, inositol is hexahydroxycyclohexane. Because of the presence of hydroxyl groups in the molecule, inositols can be considered as related to the sugars. There are nine isomers of inositol (several optically inactive forms and one pair of optically active isomers), but only the *myo*-inositol (also called *meso*-inositol or i-inositol) is biologically active and important in animal and plant metabolism. Inositol is found in nature in at least four forms: free inositol; phytin, a mixed calcium and magnesium salt of inositol hexaphosphate (phytic acid); the phospholipid phosphatidyl-inositol; and a nondialyzable, water-soluble complex. Large amounts of phytic acid (*e.g.*, in cereals and grains) in the diet form nonabsorbable complexes.

In mice a dietary deficiency causes malopecia and a failure of lactation and growth. It has sometimes been classified as a vitamin because mice require traces of *myo*-inositol in the diet. In rats a deficiency causes a "speckled-eye" condition owing to denudation around the eyes.

Inositols occur widely in the plant kingdom in whole grains and nuts and in fruits and vegetables. Considerable concentrations are present in yeast and milk.

Coenzyme Q (Ubiquinone). Coenzyme Q is so widely distributed in nature that it is appropriately called "ubiquinone." It is the collective name for a group of five crystalline homologues that differ from one another merely by the number of isoprenoid units in a side-chain. Coenzyme Q from beef heart has 10 isoprenoid units (Q_{10}); from yeast (*Saccaromyces cerevisia*), 6 units (Q_6); and from *Torula utils*, 9 units (Q_9). Coenzyme Q is quite similar in structure to vitamins K and E.

Coenzyme Q functions as an electron carrier in terminal electron transport and oxidative phosphorylation, especially in the respiratory chain linking the flavoproteins to cytochrome b. Coenzyme Q is a constituent of the phospholipids in mitochondrial membranes, where it exists in the oxidized (quinone form) under aerobic conditions and in the reduced (quinol form) under anaerobic conditions. Coenzyme Q is synthesized intracellularly but may have to be provided in the diet.

α-Lipoic Acid (Thioctic acid). α-Lipoic acid is a sulfur-containing fatty acid synthesized in adequate amounts in the mammalian cell. Both thiamine pyrophosphate and α-lipoic acid are needed for the oxidative decarboxylation of α-keto acids, such as pyruvic acid to acetate or, more properly, to acetyl coenzyme A.

The complete system for the oxidative decarboxylation of pyruvic acid involves not only thiamine and α-lipoic acid but pantothenic acid (as coenzyme A), riboflavin (as FAD), and nicotinamide derivatives (as NAD).

α-Lipoic acid occurs in a variety of foods and is active in extremely minute amounts. It has not been demonstrated to be required in the diet of higher animals. No attempt to induce a dietary deficiency of lipoic acid has been successful.

p-Aminobenzoic (PABA). A portion of the folic acid molecule is formed by PABA, but it is not certain whether it has a role in metabolism independent of folic acid. The best food sources of PABA are yeast, liver, rice, bran, and whole wheat. Since PABA exists free in food, it can be considered a dietary precursor of folic acid. It antagonizes sulfonamides.

Bioflavonoids. Extracts of lemon peel and red peppers contain a mixture of flavonoids called citrin by Szent-Györgyi in 1936. Citrin was found to be biologically active in maintaining normal capillary permeability and fragility. The active principal in citrin is hesperidin, which was designated vitamin P (for permeability), a term that has now been dropped. A number of compounds with hesperidinlike structures, including the flavanones and flavanonols, have been found to have similar physiologic activity.

Bioflavonoid deficiency has been produced in animals, resulting in a syndrome characterized by increased capillary permeability and fragility. This vitamin-C-like effect of the bioflavonoids appears to be due to an antioxidant effect that protects ascorbic acid from oxidative destruction. Their effect is therefore indirect.

At present, insufficient evidence precludes classifying the bioflavonoids as vitamins.

FURTHER READING

1. Briggs GM, Calloway DH: Bogert's Nutrition and Physical Fitness. Philadelphia, W B Saunders, 1979
2. Harper HA, Rodwell VW, Mayes PA: Review of Physiological Chemistry, 17th ed. Los Altos, California, Lange Medical Publications, 1979
3. Schneider HA, Anderson CE, Coursin DB: Nutritional Support of Medical Practice. Hagerstown, Maryland, Harper & Row, 1977

CHAPTER 73 QUESTIONS

(See P. 7 for Full Instructions)

Select the ONE best answer

1. Which of the following vitamins is the most frequent cause of moderate-to-severe toxic effects as a result of overdosage?
   A. Vitamin A
   B. Vitamin D
   C. Vitamin E
   D. Ascorbic acid
   E. Riboflavin

2. The active hormonal form of vitamin D_3 is
   A. 1,25-dihydroxyvitamin D_3.
   B. 24,25-dihydroxyvitamin D_3.
   C. 25-hydroxyvitamin D_3.
   D. cholecalciferol.
   E. dihydrotachysterol.

A = 1,2,3; B = 1,3; C = 2,4; D = 4; E = All

3. For maintaining a normal healthy physical state, one must ingest daily the recommended amount of
   1. ascorbic acid.
   2. vitamin K.
   3. vitamin A.
   4. vitamin E.

4. The correct approximate recommended daily allowance of
   1. thiamine is 1.5 mg.
   2. vitamin A is 4000 IU.
   3. niacin is 15 mg.
   4. vitamin D is 4000 IU.

5. Which of the following correctly associates a characteristic condition and the vitamin deficiency considered its cause?
   1. Pellagra—riboflavin
   2. Dementia—nicotinic acid
   3. Beri-beri—ascorbic acid
   4. Convulsions—pyridoxine

6. Mineral oil will decrease the absorption of
   1. vitamin A.
   2. vitamin D.
   3. vitamin K.
   4. vitamin C.

7. Phytylmenaquinone (vitamin K_1)
   1. deficiency causes effects that can be immediately terminated with infusion of fresh whole blood.
   2. activity is competitively antagonized by warfarin.
   3. is poorly absorbed with biliary obstruction.
   4. is an essential dietary vitamin.

74

WYATT R. HUME

Oral and Dental Pharmacology

ORAL INFECTIONS: ANTIBIOTICS AND ANTISEPTICS

The nature of the oral flora and the types of infections commonly encountered in the mouth differ significantly from those found elsewhere in the body, and therefore influence decisions on antibiotic and antiseptic use.

ORAL MICROFLORA

The normal human mouth contains more than 50 species of aerobic and anaerobic bacteria, as well as spirochetes, yeasts, viruses, protozoa, and fungi. The absolute and proportional composition of the microflora varies widely between individuals, with age, with dietary factors, and between sites in the mouth. About 50% of the organisms usually present in the adult are gram-positive cocci, mostly streptococci (*e.g.*, *Strep. sanguis*, *Strep. salivarius*), and *Veilonella*, diphtheroids, *Bacteroides*, and spirochetes also occur commonly; about 30% to 40% of the organisms are obligate anaerobes, and most of the remainder are facultative anaerobes.

Many of the usual bacterial strains adhere to the salivary protein coating of teeth, thus forming *dental plaque*. Several of these strains (most notably *Strep. mutans*) also assemble extracellular *polyglucans* from dietary sucrose. Polyglucans act as a mucilagenous cementing substance for other bacteria and as a nutrient store within dental plaque, thus facilitating the development of an anaerobic environment. Typically mixed populations of bacteria develop, adhering to the teeth and also growing in the saliva and covering the mouth's mucosal surfaces. This normal flora may be considered to some degree *protective*, inhibiting the establishment of new, invading organisms (*see* Suprainfection, Chap. 56). Most microbial infections in the oral region are mixed and are attributable to this normal flora.

DENTAL CARIES AND ITS SEQUELAE

If adequate substrate for bacterial growth and metabolism is available (dietary monosaccharides and disaccarides) a low *p*H develops in the deeper layers of mature, supragingival, dental plaque that causes demineralization and then breakdown of the enamel surface. The end-products of bacterial glycolysis continue to demineralize enamel and then dentine as the carious lesion develops; in dentine, which contains protoplasmic and intercellular proteins, proteolytic organisms contribute to the tooth breakdown. If left untreated, the inward diffusion of bacterial products and direct bacterial invasion cause inflammation of the dental pulp, which has a limited capacity to resist infection because of restricted blood flow. Pulpal necrosis commonly occurs, providing a medium for opportunistic microbial growth from the oral flora. At the apex of the tooth root, where significant defense mechanisms are available, an abscess may develop in response to these bacteria and their products.

Topical antibiotic therapy of the initial stages of this sequence is inappropriate because of the significant risk of host sensitization. Mechanical débridement is the treatment of choice (simple plaque removal before tooth breakdown as a preventive measure, and surgical removal and replacement of infected hard tissue before infection of the pulp). No antiseptic agents both effective against plaque organisms and safe for long-term use are as yet available. Use of antiseptics to treat the carious lesion of dentine involves additional insult to the pulpal tissue and is rarely practiced. Systemic antibiotics do not reach enamel or dentine in appreciable concentrations, nor are they effective in treating infected pulp, particularly in the face of overwhelming and continuing reinfection from the oral cavity. Similarly, in the management of a *periapical abscess,* no systemically administered antibiotic can reach the necrotic pulp space in adequate concentration. Thus mechanical débridement and drainage (either endodontic treatment or tooth extraction) are the prime and essential modes of treatment. Adjunct, systemic antibiotic therapy may help limit the spread of periapical infection. Since the predominant organisms in mixed pulp space infections are most likely to be gram-positive and anaerobic cocci, *penicillin V* is the drug of choice. Culture (both aerobic and anaerobic) and sensitivity testing are appropriate; if the response to penicillin V is unsatisfactory, a decision for alternate antibiotic therapy is made based on the sensitivities of the predominant strains cultivated. For patients allergic to penicillin, erythromycin (base) has proved to be a satisfactory drug of first choice for most odontogenic infections.

During mechanical débridement of the pulp space in endodontic (root canal) therapy, antimicrobial agents are used to decrease or to eliminate the bacterial population within the canal itself. Systemic antibiotic therapy is not effective because there is no remaining blood supply to the area. Topical antibiotic use carries with it the risk of host sensitization; the antiseptic sodium hypochlorite is safe and effective when used in root canal surgery.

PERIODONTAL DISEASE

Toxic bacterial products in mature dental plaque near the dentogingival junction induce chronic inflammation, local tissue breakdown, and, at the end-stage of abscess formation, eventual infection of the tissues that support the tooth. The first sign of this progressive disease (chronic marginal gingivitis) is a tendency of the gingival tissues to bleed owing to ulceration of the epithelium near the gingivodental junction. The development of defects (pockets) between the gingiva and the tooth, with periodontal ligament and bone loss and therefore loosening of the tooth, follows. Chronic periodontitis, with pus formation and recession of the gingiva, may also occur.

Fastidious mechanical plaque removal at daily intervals controls gingivitis. Topical antiseptic agents of low toxicity to the host, such as chlorhexidine and alexidine, are effective in the short term and are useful in patients with severely impaired resistance to infection. These agents are, however, unsuitable for chronic use because they *stain teeth* and *alter taste perception;* their safety in the long term has not been established. Systemic antibiotic therapy is not effective in the primary management of the disease because the causative microorganisms are outside the gingival tissue, and salivary and crevicular fluid levels of most antibiotics are ineffective. Topical antibiotic therapy is not advisable because of the risk of host sensitization.

In the treatment of chronic periodontitis, primary efforts are directed toward the mechanical control of plaque, and débridement. Systemic antibiotics may be an adjunct to surgical management, but, because the causative organisms are variable, rational antibiotic therapy is difficult. Penicillin V is advocated by some authorities, tetracycline hydrochloride by others. Metronidazole (*see* Chap. 67) is under active investigation.

Temporary remission of the acute, mixed infection of the superficial gingiva, referred to as acute necrotizing ulcerative gingivitis (ANUG;

Vincent's angina), usually follows systemic penicillin V therapy. Many topical antiseptics, and systemic antibiotics, are also effective in temporarily controlling the condition. Definitive treatment requires removal of the local bacterial irritants in the long term. The precise etiology of ANUG is not known. Probably many organisms, including *T. vincentii*, medium- and large-size spirochetes, and *B. melaninogenicus*, are involved.

ABSCESSES AND CELLULITIS

Periapical and periodontal infections may progress into deep fascial planes where, depending on the nature of the predominant organisms and the body's responses, either localized (abscess) or diffuse (cellulitis) infections are established. Penicillin V is the agent of first choice when used as an adjunct to débridement and, if the infection is localized, drainage; culture and sensitivity testing are desirable (*see* Chap. 56).

OTHER ORAL INFECTIONS

Candidiasis is discussed in Chapter 69. *Herpetic gingivostomatitis* is not amenable to antibiotic therapy; in its primary form systemic penicillin V may be administered to reduce the possibility of suprainfection.

PROPHYLACTIC ANTIBIOTIC USE

Because of the intimate relation between the bacterial flora and the gingival tissues, most operative dental procedures cause transient bacteremia. In patients where lodgement of bacteria at remote sites carries significant risks (particularly those with a history of rheumatic fever or cardiac valve prosthesis), prophylactic antibiotic administration to cover the period of dental treatment is required. Prophylactic antibiotic administration may also be advisable in contaminated facial trauma; since the organisms likely to cause infection are unknown, tetracycline hydrochloride is a reasonable choice.

JEAN HYACINTHE VINCENT, 1862–1950. French bacteriologist and epidemiologist. Discovered the bacteria that caused trench mouth and developed vaccines for typhoid and paratyphoid and sera for gas gangrene, among others. In 1894 showed that Madura foot was caused by actinomyces.

Antibiotic Prophylaxis for Preventing Bacterial Endocarditis*

- 1 million units of aqueous crystalline penicillin G mixed with 600,000 units of procaine penicillin G intramuscularly 1/2 to 1 hour before the procedure, followed by 500 mg of penicillin V orally every 6 hours for 8 doses.

or

- 2 grams of penicillin V orally every 6 hours for 8 doses, beginning 1/2 to 1 hour before the procedure.
- for patients allergic to penicillin, or for those with rheumatic fever receiving long-term penicillin, oral erythromycin, 1 g initially, followed by 500 mg every 6 hours for 8 doses.

MOUTHWASHES

Antiseptic mouthwashes are popularly used to alter breath odor. They may have a temporary effect by superimposing another odor but have no long-term influence on halitosis of systemic origin (foodstuffs, metabolic products). Halitosis of oral origin is due to breakdown of retained foods by oral bacteria or to periodontal or dentinopulpal infection. Commercially available mouthwashes may decrease salivary bacterial counts temporarily, but this is unlikely to influence the development of infective processes. The composition of commercially available mouthwashes varies widely, but representative constituents are *water*, *ethanol* (in the range 14–47%) *glycerin*, *phenol*, *menthol*, *eugenol*, *thymol*, *eucalyptol*, *saccharin*, *cetylpyridinium chloride* (a quaternary ammonium antibacterial compound), *sodium lauryl sulphate* (a detergent), and salts, buffers, and many coloring and flavoring agents. The effects of swallowing these preparations are difficult to predict but are probably benign, except for ethanol.

ANALGESICS

Either antipyretic analgesics (*see* Chap. 31), narcotic analgesics (*see* Chap. 32), or combined preparations are very commonly used to manage pain in dentistry. Dental pain is rarely of an intensity to require analgesics of greater potency than codeine–antipyretic combinations. For example, the pain of pulpitis (pri-

* American Heart Association: Prevention of bacterial endocarditis. Circulation 56:139A–143A, 1977.

marily due to local inflammation and increased intrapulpal pressure) is particularly amenable to simple antipyretic analgesic therapy. The placement of aspirin-containing tablets in the buccal sulcus adjacent to a painful tooth should be discouraged. Although some temporary relief of pain may result, the aspirin produces a characteristic ulcerative mucosal lesion.

Eugenol (5-allylguaiacol, clove oil) has been used topically to relieve pulpitis pain for hundreds of years. In low concentrations, it may inhibit prostaglandin synthetase (*see* Chap. 53) and may thus influence the inflammatory response. Its analgesic effect in the high concentrations at which it is usually applied is more likely to be due to a cytotoxic action on nerve processes.

Carbamazepine (Tegretol) is used to treat trigeminal neuralgia.

LOCAL ANESTHETICS AND VASOCONSTRICTORS

Local anesthetic–vasoconstrictor mixtures are injected in the oral region for either regional nerve block or local infiltration anesthesia. Topical local anesthetic agents may also be applied to the oral mucosa, most commonly at the site of subsequent injection. Of major concern are the risks of *toxic* and *allergic* reactions (*see* Chap. 20). The safety of the *vasoconstrictor* components of the injected mixture, particularly in patients with compromised coronary artery function, is an area of continuing medical–dental concern.

ANTIANXIETY AND SEDATIVE—HYPNOTIC AGENTS

The preoperative use of low doses of antianxiety agents such as diazepam (*see* Chap. 25) for cooperative but apprehensive adult dental patients may aid in establishing desired patterns of behavior.

"Acute conscious sedation," the use of various i.v. administered antianxiety or sedative hypnotic agents (*e.g.*, diazepam, barbiturates, hydroxyzine) often in combination with narcotic analgesics (*e.g.*, meperidine) to provide major sedation short of unconsciousness, is widely practiced in oral and periodontal surgery. The drugs are used as an adjunct to local anesthesia. There is a considerable risk of synergistic respiratory depression with sedative, analgesic, and local anesthetic combinations.

NITROUS OXIDE

Nitrous oxide is used (in combination with oxygen) at levels below those that produce unconsciousness for "relative analgesia," particularly with children. A degree of euphoria and some numbing of the oral region may aid patient management. The mechanism of its action is not known.

STAINING OF ORAL STRUCTURES

Heavy metal poisoning leads to staining of the gingival tissues for reasons that are not understood.

Teeth may be stained *externally* by bacteria that produce colored products, by pigmentation of the acquired pellicle (precipitated salivary glycoproteins), by foodstuffs and tobacco, and by many pigmented liquid drugs. *Internal* tooth staining may occur during dental development with, for example, tetracycline antibiotics, which bind to calicifying structures to form tetracycline–apatite complexes (*see* Chap. 61). Internal tooth staining may also occur with pulpal hemorrhage and with various root-filling materials.

DRUG-INDUCED XEROSTOMIA

Chronic decreased salivary flow (xerostomia) is a significant oral problem (Table 74-1). Salivary clearance of food decreases the substrate available for plaque microorganisms; salivary buffering and dilution also reduce plaque path-

TABLE 74-1. Representative Drugs with Xerostomic Potential

Class	Agent
Anticholinergic	Atropine
	Scopolamine
	Methantheline
Sedative–hypnotic	Meprobamate
	Diazepam
	Cannabis
Antidepressant	Imipramine
	Doxepin
Tranquilizer	Chlorpromazine
	Haloperidol
Antihistamine	Promethazine
	Diphenylhydramine
	Hydroxyzine
Narcotic	Meperidine
Nematocide and immune stimulant	Levamisole
Antifungal	Griseofulvin

TABLE 74-2. Medical–Dental Drug Interactions

Medical Drug	Dental Drug	Mechanism of Interaction	Possible Clinical Effect
Oral anticoagulants sodium warfarin (Coumadin, Panwarfarin); bishydroxycoumarin (Dicoumarol)	*Analgesics* particularly *salicylates* (aspirin and aspirin compounds)	Displacement from protein binding sites; also aspirin's own anticoagulant effect	Hemorrhage
	CNS depressants particularly *barbiturates* (Brevital, Pentothal, Nembutal)	Liver enzyme induction, enhanced metabolism of anticoagulant	Intravascular clotting
	Antiinflammatory enzymes, for example, papase, ananase	Unknown	Hemorrhage
	Antibiotics particularly tetracyclines, but also penicillins, cephalosporins	Decreased synthesis of vitamin K	Hemorrhage
Monoamine oxidase inhibitor (MAOI) Niamid, Marphan, Parnate, Eutonyl, others (antidepressants, sometime antihypertensives)	*Adrenergic vasoconstrictors* particularly phenylephrine, also epinephrine, norepinephrine,	Sympathetic neurotransmitter release	Severe hypertension
	CNS depressants particularly narcotics, barbiturates, tranquilizers	MAOIs inhibit liver metabolism of depressants	Enhanced CNS depression, hypotension, hyperpyrexia (meperidine)
Tricyclic antidepressants Elavil, Pentofrane, Tofranil, Aventyl, others	*Adrenergic vasoconstrictors* all	Decreased removal of vasoconstrictor from receptor area	Hypertension
	Anticholinergics atropine, scopolamine, others	Synergism	Xerostomia, acute glaucoma
Antihypertensives Guanethidine, methyldopa	*Adrenergic vasoconstrictors* all	Receptor sensitization unknown	Hypertension
Cardiac glycosides digoxin, digitoxin	*Epinephrine*	Interaction at cardiac pacemaker, β receptor	Cardiac arrhythmia
Anticonvulsants Phenytoin	*Sedatives,* for example, diazepam, chlordiazepoxide, barbiturates	Sedatives induce liver metabolism of phenytoin	Convulsions
General anesthetics Halothane, chloroform, cyclopropane	*Adrenergic amines* all	Anesthetics may sensitize myocardium	Cardiac arrhythmias
Antibiotics Penicillin	Tetracyclines, erythromycin	Inhibition of microorganism multiplication	Lessened effectiveness of penicillin
Erythromycin	Clindamycin	Unknown	Lessened effectiveness
Antacids	Tetracyclines	Decreased gastrointestinal absorption of tetracyclines	Lessened antibacterial effect
Hormones Adrenal corticosteroids	Salicylates	Synergism of ulcerogenic effects	Enhanced gastrointestinal ulceration
Oral contraceptives	Meperidine (Demerol)	Inhibition of meperidine metabolism	Enhanced effectiveness of meperidine
CNS depressants Sedatives, hypnotics, narcotics	CNS depressants	Potentiation	Enhanced depression of CNS function

ogenicity. Both dental caries and periodontal disease tend to increase markedly in xerostomia. The retention of dental prostheses and the comfort and soft tissue health of the wearer also depend on adequate salivary flow.

The autonomic control of salivary flow renders it particularly liable to modification by drugs. More than 200 drugs with xerostomic potential are known. Most of the agents are either sedative–hypnotics, antidepressants, or anticholinergics, although some have a less readily apparent mechanism of action. If chronic administration of any drug with xerostomic effects is necessary, appropriate local measures (increased fluid intake, fluoride rinses, fastidious dietary and hygienic control) should be taken to alleviate the potential oral sequelae.

DRUG-INDUCED TASTE IMPAIRMENT

Theophylline decreases taste sensitivity to sweet and bitter stimuli, presumably by modifying receptor sensitivity. Systemic lithium chloride and several topical antiseptics also modify taste, by mechanisms unknown. Penicillamine decreases the taste threshold for salt, sucrose, and acid, probably by reducing serum zinc concentration through chelation; zinc supplementation has been shown to restore taste thresholds in patients taking penicillamine. Dietary zinc deficiency may also impair taste.

FLUORIDE

Fluoride is a trace element of great importance to dental health. In the late 1930s the incidence of dental caries was linked to the concentration of fluoride ion (F^-) in water supplies; this led to the utilization F^- in drinking water and by prescription. Children who receive the optimal level of F^- from before birth to midteens experience less than half the number of carious lesions throughout life than those whose diets are deficient.

The lesion of dental caries is initiated by dissolution of the enamel surface by organic acids, the end-products of glycolysis in dental plaque bacteria (*see* above). F^- incorporation into the enamel apatite crystals at an optimal level renders them less liable to dissolution, owing to increased crystal size and to improved stacking of asymmetric units. F^- grossly in excess of the optimal level causes white or colored flecking or mottling of the enamel for reasons not understood. The optimal drinking water F^- level is about 1 ppm F^-, or 1 mg F^-/day for children over 3 years of age.

Topical F^- may reduce the initiation of dental caries through ionic transfer with the enamel surface and by inhibiting glycolysis in plaque bacteria. Adults who live in naturally or artificially fluoridated water-supply areas have less dental decay than do those with equivalent dental development who live in deficient areas. Application of F^- by mouthrinse or gel also reduces the incidence of new lesions, although generally much less than does optimal dietary intake during dental development. Acute systemic toxicity may develop if the material is ingested, since the concentrations used are several thousand times higher than those recommended for drinking water. Symptoms of acute poisoning include convulsions and eventual cardiac failure; the probable mechanism is inhibition of enzyme processes requiring heavy metal ions for activation because of the formation of fluorine-metal complexes.

The unsupervised home use of dentifrices that contain F^- reduces caries incidence in children to a slight but statistically significant degree.

ANTICANCER CHEMOTHERAPY—ORAL CARE

Anticancer drugs kill the cells of the oral epithelium. Resistance to infection thus decreases, there is an increased bleeding tendency, and the oral soft tissues tend to ulcerate. Taste perception may be impaired, and salivary flow may decrease. Common acute oral problems associated with cancer chemotherapy are candidiasis, gingival hemorrhage (exacerbated periodontal disease), and ulceration. Dental pulp tissue that is chronically inflamed before treatment may die, leading to periapical disease.

Preventive treatment to improve periodontal health and to eliminate carious lesions and compromised pulp tissue is wise but may not be possible. Antibiotic therapy for acute infections, and topical obtundents for ulceration, may also be needed.

MEDICAL—DENTAL DRUG INTERACTIONS

The important potential interactions between acutely applied dental drugs and medically prescribed agents are shown in Table 74-2.

75

MARVIN E. AMENT

Parenteral Nutrition

TOTAL PARENTERAL NUTRITION

Total parenteral nutrition (TPN) is the provision of all essential nutrients by an i.v. route. It is an excellent way to prevent or treat malnutrition in patients who do not have a functioning gastrointestinal tract. TPN will cure very few diseases other than malnutrition. However, it is an important adjunctive therapy in a number of surgical and medical conditions (Table 75-1).

The human organism needs as essential nutrients *protein*, an *energy source*, *fats*, *electrolytes*, *vitamins*, and *minerals*. Current standard TPN solutions (Table 75-2 A–D) use a balanced mixture of crystalline amino acids as the protein equivalent and, generally, hypertonic dextrose as the energy source. Added to these solutions are varying amounts of electrolytes, minerals, trace elements, vitamins, and, in certain circumstances, insulin. Intravenous fat, as either soybean or safflower oil emulsion, is given at least three times weekly to prevent essential fatty acid deficiency. This preparation may be given daily as a partial caloric source. The TPN solution usually is infused at a continuous rate either through a subclavian vein into the superior vena cava or into a peripheral vein.

TPN can be lifesaving in some disease-states; however, it is unphysiologic in that it bypasses the gastrointestinal tract, pancreas, and hepatobiliary system, which are the predominate organs of nutrient processing. The *sine qua non* for the use of TPN, therefore, is the presence of a nonfunctioning gastrointestinal tract. It is an expensive means of delivering nutrition, since a single liter of solution frequently costs from \$50 to \$75 to prepare and usually takes a pharmacist 30 minutes to formulate. If one multiplies the cost per liter by the 3 or 4 liters per patient per day times the number of patient hospital days and the cost of the infusion pump and nursing time, it becomes a considerable expense. Although TPN is safe when used by experienced hands, it is fraught with complications when administered by personnel not properly trained in its safe use.

INDICATIONS FOR TPN (TABLE 75-1)

Surgical Indications

Two weeks of preoperative TPN and postoperative TPN until gastrointestinal function recovers are indicated in patients scheduled for elec-

TABLE 75-1. Major Indications for Total Parenteral Nutrition

Surgical
- Preoperative
  1. Nutritional rehabilitation necessary in patients with a nonfunctioning gastrointestinal tract prior to elective or nonemergency surgery
- Postoperative
  1. Prolonged ileus
  2. Intraabdominal infections
  3. Wound dehiscence
  4. Enteric fistulae
  5. Short bowel syndrome

Nonsurgical
- Inflammatory bowel disease
- Pancreatitis
  1. Prolonged inflammation
  2. Pancreatic ascites
  3. Pancreatic pleural effusion
  4. Complicated pseudocyst
- Prolonged paralytic ileus
- Severe mucosal injury
- Unsafe access to gastrointestinal tract

Oncologic
- Nutritional support during therapy while the gut is nonfunctioning
- Controlled clinical trials for efficacy
- Specific organ failure
  - Acute renal failure
  - Chronic liver failure with portal systemic encephalopathy

tive or nonemergency surgery, when the patients are nutritionally deprived (defined, for the purposes of this discussion, as loss of greater than 10% body weight, serum albumin less than 3 g/dl, total lymphocyte count of less than 1200 mm^3, and a nonfunctioning gastrointestinal tract). TPN can also be used to maintain nutritional stability during prolonged ileus, intraabdominal infections, and wound dehiscence.

Parenteral nutrition has decreased mortality significantly in nonmalignant postoperative fistulas that are not secondary to inflammatory bowel disease. TPN helps under these circumstances in two ways: first, by "putting the gut to rest," there is no food stimulation of gastrointestinal secretions. Therefore, output through the fistula is decreased or eliminated, allowing the fistula a chance to heal. Second, the patient's nutritional status remains intact and may improve. Thus, if the fistula should not heal after 4 to 6 weeks of TPN and further operative repair is needed, the patient will be in better nutritional balance to undergo the operation. Occasionally, TPN may be given at home

TABLE 75-2A. Standard Neonatal Base* Total Parenteral Nutrition Solution

Ingredients	Units		Recommended Dose
Amino acids	%	2	
Dextrose	%	11	
Sodium	mEq/liter	0*	3 mEq/kg/day
Potassium	mEq/liter	0*	2.4 mEq/kg/day
Calcium	mg/dL	0*	200–600 mg/kg/day
Magnesium	mEq/liter	2	
Chloride	mEq/liter	8	
Phosphorus	mg/dL	0*	45–60 mg/kg/day
Acetate	mEq/liter	13	
Copper	mg/liter	1	
Zinc	mg/liter	2	
Available calories per liter			
Dextrose		374	
Amino acid		80	
Total		454	
Nonprotein calorie to nitrogen ratio		117	
Pharmacy formula number		N11	

* Additional electrolytes required to complete solution.

TABLE 75-2B. Standard Pediatric Total Parenteral Nutrition Solutions

		Pharmacy Formula Number*				
Ingredients	Units	*P10*	*P15*	*P20*	*P25*	*P30*
Amino acids	%	2	2	2	2	2
Dextrose	%	10	15	20	25	30
Sodium	mEq/liter	30	30	30	30	30
Potassium	mEq/liter	25	25	25	25	25
Calcium	mg/dL	20	20	20	20	20
Magnesium	mEq/liter	10	10	10	10	10
Chloride	mEq/liter	30	30	30	30	30
Phosphorus	mg/dL	23	23	23	23	23
Acetate	mEq/liter	35	35	35	35	35
Copper	mg/liter	1	1	1	1	1
Zinc	mg/liter	2	2	2	2	2
Available calories per liter						
Dextrose		340	510	680	850	1020
Amino acid		80	80	80	80	80
Total		420	590	760	930	1100
Nonprotein calorie to nitrogen ratio		106	159	212	266	319

* Columns represent, in solutions P10 through P30, the percentage of amino acids and dextrose or the mEq/liter, mg/dl, or mg/liter of each substance present.

TABLE 75-2C. Standard Adult Total Parenteral Nutrition Solutions

		Pharmacy Formula Number*				
Ingredients	**Units**	***A10***	***A15***	***A20***	***A25***	***A30***
Amino acids	%	2.25	2.25	2.25	2.25	2.25
Dextrose	%	10	15	20	25	30
Sodium	mEq/liter	35	35	35	35	35
Potassium	mEq/liter	30	30	30	30	30
Calcium	mg/dL	10	10	10	10	10
Magnesium	mEq/liter	10	10	10	10	10
Chloride	mEq/liter	35	35	35	35	35
Phosphorus	mg/dL	30	30	30	30	30
Acetate	mEq/liter	39	39	39	39	39
Copper	mg/liter	1	1	1	1	1
Zinc	mg/liter	2	2	2	2	2
Available calories per liter						
Dextrose		340	510	680	850	1020
Amino acid		90	90	90	90	90
Total		430	600	770	940	1110
Nonprotein calorie to nitrogen ratio		54	142	189	212	283

* Columns represent, in solutions A10 through A30, the percentage of amino acids and dextrose or the mEq/liter, mg/dl, or mg/liter of each substance present.

TABLE 75-2D. Standard Total Parenteral Nutrition Vitamins

Ingredients	**Units**	
Ascorbic acid	100	mg
Biotin	60	μg
Folic acid	400	μg
Niacinamide	40	mg
Pantothenic acid	15	mg
Pyridoxine HCl (B_6)	4	mg
Riboflavin (B_2)	3.6	mg
Thiamine (B_1)	3	mg
Vitamin A (retinol)	3300	IU
Vitamin B_{12}	5	μg
Vitamin D (ergocalciferol)	200	IU
Vitamin E (dl-alpha tocopherol acetate)	10	IU

for months to years if it is thought that reoperation may be more hazardous than continued i.v. feeding. TPN should be considered as supportive therapy for fistulae secondary to inflammatory bowel disease. A fistula may heal but often will recur after cessation of TPN. It is unlikely that a malignant fistula will heal without surgical intervention.

Patients with short bowel syndrome (less than 2–3 feet of small intestine) do not have enough absorptive surface to maintain nutritional health with enteral intake alone. If there are more than 2 feet of functional small intestine, it may undergo adaptive changes, such that the patient can eventually sustain life with enteral feeding. Unfortunately, complete adaptation may take as long as 1 to 2 years, necessitating long-term TPN.

Nonsurgical Indications

Inflammatory Bowel Disease. Although TPN cannot cure ulcerative colitis and Crohn's disease, it may be adjunctive in maintaining a patient's nutritional status during a flare-up. TPN may also be needed for nutritional support when treating complications of inflammatory bowel disease, such as obstruction, abscesses, fistulae, and perforations, since these complications are associated with a high rate of protein catabolism and diminished intestinal function. Additionally, 1 to 2 weeks of TPN improves immune competence and induces a positive nitrogen balance. This reduces intraoperative and postoperative morbidity and mortality.

Pancreatitis. TPN is indicated in the treatment of complications of acute and chronic pancreatitis. If pain persists or recurs after attempts at refeeding or prolonged illness, TPN should be initiated to prevent further starvation. Additionally, TPN is part of the accepted treatment for pancreatic ascites and pancreatic pleural effusion thought to be caused by pancreatic fistula. Pancreatic pseudocysts usually do not require treatment with TPN.

Prolonged Paralytic Ileus. TPN is indicated in patients with prolonged ileus whose gastrointestinal tract is unavailable for nutrient delivery. This is often seen in patients with pancreatitis, sepsis, pneumonias, and electrolyte abnormalities and in those in respirators.

Unsafe Access to the Gastrointestinal Tract. TPN should be considered if the risk of aspiration is high secondary to feeding either orally or through an indwelling feeding tube. For example, patients who require frequent postural drainage and who are either off a respirator but fully alert or who are respirator dependent should be considered for TPN.

Oncologic Indications

The use of TPN in patients with cancer is still controversial. No clinical investigation has reported increased tumor growth because of TPN. Although a number of investigators believe that TPN improves a patient's ability to tolerate anticancer therapy, no controlled trials have been done. There is no evidence that TPN improves survival in patients with malignancy. TPN should be used to treat or prevent malnutrition in patients without a functional gut and in patients likely to become malnourished as a result of anticancer therapy.

Specific Organ Failure

Patients with renal failure undergoing dialysis can use standard TPN solutions. The volumes used are usually limited by the frequency of dialysis. Special formulations of amino acids need not be used provided the patient is dialyzed daily or every other day.

Experimental work in animals and humans with chronic liver disease and encephalopathy suggests that a formula rich in branch-chained amino acids and deficient in aromatic amino acids can improve neurologic status while maintaining nutritional status. Such a solution is now available commercially.

DETERMINING NUTRITIONAL STATUS

The nutritional needs of every patient should be a fundamental part of their evaluation so as to determine whether the patient needs enteral or parenteral nutritional support. There are four key components to establishing a patient's nutritional status: nutritional history-screening, anthropometric measurements, clinical examination, and laboratory data.

Nutritional History Screening

The nutritional history screens for a nutrient deficiency from five potential causes: inadequate dietary intake, inadequate absorption, decreased use, increased loss, and increased requirement.

Anthropometric Measurement

Body weight and *height*, and *body weight per height*, are the most important anthropometric measurements, and in the presence of normal serum proteins give the most valid determinations of the patient's nutritional status.

Standard body weight–height reference graphs for adults, infants, and children are readily available and should be used routinely. Weight loss not secondary to fluid loss is an ominous sign in the hospitalized patient because it may reflect use of body protein.

Skin-fold thickness is a good indicator of body fat or caloric reserves. Skin folds are easy to measure and are likely to obviate the confusion that arises from dramatic weight changes with shifts in fluid. Triceps skin fold is a convenient site and is thought to be representative of body fat stores. The *mid-arm muscle circumference* reflects both caloric adequacy and muscle mass.

Laboratory Data

Transferrin, with a half life of 5 to 7 days, is a more sensitive indicator of the protein status of the body than serum albumin, with a half life of 14 to 19 days. The lymphocyte count is one reflection of the patient's immune status. Lymphocyte counts of less than $1200/mm^3$ are found in patients with mild to moderate malnutrition. The standard skin test antigens used to measure immune competence include tuberculosis, candida, mumps, streptokinase streptodornase, and histoplasma. In normal persons, two of these five are typically reactive. If a patient reacts to only one, he is considered to be partly anergic, and if he reacts to none he is completely anergic. If the patient is given full parenteral support and enters into positive nitrogen balance, these variables should show major improvement within 7 to 14 days.

It is unusual in everyday practice to specifically measure the serum level of certain vitamins because of the cost involved and because the tests are not readily available.

NUTRIENT REQUIREMENTS

Calorie Requirements

Calorie requirements are difficult to ascertain because marked variation occurs from person to person, and disease-states can alter calorie consumption drastically. Calorie needs of healthy, resting adults can be approximated on the basis of 30 kcal/kg of ideal body weight. Resting metabolic expenditures may increase manyfold, however, with injury or stress. Protracted fever alone will increase caloric needs by about 13% per degree Celsius; the energy cost of physical exertion will increase needs from 0% to 30% depending on whether the patient is at rest or is thrashing about. For most hospitalized adult patients, 2000 to 3000 kcal will meet daily needs. In certain patients, such as those with burns, the caloric needs can rise substantially and double or triple.

Protein Requirements

Optimal protein needs for adults range from 0.8 g/kg of body weight/day for an average healthy adult to 1 to 2 g/kg/day for a child. Larger amounts may be required under conditions of severe catabolism or of protein wastage. The typical adult patient receiving TPN is given about 1 to 2 g of protein/kg/day. The typical newborn child who requires parenteral nutrition is given about 2 g/kg/day. Restrictions on protein intake may be needed in cases of acute renal or hepatic insufficiency. Several different crystalline amino acid solutions are available for use in TPN. Virtually all contain a combination of nonessential and essential amino acids. No specific amino acid solution has been proved to be superior clinically; all may be diluted with concentrated dextrose solutions as necessary (*see* Chap. 77).

Intravenous Fat Emulsions

The human body needs from 1% to 4% of its daily caloric needs in the form of essential fatty acids. The higher percentage is needed for infants. Two preparations currently are available either as 10% or 20% emulsions that provide from 1.1 to 2.0 kcal/ml in isotonic solution. These—the soybean oil preparation and the safflower oil preparation—contain 54% and 77%, respectively, of the fatty acids in the form of linoleic acid. Both preparations contain egg phospholipids, glycerine, water, and sodium hydroxide adjusted to a *p*H of 5.5 to 9. Glycerine and the egg phospholipids suspend triglycerides in a stable emulsion and in an emulsified state with a size of 0.1 to 0.5 μm, the dimensions of chylomicrons.

Minerals

No specific recommendations can be made for electrolyte prescriptions. The average electrolyte requirements are given in Table 75-3.

Iron is not routinely included in parenteral infusions. If an iron deficiency is evident, iron may be given intravenously as Imferon in accordance with the manufacturer's instructions.

TABLE 75-3. Average Electrolyte Requirements

	Children	Adults
Sodium	3–5 mEq/kg/day	60+ mEq/day
Potassium	2–5 mEq/kg/day	60+ mEq/day
Calcium	1–4 mEq/kg/day	10–15 mEq/day
Phosphate	0.7–3 mmol/kg	20–50 mmol/day
Magnesium	0.3–2 mEq/kg	8–20 mEq/day

Trace Elements

The total number and amounts of trace elements needed for health are not fully understood. Definite syndromes have been recognized with zinc and copper deficiency, but clearly defined syndromes with chromium, manganese, and iodine deficiency have not. For premature infants, 300 μg/kg/day of zinc are recommended. One hundred μg/kg/day are recommended for full-term infants until age 5 years; thereafter adult guidelines apply. From 0.14 to 0.2 μg/kg/day of chromium, 2 to 10 μg/kg/day of manganese, and 5 μg/kg/day of iodine are recommended doses for children. For stable adults, 2.5 to 4 mg of zinc, 0.5 to 1.5 mg of copper, 10 to 15 μg of chromium, 0.15 to 0.8 mg of manganese, and 50 to 100 μg of iodine are recommended. If a patient has small bowel fluid loss, additional zinc may be needed.

Vitamins

Although the American Medical Association Committee on Nutrition has provided guidelines for the dosage of vitamins administered intravenously, data to support these values are not readily available. Commercially available vitamin preparations provide for the recommended needs of all vitamins except for vitamin K, which is generally given separately in the form of 5 to 10 mg of phytonadione weekly.

Current i.v. vitamin formulations provide 200 units of vitamin D per day. It is unknown whether this form of vitamin D can be used. However, the amount provided for children is inadequate. Children should receive 25,000 to 30,000 units of vitamin D intramuscularly/month to prevent the development of rickets.

TPN BY EITHER THE CENTRAL OR PERIPHERAL VENOUS ROUTE

Peripheral venous TPN is recommended for the following clinical situations: [1] short-term

(10–20 days) nutritional support; [2] recurring history of septic episodes; [3] presence of thrombosed subclavian veins; [4] technical difficulty or danger involved in a central venous catheter insertion; [5] need for parenteral supplementation to gastrointestinal nutrition; and [6] delay of permanent central venous line insertion.

The goal of peripheral TPN is to approximate nitrogen equilibrium in patients with mild to moderate deficits, as shown by the nutritional assessment. Peripheral TPN may be administered as a temporary measure in severely depleted patients, but only until more aggressive nutritional support can be initiated. With the availability of 20% fat emulsions, it is possible to provide a large number of calories in a small volume of solution. Peripheral TPN can be used in patients in whom there is no significant renal compromise, since renal compromise limits the volume of the infusate but cannot be used in patients who have abnormal lipid metabolism, because most of the calories are supplied by fat. It is extremely useful in patients who have excessive fluid losses when 3 to 4 liters of fluid replacement a day can easily be tolerated. A typical regimen compromises 2 liters of a 10% dextrose/4½% amino acid mixture, plus 1 liter of 10% fat emulsion infused simultaneously over 24 hours. This will supply 2100 kcal and 78 g of protein. If fat emulsion is contraindicated or fluid restriction is necessary, the osmolarity can be decreased using 2 liters of D_5W and 3½% of amino acids while still supplying 70 g of protein. Some persons have used as much as 83% of the calories in the form of fat in order to provide the necessary nonprotein calories, with 17% of the calories provided as glucose. By using a greater percentage of the calories in the form of fat, the osmolarity of the infusate is approximately 467 mOsm/liter. This compares with an osmolarity in excess of 1700 mOsm/day when glucose is the primary source of nonprotein calories, which is the typical osmolarity of a 25% dextrose solution.

FURTHER READING

1. Jeejeebhoy KN, Anderson GH, Nakhooda AF et al: Metabolic studies in total parenteral nutrition with lipid in man: Comparison with glucose. J Clin Invest 57:125–136, 1976
2. Orr G, Wade J, Boothe A Jr et al: Alternatives to total parenteral nutrition in the critically ill patient. Crit Care Med 8:29–33, 1980
3. Ikeda K, Suita S: Total parenteral nutrition using peripheral veins and surgical neonates. Arch Surg 112:1045–1049, 1977
4. Jeejeebhoy KN: Total parenteral nutrition. Ann R Coll Physicians Surg Can 9:287–300, 1976
5. Allardyce DB, Williams BJ: Parenteral solutions for nutritional support in surgical patients: A comparison of nitrogen gains employing 5% and 10% amino acid solutions. Am J Surg 133:315–318, 1977

76

JEREMY H. THOMPSON

Immunologic Agents and Active Immunization

Natural active immunity results after recovery from an infection. The objective of *active immunization* is to attempt to duplicate the beneficial effects of natural infection without the full consequences of the actual disease.

Active immunization is produced by vaccines. The resulting immunity may last a lifetime or only a few months. Vaccines are prepared from microorganisms or their products (toxins), which have been changed so that they have lost their ability to produce disease while retaining most, or all, of their antigenic potential. Reduction of pathogenicity may be produced by, for example, heat or formaldehyde inactivation (*killed vaccines*) or by the development of attenuated strains (*vaccines of live organisms*). Examples of viral vaccines include killed organisms (influenza) and live attenuated strains (poliomyelitis). Examples of bacterial vaccines include killed whole organisms (pertussis vaccine), subunit vaccines (pneumococcal polysaccharide), BCG (Bacillus Calmette–Guérin), or toxoids (diphtheria and tetanus). Typically the use of inactivated vaccines or toxoids requires several doses to achieve a complete protective antibody response. In addition, frequent "booster" injections are needed to maintain an appropriate level of immunity. With live attenuated vaccines, however, the response is more similar to that resulting from natural infection, and is therefore more long-lasting.

GENERAL PRINCIPLES

Of the immunizing agents currently available (Table 76-1), the first seven are recommended for healthy infants. Adenovirus vaccine is used by the military but is not yet licensed for general use. Tables 76-2 and 76-3 give the recommended schedules for active immunization

---

Léon Charles Albert Calmette, 1863–1933. French bacteriologist at the Institut Pasteur in Paris. Discovered a snakebite serum in the 1890s, later developed the BCG (Bacille Calmette Guérin) vaccine for tuberculosis immunization, for which mass production began in 1924.

Camille Guérin, 1872–1961. French bacteriologist, originally a veterinarian. Worked all his life on tuberculosis, including development of the BCG vaccine.

TABLE 76-1. Active Immunizing Agents

1. Diphtheria (toxoid)	11. Typhoid
2. Tetanus (toxoid)	12. Influenza
3. Pertussis antigen	13. Tularemia
4. Poliomyelitis	14. Cholera
5. Measles	15. Plague
6. Rubella	16. Vaccina
7. Mumps	17. Anthrax
8. BCG	18. Pneumococcus polysaccharide
9. Yellow fever	19. Meningococcus antigen
10. Rabies	20. Adenovirus

ALBERT BRUCE SABIN, 1906– . Russian-born American physician and microbiologist. Discovered many enteroviruses, reoviruses, and B virus and developed, as well as oral polio vaccine, vaccines against dengue and sandfly fever. Also studied experimental virally induced tumors.

JONAS EDWARD SALK, 1914– . American physician and virologist. Developed his poliomyelitis vaccine in 1954 and also worked on the immunology of influenza virus and delayed hypersensitivity.

and tuberculin testing of normal infants and children. It is more important that all children receive all immunizations recommended than an inflexible administration schedule be followed. Thus, if a scheduled dose is missed, it is *not* necessary to restart the entire schedule of vaccinations.

When contemplating the routine use of a vaccine, one should consider several specific points: the *risk* of acquiring the disease and the characteristics of *symptoms* and *treatment;* the direct and potential *benefits to the individual and to society* in preventing or attenuating the disease; the *cost, availability, efficacy,* and *safety* of the vaccine; and any alternatives to prophylactic vaccination.

Combining vaccines either at the same injection site or at different injection sites at the same time may lead to imperfect antibody response and possibly increased toxicity. However, some combinations (Tables 76-2 and 76-3) have proved both safe and efficacious.

A record of the name of the vaccine, the manufacturer, the lot or other identifying number, the dose, site and route used, and any untoward response should be noted.

There are several specific contraindications to vaccination with live vaccines: patients with immunodeficiency disorders, including a leukemia or lymphoma; those with generalized cancer; those on immunosuppressive or cytotoxic drug therapy with, for example, glucocorticosteroids or anticancer drugs, or those undergoing radiation therapy; any acute febrile illness; receipt of plasma, a blood transfusion,

TABLE 76-2. Recommended Schedule for Active Immunization of Normal Infants and Children*

2 mo	DTP†	TOPV‡
4 mo	DTP	TOPV
6 mo	DTP	§
1 yr		Tuberculin test‖
15 mo	Measles,¶ rubella¶	Mumps¶
1½ yr	DTP	TOPV
4–6 yr	DTP	TOPV
14–16 yr	Td**—repeat every 10 years	

* Based on the recommendations on immunization policies and procedures formulated by the Advisory Committee on Immunization Practices (ACIP) of the United States Public Health Service and the Committee of Infectious Diseases of the American Academy of Pediatrics.

† DTP—diphtheria and tetanus toxoids combined with pertussis vaccine.

‡ TOPV—trivalent oral poliovirus vaccine. This recommendation is suitable for breast-fed as well as bottle-fed infants.

§ A third dose of TOPV is optional but may be given in areas of high endemicity of poliomyelitis.

‖ Frequency of repeated tuberculin tests depends on risk of exposure of the child and on the prevalence of tuberculosis in the population group. For the pediatrician's office or outpatient clinic, an annual or biennial tuberculin test, unless local circumstances clearly indicate otherwise, is appropriate. The initial test should be done at the time of, or before, the measles immunization.

¶ May be given at 15 months as measles—rubella or measles—mumps—rubella combined vaccines (*see* Rubella and Mumps sections for further discussion of age of administration).

** Td—combined tetanus and diphtheria toxoids (adult type) for those older than 6 years of age, in contrast to diphtheria and tetanus (DT) toxoids, which contain a larger amount of diphtheria antigen. *Tetanus toxoid at time of injury:* For clean, minor wounds, no booster dose is needed by a fully immunized child unless more than 10 years have elapsed since the last dose. For contaminated wounds, a booster dose should be given if more than 5 years have elapsed since the last dose.

Because the concentration of antigen varies in different products, the manufacturer's package insert should be consulted regarding the volume of individual doses of immunizing agents.

Because biologics are of varying stability, the manufacturer's recommendations for optimal storage conditions (*e.g.,* temperature, light) should be followed carefully. Failure to observe these precautions may significantly reduce the potency and effectiveness of the vaccines.

or gamma globulin within the preceding 2 months; the administration of a second live vaccine (unless, of course, they have been proved safe and effective when used concomitantly); pregnancy; and a history of a hypersen-

TABLE 76-3. Primary Immunization for Children Not Immunized in Early Infancy*†

Under 6 Years of Age	
First visit	DTP, TOPV, tuberculin test
Interval after first visit	
1 mo	Measles,‡ mumps, rubella
2 mo	DTP, TOPV
4 mo	DTP, TOPV§
10–16 mo or preschool	DTP, TOPV
Age 14–16 yr	Td—repeat every 10 yr
6 years of Age and Over	
First visit	Td, TOPV, tuberculin test
Interval after first visit	
1 mo	Measles, mumps, rubella
2 mo	Td, TOPV
8 to 14 mo	Td, TOPV
Age 14–16 yr	Td—repeat every 10 years

* Physicians may choose to alter the sequence of these schedules if specific infections are prevalent at the time. For example, measles vaccine might be given on the first visit if an epidemic is underway in the community.

† Based on the recommendations on immunization policies and procedures formulated by the Advisory Committee on Immunization Practices (ACIP) of the United States Public Health Service and the Committee of Infectious Diseases of the American Academy of Pediatrics.

‡ Measles vaccine is not routinely given before 15 months of age (*see* Table 76-1).

§ Optional.

sitivity reaction to the same or a related vaccine.

ADVERSE EFFECTS

Syringes and needles should be disposed of carefully so as to minimize accidental inoculation. Side-effects of vaccination are those due to poor technique (nerve damage, sterile abscess formation) and those due to the vaccine itself (which can be local or systemic) and are usually predictable, mild, and self-limiting.

Typical local reactions at the injection site are *pain, tenderness,* and *induration.* Local reactions may rarely be severe, as, for example, after booster injections for typhoid prophylaxis. Systemic side-effects are almost invariably preceded by local reactions and usually comprise fever, skin rashes, arthralgias, general malaise and convulsions. Very rarely, a severe side-effect may be seen, such as meningoencephalitis (pertussis), permanent paralysis (influenza), anaphylactic shock (influenza, yellow fever), or even death. Anaphylaxis may develop to certain trace contaminants in vaccines grown in foreign proteins (*i.e.*, chick embryo) or to trace quantities of other "contaminants" such as antibiotics.

Parents should report any side-effects to physicians, and physicians should report any severe or unexpected reactions to local, state, or federal agencies and to the vaccine manufacturer.

SOURCES AND INFORMATION ABOUT VACCINES*

The *American Public Health Association* publishes "Control of Communicable Diseases in Man" at 5-year intervals. *The Advisory Committee on Immunization Practices* (ACIP) of the United States Public Health Service (USPHS) issues its "Morbidity and Mortality Weekly Report," directed primarily toward public health agencies. The *Committee on Infectious Diseases* of the American Academy of Pediatrics publishes the "Red Book" triannually, and revisions are issued in the Academy's *Newsletter. Local, state, and federal public health agencies* can be consulted for special problems, particularly those of a community nature, and the *package insert* and the *vaccine manufacturer* should be consulted for details on the agent itself. The *Medical Letter* evaluates new vaccines on a timely basis. Recommendations may vary slightly from source to source.

SMALLPOX

The World Health Organization (WHO) and the World Health Assembly officially declared the global eradication of smallpox in May 1980. Vaccination is now *not recommended* for civilians because of its dangers, including, rarely, death. However, vaccination is still indicated for certain populations such as the military and laboratory workers directly involved with the virus or closely related viruses, for example, monkeypox and vaccinia. VIG (Table 76-4) is a valuable adjunct in the treatment of reactions to smallpox vaccinations.

As of August 15, 1980, four nations—Demo-

* A variety of immunobiologic agents and drugs are available from the USPHS, Centers for Disease Control. These agents are listed in Tables 76-4, 76-5, and 76-6 and can be obtained by calling the Centers for Disease Control at (404) 329-3753 (8:00 a.m. to 4:30 p.m.) or (404) 329-3644 (4:30 p.m. to 8 a.m., holidays and weekends).

TABLE 76-4. Immunobiologic Agents and Drugs Procured, Distributed, and Stored by Immunobiologic Activity, Centers for Disease Control (CDC), with Information About Their Source, Licensure, and Investigational New Drug (IND) Applications

Immunobiologic	Producer or Source	Licensed or IND Status	Distributed to	Conditions for Distribution	Storage
Antitoxins					
Botulism equine antitoxin (ABE)	Connaught Laboratories, Inc.	Licensed	MD as required	Emergency	4°C
Diphtheria (equine) antitoxin	Sclavo, Inc.	Licensed	MD as required	Emergency	4°C
Globulins and plasmas					
Vaccinia immune globulin (VIG)	Hyland Laboratories	Licensed	MD as required	Emergency	4°C
Varicella-zoster immune globulin (VZIG)	Massachusetts State Health Department	IND	MD as required	Emergency	4°C
Western equine encephalitis (WEE) immune globulin	CDC	IND	MD as required	Emergency	4°C or −20°C
African hemorrhagic fever (EBOLA)	CDC	None	MD as required	Emergency	−20°C
California E.	CDC	None	MD as required	Emergency	−20°C
EEE	CDC	None	MD as required	Emergency	−20°C
Herpes simian B	CDC	None	MD as required	Emergency	−20°C
Junin (Argentinian hemorrhagic fever)	CDC	None	MD as required	Emergency	−20°C
Lassa fever	CDC	None	MD as required	Emergency	−20°C
Machupo	CDC	None	MD as required	Emergency	−20°C
Marburg (green monkey disease)	CDC	None	MD as required	Emergency	−20°C
RSSE	CDC	None	MD as required	Emergency	−20°C
SLE	CDC	None	MD as required	Emergency	−20°C
WEE	CDC	None	MD as required	Emergency	−20°C
VEE	CDC	None	MD as required	Emergency	−20°C
Vaccines or Toxoids					
Anthrax vaccine, adsorbed	Michigan State Health Laboratories	Licensed	MD as required	Prophylaxis	4°C
Botulinum toxoid, pentavalent (ABCDE)	Parke, Davis	IND	Investigators	Physician-to-physician basis	4°C
Eastern equine encephalitis (EEE) vaccine, inactivated, dried	Merrell-National Laboratories	IND	Investigators	Physician-to physician basis	−20°C
Tularemia vaccine, live, attenuated	Merrell-National Laboratories	IND	Investigators	Physician-to-physician basis	−20°C
Venezuelan equine encephalitis (VEE) vaccine	Merrell-National Laboratories	IND	Investigators	Physician-to-physician basis	−20°C

cratic Kampuchea (Cambodia), Madagascar, Djibouti and Chad—still required an up-to-date certificate of smallpox vaccination as a condition of entry but accepted smallpox vaccination waiver letters as provided in the WHO International Health Regulations.

INFLUENZA VACCINES

Vaccines are available only for types A and B influenza. Antigenic drift and antigenic shift have reduced the effectiveness of vaccines, particularly in type A disease. Vaccines against

TABLE 76-5. Recommended Dosages and Frequencies of Administration of Antitoxins Available from the Centers for Disease Control

Clinical Disease	Immunobiologic Agent	Dosage	Interval
Botulism (types A, B, E)	Botulism equine antitoxin, (A, B, E)	1 vial i.v., 1 vial i.m.	1 vial i.v. after 4 hours if signs or symptoms worsen; another vial i.v. after 12 to 24 hours
Diphtheria	Diphtheria equine antitoxin	20,000–80,000 units or more i.m. or slow i.v. drip, depending on site, severity, duration of infection	

types A and B are 60% to 70% effective if given at least 2 weeks before exposure to natural infection, are of the current antigenic strain, and are followed by an annual booster injection.

All U.S. vaccines are inactivated egg-grown products. They are usually polyvalent, containing one or several type A strains and one type B strain. "Whole" vaccines contain the complete virus, whereas "split" vaccines contain the purified antigens supposedly responsible for inducing immunity. It is not clear whether the "whole" or the "split" product is safer and more efficacious.

Local and mild systemic reactions occur frequently. Subjects with a known allergy to egg or egg products should not receive influenza vaccines. There has been considerable controversy over whether the use of influenza vaccines results in an increased incidence of the rare Guillain-Barré syndrome.

MEASLES

The current vaccine of choice for measles is an attenuated strain. Side-effects develop in about 10% to 20% of vaccinees and are usually mild. "Atypical" measles may develop in persons who received one of the early inactivated vaccines that have subsequently been proved not very effective.

GEORGES GUILLAIN, 1876–1951. French neurologist. Published the definitive account of acute polyradiculoneuritis, Guillain-Barré syndrome, with J. A. Barré and A. Strohl in 1916.

TABLE 76-6. Recommended Prophylactic Dosages and Frequencies of Administration of Antitoxins and Immune Globulins from the Centers for Disease Control

Disease Entity	Immunobiologic Agent	Dosage	Interval
Botulism (types A, B, E)	Botulism equine antitoxin, (A, B, E)	1/5 to 1 vial i.m. Details and precautions supplied with antitoxin	Single dosage; may repeat one dosage if signs or symptoms occur
Chickenpox	Varicella-zoster immune globulin (VZIG) (human)	1–5 vials	Single dosage
Complications of smallpox inoculation	Vaccine immune globulin (VIG) (human)	0.3–0.6 ml/kg i.m. (never administer i.v.	Single dosage only; may be repeated at discretion of physician
Diphtheria	Diphtheria antitoxin (purified, concentrated globulin, equine)	1000–5000 units i.m. Details and precautions supplied with antitoxin	Single dosage
Western equine encephalitis (WEE)	Western equine encephalitis (WEE) immune globulin (human)	5–10 ml i.m. (never administer i.v.)	Single dosage

RUBELLA VACCINES

Vaccine RA 27/3, grown in human cells, and licensed in 1978, is the current vaccine of choice for rubella. Despite an attempt to generate herd immunity through the widespread use of rubella vaccine, about 20% to 25% of women of child-bearing age and adult males remain susceptible to the disease. A history of previous rubella infection is worthless as a determinant of adequate immunity. Every woman of child-bearing potential should be tested serologically and then vaccinated if susceptible. Adequate precautions should be undertaken to ensure that such persons are not pregnant at the time of vaccination or do not become pregnant within 3 months of vaccination. Vaccine failure occurs in about 2% of vaccinees.

Side-effects are mild and develop in about 5% of vaccinees. Arthralgia or mild arthritis may develop rarely. To date there has been no evidence of specific vaccine-induced teratogenesis, although abortuses of women vaccinated in early pregnancy were "infected' with virus.

GAMMA GLOBULIN THERAPY

Many antibody deficiencies can be treated successfully with repeated i.m. injections of human gamma globulin. Gamma globulin is of no value in pure cellular immunodeficiencies but may be of limited value in those with combined antibody and cellular immunodeficiency.

Immune serum globulin (human), U.S.P., is prepared by alcoholic fractionation of pooled human serum from about 500 donors. Fractionation removes most other serum proteins and the hepatitis virus. Immune serum globulin is reconstituted as a sterile 16.5% solution and contains 95% IgG with trace quantities of IgA and IgM and other serum proteins. IgA and IgM globulins are therapeutically insignificant in view of their rapid half-life (about 7 days compared to about 25 days for IgG) and their low concentration. Patients on long-term gamma globulin therapy need more frequent injections during times of infection, since the rate of protein catabolism is increased.

Gamma globulin is administered intramuscularly, and in children not more than 5 ml should be given at any one site. In adults, the maximum volume per injection site can be doubled. The usual dose in adults and children is 100 mg (0.7 ml)/kg/month.

ADVERSE REACTIONS

Various manifestations of allergy may develop. Anaphylactic shock, however, is rare, and following such an occurrence the subject should be tested for the presence of hypersensitivity to gamma globulin supplied by different manufacturers. Local muscle pain, sterile abscess formation, and nerve damage may result from injection trauma.

In patients with isolated IgA deficiency, anaphylactic shock is particularly likely to occur to the trace quantities of IgA present in most gamma globulin preparations.

FURTHER READING

1. Ellis RJ: Immunobiologic Agents and Drugs Available from the Centers for Disease Control, 2nd ed. Washington, DC, U.S. DHEW, July 1979
2. Immunizations for Travelers. Med Lett 21(14):13 July 1979
3. Report of the Committee on Infectious Diseases, 18th ed. Evanston, American Academy of Pediatrics, 1977
4. Schiff GM: Active immunization for adults. Annu Rev Med 31:441–451, 1980
5. Stiehm ER, Fulginiti VA: Immunologic Diseases in Infants and Children. Philadelphia, WB Saunders, 1980

77

RAYBURN B. VRABEL

Commonly Used Intravenous Solutions and Diagnostic Agents

Intravenous (i.v.) solutions play an important role in therapy by acting as vehicles for the delivery of other drugs and in the specific correction of fluid, electrolyte, and nutritional disorders (*see* Chap. 75). Tables 77-1, 77-2, and 77-3 outline some of the commonly used standard solutions.

MAINTENANCE/REPLACEMENT SOLUTIONS

SINGLE-INGREDIENT SOLUTIONS

Dextrose

Dextrose is available in concentrations of 2.5% to 70.0%. The most commonly used is the 5% concentration, which is isotonic with plasma and used primarily as a vehicle to provide patients with their daily requirement of fluid. Since the dextrose is catabolized in the body leaving the water component, the final result is the same as if water were given alone. Water cannot be given alone because it would cause hemolysis. Nutritionally, 5% dextrose cannot provide adequate calories, although the amount provided by an average daily infusion of 5% dextrose (2000–3000 ml, 340–510 calories) is enough to prevent starvation ketosis and acidosis and to spare body protein.

Sodium

Since sodium is the principal extracellular cation, isotonic sodium chloride (0.9%, or "normal saline") solutions can be infused without affecting body fluid osmotic pressure or composition. Solutions of sodium chloride are used to provide replacement for normal daily sodium loss (about 70 mEq/day), to replace abnormal losses occurring by means of gastrointestinal fluid, urine, or sweat, and as a vehicle to administer other drugs.

Other Single-Ingredient Solutions

Other solutions are used primarily as replacement in the treatment of alkalosis (*i.e.*, ammonium chloride) and acidosis (*i.e.*, sodium bicarbonate, sodium lactate, tromethamine).

MULTIPLE-INGREDIENT SOLUTIONS

Various combinations of dextrose and sodium chloride solutions are available. Sodium chlo-

TABLE 77-1. Maintenance and Replacement Solutions

Ingredient	Concentration	Calories/liter	Millimoles/liter	Na^+	K^+	Ca^{++}	Mg^{++}	NH_4^+	Cl^-	Lactate	Other
Single-ingredient solutions	%			←				*mEq/liter*			→
Dextrose*	5.0	170	253	—	—	—	—	—	—	—	—
	10.0	340	505	—	—	—	—	—	—	—	—
Ammonium chloride	2.14	—	800	—	—	—	—	400	400	—	—
Sodium chloride											
½ normal saline	0.45	—	154	77	—	—	—	—	77	—	—
normal saline	0.9	—	308	154	—	—	—	—	154	—	—
	3.0	—	1026	513	—	—	—	—	513	—	—
	5.0	—	1710	855	—	—	—	—	855	—	—
Sodium bicarbonate	5.0	—	1190	595	—	—	—	—	—	—	595†
Sodium lactate	1.87	55	334	167	—	—	—	—	—	167	—
Tromethamine (Tham)	3.6	—	300	—	—	—	—	—	—	—	300‡
Multiple-ingredient solutions											
D5§–¼ normal saline		170	324	34	—	—	—	—	34	—	—
Dextrose	5.0										
Sodium chloride	0.2										
D5–½ normal saline		170	406	77	—	—	—	—	77	—	—
Dextrose	5.0										
Sodium chloride	0.45										
D5–normal saline		170	561	154	—	—	—	—	154	—	—
Dextrose	5.0										
Sodium chloride	0.9										
Ringer's injection		—	309	147	4	5	—	—	156	—	—
Sodium chloride	0.86										
Potassium chloride	0.03										
Calcium chloride	0.03										
Lactated Ringer's		9	272	130	4	3	—	—	109	28	—
Sodium chloride	0.6										
Potassium chloride	0.04										
Calcium chloride	0.03										
Sodium lactate	0.25										
D5/lactated Ringer's		179	524	130	4	3	—	—	109	28	—
Dextrose	5.0										
Sodium chloride	0.6										
Potassium chloride	0.04										
Calcium chloride	0.03										
Sodium lactate	0.25										

* Solutions that contain greater than 10% are used primarily in combination with amino acid solutions (*see* Table 77-3).
† Milliequivalents of bicarbonate.
‡ Milliequivalents of acid that can be neutralized.
§ D5 = dextrose 5%.

TABLE 77-2. Plasma Volume Expanders

		Electrolyte Concentration
Protein Colloid Solutions		*mEq/liter*
Albumin 5%		Sodium 130–160
Plasma protein fraction 5% (Plasmanate)		Sodium 130–160
Plasma extenders		
Hetastarch (Hespan)		Sodium 154
Contains		Chloride 154
Hetastarch	6.0%	
Sodium chloride	0.9%	
Dextran, low molecular weight (Dextran 40)		
Contains		
Dextran, LMW	10.0%	Sodium 154
Sodium chloride	0.9%	Chloride 154
or		
Dextran, LMW	10.0%	Sodium 0
Dextrose	5.0%	Chloride 0
Dextran, high molecular weight (Dextran 70)		
Contains		
Dextran, HMW	6.0%	Sodium 154
Sodium chloride	0.9%	Chloride 154
or		
Dextran, HMW	6.0%	Sodium 0
Dextrose	5.0%	Chloride 0

ride is often used in combination with dextrose to create solutions that replace needed sodium requirements while meeting the body's need for fluid and minimal amounts of carbohydrate. Typically a 5% dextrose and ¼ normal saline solution is used, since 2 to 3 liters per day of this solution satisfies the body's fluid (2–3 liters) and sodium requirements (68–102 mEq) while providing enough carbohydrate to prevent tissue breakdown.

Several multiple-ingredient solutions have been formulated that more closely approximate the concentration of major electrolytes in extracellular fluid. These solutions (Ringer's, lactated Ringer's, Dextrose 5%/lactated Ringers) are commonly used when the maintenance of electrolyte balance is more crucial (*e.g.*, postoperatively) or when gastrointestinal losses containing bicarbonate need to be replaced. The lactate in these solutions is metabolized on an equimolar basis in the body to bicarbonate, a process that requires 1 to 2 hours for persons with normal cellular oxidative activity. Because of this time delay, these solutions are not recommended if immediate correction of acid–base disturbances is needed (*e.g.*, metabolic acidosis).

PLASMA VOLUME EXPANDERS

Although it is possible to replace a small loss of blood (plasma) volume with dextrose and electrolyte solutions, significant loss secondary to shock or hemorrhage requires replacement with solutions that do not equilibrate easily with intracellular fluids. Various plasma volume expanders are available that, when infused intravenously, retain water in the central vascular compartment via their osmotic activity.

Albumin and plasma protein fraction are processed from donated blood and are prepared commercially into stabilized formulations. Although these colloid solutions are two to four times more expensive than synthetic plasma

SYDNEY RINGER, 1835–1910. Physician and physiologist at University College, London. Published classic paper on "Ringer's solution" in 1880.

TABLE 77-3A. Nutrient Solutions—Fat Emulsions

	Ingredients	Concentration	Calories/liter	Milliosmoles/liter
Intralipid		%		
10%	Soybean oil	10.0	1100	280
	Egg yolk phospholipids	1.2		
	Glycerin	2.25		
20%	Soybean oil	20.0	2000	330
	Egg yolk phospholipids	1.2		
	Glycerin	2.25		
Liposyn				
20%	Safflower oil	20.0	2000	340
	Egg yolk phospholipids	1.2		
	Glycerin	2.5		

TABLE 77-3B. Nutrient Solutions—Crystalline Amino Acid Solutions

Solution	Concentration	Millimoles/liter	Na^+	K^+	Mg^{++}	Cl^-	Acetate	Phosphate
Essential/nonessential combinations	%		←		*mEq/liter*		→	*mmol/liter*
Aminosyn								
Plain	5.0	500	—	5.4	—	—	86	—
	7.0	700	—	5.4	—	—	105	—
	8.5	850	—	5.4	—	35	90	—
	10.0	1000	—	5.4	—	—	148	—
With electrolytes	3.5	460	47	13	3	40	68	—
	8.5	1160	70	66	10	98	142	30
Travasol								
Plain	5.5	520	—	—	—	22	35	—
	8.5	860	—	—	—	34	52	—
With electrolytes	5.5	850	70	60	10	70	100	30
	8.5	1160	70	60	10	70	135	30
FreAmine	8.5	810	10	—	—	<2	74	10
Veinamine	8.0	950	40	30	6	50	50	—
Essential amino acids								
Nephramine	5.4	440	6	—	—	—	44	—

extenders (*i.e.*, hetastarch, dextran), they are preferred when significant plasma volume replacement is needed. The synthetic agents are used when dextrose and electrolyte solutions are insufficient to replace low plasma volume deficits (*e.g.*, patients requiring 1000–1500 ml/day of volume expansion). On a milliliter per milliliter basis, all plasma volume expanders produce a similar degree of plasma volume expansion. Hetastarch produces a lower incidence of allergic reactions than do dextran preparations. The dextrans, especially low molecular weight dextran, have the desirable property of decreasing platelet adhesiveness. Interference with blood cross-matching is observed in patients who receive dextrans unless the red blood cells are properly processed.

NUTRIENT SOLUTIONS

Patients unable to take nourishment orally must eventually be placed on solutions other than dextrose if they are to remain in positive nitrogen balance. Total parenteral nutrition (TPN) via i.v. hyperalimentation (*see* Chap. 75) is a method of providing these critically ill patients with basic nutritional requirements.

Using commercially available solutions of crystalline amino acids and hypertonic dextrose, it is possible to prepare an infusate that contains more than 1000 calories/liter, considerably more calories than can be achieved using the standard 5% dextrose solution (*see* above). Table 77-3 outlines some typical TPN solutions used at a large university teaching hospital. These have been formulated to meet the amino acid, calorie, and electrolyte requirements of a typical patient needing TPN. The hypertonic nature of TPN solutions requires that they be administered by means of a central venous catheter.

Intravenous fat solutions can be used as both a calorie source and a source of essential fatty acids. They are incompatible with TPN solutions and must be infused separately.

COMMONLY USED DIAGNOSTIC AGENTS

The names and purposes of the agents commonly used in diagnostic procedures are presented in Table 77-4.

Before using an agent in a test procedure, the practitioner should read and be familiar with the information contained in the package insert. Although commonly used, few of these diagnostic agents are without adverse effects, some of which may be serious. In particular, contrast media that contain organic iodine may produce serious adverse effects or even fatal anaphylactic reactions. Individuals with a history of allergy are more likely to have adverse reactions or exaggerated reactions to these compounds. Thyroid function tests may be affected by these agents for several months.

TABLE 77-3C. Nutrient Solutions—Compounded TPN Solutions*

	Na^+	K^+	Ca^{++}	Mg^{++}	Cl^-	Phosphate	Acetate	Copper	Zinc
	← *mEq/liter*				→	*mmol/liter*	*mEq/liter*	*mg/liter*	*mg/liter*
Standard adult formulation	35	30	5	10	35	9.7	39	1	2
Ingredients									
Crystalline amino acids 2.25%									
Dextrose (variable) 10–30%									
Electrolytes/minerals									

	Amino Acid/Dextrose Concentration				
Available Calories per Liter	***2.25%/10%***	***2.25%/15%***	***2.25%/20%***	***2.25%/25%***	***2.25%/30%***
Dextrose	340	510	680	850	1020
Amino acids	90	90	90	90	90
Total	430	600	770	940	1110
Nonprotein calorie to nitrogen ratio	94	142	189	236	283

	Na^+	K^+	Ca^{++}	Mg^{++}	Cl^-	Phosphate	Acetate	Copper	Zinc
	← *mEq/liter*				→	*mmol/liter*	*mEq/liter*	*mg/liter*	*mg/liter*
Standard pediatric formulation	30	25	10	10	30	7.4	3.5	1	2
Ingredients									
Crystalline amino acids 2.0%									
Dextrose (variable) 10–30%									
Electrolytes/minerals									

	Amino Acid/Dextrose Concentration				
Available Calories per Liter	***2.0%/10%***	***2.0%/15%***	***2.0%/20%***	***2.0%/25%***	***2.0%/30%***
Dextrose	340	510	680	850	1020
Amino acids	80	80	80	80	80
Total	420	590	760	930	1100
Nonprotein calorie to nitrogen ratio	106	159	212	266	319

	Na^+	K^+	Ca^{++}	Mg^{++}	Cl^-	Phosphate	Acetate	Copper	Zinc
	← *mEq/liter*				→	*mmol/liter*	*mEq/liter*	*mg/liter*	*mg/liter*
Standard neonatal base formulation*	0	0	0	2	8	0	13	1	2
* Requires additional electrolytes									
Sodium 3 mEq/kg/day									
Potassium 2.4 mEq/kg/day									
Calcium 200–600 mg/kg/day									
Phosphate 45–60 mg/kg/day (1.4–1.9 mmol/kg/day)									
Ingredients									
Crystalline amino acids 2.0%									
Dextrose 11.0%									

Available Calories per Liter	**Amino Acid/Dextrose Concentration: 2%/30%**
Dextrose	374
Amino acids	80
Total	454
Nonprotein calorie to nitrogen ratio	117

* Vitamins should be added to one bottle of TPN each day.

TABLE 77-4. Commonly Used Diagnostic Agents

Diagnostic Use	Generic Drug Name	Common Name	Route of Administration
Blood contents			
for glucose		Dextrostix	*in vitro* test
Cardiovascular function			
	Indocyanine green	Cardio-Green	i.v.
Endocrine function			
for pituitary function	L-Arginine	R-Gene 10	i.v.
	Metyrapone	Metopirone	oral, i.v.
for thyroid function	Protirelin	TRH, Thypinone	i.v.
	Thyrotropin	Thytropar	i.m.
for adrenal function	Corticotropin	ACTH, Acthar	i.v.
	Cosyntropin	Cortrosyn	i.v.
for pancreatic function	Tolbutamide sodium	Orinase	i.v.
Fecal contents			
for blood		Hematest, Hemoccult	*in vitro* test
Gastrointestinal function			
	Betazole hydrochloride	Histalog	s.c.
	D-Xylose		oral
	Histamine phosphate		s.c.
	Pentagastrin	Peptavlon	s.c.
	Sincalide	Cholecystokinin, Kinevac	i.v.
	Secretin	Secretin-Boots	i.v.
Hepatic function			
	Indocyanine green	Cardio-Green	i.v.
	Sulfobromophthalein	BSP, Bromsulphalein	i.v.
Kidney function			
	Aminohippurate sodium		i.v.
	Indigotin disulfonate sodium		i.v.
	Inulin		i.v.
	Mannitol		i.v.
	Phenolsulfonphthalein	Phenol Red	i.v.
Radiographic Contrast			
for body cavities	Iodized oil	Lipiodol	intrathecal intratracheal
	Iophendylate	Pantopaque	intrathecal
	Metrizamide	Amipaque	intrathecal
for gastrointestinal tract	Barium sulfate		oral, rectal
	Diatrizoate meglumine	Gastrographin	oral, rectal
	Diatrizoate sodium	Hypaque Sodium	oral, rectal
for gallbladder and bile ducts	Iodipamide meglumine	Chlorographin Meglumine	i.v.
	Iodipamide sodium	Cholographin Sodium	i.v.
	Iopanoic acid	Telepaque	oral
	Ipodate calcium	Oragrafin-Calcium	oral
	Ipodate sodium	Oragrafin-Sodium	oral
for pyelography and angiography	Diatrizoate meglumine	Renographin	i.v.
	Diatrizoate sodium	Hypaque sodium	i.v.
	Iothalamate meglumine	Conray	i.v.
	Iothalamate sodium	Angio-Conray	i.v.
	Methiodal sodium	Skiodan Sodium	i.v.
Urine contents			
for acetone		Acetest, Ketostix	*in vitro* test
for albumin		Albustix, Bumintest	*in vitro* test
for bilirubin		Ictotest	*in vitro* test
for blood		Hemastix	*in vitro* test
for glucose		Clinitest, Tes-Tape	*in vitro* test
Miscellaneous			
for infectious mononucleosis		Monospot	*in vitro* test
for penicillin sensitivity	Benzylpenicilloyl–polylysine	Pre-Pen	scratch, intradermal
for pregnancy		Gravindex, Pregnosis	*in vitro* test

78

RAYBURN B. VRABEL

Prolonged-Action Dosage Forms

The pharmacologic effect of a drug is based on its interaction with a site within the body to produce a particular response. This pharmacologic response is the last in a long series of steps involving the delivery of medication to its specific site of action within the body. Several steps precede this interaction: [1] delivery of the medication to the body via some type of dosage form; [2] release of the drug from the dosage form; [3] dissolution of the drug into body fluids; [4] penetration of the drug across cell walls or barriers; and [5] transport to its site of action. The composition of the drug dosage form can significantly affect the first few steps in this series of processes.

There are a variety of possible types of dosage forms in which a drug can be formulated.

1. Topical creams, ointments, or solutions
2. Oral tablets, capsules, or solutions
3. Aerosols for inhalation
4. Injectable solutions or suspensions
5. Rectal suppositories

Each of these has a profound effect on the extent to which a drug exerts its pharmacologic effect.

TOPICAL PREPARATIONS

The incorporation of drugs into topical preparations is done primarily to limit their effects to a particular external site of action. The type of ointment base can have a profound effect. Ointment bases such as petroleum jelly remain in contact with the applied area of the body for a greater time and tend to hydrate the skin. This process allows a greater penetration into the skin. Cream bases provide a less occlusive barrier, although they are much more appealing to patients, a factor that may affect compliance. Certain drugs when applied topically exert a significant systemic effect. When nitroglycerin is applied topically in an ointment formulation, a systemic vasodilatory response is produced (*see* Chap. 35). Like the sublingual route, this route avoids the primary effect of the liver on this drug's metabolism.

ORAL PREPARATIONS

The oral route is the most common route of drug administration. Among the various forms administered by this route, solutions most consistently assure the best absorption, primarily because the drug is already in solution and therefore ready for transport across the gastrointestinal tract membranes into the blood stream. When formulated into a tablet or capsule preparation, the drug's availability for absorption into the body may be affected. In the process of making a tablet or capsule, the drug is mixed with pharmacologically inert ingredients (excipients) designed to facilitate the process of manufacturing. These ingredients may interact with the drug, delaying or preventing absorption, or they may be formulated together improperly in such a way that the dosage form does not break apart (disintegrate) when it enters the gastrointestinal tract. This effect on the absorption is said to affect the *bioavailability* of the drug. For this reason the same drug dosage form manufactured by two different companies can produce quantitatively different pharmacologic effects.

Manufacturers may also intentionally mix the ingredients of a tablet in such a way as to affect the drug's bioavailability. This is often done in an effort to prolong the release of the drug, thereby prolonging its duration of effect in the body. By placing the drug in a waxy matrix, or by coating it, the time for absorption will be prolonged. The coating can be placed around whole tablets, as in the case of enteric-coated tablets, which are designed to be released only in the alkaline contents of the small intestine; or around particles of the drug, producing small pellets which are then filled into capsules. These "sustained-release" or "delayed-action" dosage forms are convenient since they allow the drug to be given less frequently.

AEROSOL PREPARATIONS

Aerosol preparations are similar to topical preparations to the extent that the medication is supplied directly to the tissue—in this case, the lung where an effect is desired. The primary problem is teaching patients to properly use the device delivering the medication, so that the maximum amount is inhaled deeply into the lungs.

INJECTABLE PREPARATIONS

Intravenous solutions provide the most effective means of delivering a drug to tissues of the body. If properly prepared and administered, all of the dose will be delivered to the patient. The problems with this route are related to these desirable properties. If the drug is injected too rapidly, the drug may exert its pharmacologic effect on certain nonprimary target organ-systems, producing undesirable effects. The local concentration of the drug close to the site of administration may affect the recipient's veins. Some drugs may be safely administered undiluted, whereas others must be diluted, or else local toxicity (*e.g.*, thrombophlebitis) may be produced.

Intramuscular injections suffer many of the same problems as oral tablet formulations. Those administered as suspensions must be dissolved into body fluids before absorption. Certain solutions administered intramuscularly will precipitate out in body fluids and therefore functionally resemble i.m. suspensions in their absorption characteristics. For these reasons, the i.m. route often produces lower, more delayed blood levels than do equivalent intravenously administered doses.

RECTAL PREPARATIONS

The rectal route, although more extensively used in Europe, is less popular elsewhere, primarily because of patient preference. It also offers a variable degree of absorption. This route is particularly affected by the release of medication from the dosage form. In addition, the proper insertion, retention, and blood flow to the area also affect the absorption of the drug into the systemic circulation.

CONCLUSION

The dosage form and route of administration can have a profound effect on the ability of a medication to reach effective concentrations in the body. The same drug administered by two different routes may exert different effects; likewise the same drug dosage form from two different manufacturers may produce markedly different patient responses. Therefore, when considering the pharmacology of a drug, one must take into account the variables associated with the drug delivery system. These dosage formulation factors may be the deciding factor in determining whether a pharmacologic effect will be seen and a therapeutic action observed.

79

DENIS O. RODGERSON

Therapeutic Drug Monitoring

The relation between the activity of a drug and its concentration in plasma was first explored by Marshall for the sulfonamides in 1940. The concept was expanded by Shannon for antimalarial drugs during World War II but did not achieve widespread acceptance until the 1970s, when interest increased rapidly primarily because of the work of Brodie. The primary goal of therapeutic drug monitoring is to assist in the rational, safe, and efficacious use of drugs. Together with pharmacokinetic techniques (*see* Chap. 5), therapeutic drug monitoring has formed a basis for designing and adjusting dosage regimens for drugs with low therapeutic indices or ambiguous clinical manifestations. Before therapeutic drug monitoring, it was, and still largely is, common medical practice to regulate drug dosage by some empirical end-point, such as the onset of nausea or other sign of toxicity. Since the action of most drugs is far removed from the quantitatable variable—the drug dose—not surprisingly there is frequently a poor correlation between the amount of drug administered and the clinical effect produced.

The recent development of many accurate, convenient, and relatively inexpensive methods for quantitating drugs has allowed the correlation of serum levels with therapeutic effects for an increasing number of drugs. These techniques show that there are optimal serum concentration ranges within which therapeutic effects can be expected in most patients receiving a particular drug. Should the serum concentration of the drug exceed the optimal therapeutic range, side-effects or toxicity can be expected in most patients. Conversely, if serum concentrations remain below the optimal therapeutic range, the desired drug effect will not be achieved for most patients. Thus the monitoring of serum drug concentrations aids in evaluating therapeutic failures to standard drug doses.

Not all drugs show a positive relation between therapeutic and toxic effects and their serum concentration. This lack of correlation may, in many cases, be due to the production of

---

BERNARD BERYL BRODIE, 1909– . British-born biochemist, living in United States. In 1944 developed a method for the determination of salicylic acid in plasma. Worked especially on drug metabolism and action mechanisms, biologic evolution, and control systems.

an irreversible reaction with receptors or other macromolecules, such that the drug effect persists beyond the time required to eliminate it and its metabolites.

Therapeutic drug monitoring can be used effectively in evaluating patient noncompliance (*see* Chap. 11), altered bioavailability (*see* Chap. 11), pharmacogenetic defects (*see* Chap. 6), variations in pharmacokinetics owing to disease (*see* Chap. 3), other drugs (*see* Chap. 8), age (*see* Chaps. 7, 11), or physiological status (*see* Chap. 11).

SERUM LEVELS OF DRUGS

Not all drugs are amenable to therapeutic monitoring. For example, drugs that act in an irreversible manner, or nonequilibrium, by binding to receptors or macromolecules cannot be evaluated, since a necessary requirement is that the drug should be in equilibrium among receptors, the extracellular water, and plasma water. Further, even among those drugs that meet the above pharmacologic and physicochemical criteria, there are only a small number for which therapeutic drug monitoring has been established as useful (Table 79-1).

Therapeutic drug monitoring is usually performed on serum. Plasma is equivalent for most assays, but the presence of anticoagulants may interfere in some assays. Whole blood is not a useful specimen in which to measure drugs because of interference by cellular components.

Most assays in common use measure the total quantity of drug in serum and do not differentiate between drug bound to proteins and free drug. Free drug quantitation may be performed for many agents by measuring their concentration in cerebrospinal fluid or saliva, where levels follow closely the concentration of free drug in plasma. Thus this sample type would be of considerable use were it not for the inappropriateness of obtaining cerebrospinal fluid routinely for the purpose of drug monitoring. Generally, the concentration of a drug in saliva is proportional to the concentration of free drug in plasma. This proportionality may, however, be distorted by variations in salivary *p*H, the active secretion of some drugs into saliva, and the binding of drugs to salivary protein.

The monitoring of free drug concentrations has not yet been established in terms of methodology or therapeutic ranges, but much progress is being made. As improvement in techniques such as ultrafiltration are achieved, free drug monitoring may increase significantly and provide important information on

TABLE 79-1. Optimal Therapeutic Drug Concentrations in Serum

Drug	Optimal Serum Concentration Range	Serum Concentration above Which Side-Effects Commonly Occur
N-Acetylprocainamide (NAPA) + procainamide	10–30 μg/ml	—
Carbamazepine	6–10 μg/ml	>15 μg/ml
Digitoxin	10–30 ng/ml	>35 ng/ml
Digoxin	0.5–2.0 ng/ml	>2.0 ng/ml
Ethosuximide	40–100 μg/ml	>100 μg/ml
Gentamicin	3–8 μg/ml	>10 μg/ml
Lidocaine	1.4–6.0 μg/ml	>9 μg/ml
Lithium	0.5–1.6 mEq/liter	>1.6 mEq/liter
Nortriptyline	50–170 ng/ml	>200 ng/ml
Phenobarbital	15–30 μg/ml	>35 μg/ml
Phenytoin	10–20 μg/ml	>25 μg/ml
Primidone	5–12 μg/ml	>15 μg/ml
Procainamide	5–10 μg/ml	10–12 μg/ml
Propranolol	40–85 ng/ml	Variable
Quinidine	2.5–5.0 μg/ml	>6.0 μg/ml
Salicylate	200–300 μg/ml	>300 μg/ml
Theophylline	5–20 μg/ml	>20 μg/ml
Valproate	50–100 μg/ml	>200 μg/ml

(Adapted from Kalman SM, Clark DR: Drug Assay: The Strategy of Therapeutic Drug Monitoring. New York, Masson Publishing, USA, 1979).

many of the interindividual variables of drug dosage, interactions, and metabolism.

ANTICONVULSANTS

Current anticonvulsant drugs are highly effective in the clinical management of epileptic patients, and monitoring serum drug levels has greatly improved seizure control and, in many patients, eliminated the requirement for multiple therapy.

PHENYTOIN

Phenytoin may be easily measured in serum since therapeutic concentrations are relatively high. The drug has a narrow therapeutic range (10–20 μg/ml) and shows considerable interpatient variation in serum levels for a given dose. Therefore, individualization of dosage is important. In addition, phenytoin exhibits saturation or zero-order kinetics near the upper limits of the therapeutic range, resulting in marked elevations of serum concentration for very small dosage increments.

Phenytoin is highly bound to plasma proteins, with slightly less than 10% of the drug in the free form. The time to achieve a steady-state is extremely variable: It is never less than 1 week but may be as long as 5 weeks. Blood samples for phenytoin should be drawn immediately before the next dose, representing the lowest or trough level of the drug.

PRIMADONE AND PHENOBARBITAL

Although a therapeutic range for serum levels of primadone is listed in Table 79-1, it may have no validity because it has not yet been established unequivocally that primadone itself has a therapeutic effect in humans. The primary therapeutic benefit of primadone may reside in its metabolites, phenobarbital and phenylethylmalonamide (PEMA). Many believe that the measurement of the derived phenobarbital provides the best basis for the individualizing of dosage. The time to steady-state for primadone is 50 to 60 hours. Blood samples should be drawn immediately before the next dose.

Phenobarbital is partially metabolized in the liver and partially excreted unchanged in the urine. It is less than 50% bound to plasma proteins, and therefore less susceptible to binding interactions than are more highly protein-bound drugs (*see* Chap. 8). The therapeutic range listed in Table 79-1 must be used only as a guide, since many patients have levels in excess of this range without toxic effects, presumably because of the development of tolerance (*see* Chap. 26). The time to steady-state for phenobarbital is 11 to 25 days in adults. Blood samples should be drawn immediately before the next dose.

SODIUM VALPROATE

It has not yet been established if valproate or one or more of its metabolites are responsible for its anticonvulsant properties. The correlation between therapeutic dose and serum concentration is poor, with considerable intersubject variation. The drug is rapidly absorbed, and steady-state is achieved within 2.5 days. Valproate is about 90% bound to plasma proteins. Reports conflict about its interactions with other anticonvulsant drugs; for example, it may displace phenytoin from its binding sites (*see* Chap. 8). Serum for valproate measurements should be obtained immediately before the next oral dose.

ETHOSUXIMIDE

Ethosuximide is rapidly and completely absorbed, with a time to steady-state of 6 to 10 days for children. It is not protein bound, and serum levels should be measured on samples drawn immediately before the next dose.

CARBAMAZEPINE

Carbamazepine is slowly absorbed, and serum concentrations do not relate well to dose, especially in patients who receive several anticonvulsants. Carbamazepine is metabolized to carbamazepine-10,11-epoxide, which may have some anticonvulsant activity. Carbamazepine is 75% protein bound, and carbamazepine-10,11-epoxide is only 50% protein bound, so that the metabolite, which can show concentrations of about half that of the parent drug, may be a very important factor in the therapeutic effect. Both the parent drug and its metabolite can be measured, although this is not commonly done. Steady-state plasma levels of carbamazepine are reached in 2 to 6 days. As with other anticonvulsants, samples for the measurement of serum carbamazepine levels are usually drawn immediately before the next dose. However, because of variability of absorption, this measurement may not reflect the lowest drug level achieved during the interval between doses. Further, carbamazepine induces its own metabolism (*see* Chap. 8) so that steady-state serum concentration falls gradually during the first 2 to 4 weeks of treatment.

ANTIARRHYTHMICS

QUINIDINE

Quinidine is metabolized to several hydroxylated derivatives, of which at least one, 3-hydroxyquinidine, has antiarrhythmic activity (*see* Chap. 34). In addition, dihydroquinidine, which is present in most formulations of the drug as a minor contaminant, is probably active in humans. Because of these factors, serum levels of quinidine must be interpreted carefully because some methods vary in their specificity with respect to dihydroquinidine and the quinidine metabolites. Therefore, definition of a therapeutic range depends on the assay used. The figures given in Table 79-1 are for quinidine-specific methods such as high-pressure liquid chromatography. Quinidine is highly protein bound and is subject to increased metabolism when administered with phenobarbital, phenytoin, warfarin-type anticoagulants, or other enzyme-inducing agents. The time to steady-state for quinidine is 20 to 35 hours. Blood samples should be obtained immediately before the next dose.

PROCAINAMIDE

Procainamide is metabolized to N-acetylprocainamide (NAPA), which has antiarrhythmic activity equal to that of the parent drug (*see* Chap. 34). The rate of metabolism depends on acetylator status (*see* Chap. 65). In rapid acetylators the serum levels of NAPA will be greater than those of procainamide, whereas in slow acetylators the ratio will be reversed. Therefore, for effective monitoring of therapy, both procainamide and NAPA levels must be measured. Procainamide is approximately 15% protein bound, and about half of an oral dose is excreted in the urine. The time to steady-state is 11 to 20 hours, with significant prolongation in patients with renal disease. Three blood samples should be drawn within one oral dosing interval—one at the time of administration and two more at equal intervals—for the measurement of procainamide and NAPA. With i.v. therapy, samples should be drawn immediately after the loading dose and thereafter at 2, 6 to 12, and 24 hours after the start of maintenance infusion.

LIDOCAINE

Lidocaine has a low therapeutic index with significant and often serious toxicity (*see* Chap. 20). It is eliminated by hepatic metabolism with one metabolite, monoethylglycine xylidide (MEGX), having antiarrhythmic properties and a second metabolite glycine xylidide (GX) potentiating the conductive convulsive effects of the parent drug and MEGX. Since lidocaine so depends on hepatic metabolism, patients with congestive heart failure or hepatocellular disease will have reduced drug clearance and may rapidly accumulate toxic levels. Lidocaine is between 60% and 70% protein bound. With continuous infusion, steady-state concentrations are usually reached after 6 to 9 hours in patients with acute myocardial infarction. However, in these patients serum lidocaine levels may continue to rise for more than 24 to 48 hours because of decreased hepatic metabolism. Blood samples should be taken 12 hours after the start of i.v. therapy and every 24 hours thereafter, or more frequently when toxicity is suspected.

PROPRANOLOL

Propranolol is extensively metabolized, and the principal one, 4-hydroxypropranolol, shares the activity of the parent drug (*see* Chap. 18). Propranolol is more than 20% bound to plasma proteins, and the time to steady-state is 10 to 30 hours for oral doses; the wide variation is due to the interindividual differences in hepatic metabolism, since the drug is subject to first-pass metabolism (*see* Chap. 4). Careful regulation of the dose along with measurement of serum concentrations can decrease the incidence of therapeutic failure. Blood samples should be drawn immediately before the next oral dose.

DIGOXIN

Considerable controversy surrounds the therapeutic value of serum digoxin concentrations. Most studies show that digoxin levels of greater than 2 ng/ml are found in patients who exhibit signs of toxicity. However, some patients with toxicity have serum digoxin levels below 2 ng/ml (the usually accepted upper limit of the therapeutic range). Similarly, in the presence of supraventricular arrhythmias, some patients require higher than usual doses of digoxin to control their cardiac rate, and such patients may have serum drug levels much greater than 2 ng/ml without signs of toxicity. This overlap between the toxic and therapeutic ranges has led some workers to conclude that serum digoxin levels are of limited usefulness. Digoxin is eliminated primarily unchanged in the urine, with only about 10% of an oral dose being metabolized. For patients with normal renal function, the time to steady-state is about 7 days. However, when renal function is compromised, steady-state may not be achieved for as long as 3 weeks. Blood samples for serum digoxin levels should be drawn at least 6 hours and preferably 8 to 12 hours after the last oral dose. Plateau levels of the drug occur 10 to 12 hours after i.m. administration, and 2 to 4 hours after i.v. injections. Serum levels must be measured in the plateau phase after i.m. or i.v. digoxin administration.

THEOPHYLLINE

The clinical efficacy and toxicity of theophylline are directly related to the serum concentration. In adults theophylline is metabolized to inactive compounds, and in neonates some of the drug is converted to caffeine, a pharmacologically active metabolite. Many of the older methods used for the quantitation of theophylline are subject to considerable nonspecificity, particularly suffering from interference by other xanthines such as theophylline metabolites, caffeine, and theobromine. In newer methods such as the homogeneous enzyme immunoassay, such interference, although considerably reduced, has not been eliminated completely. Only in chromatographic procedures can complete specificity be achieved. However, the homogeneous enzyme immunoassay has been shown to be particularly beneficial in the correlation of serum levels with therapeutic effects. The time to steady-state for oral theophylline is about 2 days in adults and 1 to 2 days in children. This time is significantly shorter in cigarette smokers and longer in patients with ventricular failure, acute pulmonary edema, chronic obstructive pulmonary disease, and liver dysfunction. Blood for serum theophylline levels should be drawn immediately before the next oral dose. When i.v. infusions are used, the therapeutic effect will not be achieved in less than 2 hours. Therefore, blood samples should be obtained 4 to 8 hours after the start of the i.v. infusion and repeated thereafter as necessary.

FURTHER READING

1. Baselt RC: Analytical Procedures for Therapeutic Drug Monitoring and Emergency Toxicology. Davis, California, Biomedical Publications, 1980
2. Evans WE, Schentag JJ, Jusko W: Applied Pharmacokineties: Principles of Therapeutic Drug Monitoring. San Francisco, Applied Therapeutics, 1980
3. Kalman SW, Clark DR: Drug Assay: The Strategy of Therapeutic Drug Monitoring. New York, Masson Publishing USA, 1979
4. Morselli P: Drug Disposition During Development: An Overview. New York, Spectrum Publications, 1977
5. Pippenger CD, Penry JK, Kuti H: Antiepileptic Drugs: Quantitative Analysis and Interpretation. New York, Raven Press, 1978
6. Wagner JG: Fundamentals of Clinical Pharmacokinetics. Hamilton, Illinois, Drug Intelligence Publications, 1975

JEREMY H. THOMPSON

80

Pharmaceutical Interactions and Incompatibilities

Pharmaceutical interactions occur when drugs are carelessly or inappropriately mixed *in vitro* in infusion bottles or syringes, or when they adsorb onto glass or plastic containers (Table 80-1). A related problem not discussed here is properly storing drugs from extremes of temperature and humidity and from exposure to sunlight or other potentially deleterious environmental conditions.

The term "incompatibility" comes from the Latin *in* (not) and *compactilis* (to join together). *Physical incompatibility* occurs if the physical state of the individual drugs in a mixture changes when the drugs are blended. Amphotericin B, for example precipitates if it is mixed with normal saline instead of 5% dextrose (*see* Chap. 69). *Chemical incompatibility* occurs when components of a drug mixture interact chemically. For example, i.v. methicillin should not be given in acidic solutions since the antibiotic is destroyed at an acid *p*H. In many instances there is observable evidence of incompatibility, such as color change, gas evolution, or formed precipitate. However, a reduced therapeutic potency may occur *without any observable signs*. While obvious evidence of incompatibility does not imply total loss of therapeutic potency, drug mixtures showing evidence of interactions should not be used. Our knowledge of physical and chemical drug incompatibilities *is* limited, and Table 80-1 represents only a partial list. Realistically, *data on compatibility of most mixtures of specific agents are not known*.

FURTHER READING

1. Hansen PD: Drug Interactions, 4th ed. Philadelphia, Lea & Febiger, 1979.
2. Trissel LA: Handbook on Injectable Drugs, 2nd ed. Washington, DC, American Society of Hospital Pharmacists, 1980

TABLE 80-1. Some Important Physical and Chemical Drug Incompatibilities

	Aminophylline	Ammonium chloride	Amobarbital sodium	Ascorbic acid	Benzyl alcohol	Calcium chloride	Calcium gluconate-glucoheptonate	Chloromycetin succinate #	Chlorpheniramine maleate	Chlortetracycline HCl	Chlorothiazide Na (Diuril Sodium)	Corticotrophin aqueous	Dextran	Dextrose	Diphenhydramine HCl (Benadryl HCl)	Diphenylhydantoin (phenytoin) Na (Dilantin Na)	Ephedrine sulfate	Epinephrine HCl (Adrenalin HCl)	Erythromycin glucoheptonate #	Heparin sodium	Hyaluronidase (Wydase)	Hydrocortisone succinate	Hydroxyzine HCl (Vistaril HCl)	Insulin, aqueous	Kanamycin sulfate	Levarterenol bitartrate	Magnesium sulfate	Meperidine HCl (Demerol HCl)	Metaraminol bitartrate (Aramine)	Methicillin sodium	Narcotic salts +	Nitrofurantoin Na (Furadantin Na)	Novobiocin sodium	Oxytetracycline HCl (Terramycin HCl)	Penicillin G, K, or Na	Pentobarbital Na	Phenobarbital sodium	Procaine HCl	Prochlorperazine maleate (Compazine)	Promazine HCl (Sparine HCl)	Protein hydrolysate	Sodium bicarbonate	Sodium iodide	Streptomycin sulfate	Succinylcholine chloride	Sulfadiazine sodium	Sulfisoxazole diethanolamine (Gantrisin)	Tetracycline HCl	Thiopental Na (Pentothal Na)	Vancomycin HCl	Vitamin B-12	Vitamin B complex with ascorbic acid	Vitamin K_1	Warfarin Na (Panwarfin Na)
Aminophylline				I												I							I					I			I			I				I	I											I		I		
Ammonium chloride																															I																I							
Amobarbital sodium															I							I	I	I		I		I			I							I						I				I		I				
Benzyl alcohol								I																																														
Blood (whole)																										I			X																								X	
Calcium chloride									I	I																																												
Calcium gluconate																											I						I						I					I										
Chlorpheniramine maleate						I																				I										I																		
Chloromycetin succinate #					I											I			I				I										I	I					I									I		I				
Chlortetracycline (Aureomycin)						I				H			I																											*	I													
Corticotrophin aqueous																																	I									I												
Dexamethasone-21-phosphate																																							I											I				
Dextran				I						I																																											I	
Dextrose																									I								I																		I			I
Dihydromorphinone HCl																																										I							I					
Dimenhydrinate (Dramamine)	I	I	I													I				I		I	I													I	I		I										I					
Diphenylhydantoin (phenytoin) sodium	I							I							I				I				I	I	I	I		I	I		I			I	I	I	I	I	I					I			I	I		I		I	I	
Ephedrine sulfate																						I														I	I												I					
Epinephrine HCl (Adrenalin HCl)																					I												I																					*
Erythromycin glucoheptonate #								I								I				I													I			I	I							I				I						
Heparin sodium																			I		I	I	I		I			I			I		I						I					I				I		I				
Hyaluronidase (Wydase)																		I		I																																		
Hydrocortisone succinate			I														I			I					I				I	I			I	I		I	I		I									I		I		I		
Hydroxyzine HCl (Vistaril HCl)	I		I					I								I				I															I	I	I										I					I		
Insulin aqueous			I								I					I																I	I			I	I					I				I	I		I					
Kanamycin sulfate (Kantrex)														I		I				I		I															I										I							
Levarterenol bitartrate (Levophed Bitartrate)			I						I		I					I																I	I			I	I					I	I	I		I	I		I					
Lincomycin HCl (Lincocin)																I																			I																			
Magnesium sulfate							I																										I					I				I												
Methicillin sodium (Dimocillin)																						I						I	I		I								I			I								I				

Metaraminol bitartrate (Aramine)																I						I							X	I					I														*					*
Morphine sulfate	I		I								I					I				I								I		I		I	I				I					I	I			I	I		I					
Narcotic salts +	I	I	I								I					I				I										I		I	I			I	I					I	I			I	I		I					
Nitrofurantoin Na (Furadantin Na)																								I		I		I			I	J						I	I		I			I				*		I				
Novobiocin sodium (Albamycin)							I	I				I		I				I	I	I		I		I		I	I				I		A					I			I			I				I		I		I		
Oxytetracycline HCl (Terramycin)	I							I								I						I												B		I	I										I							
Penicillin G, K, or Na																I							I						I										I	*								I	*	I				
Pentobarbital sodium									I						I	I	I		I			I	I	I		I		I			I			I					I	*	I	I		I	I			I		I				
Phenobarbital sodium (Luminal Na)															I	I	I		I			I	I	I	I	I		I			I			I				I	I					I				I		I				
Phenylephrine HCl (Neo-Synephrine)																I																																						
Prednisolone-21-phosphate							I																																I															
Procaine HCl	I		I								I					I											I					I	I				I					I	I			I	I		I					
Prochlorperazine maleate	I						I	I			I					I				I		I								I		I			I	I	I										I		I			I		
Promazine HCl (Sparine)										*	I																								*	*						*					*		*					*
Promethazine HCl (Phenergan HCl)	I							I			I		I			I				I		I								I		I			I	I	I										I		I			I		
Secobarbital sodium (Second Na)															I	I	I		I			I		I		I					I							I						I				I		I				
Sodium bicarbonate												I												I		I	I	I		I	I					I		I		*		E		I				I	I	I		I		
Sodium cephalothin (Keflin)																I																			I				I															
Sodium iodide																										I		I			I							I																
Streptomycin sulfate			I				I				I					I			I	I						I						I	I			I	I					I				I	I							
Succinylcholine chloride																																				I													I					
Sulfadiazine sodium																								I		I		I			I							I						I		F		I		I				
Sulfisoxazole diethanolamine (Gantrisin)		I														I							I	I	I	I		I			I			I				I	I	*				I			G	I	*	I				
Tetracycline HCl (Achromycin HCl)			I					I			I					I			I	I		I										*	I		I	I	I					I				I	I		*					*
Thiopental sodium (Pentothal Na)															I		I							I		I		I	*		I				*			I	I	*	I	I			I		*	*	D					
Tripelennamine HCl (Pyribenzamine HCl)								I								I																					I																	
Vancomycin HCl (Vancocin)	I		I					I			I					I				I		I								I		I	I		I	I	I					I				I	I					I		
Vitamin B-12 (Rubramin)				I										I																																						I	I	*
Vitamin B Complex with C (Folbesyn)	I															I						I	I										I						I			I								I	I			
Vitamin K_1 (Aqua-Mephyton)				I									I			I																																			I			
Warfarin sodium (Panwarfin)														I				*											*											*								*			*			C

(Patel JA: A guide to physical compatibility of intravenous drug admixtures. Am J Hosp Pharm 23:409, 1966)

I *Incompatible*

* Incompatible in 5% dextrose injection

Dissolve first in water for injection

X Therapeutic dose must be diluted with large volume prior to infusion

A Incompatible in dextrose 5% injection, fructose, invert sugar, lactated Ringer's, sodium lactate, ammonium chloride

B Incompatible in lactated Ringer's, sodium lactate

C Incompatible in dextrose 5% injection, fructose, invert sugar, lactated Ringer's, ammonium chloride

D Incompatible in dextrose 10% with sodium chloride, lactated Ringer's

E Incompatible in lactated Ringer's, sodium lactate, Ringer's solution

F Incompatible in fructose, invert sugar, lactated Ringer's, sodium lactate, ammonium chloride

G Incompatible in ammonium chloride

H Incompatible in lactated Ringer's, ammonium chloride, Ringer's solution.

J Incompatible in lactated Ringer's, ammonium chloride

\+ Narcotic salts; codeine phosphate, Leritine HCl, Levo-Dromoran, Bitartrate, Methadone HCl

81

JEREMY H. THOMPSON

Drug-Induced Disease

No drug escapes the stigma of causing disease (*see* Chap. 11). This chapter contains tables of drugs that have been associated with specific pathology. Diagnostic difficulties abound, however, since in many cases the pathogenesis is not clear. The references contain a more detailed presentation of this information.

FURTHER READING

1. D'Arch PF, Griffin JP: Iatrogenic Disease. New York, Oxford Medical Publications, 1972
2. Martin EW: Hazards of Medications. Philadelphia, J B Lippincott, 1971
3. Meyler L: Side Effects of Drugs, 5th ed. Princeton, Excerpta Medica Foundation, 1980

TABLE 81-1. Drugs That May Produce an Alteration in Skin Pigmentation

ACTH	Gold salts
Arsenic	Lucanthone
Bismuth	Nitrofurantoin
Bromides	Phenolphthalein
Catecholamines	Phenytoin
Chloroquine	Potassium iodide
Chlorpromazine (the "Purple People")	Quinacrine
	Quinidine
Cytotoxic agents	Silver salts
Estrogen-containing oral contraceptives (stimulate melanocytes)	Sulfonamides
	Zinc oxide

TABLE 81-2. Drugs That May Produce an Exanthematic Rash

Aminoglycosides	Methaminodiazepoxide
Anticonvulsants	Nitrofurantoin
Anticholinergics	Organic extracts
Antihistamines (H_1 type)	Para-aminosalicylic acid
Atropine	Penicillins
Barbiturates	Phenothiazines
Bromides	Phenylbutazone
Chloral hydrate	Phenytoin
Chlordiazepoxide	Primidone
Chloroquine	Quinacrine
Chlorothiazide	Quinine
Chlorpromazine	Reserpine
Diethylstilbestrol	Salicylates
Erythromycin	Serums
Gold salts	Sulfonamides
Griseofulvin	Sulfones
Insulin	Tetracyclines
Meprobamate	Thiouracil
Mercurials	

TABLE 81-3. Drugs That May Produce Contact Dermatitis

Acriflavine	Menthol
Amethocaine	Meprobamate
Aminoglycosides	Mepyramine
Antazoline	Mercurials
Antihistamines (H_1 type)	Neomycin
Arsphenamine	Nitrofurazone
Bacitracin	Para-aminosalicylic acid
Benzocaine	Parabens
Benzoyl peroxide	Penicillins
Cetrimide	Peru balsam
Chloramphenicol	Phenindamine
Chlorcyclizine	Phenol
Chlorhexidine	Potassium hydroxyquinoline sulfate
Chlorhydroxyquinoline	Procaine
Chloroxylenol	Promethazine
Chlorphenesin	Propamidine
Chlorpromazine	Pyribenazmine
Crotamiton	Quinacrine
Cyclomethycaine	Quinine
Domiphen bromide	Resorcin
Ephedrine	Salicylates
Formaldehyde	Selenium sulfide
Gold salts	Sulfonamides
Halogenated phenolic compounds	Sulfur and salicylic acid ointment
Iodine and iodides	Tetracyclines
Iodochlorhydroxyquinoline	Thiamine
Isoniazid	Thimerosal
Lanolin	

TABLE 81-4. Drugs That May Produce an Acneiform Eruption

ACTH	Iodides
Androgenic hormones	Methandrostenolone
Barbiturates	Oral contraceptives
Bromides	Phenytoin
Glucocorticosteroids	Vitamin B_{12}

TABLE 81-5. Drugs That May Cause a Fixed Drug Eruption

Acetanilid	Meprobamate
Acetarsone	Mercury salts
Acetophenetidin	Methenamine
Acetylsalicylic acid	Neoarsphenamine
Acriflavine	Opium alkaloids
Aminoglycosides	Oxophenarsine
Aminopyrine	Oxytetracycline
Amobarbital	Para-aminosalicylic acid
Amodiaquine	Penicillins
Amphetamine sulfate	Phenacetin
Anthralin	Phenobarbital
Antimony potassium tartrate	Phenolphthalein
Antipyrine	Phenylbutazone
Arsphenamine	Phenytoin
Barbital	Potassium chlorate
Barbital sodium	Pyrimidine derivatives
Belladonna	Quinacrine
Bismuth salts	Quinidine
Bromides	Quinine
Chloral hydrate	Reserpine
Chloroguanide	Saccharin
Chloroquine	Salicylates
Chlorothiazide	Santonin
Chlorpromazine	Scopolamine
Chlortetracycline	Sodium salicylate
Cinchophen	Streptomycin
D-amphetamine	Strychnine
Diallybarbituric acid	Sulfadiazine
Diethylstibestrol	Sulfaguanidine
Digilanid	Sulfamerazine
Digitalis	Sulfamethazine
Dimenhydrinate	Sulfamethoxypyridazine
Diphenhydramine	Sulfapyridine
Disulfiram	Sulfarsphenamine
Ephedrine	Sulfathiazole
Epinephrine	Sulfisoxazole
Ergot alkaloids	Sulfobromophthalein sodium
Erythrosine	Tetracyclines
Eucalyptus oil	Thiambutosine
Formalin	Thonzylamine HCl
Frangula	Tripelennamine
Gold salts	Trisodium arsphenamine sulfate
Griseofulvin	Tryparsamide
Iodine	Vaccines and immunizing agents
Ipecac	
Karaya gum (Sterculia gum)	
Magnesium hydroxide	

TABLE 81-6. Drugs That May Cause Eczematous Dermatitis

Antibiotics	Mercurials
Antihistamines	PAS
Arsenicals	Penicillins
Bromides	Quinacrine
Chloral hydrate	Streptomycin
Iodides	Sulfonamides

TABLE 81-7. Drugs That May Cause Bullous Eruptions

Acetophenetidin	Gold salts
Aminoglycosides	Griseofulvin
Aminopyrine	Insulin
Antipyrine	Iodides
Arsenicals	Mercurial diuretics
Atropine	Penicillins
Barbiturates	Phenolphthalein
Bismuth	Phenothiazines
Bromides	Phenytoin
Chloral hydrate	Quinine
Cinchophen	Salicylates
Digitalis	Streptomycin
Diuretics	Sulfonamides
Ergot	

TABLE 81-8. Drugs That May Cause Photodermatitis

Acetohexamide	Cyclamates	Monoglycerol paraamino-benzoate	Rue
Acridine dyes	Demeclocycline	Mustards	Salicylanilides
Agave lechuguilla (amaryllis)	Desipramine	Nalidixic acid	Salicylates
Agrimony	Dibenzopyran derivatives	Naphthalene	Sandalwood oil (perfume)
9-Aminoacridine	Dicyanine-A	Nortiptyline	Silver salts
Aminobenzoic acid	Diethylstilbestrol	Oral contraceptives	Stilbamidine isethionate
Angelica	Digalloyl trioleate	Oxytetracycline	Substituted benzoic acids (sun screens)
Anthracene	Dill	Para-dimethylaminoazo-benzene	Sulfonamides
Arsenicals	Diphenhydramine hydrochloride	Paraphenylenediamine	Sulfonylureas
Barbiturates	Doxycycline	Perloline	Tetrachlorsalicylanilide
Bavachi (corylifolia)	Estrone	Perphenazine	Tetracyclines
Benzene	Fennel oil	Phenanthrene	Thiazide diuretics
Benzopyrine	Fentichlor	Phenazine dyes	Thiophenes
Bergamot (perfume)	Fluorescein dyes	Phenolic compounds	Thiopropazate dihydro-chloride
Bithionol	5-Fluorouracil	Phenothiazines	Tribromosalicylanilide
Blankophores (sulfa derivatives)	Glyceryl p-aminobenzoate	Phenoxazines	Trichloromethiazide
Bromchlorsalicylanilid	Gold salts	Phenylbutazone	Triethylene melamine
Bulosemide (Jadit)	Griseofulvin	Phenytoin	Triflupromazine hydro-chloride
4-Butyl-4-chlorosali-cylanilide	Hexachlorophene	Prochlorperazine	Trimeprazine tartrate
Carbamazepine	Imipramine	Promazine hydrochloride	Trimethadione
Carbinoxamine	Isothipendyl	Promethazine hydrochloride	Trypaflavine
Carbutamide	Lantinin	Protriptyline	Trypan blue
Cedar oil	Lavender oil	Psoralens	Vanillin oils
Chlordiazepoxide	Lime oil	Pyrathiazine hydrochloride	Water ash
Chlorpromazine	Meclothiazide	Pyridine	Xylene
Chlorpropamide	Mepazine	Quinethazone	Yarrow
Chlortetracycline	9-Mercaptopurine	Quinidine	
Citron oil	Methotrimeprazine	Quinine	
Coal tar	Methoxsalen	Reserpine	
	5-Methoxypsoralen	Rose bengal perfume	
	8-Methoxypsoralen		

TABLE 81-9. Drugs That May Cause Exfoliative Dermatitis

Acetazolamide	Mesantoin
Allopurinol	Methotrimeprazine
Aminoglycosides	Nitroglycerin
Antimony compounds	PAS
Arsenicals	Penicillins
Barbiturates	Phenacetamide
Bismuth	Phenindione
Carbamazepine	Phenothiazines
Chloroquine	Phenylbutazone
Demeclocycline	Phenytoin
Furosemide	Quinacrine
Gold salts	Quinidine
Griseofulvin	Streptomycin
Hydroflumethiazide	Sulfonamides
Iodides	Sulfonylureas
Isorbide	Tetracyclines
Measles virus vaccine	Thiazide diuretics
Mercurials	Vitamin A

TABLE 81-10. Drugs That May Cause Erythema Nodosum-like Lesions

Bromides	Salicylates
Iodides	Sulfonamides
PAS	
Penicillins	

TABLE 81-11. Drugs That May Cause Stevens–Johnson Syndrome

Antipyrine	Phenytoin
Arsenicals	Quinine
Barbiturates	Salicylates
Belladonna	Smallpox vaccine
Carbamazepine	Sulfadimethoxine
Chloramphenicol	Sulfamethoxypyridazine
Chlorpropamide	Sulfisomidine
Codeine	Tetracyclines
Hydralazine	Thiacetazone
Measles vaccine	Thiazides diuretics
Mercurial diuretics	Thiouracil
Paramethadione	Trimethadione
Penicillins	Triple sulfonamides
Phenolphthalein	(sulfadiazine,
Phensuximide	sulfamethazine,
Phenylbutazone	sulfamerazine)

TABLE 8-12. Drugs That May Cause Erythema Multiforme-like Lesions

Acetophenetidin	Iodides
Aminoglycosides	Meprobamate
Aminopyrine	PAS
Antihistamines (H_1 type)	Penicillins
Antipyrine	Phenolphthalein
Arsenicals	Phenothiazines
Barbiturates	Phenylbutazone
Bismuth	Phenytoin
Bromides	Salicylates
Chloramphenicol	Streptomycin
Cinchophen	Sulfonamides
Erythromycin	Sulfonylureas
Gold salts	Thiazide diuretics

TABLE 81-13. Drugs That May Cause Toxic Epidermal Necrolysis

Acetazolamide	Neomycin sulfate
Allopurinol	Nitrofurantoin
Aminopyrine	Opium powder
Antihistamines (H_1 type)	Penicillins
Antipyrine	Phenolphthalein
Barbiturates	Phenylbutazone
Brompheniramine	Phenytoin
Chenopodium oil	Polio vaccine
Ethylmorphine HCl	Sulfonamides
Gold salts	Sulfones
Ipecac	Tetanus antitoxin
Isoniazid	Tetracyclines
Methyl salicylate	Tolbutamide

TABLE 81-14. Drugs That May Produce Lupus Erythematosus

Aminosalicylic acid	Paramethadione
Barbiturates (long term?)	Penicillamine
Chlorpromazine	Penicillins
Chlortetracycline	Phenothiazines
Digitalis (long term)	Phenylbutazone
Ethosuximide	Phenytoin
Gold compounds (long term)	Primidone
Griseofulvin	Procainamide
Hydralazine	Propranolol
Isoniazid	Propylthiouracil
Mephenytoin	Quinidine
Methsuximide	Reserpine (long term)
Methyldopa	Streptomycin
Methylthiouracil	Sulfadimethoxine
Oral contraceptives	Sulfamethoxypyridazine
(mestranol?)	Tetracycline (degraded)
Oxyphenisatin	Thiazides (long term)
Para-aminosalicylic acid	Trimethadione

TABLE 81-15. Drugs That May Cause "Collagen" Disease

Busulfan	Penicillins
Chloramphenicol	Phenylbutazone
Chlortetracycline	Phenytoin
Iodides	Pyromen
Iproniazid	Sulfonamides
Mercurial diuretics	Thiouracil

TABLE 81-16. Drugs That May Induce Acute Porphyria (A) or Cutaneous Porphyria (C) in Humans

Aminopyrine	A
Androgens	A, C
Barbiturates	A, C
Chlordiazepoxide	A
Chloroquine	C
Estrogens	A, C
Ethyl alcohol	C
Griseofulvin	A
Hexachlorobenzene	C
Meprobamate	A
Oral contraceptives	A, C
Phenytoin	A
Sulfonamides	A
Sulfonylureas	A, C

TABLE 81-17. Drugs That May Produce Purpura

Acetophenetidin	Fluoxymesterone
ACTH	Gold salts
Allopurinol	Griseofulvin
Anticoagulants	Heparin
Antihistamines (H_1 type)	Insulin
Antipyrine	Iodides
Arsenicals	Isoniazid
Arsenobenzols	Mepesulfate
Barbiturates	Meprobamate
Bismuth	Nirvanol
Bromides	PAS
Carbamides	Penicillins
Cephalosporins	Phenothiazines
Chloral hydrate	Phenylbutazone
Chloramphenicol	Phenytoin
Chlorothiazide	Quinidine
Chlorpromazine	Quinine
Chlorpropamide	Salicylates
Cinchophen	Sulfonamides
Corticosteroids	Thiazide diuretics
Digitalis	Thiouracils
Digitoxin	Trifluoperazine
Ergot	

TABLE 81-18. Drugs That May Cause Urticaria

ACTH	Mercurials
Aminoglycosides	Nitrofurantoin
Barbiturates	Opiates
Bromides	Penicillinase
Chloramphenicol	Penicillins
Dextran	Phenolphthalein
Enzymes	Phenothiazines
Erythromycin	Phenytoin
Glutethimide	Propoxyphene
Griseofulvin	Salicylates
Insulin	Sera
Iodides	Streptomycin
Iodopyracet	Sulfonamides
Liver extracts	Tetracyclines
Meperidine	Thiouracil
Meprobamate	

TABLE 81-19. Drugs That May Cause Lichenoid and Lichen Planuslike Reactions

Amiphenazole	Propylthiouracil
Chloroquine	Quinacrine
Gold salts	Quinidine
Organic arsenicals	Thiazide diuretics
PAS	

TABLE 81-20. Drugs That May Cause Alopecia

Allopurinol	Methotrexate
α-methyl dopa	Norethindrone acetate
Amphetamine	Oral contraceptives
Anticoagulants	Phenytoin
Arsenic	Propylthiouracil
Aspirin	Quinacrine
Clofibrate	Selenium sulfide
Cyclophosphamide	Sodium warfarin
5-Fluorouracil	Thallium
Gentamicin	Trimethadione
Gold salts	Triparanol
Heparin	Uracil mustard
Iodine	Vinblastine
Mepesulfate	Vincristine
Mephenytoin	Vitamin A
Methimazole	

TABLE 81-21. Drugs That May Cause Gynecomastia

Adrenocortical hormones	Heroin
Androgens	Isoniazid
Busulfan	Methyldopa
Chlortetracycline	Methyltestosterone
Cimetidine	Oral contraceptives
Diethylstilbestrol	Phenaglycodol
Digitalis	Phenelzine
Digitoxin	Phenothiazines
Estrogens	Reserpine
Ethionamide	Spironolactone
Griseofulvin	Vincristine
Haloperidol	Vitamin D_2
HCG (human chorionic gonadotropin)	

TABLE 81-22. Drugs That May Produce Serum Sickness

Antihistamines	Phenylbutazone
Arsenicals	Phenytoin
Barbiturates	Procainamide
Bismuth	Quinidine
Digitalis	Salicylates
Heparin	Sera
Hydralazine	Streptomycin
Insulin	Sulfonamides
Iodides	Thiouracils
Mercurial diuretics	Vaccines
Penicillins	

TABLE 81-23. Compounds That May Produce Hemolysis of Glucose-6-Phosphate Dehydrogenase-Deficient Red Cells

Analgesics	*Nonsulfonamide antibacterial agents*
Acetanilid	Chloramphenicol†
Acetophenetidin (phenacetin)	Furazolidone
Acetylsalicylic acid*	Furamethonol
Antipyrine	Neoarsphenamine
Pyramidone	Nitrofurantoin
Sulfonamides and sulfones	Nitrofurazone
Dapsone	Para-aminosalicylic acid
N_2-Acetylsufanilamide	*Miscellaneous drugs*
Salicylazosulfapyridine	α-Methyldopa
Sulfacetamide	Dimercaprol*
Sulfamethoxypyridazine	Hydralazine
Sulfanilamide	Mestranol
Sulfapyridine	Methylene blue*
Sulfisoxazole*	Nalidixic acid
Sulfoxone*	Naphthalene
Thiazolsulfone	Niridazole
Antimalarials	Phenylhydrazine
Chloroquine	Probenecid
Pamaquine	Pyridium
Pentaquine	Quinine‡
Primaquine	Trinitrotoluene
Quinacrine	Vitamin K (water soluble)
Quinocide	

* Slightly hemolytic in blacks or only in very large doses.
† Possibly hemolytic in whites but not in blacks or Orientals.
‡ Hemolytic in whites but not in blacks.
(Taken in part from Beutler E: Glucose-6-phosphate dehydrogenase deficiency. In Stanbury JB, Wyngaarden JB, Frederickson DS (eds): *The Metabolic Basis of Inherited Disease,* 3rd ed. New York, McGraw-Hill, 1974.

TABLE 81-24. Drugs That May Cause Blood Dyscrasias

Drug	Agranulocytosis (Leukopenia)	Aplastic Anemia	Hemolytic Anemia	Megaloblastic Anemia	Pancytopenia	Thrombocytopenia
Acetanilid			*			
Acetazolamide	*	*			*	*
Acetophenetidin		*	*		*	*
Acetylphenylhydrazine			*			
Acetylsalicylic acid	*	*	*		*	*
Allyl-isopropyl-acetylcarbamide						*
Aminopyrine	*	*	*			
Antihistamines (H_1 type)	*					
Antineoplastics	*	*			*	
Antipyrine			*			
Arsenicals	*					
Arsenobenzenes						*
Barbiturates		*		*	*	*
Busulfan					*	*
Carbamazepine	*	*				*
Cephalothin sodium			*			*
Chloramphenicol	*	*	*		*	*
Chloroquine	*		*			
Chlorothiazide	*	*			*	*
Chlorpromazine	*		*			
Chlorpropamide		*			*	*
Cinchophen	*					
Clofibrate	*					
Colchicine		*		*		
Corticotropin	*					
Cycloserine				*		
Cytarabine	*		*	*		*
Diaminodiphenylsulfone			*			
Digitalis glycosides	*	*			*	*
Dimercaprol			*			
Dipyrone	*					
5-Fluorouracil				*		
Furazolidone			*			
Gamma benzene hexachloride	*					
Glutethimide				*		
Gold compounds	*	*			*	*
Hydralazine	*					
Hydrochlorothiazide						*
Imipramine	*					
Indomethacin		*				
Iothiouracil	*					
Irradiation (radioactive drugs)		*				
Isoniazid			*			
Mepazine	*	*			*	
Meprobamate	*	*			*	
6-Mercaptopurine	*	*		*	*	*
Metformin				*		
Methiamazole	*	*			*	*
Methophenobarbital				*		
Methotrexate	*	*		*	*	*
Methyldopa	*	*	*		*	*
Methylene blue			*			
Neomycin				*		
Nitrofurantoin			*	*		
Nitrofurazone			*			

(continued)

TABLE 81-24. ***(Continued)***

Drug	Agranulocytosis (Leukopenia)	Aplastic Anemia	Hemolytic Anemia	Megaloblastic Anemia	Pancytopenia	Thrombocytopenia
Oral contraceptives				*		
Oxyphenbutazone	*					
Pamaquine			*	*		
Para-aminosalicylic acid			*	*		
Penicillin	*	*	*		*	*
Penindione	*					
Pentamidine isethionate				*		
Pentaquine			*			
Phenacetin	*					
Phenantoin		*	*		*	
Phenothiazines	*					
Phenylbutazone	*	*			*	*
Phenylhydrazine			*			
Phenytoin	*	*		*		
Primaquine			*			
Primidone				*		
Probenecid			*			
Procainamide	*					
Prochlorperazine	*					
Promazine	*					
Propylthiouracil	*					
Pyrimethamine				*		
Quinacrine	*	*	*			*
Quinidine	*	*	*		*	*
Quinine			*			*
Rifampin						*
Salicylates	*					
Stibophen			*			
Streptomycin	*	*		*		
Sulfonamides	*	*	*		*	*
Sulfoxone			*			
Tetracyclines	*		*		*	*
Thiazides	*					
Thiazolsulfone			*			
Thioridazine	*					
Thiouracil	*					*
Tolbutamide	*	*			*	*
Triamterene				*		
Trimethadione	*	*			*	
Trimethoprim				*		
Tripelennamine	*					
Vitamin K water-soluble analogues			*			

TABLE 81-25. Drugs That Cross the Human Placental Barrier and That May Endanger the Fetus During Pregnancy or in the Prenatal Period

Drug	Adverse Effect
Acetophenetidin	Methemoglobinemia
Alphaprodine	Fetal respiratory depression
Aminopterin	Abortion, anomalies, cleft palate
Ammonium chloride	Acidosis
Androgens	Advanced bone age; clitoral enlargement, labial fusion, masculinization
Anesthetics (volatile)	Depressed fetal respiration
Barbiturates	Anomalies, depressed respiration
Bishydroxycoumarin	Fetal death and intrauterine hemorrhage
Bromides	Neonatal skin eruptions (bromoderma)
Busulfan	Cleft palate
Chloral hydrate (large doses)	Fetal death
Chlorambucil	Abortion, anomalies
Chloroquine	Thrombocytopenia
Chlorpromazine	Neonatal jaundice, prolonged extrapyramidal signs, neonatal goiter
Chlorpropamide	Prolonged neonatal hypoglycemia, neonatal goiter?
Cholinesterase inhibitors	Muscular weakness (transient)
Cortisone	Cleft palate
Cyclophosphamide	Defects of extremities, stunting, fetal death
Cyclopropane	Neonatal respiratory depression
D-amphetamine sulfate	Transposition of vessels?
Estrogens	Advanced bone age, clitoral enlargement, labial fusion, masculinization, vaginal cancer (20 years later)
Ether	Neonatal apnea
Ethyl biscoumacetate	Fetal death, neonatal hemorrhage
Ganglionic blocking agents	Neonatal ileus
Heroin	Initial neonatal addiction, neonatal death, respiratory depression
Hexamethonium bromide	Neonatal ileus, death
Iodides	Goiter
Iophenoxic acid	Hypothyroidism, retardation
Iothiouracil	Neonatal goiter
Isoniazid	Retarded psychomotor activity
Levorphanol	Fetal respiratory depression
Lithium carbonate	Neonatal goiter
Lysergic acid diethylamide	Chromosomal damage, stunted offspring
Mecamylamine	Fatal neonatal ileus
Mepivacaine	Fetal bradycardia, neonatal depression
Methadone	Fetal respiratory depression
Methimazole	Neonatal goiter, hypothyroidism, mental retardation
Methotrexate	Abortion, anomalies, cleft palate
Morphine	Initial neonatal addiction, respiratory depression, neonatal death
Nicotine (smoking)	"Small for dates" neonates
Nitrofurantoin	Fetal hemolysis
Nitrous oxide	Respiratory depression
Oral progestogens	Clitoral enlargement, labial fusion, masculinization
Paraldehyde	Respiratory depression
Phenmetrazine	Multiple skeletal and visceral anomalies
Phenobarbital	Respiratory depression, death
Phenylbutazone	Neonatal goiter
Phenytoin	Anomalies
Podophyllum	Fetal resorption, deformities
Potassium iodide	Cyanosis, goiter, mental retardation, respiratory distress
Propylthiouracil	Neonatal goiter, hypothyroidism, mental retardation
Quinine	Deafness, thrombocytopenia
Radioactive iodine	Congenital goiter, mental retardation, hypothyroidism
Reserpine	Nasal block, respiratory obstruction
Salicylates	Anomalies, neonatal bleeding

(*continued*)

TABLE 81-25. (Continued)

Drug	Adverse Effects
Smallpox vaccination	Fetal vaccinia
Sodium warfarin	Intrauterine hemorrhage, fetal death
Streptomycin	Hearing loss, eighth cranial nerve damage, micromelia, multiple skeletal anomalies
Sulfonamides (long acting)	Kernicterus, hyperbilirubinemia, acute liver atrophy, anemia, neonatal goiter
Sulfonylureas	Neonatal goiter, prolonged neonatal hypoglycemia
Tetracyclines	Discolored teeth, inhibits long bone growth, micromelia, syndactyly
Thalidomide	Phocomelia, hearing defects, fetal death
Thiazides	Neonatal death, thrombocytopenia
Thiouracil	Hypothyroidism, neonatal goiter, mental retardation
Tolbutamide	Congenital anomalies and prolonged neonatal hypoglycemia
Tribromoethanol	Depressed fetal respiration
Vitamin A (large doses)	Cleft palate, congenital anomalies, eye damage, syndactyly
Vitamin D (large doses)	Hypercalcemia, mental retardation
Vitamin K analogues (large doses)	Hyperbilirubinemia, kernicterus

TABLE 81-26. Some Drugs Excreted in Human Milk

Acetaminophen	Ether	Phenacetin
Alcohol	Ethinamate	Phenaglycodol
Allergens (egg, peanuts, others)	Ethyl biscoumacetate	Phenolphthalein
Ambenonium chloride	Folic acid	Phenylbutazone
Aminophylline	Heroin	Phenytoin
Amphetamines	Hexachlorobenzene	Potassium iodide
Anthraquinone cathartics	Hydroxypylcarbamate	Prochlorperazine
Antihistamines	Hydroxyzine	Propoxyphene
Arsenical salts	Imipramine	Propylthiouracil
Aspirin	Iodine-131	Pseudoephedrine
Atropine	Iopanoic acid	Pyrimethamine
Barbiturates	Isoniazid	Quinidine
Bishydroxycoumarin	L-Propoxyphene	Quinine sulfate
Bromides	Mandelic acid	Reserpine
Brompheniramine	Mefenamic acid	Rh antibodies
Caffeine	Meperidine	Rhubarb
Calomel	Metals	Riboflavin
Cascara	Methadone HCl	Salicylates
Chloral hydrate	Methdilazine	Scopolamine
Chloramphenicol	Methimazole	Senna
Chloroform	Methocarbomal	Sodium salicylate
Chlorpromazine	Metronidazole	Streptomycin
Codeine	Morphine	Sulfadimethoxine
Copper	Narcotics	Sulfamethoxazole
Cortisone	Neomycin sulfate	Sulfanilamide
Cyclophosphamide	Niacin	Sulfapyridine
Cyclopropane	Nicotine	Sulfathiazole
Cycloserine	Nitrofurantoin	Tetracyclines
D-Amphetamine	Oral contraceptives	Thiamine
Danthron	Oxacillin	Thiazide diuretics
DDT	Oxyphenbutazone	Thiopental
Diazepam	Pantothenic acid	Thiouracil
Diphenhydramine	Papaverine	Thyroid hormones
Ephedrine	PAS	Tolbutamide
Ergot alkaloids	Penethamate hydriodide	Trifluoperazine
Erythromycin	Penicillin G	Vitamins A, B, B_{12}, C, D, E, K
Estrogens	Pentazocine	

TABLE 81-27. Drugs That May Cause Intestinal Malabsorption

Drug	Substances Involved
Alcohol (ethanol)	Folic acid, vitamin B_{12}, fat, D-xylose
Aluminum hydroxide	Tetracycline antibiotics
Bacitracin	As for neomycin
Bisacodyl	Fat, protein, potassium
Calcium carbonate	Fatty acids
Chlorothiazide diuretics	Water and sodium
Cholestyramine	Bile salts, digitalis, lincomycin, sterols, carbohydrates, iron, fat soluble vitamins, others
Clofibrate	As for cholestyramine
Colchicine	Vitamin B_{12}, cholesterol, fat, carotine, sodium, potassium, D-xylose
Contraceptives, oral	Folic acid
Ethacrynic acid	Water and sodium
5-Fluorouracil	Severe general malabsorption
Kanamycin (oral)	As for neomycin
Methotrexate	Severe general malabsorption
Neomycin	Cholesterol, disaccharides, Vitamin B_{12}, carotine, iron, potassium, sodium, chloride, nitrogen
Paromomycin	As for neomycin
PAS	Folic acid, vitamin B_{12}, cholesterol, iron, D-xylose
Phenformin	Glucose
Phenolphthaline	Fat, vitamins A, D, E, K, calcium
Phenytoin	Folic acid
Polymyxin B	As for neomycin
Potassium chloride	Vitamin B_{12}
Triparenol (MER-29)	Severe general malabsorption

DIANE ZALBA

82 Sources of Information in Pharmacology

GENERAL REFERENCES

1. *AMA Drug Evaluations*, 4th ed (Department of Drugs, American Medical Association). Acton, Massachusetts, Publishing Sciences Group, 1980
   Drug monographs of currently marketed U.S. drugs prepared by physicians. Monographs include generic/trade names, manufacturers, adverse drug reactions, dosages, dosage forms, uses, and routes of administration.
2. *American Hospital Formulary Service* (loose-leaf). Washington, DC, American Society of Hospital Pharmacy, 1969–
   A loose-leaf book that contains drug monographs arranged by pharmacologic action and therapeutic indications, which are updated regularly.
3. *Applied Therapeutics for Clinical Pharmacists*, 4th ed (Koda–Kimble MA, Katches BS, Young LY, eds). San Francisco, Applied Therapeutics, 1982
   Basic textbook of clinical pharmacy, with emphasis on the correlation between disease-state and drug therapy.
4. *Clinical Pharmacology: Basic Principles in Therapeutics*, 2nd ed (Melman KL, Morelli HF, eds). New York, Macmillan, 1978
   Clinical pharmacology textbook that emphasizes the clinical application of drug therapy, integrating physiology, pathology, and pharmacology.
5. *Facts and Comparisons* (loose-leaf) (Kastrup EK, Boyd JR). St. Louis, Facts and Comparisons, 1979, (monthly supplements)
   Contains monographs on all U.S. drugs organized by therapeutic categories and updated monthly.
6. *Martindale's Extra Pharmacopeoia*, 28th ed (Wade A, ed). London, The Pharmaceutical Press, 1982
   International drug handbook that includes information compiled from world literature. Drug monographs include synonyms, physical and chemical properties, toxic effects, drug interactions, uses, and references.
7. *The Merck Index*, 9th ed. Rahway, New Jersey, Merck and Co, 1976
   Encyclopedic listing of chemicals and drugs by generic or common chemical name. Information provided includes alternate names, trademark, formula, chemical and physical properties, structure, and more.
8. *Meyler's Side Effects of Drugs* (Dukes MNG). Amsterdam, Excerpta Medica (distributed by Elsevier–North Holland, New York), 1975–1980
   Summarizes side-effects of drugs as reported in the literature from 1975 to 1980.
9. *The National Formulary* (N.F.). Washington, DC, American Pharmaceutical Association, 1975

Official U.S. compendium designed to supplement the United States Pharmacopeia. Contains standards for the identity, quality, strength, and purity of drugs that are of therapeutic value.

10. *The Pharmacological Basis of Therapeutics*, 6th ed (Goodman LS, Gilman A, eds). Riverside, New Jersey, Macmillan, 1980
    Basic pharmacology textbook directed toward health professionals. Chapters are arranged according to therapeutic categories. Bibliographical references.
11. *The Pharmacopeia of the United States of America* (the United States Pharmacopeia: U.S.P.). Rockville, Maryland, United States Pharmacopeial Convention, 1981
    Official U.S. compendium containing standards for the quality, strength, purity, and identity of a selected group of drugs.
12. *Review of Medical Pharmacology*, 6th ed (Meyers FH, Jawetz, E, Goldfein A). Los Altos, Lange Medical Publications, 1978
    A textbook of the basic principles of medical pharmacology, emphasizing clinical aspects of drug therapy.

SPECIALTY REFERENCES

1. *Clinical Use of Drugs in Patients with Kidney and Liver Disease* (Anderson RJ, Gambertoglio JG, Schrier RW). Philadelphia, Pennsylvania, Charles C Thomas, 1981
   Information source on the pharmacokinetics and dosage adjustments of drug therapy for patients in renal failure.
2. *Clinical Toxicology of Commercial Products*, 4th ed (Gleason MN et al, eds). Baltimore, Williams & Wilkins, 1977
   A comprehensive guide to the treatment of accidental poisonings involving commercial products.
3. *Drug Interactions*, 4th ed (Hansten PD). Philadelphia, Lea & Febiger, 1979
   Documents the clinical significance of drug-drug interactions and drug effects on clinical laboratory results.
4. *Handbook of Nonprescription Drugs*, 6th ed. Washington, DC, American Pharmaceutical Association, 1982
   Guide to over-the-counter medications, each chapter organized on the basis of therapeutic classes of drugs.
5. *Pediatric Dosage Handbook* (Shirkey HC). Washington, DC, American Pharmaceutical Association, 1980
   Contains information on the dosing of drugs in the pediatric patient.
6. *The Use of Antibiotics*, 3rd ed (Kucers A, Bennett NM). London, William Heinemann Medical Books, 1979
   Comprehensive review of antibiotic therapy with emphasis on clinical application.

RELEVANT JOURNALS

1. *Annual Review of Pharmacology and Toxicology*. Palo Alto, Annual Reviews, 1932—annual.
2. *Archives Internationales de Pharmacodyamie et de Thérapie*. Ghent, Heymans Institute of Pharmacology, 1894—monthly.
3. *Biochemical Pharmacology*. New York, Pergamon Press, 1958—24X a year.
4. *British Journal of Pharmacology*. London, Macmillan Journals, 1946—monthly.
5. *Clinical Pharmacology and Therapeutics*. St. Louis, C V Mosby, 1960—monthly.
6. *Drug Intelligence and Clinical Pharmacy*. Hamilton, Illinois, Drug Intelligence and Clinical Pharmacy, 1967—monthly.
7. *Drugs*. Balgowlah, Australia, ADIS Press Australasia Pty, 1971—monthly.
8. *European Journal of Pharmacology*. Amsterdam, Elsevier-North Holland Biomedical Press, 1967—24X a year.
9. *Journal of the American Medical Association*. Chicago, American Medical Association, 1883—weekly.
10. *Journal of Pharmacology and Experimental Therapeutics*. Baltimore, Williams & Wilkins, 1909—monthly.
11. *Journal of Pharmacy and Pharmacology*. London, Pharmaceutical Society of Great Britain, 1949—monthly.
12. *The Medical Letter on Drugs and Therapeutics*. New Rochelle, New York, The Medical Letter, 1959—fortnightly.
13. *Molecular Pharmacology*. New York, Academic Press, 1965—6X a year.
14. *Naunyn-Schmiedebergs Archives of Pharmacology*. Wurzberg, Springer International, 1873—3 volumes a year.
15. *New England Journal of Medicine*. Boston, Massachusetts Medical Society, 1812—weekly.
16. *Pharmacological Reviews*. Baltimore, Williams & Wilkins, 1951—4X a year.
17. *Toxicology and Applied Pharmacology*. New York, Academic Press, 1959—monthly.
18. *Toxicon*, Elmsford, New York, Pergamon Press Journals Division, 1962—bimonthly.

DESMOND J. FITZGERALD
KEVIN O'MALLEY

Therapeutic Agents Available in Europe That Have Not Been Released in the United States

83

There has been an increasing awareness over the past 20 years of the potential of drugs to cause harm, the main catalyst being the thalidomide disaster. The reaction in Western countries was to establish drug regulatory agencies, the responsibility of which was to oversee the introduction of new drugs. The approaches of these agencies vary considerably: Some have quite liberal policies, whereas others, such as the Food and Drug Administration (FDA), have a more conservative attitude. One result is that many drugs available in various parts of the world are not available in the United States.

More new drugs are available in Europe than in America.

One aspect of this difference is the so-called drug lag—the time between drugs being introduced in Europe and in the United States. Thus one can forecast that many drugs now on the market in Europe will in time be marketed in the United States. Many of these drugs are also of pharmacologic interest. We discuss herein the most important of these drugs.

ANTIHYPERTENSIVE DRUGS

LABETALOL

Labetalol is a combined alpha- and beta-adrenoceptor antagonist. With respect to its beta-blocking propensities, labetalol resembles propranolol in its nonselectivity but with only one third of its potency. With regard to the alpha-receptors, it has one tenth the potency of phenoxybenzamine. Labetalol has no intrinsic sympathetic activity. It is a more potent beta- than alpha-adrenoceptor blocking drug. Its blood pressure lowering effect does not depend on beta-blockade alone because it lowers blood pressure in patients already receiving beta adrenoceptor antagonists. Labetalol causes decreased peripheral resistance without a compensatory tachycardia or increased cardiac output presumably because of its beta-blocking effect.

Labetalol is well absorbed, but, because of first-pass metabolism, bioavailability is only

40%. Peak levels are achieved in 1 to 2 hours, and 50% of the drug is protein bound. The metabolites and also the unchanged drug (5%) are excreted by the kidney. The plasma T½ is 3.5 to 4.5 hours, although it may be longer in patients with hepatic disease. Labetalol is as effective as methyldopa alone or the combination of hydralazine and a beta blocker in the treatment of hypertension. The fall in blood pressure begins at 2 hours and is maximum at 4 hours. Other beta-blockers require considerably more time for the full effect to be seen. Labetalol has been used to control severe hypertension. In large doses, it is effective in controlling the blood pressure of patients with pheochromocytoma. Labetalol may be given intravenously for the urgent control of blood pressure, although its rapid effect when given orally may make i.v. therapy unnecessary. The most frequent side-effect is postural hypotension, which occurs in 3% to 8% of patients receiving 800 mg per day or less. At higher doses, this adverse effect occurs more frequently. Other side-effects are rare. Labetalol is less likely than propranolol to precipitate asthma. It may cause lethargy and failure of ejaculation. Dosage begins at 300 mg daily in divided doses, rising to 2400 mg in severely hypertensive patients or in patients with a pheochromocytoma.

INDAPAMIDE

Indapamide, a chlorosulphamide derivative, is structurally related to the thiazide diuretics. It has both diuretic and vasodilator properties, the latter effect possibly being due to a reduced calcium ion flux across the cell membrane of vascular smooth muscle. It is thought to exert its blood pressure lowering effect by peripheral vasodilation, although it also causes a diuresis. However, its antihypertensive action is not associated with the reflex sympathetic changes usually associated with vasodilator therapy. With chronic administration its duration of action is extremely long; this is not explained by a long half-life alone, since the blood pressure may not return to baseline until weeks after therapy has been discontinued.

After an oral dose, peak concentrations are reached in ½ to 1 hour. Indapamide is metabolized in the liver, and metabolites and active drug (5%) are excreted by the kidney. Its plasma T½ is about 18 hours. Indapamide lowers blood pressure gradually, and the full effect may not be seen for 6 weeks. It is as effective as chlorothiazide and frusemide when used alone and is useful as adjunctive therapy in patients not controlled on a beta-blocker alone. During therapy, serum potassium may fall and uric acid rise, although rarely do they achieve abnormal levels. The dose of the drug is 2.5 or 5.0 mg daily as a single dose. Doses above this level have little additional antihypertensive effect. Even at 5.0 mg daily, the thiazidelike pattern of unwanted effects may be seen.

XIPAMIDE

Xipamide is a diuretic that structurally resembles chlorthalidone. It is as effective as frusemide but with a less abrupt and more prolonged duration of action. It acts on the distal tubule but may have an effect on the loop of Henle also. After an oral dose, peak plasma concentrations are reached in 2 hours. Xipamide has a plasma half-life of 5 to 8 hours, but the diuresis continues for 12 hours and its antihypertensive effect lasts for 24 hours. It is as effective in controlling blood pressure as are the beta-blockers. It can, however, cause a marked fall in serum potassium level, which makes it unsuitable as a first-line drug in the long-term treatment of hypertension. Other adverse effects include hyperuricemia and decreased glucose tolerance. It is given in a dose of 20 mg.

INDORAMIN

Indoramin is a novel antihypertensive agent that combines a postsynaptic alpha-adrenoceptor blocking effect with a quinidine-like cardioinhibitor effect. Because of its specific alpha-1-adrenoceptor blocking property, it resembles prazosin and does not cause a reflex tachycardia or postural hypotension. Its cardioinhibitory action prevents a rise in cardiac output associated with peripheral vasodilation. However, cardiac failure may be precipitated in susceptible subjects. Further, its quinidine-like membrane stabilizing effect leads to the abolition of some experimental arrhythmias. After an oral dose, the maximum fall in blood pressure occurs at 2 hours, with a return to baseline at 5 hours. Indoramin may be used to treat mild to moderate hypertension. Side-effects include sedation, particularly with doses greater than 150 mg/day, and failure to ejaculate, which may occur in up to two thirds of patients. Fluid retention has been observed. The drug is given in doses of 60 to 150 mg daily in three divided doses.

SULPHONYLUREAS

As elsewhere, biguanides have fallen into disrepute in Europe, and only one agent, metformin, is available. In the United States, 2 million treatment years of oral hypoglycemics were prescribed in 1975 for an adult-onset diabetic population of 3.84 million. The large market worldwide has stimulated the development of a second generation of sulphonylureas, which differ from their parent drugs, tolbutamide and chlorpropamide, in their pharmacokinetics and unwanted effects. Newer agents (*see* Table 83-1) are more potent than their predecessors, although the maximum reduction in blood glucose is no greater. Increased potency does not confer advantage in this context. Sulphonylureas are indicated in the treatment of adult-onset insulin-resistant diabetes, and the choice of agent is determined by their duration of action and mode of elimination. In elderly subjects, longer-acting drugs may accumulate, resulting in hypoglycemia. Therefore, drugs with a short half-life, such as glipizide, are preferred. Where there are doubts about compliance, a long-acting drug such as glibenaclamide may be appropriate. Concurrent renal or hepatic illness will further affect the choice of drug.

GLIBENCLAMIDE

Glibenclamide (presently under investigation in the United States as glyburide) is a potent second-generation sulphonylurea analogous to chlorpropamide. Like other sulphonylureas, it acts both on pancreatic endocrine tissue and peripherally. Glibenclamide suppresses glucagon secretion. Peripherally it increases insulin receptor numbers partly by attenuating insulin-mediated receptor loss. The drug is almost completely absorbed and undergoes hepatic metabolism to hydroxy derivatives, which are excreted in the urine. One of these, 4-trans hydroxy glibenclamide, has hypoglycemic activity in animals. The plasma T½ of glibenclamide varies considerably and increases after 2 weeks of treatment. Glibenclamide is 450 times more potent than tolbutamide and is the most potent of all the sulphonylureas. However, the maximum hypoglycemic effect of glibenclamide does not exceed that of tolbutamide. Because it is extensively metabolized, glibenclamide may be used in renal disease without dose adjustment.

Side-effects are common, with hypoglycemia occuring in 6% of patients and gastrointestinal disturbances in 2%. Skin rash, hypersensitivity reactions, and, rarely, thrombocytopenia or leukopenia may occur.

TABLE 83-1. Comparison of Newly Available Sulphonylureas

	Time to Peak Plasma Concentration	Elimination Half-Life	Rate of Elimination	Daily Dose (Average)	Doses per Day
	hr	*hr*			
Glibenclamide	2–5	10–16	Hepatic metabolism. Renal excretion of less active metabolite	5–10 mg	1
Glipizide	1–2	3–7	Hepatic metabolism. Renal excretion of inactive metabolites	2.5–20 mg	1–2
Gliclazide	2	12	Hepatic metabolism	80–240 mg	1–2
Glisoxepide	1–5	1.7–3	Hepatic metabolism (55%). Renal excretion (43%)	2–16 mg	2–3
Gliborunide	2–4	5.4–10.9	Hepatic metabolism. Renal elimination of less active metabolites	12.5–75 mg	1–2
Glymidine	?	4–8	Renal excretion of active metabolites	0.5–2 g	2–3

The dose is 5 to 10 mg once daily. As the drug's plasma T½ tends to lengthen, after 2 to 3 weeks the dose should be reduced.

GLIPIZIDE

Glipizide is a potent sulphonylurea that resembles tolbutamide in its pharmacokinetic profile. It is rapidly absorbed in the fasting state, is highly protein bound, and is extensively metabolized in the liver, with only 2% to 3% excreted as unchanged drug. Food reduces the rate but not the extent of absorption. It has a short half-life (*see* Table 83-1), so that the dose can be titrated rapidly. The most common side-effects are hypoglycemia (3.4%) and gastrointestinal complaints (2.2%). Because it is rapidly inactivated by hepatic metabolism, glipizide is useful in patients with renal disease.

GLICAZIDE

Glicazide has attracted attention because, in addition to a hypoglycemic effect, it has antiplatlet properties. There is increasing evidence that platelet aggregability is increased both *in vivo* and *in vivo* in diabetic subjects, particularly in patients with vascular complications. In animal studies, hyperaggregability of platelets precedes the onset of vascular lesions, suggesting that this is a primary defect. The hyperaggregability may be due to an imbalance of prostacyclin (PGI_2), an antiaggregant, and thromboxane A_2, a proaggregant. Glicazide reduces platelet adhesiveness and aggregability to ADP and adrenaline in humans, the effect increasing with the duration of treatment. How glicazide achieves this is not known, but it may inhibit membrane phospholipase and therefore reduce the availability of the precursor to thromboxane A_2. Further, some evidence suggests that diabetic retinopathy may be prevented or improved by treatment with glicazide, although much work remains to be done on the effect of antiplatelet agents alone in the treatment of diabetes.

Glicazide is 10 to 20 times more potent than tolbutamide. Absorption is variable—fast and slow absorbers have been identified. Glicazide is hydroxylated, with less than 20% excreted unchanged in the urine. Its side-effects are similar to those of other sulphonylureas. It has a duration of action of up to 12 hours, and it is generally given in two doses/day.

GLYMIDINE

Glymidine is a sulphapyrimidine derivative. Because it has a very different structure, it does not cross-react with other sulphonylureas and is useful in patients who develop hypersensitivity reactions to these drugs. After complete absorption, it is rapidly metabolized in the liver by demethylation and oxidation. Some of its metabolites have hypoglycemic potency in animals that may prolong the effect of the drug beyond that predicted by its half-life.

ANTIANGINAL DRUGS

Nifedipine has recently become available in the United States for the treatment of angina. Perhexiline has been available in Europe for some time and will be discussed here. Beta blockers are dealt with separately.

PERHEXILINE MALEATE

Perhexiline is a chemical analogue of hexadylamine, a piperdine derivative that is a coronary vasodilator. Perhexiline acts as a coronary and peripheral artery vasodilator probably by antagonizing calcium ion flux through an action on the transmembrane calcium ion carrier. It has a greater effect on coronary artery smooth muscle cells than on myocardial fibers. It has little effect on atrial tissue, although it suppresses ventricular ectopic activity. In animals it decreases conduction between the atria and ventricles, although not to the same extent as verapamil. Perhexiline decreases the tachycardia induced by exercise by an effect that appears independent of any alteration in autonomic innervation of the heart.

Perhexiline is well absorbed and is hydroxylated in the liver to metabolites that are excreted through the kidney. It has a long plasma half-life, calculated in some studies to be 2 to 6 days, although it may be as long as 30 days. Considerable time is required to achieve therapeutic tissue levels, and doses should not be altered at periods less than 1 to 2 weeks. Side-effects include gastrointestinal discomfort, which subsides with treatment, and weight loss. Central nervous system toxicity is common and presents as dizziness, nystagmous, ataxia, and tremor. Hyperglycemia occurs and may be symptomatic. Hepatotoxicity of some degree occurs in 20% of patients, but in most cases this is comprised of small increases in transaminases that revert to normal on withdrawal of the drug. Peripheral neuropathy of a mixed sensory–motor type has been reported particularly in doses greater than 200 mg/day and in patients who are genetically slow metabolizers of the drug. Such patients are also slow metabolizers of debrisoquine. The neuropathy associated with perhexilene may be accompanied by bilateral papilledema and usually resolves on drug withdrawal.

Indications for perhexiline are not clearly defined, but the drug may be useful in the treatment of angina where other therapy has failed or where beta-blockers are contraindicated, as in cardiac failure. In view of the dose-dependent side-effects, the drug should be administered in doses not exceeding 200 mg/day.

ANTICONVULSANTS

ETHOSUXIMIDE

Ethosuximide is a succinimide derivative effective in petit mal epilepsy. In animal studies ethosuximide prevents the seizures induced by pentylenetetrazole. It also reduces synaptic transmission to low-frequency electrical stimulation. Thus it is effective in absence seizures characterized by three per second discharges seen during electroencephalography.

Ethosuximide is well absorbed, with 100% bioavailability, and is not protein bound. It is metabolized in the liver, and only 10% to 20% of unchanged drug is excreted in the urine. Unlike methsuximide, ethosuximide has no active metabolites. The rate of elimination of ethosuximide is higher in children than in adults. In children, the plasma half-life is about 30 hours, increasing to 60 hours in adults.

Ethosuximide is effective in the treatment of absence seizures and is now considered to be the drug of first choice in this disorder. It has been suggested that ethosuximide be combined with phenytoin or some other agent effective in grand mal seizures because these seizures may be activated by ethosuximide. Unwanted effects are infrequent and usually minor, including gastrointestinal disturbances and drowsiness. At excessive doses, dizziness and ataxia occur. Other side-effects include erythema multiforme, headaches, and hiccups. Because leukopenia, thrombocytopenia, and agranulocytosis have been reported occasionally during long-term treatment, regular blood counts are necessary, and the drug should be withdrawn if hematologic abnormalities develop.

The drug is taken in two to four divided doses. Therapy can be monitored by plasma drug levels, although there is a poor relation between plasma levels and side-effects. As this drug has a long plasma $T\frac{1}{2}$, steady-state plasma and tissue levels are achieved only after 1 week of drug administration so that dose adjustments should not be made at shorter periods.

SULTHIAME

Sulthiame is an effective anticonvulsant in the treatment of grand mal epilepsy and as an adjuvant to other treatment regimens in the control of psychomotor epilepsy. However, much of the beneficial effect of sulthiame may be due to its interaction with phenytoin, with which it is often combined. Sulthiame inhibits hepatic metabolism of phenytoin and thereby increases phenytoin plasma levels. It is well absorbed and 29% protein bound. Sulthiame undergoes both renal and hepatic elimination, 60% to 70% being excreted by the kidney as unchanged drug. In patients with renal failure, the plasma half-life of the drug, normally 30 hours, is lengthened and the dosing interval should be increased.

Sulthiame is a drug of second choice in the treatment of grand mal epilepsy and is usually used in combination with a first-line drug such as phenytoin or phenobarbitone. It has been found to improve behavior in epileptic children, and some evidence suggests that an anticonvulsant drug such as sulthiame may be effective in behavioral disorders associated with cerebrovascular disease in elderly persons. Side-effects are uncommon and include drowsiness, headaches, and irritating paresthesia in the extremities. Sulthiame is given in a daily dose of 200 to 1200 mg in two or three divided doses.

OTHER ANTICONVULSANTS

Ethotoin and *methoin*, hydantoins similar to phenytoin, are used to treat grand mal epilepsy. Their side-effects are similar to those of phenytoin. Side-effects are less frequent with ethotoin, but this drug is also less effective in controlling seizures. Methoin causes fewer minor side-effects than does phenytoin, but severe reactions are more common. It may be used instead of phenytoin when phenytoin is ineffective.

Beclamide is a weak anticonvulsant with minimal side-effects. It is of some value as adjuvant therapy in epileptic children with behavioral disorders.

ANTIDEPRESSANTS

TETRACYCLIC AGENTS

Maprotiline

Maprotiline, a tetracyclic compound, is distinguished from the tricyclics by the rigid skeleton of its molecular structure. It has a secondary amine side-chain similar to that seen in the demethylated metabolites of imipramine and amitriptyline. It blocks noradrenaline uptake selectively, having little effect on serotonin reuptake. In animals, maprotiline has no effect on serotonin metabolism in the central nervous system and in humans has negligible effects on the cardiovascular system. The potency of maprotiline is similar to that of imipramine and amitriptyline. Maprotiline is completely although slowly absorbed, with a bioavailability of 37% to 67%. It is slowly eliminated, partly as active metabolites, and its plasma half-life is about 2 days, so that steady-state plasma levels are reached after about 1 week. Maprotiline is as effective as any currently available tricyclic, although sedative and anticholinergic side-effects are less frequent. Skin rashes are common (5%), and 25% of patients who overdose with maprotiline experience convulsions.

Mianserin

Mianserin is a tetracyclic antidepressant with a 6-7-6 structure to which is added a six-membered ring in the plane of the seven-membered ring. The profile of pharmacologic effects of this drug differs from that of tricyclic antidepressants. It has presynaptic alpha-adrenoceptor blocking activity combined with an antihistamine action but little effect on serotonin or noradrenaline uptake. It is less cardiotoxic in animals than are tricyclics or maprotiline; this also appears to be the case in human overdose.

Mianserin is readily absorbed but undergoes considerable first-pass metabolism such that its bioavailability is only 30%. It is widely distributed and enters the central nervous system readily. Mianserin is extensively metabolized, and only 4% to 7% is excreted by the kidney as unchanged drug. Its plasma half-life is 11 to 17 hours. Steady-state levels are achieved after 2 weeks of drug administration. It is as effective as standard tricyclic antidepressants. Mianserin may have an additional anxiolytic effect. Anticholinergic symptoms rarely occur, and mianserin is well tolerated in elderly patients and in patients with cardiovascular disease.

BICYCLIC AGENTS

Viloxazine

Viloxazine is a bicyclic (two-ringed) antidepressant related structurally to beta-adrenoreceptor antagonists. It has similar, although weaker, effects on catecholamine uptake than does desipramine. Viloxazine has some amphetamine-like effects that partly explain its antidepressant action, although dependence has not been reported. The drug has minimal peripheral anticholinergic properties.

Viloxazine is rapidly and almost completely absorbed and is extensively metabolized to inactive compounds excreted by the kidney. It has a plasma half-life of 2 to 5 hours. It is as effective as tricyclics but causes fewer sedative and anticholinergic side-effects. Nausea and vomiting are frequent, however, and may limit its use, especially in elderly subjects. Viloxazine may also provoke migraine. Cardiotoxicity has not been reported in cases of drug overdose.

Zimelidine

Zimelidine differs from traditional antidepressants in that it selectively blocks the uptake of serotonin with little effect on catecholamine uptake. It is almost completely demethylated to an active metabolite, the half-life of which is 15 hours. Zimelidine may distinguish serotonergic from noradrenergic types of depression. Further, it may replace the use of serotonin precursors such as tryptophan.

DIBENZOXAZEPINES

Amoxapine

Amoxapine, a new antidepressant drug, belongs to the second generation of tricyclic antidepressants. It is a variant of the 6-7-6 ring structure of the tricyclic compounds. The only chemical difference between this drug and loxapine, an effective antipsychotic agent, is the absence of a methyl group on the piperazide side-chain. Thus amoxapine has many of the pharmaceutical properties of antidepressants while retaining a degree of postsynaptic dopamine blockade. However, it does not cause parkinsonism or tardive dyskinesia, although

TABLE 83-2. Comparison of New Antidepressant Drugs

	Predominant Biochemical Effects	Metabolites	Half-Life	Predominant Side-Effects	Daily Dose
			hr		*mg*
Dibenzoxazepines					
Amoxapine	Dopamine blockade, catecholamine uptake decreased		?	Dry mouth, sexual disturbances	150–300
Tetracyclics					
Maprotilene	Catecholamine uptake decreased	Nonactive	48	Mild sedative and anticholinergic	75–300
Mianserin	Presynaptic alpha-adrenoceptor blockade. Antihistamine	Nonactive	11–27		30–120
Bicyclics					
Viloxazine	Amphetamine-like effect. Catecholamine uptake decreased	Nonactive	2–5	Nausea and vomiting	100–300
Zimelidine	Serotonin uptake decreased	Active	5*	Headache, nausea	100–300
Tricyclics					
Clomipramine	Catecholamine uptake decreased	Active	12–40	Mild sedative and anticholinergic	75–300

* Active metabolite, T½, 15 hours.

galactorrhea-amenorrea syndrome has been reported. Further, it is not known if this drug would be beneficial in schizoaffective disorders with associated depression. In clinical trials it is as effective as amitriptyline and imipramine, although only half as potent. The major clinical difference from standard tricyclics is a more rapid onset of effect seen in the first 2 weeks of treatment. Although it causes fewer sedative effects than do tricyclics, constipation and sexual dysfunction occur more frequently, sexual dysfunction being consistent with its dopamine-receptor blocking action. It is also thought to be less cardiotoxic.

OTHER ANTIDEPRESSANT DRUGS

Nomifensine

Nomifensine, a tetrahydroisoquinoline derivative, is not chemically related to tricyclics or monoamine oxidase inhibitors. It resembles amphetamines and blocks the reuptake of noradrenaline and dopamine with little effect on serotonin. It has only mild sedative, anticholinergic, and cardiotoxic activity. Immune hemolytic anemia has been reported in one patient.

The drug is well absorbed and has active metabolites. It is present in the plasma mainly as the glucoronide. Ninety-seven percent of the drug is excreted in the urine, and its plasma half-life is 2 to 4 hours, being prolonged in severe renal failure. In clinical trials it is as effective as tricyclics and causes fewer anticholinergic side-effects. Nomifensine is claimed to have a more rapid onset of effect. Because it blocks dopamine uptake, it may aggravate psychotic conditions.

Trazodone

Trazodone, a triazolopyridine derivative, is unrelated to previous antidepressants. It has little of the pharmacologic properties of most other antidepressants. It blocks serotonin uptake in animals, but its mode of action in humans is uncertain. Its anticholinergic activity is less than that seen with tricyclic antidepressants. Trazodone has fewer cardiotoxic effects than do tricyclics in humans and animals. However, it has not been compared with tetracyclic or bicyclic antidepressants.

Trazodone is well absorbed, although absorption may be delayed by food. The drug is extensively metabolized, only 1% being excreted as unchanged drug, with a plasma half-life of 6.3 hours. It is as effective as tricyclics with a similar delay in onset of effect. Side-effects occur less frequently in both old and young patients. A previous member of this class, oxypetrine, had both antipsychotic and anxiolytic effects. It is unknown whether trazodone is effective in psychotic depressions.

TRICYCLIC ANTIDEPRESSANT DRUGS

A number of new tricyclic compounds are formed by small substitutions on the basic 6-7-6 structure or its side-chain, including butryptiline, clomipramine, and trimipramine. These compounds seem to have no important advantages over other available drugs.

BRONCHODILATORS AND OTHER DRUGS USED TO TREAT ASTHMA

BETA$_2$-ADRENOCEPTOR-AGONIST AGENTS

The drugs available in Europe and in the United States differ, as do the routes by which drugs may be given. Salbutamol is marketed as an inhaler in the United States but in Europe is also available as i.v. and oral preparations.

Rimiterol

Rimiterol is a β_2-adrenoceptor–agonist effective by the i.v. route and by inhalation. Unlike many new β_2-adrenoceptor–agonists, rimiterol has the catechol moiety and is therefore metabolized by catechol-O-methyltransferase. Inhaled or i.v. rimiterol causes bronchodilatation and reverses histamine- and acetylcholine-induced bronchospasm. It is as potent as salbutamol but with fewer cardiac effects. After an i.v. bolus, rimiterol is rapidly metabolized to a 3-O-methyl derivative, the half-life of the parent drug being only 5 minutes. After oral administration, 50% is excreted as unchanged rimiterol, but after i.v. bolus most is excreted as metabolites in the urine. It also appears to be metabolized by the lung. After inhalation, bronchodilatation begins in 1 minute and lasts 90 to 180 minutes, which is a shorter duration of action than that of salbutamol or terbutaline. A significant rise in heart rate occurs after inhalation of salbutamol or isoprenaline, 500 to 1000 μg, but not after an equipotent bronchodilatory dose of rimiterol. Rimiterol is available in pressurized aerosols that deliver 200 μg of drug in each dose and, as an i.v. preparation, is given in a dose of 0.05 to 0.2 μg/kg/min.

Hexoprenaline

Hexoprenaline, a selective β_2-adrenoceptor–agonist, comprises two noradrenaline molecules joined by a hexamethylene chain through their aminogroups. It therefore retains the catechol moiety and is metabolized by catechol-O-methyltransferase. It has a longer duration of action than other catechol-containing bronchodilators such as rimiterol or isoprenaline. Hexoprenaline causes bronchodilatation and protects against histamine-, acetylcholine-, and allergen-induced bronchoconstriction. It can cause a tachycardia when used as an inhaler but usually at doses greater than those required for bronchodilatation. After i.v. injection, hexoprenaline causes a tachycardia, although to a lesser degree with repeated administration. In studies in asthmatic patients with concomitant cardiovascular disease, hexoprenaline caused no adverse effects. Other actions include inhibition of uterine contractions, glycogenolysis, and lipolysis.

Hexoprenaline is active by the oral and i.v. routes and by inhalation. It is slowly metabolized, partly to the 3-O-methyl derivative, which is also an effective bronchodilator and may add to the duration of action of hexoprenaline. Excretion of unchanged drug and metabolites is through the kidney. Hexoprenaline is used in asthmatic patients and in those with chronic obstructive airway disease. It appears to be more selective than orciprenaline or salbutamol, causing fewer cardiac effects for a similar degree of bronchodilatation. It is more effective than trimetoquinol and equieffective with orciprenaline. Side-effects occur less frequently than with fenoterol or orciprenaline and include tachycardia, tremor, sweating, and dizziness. Hexoprenaline is given by aerosol in doses of 200 to 400 μg four or five times daily. It may also be given by compressed air or ultrasound inhalers or through air-humidifying devices. Oral doses range from 0.5 to 1.0 mg three times daily.

Fenoterol

Fenoterol, a 4-hydroxyphenyl derivative of orciprenaline, is a highly selective β_2-adrenoceptor–agonist with a prolonged duration of action. It is effective when given orally or by inhalation. It differs from isoprenaline in having an hydroxyphenyl residue on the isopropyl ring and a resorcinol nucleus that bestows longer activity because it is not metabolized by catechol-O-methyl transferase. In animals fenoterol is highly selective for β_2-receptors and increases ciliary activity. It is superior to isoprenaline, hexoprenaline, and salbutamol in protecting against spasmogenic agents and has minimal cardiac effects after inhalation. After rapid absorption fenoterol is conjugated with sulfuric acid and is excreted rapidly by the kidneys and liver, mainly in this conjugated form. Clinical studies show it to be as effective as salbutamol, orciprenaline, and terbutaline. A mean maximum increase of 20% in forced expiratory volume in 1 second has been reported, most of the increase occurring in 10 to 15 minutes. Side-effects such as tremor, palpitations, and nervousness occur more often after oral administration than after inhalation. The amount of drug administered by metered aerosol is 200 μg per puff, the standard dose being 2 puffs two or three times daily.

ANTICHOLINERGIC BRONCHODILATOR DRUGS

Ipratropium bromide

Muscarinic blocking drugs depress bronchial secretions and induce bronchodilatation. However, they cause excessive drying of secretions, leading to difficulty in expectoration. Ipratropium is a congener of methylatropine that produces bronchodilatation by inhibiting cholinergic bronchomotor tone. As expected, it has little effect on serotonin- or histamine-induced bronchospasm but offers protection against a cholinergic challenge. It is more effective in reversing bronchospasm in patients with chronic bronchitis than in those with allergic asthma. Fifty percent of the response after inhalation is seen within a few minutes, although its maximum effect may be delayed for 2 hours. The duration of effect varies between 4 and 6 hours. The maximum effective dose is 20 to 40 μg, doses in excess of 40 μg having little additional effect. Mucociliary clearance and the volume and viscosity of the sputum are not altered by ipratropium, and, after inhalation of the usual therapeutic dose, cardiovascular effects are not seen.

After oral administration, 30% of the drug is absorbed. A smaller fraction is absorbed after inhalation. At equieffective bronchodilator doses, the plasma concentration is 1000 times greater after the oral dose. Peak plasma concentrations are achieved at 3 hours. Ipratropium is metabolized in the liver and excreted in the feces and by the kidney. Its plasma half-life is about 3.5 hours. In clinical trials, ipratropium is less effective than salbutamol or fenoterol in asthmatic patients. In patients with chronic bronchitis, it has been as effective as β_2-adrenoceptor–agonists. Interestingly, it has been equally effective in atopic and nonatopic asthmatic patients, whereas β-adrenoceptor–agonists exert a greater bronchodilator effect in atopic persons. In some studies, the response to ipratropium increased after several months of treatment, and combination therapy with β_2-adrenoceptor–agonists was more effective than therapy with either drug alone. Adverse effects are usually transient and local and include a dry mouth and bad taste. The usually prescribed dose is 20 to 40 μg (1–2 puffs) at 8 to 12 hourly intervals.

DRUGS USED TO PREVENT ASTHMATIC ATTACKS

Ketotifen

Ketotifen is the first oral preparation for the prevention of allergic-type asthmatic attacks. It is chemically related to pizotifen, which is used in the prevention of migraine. Like disodium chromoglycate, ketotifen prevents the liberation of histamine and other mediator substances from mast cells. It is also an H_1-receptor antagonist and inhibits phosphodiesterase. Ketotifen has no effect on acetylcholine or serotonin. It is well absorbed and has a duration of effect of 12 hours. Unlike disodium chromoglycate, which has an early onset of action, ketotifen's maximum effect takes several weeks. It may be as effective as disodium chromoglycate and more effective than antihistamines in preventing allergic asthma. It is not intended for use in nonallergic asthma or for children. Side-effects include drowsiness, which may be marked, and patients should be warned about driving or operating machinery. Other side-effects are dry mouth, headache, and dizziness. The dose is 1 to 2 mg every 12 hours.

BETA-ADRENOCEPTOR BLOCKING DRUGS

ACEBUTALOL

Acebutalol is both a cardioselective β-adrenoceptor antagonist and a membrane stabilizer. However, at therapeutic concentrations, membrane stabilizing activity is probably of no clinical importance. It is well absorbed but undergoes first-pass metabolism, reducing bioavailability to 20% to 60%. It has a long half-life. Acebutalol is partly metabolized to acetyl-acebutalol (28%), which is active and which rises to levels in excess of the parent drug, and thus may have important beta-blocking and antiarrhythmic properties. Elimination of metabolites and unchanged drug (15%) is through the kidneys. Side-effects are similar to those for beta-blockers generally.

PINDOLOL

Pindolol is a nonselective beta-blocker with marked intrinsic sympathetic activity, that is, it induces a tachycardia in animals depleted of noradrenaline. It causes a fall in blood pressure with little change in plasma renin activity after acute administration, suggesting a dissociation between its blood pressure lowering effect and changes in plasma renin. Beta-blockers with intrinsic sympathetic activity such as pindolol may be useful in patients with asthma or cardiac failure when beta-adrenoceptor blocking drugs are needed. Interestingly, in overdose, this drug may cause hypertension; otherwise the side-effects are similar to those of propranolol, although pindolol seems to have a propensity to cause nightmares. The average dose is 15 mg daily in divided doses.

PENBUTOLOL

Penbutolol is a nonselective beta-blocker that, like pindolol, has some intrinsic sympathetic activity. It has a long duration of action, with a significant fall in heart rate persisting for 24 hours after a single dose. However, whether angina would be controlled by penbutolol for this length of time is not known. Penbutolol is rapidly absorbed, and unlike *sotalol* and *alprenolol,* two other nonselective beta-blockers available in Europe, has a high bioavailability (100%). It is extensively metabolized and excreted mainly as the glucoronide of the parent drug. One of its metabolites, 4-hydroxy penbutolol, is active although its contribution to the clinical effect is not known. The parent drug has a long plasma half-life (26 hours) and is thus suitable for once daily administration. Penbutolol has a flat dose-response curve suitable for rapid titration, and a further fall in blood pressure is rarely seen in doses in excess of 40 mg.

The profile of side-effects seen with penbutolol is similar to propranolol, although nightmares and hallucinations may be less frequent. The dose is 20 to 40 mg once or twice daily.

OTHER β-ADRENOCEPTOR BLOCKING DRUGS

Sotalol, a nonselective beta-blocker with a long half-life (5–13 hours), lacks a membrane stabilizing effect or intrinsic sympathetic activity but has effects on ventricular repolarization and refractoriness not seen with propranolol at usual doses. Thus it may have additional antiarrhythmic properties. It is excreted mainly unchanged in the urine (75%), and its half-life is prolonged in renal impairment. *Timolol* is available for the treatment of glaucoma and hypertension. It is a potent nonselective beta-blocker with little agonist activity. It has a high bioavailability (75%) and is metabolized in the liver. Metabolites and active drug (10%) are excreted in the urine. Its half-life is 4 to 5 hours. *Alprenolol* is another nonselective beta-blocker that, like propranolol, is highly lipid soluble.

TABLE 83-3. Comparison of Beta-Adrenergic Blocking Drugs

	β-Blocking Potency (Propranolol = 1)	Cardioselectivity	ISA*	Membrane Stabilizing Effect	Plasma Half-Life	Daily Dose
					hr	*mg*
Acebutalol	0.3	+	+	+	8	200–600
Alprenolol	0.3	0	++	+	2–3	10
Oxprenolol	0.5–1	0	++	+	2–3	160–320
Pindolol	6.0	0	+++	+	3–4	10–15
Sotalol	0.3	0	0	0	15–17	160–240
Timolol	6.0	0	±	0	4–5	20–30
Penbutolol	4.0	0	++	+	26	20–40

* ISA = intrinsic sympathomimetic activity.

ANTIARRHYTHMIC DRUGS

TOCAINIDE

Tocainide is a new antiarrhythmic drug structurally similar to lidocaine except that it is active after oral and parenteral administration. Tocainide does not have the two ethyl groups of lidocaine; thus it does not have a high first-pass

LIDOCAINE

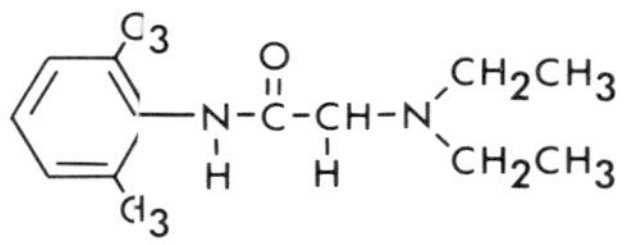

TOCAINIDE

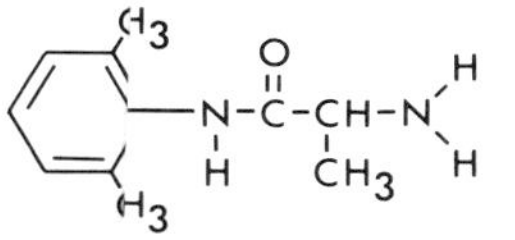

MEXILETINE

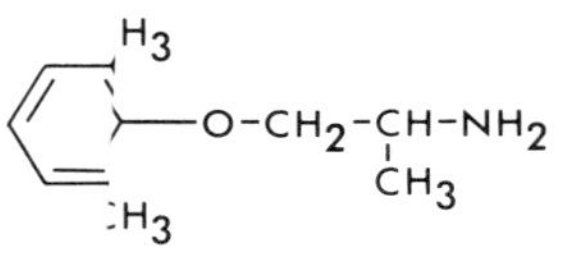

metabolism, and bioavailability is high. Like lidocaine, it is a class 1b antiarrhythmic in that it reduces the rate of depolarization of Purkinje and ventricular myocardial muscle fibers with little effect on atrioventricular conduction or atrial myocardium. It causes a rise in systemic vascular resistance and blood pressure with little effect on cardiac output or left ventricular end-diastolic pressure. Tocainide is rapidly absorbed and, unlike lidocaine, has a long half-life (12–15 hours). Peak levels of the drug occur at 60 to 90 minutes. Sixty percent of the drug is metabolized by the liver, and 40% is excreted unchanged in the urine. As with lidocaine and mexiletine, elimination is erratic after myocardial infarction and is reduced in cardiac failure.

Tocainide is used to treat ventricular ectopic beats and ventricular tachyarrhythmias after myocardial infarction, its use in this situation being similar to that of lidocaine. Because of a prolonged half-life, however, tocainide lacks the flexibility of the parent compound during acute therapy. One advantage is that once the arrhythmia has been controlled by parenteral treatment, the patient can be maintained on oral tocainide therapy. Tocainide is also used in the long-term management of chronic ventricular arrhythmias. Side-effects are uncommon except during i.v. loading, when signs of central nervous system toxicity (dizziness, tremor, nystagmus) may occur transiently. More recently hematologic abnormalities have been described during chronic administration. Tocainide is usually given in a dose of 400 to 800 mg at 8-hour intervals.

MEXILETINE

Mexiletine is a primary amine structurally related to lidocaine but, unlike it, is active orally. It is a class 1b drug with little effect on the atrial myocardium or on atrioventricular conduction. It may cause hypotension and bradycardia and has little effect on myocardial contractility. Mexiletine is well absorbed, achieving peak concentration in 2 to 4 hours, and has a bioavailability of 88%. It is metabolized in the liver, 10% being excreted as unchanged drug, although this decreases in the presence of an alkaline urine. Its plasma T½ is 10 to 12 hours in normal subjects, becoming more prolonged in heart disease. Following a loading dose, mexiletine may be given intravenously by infusion. It is used to treat acute and chronic ventricular arrhythmias and is as effective as lidocaine in postmyocardial infarction arrhythmias.

Mexiletine has few side-effects and thus is useful for the long-term treatment of cardiac arrhythmias. Side-effects occur most frequently during i.v. loading and are minimized by slow administration. Neurologic side-effects include dizziness, tremor, nystagmus, and ataxia. Hypotension and bradycardia may occur in as many as 14% of cases. Thrombocytopenic purpura and the development of a positive antinuclear factor have been reported during oral therapy. Peak plasma levels after oral therapy are delayed, so that i.v. loading may be indicated if a rapid effect is needed. The loading dose is 400 to 600 mg followed by a maintenance therapy of 200 to 400 mg every 8 hours.

AMIODARONE

The clinical observation that few hypothyroid patients suffer from angina or cardiac arrhythmias stimulated the development of a drug structurally related to thyroxine. Amiodarone is a benzfuran derivative first introduced as an antianginal agent in Europe in 1967 but later noted to have antiarrhythmic properties. It is a class-3 antiarrhythmic drug in that it prolongs the refractory period. It acts on both atrial and ventricular myocardium and depresses atrioventricular conduction. At higher doses, amiodarone depresses myocardial contractility. It decreases cardiac work and myocardial oxygen consumption, which, combined with a direct vasodilator effect on coronary arteries, explains its antianginal effect. It also has weak alpha- and beta-adrenergic receptor blocking effects and reduces heart rate and blood pressure.

Amiodarone, 50% absorbed from the gastrointestinal tract, achieves peak plasma levels at 4 to 6 hours, which is too slow for the treatment of acute life-threatening arrhythmias, in which case it can be given intravenously. Amiodarone binds strongly to many tissues and is excreted slowly, the plasma half-life being about 2 weeks. Therefore a therapeutic tissue level is slowly achieved during initial therapy, and it may take several weeks for the full antiarrhythmic effect to be seen. Similarly, after treatment has been discontinued, the drug may continue to be effective for weeks.

Amiodarone has long-term side-effects that make it unsuitable as a first choice in treating chronic cardiac arrhythmias. It is most useful in treating arrhythmias resistant to less toxic agents. Amiodarone is effective in treating ventricular ectopic beats and ventricular tachyarrhythmias. It is of value in the long-term prevention of reentrant nodal tachycardias associated with the Wolff–Parkinson–White (WPW) syndrome, especially in patients who develop fast atrial arrhythmias (atrial fibrillation, atrial flutter) that, in the presence of a drug-induced decrease in conduction at the atrioventricular node, may be conducted down the accessory pathway. Because there is no natural delay in the accessory pathway, a rapid ventricular rate with an increased risk of ventricular tachycardia and fibrillation result. Amiodarone decreases conduction of the accessory pathways as well as the atrioventricular node and thus prevents a fast ventricular response to atrial tachyarrhythmias.

Amiodarone is well tolerated by patients and causes few gastrointestinal symptoms. The most consistent side-effect is reversible microdeposits of yellow-brown pigment in the cornea that may interfere with vision. Deposits may also occur in the skin, causing a bluish discoloration that resolves when the drug is withdrawn. Electron microscopy demonstrates the presence of histiocytes that contain melanin and lipofuscin. In patients with conduction defects, heart block may occur. Thyroid function tests are altered in some patients, with a rise in serum T_4 and a fall in T_3 owing to depression of the peripheral conversion of T_4 to T_3. Protein-bound iodine is also increased. Hypothyroidism and hyperthyroidism have been reported, but biochemical changes in the absence of clinical disease is more common. The dose of the drug is 200 to 800 mg as a once-daily dose. For rapid control of arrhythmias, 5 to 10 mg of amiodarone is given by slow i.v. injection.

APRINDINE

Aprindine, developed in Belgium, is a class-1b antiarrhythmic with a prominent local anesthetic action. It is currently under investigation in the United States. Like all class-1b drugs, aprindine depresses the rate of depolarization in myocardial cells, and in this respect is more effective than lidocaine. It differs from other class-1b drugs in prolonging conduction at the atrioventricular node and the His bundle. Aprindine acts on both atrial and ventricular muscle, blocking conduction in accessory bundles of patients with WPW syndrome. Myocardial contractility is mildly depressed by this drug, and widening of the QRS of the electrocardiogram may occur.

Generally, aprindine is well absorbed, although absorption may be erratic in postinfarction patients. Aprindine is 85% to 95% protein bound, and after hydroxylation in the liver the metabolites are eliminated in the urine (65%) and feces (35%) as glucuronides, only 1% of the drug being excreted unchanged. Its plasma half-life is long and variable, the average being about 28 hours. Aprindine is more effective than disopyramide in treating ventricular ectopics and is effective in treating ventricular tachyarrhythmias even when they have failed to respond to lidocaine or quinidine. It prevents the reentrant nodal tachycardias of WPW syndrome and, because it blocks the accessory pathways, can be used in patients with associated atrial tachyarrhythmias.

Aprindine has a small toxic therapeutic ratio, and central nervous system and gastrointestinal side-effects may occur even at therapeutic plasma levels. Central nervous system side-effects, including tremor, dizziness, and ataxia, are seen in 20% of patients. Gastrointestinal symptoms (nausea, vomiting, diarrhea) occur less frequently. More disturbing are reports of agranulocytosis and cholestatic jaundice. Agranulocytosis occurs infrequently and is usually reversible after withdrawal of the drug. It is not dose related and appears to be an idiosyncratic reaction. However, this potentially fatal side-efft restricts the use of aprindine to patients vh life-threatening arrhythmias that do not spond to less toxic agents. The dose of the ug is 100 to 200 mg once daily, after a loadz dose of 200 to 400 mg. For rapid control o tachyarrhythmias, 80 to 160 mg may be ;en intravenously in increments of 20 mg 2-minute intervals.

NONSTEROID. ANTIINFLAMMATORY DRUGS

The modern era antirheumatic drugs began with the develoрnt of aspirin by Felix Hoffman in 1893 anoday has mushroomed into a bewildering groı of agents. The benefit of a wide range of ısteroidal antiinflammatory drugs lies in thect that patients' responses to therapy are unıdictable, and many agents may be tried bre any clinical response is seen. Generally,ewer agents have fewer side-effects, particuly gastrointestinal, and in many cases theplasma half-lives are longer such that onceaily administration is sufficient. Althoughost of the newer drugs (Table 83-4) induce gric erosions and intestinal blood loss less quently than does uncoated aspirin, they h: rarely been compared with enteric-coated ;irin.

PROPIONIC AC DERIVATIVES

Propionic acid rivatives act, at least partly, by supressing ›staglandin synthesis. Newer drugs in this gıp are similar in most respects to the originalugs naproxyn and ibuprofen. Generally, the re better tolerated than aspirin and do noterfere with oral anticoagulants. Fenoprn, flurbiprofen, and fenbufen are not yet avıble in the United States.

FENOPROFEN

Fenoprofen hantiinflammatory, antipyretic, and analgesicoperties in animal models and in humans. Inhibits collagen-induced, but not ADP-indud, platelet aggregation and inhibits prostandin synthesis. In animal models, fenofen causes less gastrointestinal blood loss thdoes aspirin. Absorption is reduced by foodd aspirin, and the calcium salt is less well arbed than the sodium salt. Fenoprofen is 99rotein bound but binds to a different site tı do oral anticoagulants, and therefore doaot displace them. This drug is extensively metabolized and has a short plasma T½—2 to 3 hours. Fenoprofen is as effective as aspirin in the treatment of rheumatoid arthritis. It is also effective in gout and osteoarthritis. Side-effects include dyspepsia, nausea, and skin rashes, which occur more frequently than with naproxen.

FLURBIPROFEN

Like fenoprofen, flurbiprofen has antipyretic, antiinflammatory, and analgesic properties. It is a potent inhibitor of prostaglandin synthesis possibly by inhibiting endoperoxygenase, which catalyzes the conversion of arachidonic acid to cyclic endoperoxide. Flurbiprofen inhibits collagen, adrenaline, and ADP-induced platelet aggregation without prolonging the bleeding time. It is readily absorbed, with peak plasma concentrations at 1.5 to 3 hours. Synovial fluid concentration exceeds plasma concentration at 12 hours, which may prolong the duration of action of the drug. Glucoronide and sulfate conjugates and free drug (20–25%) are excreted in the urine, the plasma T½ being 3.5 hours. It is as effective as aspirin or indomethacin in rheumatoid arthritis, although it causes fewer abdominal or central nervous system complaints than either drug. Flurbiprofen is also useful in treating osteoarthritis. As with all these drugs, flurbiprofen is given under supervision to patients with gastrointestinal complaints and avoided in patients with active peptic ulceration.

Fenbufen has a longer T½—10 hours—and is therefore suitable for once- or twice-daily administration. Otherwise its side-effects and indications are similar to those of fenoprofen and flurbiprofen.

FENAMATES

The fenamates are structurally related to salicylates but have the unique property of blocking the action of formed prostaglandins as well as inhibiting their synthesis. Flufenamic acid and meclofenamate sodium are not available in the United States.

FLUFENAMIC ACID

Flufenamic acid is well, although slowly, absorbed, achieving peak plasma levels at 6 hours. It is extensively metabolized and excreted through the kidney as metabolites and

TABLE 83-4. Nonsteroidal Antiinflammatory Drugs

	Analgesic	Antiinflammatory	Half-Life	Da Dose	Doses per Day
			hr	*mg*	*no.*
Propionic acid derivatives					
Fenoprofen	++	+++	2–3	12C2400	3–4
Flurbiprofen	++	+++	3–5	15300	3–4
Fenbufen	++	+++	10	60900	2
Fenamates					
Flufenamic acid	++	++	9	40600	2–3
Meclofenamate sodium			?	20400	3
Phenylacetic acid derivatives					
Diclofenac	++	+++	1–12	5150	3
Fenclofenac			12–21	601200	1–2
Piroxicam	++	++	40	160	1
Pyrazole derivatives					
Feprazone			24	20000	3
Azapropazone	++	+++	12	120(	4
Salicylate derivatives					
Diflunisal	++	+	5–11	500000	2
Benorylate	++	+	?	4000000	3

unchanged drug (21%). Both flufenamic and mefenamic acids are protein bound, where they displace oral anticoagulants. By increasing the plasma level of free anticoagulant, they potentiate its action and thus are relatively contraindicated in patients who need anticoagulant therapy. Flufenamic acid is used to treat rheumatoid and other inflammatory arthritides. Side-effects include gastrointestinal disturbances, particularly diarrhea, although this is not as troublesome as it is with mefenamic acid. Central nervous system complaints are infrequent and include headaches and dizziness. Hematologic abnormalities have not been reported as they have with mefenamic acid.

PHENYLACETIC ACID DERIVATIVES

Diclofenac sodium and *fenclofenac* are derived from phenylacetic acid; both are effective antiinflammatory analgesics. They act by irreversible inhibition of prostaglandin synthesis, and in animal studies their antiinflammatory effect exceeds aspirin and naproxen. *In vitro*, diclofenac inhibits platelet oxygenation, but this does not occur at the usual oral dose. In healthy subjects gastric mucosal changes occur less with these drugs than with aspirin or naproxen. Both drugs are well absorbed and undergo hepatic metabolism. The plasma T½ of diclofenac (1.5 hours) is short compared with that of fenclofenac (12–21 hours), which may be given once or twice dai These drugs are recommended in the treatnt of less severe rheumatic conditions. Theiде-effects include gastrointestinal disturbanc skin rashes, and headache. A slow release paration of diclofenac is now available that l reduce the need for frequent doses. A thi member of this group, *aclofenac*, has sinr properties but may cause severe skin rasl.

PYRAZOLE DERIVATIVES

Feprazone and *azapropazc* have chemical structures similar to that ohenylbutazone. Both are well absorbed arhave prolonged plasma T½ suitable for oncer twice-daily administration of the drugs. Aropazone is excreted largely as unchangeшug (60%); thus the dose should be reduced iatients with impaired renal function. Thedrugs have the same antiinflammatory acti as do propionic acid derivatives, and indicans for their use are the same. Side-effects inde gastrointestinal discomfort and skin ra Unlike phenylbutazone, marrow toxicity s not been reported.

PIROXICAM

Piroxicam, a recently develd nonsteroidal antiinflammatory analgesic, not chemically related to other drugs in thisoup. It causes less gastrointestinaod loss than does uncoated aspirin in ail models. It reversibly inhibits the cyclooxase step of arachidonic acid metabolism ahe secondary phase of platelet aggregatioduced by collagen and ADP. It is well absd orally and rectally and is extensively metzed to inactive metabolites. Its plasma Ts long (40 hours); thus once daily adminison is sufficient. Steady-state levels are nchieved in less than 1 week, and therefoiration of the dose should be carried out slowPiroxicam is as effective as indomethacin ibuprofen in treating rheumatoid arthrind has been found useful in managing goud osteoarthritis. Side-effects are dose rel but at commonly used doses occur less juently than with indomethacin and asp Piroxicam is contraindicated in asthmatatients who cannot tolerate aspirin.

SALICYLATE DEFTIVES

Although not neroidal antiinflammatory agents, salicylatéivatives are included here because they ared in the same conditions. Two salicylate datives available in Europe but not in the Ud States are diflunisal and benorylate. Bothgs cause less gastrointestinal blood loss anscomfort than does aspirin. *Diflunisal* has ag plasma T½ (12 hours), which allows twdaily dosage. It has slight antiinflammatos well as analgesic properties but does naffect platelet function or bleeding time. I/8% protein bound and may displace proteinding of oral anticoagulants. Diflunisal is beitolerated than aspirin. Because it is partlycreted unchanged, the dose should be redu in patients with renal impairment.

Benorylate ietabolized to aspirin and paracetamol, a high circulating levels of salicylate may ur, causing signs and symptoms of salicyli Further, in overdose, paracetamol plasnlevels sufficient to cause hepatic toxicityay occur.

NEUROLEPTS (MAJOR TRANQUILIZS)

DIPHENYLBUT'IPERIDINES

Pimozide

Pimozide is throtootype of the diphenylbutylpiperidines, a mical class separate from the butyrophenones and phenothiazines. It acts by blocking dopamine receptors but has no adrenoceptor blocking properties. Animal behavioral tests show that it resembles haloperidol.

In clinical studies pimozide is as effective as fluphenazine. Thought disorder and apathy tend to improve while the drug is being taken, although violence and excitement may worsen. Side-effects are as common as with fluphenazine, with about half the patients developing extrapyramidal side-effects. Facial edema and disorganized psychotic behavior may also occur. It is given orally as a once-daily dose of 10 mg.

Fluspirilene

Fluspirilene is a long-acting injectable neuroleptic belonging to the diphenylbutylpiperidine group. It acts as a central dopamine receptor antagonist and has little effect on central adrenoceptors. It is a potent histamine antagonist but has no effect on cholinergic or serotonin receptors. Fluspirilene is injected intramuscularly as a microcrystalline aqueous suspension, and its slow absorption from the injected site ensures a long duration of action. Previously available depot neuroleptics are released by gradual hydrolysis of the fatty acid ester of the active drug, and plasma concentrations tend to vary between patients. In contrast, fluspirilene absorption depends on the solubility of the drug, and plasma concentrations tend to be more consistent between patients. Plasma concentrations are maximal at 24 hours and begin to decline after 3 days. Clinical trials suggest that the effects of a single injection lasts about 8 days. It is as effective as depot injections of fluphenazine or oral trifluoperazine in treating schizophrenia, and fluspirilene alleviates symptoms of withdrawal and apathy. Side-effects are similar to those that occur with existing neuroleptics but are less frequent. Extrapryamidal effects occur between 12 and 48 hours after each injection. Fatigue and subcutaneous nodules at the site of injection may also occur. The drug is given in a dose of 2 to 8 mg once per week.

CHEMOTHERAPEUTIC AGENTS: ANTICANCER DRUGS

ETOPOSIDE

Etoposide is a semisynthetic glucosidic derivative of podophyllotoxin, the main active constituent of podophyllin. Etoposide is insoluble in water and is dissolved in a detergent mixture that includes polyethylene glycol and ethanol to give an oily solution. It acts by arresting cells in the G2 (premitotic) phase of the cell cycle, and this persists despite removal of the drug from the bathing fluid. It also induces single-strand breaks in DNA, which appears to be an important mechanism in the antitumor activity of the drug, at least in laboratory animals. The drug prevents the cell uptake of thymidine and uridine, although at low concentrations uridine uptake is enhanced. Unlike podophyllotoxin, it has no effect on the *in vitro* assembly of microtubules.

After i.v. administration of the drug, 60% is excreted over the next 72 hours, the fate of the remaining 40% being uncertain. Forty-four percent of the drug is excreted in the urine, mostly unchanged. The drug is also available in oral form, a large gelatin capsule that some patients find difficult to swallow. Bioavailability studies have not been carried out, but clinical data suggest that absorption is about 50% of the oral dose.

Clinical trials have shown that etoposide is one of the most active agents tested against small-cell lung cancer. It has been combined successfully with cisplatin to treat squamous cell carcinoma of the lung. Other responsive malignancies include nonseminomatous testicular cancers, acute leukemia, particularly when there is a monocytic component, and both Hodgkin's and non-Hodgkin's lymphomas.

Dose-related side-effects include nausea and vomiting (25%), both more likely with the oral preparation. Alopecia occurs in 35% of patients. Dose-related myelosuppression presents as neutropenia after 8 to 10 days of administration, and thrombocytopenia occurs 2 to 3 days later. At doses of 170 mg/m²/week, neutropenia is seen in 100% of patients and thrombocytopenia in 13%. However, septicemia occurs infrequently, and marrow recovery is complete by Day 20. Stomatitis has also been reported, and transient hypertension may occur as a reaction to the solvent mixture used in the i.v. preparation. Generally, side-effects are fewer than those with many currently available agents. Dose-scheduling studies have not indicated any particular regimen as being superior. Usually 60 mg/m², is given once daily for 5 days intravenously, and this is repeated for 2 to 3 weeks. The oral dose is 120 mg/m². Precautions include a test dose to guard against a hypersensitivity reaction and repeated blood screening.

RAZOXANE

Razoxane is a pipera derivative of the chelating agent EDTA. ‹ests the cell cycle between the premitotic and early mitotic (M) phases of the cell cy It suppresses metastases in some animal ors and is synergistic with other antimitoti gs. Razoxane potentiates radiotherapy aby depressing B-cell function, has some i nosuppressive properties. Clinical trials ve been carried out mainly in patients esponsive to other chemotherapeutic ag and thus its role has not been established. is effective in non-Hodgkin's lymphoma Kaposi hemangiosarcoma unresponsive other therapy. Combined with radiothera may reduce the size of sarcomas or induce emission. Razoxane has also been shown to e antipsoriatic properties but has not, as ye en approved for use in psoriasis.

Side-effects includ ose-related leukopenia, which resolves n the drug is withdrawn. Skin reactions radiotherapy occur more frequently in pat s taking razoxane, and late complications lude pneumonitis, subcutaneous fibrosis, a sophagitis, if these areas are irradiated.

MISCELLANEOUS DGS

LEVAMISOLE

Levamisole is a levo-isor of tetramisole, an effective anthelmintic a . Levamisole has been used to treat variou festations, including ascaris lumbricoide nd dipetalonema perstans, a filarial paras More recently, it has been shown to hav munomodulating properties that may be xploited to treat immune disorders and so malignancies. Levamisole stimulates paras pathetic and sympathetic ganglia and, by i iting norepinephrine uptake, may have antidepressant effect. In nematodes suc ascaris lumbricoides, it inhibits fumarat ductase. Most attention, however, is no focused on the changes in the immune sy m induced by levamisole. Animal studie uggest that, depending on the dose of t rug, levamisole may act either as an immu timulant or as an immunosuppressant. It in ses the number of activated T lymphocytes aving B-lymphocyte activity unchanged. L misole also augments macrophage chemo s, mobility, and phagocytosis. Although tot ntibody production is unaltered, early synthesis of IgG antibodies in response to an antigen is triggered. Further, neutrophil mobility, adherence, and chemotaxis are increased. The immunopotentiation of levamisole may be due to the release of a serum factor that resembles thymic hormones in stimulating T-cell differentiation. Levamisole also has dose-dependent immunosuppressive effects against various antigens.

Levamisole is rapidly absorbed, peak plasma levels occurring within 2 to 4 hours. The drug is extensively metabolized in the liver, and only 5% is excreted unchanged. One of its metabolites, dl-2-oxo-3-(2-mercaptoethyl)-5-phenylimidazolidine, may be important in enhancing leukocyte function by protecting leukocytes from auto-oxidative necrosis.

Levamisole is used as an anthelmintic, usually as a single dose of 120 mg or in combination with other anthelmintics. Its role in such conditions as Crohn's disease, sarcoidosis, and rheumatoid arthritis is currently under investigation. Side-effects include severe nausea and vomiting (0.5%), allergy, and a disulfiramlike reaction with alcohol. Agranulocytosis has been reported in patients with rheumatoid arthritis treated with levamisole and is reversible on withdrawal of the drug.

CALCIUM CARBIMIDE

Like disulfiram, calcium carbimide is an inhibitor of hepatic aldehyde-NAD oxidoreductase (ALDH), causing increased plasma acetaldehyde levels after ingestion of alcohol. Unlike disulfiram, inhibition of ALDH is rapid and reversible, with 80% of activity restored within 24 hours of administration. Thus calcium carbamide sensitizes the patient to alcohol by inhibiting the metabolism of acetaldehyde. The extent of the carbimide reaction depends on the dose of alcohol ingested. With small doses of alcohol, patients experience flushing, tachycardia, tachypnea, and dyspnea lasting 30 minutes. Higher doses of ethanol induce vomiting and nausea, and the symptoms are more prolonged. The prospect of this unpleasant reaction either deters alcohol consumption or reduces intake.

Calcium carbimide is rapidly absorbed after hydrolysis to carbimide in the gastrointestinal tract. Little is known of its pharmacokinetics but in view of its short duration of action metabolism must be extremely rapid. No rigorous studies of the efficacy of calcium carbimide have been reported. The intensity of the carbimide reaction varies between patients and in the same patient on different occasions. Tolerance to the reaction can develop with repeated ethanol ingestion, but with abstinence this tolerance wanes. Carbimide causes fewer side-effects than does disulfiram during long-term administration. Unlike disulfiram, carbimide does not inhibit dopamine-β-hydroxylase and thus does not cause behavioral changes or drowsiness. Peripheral neuropathy and hepatocyte inclusions have been described. High doses may cause nausea, vomiting, and headaches. Carbimide does not inhibit the metabolism of phenytoin and may be preferable to disulfiram when concomitant anticonvulsant therapy is required. The dose of carbimide is 50 mg twice daily.

NEFOPAM

Nefopam belongs to a new class of analgesics, the benzoxazocines, related to orphenadrine but with little antihistaminic effect. Its mode of action is unknown. It does not cause respiratory depression and is not antagonized by naloxone. Nefopam has no effect on prostaglandin synthesis and is not an antiinflammatory drug. It has clinically significant anticholinergic and sympathomimetic effects. Animal studies suggest that nefopam has no abuse potential; however, it does have mild amphetaminelike effects and has not been available for sufficient time to assess the risk in patients. Nefopam has about 0.2 to 0.6 times the analgesic potency of morphine. As with many analgesics, a ceiling occurs in analgesic effect with increasing doses, and maximum response is seen with 60 mg as a single oral dose.

Nefopam is well absorbed from the gastrointestinal tract, reaching peak plasma levels at 1 to 3 hours. It is 75% protein bound and is extensively metabolized, only 5% being excreted in the urine unchanged. The plasma $T\frac{1}{2}$ of nefopam is about 4 hours and is not altered after repeated administration. Clinical studies have shown it to be effective in postoperative pain and pain due to malignancy, giving good or excellent relief in up to 85% of patients. It compares favorably with dextropropoxyphene and pentazocine.

Side-effects include nausea and sweating (10–30%), sedation (20–30%), and pain at the injection site. Nefopam causes less gastrointestinal blood loss than does aspirin. Respiratory depression does not occur in healthy subjects; however, it has not been assessed in patients with chronic respiratory diseases. Dry mouth may occur because of nefopam's anticholinergic effect, which may also precipitate glaucoma and urinary retention in susceptible patients. The starting dose is 30 mg three or four times daily. The dose can be increased to 60 mg and the intervals between doses shortened if pain has not been relieved. Parenteral doses are one third those recommended for oral use.

PIZOTIFEN

Pizotifen is structurally related to cyprohepatidine and has strong antiserotonin, antihistaminic, antitryptaminic, and anticholinergic actions. It is recommended for prophylaxis in migraine headache. Pizotifen is well absorbed and has an average T½ of 20 hours. In clinical studies it reduced the number of migraine attacks as effectively as methysergide, an effect that persists on long-term treatment. Unwanted effects include drowsiness and weight gain owing to an increased appetite. As with methysergide, muscle pain occurs, but the serious side-effects associated with methysergide have not been reported with pizotifen. It can be used in combination with drugs effective in aborting or relieving acute attacks. Pizotifen is given in doses of 0.5 mg three times daily, increasing to a maximum of 6 mg/day.

FAZADINIUM

Fazadinium bromide is a nondepolarizing neuromuscular blocking drug. It is a bisquarternary azapyridine and has a distinctive yellow color. Animal studies have shown that fazadinium does not depolarize the muscle end-plate but causes competitive neuromuscular blockade easily reversed by anticholinesterases. Its effects are partly antagonized by depolarizing drugs such as suxemethonium. In animals, fazadinium has a rapid onset of action and is short acting because it is rapidly hydrolyzed. In humans, it has a similarly rapid onset but a more prolonged action, since it is slowly hydrolyzed. Fazadinium is excreted by the kidney and may accumulate in patients with renal impairment. The rapidity of onset and duration of muscular relaxation are dose dependent. At higher doses, rapid and complete reversal may not always follow injections of neostigimine. Fazadinium has the advantage over depolarizing muscle relaxants in having fewer side-effects and in being rapidly reversed by neostigimine. Further, in patients in whom muscle relaxation is required for a short period after intubation, fazadinium can be used alone instead of with a combination of suxamethonium and tubocurarine. Side-effects include tachycardia, even at doses sufficient to produce paralysis, and occasionally urticaria and wheezing.

MINOR TRANQUILIZERS AND HYPNOTICS

BENZODIAZEPINES

More than 2000 benzodiazepines have been synthesized, and many of these have been introduced into European markets but are not yet available in the United States. Many of these drugs are prodrugs that form active metabolites on which their clinical effects depend. Indeed many new drugs such as chlorazpeate and ketazolam resemble diazepam in that they are rapidly converted to the same metabolite, desmethydiazepam (nordiazepam). Some of these newer drugs should therefore differ little from diazepam. Other new benzodiazepines are metabolites of diazepam, such as temazepam, and have shorter half-lives that make them suitable as hypnotics, since they have little hangover effect. Although there is some evidence on the basis of EEG patterns and alterations in the stages of sleep that hypnotic and antianxiety effects of newer drugs can be differentiated, all benzodiazepines have sedative, hypnotic, anticonvulsant, and muscle-relaxant properties. Indeed, the effect seen may depend largely on the dose used and time of administration. For example, temazepam is recommended in the United Kingdom as a hyp-

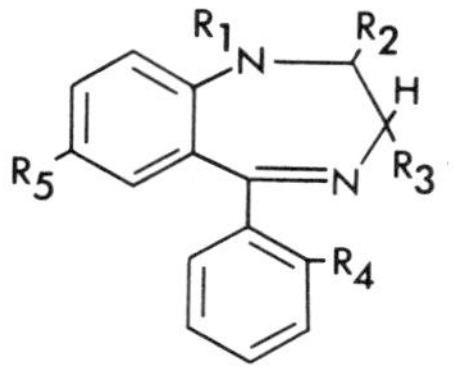

BASIC STRUCTURE 1,4 BENZODIAZEPINES

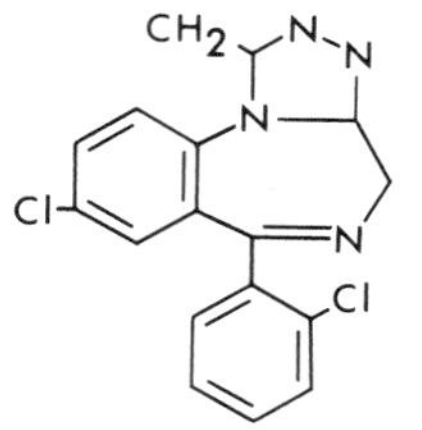

TRIAZOLAM

TABLE 83-5. Comparison of Pharmacokinetics of Benzodiazepines

Drug	Time to Peak	Plasma Half-Life	Active Metabolites	Dose	Doses per Day
	hr	*hr*		*mg*	*no.*
Desmethydiazepam		51–100	Oxazepam		
Temazepam	0.8–1.4	7.3–8.3	Oxazepam	10–30	Nocte*
Clobazam	1–4	9–30	N-Desmethylclobazam	20–30	1–2
Clorazepate	1–2	1–2	N-Desmethyldiazepam	15–30	Nocte
Nitrazepam	2	18–31	Unknown	5–10	Nocte
Triazolam	1–3	2.2	α-hydroxy-triazolam	0.25–0.5	Nocte
Medazepam	1–2	1–2	Diazepam Nordiazepam Temazepam Oxazepam	5–10	2–3
Bromazepam	Rapid	8–24	None	3–6	2–3
Ketazolam	Rapid	?	N-Desmethyldiazepam	15–30	Nocte

* At night.

notic but has been used at a lower dose in Italy as a sedative. The benzodiazepines are listed in Table 83-5, along with data on pharmacokinetics. Some of these agents are discussed in detail, particularly those for which special properties have been claimed.

CLOBAZAM

Clobazam is a 1,5 benzodiazepine that differs structurally from existing compounds that are 1,4 benzodiazepines. In animals, clobazam has antianxiety and anticonvulsant properties at doses considerably lower than those required for muscle relaxation. In human studies, it impairs psychomotor performance less than equivalent therapeutic doses of diazepam or lorazepam. Clobazam is well absorbed, with peak plasma levels occurring at 1 to 4 hours. Through an unknown effect, its bioavailability is increased by 50% with concomitant administration of alcohol. It is metabolized to N-desmethylclobazam, an active metabolite, the plasma concentration of which is eight times that of the parent drug when steady-state has been achieved. Although N-desmethylclobazam is less active than clobazam, it may have important sedative and anticonvulsant properties in the concentration achieved. Clobazam forms eight other metabolites; although the plasma T½ of the parent drug is 18 hours, the plasma T½ of some metabolites is 50 hours.

Clobazam is as effective as diazepam in treating neurotic anxiety or anxiety associated with organic disease. Diazepam is more effective in relieving muscular symptoms. Clobazam is also effective in treating alcohol withdrawal and relieves insomnia as part of a generalized antianxiety effect. Side-effects of drowsiness, sedation, and hangover are common, as with diazepam. The dose is 20 to 30 mg once daily, preferably at bedtime.

TRIAZOLAM

Triazolam, a triazolobenzodiazepine, is characterized by the inclusion of a triazol ring in the benzodiazepine structure. It has a prominent hypnotic effect in animals and, in sleep-laboratory studies in humans, causes dose-dependent changes in sleep stages claimed to be typical of other hypnotic benzodiazepines. Neither tolerance nor rebound insomnia occurs. At low doses (0.25–0.5 mg) REM sleep is not suppressed, but at higher doses suppression may occur with a rebound increase in REM sleep after drug withdrawal. Unlike flurazepam and nitrazepam, psychomotor and cognitive tests are not impaired beyond 10 hours after ingestion of 0.25 mg to 0.5 mg.

Triazolam is rapidly absorbed, achieving peak plasma concentration at 1.3 hours. Like almost all benzodiazepines, it is highly protein bound. Triazolam is metabolized extensively, and one of its metabolites, α-hydroxytriazolam, is active *in vitro*. However, because it is present in the plasma only in a conjugated form, it probably does not contribute to the pharmacologic effect. Triazolam is excreted in the urine as metabolites and has a plasma T½ varying from 2 to 7 hours.

In view of its relatively short plasma T½, triazolam probably has no hangover effect. It should thus be a suitable hypnotic in patients with sleep disorders unrelated to neurotic anxiety. In anxiety states a drug with continued sedative effect during the day may be more suitable. Triazolam is as effective as flurazepam and nitrazepam in treating chronic insomnia. In elderly persons, triazolam has not caused paradoxical agitation or a hangover effect. It induces sleep more quickly and for longer than does flurazepam. Side-effects include residual drowsiness, which is dose dependent and infrequent at doses lower than 0.5 mg, headache, dizziness, and dry mouth.

TEMAZEPAM

Temazepam is an active minor metabolite of diazepam and is used as a hypnotic. It is rapidly absorbed, achieving peak plasma concentrations in about 1 hour. It is metabolized mainly to inactive metabolites, 5% being excreted in the urine as oxazepam. Thus temazepam differs from existing benzodiazepines in not forming active metabolites with different half-lives. The plasma T½ is short relative to those of diazepam and nitrazepam—7.3 to 8.3 hours—and temazepam is therefore more suitable for use as a hypnotic. In clinical trials, 20 mg prolongs sleep by 1 hour without altering REM sleep. The onset of sleep is only slightly faster than with a placebo. In psychiatric patients there was no difference in hypnotic efficacy between temazepam and nitrazepam. Behavioral impairment tends to be less with temazepam. Because it has a short duration of action, temazepam may be less suitable for sleep disorders associated with anxiety states in patients with early morning wakening. The usual dose is 10 to 30 mg at bedtime.

CLORAZEPATE

Clorazepate resembles medazepam and diazepam in that it is a prodrug converted by acid hydrolysis in the stomach or during absorption to the active metabolite desmethyldiazepam. After i.m. injection, clorazepate reaches peak plasma concentration at 2 hours and is also converted into desmethyldiazepam. Although the plasma T½ of clorazepate is 1 to 2 hours, desmethyldiazepam has a T½ of 51 to 100 hours; thus the effective plasma T½ of the drug is prolonged, and accumulation of desmethyldiazepam proceeds for up to 2 weeks with repeated administration. Clorazepate is as effective as diazepam in treating anxiety states. Because it has a prolonged effect, chlorazepate is used to treat sleep disorders secondary to anxiety. It is given in a dose of 15 to 30 mg once daily, preferably at bedtime.

KETAZOLAM

Ketazolam, a 1,4 benzodiazepine, resembles clorazepate in that it is a prodrug and is rapidly metabolized to desmethyldiazepam. Thus it is similar to clorazepate and diazepam in its clinical use, side-effects, and contraindications. Ketazolam is given in a dose of 15 to 30 mg daily, preferably at bedtime.

ALPRAZOLAM

Alprazolam is, like triazolam, a triazolobenzodiazepine that will become available in Europe shortly. Animal studies suggest that this drug has similar anxiolytic and hypnotic effects to diazepam, although it is more potent. Alprazolam also has a muscle relaxant effect at higher doses but without causing significant depression of the respiratory or circulatory systems. In human studies using EEG and analysis of sleep stages, alprazolam has been shown to have a predominantly anxiolytic effect. It is as effective as diazepam in allaying anxiety. In addition, in one study it was found to have antidepressant effects equivalent to imipramine. If an antidepressant effect is confirmed, this would be an important departure from currently available benzodiazepines.

ANTIBIOTICS

PENICILLINS

Pivampicillin and *bacampicillin* are esters of ampicillin that, like talampicillin, are converted into ampicillin in the body. They have the same spectrum of antibiotic activity as ampicillin, their only advantage being that, like amoxicillin, they are well absorbed and less likely to cause diarrhea. Pivampicillin liberates pivalic acid and formaldehyde, which are further metabolized. Bacampicillin releases ethanol. Both drugs have a plasma T½ of just under 1 hour. Because 70% to 100% of these drugs are absorbed and excreted unchanged in the urine, they may have greater efficacy in urinary tract infections. However, the amount of ampicillin absorbed after a standard dose (30% of the oral dose) gives a concentration sufficient to inhibit pathogens. A side-effect of ampicillin esters is nausea, although with newer preparations this is less frequent.

Mecillinam and *pivmecillinam* are the first of a new group of amidino-penicillins. They differ in having the side-chain joined to the β-lactam ring by a β-amidino group rather than by a β-acylamino group, which results in their having different properties. Unlike other penicillins, these drugs act on only one enzyme in the biosynthesis of the bacterial cell wall. Pivmecillinam is the ester of mecillinam and is converted after absorption to mecillinam, which is active only when given parenterally. The drug is excreted by renal tubular excretion and in the bile as active mecillinam so that the dosage should be adjusted in renal failure. The T½ plasma is 1 hour. Its antibiotic spectrum includes most aerobic gram-negative rods such as *Escherichia coli* and *Klebsiella*. However, *Pseudomonas, Hemophilus influenzae*, and anaerobes are resistant. It is inactive against gram-positive organisms. Thus the clearest indication for their use is urinary tract infection caused by resistant gram-negative bacteria. Side-effects include gastrointestinal discomforts, vomiting (6%), and penicillinlike hypersensitivity reactions. The daily dose is 800 mg in four divided doses.

CARBENICILLIN-RELATED PENICILLINS

Mezlocillin is a semisynthetic penicillin for parenteral use. It embraces the spectrum of ampicillin and carbenicillin. *In vitro*, it is more potent than ampicillin or carbenicillin against *E. coli, Klebsiella*, indole-positive *proteus* and *Serratia*. It is hydrolyzed by the β-lactamase found in ampicillin- and carbenicillin-resistant *E. coli*. Mezlocillin is twice as active as carbenicillin against *Pseudomonas aeruginosa* and may be active against some ticarcillin- and carbenicillin-resistant strains. It has no advantage over penicillin or ampicillin against *Staphylococcus aureus*. Its plasma T½ (1 hour) is shorter than that of ticarcillin. Six hours after receiving 5 g as an i.v. bolus, the patient's plasma drug levels are below the minimal inhibitory concentration (MIC). It is therefore given as a 5-g bolus every 4 hours. Sixty percent is excreted in the urine, and the rest is eliminated in the bile, where it is concentrated. In renal failure, the T½ is little increased until the glomerular filtration rate falls below 10 ml/min. Side-effects are rare, although allergy may occur. Mezlocillin is used to treat *Pseudomonas* infections and, because aminoglycosides act synergistically with mezlocillin against gram-negative organisms, in the "blind" treatment of severe infections when these organisms are suspected.

Azlocillin is a new parenteral acylureido-penicillin similar in spectrum and structure to mezlocillin. It is used to treat *Ps. aeruginosa* infections and in combination therapy for "blind" treatment of serious infections when *Pseudomonas* is a possible cause. It is two to four times more potent than mezlocillin against *Pseudomonas* organisms *in vitro* and is active against resistant strains. It is less active than mezlocillin against *E. coli* and *Klebsiella* species. As with mezlocillin, synergy occurs with aminoglycosides against gram-negative organisms. It is inactivated by β-lactamase-producing organisms. Its T½ is 5.5 hours, and azlocillin is excreted largely unchanged. Azlocillin has been used successfully to treat *Pseudomonas* infections resistant to other antibiotics, and perhaps it should be reserved for this, since azlocillin-resistant strains have appeared in children with cystic fibrosis.

CEPHALOSPORINS

With the isolation of the active nucleus of cephalosporin, it has become possible, by the addition of side chains, to produce semisynthetic compounds with a wider spectrum of antibacterial activity than the parent compound, so-called second- and third-generation cephalosporins.

Cefuroxime

Cefuroxime is a new second-generation cephalosporin that must be administered parenterally. It is active against gram-negative bacilli and staphylcocci and particularly active against *Hemophilus influenzae* and gonococci, even when they are penicillin resistant. Metabolism is negligible, the parent compound appearing unchanged in the urine. The plasma T½ is 1.1 to 1.4 hours. It is partially excreted in the bile, where it is concentrated. The concentration achieved in the sputum and pleural fluid on usual doses exceeds the MIC for *H. influenzae, Strep. pneumoniae*, or *Staph. aureus*. Cefuroxime is used to treat lower respiratory tract infections, including exacerbations of chronic bronchitis, and to treat penicillin-resistant gonorrhea. Side-effects include thrombophlebitis, pain at injection sites, and nephrotoxicity, although to a lesser degree than with earlier cephalosporins. With normal renal function, the dose is 2 g every 8 hours, the interval between injections being extended in renal failure.

Cefotaxime

Cefotaxime, a semisynthetic third-generation cephalosporin similar to earlier cephalosporins, is active against gram-positive microorganisms and a wide range of gram-negative bacilli. It is distinguished by being active against *Ps. aeruginosa,* including aminoglycoside-resistant strains and indole-positive *Proteus* species. It is less active against *Staph. aureus* than is cephalothin. Cefotaxime is not active orally and must be given parenterally. It is rapidly distributed in the body and slowly excreted in the urine. It is largely metabolized to a desacetyl derivative. Side-effects include night sweats, fatigue, and loose stools.

Other Cephalosporins:

Ceforamide is administered parenterally. It is less active against *Staphylococci* than is cephalothin but equally active to cefamandole against gram-negative bacilli. It has a plasma T½ of 3 hours. *Cephacetrile* is a semisynthetic agent with similar antibacterial, pharmacologic, and toxic properties to earlier cephalosporins. *Cefatrizine* is active orally. *In vitro* it is more active against *H. influenzae* than is cephalexin or cephadrine and more active against *Staph. aureus,* group A streptococci, and enterobacteriae than previously available cephalosporins.

AMINOGLYCOSIDES

Sisomycin

Sisomycin is a recently developed aminoglycoside isolated from *Micromonospora inyoensis.* It is closely related to gentamicin and must be given parenterally. It is excreted in the urine, with a plasma T½ of 3.5 hours, falling to 0.01 in anuric subjects. Sisomycin has a similar antibacterial spectrum and toxicity to gentamicin and tobramicin and thus offers no clinical advantage over these drugs.

URINARY TRACT ANTISEPTICS

Cinoxacin

Cinoxacin, a derivative of cinnolinic acid, is chemically related to nalidixic acid and oxolinic acid. It is active against gram-negative urinary pathogens and gram-positive cocci, including *Strep. faecalis* and staphylococci. Most organisms resistant to nalidixic acid are also resistant to cinoxacin. The MIC of cinoxacin in the urine is between 4 and 8 mg/liter, lower than the MIC of nalidixic acid. It is active orally, the peak concentration occurring 1 hour after an oral dose of 500 mg. Its plasma T½ is 1 to 1.5 hours. Cinoxacin is rapidly excreted by the kidney and concentrated in the urine, peak urinary concentrations occurring at 2 to 4 hours, falling to 12 mg/liter at 10 to 12 hours. Thus cinoxacin is effective in a twice-daily regimen. Whereas only 20% of nalidixic acid is excreted in the active form in the urine, 60% of cinoxacin is excreted unchanged. Cinoxacin compares favorably with co-trimoxazole and nitrofurantoin in the treatment of urinary tract infections. Cinoxacin eradicates urinary tract infections more commonly than does nalidixic acid. Further, fewer resistant strains develop during treatment with cinoxacin. Side-effects include gastrointestinal discomfort and hypersensitivity reactions and are less frequent than those for nalidixic acid. The dose is 500 mg every 12 hours, which may improve compliance over nalidixic acid, usually given every 6 hours.

H_2-RECEPTOR ANTAGONISTS

RANITIDINE

Ranitidine has been found in animal and human studies to be 4 to 12 times more potent than cimetidine. By selectively blocking H_2-receptors it inhibits gastric acid secretion induced by food, histamine, and pentagastrin. Animal studies show that it may also have a cytoprotective action independent of its effects on acid secretion, since it prevents the gastric erosions induced by aspirin in the presence or absence of gastric acid.

Ranitidine has no antiandrogenic properties, unlike cimetidine (Table 83-6), which displaces dihydrotestosterone from androgen-binding sites and, during high-dose treatment in humans, may cause gynecomastia. Further, ranitidine has no effect on the hypothalmic–pituitary–testicular axis. Hyperprolactinemia, which occurs with high doses of cimetidine, has not been reported.

Ranitidine possesses a furan ring in place of the imadazole ring present in cimetidine. The imidazole ring is thought to bind with cytochrome P-450 and inhibit hepatic oxidative metabolism. This decreases the rate of metabolism of some drugs (benzodiazepine, oral anticoagulants, and probably many others). Cime-

TABLE 83-6. Comparison of Ranitidine and Cimetidine

	Ranitidine	Cimetidine
Structure	Furan ring	Imidazole ring
Potency	++++	+
Half-life, *hr*	2	2
Duration of effect, *hr*	8–12	4–6
Antiandrogenic	–	+
Hyperprolactinemia	–	+ (high doses)
Oxidative metabolism	–	Reduced
Liver blood flow	–	Reduced
Gynecomastia	–	+
Daily dose, *mg*	150–300	800–1000
Dose frequency per day	2–3	4

tidine is also more lipid soluble than ranitidine, which may augment its potential to alter microsomal drug metabolism. Cimetidine reduces liver blood flow such that the clearance of a drug whose metabolism is liver-blood-flow dependent, such as propranolol, is reduced if taken with cimetidine. Ranitidine, however, does not alter liver blood flow. Finally cimetidine blocks cardiac H_2-receptors, resulting in a fall in heart rate. This effect has yet to be demonstrated with ranitidine.

Ranitidine is well absorbed, with a bioavailability of 88%. Between 50% and 70% is excreted unchanged in the urine, and it would thus be expected that lower doses would be needed in severe renal impairment. The plasma $T\frac{1}{2}$ of ranitidine is about 2 hours, similar to that of cimetidine. The clearance of cimetidine is age dependent, decreasing in elderly patients presumably because of diminished handling by the liver. It is not known if the decrease in renal function associated with aging significantly increases the plasma $T\frac{1}{2}$ of ranitidine. Although the half-lives of ranitidine and cimetidine are similar, ranitidine has a longer duration of action (8–12 hours with a standard dose) and thus may be given less frequently. Ranitidine has been found to enter the CSF in healthy subjects, but only in small amounts. Cimetidine also enters the CNS and, in patients with renal and hepatic impairment, may cause confusion. As yet, ranitidine has not been tested in these subjects.

Cimetidine and ranitidine have been compared in the treatment of peptic ulcer. Both induce a similar rate of healing, and the remission rate is similar on both drugs. Ranitidine, however, suppresses nocturnal acidity to a greater extent even when given as a twice-daily dose. Ranitidine has been shown to be useful in the Zollinger–Ellison syndrome even in patients who have failed to respond to cimetidine. The daily dose of ranitidine is 150 to 300 mg in two or three divided doses.

Appendix A: Contents of Typical Emergency Drug Tray

CONTENTS OF TYPICAL EMERGENCY DRUG TRAY FOR ADULTS

Aminophylline (25 mg/ml)	500 mg/20 ml vial (2)
Atropine (0.1 mg/ml)	1 mg/10 ml PLS (3)
Bretyllium tosylate (50 mg/ml)	500 mg/10 ml ampule (3)
Calcium chloride 10% (0.1 g/ml)	1 g/10 ml PLS/IC (4)
Calcium gluconate 10% (100 mg/ml)	1 g/10 ml ampule (2)
Dextrose (0.5 g/ml)	25 g/50 ml PLS (1)
Diazepam (5 mg/ml)	10 mg/2 ml PLS (2)
Digoxin (100 μg/ml)	0.5 mg/2 ml ampule (6)
Diphenhydramine (50 mg/ml)	50 mg/1 ml PLS (4)
Dobutamine (250 mg/vial)	250 mg/vial (1)
Dopamine (40 mg/ml)	200 mg/5 ml ampule (5)
Epinephrine 1:10,000 (0.1 mg/ml)	1 mg/10 ml PLS/IC (3)
Furosemide (10 mg/ml)	20 mg/2 ml ampule (2)
Furosemide (10 mg/ml)	100 mg/10 ml ampule (4)
Heparin sodium (1,000 units/ml)	10,000 units/10 ml vial (1)
Hydrocortisone (50 mg/ml)	100 mg/2 ml vial (4)
Isoproterenol (0.2 mg/ml)	1 mg/5 ml ampule (5)
Levarterenol (1 mg/ml)	4 mg/4 ml ampule (4)
Lidocaine (20 mg/ml)	100 mg/5 ml PLS (3)
Lidocaine (200 mg/ml); for i.v. additive 2 g/10 ml	PLS (3)
Metaraminol (10 mg/ml)	100 mg/10 ml vial (1)
Naloxone (0.4 mg/ml)	0.4 mg/1 ml ampule (4)
Nitroprusside (20 mg/ml)	200 mg/10 ml vial (2)
Phentolamine (5 mg/ampule)	5 mg/ampule (1)
Phenylephrine (10 mg/ml)	10 mg/1 ml ampule (2)
Phenytoin (50 mg/ml)	250 mg/5 ml ampule (4)
Procainamide (100 mg/ml)	1 g/10 ml vial (2)
Propranolol HCl (1 mg/ml)	1 mg/1 ml ampule (5)
Sodium bicarbonate (0.9 mEq/ml)	44.6 mEq/50 ml PLS (5)

CONTENTS OF TYPICAL EMERGENCY DRUG TRAY FOR PEDIATRIC PATIENTS

Aminophylline (25 mg/ml)	500 mg/20 ml vial (2)
Atropine (0.1 mg/ml)	1 mg/10 ml PLS (3)
Bretyllium tosylate (50 mg/ml)	500 mg/10 ml ampule (3)
Calcium chloride 10% (0.1 g/ml)	1 g/10 ml PLS/IC (4)
Calcium gluconate 10% (100 mg/ml)	1 g/10 ml ampule (2)
Dextrose 50% (0.5 g/ml)	25 g/50 ml PLS (1)
Diazepam (5 mg/ml)	10 mg/2 ml PLS (2)
Digoxin (100 μg/ml)	100 μg/1 ml ampule (6)
Diphenhydramine (50 mg/ml)	50 mg/1 ml PLS (4)
Dobutamine (250 mg/vial)	250 mg/vial (1)
Dopamine (40 mg/ml)	200 mg/5 ml ampule (5)
Epinephrine 1 : 10,000 (0.1 mg/ml)	1 mg/10 ml PLS/IC (3)
Furosemide (10 mg/ml)	20 mg/2 ml ampule (2)
Furosemide (10 mg/ml)	100 mg/10 ml ampule (4)
Heparin sodium (1,000 units/ml)	10,000 units/10 ml vial (1)
Hydrocortisone (50 mg/ml)	100 mg/2 ml vial (4)
Isoproterenol (0.2 mg/ml)	1 mg/5 ml ampule (5)
Leverterenol (1 mg/ml)	4 mg/4 ml ampule (4)
Lidocaine (20 mg/ml)	100 mg/5 ml PLS (3)
Lidocaine (200 mg/ml); for i.v. additive 2 g/10 ml	PLS(3)
Metaraminol (10 mg/ml)	100 mg/10 ml vial (1)
Naloxone (0.4 mg/ml)	0.4 mg/1 ml ampule (4)
Nitroprusside (20 mg/ml)	200 mg/10 ml vial (2)
Phentolamine (5 mg/ampule)	5 mg/ampule (1)
Phenylephrine (10 mg/ml)	10 mg/1 ml ampule (2)
Phenytoin (50 mg/ml)	250 mg/5 ml ampule (4)
Procainamide (100 mg/ml)	1 g/10 ml vial (2)
Propranolol HCl (1 mg/ml)	1 mg/1 ml ampule (5)
Sodium bicarbonate (0.9 mEq/ml)	44.6 mEq/50 ml PLS (4)
Sodium bicarbonate (1 mEq/ml)	10 mEq/10 ml PLS (3)

Appendix B: Approximate Metric and Apothecaries' Equivalents

The metric system is used throughout essentials of pharmacology, and the physician is strongly urged to use these measures exclusively for writing prescriptions. The following tables are included because, on occasion, they may prove useful. It is imperative that no confusion exist between grams (g) and grains (gr).

Approximate Metric and Apothecaries' Equivalents of Household Measures

Household Measure	Metric	Apothecaries'
1 drop	0.06–0.1 milliliter	1–1.5 minims
1 teaspoonful	5 milliliters	1 fluid dram
1 dessertspoonful	8 milliliters	2 fluid drams
1 tablespoonful	15 milliliters	0.5 fluid ounce
1 water glass	250 milliliters	8 fluid ounces

Approximate Metric and Apothecaries' Equivalents

Metric	Apothecaries'
1 milligram	1/60 grain
1 gram	15 grains
1 kilogram	2.20 pounds (avoirdupois)
1 milliliter	15 minims
1 liter	1 quart
1 liter	34 fluid ounces
1 grain	60 milligrams
1 dram	4 grams
1 ounce	30 grams
1 minim	0.06 milliliter
1 fluid dram	4 milliliters
1 fluid ounce	30 milliliters
1 pint	500 milliliters
1 quart	1000 milliliters

Apothecaries' System of Equivalent Weights and Measures

Weights	
20 grains	1 scruple
60 grains	1 dram
480 grains (8 drams)	1 ounce troy
5760 grains (12 ounces)	1 pound troy
Measures	
60 minims	1 fluid dram
480 minims (8 fluid drams)	1 fluid ounce
7680 minims (16 fluid ounces)	1 pint
32 fluid ounces	1 quart

Appendix C: The Top 200 Prescription Drugs in the United States—1980

The top 200 listings and related tabulations are supplied by Pharmaceutical Data Services, Phoenix, Arizona, subsidiary of Foremost—McKesson, Inc. PDS provides various marketing research and sales analyses to the pharmaceutical industry and government. The data are derived from a subsample of more than 700 pharmacies located in 42 states. Accuracy of the data has been validated by large and medium pharmaceutical houses.

Two "Top 200" listings are presented—one covering all prescriptions new and refilled dispensed in community pharmacies in the United States 1980, the other covering new prescriptions only. PDS reports prescriptions as actually dispensed. Participating pharmacies provide NDC numbers; hence, PDS is able to report manufacturers' names for generic as well as branded products. Each name covers all strengths of the drug product involved.

As would be expected, medications for acute conditions show up more prominently in the new-only listing than in the combined listing for new and refilled drugs. For example, such antibiotics as cephalexin (Keflex), erythromycin ethylsuccinate (E.E.S.), amoxicillin (Amoxil), penicillin VK (V-Cillin-K), ampicillin (Amcill), doxycycline (Vibramycin), erythromycin (E-Mycin), ampicillin (Omnipen), and tetracycline (Achromycin-V) all have higher rankings in the listing of new prescriptions than in the new-and-refill compilation.

Conversely, long-term medications tend to have lower rankings in the new-drug list than in the combined list, for example, propranolol, digoxin, cimetidine, ibuprofen.

Altogether, the top 200 products, new and refill combined, account for 64.6% of all new and refilled prescriptions. The top 100 account for 50.3%, the top 50 for 36.3%.

With 15 each, Merck and Parke-Davis lead in numbers of products but not necessarily in number of prescriptions. Wyeth follows, with 11; Burroughs-Wellcome with 10; Roche with 9; SK & F and Upjohn with 8 each; and Searle and Squibb with 7 each.

THE TOP 200—NEW AND REFILL COMBINED

Rank	Drug Product: Generic Name (Trade Name)	Manufacturer
1.	Diazepam (Valium)	Roche
2.	Propranolol (Inderal)	Ayerst
3.	Triamterene/Hydrochlorothiazide (Dyazide)	SKF
4.	Digoxin (Lanoxin)	BW
5.	Acetaminophen/Codeine (Tylenol w/Codeine)	McNeil
6.	Furosemide (Lasix)	Hoechst
7.	Brompheniramine Compound (Dimetapp)	Robins
8.	Ibuprofen (Motrin)	Upjohn
9.	Cimetidine (Tagamet)	SKF
10.	Propoxyphene Napsylate/Acetaminophen (Darvocet-N)	Lilly
11.	Flurazepam (Dalmane)	Roche
12.	Methyldopa (Aldomet)	MSD
13.	Norethindrone/Mestranol (Ortho Novum)	Ortho
14.	Pseudoephedrine/Triprolidine (Actifed)	BW
15.	Cephalexin (Keflex)	Dista
16.	Potassium Chloride (Slow-K)	Ciba
17.	Aspirin/Codeine (Empirin w/Codeine)	BW
18.	Estrogens, Conjugated (Premarin)	Ayerst
19.	Diphenhydramine (Benadryl)	Parke-Davis
20.	Phenytoin (Dilantin)	Parke-Davis
21.	Erythromycin Ethylsuccinate (E.E.S.)	Abbott
22.	Sulindac (Clinoril)	MSD
23.	Indomethacin (Indocin)	MSD
24.	Levothyroxine (Synthroid)	Flint
25.	Chlorthalidone (Hygroton)	USV
26.	Amoxicillin (Amoxil)	Beecham
27.	Hydrochlorothiazide (Hydrodiuril)	MSD
28.	Isosorbide Dinitrate (Isordil)	Ives
29.	Penicillin VK (V-Cillin K)	Lilly
30.	Chlorazepate (Tranxene)	Abbott
31.	Naproxen (Naprosyn)	Syntex
32.	Belladonna/Phenobarbital (Donnatal)	Robins
33.	Thioridazine (Mellaril)	Sandoz
34.	Oxycodone/Aspirin (Percodan)	Endo
35.	Chlorpropamide (Diabinese)	Pfizer
36.	Ampicillin (Amcill)	Parke-Davis
37.	Butalbital/Aspirin Compound (Fiorinal)	Sandoz
38.	Dexbrompheniramine/Isoephedrine (Drixoril)	Schering
39.	Amitriptyline (Elavil)	MSD
40.	Ethinyl Estradiol/Norgestrel (Ovral)	Wyeth
41.	Methyldopa/Hydrochlorothiazide (Aldoril)	MSD
42.	Ethinyl Estradiol/Norgestrel (Lo/Ovral)	Wyeth
43.	Thyroid	Armour
44.	Allopurinol (Zyloprim)	BW
45.	Tetracycline (Achromycin V)	Lederle
46.	Dipyridamole (Persantine)	Boehringer
47.	Erthromycin (E-Mycin)	Upjohn
48.	Doxycycline (Vibramycin)	Pfizer
49.	Triamcinolone/Neomycin Compound (Mycolog)	Squibb
50.	Spironolactone/Hydrochlorothiazide (Aldactazide)	Searle
51.	Lorazepam (Ativan)	Wyeth
52.	Chlordiazepoxide (Librium)	Roche
53.	Metoprolol (Lopressor)	Geigy
54.	Ampicillin (Omnipen)	Wyeth
55.	Miconazole (Monistat)	Ortho
56.	Norethindrone/Mestranol (Norinyl)	Syntex
57.	Amitriptyline/Perphenazine (Triavil)	MSD
58	Chlordiazepoxide/Clidinium (Librax)	Roche

THE TOP 200—NEW AND REFILL COMBINED

Rank	Drug Product: Generic Name (Trade Name)	Manufacturer
59.	Diphenoxylate/Atropine (Lomotil)	Searle
60.	Meclizine (Antivert)	Roerig
61.	Hydroxyzine (Atarax)	Roerig
62.	Erythromycin Estolate (Ilosone)	Dista
63.	Tetracycline (Sumycin)	Squibb
64.	Reserpine/Apresoline/Hydrochlorothiazide (Ser-Ap-Es)	Ciba
65.	Ampicillin (Principen)	Squibb
66.	Tetracycline	Parke-Davis
67.	Phenylbutazone/Antacid (Butazolidin Alka)	Geigy
68.	Chlorpheniramine/Phenylpropanolamine Compound (Naldecon)	Bristol
69.	Timolol (Timoptic)	MSD
70.	Doxepin (Sinequan)	Pfizer
71.	Phenobarbital	Lilly
72.	Penicillin VK (Pfizerpen VK)	Pfipharmecs
73.	Propoxyphene/Aspirin Compound (Darvon Comp 65)	Lilly
74.	Sulfamethoxazole/Trimethoprim (Bactrim DS)	Roche
75.	Prazosin (Minipress)	Pfizer
76.	Amoxicillin (Larotid)	Roche
77.	Nitroglycerin (Nitro-Bid)	Marlon
78.	Chlorzoxazone/Acetaminophen (Parafon Forte)	McNeil
79.	Nitrofurantoin (Macrodantin)	Norwich
80.	Penicillin VK (Pen-Vee K)	Wyeth
81.	Hydrocortisone/Neomycin Compound (Cortisporin Otic)	BW
82.	Clotrimazole (Gyne-Lotrimin)	Schering
83.	Sulfamethoxazole/Trimethoprim (Septra DS)	BW
84.	Promethazine Compound/Codeine (Phenergan w/Cod)	Wyeth
85.	Hydralazine (Apresoline)	Ciba
86.	Dihydrocodeine/Promethazine Compound (Synalgos-DC)	Ives
87.	Warfarin (Coumadin)	Endo
88.	Acetaminophen/Codeine (Phenaphen w/Cod)	Robins
89.	Erythromycin	Abbott
90	Chlorothiazide (Diuril)	MSD
91.	Haloperidol (Haldol)	McNeil
92.	Ethynodiol Diacetate/Ethinyl Estradiol (Demulen)	Searle
93.	Terbutaline (Brethine)	Geigy
94.	Fenoprofen (Nalfon)	Dista
95.	Ampicillin (Pen A)	Pfipharmecs
96.	Theophylline (Theo-Dur)	Key
97.	Betamethasone (Valisone)	Schering
98.	Papaverine (Pavabid)	Marion
99.	Caramiphen/Chlorpheniramine Compound (Tuss-Ornade)	SKF
100.	Reserpine/Hydrochlorothiazide (Hydropres)	MSD
101.	Prednisone (Deltasone)	Upjohn
102.	Ethynodiol Diacetate/Mestranol (Ovulen)	Searle
103.	Tolbutamide (Orinase)	Upjohn
104.	Oxazepam (Serax)	Wyeth
105.	Butalbital/Aspirin Compound/Codeine (Fiorinal w/Codeine)	Sandoz
106.	Clonidine (Catapres)	Boehringer
107.	Tolmetin (Tolectin)	McNeil
108.	Nitroglycerin (Nitrostat)	Parke-Davis
109.	Doxylamine/Pyridoxine (Bendectin)	Merrell
110.	Dicyclomine (Bentyl)	Merrell
111.	Norethindrone/Ethinyl Estradiol (Modicon)	Ortho
112.	Ergoloid Mesylates (Hydergine)	Sandoz
113.	Penicillin VK (Ledercillin VK)	Lederle
114.	Chlorpromazine (Thorazine)	SKF
115.	Metronidazole (Flagyl)	Searle
116.	Pentazocine (Talwin)	Winthrop

THE TOP 200—NEW AND REFILL COMBINED

Rank	Drug Product: Generic Name (Trade Name)	Manufacturer
117.	Hydrochlorothiazide (Esidrex)	Ciba
118.	Sulfamethoxazole/Trimethoprim (Septra)	BW
119.	Amoxicillin	Parke-Davis
120.	Triamcinolone (Kenalog)	Squibb
121.	Diethylpropion (Tenuate)	Merrell
122.	Isosorbide Dinitrate (Sorbitrate)	Stuart
123.	Clofibrate (Atromid-S)	Ayerst
124.	Prochlorperazine (Compazine)	SKF
125.	Neomycin Compound (Neosporin)	BW
126.	Methyclothiazide (Enduron)	Abbott
127.	Tolazamide (Tolinase)	Upjohn
128.	Penicillin VK	Parke-Davis
129.	Promethazine Compound/Codeine (Phenergan VC w/Codeine)	Wyeth
130.	Cefaclor (Ceclor)	Lilly
131.	Potassium (K-Lyte)	Mead Johnson
132.	Beclomethasone (Vanceril)	Schering
133.	Pseudoephedrine/Triprolidine/Codeine/Guaifenesin (Actifed-C)	BW
134.	Lindane (Kwell)	Reed & Carnrick
135.	Hydrochlorothiazide	Lederle
136.	Hydroxyzine (Vistaril)	Pfizer
137.	Theophylline (Slo-Phyllin)	Rorer
138.	Metaproterenol (Alupent)	Boehringer
139.	Cyclobenzaprine (Flexeril)	MSD
140.	Chlordiazepoxide/Amitriptyline (Limbitrol)	Roche
141.	Minocycline (Minocin)	Lederle
142.	Amoxicillin (Trimox)	Squibb
143.	Meprobamate/Ethoheprazine/Aspirin (Equagesic)	Wyeth
144.	Isopropamide/Prochlorperazine (Combid)	SKF
145.	Sulfamethoxazole/Trimethoprim (Bactrim)	Roche
146.	Sulfisoxazole (Gantrisin)	Roche
147.	Disopyramide (Norpace)	Searle
148.	Nitroglycerin	Lilly
149.	Cyproheptadine (Periactin)	MSD
150.	Trimethobenzamide (Tigan)	Beecham
151.	Erythromycin (Erythrocin)	Abbott
152.	Spironolactone (Aldactone)	Searle
153.	Oxtriphylline (Choledyl)	Parke-Davis
154.	Butabarbital (Butisol)	McNeil
155.	Trifluoperazine (Stelazine)	SKF
156.	Phentermine (Ionamin)	Pennwalt
157.	Multivitamins w/Fluoride (Poly-Vi-Flor)	Mead Johnson
158.	Orphenadrine/Aspirin Compound (Norgesic Forte)	Riker
159.	Methocarbamol (Robaxin)	Robins
160.	Aminacrine/Sulfanilamide/Allantoin (AVC)	Merrell
161.	Fluocinonide (Lidex)	Syntex
162.	Methylphenidate (Ritalin)	Ciba
163.	Benztropine (Cogentin)	MSD
164.	Hydroxyzine/Ephedrine (Marax)	Roerig
165.	Diphenhydramine (Benylin)	Parke-Davis
166.	Carbidopa/Levodopa (Sinemet)	MSD
167.	Isoxsuprine (Vasodilan)	Mead Johnson
168.	Bismuth Compound/Hydrocortisone (Anusol-HC)	Parke-Davis
169.	Phenobarbital	Parke-Davis
170.	Imipramine (Tofranil)	Geigy
171.	Methylprednisolone (Medrol)	Upjohn
172.	Promethazine (Phenergan)	Wyeth
173.	Pilocarpine (Isopto Carpine)	Alcon
174.	Sulfacetamide (Sodium Sulamyd)	Schering

THE TOP 200—NEW AND REFILL COMBINED

Rank	Drug Product: Generic Name (Trade Name)	Manufacturer
175.	Metolazone (Zaroxolyn)	Pennwalt
176.	Phenazopyridine (Pyridium)	Parke-Davis
177.	Pseudoephedrine (Sudafed)	BW
178.	Noscapine (Tusscapine)	Fisons
179.	Penicillin VK (Veetids)	Squibb
180.	Chlorpheniramine (Chlor-Trimeton)	Schering
181.	Phentermine (Fastin)	Beecham
182.	Hydralazine/Hydrochlorothiazide (Apresazide)	Ciba
183.	Dexamethasone (Decadron)	MSD
184.	Quinidine Sulfate	Parke-Davis
185.	Medroxyprogesterone (Provera)	Upjohn
186.	Procainamide (Pronestyl)	Squibb
187.	Hydrocodone/Phenyltoloxamine (Tussionex)	Pennwalt
188.	Thiothixene (Navane)	Roerig
189.	Meprobamate (Equanil)	Wyeth
190.	Trihexyphenidyl (Artane)	Lederle
191.	Norethindrone Acetate/Ethinyl Estradiol/Ferrous Sulfate (Norlestrin FE)	Parke-Davis
192.	Ampicillin (SK-Ampicillin)	SKF
193.	Quinine Sulfate (Quinamm)	Merrell
194.	Erythromycin Stearate	Lederle
195.	Loperamide (Imodium)	Ortho
196.	Tetracycline (Panmycin)	Upjohn
197.	Chlorthalidone/Reserpine (Regroton)	USV
198.	Erythromycin	Parke-Davis
199.	Theophylline/Guaifenesin (Quibron)	Mead Johnson
200.	Fluocinolone (Synalar)	Syntex

THE TOP 200—NEW PRESCRIPTIONS ONLY

Rank	Drug Product: Generic Name (Trade Name)	Manufacturer
1.	Acetaminophen/Codeine (Tylenol w/Codeine)	McNeil
2.	Diazepam (Valium)	Roche
3.	Brompheniramine Compound (Dimetapp)	Robins
4.	Cephalexin (Keflex)	Dista
5.	Aspirin/Codeine (Empirin w/Codeine)	BW
6.	Erythromycin Ethylsuccinate (E.E.S.)	Abbott
7.	Propoxyphene Napsylate/Acetaminophen (Darvocet-N)	Lilly
8.	Amoxicillin (Amoxil)	Beecham
9.	Furosemide (Lasix)	Hoechst
10.	Triamterene/Hydrochlorothiazide (Dyazide)	SKF
11.	Digoxin (Lanoxin)	BW
12.	Flurazepam (Dalmane)	Roche
13.	Pseudoephedrine/Triprolidine (Actifed)	BW
14.	Propranolol (Inderal)	Ayerst
15.	Ibuprofen (Motrin)	Upjohn
16.	Penicillin VK (V-Cillin K)	Lilly
17.	Oxycodone/Aspirin (Percodan)	Endo
18.	Cimetidine (Tagamet)	SKF
19.	Diphenhydramine (Benadryl)	Parke-Davis
20.	Ampicillin (Amcill)	Parke-Davis
21.	Doxycycline (Vibramycin)	Pfizer
22.	Erthromycin (E-Mycin)	Upjohn
23.	Ampicillin (Omnipen)	Wyeth
24.	Indomethacin (Indocin)	MSD
25.	Tetracycline (Achromycin V)	Lederle
26.	Miconazole (Monistat)	Ortho

THE TOP 200—NEW PRESCRIPTIONS ONLY

Rank	Drug Product: Generic Name (Trade Name)	Manufacturer
27.	Triamcinolone/Neomycin Compound (Mycolog)	Squibb
28.	Sulindac (Clinoril)	MSD
29.	Erythromycin Estolate (Ilosone)	Dista
30.	Ampicillin (Principen)	Squibb
31.	Estrogens, Conjugated (Premarin)	Ayerst
32.	Norethindrone/Mestranol (Ortho Novum)	Ortho
33.	Penicillin VK (Pfizerpen VK)	Pfipharmecs
34.	Chlorazepate (Tranxene)	Abbott
35.	Diphenoxylate/Atropine (Lomotil)	Searle
36.	Belladonna/Phenobarbital (Donnatal)	Robins
37.	Methyldopa (Aldomet)	MSD
38.	Amoxicillin (Larotid)	Roche
39.	Butalbital/Aspirin Compound (Fiorinal)	Sandoz
40.	Dexbrompheniramine/Isoephedrine (Drixoril)	Schering
41.	Phenylbutazone/Antacid (Butazolidin Alka)	Geigy
42.	Hydrocortisone/Neomycin Compound (Cortisporin)	BW
43.	Tetracycline	Parke-Davis
44.	Potassium Chloride (Slow-K)	Ciba
45.	Naproxen (Naprosyn)	Syntex
46.	Penicillin VK (Pen-Vee K)	Wyeth
47.	Tetracycline (Sumycin)	Squibb
48.	Sulfamethoxazole/Trimethoprim (Bactrim DS)	Roche
49.	Chlorthalidone (Hygroton)	U.S.V.
50.	Erythromycin	Abbott
51.	Levothyroxine (Synthroid)	Flint
52.	Promethazine Compound/Codeine (Phenergan w/Cod)	Wyeth
53.	Sulfamethoxazole/Trimethoprim (Septra DS)	BW
54.	Dihydrocodeine/Promethazine Compound (Synalgos-DC)	Ives
55.	Hydroxyzine (Atarax)	Roerig
56.	Ampicillin (Pen A)	Pfipharmecs
57.	Chlorpheniramine/Phenylpropanolamine Compound (Naldecon)	Bristol
58.	Clotrimazole (Gyne-Lotrimin)	Schering
59.	Lorazepam (Ativan)	Wyeth
60.	Acetaminophen/Codeine (Phenaphen w/Cod)	Robins
61.	Chlordiazepoxide (Librium)	Roche
62.	Metronidazole (Flagyl)	Searle
63.	Chlorpheniramine Compound (Ornade)	SKF
64.	Penicillin VK (Ledercillin VK)	Lederle
65.	Chlorzoxazone/Acetaminophen (Parafon Forte)	McNeil
66.	Amitriptyline (Elavil)	MSD
67.	Hydrochlorothiazide (Hydrodiuril)	MSD
68.	Amoxicillin	Parke-Davis
69.	Nitrofurantoin (Macrodantin)	Norwich
70.	Phenytoin (Dilantin)	Parke-Davis
71.	Chlordiazepoxide/Clidinium (Librax)	Roche
72.	Neomycin Compound (Neosporin)	BW
73.	Meclizine (Antivert)	Roerig
74.	Penicillin VK	Parke-Davis
75.	Thioridazine (Mellaril)	Sandoz
76.	Caramiphen/Chlorpheniramine Compound (Tuss-Ornade)	SKF
77.	Cefaclor (Ceclor)	Lilly
78.	Propoxyphene/Aspirin Compound (Darvon Comp 65)	Lilly
79.	Lindane (Kwell)	Reed & Carnrick
80.	Amoxicillin (Trimox)	Squibb
81.	Isosorbide Dinitrate (Isordil)	Ives
82.	Prednisone (Deltasone)	Upjohn
83.	Butalbital/Aspirin Compound/Codeine (Fiorinal w/Codeine)	Sandoz
84.	Promethazine Compound/Codeine (Phenergan VC w/Codeine)	Wyeth

THE TOP 200—NEW PRESCRIPTIONS ONLY

Rank	Drug Product: Generic Name (Trade Name)	Manufacturer
85.	Chlorpropamide (Diabinese)	Pfizer
86.	Sulfamethoxazole/Trimethoprim (Septra)	BW
87.	Betamethasone (Valisone)	Schering
88.	Pseudoephedrine/Triprolidine/Codeine/Guaifenesin (Actifed-C)	BW
89.	Allopurinol (Zyloprim)	BW
90.	Prochlorperazine (Compazine)	SK&F
91.	Ethinyl Estradiol/Norgestrel (Lo/Ovral)	Wyeth
92.	Diethylpropion (Tenuate)	Merrell
93.	Methylphenidate (Ritalin)	Ciba
94.	Erythromycin (Erythrocin)	Abbott
95.	Phenobarbital	Lilly
96.	Thyroid	Armour
97.	Cyclobenzaprine (Flexeril)	MSD
98.	Amitriptyline/Perphenazine (Triavil)	MSD
99.	Doxepin (Sinequan)	Pfizer
100.	Trimethobenzamide (Tigan)	Beecham
101.	Pentazocine (Talwin)	Winthrop
102.	Sulfisoxazole (Gantrisin)	Roche
103.	Ethinyl Estradiol/Norgestrel (Ovral)	Wyeth
104.	Sulfamethoxazole/Trimethoprim (Bactrim)	Roche
105.	Metoprolol (Lopressor)	Geigy
106.	Aminacrine/Sulfanilamide/Allantoin (AVC)	Merrell
107.	Triamcinolone (Kenalog)	Squibb
108.	Fenoprofen (Nalfon)	Dista
109.	Nitroglycerin (Nitrostat)	Parke-Davis
110.	Norethindrone/Mestranol (Norinyl)	Snytex
111.	Dicyclomine (Bentyl)	Merrell
112.	Minocycline (Minocin)	Lederle
113.	Spironolactone/Hydrochlorothiazide (Aldactazide)	Searle
114.	Sulfacetamide (Sodium Sulamyd)	Schering
115.	Penicillin VK (Veetids)	Squibb
116.	Methyldopa/Hydrochlorothiazide (Aldoril)	MSD
117.	Doxylamine/Pyridoxine (Bendectin)	Merrell
118.	Phentermine (Ionamin)	Pennwalt
119.	Meprobamate/Ethoheprazine/Aspirin (Equagesic)	Wyeth
120.	Phenazopyridine (Pyridium)	Parke-Davis
121.	Methylprednisolone (Medrol)	Upjohn
122.	Orphenadrine/Aspirin Compound (Norgesic Forte)	Riker
123.	Tolmetin (Tolectin)	McNeil
124.	Ampicillin (SK-Ampicillin)	SK&F
125.	Dipyridamole (Persantine)	Boehringer
126.	Meperidine (Demerol)	Winthrop
127.	Promethazine (Phenergan)	Wyeth
128.	Oxazepam (Serax)	Wyeth
129.	Cyproheptadine (Periactin)	MSD
130.	Dexamethasone (Decadron)	MSD
131.	Diphenhydramine (Benylin)	Parke-Davis
132.	Erythromycin Stearate	Lederle
133.	Oxycodone/Acetaminophen (Percocet)	Endo
134.	Theophylline (Theo-Dur)	Key
135.	Isopropamide/Prochlorperazine (Combid)	SK&F
136.	Erythromycin	Parke-Davis
137.	Methaqualone (Mequin)	Lemmon
138.	Ampicillin	Lederle
139.	Hydroxyzine (Vistaril)	Pfizer
140.	Erythromycin (Wyamycin)	Wyeth
141.	Warfarin (Coumadin)	Endo
142.	Bismuth Compound/Hydrocortisone (Anusol-HC)	Parke-Davis

THE TOP 200—NEW PRESCRIPTIONS ONLY

Rank	Drug Product: Generic Name (Trade Name)	Manufacturer
143.	Noscapine (Tusscapine)	Fisons
144.	Haloperidol (Haldol)	McNeil
145.	Phentermine (Fastin)	Beecham
146.	Methocarbamol (Robaxin)	Robins
147.	Medroxyprogesterone (Provera)	Upjohn
148.	Chlordiazepoxide/Amitriptyline (Limbitrol)	Roche
149.	Antipyrine/Benzocaine (Auralgan)	Ayerst
150.	Hydrocodone/Phenyltoloxamine (Tussionex)	Pennwalt
151.	Penicillin VK (SK-Penicillin VK)	SK&F
152.	Cloxacillin (Tegopen)	Bristol
153.	Reserpine/Apresoline/Hydrochlorothiazide (Ser-Ap-Es)	Ciba
154.	Prazosin (Minipress)	Pfizer
155.	Oxycodone/Acetaminophen (Tylox)	McNeil
156.	Nystatin (Mycostatin)	Squibb
157.	Promethazine Compound (Phenergan VC Plain)	Wyeth
158.	Brompheniramine (Dimetane)	Robins
159.	Nitroglycerin	Lilly
160.	Terbutaline (Brethine)	Geigy
161.	Loperamide (Imodium)	Ortho
162.	Opium/Kaolin/Pectin/Belladonna (Donnagel PG)	Robins
163.	Chlorpromazine (Thorazine)	SK&F
164.	Amoxicillin (Wymox)	Wyeth
165.	Triple Sulfonamide (Sultrin)	Ortho
166.	Amoxicillin (Polymox)	Bristol
167.	Tetracycline (Panmycin)	Upjohn
168.	Brompheniramine Compound/Codeine (Dimetane DC)	Robins
169.	Fluocinonide (Lindex)	Syntex
170.	Nitroglycerin (Nitro-Bid)	Marion
171.	Timolol (Timoptic)	MSD
172.	Sulfisoxazole/Phenazopyridine (AzoGantrisin)	Roche
173.	Brompheniramine Compound/Codeine (Ambenyl)	Marion
174.	Penicillin VK (Robicillin VK)	Robins
175.	Promethazine (Phenergan)	Wyeth
176.	Chlorothiazide (Diuril)	MSD
177.	Hydrochlorothiazide (Esidrex)	Ciba
178.	Theophylline (Slo-Phyllin)	Rorer
179.	Tetracycline	Wyeth
180.	Fluocinolone (Synalar)	Syntex
181.	Hydralazine (Apresoline)	Ciba
182.	Hydrocortisone (Hytone)	Dermik
183.	Desoximetasone (Topicort)	Hoechst
184.	Prenatal Vitamins (Stuartnatal 1 + 1)	Stuart
185.	Propoxyphene/Acetaminophen (Wygesic)	Wyeth
186.	Butabarbital (Butisol)	McNeil
187.	Clonidine (Catapres)	Boehringer
188.	Ethynodiol Diacetate/Ethinyl Estradiol (Demulen)	Searle
189.	Iodochlorhydroxyquin/Hydrocortisone (Vioform HC)	Ciba
190.	Chlorpheniramine/Phenylephrine (Demazin)	Schering
191.	Tetracycline (Robitet)	Robins
192.	Tretinoin (Retin A)	Johnson & Johnson
193.	Metaproterenol (Alupent)	Boehringer
194.	Trifluoperazine (Stelazine)	SK&F
195.	Norethindrone/Ethinyl Estradiol (Modicon)	Ortho
196.	Estrogens, Conjugated, Vaginal (Premarin Vaginal)	Ayerst
197.	Benztropine (Cogentin)	MSD
198.	Methyclothiazide (Enduron)	Abbott
199.	Betamethasone (Diprosone)	Schering
200.	Theophylline/Guaifenesin (Quibron)	Mead Johnson

47 COMPANIES MARKET THE TOP 200 DRUGS (NEW AND REFILL COMBINED)

Number of Products	Company
15	Merck Sharp & Dohme, Parke-Davis
11	Wyeth
10	Burroughs-Wellcome
9	Roche
8	Smith Kline & French, Upjohn
7	Searle, Squibb
6	Ciba, Lederle, Lilly, Schering
5	Abbott, McNeil, Merrell, Pfizer
4	Geigy, Mead Johnson, Ortho, Robins, Roerig, Sandoz, Syntex
3	Ayerst, Beecham, Boehringer, Dista, Pennwalt
2	Endo, Ives, Marion, Pfipharmecs, U.S.V.
1	Alcon, Armour, Bristol, Fisons, Flint, Hoechst, Key, Norwich, Reed & Carnrick, Riker, Rorer, Stuart, Winthrop

THE TOP 100 DRUGS ACCOUNT FOR HALF OF ALL NEW AND REFILL PRESCRIPTIONS

Quartile	Percent	Cumulative Percent
1 (Top 50)	36.3%	36.3%
2 (Second 50) . .	14.0%	50.3%
3 (Third 50) . . .	8.5%	58.8%
4 (Last 50) . . .	5.8%	64.6%

PRESCRIPTION DRUG TRENDS

December 1980: 5 Leading Categories and All Rxs, New and Refills

	Number of Rxs (+000)	% Chg Vs Previous Month	Dollar Volume (+000)	% Chg Vs Previous Month
Antiarthritics	5,009	− 5.5	52,188	− 4.0
Antibiotics	18,612	+17.7	80,927	+14.1
Cardiovasculars	14,259	− 1.3	94,783	− 0.6
Cough/cold drugs	11,519	+28.2	31,263	+25.0
Tranquilizers	7,208	− 2.2	43,584	− 2.7
5 categories combined .	56,607	+ 9.1	302,745	+ 4.2
All Rxs	126,329	+ 2.5	646,623	+ 1.3

OUTPATIENT DRUG INDEX

(Average retail price and dosage units per Rx for a representative group of 100 drugs. Data are for months in 1980. Index base = January 1980)

	Avg Rx Price	Index	Dosage Units/Rx	Index
January	$8.49	100.0	56.89	100.0
March	$8.52	100.3	56.90	100.0
June	$8.90	104.7	57.58	101.2
September	$9.02	106.2	56.39	99.1
October	$9.09	107.0	56.51	99.3
November	$9.18	108.0	56.76	99.8
December	$9.20	108.4	57.01	100.2

ANSWERS TO REVIEW QUESTIONS THAT APPEAR AT THE END OF CHAPTERS

Chapter 2
1. C
2. D
3. C
4. B
5. B

Chapter 3
1. D
2. C
3. D
4. C
5. A
6. B
7. A
8. A

Chapter 4
1. C
2. E
3. D
4. A
5. A
6. A
7. A

Chapter 5
1. C
2. A
3. E
4. D
5. E
6. B
7. B
8. C
9. E

Chapter 6
1. C
2. B
3. B
4. B
5. E

Chapter 7
1. C
2. C
3. B

Chapter 8
1. B
2. E
3. B
4. B
5. E
6. C
7. B
8. D

Chapter 9
1. D
2. D
3. B
4. C

Chapter 11
1. D
2. D
3. C
4. C
5. A
6. E
7. E
8. B
9. E
10. A

Chapter 13
1. D
2. C
3. A
4. D
5. B
6. B
7. B
8. B
9. A

Chapter 14
1. B
2. C
3. D
4. B
5. E
6. A
7. C
8. B

Chapter 15
1. C
2. C
3. B
4. A
5. A
6. E
7. D
8. A

Chapter 16
1. E
2. D
3. C
4. E
5. A
6. A
7. B
8. A

Chapter 17
1. B
2. C
3. C
4. D
5. D
6. A
7. A
8. B

Chapter 18
1. C
2. B
3. B
4. C
5. A
6. E
7. D
8. D

Autonomic Pharmacology Review Items
1. C
2. D
3. C
4. D
5. C
6. A
7. D
8. B
9. B
10. B
11. D

Chapter 19
1. E
2. D
3. C
4. C
5. B
6. E
7. A
8. A

Chapter 20
1. E
2. C
3. A
4. B
5. E
6. C

Chapter 21
1. C
2. B
3. A

Chapter 22
1. B
2. C
3. E
4. B
5. C
6. D
7. A

Chapter 23
1. C
2. C
3. C
4. B

Chapter 24
1. E
2. A
3. A
4. B
5. D
6. E
7. B
8. B

General Questions on Neuroleptic Drugs
1. E
2. C
3. C
4. E
5. B
6. C
7. C
8. B

Chapter 25
1. D
2. C
3. B
4. E
5. A
6. C
7. A
8. A
9. B

Chapter 26
1. B
2. B
3. A
4. B
5. B
6. A
7. A
8. C
9. C
10. B

Chapter 27
1. E
2. C
3. E
4. D
5. A
6. A
7. B
8. B
9. A

Chapter 28
1. E
2. D
3. D
4. D
5. D
6. C
7. C
8. E
9. A
10. A

Chapter 29
1. B
2. B
3. B
4. B
5. C
6. E
7. A
8. A
9. B
10. D
11. E

Chapter 30
1. D
2. E
3. C
4. D
5. B
6. B
7. E
8. A

Chapter 31
1. D
2. E
3. D
4. C
5. E
6. C
7. B
8. B
9. E
10. D

Chapter 32
1. D
2. B
3. C
4. E
5. B
6. B
7. A
8. E
9. A
10. E

Chapter 33
1. D
2. D
3. B
4. A
5. D
6. E
7. A
8. C
9. A
10. B

Chapter 34
1. D
2. E
3. D
4. B
5. C
6. A
7. E
8. E
9. E
10. D

Chapter 35
1. C
2. A
3. D
4. C
5. B
6. C
7. C

Chapter 36
1. C
2. D
3. E
4. D
5. A
6. C
7. A
8. E
9. E
10. C

Chapter 37
1. C
2. B
3. C
4. D
5. C
6. D
7. C
8. A
9. A

Chapter 38
1. C
2. B
3. B
4. D
5. B
6. C
7. A
8. A
9. C
10. A

Chapter 39
1. C
2. E
3. C
4. C
5. B
6. A

Chapter 40
1. A
2. C
3. D
4. B
5. A
6. E
7. B
8. B
9. B
10. C
11. A
12. C

Chapter 41
1. A
2. C
3. B
4. D
5. B
6. D
7. E
8. C

Chapter 42
1. E
2. D
3. D
4. D
5. A
6. B
7. D
8. B

Chapter 43
1. C
2. C
3. A
4. B
5. C
6. E

Chapter 44
1. D
2. B
3. C
4. E
5. C
6. B
7. E
8. C

Chapter 45
1. D
2. E
3. D
4. C
5. A
6. D

Chapter 46
1. E
2. B
3. C
4. A
5. D
6. D
7. C
8. C

Chapter 47
1. D
2. D
3. D
4. C
5. A
6. E
7. A
8. A
9. C

Chapter 48
1. B
2. D
3. E
4. B
5. B
6. A
7. E
8. E
9. C
10. E

Chapter 49
1. E
2. B
3. D
4. A
5. C
6. B
7. C

Chapter 50
1. B
2. C
3. D
4. B
5. A
6. C

Chapter 51
1. E
2. D
3. B
4. B
5. C
6. E
7. C
8. E
9. B
10. B
11. B

Chapter 52
1. C
2. D
3. A
4. E
5. A
6. B
7. A
8. A
9. A
10. A

Chapter 53
1. A
2. E
3. C
4. A
5. B
6. E
7. A

Chapter 54
1. D
2. D
3. C
4. A
5. C
6. B

Chapter 55
1. B
2. A
3. C
4. B
5. B
6. A

Chapter 56
1. D
2. D
3. A
4. B
5. E
6. D
7. E
8. A
9. A
10. D
11. D
12. D
13. A
14. A
15. A
16. B

Chapter 57
1. D
2. A
3. C
4. A
5. D
6. D
7. D
8. A
9. E
10. D
11. A
12. E
13. E
14. A
15. D

Chapter 58
1. B
2. E
3. C
4. A
5. B
6. A
7. A
8. C
9. C

Chapter 59
1. B
2. B
3. E
4. B
5. C
6. E
7. A
8. B
9. C
10. A
11. A

Chapter 60
1. B
2. C
3. B
4. D
5. E
6. A
7. D
8. C
9. E
10. E
11. A
12. B
13. A

Chapter 61
1. D
2. A
3. B
4. D
5. E
6. D
7. A
8. C
9. E
10. E
11. E

Chapter 62
1. B
2. C
3. D
4. E
5. A
6. C
7. E

Chapter 63
1. C
2. A
3. C
4. B
5. E
6. A
7. E

Chapter 64
1. B
2. A
3. C
4. B
5. D
6. A
7. E
8. C
9. A
10. B
11. A
12. E
13. B

Chapter 65
1. A
2. B
3. C
4. C
5. B
6. C
7. A
8. B
9. D
10. E
11. E
12. C
13. A
14. D
15. C
16. C
17. E

Chapter 66
1. C
2. D
3. B
4. E
5. A

Chapter 67
1. C
2. B
3. B
4. D
5. B
6. B
7. E
8. A
9. B
10. C

Chapter 68
1. B
2. B
3. A
4. C
5. B
6. A
7. B
8. A

Chapter 69
1. E
2. B
3. C
4. B
5. C
6. B
7. B
8. C
9. B
10. A
11. A
12. A
13. D
14. C
15. D
16. C
17. B
18. A
19. D
20. C
21. A
22. A
23. A
24. A

Chapter 70
1. A
2. D
3. C
4. C
5. E
6. A
7. D
8. E
9. A
10. A
11. C
12. C
13. C
14. B

Chapter 71
1. C
2. E
3. E
4. A
5. B
6. B
7. C
8. C
9. A
10. B

Chapter 72
1. D
2. A
3. A
4. D
5. C
6. C
7. B
8. B
9. E
10. A

Chapter 73
1. B
2. A
3. B
4. A
5. C
6. A
7. A

Subject Index

The Subject Index is followed by a Drug Index, in which all drugs are listed by name. Drug families can be found in the Subject Index.

Drug Index

This index contains specific drugs. Drug families can be found in the preceding Subject Index.